HANDBOOK OF
BIOMATERIALS
EVALUATION

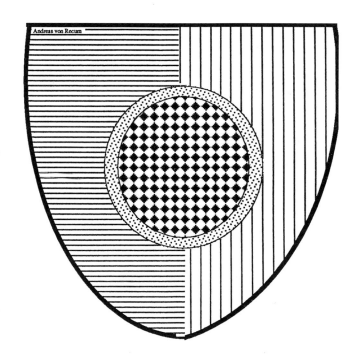

E D I T O R

Andreas F. von Recum,
D.V.M., Dr. med. vet., Ph.D., FBSE

Professor of Experimental Surgery,
Oral Surgery and Biomedical Engineering
Associate Dean of Veterinary Research
College of Veterinary Medicine
The Ohio State University
1900 Coffey Road
101 Sisson Hall
Columbus, OH 43210

S E C T I O N   E D I T O R S

James M. Anderson
Stephen R. Ash
Francis W. Cooke
Ulrich M. Gross
Martine LaBerge
W. Homer Lawrence
Antonios G. Mikos
William A. Morton
Andreas F. von Recum
Richard F. Wallin

A S S I S T A N T   E D I T O R

Jane E. Jacobi

HANDBOOK OF BIOMATERIALS EVALUATION

Scientific, Technical, and Clinical Testing of Implant Materials

Second Edition

USA	Publishing Office:	Taylor & Francis
		325 Chestnut Street
		Philadelphia, PA 19106
		Tel: (215) 625-8900
		Fax: (202) 625-2940
	Distribution Center:	Taylor & Francis
		47 Runway Road, Suite G
		Levittown, PA 19057-4700
		Tel: (215) 269-0400
		Fax: (215) 269-0363
UK		Taylor & Francis
		1 Gunpowder Square
		London EC4A 3DE
		Tel: 44 171 583 0490
		Fax: 44 171 583 0581

HANDBOOK OF BIOMATERIALS EVALUATION: Scientific, Technical, and Clinical Testing of Implant Materials

2 3 4 5 6 7 8 9 0

Printed by Edwards Brothers, Ann Arbor, MI, 1998

A CIP catalog record for this book is available from the British Library.
∞ The paper in this publication meets the requirements of the ANSI Standard
Z39.48-1984 (Permanence of Paper)

Library of Congress Cataloging-in-Publication Data

Handbook of biomaterials evaluation : scientific, technical, and clinical testing
  of implant materials / editor, Andreas F. von Recum. — 2nd ed.
     p.   cm.
  Includes bibliographical references and index.
  ISBN 1-56032-479-1 (alk. paper)
  1. Biomedical materials—Evaluation—Handbooks, manuals, etc.
  2. Biomedical materials—Testing—Handbooks, manuals, etc. I. Von
Recum, Andreas.
R857.M3H35   1999
610′.28—dc21   98-36552
                                     CIP

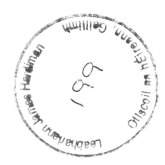

ISBN 1-56032-479-1

Contents

SECTION FIVE   ACTIVE IMPLANTS
Introduction: *Antonios G. Mikos, Editor*

SECTION SIX   IMPLANTOLOGY
Introduction: *Andreas F. von Recum, Editor*

SECTION TEN   CLINICAL TRIALS
Introduction: *Stephen R. Ash, Editor*

Contributors

JAMES M. ANDERSON, PhD, MD, FBSE
Professor of Pathology
Institute of Pathology
University Hospital of Cleveland
Case Western Reserve University
2074 Abington Road
Cleveland, OH 44106-2622

STEPHEN R. ASH, MD
Chairman and Director of R & D
HemoCleanse, Inc.
Purdue Research Park
2700 Kent Avenue
West Lafayette, IN 47906

NORMAN R. BAYNE, DVM, MS
Pfizer, Inc.
North American Animal Health
    Division
One Pfizer Way
Lee's Summit, MO 64081-2998

SCOTT BECKER
Attorney
Ross and Hardies
150 N. Michigan Avenue
Suite 2500
Chicago, IL 60601

CAROLYN E. BROWN, MS
Becton Dickinson Infusion Therapy Systems
9450 South State Street
Sandy, Utah 84070

KAREN J. L. BURG, PhD
Bioengineering Fellow
Department of General Surgery
Cannon Research Building
Room 406
Carolinas Medical Center
Charlotte, NC 28232-2861

KARIN D. CALDWELL, PhD
Professor
Center for Surface Biotechnology
Uppsala University
BMC PO Box 577
S-75123 Uppsala
Sweden

JOHN N. CAMMACK, PhD
Research Scientist
Baxter Healthcare Corporation
Route 120 & Wilson Road
Round Lake, IL 60073

LAURIE C. CARTER, DDS, MA
Assistant Professor
Department of Stomatology
School of Dental Medicine
SUNY at Buffalo
114 Squire Hall
Buffalo, NY 14214

VIRGINIA C. CHAMBERLAIN, PhD
Biometric Research Institute
Quality Regulatory Alliance, Inc.
5009 Alta Vista Court
Bethesda, MD 20814

NEAL CHOLVIN, PhD, DVM
Consultant
1910 Edgemont Place West
Seattle, WA 98199-3915

ARTHUR A. CIARKOWSKI, MSE, MPA
Associate Director
Division of Cardiovascular, Respiratory and
    Neurological Devices
Center for Devices and Radiological Health at
    FDA
9200 Corporate Boulevard
Rockville, MD 20850

ALEXIS CLARE, PhD
Associate Professor of Glass Science
Site Director
NSF Industry/University Center for Biosurfaces
New York State College of Ceramics
Alfred University
224 Binns-Merrill
Alfred, NY 14802

FRANCIS W. COOKE, PhD
Research Director
Orthopaedic Research Institute
St. Francis Hospital
929 N. St. Francis
Wichita, KS 67214

ROBERT G. CRAIG, PhD, FBSE
Professor Emeritus
(Department of Dental Materials
University of Michigan
School of Dentistry)
1011 N. University Avenue
Ann Arbor, MI 48109-1078

JAMES T. DALTON, PhD
Assistant Professor
Department of Pharmaceutical Sciences
College of Pharmacy
The Health Science Center
University of Tennessee, Memphis
874 Union Avenue
Memphis, TN 38163

MELVIN B. DENNIS, DVM
Professor and Chair
Department of Comparative Medicine
School of Medicine
University of Washington
Box 357190
Seattle, WA 98185

SCOTT P. DOWNING
Attorney
Ross and Hardies
150 N. Michigan Avenue
Suite 2500
Chicago, IL 60601

DIETER ESCHBERGER, MD, PhD
Professor
Ludwig Boltzmann Institute for Osteology at
    Vienna Meidling Trauma Center
Lorenz Böhler Trauma Center
Donaueschingenstr. 13
Vienna A-1200
Austria

JOSEF ESCHBERGER, MD
Ludwig Boltzmann Institute for Osteology at
    Vienna Meidling Trauma Center
Lorenz Böhler Trauma Center
Donaueschingenstr. 13
Vienna A-1200
Austria

MARIEN E. EVANS, JD
Attorney
9 South Street, #2
Brighton, MA 02135

STEVEN L. GOODMAN, PhD
Center for Biomaterials
University of Connecticut Health Center
263 Farmington Avenue
Farmington, CT 06030

DAVID W. GRAINGER, PhD
President
Gamma-A Technologies
520 Huntmar Park Drive, Suite 101
Herndon, VA 22070

ULRICH M. GROSS, MD, PhD, FBSE
Professor
Institut für Pathologie UK BF
Medizinische Fakultät
Freie Universität Berlin
Hindenburgdamm 30
D-12200 Berlin
Germany

ROBERT GUIDOIN, Dsc
Laboratoire de Chirurgie
    Experimentale
Université Laval
2450, boul. Hochelaga
Québec, Québec G1K 7P4
Canada

KEVIN E. HEALY, PhD
Associate Professor
Division of Biological Materials
Northwestern University
311 E. Chicago Ave.
Chicago, IL 60611-3008

MARK A. HELLER, ESQ.
Patton, Bloggs & Blow
2550 M Street NW
Washington, DC 20037

JULIE M. HIGASHI
Department of Biomedical Engineering
Case Western Reserve University
Cleveland, OH 44106

LOUISE N. HOWE
Patton, Bloggs & Blow
2550 M Street NW
Washington, DC 20037

YOSHITO IKADA, PhD
Professor
Institute for Frontier Medical Sciences
Kyoto University
Kawahara-Cho, Shogoin
Sakyo-Ku
Kyoto, 606–8507
Japan

JOHN A. JANSEN, DDS, PhD
Professor and Head
Department Oral Function/Biomaterials
Katholieke Universiteit Nijmegen
Faculty of Medical Sciences
P.O. Box 9101
6500 HB Nijmegen
The Netherlands

MICHELLE E. JENKINS, MS
1012 South 7th St. #4
Springfield, IL 62703

WEIYUAN JOHN KAO, MSE
Department of Macromolecular Science
Case Western Reserve University
10900 Euclid Avenue
Cleveland, OH 44106-4907

MARTINE LABERGE, PhD
Associate Professor
Department of Bioengineering
Clemson University
501 Rhodes Engineering Research Center
Clemson, SC 29634-0905

WILLIAM LACEFIELD, PhD
Professor and Acting Chair
Department of Biomaterials
School of Dentistry
University of Alabama at Birmingham
Box 49SDB
Birmingham, AL 35294

BYRON J. LAMBERT, PhD
Manager, Quality Service Systems
Guidant Corp.
Advanced Cardiovascular Systems
26531 Ynez Road
Temecula, CA 92591-4628

ROBERT A. LATOUR, JR., PhD
Associate Professor of Bioengineering
and of Materials Science and Engineering
Clemson University
501 Rhodes Engineering Research Center
Clemson, SC 29634-0905

W. HOMER LAWRENCE, PhD
Professor Emeritus
(Pharmaceutical Sciences
University of Tennessee, Memphis)
1725 Regency Street
Malvern, AR 72104

JACK LEMONS, PhD
Professor and Director
Laboratory for Surgical Implant Research
Schools of Dentistry and Medicine
University of Alabama at Birmingham
1919 Seventh Avenue South, UAB Station
Birmingham, AL 35294-0007

LINDA C. LUCAS, PhD
Professor and Chair
Department of Biomedical Engineering
College of Engineering
University of Alabama at Birmingham
1150 10th Avenue South, BEC 256
Birmingham, AL 35294-4461

DONALD J. LYMAN, PhD, FBSE
Professor Emeritus
(Materials Science and Bioengineering)
University of Utah
P. O. Box 5314
Lacey, WA 98509-5314

SURYA K. MALLAPRAGADA, PhD
Professor
Department of Chemical Engineering
Iowa State University of Science and
    Technology
1035 Sweeney Hall
Ames, IA 50011-2230

ROGER E. MARCHANT, PhD
Associate Professor
Department of Biomedical Engineering
College of Engineering
Case Western Reserve University
Cleveland, OH 44106

YVES MAROIS, MSC
Department of Surgery
Université Laval
2450, boul. Hochelaga
Québec, Québec G1K 7P4
Canada

BARBARA F. MATLAGA, BS, MBA
Section Manager
Corporate Products Characterization
Ethicon Inc.
P.O. Box 151 (US Highway 22)
Sommerville, NJ 08876

JOHN B. MEDLEY, PhD, P ENG
Associate Professor
Department of Mechanical Engineering
University of Waterloo
Waterloo, Ontario N2L 3G1
Canada

H. VINCE MENDENHALL, DVM, PhD
Senior Research Surgeon
GTC/TSI Mason Laboratories
57 Union St.
Worcester, MA 01608

KATHARINE MERRITT, PhD
Research Biologist
FDA/OST
12709 Twinbrook Parkway, MS HFZ 100
Rockville, MD 20852

ANNE E. MEYER, PhD
Principal Research Scientist
Industry/University Cooperative Research
   Center for Biosurfaces
SUNY at Buffalo
110 Parker Hall
Buffalo, NY 14214-3007

ANTONIOS G. MIKOS, PhD
T. N. Law Associate Professor
John W. Cox Laboratory for Biomedical
   Engineering
Institute of Biosciences and
   Bioengineering–MS 144
Rice University
P. O. Box 1892
Houston, TX 77251

DIANE E. MINEAR
Regulatory Affairs Consultant
Medical Device Consultants, Inc.
49 Plain Street
N. Attleboro, MA 02760

WILLIAM A. MORTON, BS, RAC
President
Medical Device Consultants, Inc.
49 Plain Street
North Attleboro, MA 02760

EDWARD P. MUELLER, PhD
Director, Division of Mechanics and Material
   Science
Office of Science and Technology
Center for Devices and Radiological
   Health
12200 Wilkins Ave
Rockville, MD 20852

BALAJI NARASIMHAN, PhD
Assistant Professor
Department of Chemical and Biochemical
   Engineering
Rutgers University
98 Brett Road
Piscataway, NJ 08854-8058

JOSEPH R. NATIELLA, DDS
Professor
Department of Oral Diagnostic Sciences
SUNY at Buffalo
355 Square Hall
Buffalo, NY 14214-3008

JENNIFER A. NEFF, BS
Department of Bioengineering
College of Engineering
University of Utah
194 BPR Building
Salt Lake City, UT 84112

SHARON J. NORTHUP, PhD, DABT
Managing Associate
The Weinberg Group, Inc.
1220 Nineteenth Street, NW
Suite 300
Washington, DC 20036-2400

THOMAS A. O'CONNOR, PhD
Professor
Department of Mathematics
University of Louisville
Louisville, KY 40292

PATRICK J. PARKS, MD, PhD
Staff Scientist
Biomaterials Technology Center
3M, 3M Center, 270-2A-08
St. Paul, MN 55144-1000

J. BARRY PHELPS, BS
Section Manager
In Vitro Toxicology
North American Science Associates
2261 Tracy Road
Northwood, OH 43551

ROBERT M. PILLIAR, PhD, FBSE
Professor
Centre for Biomaterials
University of Toronto
124 Edward Street #464
Toronto, Ontario M5G 1G6
Canada

ROBERT J. PRISTAVE, JD
Attorney
Ross and Hardies
150 N. Michigan Avenue
Suite 2500
Chicago, IL 60601

BERTON A. RAHN, MD, PhD
Professor
AO Research Institute
Clavadelerstrasse
CH 7270 Davos
Switzerland

W. MONTY REICHERT, PhD
Associate Professor
Department of Biomedical Engineering
College of Engineering
Duke University
Durham, NC 27708-0281

JONETTE M. ROGERS-FOY, PhD
Assistant Professor
Department of Engineering Science and
    Mechanics
Virginia Polytechnic Institute and State
    University
Blacksburg, VA 24061

THOMAS N. SALTHOUSE, F.I.M.L.S.,
F.R.P.S., FBSE
714 Teakwood Court
West Columbia, SC 29169

SUNEETI SAPATNEKAR, MD, PhD
Resident in Pathology
Institute of Pathology
Case Western Reserve University
and University Hospitals of Cleveland
Cleveland, OH 44106

FREDERICK J. SCHOEN, MD, PhD, FBSE
Professor of Pathology, Harvard Medical
    School
Vice Chair, Department of Pathology
Director, Cardiac Pathology
Brigham & Women's Hospital
75 Francis Street
Boston, MA 02115

MICHAEL V. SEFTON, PhD, FBSE
Professor
Institute of Biomedical Engineering
University of Toronto
4 Taddle Creek Rd., Rm 407
Toronto, Ontario M5 S1 A4
Canada

SHALABY W. SHALABY, PhD
President
Poly-Med, Inc.
6309 Highway 187
Anderson, SC 29625

CLARE SHANNON, MS
Project Manager
Device Development
Encelle, Inc.
2408 S. Charles St., Suite 4
Greenville, NC 27834

A. ADAM SHARKAWY, MS, PhD
Director, Clinical Science and Engineering
Ventrica, Inc.
985 University Avenue, Suite 35
Los Gatos, CA 95032

MOLLY S. SHOICHET, PhD
Assistant Professor
Department of Chemical Engineering and
    Applied Chemistry
and Centre for Biomaterials
University of Toronto
Toronto, Ontario M5S 3E5
Canada

PIPPA M. SIMPSON, MSC
Consultant Statistician
2536 Ransdell Avenue
Louisville, KY 40204

ROGER W. SNYDER, PhD
Manager, Technical Services and Regulatory
    Affairs
L. VAD Technology, Inc.
300 River Place, Suite 6850
Detroit, MI 48207

FUH-WEI TANG, PhD
Senior Material and Radiation
    Engineer
Guidant Corp.
Advanced Cardiovascular Systems
26531 Ynez Road
Temecula, CA 92591-4628

ALLAN F. TENCER, PhD
Associate Professor and Director
Biomechanics Laboratory
Department of Orthopaedics
Harborview Medical Center
University of Washington
325 Ninth Avenue (ZA-48)
Box 35979
Seattle, WA 98104

JOHN A. THOMAS, PhD
Vice President for Academic Services
Professor, Department of Pharmacology
Health Science Center at San Antonio
The University of Texas
7703 Floyd Curl Drive
San Antonio, TX 78284-7722

PAUL UPMAN, BA
Senior Scientist
North American Science Associates
2261 Tracy Road
Northwood, OH 43619

RAMAKRISHNA VENUGOPALAN, BE, MS
Department of Biomedical Engineering
University of Alabama at Birmingham
1150 10th Avenue South, BEC 256
Birmingham, AL 35294-4461

ANDREAS F. VON RECUM, DVM, DR.
MED. VET., PhD, FBSE
Associate Dean for Research
and Professor of Veterinary Medicine
College of Veterinary Medicine
The Ohio State University
1900 Coffey Road, 101 Sisson Hall
Columbus, OH 43210

HORST A. VON RECUM, MCHE
Center for Controlled Chemical Delivery
Building #205
University of Utah
Salt Lake City, UT 84112

RICHARD F. WALLIN, DVM, PhD
President
North American Science Associates
2261 Tracy Road
Northwood, OH 43619

RICHARD A. WARD, PhD
Professor, Kidney Disease Program
School of Medicine
University of Louisville
615 S. Preston
Louisville, KY 40292

RONALD L. WATHEN, MD, PhD
Professor of Medicine
General Internal Medicine
College of Medicine
University of Louisville
3rd Floor ACB
Louisville, KY 40292

STEPHEN C. WOODWARD, MD
Professor of Pathology
Vanderbilt University
Chief, Pathology and Laboratory
   Medicine Service
VAMC
1310 24th Avenue South
Nashville, TN 37203

MICHAEL J. YASZEMSKI, PhD
Associate Professor
Department of Orthopedic Surgery
Mayo Clinic and Mayo Medical School
200 First Street SW
Rochester, MN 55905

NICHOLAS P. ZIATS, PhD
Institute of Pathology
Case Western Reserve University
10900 Euclid Avenue
Cleveland, OH 44106-4907

Preface

While prosthetic materials have been implanted for centuries, the professional discipline of Biomaterials Science and Engineering has only begun to evolve recently. Exciting progress has taken place in just the last ten years, as can be seen by a quick comparison of the tables of contents of this second edition of the handbook with that of the first edition. While implant performance and biocompatibility are still being improved by means of more traditional approaches such as tribology studies, surface topographic designs, and surface electrochemical modifications, newer approaches are now evolving such as the design of the surface chemistry on a molecular level (allowing chemical interactions with the contacting tissues and cells), purposeful incorporation of material-triggered biological responses (such as preventing blood coagulation in catheters and vascular grafts, or providing specific adhesion molecules for attaching tissues and cells), or the use of prosthetic biomaterials with living biological substrates (as for example meniscus replacement grafts contacting cartilage cells or implants containing insulin producing living cells). This new edition addresses both the traditional and newer methods of evaluation.

This handbook is the result of a multidisciplinary collaboration on evaluating biomaterials as they are designed for prosthetic and therapeutic implants. The chapters of this handbook reflect a variety of research fields and professional expertise spanning basic sciences, engineering bio-medical sciences, and clinical medicine and surgery. Each chapter in this handbook describes a small part of the body of knowledge required to evaluate materials and implants for their effective and safe use as prosthetic or therapeutic implants.

The logo accompanying each section illustrates the multidisciplinary field of biomaterials as a puzzle, in which each piece is an essential part, but in which only the assembly of all of the pieces in their proper order reveals the meaning of the entire picture. The purpose of this handbook is to assemble the puzzle pieces in such a way as to make the complex process of biomaterials evaluation understandable to the reader.

The editor of this handbook and many of his editorial board members have been privileged to participate in the evolution of the field of biomaterials from its beginnings. It is their hope that this handbook continues to contribute to the education of coming generations of biomaterials scientists and engineers and to serve as a reference to those practicing in the field.

Acknowledgments

The catalyst for the first edition of this Handbook was a Biocompatibility Gordon Conference in New Hampshire in 1980, when biocompatibility was nothing but a research interest shared by investigators from many disciplines. It took six years for the book concept to crystallize and the manuscript to get published by Macmillan Publishing Company. For the second edition it was Richard O'Grady with Taylor & Francis Publishers who in November 1995 urged me to update and re-publish the Handbook. It is due to Richard's insistence that the second edition came about and I thank him for that.

I am grateful to the section editors who defined the scope and contents of their sections. They assured that this Handbook remain a multidisciplinary effort focused on methodology. I am indebted to the many authors who toiled to deliver chapters written to the specifications of this book. I am also grateful for my fellow faculty members, for staff, and graduate students in the Department of Bioengineering at Clemson University who supported this project in many ways. I specifically thank my graduate student Matthew Gevaert who helped me draw the puzzle as an illustration. Finally I am grateful to Jane E. Jacobi who assisted in every phase of the evolution of this second edition.

I am most grateful to my family who patiently supported me throughout this project and saw my time and energy being spent on both Handbook editions as if they were my seventh and eighth children.

A. v. R.

Introduction: Biomaterials and Biocompatibility

Andreas F. von Recum
Michelle E. Jenkins
Horst A. von Recum

DEFINITIONS

To discuss the notion of successful implantation of a prosthetic material into the human body, we must first elucidate, as much as possible, the terms **biomaterial** and **biocompatibility**. Both words have been exhaustively defined, and several consensus definitions are currently accepted. Williams, reporting the result of a consensus conference, defined biomaterials as "nonviable materials used in a medical device, intended to interact with biological systems" [1]. Black included the use of living tissue in his definition of biomaterials as "materials of natural or manmade origin that are used to direct, supplement, or replace the functions of living tissues" [1]. Natural materials could include cells and tissues designed and grown for implantation.

One difficulty in defining biocompatibility is its purely qualitative character. Biocompatibility, a term that evolved from descriptive morphological histopathology, represents a global and biased statement on how well body tissues interact with a material and how this interaction meets the designed expectations for a certain implantation purpose and site. Biocompatibility, therefore, is an ideal and as such is never completely realized. It is intangible and unmeasurable. A better term would be "biomaterial performance." Biocompatibility in that sense represents a summary statement that may be based on many qualitative, semiquantitative, and/or quantitative observations and measurements. These observations may include data on surface corrosion or abrasion products, changes in bulk properties including mechanical stability, changes in surface properties including protein adsorption, histological and histochemical definition of inflammation, identification of specific inflammatory cells, or measurements of enzyme and other reactive biological molecule levels. Biocompatibility thus defined in terms of biomaterial performance still remains largely a matter of interpretation.

Another difficulty in defining biocompatibility is the paucity of well-documented reference standards of materials, methods, and responses. Biocompatibility cannot be absolute; obviously there exist varying degrees of beneficial and deleterious reactions. Therefore it remains the task of the various contributing disciplines to generate characteristic and application-specific parameters that can describe interactions in a quantitative, reproducible, and informative way. And indeed, many such efforts have been published, including the very noteworthy "Guide to the Study of Blood-Tissue-Material Interactions" [1] which was initiated and has been revised repeatedly over the past two decades under the leadership of the former Devices and Technology Branch (now called the Bioengineering Research Group) of the National Heart, Lung and Blood Institute.

The definition of biocompatibility must account for a host's response to a material, as well as the physiological environment's effects on the material. It is difficult to separate

1

these two interactions. They will change with respect to each other due to the passage of time, alterations in the physical condition of the host, or material degradation. For a material to be termed biocompatible, it must be beneficial to the function of the tissue(s) that it is augmenting or replacing; in addition it must not cause harm to other tissues.

In the past biomaterials were selected on a trial-and-error basis. Clinical and histopathological observations with these off-the-shelf materials led to use of the term "biocompatibility" for describing the performance of these implanted materials in light of the researchers' expectations. With time and increasing therapeutic successes, expectations increased and assessment methods were refined. The term biocompatibility soon became insufficiently descriptive. Current material development needs to rely upon an engineering, or design, approach considering the functional requirements, environmental conditions, and tissue regenerative processes at the interface between the living and the prosthetic material at molecular levels. New insights and technologies in molecular biology, surface sciences, and materials science offer biomaterial engineers and scientists increasing opportunities for the design of biocompatible materials. In fact, the ultimate goal of biomaterials research must be to replace lost organ or tissue function without introducing undesirable side effects.

In our opinion biocompatibility implies merely a degree of mutual toleration of a biomaterial in its implantation site. Our new aims should be directed towards the development of "bio-cooperative" implant materials which actively cooperate with the implantation site tissues in the physiological maintenance of function and homeostasis.

BIOCOMPATIBILITY DESCRIBED BY INTERACTIONS AT INTERFACES

Whatever the origin of materials used, once they are implanted into the body they interface with living tissues. It is the interface between foreign, man-made, non-living material and living tissue that is of the greatest concern for biocompatibility studies. This interface is schematically presented in the logo of this handbook as shown in Figure 1.

Interactions at Interfaces

The biomaterial will encounter the body's physiological environment which presents many forces capable of damaging or destroying the implanted material. Extracellular fluid, an electrolyte solution similar to serum, promotes corrosion and degradation. Proteins and lipids from extracellular fluid and adsorbed to the material surface can trigger changes in chemical and mechanical properties of the bulk material by oxidative and/or hydrolytical reactions. Relative motion between tissues and the implant allows wear of the material surface and the interfacing tissue components and thus promotes chronic inflammation leading to an even harsher chemical environment. Finally, repetitive or cyclic forces on the implant below the fracture stress can lead to failure by dynamic fatigue where implant location determines in part what mechanical forces will be experienced.

Normally the body's physiology is carefully monitored and controlled to maintain homeostasis. This control includes constant adaptation and regeneration of body tissues. Implantation of a tissue-foreign material results in tissue injury which leads to acute inflammation, the first step of wound healing and subsequent re-establishment of homeostasis. The presence of the implant, however, interferes with the normal progression of wound healing; the body then responds with chronic inflammation. Accumulating chronic inflammatory cells produce many dissolving enzymes. The enzyme activity then causes a drop

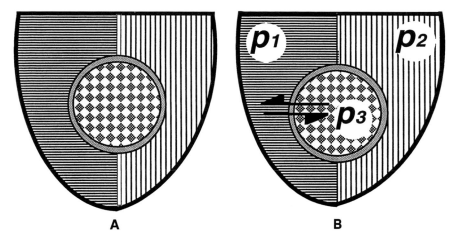

A   **B**

Figure 1 The concept of biocompatibility as an interfacial phenomenon: (A) An implanted BIO-MATERIAL (checkered center field) interfaces with internal body tissues (striated fields). The interfacing substrata interact chemically and physically across their respective boundaries (dotted space around implant); (B) Quantitative EVALUATION of these interactions (symbolically represented here by vectors and material properties p_n) enables the biomaterials scientist and engineer to design implants and to predict their performance.

in local pH and subsequent acidic destruction of tissue components and possibly implanted materials. This enzyme activity perpetuates chronic inflammation as long as the implant persists. This means that the presence of the implant prevents the body from re-establishing pre-implantation homeostasis at its interface with the implant. It seems, then, that the body cannot integrate foreign materials into its balance of homeostasis; consequently the inflammatory response represents the body's compensatory effort to isolate the foreign material from body tissues.

Design Considerations for the Interface

Generally speaking, the body seems to have two physiological means of dealing with (biological) interfaces:

A. **Integration** of tissues at interfaces both physically and functionally by forming extracellular matrix and cellular bonds (connective tissue links between various different tissues in general such as bone-tendon, tooth-bone, or blood vessel connections with other tissues) and thus achieving functional interactions.

B. **Barrier formation** through epithelia which negotiate all physiological challenges at interfaces including physical and functional separation of tissues from compartments, communication across such interfaces, and friction, wear, renewal, resorption, and cleansing of the interfacial space.

Tissues respond to foreign materials with different rejection mechanisms. The most frequently observed histopathological response to an implant is encapsulation: a fibrous or granulous tissue capsule forms around the implant and isolates it from the rest of the body environment, as shown schematically in Figure 2.

Even though encapsulation was not a design goal but the observed result around every implant, it served many implants adequately, especially if the implant did not require a functional integration with the tissues surrounding it (pumps or pacemakers may serve as

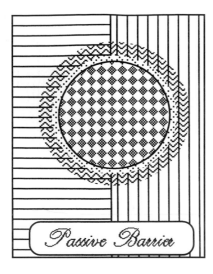

Figure 2 Implant encapsulation. An implant (checkered center) that is implanted in tissue (striated area) is encapsulated with fibrous or granulous tissue (cross-hatched ring), creating a dead space between it and the implanted material.

examples). Encapsulation and its consequences do pose problems when morphological or functional integration are key design criteria (vascular grafts, intraocular lenses, or breast implants may serve as examples here).

If one would apply to the tissue/biomaterials interface the earlier described physiological solutions for biological interfaces, there seem to be two theoretical scenarios: an active integration (Figure 3A) or an active barrier (Figure 3B).

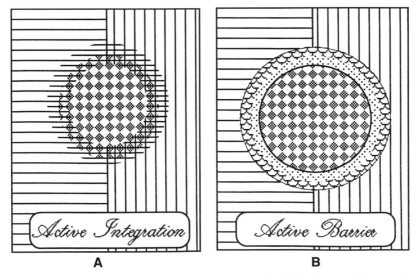

A   **B**

Figure 3 Integration versus barrier: alternative design goals. (A) An implant (circular checkered field) is shown inside the tissue (striated square). The design goal of functional integration is the formation of a functional or connective tissue bond between tissue and implant, allowing or promoting integrated function. Clear demarcations disappear. (B) The design goal of a functional barrier is the formation of a capsule which has epithelial function (capsule lined with epitheloid cells at its luminal side) which controls the dead space (dotted space) between the capsule and the clearly demarcated implant.

Implant design efforts have concentrated on the design goal of "integration," that is, the integration of tissue and material at their interfaces at least morphologically if not also functionally. If adherence of tissue components to the material is the specific goal, then the following are important design criteria: porous or textured surfaces to create mechanical interlocking, and chemically modified surfaces to affect chemical bonding. But actual integration, morphological or functional, has not yet been achieved.

We propose the formation of an "active barrier" as an alternative design goal: barrier formation follows the principle of encapsulation (tissue capsule formation) but incorporates active biological control over the interfacial space. This might be achieved with tissue engineering principles. One could consider adding epithelial tissues or functions to the implant material surface. Epithelia are capable of combatting the effects of friction and wear with (epithelial) self-renewal characteristics such as in epidermis, mucosa at body openings, or epithelia of the intestinal tract, vagina, esophagus and trachea; with lubricant secretion such as in joint capsular mucosa or epithelia from the alimentary and respiratory tract; with cleansing agent production such as in tear glands; or with the capacity of resorbing accumulated waste products at the interface such as is known for the dental sulcus or mesothelia of the major cavities.

Traditional approaches to biomaterial design and selection will likely continue and be justified in future implants because of their undeniable clinical successes. However, they will only lead to "biocompatible" implants, tolerated by tissues at best. Further progress in understanding the mechanisms of tissue/material interactions may lead to physiologically interactive "bio-cooperative" interfaces such as our above-described concept of the "active barrier." This will necessitate reliance upon newer and much more expensive technologies to tailor design materials on the molecular level and to design cell/material composites. Intensive multi-disciplinary collaboration will be essential in realizing these goals.

BIOCOMPATIBILITY AS A FUNCTION OF MATERIAL PROPERTIES, TIME, AND IMPLANT LOCATION

Biocompatibility evaluations should pay careful attention to implantation timelines. The initial response of a host to an implanted material, and vice versa, occurs at the interface between surfaces of the material and the tissue. The molecular configuration of the material, as well as surface energetics, charge and other properties, influence the molecular reaction with the tissue constituents. Currently it is thought that proteins are the first biomolecules to adsorb to a surface. Protein adsorption is followed by a cellular response, the type of which depends on numerous properties including material properties previously mentioned, as well as implant location. For example, polymers exposed to blood in vascular prostheses, artificial hearts, or dialyzer fibers will likely adsorb complement proteins. Following adsorption the activated protein fragments signal platelets at the blood side and inflammatory cells such as macrophages at the connective tissue side of the implant material.

The blood-material response differs in protein and cellular makeup from a connective tissue-material response and again from a hard tissue-material response. While bone is actively resorbed and deposited in response to trauma and implantation, replacement of any soft tissue like muscle is generally by fibrous connective tissue which has different functional capabilities than those of muscle.

It should be re-emphasized that the interfacial layer is not static; proteins are cleaved and replaced by others as a function of time. Cells die and are replaced at a yet-unknown rate. This creates additional questions in designing biocompatible surfaces. What surface characteristics are most influential in protein adsorption? Do proteins that initially adsorb alter a material surface in such a way that subsequent protein adsorption or cellular inter-action is affected? If so, is it even possible to predict a "final" cellular response at such a dynamic interface?

BIOCOMPATIBILITY ASSESSMENT

Biocompatibility should be evaluated in terms of local and systemic responses to material implantation. In both cases it is important to distinguish between a body's reaction to a surgical insult and a biocompatibility response with respect to the implanted material. Experts in the fields of toxicology, immunology, and cell and molecular biology should be consulted concerning systemic reactions. Histological testing of retrieved implants allows researchers to document actual and overall patient responses while in vitro analyses allow for more general predictions of population responses to a material. In culture it is possible to isolate the target tissues or cells and study their reactions to a material without interference from the body's inflammatory and immune systems. In addition, in vitro testing provides less expensive estimates of patient responses.

Evaluations must consider infection, which may drastically alter the local response to implants and often results in additional systemic catastrophies. The presence of a (foreign) biomaterial has been shown to alter the natural tissue defense mechanisms in such a way that the presence of even a few contaminating bacteria can lead to full-fledged and treatment-resistant infections.

Initially in the design process bulk materials are selected for an application based on desired properties such as mechanical strength, elasticity, and thermal and oxidative stabilities. The next logical evaluation step is the consideration of compatibility with sur-rounding tissue in terms of compliance match or mismatch, possibility of wear debris and degradation products.

The biomaterials scientist should not overlook the compatibility of bulk materials placed together in a device. For example, galvanic corrosion occurs when two dissimilar metals are present in the same aqueous environment [1]. Due to such a corrosion effect, both metals will be affected, and the metal which is more anodic in the galvanic series will be degraded, leading to implant failure. Adhesion of two different materials often leads to delamination in the implantation site due to differing molecular responses of the different materials at the material/material interface. The potential dead space created by the delaminated surfaces becomes its own source of undesirable biological consequences.

EVALUATIONS ON A MOLECULAR LEVEL

From the realm of immune histochemistry, staining of specific biological molecules al-lows the precise definition of extracellular and intracellular molecules participating in the material/tissue interactions. Detailed understanding of these molecular interactions pro-vides avenues to incorporate design criteria for biomaterial development. From the realm of biochemistry, molecular biology provides an avenue for studying the effects of material implantation on proteins and DNA. Gene therapy involves changing the coding sequence of a gene along with its regulatory regions in order to change the amount and/or func-tional properties of its corresponding protein product. This may lead to an ability to modify tissue responses to implant materials. In fact it has been shown that the standard heal-ing response, which is the replacement of injured tissue by fibrous (granulation or scar) tissue, can be altered to actual replacement of the injured tissue. This has opened doors for the engineering of biological solutions to replace tissue function. While in the past one of the design goals was minimization of the inflammatory response, novel approaches incorporate material designs that elicit specific cellular responses, such as circumvention of inflammation.

THE PLAYERS IN BIOMATERIALS EVALUATION

This topic is represented as a puzzle (Figure 4), whose pieces themselves, representing fields of expertise, can be considered as composed of many small pieces of pressed chips, representative of the knowledge that has been compiled by hundreds of physicians, scientists, and engineers in that field. Very many of them are appropriately quoted in the references of this handbook. There are a few investigators whose work will be remembered as giant contributions toward the progress of the field of biomaterials. They include Leo Vroman, a forerunner of the evolution in the approach to blood-surface interactions [2]; S. Adam

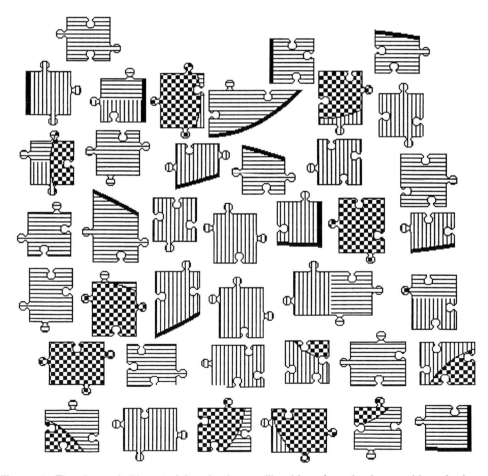

Figure 4 The players in biomaterial evaluation are like chips of puzzle pieces, with each piece representing a field of expertise. When all fields are assembled together they constitute the discipline of Biomaterials Science and Engineering.

Wesolowski (later named Wesolow), whose basic research of tissue formation in pores became the scientific basis for vascular graft development; Tom Salthouse, who quantified healing around implants and discovered the independent effect of implant morphology on tissue response (see Section VII); Willem J. Kolff, who pioneered the principles and practice of extracorporeal hemodialysis and of implantable blood pumps; John Charnley, who pioneered the principles and design of hip joint replacement and the use of bone cement; David Williams, who contributed with his extensive reviews and critical analyses of the published literature; and William C. Hall, who recognized the critical importance of peer review in biomaterials research and who guided the biomaterials community through the establishment of scientific meetings and the formation of the Society for Biomaterials [2].

The past fifty years have seen the ingenious but daring implant trials of pioneering surgeons supplemented gradually with professional multidisciplinary teams of experts who are bound to assure effectiveness and safety of implants. Today there are a number of respectable scientific journals and textbooks available to the expert and the student of the discipline of Biomaterials Engineering and Science. Professional standards and governmental regulations assist in the evaluation of biomaterials and implants and control their use in patients.

REFERENCES

1   von Recum AF, LaBerge M. Educational goals for biomaterials science and engineering: Prospective views. *J Appl Biomat*, 6 (1995), 137–144.
2   von Recum AF. The academic environment of biomaterials science and engineering. *J Appl Biomat*, 3 (1992), 61–73.
3   Williams DF (Ed.). *Definitions in Biomaterials: Proceedings of a Consensus Conference of the European Society for Biomaterials, Chester, England.* Amsterdam: Elsevier, 1987.
4   Black J. *Biological Performance of Materials: Fundamentals of Biocompatibility*, 2nd ed. New York: Marcel Dekker, Inc., 1992.
5   Harker LA, Ratner BD, Didisheim P. Cardiovascular biomaterials and biocompatibility. *Cardiovascular Pathology*, 2:3 (1993; Suppl.).
6   Park JB, Lakes RS. *Biomaterials : An Introduction*, 2nd ed. New York: Plenum Press, 1992.
7   Alberts B, Bray D, Lewis J, Raff M, Roberts K, Watson JD. *Molecular Biology of the Cell*, 2nd ed. New York: Garland Publishing, Inc., 1989.
8   Leonard EF. *Leo Vroman, scientist: An appreciation.* In Bamford CH, Cooper SL, Tsuruta T. *The Vroman Effect.* Utrecht, The Netherlands: VSP, 1992, v–vii.
9   Hulbert SF. Dr. C. W. Hall eulogy. *J Biomed Mat Res*, 27 (1993), 1–2.

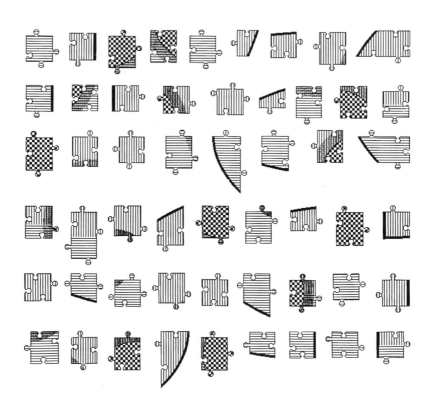

Section One

Bulk Characterization

Francis W. Cooke

INTRODUCTION

Section I is devoted to an overview of the materials which are important for surgical implants and other medical applications involving tissue contact, i.e., biomaterials. The first three chapters cover the three great classes of materials: metals, polymers, and composites. The treatment of ceramic materials which play a lesser role as biomaterials has been incorporated into Chapter One. Other chapters deal with materials used in special medical applications: dental materials (Chapter 4), textiles (Chapter 5), and absorbable materials (Chapter 6).

The subject material in each chapter is described in terms of its composition, structure, properties, manufacture, and use in implant surgery. In each case, representative values of the important physical and mechanical properties are given. Following these descriptive sections, each chapter concludes with a survey of the most important methods of testing and evaluation. For the most part, these physical and mechanical tests are the same as those commonly used in engineering practice. Special tests intended to evaluate a materials performance in the biological environment have been reserved for subsequent sections of this handbook.

It should be carefully noted that the procedures described in Sections I and II represent the spectrum of testing and evaluation to which every material should be subjected before it is evaluated and used as an implanted biomaterial. It is one of the main objectives of this handbook to underscore the necessity for thoroughly characterizing a material in terms of its engineering and physical properties before it is subjected to implant or other biocompatibility testing. Failure to adequately describe a material can mean that subsequent in vitro or in vivo evaluations may be uninterpretable and may significantly impede the development of the material for implantation or other medical applications.

ADDITIONAL READING

1   Black J. *Biological Performance of Materials: Fundamentals of Biocompatibility*, 2nd ed. New York: Marcel Dekker, 1992.
2   Black J. *Orthopaedic Biomaterials in Research and Practice*. New York: Churchill Livingston, 1988.
3   Hench LL, Ethridge EC. *Biomaterials*: An Interfacial Approach. New York: Academic Press, 1982.
4   Kambic HE, Yokobori AT (Eds) *Biomaterials Mechanical Properties*. ASTM STP 1173. W. Conshohocken, PA: American Society for Testing Materials, 1994.
5   Park JB, Lakes RS. *Biomaterials*. 2nd ed. New York: Plenum Press, 1992.
6   Williams D (Ed.). *Concise Encyclopedia of Medical and Dental Materials*. Cambridge, MA: The MIT Press, 1990.

Chapter 1
Metals, Alloys, and Ceramics

Robert M. Pilliar

Implantable devices intended for major load-bearing applications (primarily in orthopedics and dentistry) are made mainly from metals or ceramics, ultrahigh molecular weight polyethylene being a notable exception. This is due to intrinsic factors related to the interatomic bonding acting in these classes of materials as well as the microstructures that result during implant processing. This chapter briefly reviews metal and ceramic structures before discussing processing and property characterization of metallic and ceramic biomaterials. Material testing represents an important step in the design and fabrication of effective implants. Final pre-clinical testing should include performance testing of whole implants in the laboratory. Continued monitoring of devices during clinical use as well as assessment of retrieved devices represents the final important stage of biomaterial and implant characterization.

THE STRUCTURE OF METALS AND CERAMICS

Interatomic Bonding

Interatomic bonding in solids involves primary and secondary bonds, the former represented by strong ionic, covalent, and metallic bonds and the latter being weaker van der Waals and hydrogen bonds. For metals, ceramics and glasses, primary bonding results in their high melting points, high elastic moduli, and usually high strengths (although processing conditions are important in ensuring this last property). In all cases, the resulting forces acting between atoms are due to interactions involving outer orbit or valence electrons (the highest-energy, most loosely-bound electrons). Metals are characterized by non-directional metallic bonding with valence electrons being "pooled" and shared by all atoms. A consequence of this electron "pooling" is the ability of atoms to be displaced relatively readily from one lattice site to an adjoining site during force application. This translates into ductile behavior, a characteristic that is important in certain implant applications. Additionally, dense atom packing and electron sharing in metals leads to formation of partially filled outer electron "bands" [4]. This in turn results in the high electrical conductivity of metals, an important feature in conducting leads for neuromuscular stimulators (e.g., cardiac pacing leads). Ceramics and glasses are characterized by ionic and/or covalent bonding, resulting in very different intrinsic material characteristics. Ionically bonded ceramics (such as Al_2O_3 and ZrO_2) rely on electrostatic interactions between oppositely charged ions, and while this results in close ionic packing and high coordination numbers (i.e., number of immediately surrounding neighbor atoms), the need for nearest neighbors to be of opposite electrical charge leads to resistance for ion displacements and, hence, low ductility. Covalently bonded materials such as the silicate glasses with $(SiO_4)^{4-}$ networks form directional bonds (involving hybrid shared valence electron orbitals), thereby resulting in limited ductility and brittle behavior. These intrinsic characteristics related to interatomic bonding dictate both processing and design of components for all applications.

Strength of Materials

The strength of materials in the bulk depends directly on the strengths of the interatomic bonds (as well as other structural features still to be discussed). Strength is determined in standardized tests in which force is applied to specimens of uniform size and shape. In order to separate the effects of specimen geometry from those due to intrinsic material properties, force is normalized by dividing by specimen cross-sectional area to give *stress*. In tension (and compression), the applied force divided by the cross sectional area normal to the force application direction is called tensile (or compressive) stress, $\sigma = F/A_n$. A tensile stress will deform the specimen, causing it to elongate. (A compressive stress results in the opposite effect, causing specimen contraction parallel to the loading direction.) The increase in length due to a tensile force, Δl, divided by the original length, l_o, is defined as the tensile strain, $\varepsilon = \Delta l/l_o$. If one plots tensile stress, σ, versus tensile strain, ε, a stress-strain diagram will result. Initially, for metals and ceramics, the relationship is linear and strain is proportional to stress. Therefore, one can write $\sigma = E\varepsilon$ where E, the proportionality constant (called the *Young's modulus*) is a measure of the material's resistance to *elastic* deformation. At higher stress levels, this linear relationship breaks down. Either the specimen fractures without significant nonelastic deformation (brittle fracture), or nonlinear *plastic* deformation (involving shear deformation) commences. Similarly, a standardized specimen can be subjected to a shearing force where shear stress, τ, is equal to the applied load divided by the specimen area parallel to the force direction ($\tau = F/A_p$); the resulting shear strain, γ, is given by $\gamma = x/y = \tan\theta$ where θ is the angle through which the face of a cube unit of the specimen is displaced relative to the adjacent face as a result of the applied shear stress.

As with tensile loading, τ and γ are proportional initially (for metals and ceramics) with $\tau = G\gamma$ where G is another intrinsic material elastic property, the *Shear modulus*. Ultimately, the specimen will either deform plastically prior to failure or fail in a brittle manner. The shear stress versus shear strain curve for a given material is similar in shape to the stress-strain curve generated in response to tensile loading. A third elastic constant, Poisson's ratio (υ), is the ratio of radial contractile strain to axial strain: $\upsilon = -\varepsilon_{radial}/\varepsilon_{axial}$. The three elastic constants (E, G, υ) are not independent and for isotropic materials, $E = 2G(1+\upsilon)$.

The elastic relationships may be summarized as shown in Table 1-1.

Interatomic Forces, Elastic Moduli, and Crystal Lattices

For any material under given conditions, a characteristic three-dimensional atomic structure with a specific interatomic spacing (the equilibrium spacing) will form. This structure may be regular and repeating, in which case the material is crystalline or it may consist of a random arrangement of atoms or ions, thus defining an amorphous or glassy structure. For all solids, there is a characteristic interatomic spacing corresponding to a minimum energy state

Table 1-1 Elastic Relationships for Tension, Compression and Shear

	Tensile/compressive	Shear
Stress	$\sigma = F/A_n$	$\tau = F/A_p$
Strain	$\varepsilon = \Delta l/l_o$	$\gamma = x/y = \tan\theta$
Modulus	$E = \sigma/\epsilon$	$G = \tau/\gamma$

for the solid under prescribed external conditions. This equilibrium atomic configuration can be determined using x-ray or electron diffraction techniques. The slope of the interatomic force-versus-distance curve at the equilibrium spacing position is related to the elastic constants for the material [1–4]. Material processing has very little influence on this force-versus-displacement relation so that E, G and v represent intrinsic material properties independent of processing. They are dependent on atomic spacing and packing and, hence, the interatomic force-displacement relations. Thus, they are expected to change as materials transform from one crystallographic form to another. The different elastic constants for $(\alpha + \beta)$-Ti and the 100% β-Ti alloys (110 GPa versus 70 GPa) illustrate this effect.

The three-dimensional regular atomic arrangements characteristic of crystalline materials can be described by repeating units (unit cells) of which there are 14 different forms. The closest atom packing (highest coordination number) corresponds to structures with 12 nearest neighbors. The face-centered cubic (fcc) and hexagonal close-packed (hcp) unit cells represent such high coordination number structures and, along with body-centered cubic structures (coordination number $= 8$), they represent the most commonly occurring crystal structures for metallic biomaterials. Thus, the Co-based alloys are either fcc or hcp (dependent on temperature and composition), while Ti and its alloys form either hcp or bcc structures. Ceramics form somewhat more complex structures (hexagonal-rhombohedral for Al_2O_3 and cubic, tetragonal, or monoclinic for ZrO_2-based ceramics). Formation of amorphous structures by cooling from the melt is more easily achieved with the more complex non-metallic compounds such as the silicate-based glass materials.

Atomic Bonding and Plastic Deformation

Metals can display high degrees of ductility if appropriately processed. This, as already noted, is an intrinsic characteristic of metals resulting from the nature of the metallic bond and is responsible for the deformation behavior. In contrast, most ceramics display brittle behavior with very little plastic deformation prior to fracture. This is due to the fact that ionic bonding inhibits the movement of the ions relative to their nearest neighbors. If such movement occurred, it would violate the requirement that each ion be surrounded by ions of opposite charge.

Covalent bonding involves the sharing of valence electrons through the formation of hybrid electron orbitals between atoms. As a result, such bonding is directional, making plastic deformation difficult. A number of inorganic polymers form such bonds, and these represent an interesting group of ceramics and glasses currently being investigated for biomaterial applications. Included are various silicate-based glasses (based on covalently bonded $(SiO_4)^{4-}$ tetrahedra) and calcium polyphosphates (based on $(PO_4)^{3-}$ tetrahedra).

Phase Transformations—Diffusive and Displacive

The three-dimensional spatial arrangement of atoms and ions in solids is determined by factors such as atomic size, valence, and chemical affinity between elements under specific extrinsic conditions (i.e., temperature, pressure). For given conditions, the stable state of matter is determined by the structure displaying the minimum free energy [2]. The free energy, G, is related to the enthalpy, H, (heat of formation), and entropy, S, by the relation $G = H - TS$, where T is the absolute temperature. Changes in state or phase transformations in solids are possible if the reaction results in a decrease in G (i.e., $\Delta G = \Delta H - T\Delta S < 0$). At room temperature, therefore, if the system is at equilibrium, the structure with the lowest free energy will exist. Upon heating, the free energy of all possible phases will increase but may increase more rapidly for one phase than another. At some higher temperature, a new phase may form because it represents the lowest free energy form of the material at that temperature.

While this reduction in G represents a necessary condition for a phase change, it is not sufficient since the required atomic or ionic rearrangement to form the new phase depends on atomic or ionic transport processes occurring in reasonably short time periods. That is, kinetic as well as energy criteria must be satisfied. For most solid state phase transformations in metals and ceramics, structural rearrangements occur through thermally controlled atom diffusion (diffusive transformations). In some cases, phase transformations can occur by diffusionless processes (displacive transformations) that are not thermally controlled. Nearly all phase transformations of interest in the biomaterials field are of the diffusive type. However, the shape-memory alloy, NiTi, for example, undergoes a displacive (martensitic) transformation that results in its special characteristics. Martensitic transformations can occur during rapid cooling of Ti alloys from elevated temperatures ($>1000°C$). In addition, a strain-induced phase transformation occurs with stabilized ZrO_2 ceramics that is diffusionless and contributes to the observed high fracture toughness properties of this ceramic.

Atomic diffusion is important in many processes that occur during the production of metallic and ceramic implants. These include crystal formation from the melt; grain growth (during elevated temperature heating); the precipitation and growth of second phases; sintering of particles to form porous coatings; bonding of films to substrates; recrystallization in which relatively strain-free crystals nucleate and grow, replacing mechanically deformed crystals; and the formation of protective oxides over metal substrates (passive film growth). Bulk diffusion involves either interstitial or vacancy migration. In interstitial migration, small atoms move through interstitial spaces within crystal lattices. Because of the relatively low energy barriers for this process, interstitial diffusion rates are much higher than those for diffusion of large atoms. Diffusion of larger atoms, i.e., atoms of approximately the same size as the atoms of the crystal through which diffusion is occurring, depends on the presence of empty lattice sites or vacancies. For these large atoms, diffusion occurs by the stepwise exchange of positions of the diffusing atom and an adjacent vacant lattice site. This exchange requires a higher activation energy than does interstitial diffusion, and vacancy diffusion rates are consequently lower. Rapid interstitial diffusion can, in some cases, create problems. For example, the rapid diffusion of hydrogen into Ti-based alloys can result in the formation of brittle hydride phases. The diffusion of Cr atoms through the Fe crystal lattice of stainless steel is an example of vacancy diffusion. Note that the Cr atom is only 0.6% larger than the atoms of the iron lattice. Diffusion rates fall exponentially with temperature so that at some lower temperature, diffusion-driven structural changes will not occur in practical time periods even though they are energetically favored by ΔG considerations (i.e., $\Delta G < 0$). As a result, metastable structures can exist at ambient temperatures for some solids. The retention of fcc-structured phases in Co-based alloys is an example of this. The fcc phase is stable above about $900°C$; below this temperature, the hcp phase should form. However, the slow diffusion of Co, Cr, and Mo atoms at these lower temperatures prevents the ready formation of the hcp phase. The reaction is described as "sluggish" and only under special circumstances does the stable hcp phase form [5].

The formation of well-developed crystals requires the movement of atoms (or ions) to specific lattice sites during solidification from the melt (or during other types of solid formation reactions such as chemical or physical vapor deposition processes, methods that are being studied for making biomaterial films and coatings). Again, should rates of cooling be too great, the ordered positioning of atoms or ions cannot occur through diffusion and, instead, disordered or amorphous structures will develop. For ionically-bonded ceramics, this is more likely because of the relatively lower diffusion rates in the more complex ionically-bonded compounds (silicate glasses, for example).

Structure-Property Relations: Yield Strength and Dislocations

Point defects (vacancies), planar defects (grain boundaries), as well as line defects (dislocations) significantly affect the mechanical behavior of solids and are responsible for the various phenomena associated with plastic deformation [6]. These line defects extend from one surface of a crystal or grain to another. They have a surprising property: they can move or glide quite readily through the crystal under the influence of an applied shear stress. The onset of plastic deformation is identified by a material's yield strength. Yielding refers to the permanent deformation that occurs through shearing of atom planes relative to one another during the application of a shear force. Lattice shearing occurs along certain preferred crystallographic planes (close-packed planes oriented nearest to the maximum resolved shear force direction). The "glide" of dislocations along these close-packed planes results in material "slip" and irreversible plastic deformation. Microstructural features such as grain boundaries, impurity or alloying elements, and other dislocations act as barriers to dislocation movement, thereby explaining the observed effects of grain size, alloying, and mechanical deformation (work-hardening) on a material's stress-strain curve. A crystal yields when an applied force exceeds the force-resisting dislocation movement. For polycrystalline materials in which not all grains have close-packed planes ideally oriented for easy "glide" of dislocations, yielding will occur initially in the more favorably-oriented grains [6]. The tensile or compressive yield strength, σ_y, for a polycrystalline material is related to the shear yield stress, τ_y, by the relation $\sigma_y = 3\tau_y$. Thus, the tensile (and compressive) yield strengths are affected by structural features in the same way as τ_y. For metals, σ_y increases as grain size decreases ($\sigma_y \propto d^{-1/2}$ where d = grain size), illustrating the importance of grain size control on tensile yield strength of metals.

A further consideration in the selection and processing of materials for load-bearing applications is the effect of structure on fracture resistance. For metals, increasing the load during tensile testing results in increasing resistance to continued dislocation glide because of dislocation interactions with grain boundaries and other lattice imperfections, including other dislocations. This results in a strain hardening effect that increases to the point of local interatomic disruption and microvoid formation. These can grow and coalesce, leading eventually to gross sample fracture. An important determinant of how readily these phenomena will occur is the material's intrinsic ability to resist growth and coalescence of microvoids. Both internal microvoids formed through deformation and other pre-existing voids and defects due to material processing or component fabrication act similarly in determining fracture susceptibility. Fracture resistance can be described by the fracture energy, G_c, or fracture toughness, K_c, (critical stress intensity factor) for a material. G_c, (units of J-m^{-2}), is a measure of the maximum strain energy that can be applied at a stress concentration site, be it an internal or surface discontinuity. K_c, (units MN-m$^{-3/2}$), represents the critical stress concentration or stress intensity factor that can be tolerated at such a structural discontinuity prior to its unstable growth. The parameters G_c and K_c are related such that $K_c = (EG_c)^{1/2} = Y\sigma_f(\pi a)^{1/2}$ (for the case of plane stress deformation), where E and v are elastic constants as already defined, σ_f is the fracture strength, a is the length of the flaw resulting in the stress concentration, and Y is a function of flaw length and sample geometry. K_c and G_c are intrinsic material properties. The fracture strength of a material is determined by both this intrinsic material property and the geometry of structural discontinuities associated with the material. Both size and shape of the discontinuity are important in determining the local stress intensity. Very sharp flaws result in high local stress intensities for a given applied force. The ability of metals to deform plastically has a very profound effect on fracture resistance since plastic flow can blunt sharp discontinuities, thereby reducing local stress intensification. In contrast, brittle metals and ceramics, due to their limited ability to deform plastically, are very sensitive to the presence of stress-concentrating defects. Typically, metals used for biomaterial applications have fracture toughness values that are an order of magnitude or so higher than the highest values reported for bioceramics. As discussed below, the ability to form bioceramic components with diminutive flaws or defects is critical to the development of components that can be used reliably in certain load-bearing implant applications. Test methods based on fracture mechanics principles are used for quality control of bioceramic components [7]. The use of ceramic components is normally restricted to components that are expected to bear primarily compressive stresses, in which case this susceptibility to flaw growth due to high stresses acting locally is dramatically reduced. The fracture strengths of ceramics are typically 15 times greater in compression than in tension.

Metallic and Ceramic Biomaterials

Relatively few metals and ceramics are used as biomaterials (Table 1-2). These materials are used to form both bulk structures and coatings over appropriate substrates. It is important that processing conditions are carefully controlled to ensure desired component characteristics.

Metals (General)

A number of review articles describing the processing and properties of metallic biomaterials are available [5, 8–11]. The compositions most commonly used for orthopedic implant fabrication consist of stainless steels (primarily for temporary fracture fixation devices), Co-based alloys (cast or wrought), and, increasingly, thermomechanically processed Ti alloys. Recently, there has been increasing interest in some β-phase Ti alloys (because of the lower Young's moduli of these bcc metals, $E \approx 70$ GPa), and the shape memory alloy (TiNi) because of both its shape memory property (a characteristic that results in the component returning to a prior shape on reaching body temperature, for example), and its pseudoelastic property (i.e., $E_{\text{effective}} \approx 40$ GPa, a benefit in forming low stiffness, high springback orthodontic wires, for example). Current dental implants are made of commercial purity (cp) Ti or Ti alloys while the noble metals (Pt, Pt-Ir) find use as electrodes in cardiac pacing and other neuromuscular stimulatory devices. Relatively few metals are used for fabricating implantable devices (Tables 1-2 and 1-3), due principally to concerns over metal corrosion and the effects of degradation products on biocompatibility [14, 15] (see Chapter 14). In addition, the noble metals and alloys used as electrodes for neuromuscular stimulation are included in Table 1-2.

In order to achieve a required final metal implant shape, current practice utilizes either cast or wrought processing routes along with machining [11]. All metals are initially produced from the melt as cast billets that can be subsequently mechanically formed (e.g., forged, extruded or rolled) to a wrought product (bar or rod) from which final shapes can be made by further thermomechanical processing. Alternatively, implants can be formed directly by casting (usually with some additional machining, honing, and/or polishing). By casting, the higher costs of machining a shape from wrought bar stock can be avoided. Mechanical properties are not as high, however, as for wrought products (see Table 1-4).

Table 1-2 Selected Metals and Ceramics for Implant Fabrication

	Metals				Ceramics
	Ti-Based	**Co-Based**	**Fe-Based**	**Other**	
In clinical use	Ti (cp) Ti6Al4V Ti6Al7Nb Ti5Al2.5Fe	CoCrMo (*cast*) CoCrMo (*wr*) CoCrW (*wr*) CoNiCrMo (*wr*) CoNiCrFeMo (*wr*)	316L (*ss*) High N-Cr (*ss*)	Pt Pt-Ir Ta	Al_2O_3 Stabilized ZrO_2 Carbon Calcium Phosphate (HA, TCP) Bioglass AW Glass-Ceramic
Experimental	TiZrAlV TiZrNbTaPd TiSnNbTaPd NiTi TiNbZr		FeCrAl FeCrNiMoN	Nb ZrNb	Ca(Na)polymetaphosphates Monoclinical Al_2O_3/ZrO_2 Tera $Al_2O_3/ZrO_2/Y_2O_3$ Aluminium oxynitride

cp, commercial purity
wr, wrought
ss, stainless steel

Table 1-3   Compositions of Metal Alloys Used for Implant Fabrication

Element	Ti-based Tb (cp)	Ti6Al4V	Ti6Al7Nb	Ti5Al2.5Fe
H	0.0125–0.015	0.0125max	0.009max0.012	0.0125max
C	0.010max	0.08max	0.08max	0.08max
O	0.18–0.40	0.13max	0.20max	0.20max
N	0.03–0.05	0.05max	0.05max	0.05max
AL	–	5.5–6.5	5.5–6.5	4.5–5.5
V	–	3.5–4.5	–	–
Nb	–	–	6.5–7.5	–
Fe	0.30–0.50	0.25max	0.25max	2.0–3.0
Ti	Bal	Bal	Bal	Bal

	Co-Based Cast F75	Forged F75	p/m HIP F75	Wrought F90	Wrought F562	Wrought F563
C	0.35max	0.05max	0.23	0.05–0.15	0.025max	0.05max
Cr	27–30	26–28	28.8	19–21	19–21	18–22
Fe	0.75max	0.75max	0.15	3.0max	1.0max	4.0–6.0
Mo	5.0–7.0	5.0–7.0	5.81	–	9.0–10.5	3.0–4.0
Mn	1.0max	1.0max	0.4	2.0max	0.15max	1.0max
Ni	2.5max	1.0max	0.14	9.0–11.0	33–37	15–25
W	–	–	–	14–16	–	–
Si	1.0max	1.0max	0.7	–	0.15max	0.50max
Ti	–	–	–	–	–	0.5–3.5
Co	Bal	Bal	Bal	Bal	Bal	Bal

	Fe-Based 316L F55	316L F138	Rex 734
C	0.03max	0.03max	0.05
Cr	17.0–19.0	17.0–19.0	21.4
Mo	2.0–3.0	2.0–3.0	2.7
Mn	2.0max	2.0max	3.7
Ni	12.0–14.0	12.0–14.0	9.3
P	0.03max	0.025max	0.017
S	0.03max	0.01max	0.003
Si	0.75max	0.75max	0.19
Cu	0.50max	0.50max	–
N	0.10max	0.10max	0.39
Nb	–	–	0.28
Fe	Bal	Bal	Bal

cp, commercial purity

One other method of forming bulk metallic products has been considered for implant manufacture, namely consolidation of metal powders to form full density parts [11, 16]. The approach offers some advantages over the more conventional casting or forging and machining processes (i.e., finer grain size and retention of finely dispersed, nonmetallic phases), but the higher costs associated with processing have limited its use to certain components with special requirements.

The production of many implant components includes surface modification treatments such as coating metal surfaces with metal powders, wires, or fibers using high-temperature sintering to form porous coated, textured components for tissue (usually bone) ingrowth [17, 18]. Plasma-sprayed metal powders are used to form irregular surface geometries, again to allow tissue interlocking for implant fixation [19, 20], and different processes

Table 1-4 Mechanical Properties of Metals Used for Implant Fabrication

Treatment	Young's modulus (GPa)	Yield strength (MPa)	Ult strength (MPa)	% Elong	Fat strength (MPa) $R = -1$
Co-Based					
Cast F75	210–220	450–490	731–889	11.0–17.0	250
Forged F75	"	890–1030	1410–1510	28	790–970
p/m HIP F75	"	840	1280	14	725
Wrought F90	"	1180–1610	1350–1900	10.0–22.0	490–590
Wrought F562	"	650–1900	1000–2050	10.0–20.0	405–435
Wrought F563	"	828	1000	18	
Ti-Based					
cpTi (low O)	116	170	240	24	–
cpTi (high O)	"	485	550	15	–
Ti6Al4V	≈110	1050	1150	13	625
Ti6Al7Nb	"	900–1000	1000–1100	13	500–600
Ti5Al2.5Fe	"	820–920	940–1050	13–17	600
Fe-Based					
316L (annealed)	190–200	170–205	480–645	40–68	207
316L (cold worked)	"	655–1160	655–1260	6–28	440
316L (high N anneal)	"	–	–	–	270
Rex734	"	810	1150	15	583

(plasma spraying, sputtering, precipitation from solution, sol-gel wet chemistry) are used for placement of coatings of so-called bioactive ceramics (calcium hydroxyapatite and other calcium phosphate phases) over metallic substrates [21, 22]. Surface modification treatments involving physical or chemical vapor deposition processes (PVD or CVD, respectively) are also used for enhancing the wear and corrosion resistance of implants [23, 24]. These processes include ion implantation (with N^+ and other elements) [25, 26] and TiN coatings formed by plasma ion plating [24]. The application of diamond-like coatings (DLC) on Ti alloy substrates represents a more recent approach for developing superior wear-resistant Ti alloy surfaces [27].

Testing and Evaluation of Metals for Biomaterials Applications

The major advantage offered by metals for implant fabrication is their ductility and high fracture toughness. Their major disadvantage is their susceptibility to corrosion, resulting in concerns over ion release and effects on cells and tissues as well as effects on long-term mechanical properties. Thus, test methods for evaluating metals to be used for implant fabrication should assess mechanical properties and corrosion resistance as well as the effects of mechanical loading in corrosive environments that simulate in vivo conditions.

Mechanical Testing of Metallic Biomaterials

Static Tests: Stress-Strain Diagrams The initial linear portion of the σ-ε curve represents elastic behavior and, as already noted, is related to the interatomic forces. Metals typically display such linear elastic behavior. Young's moduli for metallic biomaterials range from about 40 GPa (inclusive of pseudoelastic behavior) to 210 GPa, values that are an order of magnitude or so greater than the values for bone ($E_{cortical\ bone} \approx 10-20$ GPa; $E_{cancellous\ bone} \approx 1-5$ GPa). Increasing the stress beyond the Proportional Limit (the maximum stress for which σ is linearly related to ε) results in a nonlinear σ versus ε relation corresponding to plastic deformation. For specimens loaded within the elastic range, unloading results in complete reversal of the deformation (strain returns to zero). The stress at which noticeable plastic deformation initiates is defined as the yield strength, σ_y, or proof stress corresponding to the stress required to cause an arbitrarily selected level of strain, usually 0.1% ($\sigma_{0.1}$) or 0.2% ($\sigma_{0.2}$).

Stress-strain curves should be determined using test specimens loaded at prescribed rates (ASTM E8 and E8M—tensile testing; ASTM E9—compressive testing) in well-defined test environments with controlled atmospheric and temperature conditions. Loads are measured using load cells, devices that determine mechanical force amplitudes through measurements of changes in electrical resistance of elements within the cell, while displacements are accurately measured using strain gauges or extensometers attached to the surface of the test specimen. These measure changes in electrical impedance that can be related to displacements. These instruments can give accurate determinations of extension to within 0.1 μm, and should be used when determining elastic constants of metals (see ASTM E83 for classifications of extensometers). At higher strains, cross-head displacement can be used to determine strains. For certain specialized applications in which very small specimen dimensions occur, non-contacting methods for measuring displacement are possible. These utilize laser optical methods for measuring displacements. Displacements less than 0.1 μm can be detected with the more sophisticated laser telemetry systems that are currently available. This is not normally required for testing standard metallic specimens but could be important when evaluating properties of fine wires, fibers, or films, for example. In addition, other methods involving the measurement of the velocity of an ultrasonic wave propagating through a sample [28], or of the vibration frequency of thin reed-like specimens [29] can be used to determine elastic constants.

Plastic deformation occurs at stresses above σ_y, so unloading leaves the specimen permanently deformed. Upon subsequent re-loading, an increased stress is required for further plastic deformation, a phenomenon known as strain hardening or work hardening. This increase reflects the higher shear stress needed for additional slip by dislocation glide.

The ductility of a material can be approximated by fitting the halves of a fractured specimen back together and then measuring the overall length, l_{final} of the sample. The change in length, Δl, is equal to $l_{final} - l_{initial}$ and the percent ductility is equal to $\Delta l / l_{initial} \times 100$. An additional quantity that is often reported as a measure of ductility is the % Reduction in Area. This is equal to the change in cross-sectional area/original cross-sectional area, ($\Delta A / A_i \times 100$ for the test specimen, with the final cross-sectional area being determined at fracture.

While the σ-ε relationship of the metals currently used for implant fabrication is not affected greatly by the rate of loading (or strain rate), other metals, particularly those that rely on interstitial atoms for solid solution strengthening (like mild steel), display significant strain rate sensitivity. Strain or loading rates should always be included in reports of static load tests.

The determination of resistance to shear forces can be achieved using appropriate test specimens (ASTM E143) and machines fitted with load cells to measure applied torque (force $\times$ moment arm) for varying angular displacements. Torque versus angular displacement (normalized to give shear stress, τ, versus shear strain, γ) curves can be used to determine G, τ_y, τ_{ult} and γ_{max}.

In some cases, it is more convenient to assess elastic properties using bending rather than axial loading. Often, difficulties in making samples with reduced cross-sectional gauge length regions necessitate the use of simple rectangular cross-sectional bars or cylinders that are deformed by 3- or 4-point loading or other configurations such as cantilever loading (ASTM E855). Loading results in tensile stressing of one surface (the convex surface) and compressive stressing of the opposing (concave) surface. Relations between surface stress and deflection for given span lengths and specimen dimensions within the elastic strain region are readily determined. It should be noted that these relations are only valid within the elastic range of deformation. Hence, they are used primarily with brittle materials (such as ceramics) but find use in metals as well if the metallic samples display limited ductility. This is the case with metal-powder-based samples in the so-called "green" state (prior to sintering) (ASTM B312). Such tests can be used to determine E and the transverse rupture strength, TRS (also referred to as the Modulus of Rupture which is just the calculated outer fiber tensile stress at fracture). The test is used to a greater extent with ceramics (ASTM C674).

Hardness Testing

One of the most convenient tests for characterizing the yield strength of metals is the hardness test. The test consists of pressing a pyramidal (diamond) or spherical-shaped (hardened steel) indenter into a flat, polished surface of a material and then measuring the dimensions of the resulting indentation. The hardness, H, is defined as the force, F, applied to the indenter divided by the projected area of the indent, $H = F_{applied}/A_{projected}$. Hardness is related to the yield strength, σ_y, for many metals; $H = 3\sigma_y$ assuming no work hardening during indentation, a condition that is rarely satisfied [1]. The test provides a non-destructive method for assessing the effect of processing on σ_y, for example, or for comparing materials. Microhardness testing (ASTM E384) allows very localized regions to be characterized so that variations in properties from one region to another can be determined at the micron-range of spatial resolution. Recently, nano-hardness testing machines have been developed that allow assessment of hardness of very thin surface films with a spatial resolution of 100 nm [30]. This could prove of great value in characterizing properties of thin films placed over metallic or ceramic substrates to form surface-modified implant materials. (This test method is also useful for assessing hardness properties of softer materials such as polymers and elastomers.)

Fracture Toughness Testing

Measurement of the area under the elastic portion of a σ-ε curve provides a measure of the energy of elastic deformation $= 1/2(\sigma\varepsilon)$ (assuming linear σ-ε behavior). This quantity is commonly considered an indicator of a material's toughness, although it should be recognized that, for most metals, the major portion of strain energy resulting in fracture involves plastic deformation. Even then, the area under a σ-ε curve to fracture does not necessarily reflect the fracture resistance of a material. This is because for most materials (metals and ceramics included), local regions of stress concentration due to structural flaws occur and these regions determine the fracture characteristics.

Test specimens with a variety of geometries used for assessing the fracture toughness parameter, are K_{Ic}. Standard test specimens (ASTM E399 and E1304) containing a fatigue pre-crack of specified length are normally used. These specimens are loaded in a crack opening mode for which the local stress intensity acting at the crack tip can be determined using available relations. The maximum load, P_c, to cause initiation of unstable growth of this pre-crack is measured and used to calculate K_{Ic}, the plane strain fracture toughness. Typically, alloys designed for load-bearing applications display K_{Ic} values $\approx$100 MN-m$^{-3/2}$. This is in contrast with the highest K_{Ic} values reported for ceramics $\approx$15 MN-m$^{-3/2}$ and more usually $\approx$1–5 MN-m$^{-3/2}$. The tests are limited to materials that display limited ductility such that the plastic zone size associated with the crack tip is small compared with the specimen dimensions. For metals displaying general yielding at the crack tip, more complex elastic-plastic testing procedures and analysis methods are required [31]. These are not commonly used in characterizing metallic biomaterials.

Dynamic Testing: Fatigue

While static test methods as described above are useful in selecting metals for load-bearing applications, in most cases metallic components are used in situations involving repeated or cyclic loads. Mechanical failure is most likely to occur by metal fatigue. Thus, it is important that fatigue testing is undertaken as part of a program for selecting metals for load-bearing implant applications.

Tests for fatigue are designed to determine the number of load cycles that a standard test specimen can tolerate prior to failure. The direction of force application during testing can be the same as for static testing (axial, torsion, or bending). Bend tests using rotating beam specimens (circular cross sections) or axial test specimens (circular or rectangular cross-sections) are most often used (ASTM E466). The surfaces of rotating beam specimens are subjected to alternating tensile and compressive stresses. The rotating beam fatigue specimens give a fatigue ratio, R, (minimum/maximum stress) $=$ 1. Using axial fatigue specimens, different R values can be used and should be reported with test data. Care must be taken to properly align axial fatigue specimens to avoid bending moments superimposed on the intended axial forces. The problem of bending becomes especially critical for testing with $R < 0$, since specimen instability by buckling can occur.

Fatigue testing is conducted at selected test frequencies and under fixed test conditions (environment, temperature). Test specimen surface preparation is critical for ensuring reliable and reproducible test results. Fatigue is a two-stage process involving i) initiation and ii) propagation of cracks. Thus, any inadvertent surface flaw due to machining or poor polishing can severely affect results through introduction of preformed stress concentrations that will readily promote crack initiation. Other tests in which surface notches are purposely added are sometimes used to assess the notch fatigue sensitivity of metals [32, 33]. Care must be taken to ensure that the notch root radius in such test specimens is constant from one test specimen to another since this will affect the local stress concentration and, therefore, crack initiation at the notch root.

In conducting fatigue tests, the stress amplitude, $\Delta\sigma = (\sigma_{max} - \sigma_{min})$, the mean stress, $\sigma_m = (\sigma_{max} + \sigma_{min})/2$, and mean stress amplitude, $\sigma_a = (\sigma_{max} - \sigma_{min})/2$ should be specified. Results of tests are normally plotted as $\Delta\sigma$ versus log N(N = number of cycles to failure). Such a plot allows the identification of either a fatigue limit (stress below which failure is unlikely regardless of the number of load cycles, assuming a constant environment and test frequency or an endurance limit for a certain number of cycles (e.g., 10^7 or 10^8 cycles). This latter approach is used with materials that do not display a well-defined fatigue limit.

Fatigue life is a function of the shape of the imposed cyclic load pattern as well as the mean load and load amplitude. Most often, sinusoidal load patterns of constant amplitude and mean load are used during testing. However, modern computer-controlled, servo-hydraulic testing machines allow the use of complex load patterns that can be more representative of expected in-service loading. While this is not common for implant testing at present, it represents fairly standard practice in other fields such as the automotive and aircraft industries. Even for simpler waveforms, with a fixed amplitude, differences in the mean load will affect specimen lifetime. Mean stress and stress amplitude should always be reported with results of fatigue testing.

Fatigue of metals is divided into two regimes depending on the stress amplitude used during testing and the resulting number of cycles to failure. Specimens that are loaded at σ_{max} above the nominal (general) yield stress (i.e., the average stress ignoring local stress concentrations), will fail normally in $<10^4$ cycles or so. This is referred to as low cycle fatigue (LCF). During low cycle fatigue, the specimen lifetime is divided more or less equally between initiation and propagation of fatigue cracks. For specimens loaded at stresses below the general yield stress, most of the fatigue lifetime involves initiating fatigue cracks that then propagate to cause failure (i.e., $N_{init} \approx 0.9N_{total}$). This is known as high cycle fatigue (HCF). Since the process of fatigue crack initiation represents a statistical event, fatigue lifetimes, particularly in cases of HCF, will vary over a range (typically an order of magnitude), assuming all other factors are constant. For this reason, it is important that a sufficient number of specimens be tested for statistically significant S-N curves to be plotted (34) and that data is presented in accordance with recommended practice (ASTM E468).

The results of fatigue tests are dependent on environmental conditions and test frequency as already stated. Because of the nature of fatigue mechanisms, these environmental factors are especially critical. The process of fatigue can involve lengthy periods of specimen testing so that interactions between the specimen surface and the test environment can profoundly affect the initiation and propagation of fatigue cracks. After initiation of cracks, test frequency becomes particularly important since it will determine the time of exposure to the testing environment of a freshly-formed surface at the crack tip. For metals such as Ti and its alloys that react strongly with H^+ and O^{2-} ions upon exposure of native surfaces, this can be extremely important [35].

In addition to determination of overall fatigue lives by cyclic testing, crack propagation rates can also be determined using standard test methods (ASTM E647). This represents a fracture mechanics approach to assessing the rate at which a crack will propagate through a test specimen during cyclic loading under set conditions (environment, frequency). Test specimens similar to those used for fracture toughness testing are used. In this case, however, the rate of crack growth as a function of load cycles is measured using either optical methods or measurements of changes in electrical resistivity or specimen compliance (determined using strain gauges or extensometers attached to the specimen). The results are plotted as log-log plots of da/dN versus ΔK, where a = crack length, N = number of cycles, and ΔK = stress intensity range = $K_{max} - K_{min}$ during each cycle of loading. The test provides a convenient method for determining the effect of environment on crack propagation since the specimen can be mounted in a fatigue testing machine with the crack tip region exposed to a particular solution of known pH, temperature or composition [35].

Microstructural Characterization

Properties of materials are inextricably related to structure at the atomic (10^{-10} m), nano- (10^{-7} to 10^{-9} m), and microscale ($>10^{-7}$ m) (4). Microscopic characterization of metals (and other materials) at the submicron and micron level represents a valuable approach for understanding processing effects on material performance.

For studying bulk structures of metallic samples, metallographic techniques involving grinding and polishing of sample surfaces and their subsequent examination in either the unetched or etched condition represents common practice for determination of grain size (ASTM E112), identification and determination of distribution of phases (ASTM E1382), and other microstructural features such as twins, stacking faults, precipitates, and non-metallic inclusions (ASTM E1245). Identification of precipitates and inclusions is most commonly achieved by X-ray diffraction. Fractographic analysis using either relatively low magnification optical ($<50 \times$) or high resolution scanning electron microscopic (20 to 20000 $\times$) methods are extremely useful in identifying modes and causes of part failure. At the experimental phase of material study, transmission electron microscopy of thin metal foil samples is used to investigate deformation mechanisms, phase transformations, and many other fundamental phenomena that determine material properties.

Ceramics (General)

The ceramics used for implant fabrication are listed in Table 1-5. In addition to the excellent *in vivo* corrosion and wear resistance of the bulk "inert" ceramics (Al_2O_3, ZrO_2), surface reactive and biodegradable ceramics and glasses described as "bioactive" have been developed [12, 13]. These materials appear capable of allowing (perhaps promoting) tissue bonding or, at least, close tissue apposition, resulting in better attachment of living tissues to implants through mechanical or chemical interactions [36–38]. Widespread use of these materials for load-bearing applications remains limited, however, because of their low fracture toughness and consequent concerns about in vivo fracture [39, 40]. This limitation must be considered in designing ceramic (or glass) implant components.

Most "inert" ceramic implant components are formed by consolidating powders using high-temperature sintering and pressure [2, 3]. Melt forming is not feasible commercially

Table 1-5   Properties of Some Glass and Ceramic Biomaterials

Material	Young's Modulus (GPa)	Strength Comp (MPa)	Bend Strength (MPa)	Hardness	Density (g/cm³)	KIc (MPa-m$^{1/2}$)
Inert						
Al_2O_3	380	4000	300–400	2000–3000 (HV)	>3.9	5.0–6.0
ZrO_2 (PS)	150–200	2000	200–500	1000–3000 (HV)	≈6.0	4.0–12.0
C-(Graphite)	20–25	138			1.5–1.9	—
C-(LTI pyrolitic)	17–28	900	270–550		1.7–2.2	—
C-(Vitreous)	24–31	172	70–207	150–200 (DPH)	1.4–1.6	—
Bioactive						
HA	73–117	600	120	350	3.1	<1
Bioglass	≈75	1000	50	—	2.5	0.7
AW Glass-Ceramic	118	1080	215	680	2.8	≈2

N.B. The variation in Young's Modulus noted for some of the materials listed is due to variations in density of test specimens. PS, partially stabilized; HA, hydroxy apatite; AW, apatite–wollanstonite; HV, Vickers hardness; DPH, diamond pyramid hardness.

because of the high melting points of these materials. Powders are first compacted to a starting shape with or without the use of a binder to give a "green" compact. This unsintered part should be strong enough to be handled and transferred to a furnace or hot press for further processing. Pressureless sintering causes particles to bond together by the growth of interparticle "necks," thereby reducing total surface area and increasing density of the component. Sintering rates increase with higher sintering temperatures (as expected for a diffusion-controlled process) and decreasing particle size. Hence, the use of very fine starting powders is favored for achieving full-density components with sintering temperatures being as high as practical. Nevertheless, even when such steps are taken, some residual porosity remains even after very long (and economically impractical) sintering times. These residual pores represent structural flaws or defects that can have a very detrimental effect on fracture strength of ceramics and glasses. Thus, hot pressing (using either axial or isostatic compression) is favored in order to achieve the highest density possible (>99.99% full density). This is important in developing high-performance ceramics such as those required for the articulating surfaces of orthopedic joint replacement implants, since any internal voids or surface irregularities will act as stress concentrators and potential sites for initiation of component fracture. Ceramics (crystalline and amorphous) are intrinsically brittle because of the ionic and/or covalent nature of their interatomic bonds and because of their complex lattice structures that do not allow easy plastic flow by dislocation glide. Thus, the intensity of these stress concentrators cannot be reduced by plastic flow and crack tip blunting, as occurs with ductile metals. The fracture strength of ceramics can be described using fracture mechanics (i.e., tensile or fracture strength, $\sigma_{ts} \propto K_{Ic}/(\pi a)^{1/2}$). This relation predicts that materials with smaller intrinsic flaws (i.e., lower "a") will have higher σ_{ts}. Therefore very fine powders and well-controlled processing should be used to limit the number and size of internal pores or voids within a component, and careful finishing operations should be conducted to avoid significant machining marks or other surface features that could act as critical stress concentrators.

Carbon

Chemical vapor deposition processes and direct pyrolysis of polymeric preforms are used to form carbon-based ceramics. Carbon in its various forms (diamond, graphite, pyrolitic low temperature isotropic (LTI) and ultra-low temperature isotropic (ULTI) carbon, and vitreous carbon) is covalently bonded with weaker secondary bonds (van der Waals) also contributing to the structure of all but the diamond form. The nature of the interatomic bonding and combined covalent-van der Waals bonds strongly influence final properties. These carbon-based materials are highly suitable for many tissue-interfacing applications (e.g., disc occluders in heart valves). They do not normally invoke undesirable host responses. Caution must be used, however, in their use in major load-bearing applications, again because of their intrinsic brittleness and low tensile strength [41].

Glasses

While crystalline solids have very well-defined melting and freezing temperatures, glasses tend to soften upon heating and become viscous prior to becoming liquid. The temperature at which a material becomes viscous (on heating) or rigid (on cooling) is defined as the glass temperature, T_g. It is the temperature at which an arbitrarily-selected viscosity (typically 10^{-7} poise) is reached. The determination of T_g should be included in characterizing glasses in order to allow proper processing and use of glassy implants. As with crystalline ceramics, glasses are brittle so that the same considerations concerning the effects of surface flaws and internal structural defects apply. Assessment of fracture resistance and fracture toughness should be included in glass characterization.

Melting and casting of silicate-based glass components represents a commercially practical processing route because of the relatively low melting temperatures of these materials. Alternatively, glass particles (or frit) formed by ball milling coarser particles can be consolidated by sintering at above T_g to form final shapes.

Testing and Evaluation of Bioceramics

While fatigue and yield strength are properties of prime importance in the design of metallic load-bearing components, fracture resistance is the primary design consideration for ceramics. Many of the test methods used for characterizing metallic biomaterials are applicable to bioceramics, but their intrinsic brittleness makes some of these methods impractical. In general, electrochemical corrosion is insignificant with these materials since they are electrical insulators, although they are susceptible to localized chemical attack. While corrosion assessment is not as critical for ceramics as for the metals, due consideration must be given to possible chemical degradation and its effects on other properties (i.e., mechanical strength and fracture resistance).

Static Testing

The intrinsic brittle nature of ceramics and glasses introduces certain difficulties in the mechanical testing of these materials. Thus, the use of axial tensile testing is not usual with ceramics since major problems are encountered in gripping specimens with stress concentrations at the specimen grip junctions, resulting in crack initiation and propagation at this point. By using bending tests (either 3- or 4-point loading) of rectangular cross-sectioned bars, this problem can be avoided. This test is used to determine elastic modulus, flexure strength or Modulus of Rupture (MOR), and maximum deflection prior to fracture (ASTM C674). Four-point bending offers the advantage of not forcing fracture at the mid-span position since a constant bending moment applies between the two inner points of load application. The flexure strength (or MOR) is given by $\sigma_{flex} = 6Fl/bh^3$ where b is the width of the specimen and F is the load at fracture. Young's modulus, E, is given by $E = (Fa/2bh^3 S)(3l^2 - 4a^2)$ where S is the maximum deflection. Using a disk-shaped ceramic specimen loaded in flexure with a point load in the center of the disk and 3-point- or ring-loading near its circumference, a biaxial flexure strength can be determined (ASTM F394). This geometry is often more convenient in terms of specimen preparation and testing. An alternate method for determining Young's modulus of ceramics is the use of ultrasonics, in which the velocity of sound in the material in a specific direction, v_x, is measured and E is determined using the relation $v_x = (E/\rho)^{1/2}$ where $\rho =$ density of the material being tested [1]. The method is reliable and convenient, assuming that the percentage of internal voids is low, thereby allowing relatively unscattered transmission of sound waves through the test sample. Determination of elastic moduli can also be determined by resonance testing of rod-shaped specimens (ASTM C848, C623).

Another simple and convenient test for determining the fracture strength, σ_{ts}, of completely brittle materials is the diametral compression test [42] in which a cylindrical test specimen is loaded along its diameter until it fails. For this test, $\sigma_{ts} = 2F/\pi Dt$ where $F =$ applied load, $D =$ specimen diameter, $t =$ specimen thickness.

The importance of the low fracture toughness and presence of a distribution of internal flaws of varying size, shape, and orientation within test specimens introduces a further complication in the mechanical testing of ceramics and glasses. Since, as noted above, $\sigma_{ts} \propto K_{Ic}/(\pi a)^{1/2}$, the largest favorably-oriented flaw within the test specimen will determine its fracture strength. Thus, some scatter in measured strengths is expected for a population of test specimens. The degree of scatter represents an important material characteristic reflecting both an intrinsic material parameter, K_{Ic}, and processing conditions (flaw characteristics). It is characterized quantitatively by use of the Weibull distribution function, in which, for a volume of material, V_o, the survival probability, $P\sigma(V_o) = \exp\{-(\sigma/\sigma_o)^m\}$, where σ_o is the tensile stress at which $1/e(= 0.37)$ of the specimens survive and m is a constant, the Weibull modulus, related to the degree of scatter in σ_{ts} [1]. A population of test specimens exhibiting very little scatter will have a high value of m while low values will result for samples displaying large variations in properties. A plot of $\ln\{\ln(1/P\sigma(V_o))\}$ vs $m \ln(\sigma/\sigma_o)$ allows the constant m to be determined as the slope of the resulting straight line. Sufficient test samples should be included in assessing fracture strengths of these brittle materials to provide the required degree of confidence in designing ceramic implants. Test environment and specimen volume can also affect these parameters.

Hardness Testing

Hardness testing represents a common method for characterizing ceramics. It is used as a means of predicting wear resistance and assessing fracture toughness using the indentation fracture toughness test (see below). Because of their high hardness, diamond indenters are usually used for the testing of ceramics and glasses. The Vickers hardness test utilizing a diamond pyramidal indenter is commonly used. Test procedures are similar to those used with metals. Knoop hardness testing of ceramics (ASTM C849) and glass (ASTM C730) is also used.

Fracture Toughness Testing

The use of compact tension or 3-point bend tests (ASTM E-399) for assessing K_{Ic} of metals requires the introduction of a fatigue pre-crack. Ceramics and glasses pose a problem in forming controlled fatigue pre-cracks because of their brittle nature, but because of this intrinsic brittleness, fatigue pre-cracking is not as critical prior to fracture toughness testing. Rather, a sharp machined notch can be used as a reproducible stress concentrator suitable for conducting the test. Given the specimen dimensions and an empirically-derived compliance calibration factor, K_{Ic} is then determined from the critical load, P_c, corresponding to the onset of unstable crack growth. Even so, the preparation of notched specimens can be troublesome with hard ceramics and glasses. An alternative fracture toughness test for these difficult-to-machine materials is the indentation fracture toughness test. This test utilizes a diamond pyramidal indenter loaded so that cracking occurs from the corners of the indenter. The lengths of the radial cracks are measured and an empirical relation is used to relate these and the indenter parameters to K_{Ic} [43]. The method appears to give reliable results at least for those materials that are homogenous, isotropic, and brittle. This test has also been used to assess other biomaterials including bone and enamel.

Dynamic Testing-Fatigue

Because of the limited ductility and relatively low fracture toughness of ceramics and glasses, they do not normally fail in fatigue by mechanisms assumed to act in metals involving plastic deformation and slip causing crack initiation and propagation. For brittle materials, crack growth can occur during sustained static loading as well as during cyclic loading. Crack progression results in increased stress intensities at the crack tip, leading to eventual catastrophic fracture of the material. Progressive crack growth under static loading conditions is referred to as static fatigue while cyclic loading results in flaw or crack growth due to dynamic fatigue. In both cases, knowledge of crack growth rates, da/dt (or da/dN) as a function of local stress intensity, K, or stress intensity range, ΔK, allows an estimate of lifetime to fracture. However, even under the most stringent quality-control conditions, some degree of uncertainty remains in predicting performance of these brittle materials in load-bearing implant applications [7].

Microstructural Characterization

The methods for characterization of structures and physical properties of ceramics and glasses are similar to those used with metals. Despite their high chemical stability, ceramics can degrade in physiological solutions.

Characterization of Porous and Other Surface Coatings

In order to satisfy quite diverse bulk and surface property requirements, some implants are dual-structured, having surface coatings or films to satisfy certain requirements (e.g., tissue ingrowth or bonding, corrosion resistance, wear resistance) over substrates satisfying other needs (e.g., load-bearing, electrical conduction). The assurance of reliable coating-substrate bonding represents a common requirement for all such systems with other parameters, such as geometric features of the coatings or films (throughout or at the surface) being specific to the application. This section will focus on the methods for characterizing coatings (metal, ceramic, or polymer-based) applied to metal or ceramic substrates.

Coatings for Implant Fixation

Porous coatings for implant stabilization by tissue ingrowth can be formed by sintering metal, ceramic or polymeric powders, wires (single strand or in mesh form), or fibers onto solid substrates, thereby creating a three-dimensional, interconnected array of pores throughout the coating thickness [18]. Additionally, plasma-sprayed metallic coatings are described as "porous" although the porosity resulting in some of these coatings is not as extensive or interconnected as with sintered coatings. Notwithstanding this distinction between sintered and plasma-sprayed coatings, both appear effective in fixing implants to bone, the sintered systems by a three-dimensional ingrowth and interconnection, and the plasma-sprayed systems by bone formation within available undercut regions and other surface irregularities. The effectiveness of both types of coatings is strongly dependent on the geometric characteristics of the coating layer as well as the mechanical integrity of the coating and its bonding to the underlying substrate. Because of the high surface area that such coatings normally present (typically 5 to 10 times that of a smooth, non-porous-coated surface), corrosion properties and possible higher rates of metal ion release should be considered. Also, the geometric features resulting at the junction of the coating elements to the solid substrate introduce regions of stress concentration that can affect mechanical properties of the substrate; this emphasizes the need for mechanical testing of porous-coated test specimens [22]. The processing to form well-bonded coatings may also involve special heat treatments that alter microstructures and mechanical properties of substrates.

While the bioactive glass, ceramic, and glass-ceramic compositions evoke desirable tissue reactions at their surfaces (promote attachment or bonding), the low tensile strength and poor fracture resistance of these materials make them unsuitable for forming mono-lithic load-bearing implants. They can, however, be used effectively as surface coatings. Plasma-sprayed calcium hydroxyapatite coatings have found the greatest application in this regard, although studies with other bioactive coatings (silicate-based bioglass, apatite-wollastonite-containing glass-ceramics) formed by other methods (sintering, dipping, wet chemical methods, electrodeposition, sol-gel coating, sputtering) have also been reported [18]. A common concern with all these methods is assurance that suitable coating-substrate bonding occurs in order to avoid delamination and debris generation during in vivo use. Appropriate testing to ensure reliable coating integrity should be included in characterizing these systems. The very thin films that result with some of these methods (submicron-thick-sputtered and sol-gel-formed films, for example) require special testing methods.

The use of bioactive coatings as a temporary layer to accelerate the rate of bone for-mation on the surface of porous-coated metallic implants has been studied by a number of investigators [9, 18, 44]. The approach seeks benefits from the demonstrated osteoconduc-tive properties of plasma-sprayed hydroxyapatite. In this application, the bond strength of the hydroxyapatite to the substrate is supposedly of less concern, but it should be noted that coating delamination and fragmentation over the short term or even during implant insertion represents a potential source of particulate debris that could act as wear particles (3-body wear) or invoke undesirable inflammatory responses. Hence, the need for coatings with good substrate attachment remains.

Other Coatings

Wear and corrosion resistance of implants can be improved potentially through the application of coatings such as flame-sprayed Al_2O_3 [45], sol-gel-formed ZrO_2 thin films [46], and TiN ion-plated layers [24, 47]. Characterization of wear, corrosion, fatigue and other properties should be undertaken as with uncoated materials. The characterization of coating-to-substrate bonding, as with the bioactive films noted above, require special test methods. This becomes particularly important since the formation of cracks within the coating layer can result in accelerated corrosion, fatigue, or wear compared with uncoated substrates.

CHARACTERIZATION OF COATINGS

Stereomicroscopy

If the principal reason for use of coatings is to allow reliable implant-tissue fixation by tissue (usually bone) ingrowth, geometric characterization of the coating is important [48–50]. Volume percent porosity, mean pore size and pore size distribution throughout the coating thickness, and shape and interconnectedness of pores are parameters that will affect tissue interactions and interfacial fixation strength. Similarly, interparticle neck diameters (for sintered powders, wires, or fibers), and local radii of curvature of surface discontinuities (for plasma-sprayed layers) are parameters that will affect the strength of the coating itself and the coating-substrate complex. These parameters can be determined by reflected light and scanning electron microscopic examination of ground and polished sections prepared transverse to the coating thickness. Additionally, the size and distribution of openings available for tissue ingrowth can be determined directly by mercury intrusion porosimetry (with due recognition of its limitations for assessing properties of thickness-limited coatings) or scanning electron microscopic examination of structures viewed normal to the coated surface.

Mechanical Properties (Interfacial Shear and Tensile Strengths—Static and Fatigue)

In situations of implant-to-bone fixation, significant forces can act at the coating-substrate interface especially where the coating and substrate have significantly different elastic moduli, (e.g., ceramic or glass on metal). Such combinations can lead to coating delamination. Thus, knowledge of the mechanical strength of this interface, both for static and dynamic loading is important. Methods for assessing the coating-substrate interface strength for sintered porous coatings have been established (ASTM F1044 for interfacial shear strength, ASTM F1147 for tension testing), although it should be recognized that other test methods may be equally acceptable. Similar methods should be appropriate for testing plasma-sprayed coating-substrate interfaces. These methods can be adapted for characterization of interfacial shear *fatigue* strengths. Determination of interfacial tensile fatigue strengths, however, is not straightforward, and development of reliable test methods continues to present a challenge. Following testing, the nature of the fracture (adhesive or cohesive) can be characterized by examination of failed surfaces using scanning electron microscopy.

While shear and tensile strength testing of thicker coatings ($>20 \ \mu$m) is possible using the methods described above, characterizing the interfacial strength for "thin" coatings ($<1 \ \mu$m thick) on solid substrates is difficult since the use of shearing collars or adhesives for forming lap shear tests or interfacial tensile strength test samples is either impractical or fraught with possible artifacts due to the thinness of the coating or film. The methods that have been used with biomaterials include bend testing of specimens to determine deflections (and interfacial shear stresses) at which delamination of coatings initiates [51], scratch testing [52, 53], and shear lag testing, a method based on composite theory and determination of stress transfer distances between substrate and coating to determine interfacial shear strengths [54, 55]. Filiaggi [46, 54] has recently reported on the successful use of a shear-lag test method for assessing the interfacial shear strength of thin ZrO_2 sol-gel-formed coatings ($\approx$100 nm thick) on Ti alloy substrates. In general, there remains a need for the development of novel and easy-to-apply test methods for assessing the mechanical integrity and bonding properties of such thin coatings. The topic has received attention in recent years, primarily because of its importance in other areas of materials science (e.g., optoelectronics).

Mechanical Properties of Coated Specimens

In addition to characterization of coating-substrate interface strengths, static (tensile) and fatigue strengths of coated specimens should be determined using standard test methods. These tests can be used to assess the effect of surface or substrate-coating interface features that may introduce significant stress concentrators, thereby lowering mechanical properties.

Other characterization methods such as corrosion testing and general microstructural characterization of coated specimens should be included when characterizing coatings on implants. The assessment methods can be the same as noted previously for uncoated metals and ceramics.

REFERENCES

1   Ashby MF, Jones DR. *Engineering Materials 1: An Introduction to Their Properties and Applications.* London: Pergamon Press, 1980.

2   Ashby MF, Jones DR. *Engineering Materials 2: An Introduction to Microstructures, Processing and Design.* London: Pergamon Press, 1980.

3   Kingery WD, Bowen HK, Uhlmann DR. *Introduction to Ceramics.* 2nd ed. London: John Wiley & Sons, 1976.

4   Newey C, Weaver G. *Materials Principles and Practice.* Butterworth Scientific Ltd., 1990.

5   Pilliar RM, Weatherly GC. Developments in implant alloys. *CRC Critical Reviews in Biocompatibility,* 1 (1986), 371–403.

6   John BV. *Introduction to Engineering Materials.* 2nd ed. New York: Macmillan Publishing Co., 1983.

7   Ritter JE, Jr., Greenspan DC, Palmer RA, Hench LL. Use of fracture mechanics theory in lifetime predictions for alumina and Bioglass-coated alumina. *J Biomed Materials Res,* 13 (1979), 251–263.

8   Pilliar RM. Modern metal processing for improved load-bearing surgical implants. *Biomaterials,* 12 (1991), 95–100.

9   Kohn DH, Ducheyne P. Materials for bone and joint replacement. In Williams DF (Ed.), *Materials Science and Technology: A Comprehensive Treatment,* Vol. 14., VCH Publ, 1992, 31–101.

10 Heimke G. Structural characteristics of metals and ceramics. In Ducheyne P, Hastings GW (Eds.), *Metal and Ceramic Biomaterials,* Vol. 1. Boca Raton, FL: CRC Press, 1984, 7–62.

11 Pilliar RM. Manufacturing processes of metals: The processing and properties of metal implants. In Ducheyne P, Hastings GW (Eds.), *Metal and Ceramic Biomaterials,* Vol. 1. Boca Raton, FL: CRC Press, 1984, 79–105.

12 Christel P. Ceramics for joint replacement. In Morrey BF (Ed.), *Biological, Material, and Mechanical Considerations of Joint Replacement.* Raven Press Ltd., 1993, 303–317.

13 Rawlings RD. Bioactive glasses and glass-ceramics. *Clin Mater,* 14 (1993), 155–179.

14 Williams DF. Electrochemical aspects of corrosion in the physiological environment. In Williams DF (Ed.), *Fundamental Aspects of Biocompatibility,* Vol. 1. Boca Raton, FL: CRC Press, 1981, 11–42.

15 Kruger J. Fundamental aspects of corrosion of metallic implants. In Syrett BC, Achrya A (Eds.), *Corrosion and Degradation of Implant Materials*, ASTM STP 684. Philadelphia, PA: American Society for Testing and Materials, 1979, 107, 127.

16 Bardos DI. High-strength Co-Cr-Mo alloy by hot isostatic pressing of powder. *Biomater Med Devices Artif Organs*, 7:1 (1979), 73.

17 Pilliar RM. Porous-surfaced metallic implants for orthopedic applications. *J Biomed Mater Res: Appl Biomater*, A1 (1987), 1–33.

18 Spector M. Bone ingrowth into porous metals. In Williams DF (Ed.), *Biocompatibility of Orthopedic Implants*, Vol. I. Boca Raton, FL: CRC Press, 1982, 89–128.

19 Hahn H, Lare PJ, Rowe RH, Jr., Fraker AC, Ordway F. Mechanical properties and structure of Ti6Al4V with graded-porosity coatings applied by plasma spraying for use in orthopaedics. In Fraker AC, Griffin CD (Eds.), *Corrosion and Degradation of Implant Materials*, ASTM STP859. Philadelphia, PA: American Society for Testing and Materials, 1985, 179–191.

20 Luckey HA, Lamprecht EG, Walt MJ. Bone apposition to plasma-sprayed cobalt-chromium alloy. *J Biomed Mater Res*, 26 (1992), 557–575.

21 de Groot K, Geesink R, Klein CPAT, Serekian P. Plasma-sprayed coatings of HA. *J Biomed Mater Res*, 21 (1987), 1375–1381.

22 Pilliar RM, Filiaggi MJ. New calcium phosphate coating methods. In Ducheyne P, Christiansen D (Eds.), *Bioceramics*, Vol. 6. Butterworth–Heinemann Ltd., 1993, 165–171.

23 Wisbey A, Gregson PJ, Tuke M. Application of PVD TiN coating to Co-Cr-Mo based surgical implants. *Biomaterials*, 8 (1987), 477–480.

24 Rieu J. Ceramic formation on metallic surfaces (ceramization) for medical applications. *Clin Mater*, 12 (1993), 227–235.

25 Sioshansi P. Medical applications of ion beam processes. *Nucl Instrum Methods Phys Res*, Sect. B, B19–12, pt. 1, 19/20 (1987), 204–208.

26 Williams JM, Buchanan RA. Ion implantation of surgical Ti6Al4V alloy. *Mater Sci Eng*, 69 (1985), 237–247.

27 Dearnaley G. Diamond-like carbon: A potential means of reducing wear in total joint replacements. *Clin Mater*, 12 (1993), 237–244.

28 Gilmore RS, Katz JL. Elastic properties of apatites. *J Mater Sci*, 17 (1982), 1131–1141.

29 Maddalena A. Determination of Young's modulus of thin films. *J Am Ceram Soc*, 75 (1992), 2915–2917.

30 Hainsworth SV, Page TF. Nanoindentation studies of the chemomechanical effect in sapphire. *J Mater Sci*, 29 (1994), 5529–5540.

31 Ewalds HL, Wanhill RJH. *Fracture Mechanics*. Edward Arnold, 1984.

32 Hughes AN, Jordan BA, Orman S. The corrosion fatigue properties of surgical implant materials. Third progress report—May 1973. *Eng in Medicine*, 7 (1978), 135–141.

33 Eylon D, Pierce CM. Effect of microstructure on notch fatigue properties of Ti6Al4V. *Met Trans A*, 7A (1976), 111–121.

34 *A Guide to Statistical Testing and the Statistical Analysis of Fatigue Data*, ASTM STP 91-A. Philadelphia, PA: American Society for Testing and Materials, 1963.

35 Ryder JT, Krupp WE, Pettit DE, Hoeppner DW. Corrosion-fatigue properties of recrystallization annealed Ti6Al4V. In Craig HL, Jr., Crooker TW, Hoeppner DW (Eds.), *Corrosion-Fatigue Technology*, ASTM STP 642, Philadelphia, PA: American Society for Testing and Materials, 1978, 202–222.

36 Hench LL. Bioactive ceramics: Theory and clinical applications. In Andersson OH, Yli-Urpo A (Eds.), *Bioceramics*, Vol. 7. Butterworth-Heinemann Ltd., 1994, 3–14.

37 Davies JE, Pilliar RM, Smith DC, Chernecky R. Bone interfaces with retrieved alumina and hydroxyapatite ceramics. In Bonfield W, Hastings GW, Tanner KE (Eds.), *Bioceramics*, Vol. 4. Butterworth-Heinemann Ltd., 1991, 199–204.

38 Jarcho M, Kay JF, Gumaer KI, Doremus RH, Drobeck HP. Tissue, cellular and subcellular events at the bone-ceramic hydroxyapatite interface. *J Bioeng*, 1 (1977), 79–92.

39 Santos JD, Morrey S, Hastings GW, Monteiro FJ. The production and characterisation of a hydroxyapatite ceramic material. In Bonfield W, Hastings GW, Tanner KE (Eds.), *Bioceramics*, Vol. 4. Butterworth- Heinemann Ltd., 1991, 71–78.

40 Planell JA, Vallet-Regi M, Fernandez E, Rodriguez LM, Salinas A, Bermudez O, Baraduc B, Gil FJ, Driessens FCM. Fracture toughness evaluation of sintered hydroxyapatite. In Andersson OH, Yli-Urpo A (Eds.), *Bioceramics*, Vol. 7. Butterworth-Heinemann Ltd., 1994, 17–22.

41 Dauskardt RH, Ritchie RO, Brendzel AM. Role of small cracks in the structural integrity of pyrolitic carbon heart-valve prostheses. In Ducheyne P, Christiansen D (Eds.), *Bioceramics*, Vol. 6. Butterworth Heinemann Ltd., 1993, 229–236.

42   Rudnick A, Hunter AR, Holden FC. An analysis of the diametral-compression test. *Materials Res and Standards*, 3 (1963), 283–289.

43   Anstis G, Chantikul P, Lawn B, Marshall D. A critical evaluation of indentation techniques for measuring fracture toughness: I. Direct crack measurements. *J Am Ceram Soc*, 64 (1981), 533–538.

44   Jarcho M. Calcium phosphate ceramics as hard tissue prosthetics. *Clin Orthop Rel Res*, 157 (1981), 259–278.

45   Baldwin CM, Mackenzie JD. Flame-sprayed alumina on stainless steel for possible prosthetic applications. *J Biomed Mater Res*, 10 (1976), 445.

46   Filiaggi M. Evaluating sol-gel ceramic thin films for metal implant applications. A study on the processing and mechanical properties of zirconia films on Ti6Al4V, PhD thesis, University of Toronto, Toronto, Ontario, Canada, 1995.

47   Davidson JA, Mishra AK. Surface modification issues for orthopaedic implant bearing surfaces. In Sudarshan TS, Braza JF (Eds.), *Surface Modification Technologies V*. Cambridge: The University Press, 1992, 1–14.

48   Hamman G. Comparison of measurement methods for characterization of porous coatings. In Lemons JE (Ed.), *Quantitative Characterization and Performance of Porous Implants for Hard Tissue Applications*, ASTM STP953. Philadelphia, PA: American Society for Testing and Materials, 1987, 77–91.

49   Smith TS. Morphological characterization of porous coatings. In Lemons JE (Ed.), *Quantitative Characterization and Performance of Porous Implants for Hard Tissue Applications*, ASTM STP953. Philadelphia, PA: American Society for Testing and Materials, 1987, 92–102.

50   Shors EC, White EW, Edwards RM. A method for quantitative characterization of porous biomaterials using automated image analysis. In Lemons JE (Ed.), *Quantitative Characterization and Performance of Porous Implants for Hard Tissue Applications*, ASTM STP953. Philadelphia, PA: American Society for Testing and Materials, 1987, 347–358.

51   Ting B-Y, Winer WO, Ramalingam S. A semi-quantitative method for thin film adhesion measurement. *Trans ASME*, 107 (1985), 472–477.

52   Bull SJ. Failure modes in scratch adhesion testing. *Surf Coat Technol*, 50 (1991), 25–32.

53   Cotell CM, Chrisey DB, Grabowski KS, Sprague JA. Pulsed laser deposition of hydroxyapatite thin films on Ti6Al4V. *J Appl Biomater*, 3 (1992), 87–93.

54   Filiaggi MJ, Pilliar RM. Evaluating sol-gel ceramic thin films for surface modification of metallic implants: Film adhesion and the ZrO2Ti6Al4V system. *Trans 21st Annual Meeting Soc for Biomater*, San Francisco, CA, March 1995, 430.

55   Chandra L, Clyne TW. Characterization of the strength and adhesion of diamond films on metallic substrates using a substrate plastic straining technique. *Diamond and Related Mater*, 3 (1994), 791–798.

ADDITIONAL READING

1   Smith WF. *Principles of Materials Science and Engineering*, 2nd ed. New York: McGraw-Hill, 1990.

2   Reed-Hill RE. *Physical Metallurgy Principles*, 3rd ed. Boston: PWS-Kent Publishing Co., 1991.

3   Callister WD, Jr. *Materials Science and Engineering. An Introduction*, 3rd ed. New York: John Wiley & Sons, Inc., 1994.

4   Hertzberg RW. *Deformation and Fracture Mechanics of Engineering Materials*, 4th ed. New York: John Wiley & Sons, Inc., 1995.

Chapter 2

Polymers

Donald J. Lyman

STRUCTURE-PROPERTY RELATIONSHIPS

By definition, a polymer is a material composed of high molecular weight, chain-like molecules whose atoms are linked together through covalent bonds. The high viscosity of the molten polymer and the strength and long-range elastic properties associated with polymers are a direct consequence of the size and structure of the molecules which make up the bulk material. The atoms which make up a polymer molecule are combined in distinct, simple repeat units which link to form long chains–hence the combination of "poly" (meaning "many") and "mer" (meaning "unit") for the name of this class of materials. For example, polyethylene is made up of repeating units of ethylene, i.e., $(-C_aH_2-CH_2-)_n$, where n is called the degree of polymerization (DP). At low DPs, most organic materials are liquids, waxy solids or friable powders. As the DP increases, these materials rapidly develop strength and mechanical properties, until at some high molecular weight, the properties plateau; thereafter, further increases in molecular weight generally cause only slight increases in properties. However, melt viscosity of a polymer continues to increase rapidly; at some point this becomes a limiting factor in extrusion or injection molding of polymers. All polymers show this type of behavior. However, the molecular weight at which this plateau begins and the material exhibits properties associated with polymers does vary for each class of polymer (e.g., the molecular weight for polyamides is about 10,000 daltons while that for polyhydrocarbons is hundreds of thousand daltons). This is due to differences in the types and arrangements of atoms in the polymer chain which influence the attractive forces between neighboring chains, the chain shape (configuration) and chain flexibility.

The repeat units of a polymer usually link to give a linear chain structure. However, the repeat units can link to form branched, non-linear structures or the branches may interconnect to form a three-dimensional, cross-linked network. The type of structure formed depends on the intermediates used to make the polymer, the synthesis conditions, or the post-treatment of the bulk material. Based only on these changes in macroscopic structure, polymers can be grouped into two broad property categories. The linear and branched structures are, in general, thermoplastic materials (those which can be melted or dissolved); the cross-linked structures are thermoset materials (those which are infusible and insoluble). Branching can also affect the physical and mechanical properties of the polymer. For example, polyethylene prepared by a free radical process is branched due to the mechanism of this reaction. The branches keep the polymer chains from packing closely and lower the density (this material has a density of 0.910 g/cm^3 and is called low-density polyethylene, LDPE). Since the effective intermolecular forces are reduced by this chain separation, the material softens at 88–100° and melts at 104°C. In contrast, polyethylene made by organometallic catalysis is non-branched (i.e., linear) and has a higher density, 0.965 g/cm^3, and is called high-density polyethylene (HDPE). The closer packing of the linear polymer chains increases the effective intermolecular forces, and HDPE softens and melts at higher temperatures (112–132° and 135°C respectively). Thus a part made from

LDPE would be distorted by steam autoclaving, while an identical part made from HDPE would maintain its shape.

The properties of polymers are primarily controlled by the kinds of atoms and their arrangement along the polymer chain and the effect that this has on intermolecular forces, chain shape (configuration) and chain flexibility [1]. For example, the introduction of amide linkages (-NH-OC-) into a linear polyethylene chain increases the intermolecular forces and thus increases the melting temperature. HDPE ($-CH_2CH_2-)_n$, melts at 135°C, whereas 66 nylon, $[-NHO-C-(CH_2)_4-C-ONH-(CH_2)_6]_n$, melts at 255°C. In addition, the tensile strength and modulus of 66 nylon is almost triple that of HDPE because of the amide groups [2]. The water absorption, Rockwell Hardness, heat deflection temperature and solubility also increase, while electrical resistivity decreases.

The properties of a homopolymer (a polymer which has a single type of repeat unit) can be modified by copolymerization. A copolymer has two or more types of repeat units in the polymer chain. The properties of the copolymer will be affected by the structure and concentration of the second repeat unit and its distribution along the copolymer chain. In most copolymerizations, the distribution of the repeat units is random. However, it is possible to modify the synthetic procedure to form block copolymers (or segmented copolymers) in which one repeat unit forms a long block followed by a long block of the second repeat unit. For example, ionic copolymerizations of styrene and isoprene have allowed the formation of $(A)_n-(B)_p$ and $(A)_n-(B)_p-(A)_n$ block copolymers where the A represents a high molecular weight polystyrene block and the B represents a high molecular weight polyisoprene block. The presence of these two incompatible polymers linked together by a covalent bond causes a phase separation [3]. Depending on the relative size of the blocks, several phase-separated structures can be formed. The lower concentration block usually separates into domains within a matrix of the higher concentration block. When the concentrations of the blocks are more equivalent, a lamellar phase-separated structure forms. The crystallinity of a polymer block can also influence the phase separation. The linear, urethane elastomers represent a class of phase-separated copolymers having multiple, smaller blocks along the copolymer chain [3].

While polymers derive their wide range of properties from the factors described above, variations in some properties can result from changes in their physical state defined in terms of the intermolecular packing or morphology of the polymer chains. For example, the strength and toughness of fibers, such as those made from polyethylene terephthalate, polyamides, or polypropylene, can be increased by drawing (stretching) the fiber to orient the polymer chains along the fiber axis. However, if a drawn fiber is melted to bond it to another material, the orientation is lost and the material often becomes brittle. The polymer may also be formed into porous or foam-like structures. The pores, or cells, in the material may be open or closed and be of differing sizes and concentration. This can result in varying degrees of softness, flexibility or compressibility of the material. The pores can be formed by blowing agents (CO_2 or easily vaporized solvents) during the polymerization reaction, by using extractable salts, or by biaxial stretching of a film (such as forming expanded polytetrafluoroethylene).

BIOMEDICAL POLYMER DEVELOPMENT

After World War II, with the expanding polymer industries, a wide variety of polymers became available as solids, tubes, fibers, films and textiles; biomedical researchers explored these materials in implant and device studies. However, by the 1960s, researchers began to realize that new materials developed specifically for biomedical applications were needed.

With early research support coming primarily from the artificial kidney and artificial heart programs, much effort was focused on surface modification of polymers to improve blood compatibility (see Chapter 12). This led to rapid advances in many biomedical applications and, in turn, to an explosive growth in the medical products industry. As with any new advance, there were occasional problems which became highly publicized. In 1969, President Nixon established the Cooper Committee to study medical device regulation. This became the basis for the Medical Device Amendments of 1976 which set up, under the FDA, premarket requirements for medical implants and devices. An F-4 committee on Medical and Surgical Materials and Devices was also established by the American Society for Testing and Materials.

THE BIOMATERIALS CRISIS

Increasing regulatory costs have become an important factor in the changing market place, especially for Class III devices (see Chapter 50) where there is a potential for serious risk to the health, safety, or welfare of a subject. With Class III devices, premarket approval is not given until a device is completely developed and extensive in vitro and in vivo (animal) testing and human clinical trials have been completed (see Chapters 50 and 51) [4].

A more serious problem has now arisen. Modern society appears to expect that biomedical devices should restore an ailing individual to a state of health equal to that of a healthy individual. Also, the public believes that the implant (unlike natural tissues or organs) should never fail. This expectation, coupled with U.S. product liability laws, the litigious nature of the U.S. population and the willingness of juries to award substantial damages even when the material and implant are based on the best science available, has brought on a crisis situation in the 1990s. In late 1992, the DuPont Corporation notified all vascular graft manufacturers that it would cease shipment of polyester yarn by January 1993. A number of other polymers (including the polyesters, polyfluorocarbons, polyacetals, silicone elastomers, nylon and some polyurethanes) were also withdrawn from use in medical implants by DuPont and other suppliers [5]. A search for new sources for materials has not been very successful, again because of U.S. product liability laws and the general litigious environment. The relatively low dollar value of the materials purchased by the medical product industry compared to the size of the non-medical commercial markets for these same materials make many suppliers unwilling to assume the liability risks. To help correct this problem, Senator Lieberman introduced the Biomaterials Access Assurance Act into the U.S. Senate in 1994 as part of the Product Liability Fairness Act; unfortunately, it was not enacted. The impact of this loss of materials may not be fully noticed for several years since many companies had stockpiled some of these polymers. However, there are no known polymers suitable for replacing the withdrawn materials. Therefore, if the biomaterials crisis is not solved quickly, one may soon see the relocation of medical product businesses overseas, and worse, the unavailability of implants and devices needed for the treatment of millions of American patients [5].

SOLID STATE CHARACTERIZATION

The variety of end-use applications of polymers in orthopedics, ophthalmology, plastic and reconstruction surgery, dentistry, cardiovascular surgery, and neurosurgery plus their use in extracorporeal artificial organs, is indicative of the need for a wide spectrum of polymers (see Table 2-1). While some of these materials have applications as short-term implants (such as some catheters, shunts and degradable implants), most are intended for long-term

Table 2-1 Synthetic Polymers Used in Biomedical Applications

Polymer	Repeat unit	Applications
Polyethylene (PE)	$(-CH_2CH_2-)$	hip, knee, shoulder joints (UHMW), catheters
Polypropylene (PP)	$\overset{\displaystyle CH_3}{(-CHCH_2-)}$	sutures, reinforcing meshes, catheters
Polyvinyl chloride (PVC)	$\overset{\displaystyle Cl}{(-CHCH_2-)}$	catheters, shunts, tubing
Polytetrafluoroethylene (PTFE)	$(-CF_2CF_2-)$	vascular grafts, felts, membranes
Polymethyl methacrylate (PMMA)	$\overset{\displaystyle CH_3}{\underset{\displaystyle COOCH_3}{(-CH_2C-)}}$	bone cement, intraocular lenses, artificial teeth
Polyhydroxyethyl methacrylate (PHEMA)	$\overset{\displaystyle CH_3}{\underset{\displaystyle COOCH_2CH_2OH}{(-CH_2C-)}}$	contact lenses, membranes, drug delivery, coatings
Polymethyl 2-cyanoacrylate	$\overset{\displaystyle C\equiv N}{\underset{\displaystyle COOCH_3}{(-CH_2C-)}}$	surgical adhesive
Polyethylene terephthalate (PET)	$(-CH_2CH_2-O\overset{\displaystyle O}{\overset{\|}{C}}\bigcirc\overset{\displaystyle O}{\overset{\|}{C}}O-)$	sutures, vascular grafts, meshes, sewing rings
Poly β-hydroxybutyrate	$\overset{\displaystyle CH_3}{(-CHCH_2\overset{\displaystyle O}{\overset{\|}{C}}O-)}$	sutures
Polylactide	$\overset{\displaystyle CH_3}{\underset{\displaystyle \overset{\|}{O}}{(-CHC-)}}$	sutures, scaffolding
Polyglycolide	$\underset{\displaystyle \overset{\|}{O}}{(-CH_2C-)}$	sutures, scaffolding
Polyether-ether ketone (PEEK)	$(-\bigcirc\overset{\displaystyle O}{\overset{\|}{C}}\bigcirc O\bigcirc O-)$	composite joints
Polyamide (Nylon 66)	$[-NH(CH_2)_6NH\overset{\displaystyle O}{\overset{\|}{C}}(CH_2)_4\overset{\displaystyle O}{\overset{\|}{C}}-)$	sutures
Polyamide (Nylon 6)	$[-NH(CH_2)_5\overset{\displaystyle O}{\overset{\|}{C}}-)$	sutures
Polyurethane-ureas (PUU)[1]		vascular grafts, intraaortic balloons, pacemaker leads, tubing, artificial heart and left ventricular assist devices
Polysiloxanes[2]	$\overset{\displaystyle R}{\underset{\displaystyle R'}{(-O-Si-)}}$	finger joints, maxiofacial implants, heart valves, tubing shunts, adhesives, membranes

1. $[-R-NH\overset{O}{\overset{\|}{C}}O-R''-O\overset{O}{\overset{\|}{C}}NH-R-NH\overset{O}{\overset{\|}{C}}NH-R'-NH\overset{O}{\overset{\|}{C}}NH-]$, where R is aromatic or alicyclic; R' is aliphatic; R'' is ether, ester or hydrocarbon oligomers.

2. Usually crosslinked gels and solids where R and R' are methyl, phenyl or ethylenic.

Table 2-2   Properties of Polymers Used as Implants[1]

Property	HDPE	UHMWPE	PMMA	Silcone	PTFE	PEEK
Tensile strength, MPa[2]	23–40	21	21	5.8–8.2	7-28	92
Tensile modulus, GPa	0.6–1.8	1.0	3.5–4.5	–	0.4	3.7
Elongation, %	400–500	450	2.5–5.4	350–600	100–200	50
Izod impact strength, J/m	0.7–20	NB[3]	0.3–2.5	–	160	NB[3]
Hardness	D60–D70	D65	M80–M105	A25–A75	D50–D65	R126
Compressive strength, MPa	18–25	25–28	75–144	–	11.7	–
Density, g/cc	0.96–0.97	0.94	1.18	1.1–1.23	2.2	1.32
Water absorption, %	0.01	0.01	0.1–0.4	–	–	–

1. Data from refs. 2, 39.
2. MPa to psi, multiply by 145.
3. NB means no break (PEEK sample was unnotched).

implantation. Some properties of selected materials are shown in Table 2-2. For comparison, the mechanical properties of various tissues are shown in Table 2-3. Each end-use requires a different balance of properties, and this complicates the evaluation of a polymer for a particular implant. However, some characterizations should be done on any potential biomaterial. Initially, characterizations give information about the structure and purity of the polymer being investigated and its basic physical and mechanical properties. These are important both for new materials as well as for ascertaining batch-to-batch reproducibility of materials in continuing use. A second level of characterizations is then made on suitable candidates to determine the polymer's response to fabrication, sterilization and simulated

Table 2-3   Physical Properties of Rigid and Soft Human Tissue[1]

Tissue type	Tensile strength (MPa)[2]	Ultimate elongation (%)	Compression strength (MPa)[2]	Modulus of elasticity (GPa)
Bone, Tibia	140	1.5	159	18.1
Bone, Femur	12.1	1.4	167	17.2
Tendon	53.0	9.4		
Skin	7.60	78		
Heart valve (tricuspid)				
radial	0.97	14		
circumferential	1.53	15.8		
Heart valve (aortic)				
radial	0.45	15.3		
circumferential	2.62	10		
Aorta, transverse	1.07	77		
longitudinal	0.069	81		
Vena Cava, transverse	3.03	51		
longitudinal	1.17	84		
Ureter, transverse	0.47	98		
longitudinal	1.03	36		

1. Data from ref. 39.
2. MPa to psi multiply by 145.

in vivo exposure, including hydrolytic degradation and dynamic loading. A third level of characterization involves the interaction between the implant (particularly its surface) and the physiological environment.

One must know how a polymer is to be used so that the tests conducted are appropriate for its application. To determine initial property levels and batch-to-batch variation, the standard ASTM test methods are satisfactory. However, since the implant functions in an aqueous, oxidizing environment (containing salts and fatty materials) at 37°C, mechanical testing should also be conducted under these conditions.

Initial Screening for Verification of Polymer Structure and Properties

Infrared At room temperature, thermal excitation causes vibrational motions in the various bonds in polymer molecules. The frequency of vibration is characteristic of the bond, the mode of vibration (e.g. stretching, bending, twisting) and the environment around the bond (e.g., other atoms or functional groups attached to or interacting with the bond (e.g., hydrogen bonds)). If a sample of the polymer is exposed to infrared radiation, the energy at the characteristic frequencies of these bonds will be absorbed, thereby indicating their presence. Thus, absorption at a series of characteristic frequencies or wave numbers, v (v = 1/wave length (cm)) provides a clear identification of the chemical structure of the polymer [6] as well as providing qualitative identification of possible additives or unwanted contaminants present in the material. In addition, comparison of spectra of different batches of the same general type of polymer allows detection of differences in copolymer composition, blend composition, polymer branching, and stereo-conformational changes (i.e., the geometric arrangement of groups along the polymer chain) [7]. The spectrum of a polymer is taken at wave numbers from 700 to 4000 cm^{-1} at a resolution of either 8 or 4 cm^{-1}. Spectral measurements can be made on a variety of sample types: powder, films or sheets, fibers, and solid pieces. The best spectra are usually obtained by transmission of the IR beam through a thin film of the material. A finely powdered polymer may be compressed in a KBr pellet to obtain a spectrum in a similar manner. With polymer solutions, a thin film can be cast onto a NaCl crystal. However, with some polymers (such as the copolyurethane-ureas) there can be an interaction of the solvent with the salt crystal which may alter the IR spectrum of the polymer [8]. Internal reflection spectroscopy (IRS) provides an alternative in which the powder, fiber, or thick piece of film or sheet is placed on an IRS crystal positioned in the IR beam. A 45° ZnSe crystal and a 45° IR beam angle allow good penetration by the incident wave of the IR beam into the sample. Spectra can also be obtained on powders and solid chips using diffuse spectroscopy. The use of known reference materials (see Chapter 11) or spectral libraries can greatly assist in these analyses.

Density Variations in the density of a polymer can reflect changes in crystallinity and stereoregularity; with filled polymers it can reflect differences in the loading of the material. Thus density measurements can be used as a simple screening test for comparing different samples of the same general type. Density measurements can be made by a water displacement method using a pycnometer [9] or with a density-gradient column [10].

Stress-Strain Properties While the mechanical stresses imposed on polymer implants are usually small, the uniaxial tensile stress-strain curves do indicate the limits of a material's use in an implant. The ASTM standard method for tensile testing [11, 12] enables

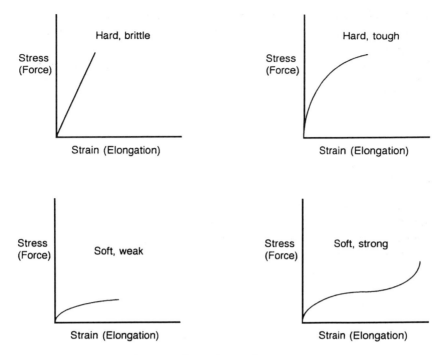

Figure 2-1 Typical stress-strain curves for various polymer types.

one to measure tensile strength, modulus of elasticity and percent elongation of a polymer. A dog-bone-shaped sample is clamped in the jaws of a tensile tester which moves the jaws apart at a constant and specified rate. The force, measured by a load cell, is recorded versus elongation. The Young's or tensile modulus (or stiffness) of the material is the initial slope of the curve. The point at which the sample breaks determines the tensile strength and percent elongation. Since most polymers exhibit viscoelastic behavior, these properties vary with the rate of deformation. Thus, the strain rate used should also be reported (for a more detailed discussion see Chapter 1). Typical stress-strain curves shown by various polymers are shown in Figure 2-1. Stress-strain testing done on dry samples is suitable for initial property evaluation and for determining batch-to-batch reproducibility. However, since implants usually function in a wet environment, the dog-bone samples should at least be conditioned in water and tested while wet; testing under wet conditions at 37°C would be preferred. For some materials, water may plasticize the polymer, making it softer and weaker. For materials with glass-brittle transition temperatures near body temperature, significant changes in properties associated with this transition may be observed when testing at 37°C. These changes in tensile properties can affect the performance of a material. In a second level of tensile testing, tests should be made on a sample of the material in the actual structural form in which it will be used in the final implant.

Molecular Weight and Molecular Weight Distribution   Many properties of polymers (such as strength, toughness and melt viscosity) are dependent on the molecular weight of the polymer. Unlike small organic molecules, polymer molecules have a distribution of chain lengths, and so in any material there is a distribution of molecular weights. Thus, the measured value of molecular weight represents an average for the polymer. The distribution of molecular weights can also affect the properties since lower molecular weights can act as plasticizers and soften the material, increase its creep, etc. Therefore, it is necessary to determine both the average molecular weight of a polymer and the molecular weight distribution.

Gel permeation chromatography (GPC) is one common method for determining the average molecular weight of a polymer [1, 13, 14]. This is accomplished by letting the dissolved polymer flow through a rigid porous gel. Since the larger molecules will not penetrate into the gel pores as readily as the smaller molecules, the larger molecules will pass through the column faster. Thus, the different molecular sizes are eluted from the GPC column in order of their molecular size. By calibrating the column with known molecular weight polymer samples (whose molecular weights have been determined by an absolute method), one can calculate the molecular weight of the unknown material. The molecular weight determined in this manner is termed the weight average molecular weight (Mw).

Intrinsic viscosity measurements (1, 15) can also be used to determine the molecular weight, in this case a number average molecular weight (M_n) of the polymer. The ratio of M_w to M_n provides a measure of the molecular weight distribution of the material [1, 13, 14]. For a monodispersed polymer, i.e., one in which all chains are the same size, the ratio equals 1. For many commercial polymers, the ratio ranges from as low as 2 to as high as 50 depending on the method of polymerization [1]. In addition, solution viscosity measurements such as Inherent Viscosity [15], where solvent, solution concentration and temperature are kept constant, can be useful for monitoring variances in molecular weights of different batches of nominally identical polymers. Cross-linked polymers are effectively three-dimensional networks of infinite molecular weight and are not soluble. Thus molecular weights are not determined. However, solvent swelling data may be of value since they can indicate the degree of cross-linking in the material.

Hardness   The hardness of a polymer is defined as its resistance to local deformation and relates to its compression modulus and compression yield strength. In some cases hardness may correlate with a polymer's abrasion or wear resistance. Hard materials such as glassy polymers or reinforced polymers may be characterized using a Barcol Impressor test [16] or a Rockwell hardness test [17]. In these tests, the force required to produce a given indentation in the material is measured. The test method for soft, elastomeric materials is the Durometer test [18]. It is similar to the Rockwell test except that the indenter is spring-loaded. An equilibrium indentation load-indentation depth establishes the hardness of the material. The thermal history of a polymer as well as the concentration of any additives can affect the test results.

Porosity   A measure of water porosity is often important for foamed polymers, for open pore implants such as the vascular grafts of expanded polytetrafluoroethylene or polyurethane, and for membranes. The porosity of vascular grafts can be measured using techniques described in Chapter 5; membranes can be characterized using techniques described in the hemodialyzer manual [19]. Occasionally, there are situations where the pore (or void) density and size distribution is critical to the success of an implant. Pore volume and pore size distribution can be measured by mercury intrusion porosimetry [20]; the pressure required to force mercury into the pores gives a measure of the interconnecting pore size and the volume of mercury intruded provides a measure of pore volume.

Thermal Analysis   The behavior of a polymer during a controlled heating process characterizes its thermal history, potential for crystallization, glass-rubber transition temperature (T_g) and melting temperature [21]. T_g is an important consideration in new catheter materials which are stiff at room temperature, but become soft and flexible at body temperature after insertion. Differential thermal analysis (DTA) is a measurement of the change in temperature of a polymer (compared to a reference material) as it is heated at a constant rate of heat input from a temperature within its glassy region to above its melting point. The change in the polymer heat capacity, noted by a change in the slope of the time-temperature plot, is a result of some phase change such as T_g, crystallization or melting. Differential scanning calorimetry (DSC) measurements allow similar data to be obtained by measuring the energy difference required to maintain the polymer at the same temperature as a reference material when both are heated at a uniform rate. Since DSC is a faster and more accurate method, it appears to be replacing DTA as the method of choice.

Second-Level Testing for Properties Related to Fabrication and End-Use Performance

Solvent Response   The solubility or solvent-sensitivity of a polymer is important in regards to its characterization, fabrication into test specimens and implants, possible post-fabrication treatments (such as the swelling of tubing for insertion of lead wires or for bonding two materials) and for surface cleaning. Typical polymer solvents are given in Ref. 22. Some solvents may only cause a polymer to swell. However, since the morphology of a polymer (and thereby its physical and mechanical properties) may be modified by the swelling process, tests must be made to ensure that adverse property changes have not occurred.

Extractables   Polymers often contain a variety of contaminants from their synthetic procedures (solvents, unreacted reagents, low molecular weight fractions, catalysts, etc.) as well as from polymerization vessels and processing equipment (such as lubricants on fibers from spinning equipment). In addition, additives such as plasticizers, stiffeners (e.g., carbon blacks), antioxidants and UV stabilizers may be present. Since these may be extracted by and may react with the physiological environment, it is important to determine their presence. Also, different batches of supposedly identical polymers can have different kinds and amounts of extractables. While the IR spectrum of the polymer may provide useful information on possible contaminants, solvent extraction is a better way to identify contaminants. Extractions of both fat-soluble and water-soluble components can be carried out using an aqueous alkaline emulsion of oleic acid/sodium oleate containing 150 mM NaCl medium [23]. Acidification and separation of the mixture followed by IR or chromatographic analysis allows identification of the extracted components. Other extraction media include water and vegetable oil [24].

Degradation   Originally it was believed that degradation of polymers in the body was hydrolytic and thus limited to polymers having hydrolyzable linkages (amide, ester, etc.). However, studies with radio-tagged polymers such as polystyrene and polymethyl methacrylate have shown that non-hydrolyzable polymers were degraded oxidatively in the body. Similar results were obtained in vitro using aqueous peracetic acid solutions [25]. With hydrophobic polymers, degradation is generally a surface phenomenon with a slow erosion of the polymer; with hydrophilic polymers the degradation usually occurs throughout the bulk of the sample. Thus any treatment which could alter a polymer's hydrophobicity, such as orientation and crystallinity, could affect its rate of degradation.

While most implants require a material to be stable for long-term implantation, some applications (e.g., sorbable sutures and implantable drug delivery systems) require the material to degrade at known rates (see Chapter 6). Also, some new approaches to long-term implants utilize polymers which act as biosorbable scaffolding for controlled regeneration of natural tissue (see Section V).

It is important to determine the stability of a polymer in the physiological environment. Since hydrolysis is the primary mechanism of degradative failure in both steam sterilization (see Chapter 15) and implantation, the stability of the polymer in an aqueous environment can be determined first. Later tests can be used to determine stability in an oxidative aqueous environment. Enzymatic effects on degradation appear to be relatively minor compared to hydrolytic and oxidative effects.

Dynamic Mechanical Properties   The stability of the mechanical properties of an implant during use is important for maintaining satisfactory long-term performance. During use, a number of static and dynamic loads are imposed on implants. While these loads are especially severe for joint replacement components, the performance of any implant may be affected. Current in vitro tests can give relative comparisons between candidate polymers. These include static tests such as creep and stress relaxation, and dynamic tests such as impact, fatigue, fracture toughness and dynamic mechanical spectroscopy.

Creep   Most polymers exhibit some time-dependent deformation, or creep, under load. Since this appears to be related to the relatively weak intermolecular forces between chain segments, factors such as crystallinity and crosslinking can reduce a material's creep. The ability of a polymer to withstand the load to which it will be exposed during use should be a factor in its selection. Creep is easily measured by applying a force to the sample and measuring the displacement over time [26]. To obtain reproducible creep measurements for elastomeric materials, the samples should be conditioned prior to testing by a series of creep and recovery cycles.

A related test is stress relaxation. In this test a sample is rapidly strained to a constant strain, and the decay of stress is monitored as a function of time.

Impact Strength   The resistance of a polymer to high strain rate loading (impact toughness) is measured by striking a sample, usually notched to provide a standardized weak point for the initiation of fracture, with a rapidly moving weight. In the Charpy method, the sample is supported on both ends and is struck in the middle. In the Izod method, the sample is supported at one end, cantilever-style. The results are usually reported in joules/meter or foot-pounds of energy absorbed per inch of notch [27]. Viscoelastic effects can increase the impact strength of some polymers since the sample can yield in shear.

Fracture Toughness   Recently a fracture toughness parameter, K_{IC}, (Chapter 1) has found some use in the development and utilization of brittle polymers for implant applications [28, 29]. Values of K_{IC} for selected materials are listed in Table 2-4. Besides providing a measure of the inherent toughness of a material, these techniques can be used to determine crack propagation rates in various environments and to analyze the fatigue behavior of some polymers.

Fatigue   Fatigue refers to material failure due to repeated loading at stresses below the single cycle failure stress. Since fatigue is by far the most common mode of service failure of components that undergo movement [30], it should be a major design consideration for biomedical polymers, especially those used for load-bearing implant applications such as prosthetic joints (e.g., UHMWPE and PMMA) and heart valves (e.g. polysiloxanes). Unfortunately, only limited data are available for these materials [31–33] and few standards

Table 2-4   Plane Strain Fracture Toughness for Selected Materials

Material	$K_{IC}(MPm^{-1/2})$
Epoxies	0.6–1.7
Methacrylate Bone Cement	1.3–1.6
PMMA (commercial)	0.9–1.7
Wet Compact Bone	1.6–3.5
Polystyrene	2.0
Nylon	3.5
Aluminum Oxide (Al_2O_3)	3.5
Titanium Alloys	55–115

have been established for the fatigue testing of polymers [34, 35]. Currently, because of the high degree of variability exhibited by fatigue data, it is necessary to test large numbers of specimens at each stress level and to treat the results statistically in order to determine the fatigue life of the material in terms of survival probability [36]. The fatigue behavior of polymers is particularly sensitive to loading frequency because their high mechanical hysteresis leads to a temperature rise as the frequency is increased. Test frequencies and environments should, therefore, be the same as those to be encountered in service. Loading range, loading mode and the presence of defects can also affect polymer fatigue resistance.

Dynamic Mechanical Spectroscopy (DMS)   Viscoelastic properties, such as the dynamic modulus and the mechanical damping of a polymer sample under oscillatory load as a function of temperature and frequency, can be determined by DMS [37]. This enables one to determine the glass-rubber plateau regions of a polymer, the T_g and rubbery flow temperature of the polymer under various conditions. With the segmented urethane copolymers, phase separation can also be determined.

Special Characterization Methods

Wide-Angle X-Ray   Wide-angle X-ray analysis of formed components such as fibers and films can give information on the crystallinity and orientation of the polymer chains and on structural changes in a material as a result of processing steps. However, DTA and DSC can give results that agree well with those from X-ray diffraction techniques.

Nuclear Magnetic Resonance (NMR)   High-resolution NMR spectroscopy can be used to quantitatively identify nuclei and their environments in a polymer molecule [7]. The most common technique is proton NMR. Information on chemical structure as well as polymer conformation, stereochemistry, copolymer composition and the types of additives present can be obtained from polymer solutions.

CRITICAL PROBLEMS AND DIRECTIONS FOR FUTURE EVALUATION

In vitro mechanical tests on the bulk polymer are suitable for relative comparisons of properties of candidate materials. However, there is a need for developing more reliable in vitro mechanical tests conducted under conditions more closely related to end-use conditions. This is especially needed for cyclic fatigue testing.

Degradation studies must include testing under both static and dynamic stress conditions. For both the degradation studies and the mechanical testing, standardized "physiological media" should be established which will simulate the environment that the implant material will encounter in its use.

Retrieval of implants (both successful and failed) from animal studies have guided researchers in refining biomaterials, implant design and surgical implantation techniques. This information has also shown that variations in response do occur within an animal species. Recently, retrieval and analysis of implants which have failed (in their intended clinical function) have begun [38]. These procedures will help to build an improved data base on both clinical implant function and human versus animal responses to implants and materials. However, to give a more balanced picture, this program must be expanded to include the retrieval of successful implants from patients dying from other causes. A number of potential problems [38] must also be addressed: how should implants be retrieved; how can medical and life style information on implant recipients be obtained; to what evaluations should the implant and surrounding tissue be subjected; how can investigators be guarded against biohazards; and how are questions of logistics and legal liability to be resolved?

The urgent need for new sources of polymers in current use by the medical products industry as well as the continuing development of new polymers appears to be at a critical state. A first step toward alleviating this crisis would be enactment of legislation on biomaterials and tort reform. Ultimately, the public expectation that implants should be totally effective and failure-free and the judicial view that failure is solely the fault of the material or the implant must be corrected. The responsibility for effecting these changes falls on the entire biomedical community.

REFERENCES

1   Billmeyer FW, Jr. *Textbook of Polymer Science*, 3rd ed. New York: Wiley-Interscience, 1984.
2   Brandrup J, Immergut EH. *Polymer Handbook*, 3rd ed. New York: Wiley-Interscience, 1989.
3   Allport DC, Janes WH (Eds.). *Block Copolymers*. New York: John Wiley, 1973.
4   Boretos JW, Eden M (Eds.). *Contemporary Biomaterials*. Park Ridge, NJ: Noyes Publications, 1984, Chapter 32.
5   Benson JS, Boretos JW. Biomaterials and the future of medical devices. *Med Device Diagnostic Ind* 17 (1995), 32–37.
6   Bellamy LJ. *The Infrared Spectra of Complex Molecules*, Vol. 1, 3rd ed. New York: John Wiley, 1975.
7   Koenig JL. *Spectroscopy of Polymers*. Washington, DC: American Chemical Society, 1992.
8   Lyman DJ, Gower LA. The effect of IR salt crystals on the spectra of copolyether-urethane-urea films. *Vibrational Spectroscopy*, 9 (1995), 203–207.
9   Test methods for specific gravity (relative density) and density of plastics by displacement. *Annual Book of ASTM Standards*, Vol. 08.01. Philadelphia, PA: American Society for Testing and Materials, 1995, D792-891.
10 Test method for density of plastics by the density-gradient technique. *Annual Book of ASTM Standards*, Vol. 08.01. Philadelphia, PA: American Society for Testing and Materials, 1995, D1505-1585.
11 Test method for tensile properties of plastics. *Annual Book of ASTM Standards*, Vol. 08.01. Philadelphia, PA: American Society for Testing and Materials, 1995, D638-694 and B639M-694 (metric).
12 Test method for tensile properties of plastics by use of microtensile specimens. *Annual Book of ASTM Standards*, Vol. 08.01. Philadelphia, PA: American Society for Testing and Materials, 1995, D1708-1793.
13 Test method for molecular weight averages and molecular weight distribution of polystyrene by liquid exclusion chromatography (gel permeation chromatography–GPC). *Annual Book of ASTM Standards*, Vol. 08.02. Philadelphia, PA: American Society for Testing and Materials, 1995, D3536-3580.
14 Standard test method for molecular weight averages and molecular weight distribution of polystyrene by high performance size-exclusion chromatography. *Annual Book of ASTM Standards*, Vol. 08.03. Philadelphia, PA: American Society for Testing and Materials, 1995, D5296-5392.

15 Test method for determining inherent viscosity of poly(ethylene terephthalate) (PET). *Annual Book of ASTM Standards*, Vol. 08.03. Philadelphia, PA: American Society for Testing and Materials, 1995, D4603-4691.

16 Test method for indentation hardness of rigid plastics by means of a barcol impressor. *Annual Book of ASTM Standards*, Vol. 08.02. Philadelphia, PA: American Society for Testing and Materials, 1995, D2583-2593.

17 Test method for Rockwell hardness of plastics and electrical insulating materials. *Annual Book of ASTM Standards*, Vol. 08.01. Philadelphia, PA: American Society for Testing and Materials, 1995, D785-793.

18 Bikales NM (Ed.). *Mechanical Properties of Polymers*. New York: Wiley-Interscience, 1971.

19 *Evaluation of Hemodialyzers and Dialysis Membranes*. Report of Study Group for NIAMDD, DHEW Pub. No. (NIH) 77–1294.

20 Test method for interior porosity of poly(vinyl chloride) (PVC) resins by mercury intrusion porosimetry. *Annual Book of ASTM Standards*, Vol. 08.02. Philadelphia, PA: American Society for Testing and Materials, 1995, D2873-2894.

21 Bikales NM (Ed.). *Characterization of Polymers*. New York: Wiley-Interscience, 1971.

22 Practice for dissolving polymer materials. *Annual Book of ASTM Standards*, Vol. 08.03. Philadelphia, PA: American Society for Testing and Materials, 1995, D5226-5292.

23 *Guidelines for Blood-Material Interactions*. Report of the NHLBI Working Group, NIH Publication No. 85-2185, USDHHS.

24 Standard practice for extraction of medical plastics. *Annual Book of ASTM Standards*, Vol. 13.01. Philadelphia, PA: American Society for Testing and Materials, 1995, F619-679 (1991).

25 Lyman DJ. Biomedical polymers. *Revs Macromol Chem*, 1 (1966), 355–391.

26 Test methods for tensile, compressive, and flexural creep and creep rupture of plastics. *Annual Book of ASTM Standards*, Vol. 08.02. Philadelphia, PA: American Society for Testing and Materials, 1995, D2990-2993a.

27 Test methods for impact resistance of plastics and electrical insulating materials. *Annual Book of ASTM Standards*, Vol. 08.01. Philadelphia, PA: American Society for Testing and Materials, 1995, D256-281.

28 Pilliar RM, Vowles R, Williams DF. Fracture toughness testing of biomaterials using a mini-sheet rod specimen design. *J Biomed Mats Res*, 21 (1987), 145–154.

29 Rimnac CM, Wright TM, McGill DC. Effect of centrifugation on the fracture properties of acrylic bone cements. *J Bone Joint Surg*, 68A (1986), 281–287.

30 Meyers MA, Chawla KK. *Mechanical Metallurgy, Principals and Applications*. Englewood Cliffs, NJ: 1984, 688.

31 Krause WR, Mathis RS. Fatigue of acrylic bone cement: A review of the literature. *J Biomed Mats Res*, 22 (1988), 37–53.

32 Li S, Burstein AH. Current concepts review: Ultra high molecular weight polyethylene. *JBJS*, 76A (1994), 1080–1090.

33 Hwang NHC, Nan XZ, Gross DR. Prosthetic heart valve replacements. *CRC Crit Rev Biomed Eng*, 9 (1983), 99–132.

34 A guide for fatigue testing and the statistical analysis of fatigue data. *Annual Book of ASTM Standards*, STP 91-A. West Conshohocken, PA: American Society for Testing and Materials, 1963.

35 Krause WR, Mathis RS, Grimes LW. Fatigue properties of acrylic bone cement: S-N, P-N, and P-S-N data. *J Biomed Mats Res*, 22 (1988), 221–244.

36 Test method for flexural fatigue of plastics by constant-amplitude-of-force. *Annual Book of ASTM Standards*, Vol. 08.01. West Conshohocken, PA: American Society for Testing and Materials, 1987, D071-087.

37 Murayama T. *Dynamic Mechanical Analysis of Polymeric Materials*, 2nd ed. Amsterdam, The Netherlands: Elsevier, 1982.

38 Freiherr G. Explanting information: Database proposals pose dilemma for implantable device community. *Med Device Diagnostic Ind*, 17 (1995), 92–96.

39 Boretos JW. *Concise Guide to Biomedical Polymers*. Springfield, IL: C.C. Thomas, 1973.

ADDITIONAL READING

1 Billmeyer FW, Jr. *Textbook of Polymer Science*, 3rd ed. New York: Wiley-Interscience, 1984.

2 Boretos JW, Eden M (Eds.). *Contemporary Biomaterials*. Park Ridge, NJ: Noyes Publications, 1984.

3 Cooper SL, Bamford CH, Tsuruta T. *Polymer Biomaterials in Solution, as Interfaces and as Solids*. Utrecht, The Netherlands: VSP, 1995.

4 Szycher M (Ed.). *High Performance Biomaterials, A Comprehensive Guide to Medical and Pharmaceutical Applications*. Lancaster, PA: Technomic, 1991.

Chapter 3

Composites

Robert A. Latour, Jr.

INTRODUCTION

Composites are engineered, multicomponent materials which can be designed to possess a much broader range of properties than can be achieved with individual homogeneous materials alone. Fiber-reinforced polymers (FRP) are the most widely investigated composites for medical device applications. These applications have included the development of low stiffness femoral components for hip joint arthroplasty [1–3], radiolucent and biodegradable fracture fixation devices [4–6], fracture-resistant bone cements [7–9], and wear-, creep-, and fracture-resistant articulation components [10].

It is the objective of this chapter to provide a general overview and guide to the accepted techniques which have been developed for the evaluation of FRP composite materials. The evaluation of FRP composite materials is addressed in six sections: the mechanical evaluation of constituent materials of the composite (fiber, polymer matrix, fiber/matrix bond), the mechanical properties of the composite material itself, the physical evaluation of composite architecture (fiber orientation and distribution within the matrix), nondestructive evaluation, fractography, and environmental exposure.

Evaluation of Constituent Material Properties

The evaluation of constituent properties will be addressed only briefly in this chapter with references provided for the specific evaluation methods (see also Chapter 2). Bulk material properties for fibers and polymers are determined by standard test methods published by the American Society for Testing and Materials (ASTM), West Conshohocken, PA (formerly from Philadelphia, PA) [11, 12]. Approximate room temperature mechanical properties for selected fibers, polymers, and composite materials are presented in Table 3-1 along with other relevant materials for comparison purposes [13–23].

Density, strength, modulus, toughness, Poisson's ratio, failure strain, and creep are some of the most important bulk properties to be evaluated for polymer matrices. These properties are determined following methods described in ASTM specifications D 792 (density), D 638 (tension), D 695 (compression), and D 2990 (creep). Fiber properties of primary importance are density, strength, and modulus which are described for single filaments in ASTM D 3800 (density) and D 3379 (strength, modulus), and for carbon and glass fiber yarns/tows in ASTM D 2343 and D 4018, respectively. Although not published as ASTM standards, three basic techniques are primarily used for interfacial bond strength evaluation (Figure 3-1): the single fiber pull-out test [24, 25], the fiber fragmentation (critical-length) test [26, 27], and the single fiber push-out test [28]. In addition, fractographic evaluation can be used to qualitatively assess bond strength in fractured composite specimens, and is further discussed below.

Table 3-1   Approximate Room Temperature Mechanical Properties of selected materials

Material	Properties			
	Elastic modulus (GPa)	Yield strength (MPa)	Ultimate strength (MPa)	Elongation (%)
Cortical Bone (axial)	18	130	140	1.0
METALS:				
Ti6Al4V (ASTM F136) [13]	110	800	860	10.0
Co-Cr-Mo (ASTM F75) [14, 15]	240	450	660	8.0
POLYMERS				
UHMWPE [14, 15]	2.2	35	–	>250
Bone Cement (PMMA) [14, 15]	2.2	29	–	2.0
PSF [16]	2.5	70	–	75
PEEK [17]	3.6	92	–	50
PAEK [18]	4.0	104	–	50
FIBERS				
Carbon [19]	214	–	4,000	1.6
Silica Glass [20]	72	–	1,900	2.6
Aramid [21]	117	–	2,700	2.5
UHMWPE [22]	120	–	2,300	2.7
COMPOSITE				
AS4/APC2 (61% fiber by volume) [23]				
0° fiber orientation	138	–	2,100	1.5
90° fiber orientation	10	–	86	0.9

Evaluation of Composite Mechanical Properties

The ASTM D20 Committee (Plastics) and D30 Committee (High Modulus Fibers and Their Composites) have developed a large number of test methods for composite materials which are suited for both continuous and for discontinuous composite materials evaluation. These evaluation methods describe tests to determine basic material properties of composites,

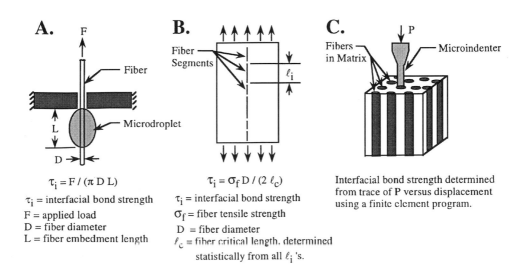

Figure 3-1   Fiber/matrix interfacial bond strength tests, showing (A) fiber pull-out test, (B) fiber fragmentation test, and (C) fiber push-out test.

but are often not directly applicable for structural testing of actual composite devices for medial applications. Although much work has been conducted to develop specific methods for the evaluation of composite-based medical devices, the complexities involved have made it difficult to develop standardized test methods. Several of the test methods which have been developed and utilized are published in the ASTM Special Technical Publication 1178, *Composite Materials for Implant Applications in the Human Body* [29]. The ASTM F04.14 Subcommittee (Composites) of the F04 Committee (Medical Devices) is currently developing accepted test standards for specific composite-materials-based medical devices. At the time this chapter was written, however, these standards had not yet been finalized for publication. Therefore, in this chapter, emphasis will be placed upon providing an overview of accepted general composite test methods which are pertinent to basic composite materials evaluation in support of medical device design and development.

The basic composite mechanical property test methods determine tensile, compressive, shear, and flexural properties of composite materials. Relevant tensile, compressive, and shear test methods have been developed primarily for flat-plate laminated coupon specimens to determine both in-plane and out-of-plane material property values (see Figure 3-2), while flexural tests have been developed to provide information on structural performance, versus actual material properties, of composite bars and plates with rectangular cross-sections. Referring to Figure 3-2, in-plane mechanical properties of a laminate are the strengths: $\sigma_{xx}^*, \sigma_{yy}^*,$ and τ_{xy}^* (asterisk designating stress level causing failure); moduli: $E_x, E_y,$ and G_{xy} (elastic moduli in the x and y direction, and the shear modulus in the x-y plane, respectively); and Poisson's ratio in the x-y plane, υ_{xy}. Out-of-plane mechanical properties of a laminate are the strengths: $\sigma_{zz}^*, \tau_{zx}^*,$ and τ_{zy}^* (asterisk designating stress level causing failure); moduli: $E_z, G_{zx},$ and G_{zy} (elastic modulus in the z direction, and the shear moduli in the z-x and z-y planes), and Poisson's ratios in the z-x and z-y planes, υ_{zx} and υ_{zy}, respectively. The out-of-plane elastic properties ($E_z, G_{zx}, G_{zy}, \upsilon_{zx}, \upsilon_{zy}$) are more difficult to determine than the in-plane elastic properties ($E_x, E_y, G_{xy}, \upsilon_{xy}$). However, these out-of-plane properties can

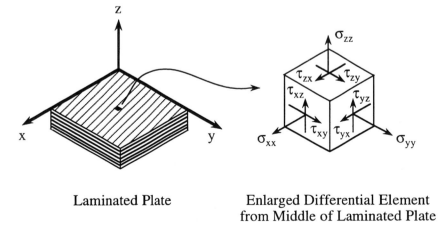

Laminated Plate   Enlarged Differential Element
                           from Middle of Laminated Plate

Figure 3-2 In-plane and out-of-plane properties of a laminated composite plate. Diagram shows a multi-ply laminated plate with plies oriented in x-y plane. A 3-D differential element is shown with the nine components of stress with σ_{xx}, σ_{yy}, and $\tau_{xy} = \tau_{yx}$ representing in-plane stresses, and σ_{zz}, $\tau_{zx} = \tau_{xz}$, and $\tau_{zy} = \tau_{yz}$ representing out-of-plane stresses. σ_{ii} represents the normal stress pointing in the i-direction and acting on the i-face (outer normal of face pointing in the i-direction), and τ_{ij} represents the shear stress pointing in the j-direction and acting on the i-face, where i and j each represent one of the x, y, or z coordinates.

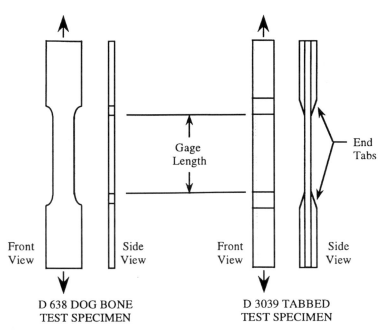

Front   Side   Front   Side
View   View   View   View

D 638 DOG BONE   D 3039 TABBED
TEST SPECIMEN   TEST SPECIMEN

Figure 3-3   Tensile test specimens.

be determined ultrasonically by the correlation which exists between the elastic properties and the velocity of ultrasonic wave propagation in various directions within a material [30].

Tensile Test Methods

ASTM static tensile test methods (Figure 3-3) are designated as D 638 and D 3039, with a tensile fatigue test method designated as D 3479. These test methods are recommended for evaluating in-plane properties of tensile strength, tensile modulus, and in-plane Poisson's ratio, where the composite coupon to be characterized can be cut such that the tensile properties in any desired in-plane direction can be evaluated. D 638 specifies a dog-bone-shaped, untabbed specimen which is particularly suited for evaluating the properties of discontinuous, fiber-reinforced polymer composites, but should not be used for highly oriented composite materials because of their tendency to split longitudinally at the neck-down region of the specimen. D 3039 should be utilized for highly oriented specimens and specifies a straight-sided, rectangular test specimen with end tabs for gripping. D 3479 utilizes the same test specimen geometry as D 3039, with the standard primarily focusing upon the appropriate procedures for applying cyclic versus quasistatic loading.

Compression Test Methods

In-plane compressive properties of static and fatigue strength, modulus, and Poisson's ratio can be determined using either ASTM D 695 or D 3410 test methods (Figure 3-4). D 3410 is recommended only for unidirectional, continuous, orthotropic fiber-reinforced polymer composites (i.e., 0°, 90°, or 0°/90° [cross-ply] laminates), while D 695 can be used with any fiber-reinforced polymer composite material. Each of these test methods requires special fixturing with specifications for test fixture fabrication provided in the ASTM test method. D 3410 utilizes a tabbed test specimen with a short unsupported gage length where

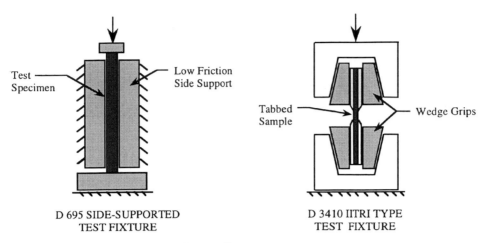

Test Specimen — Low Friction Side Support

Tabbed Sample — Wedge Grips

D 695 SIDE-SUPPORTED
TEST FIXTURE

D 3410 IITRI TYPE
TEST FIXTURE

Figure 3-4 Schematic of compression test fixtures.

compressive failure should ideally occur. In this method, loading is applied via a side-supported, wedge-gripping system to transfer load to the gage section. Because the gage section is unsupported, careful techniques must be used to ensure the specimens actually fail under uniform compression instead of compression-induced bending or buckling. The best method for determining that the proper state of loading is achieved in the test is to do preliminary testing with representative samples which are strain gaged on both the front and back. These samples should then be tested to failure and the percent difference between the front and back strain gage signals compared [31, 32]. If the percent difference in strain (ε) between these gages is 10% or less, or

$$\frac{(\varepsilon_f - \varepsilon_b)}{\frac{1}{2}(\varepsilon_f + \varepsilon_b)} \le 0.10$$

where ε_f is the strain on the front face of the coupon and ε_b is the strain on the back face, then the fixture and sample combination can be considered to be appropriate for compressive strength determination; if the percent difference is greater than 10%, excessive bending is occurring during the test. This problem can usually be corrected by realigning the test fixture, using a thicker test specimen, or shortening the gage length of the sample. D 695 can be used with either a tabbed or untabbed specimen and involves an end-loaded side-supported fixture to inhibit global buckling of the samples. This method can be unsuitable for highly oriented, high-compressive-strength samples which may fail by the crushing of the sample ends versus true compressive failure in the gage section.

Shear Test Methods

In-plane static shear properties of strength and modulus can be determined by ASTM D 3518 ($\pm 45°$ coupon tension) and ASTM D 5379 (V-Notch/Iosipescu shear) (Figure 3-5). As with the compressive test methods, D 5379 requires the use of a special test fixture with dimensions for fixture fabrication provided in the test method. Each of these methods uses a flat-plate composite specimen.

Out-of-plane (or through-the-thickness) static shear strength can be approximated by ASTM D 2344 and D 3846 (Figure 3-5). D 2344 is a short-beam shear test method which is recommended for the measurement of interlaminar shear strength in laminated FRP

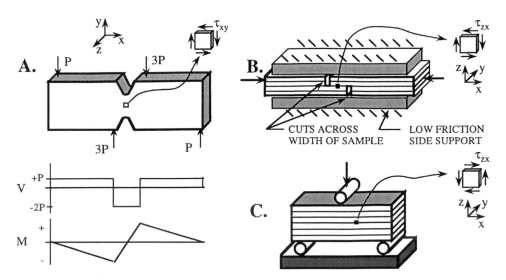

Figure 3-5 Illustration of three shear test methods: (A) D 5379, V-notch (Iosipescu) shear test, resultant shear force (V) and moment (M) diagrams shown for applied load; (B) D 3846, interlaminar shear test; and (C) D 2344, short beam shear test. In each example, samples shown with plies lying in the x-y plane. As shown by the indicated differential elements, illustration A indicates the measurement of in-plane stress τ_{xy}, and illustrations B and C indicate the measurement of the out-of-plane stress, τ_{zx}.

composites, whereas D 3846 can be used with any flat-plate composite material. Out-of-plane shear properties are particularly difficult to determine because of the complex stress fields and stress concentrations induced by the test method. Therefore, these test methods are useful primarily for obtaining comparative data between different composite materials rather than providing actual material properties.

Flexural Test Methods

Static and fatigue flexural properties (strength and modulus) of rectangular, cross-sectioned composite bars (either directly fabricated or cut from plates) can be determined by ASTM D 790. D 790 presents the methods for properly conducting both 3-point and 4-point bending tests. Failure under flexural testing can be due to tensile, compression, or shear properties, either singly or in combination, and thus does not provide actual material property data. A bending test does provide structural data which are dependent upon both the material and the test specimen geometry, and thus can provide useful data if the test accurately simulates the geometry and mode of loading in a given application. There is currently no ASTM test method to determine the flexural behavior of composite tubes. However, the F04.14 Subcommittee of ASTM is currently working on such a document primarily for the purpose of evaluating support structures for external fracture fixation applications.

Test Methods for Creep

Like bulk polymers, polymer matrix composite materials, depending upon their design, may undergo significant amounts of permanent deformation following long-term exposure to even relatively low levels of load, and this behavior may be strongly influenced by exposure to moisture and/or organic molecules such as lipids. Thus, creep behavior characterization in environments simulating in vivo conditions is important when designing composite-material-based implant devices. Tensile, compressive, and flexural creep and creep-rupture of composite materials may be determined by test methods presented in ASTM D 2990. The tensile creep test, however, should not be used for highly oriented composite materials because creep between the test specimens and grips can significantly confound test results.

Evaluation of Physical Properties

Composite materials do not have inherent internal organization but require the designer to engineer the material's internal structure. Because of this, evaluation of the internal design of a given composite material is just as important as its mechanical characterization. The internal design can be broken down into three basic categories: volume fractions (fiber, matrix, and void), fiber distribution, and fiber orientation.

Component Volume Fractions

ASTM provides four test methods for the determination of fiber and matrix volume fractions: C 613, D 2584, D 3171, and D 3529. C 613 and D 3529 are solvent extraction methods using Soxhlet and boiling solvent techniques, respectively, in which the matrix is removed from the fiber by dissolving it in a suitable solvent which does not interact with the reinforcement phase of the composite. D 3171, on the other hand, is a matrix digestion method using a strong oxidizing agent (such as nitric acid) to remove the matrix. In each of these methods, the remaining reinforcement phase is dried and weighed, and fiber volume fraction and matrix volume fractions are then determined based upon the "before" and "after" weight determinations and the densities of the constituent phases. D 2584 is a "burn-off" technique in which the matrix is burned away, leaving behind the reinforcement. This technique, of course, can only be used if it is known a priori that the reinforcement is stable at the temperature used.

Composite void volume fraction can be determined by ASTM D 2734. In this method, the densities of the matrix, reinforcement, and composite are first measured. The matrix weight fraction is then measured by methods described in the preceding paragraph, following which a theoretical zero void content density is calculated for the composite and compared to the measured composite density. The difference between these two density values is representative of the void volume fraction within the actual composite.

Reinforcement Architecture

In continuous FRP composite materials, fiber organization is determined and directly controlled by the material's designer prior to fabrication. The composite architecture is defined by describing the fiber orientation, layer thickness, and orientation sequence of each ply or wrap within the material. Discontinuous reinforced composites, however, are more difficult to characterize because fiber orientation and length distribution are not directly controlled by the designer, but rather are indirectly determined by flow fields induced during component fabrication [33]. A microscope-based image analysis system is therefore essential equipment for evaluating the organization of discontinuous FRP composites.

Two-dimensional characterizations for discontinuous FRP composites are determined by sectioning and polishing a composite material specimen followed by microscopic visualization of selected portions of the cross-section [33]. Each fiber filament within the microscope field of view is measured for length and angle of orientation with respect to

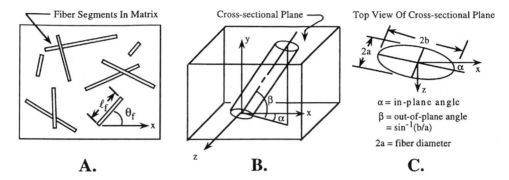

Figure 3-6 Evaluation of fiber orientation and length distribution in discontinuous composites: (A) Evaluation of 2-D fiber length (l_f) and orientation (θ_f) distribution for cross section; (B) illustration of 3-D orientation of fiber segment with respect to cross section; (C) evaluation of out-of-plane angle (β) from planar view of fiber cross section.

a defined global coordinate system (Figure 3-6), and histograms are then created for both fiber length and fiber orientation to map out these distributions. If fully three-dimensional fiber orientation is present and fibers are known to have circular cross-sections, the angle of the fiber in the out-of-plane direction can be determined by the elliptical cross-section of the fiber in the plane of the specimen cross-section [33], as shown in Figure 3-6.

NONDESTRUCTIVE EVALUATION

Unlike homogeneous materials which typically fail by the initiation of distinct surface cracks which can then propagate through the material, composite materials, due to their complex heterogeneous nature, typically fail by the development of zones of dispersed internal damage. These damage zones can occur within the material during processing or be induced by post-processing treatment. If the damage is internal, it may not be evident by visual inspection of the external surface of the material. Several techniques have therefore been developed for the nondestructive evaluation (NDE) of composite materials which allow the extent of internal damage to be monitored and evaluated. Four of the most common methods of NDE employed for composite materials evaluation are stiffness monitoring, ultrasonic imaging, dye-penetrant/radiography, and acoustic-emission [34].

Nondestructive Evaluation Techniques

Because damage within a composite material slowly reduces the deformation resistance of the material to applied loads, damage accumulation can be evaluated by monitoring stiffness [34]. This technique is particularly suited for detecting damage development during fatigue testing in which the stiffness is either continuously monitored or checked following set intervals of fatigue cycles. While very informative, this technique does not provide information regarding the type and location of damage which occurs within the material, and thus additional NDE techniques are required along with stiffness monitoring to provide this type of information.

Ultrasonic techniques (C-scan and A-scan modes) are the most frequently employed and useful methods of nondestructive evaluation for locating internal zones of damage within composite materials [34]. The C-scan mode utilizes an ultrasonic transducer/receiver to locate defects by scanning the entire surface of a composite plate while monitoring the attenuation of reflected waves, with wave attenuation being related to the severity of damage within the plate. C-scanning has been extensively used to evaluate the integrity of components following manufacturing processes, and to monitor damage induced by mechanical loading. The A-scan mode provides through-the-thickness depth profiling data regarding the depth of subsurface damage. In this mode, the transducer/receiver system is used to monitor the time of echo return as the ultrasonic wave is reflected by areas of discontinuity (i.e., delamination) within the composite material. The time between wave generation and echo return is then correlated with the material's thickness to determine the depth of the delamination surface which reflected the wave.

Radiography is another NDE technique which provides detailed information on the state of damage developed within a composite material [34]. In this method, a radiopaque penetrating dye is used to highlight microscopic cracks within the material, following which X-ray radiographs are taken to visualize the damage areas as a function of dye concentration. Diiodobutane and zinc-iodide-water solutions have been found to perform very well as dye penetrants for this technique.

Acoustic emission (AE) is a technique to detect real-time fracture events which occur within a material due to the energy waves generated as the material fractures [34]. AE involves the use of two acoustic receivers separated by a designated distance over a span of the material. The difference between the times when a given event is sensed by each of the two transducers provides the general location of the event within the material. In addition to damage location, AE has also been used to discriminate between the types of fracture events occurring within the material, with matrix cracking, fiber fracture, and delamination potentially providing discernibly different acoustic signatures.

Fractography

Fractography is the art of qualitatively interpreting the mechanisms of fracture that occur in a specimen by microscopic examination of fracture surface morphology [35–38]. Fractography of composite materials will only be briefly discussed here with the indicated references [35–38] providing a photographic guide for readers interested in in-depth treatments of this type of evaluation.

In continuous fiber-reinforced polymer composites [35, 36], fracture types can be separated into three categories: intralaminar, interlaminar, and translaminar (Figure 3-7) [35]. Intralaminar and interlaminar fractures typically occur within the matrix or fiber/matrix

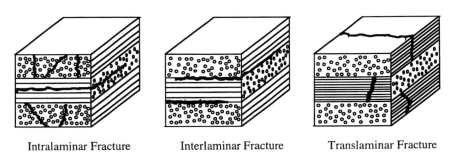

Intralaminar Fracture   Interlaminar Fracture   Translaminar Fracture

Figure 3-7 Illustration of primary fracture modes in laminated composite.

interfaces with little or no involvement of fiber fracture, while translaminar fracture primarily involves fiber fracture. Fractures in discontinuous fiber-reinforced composites involve processes which are somewhat different from those in continuous fiber-reinforced composites, since stress concentrations at fiber ends and at voids typically are the initiators of failure, with the initiated damage zones then growing and coalescing to cause final failure [37, 38]. The fracture behavior in these materials thus tends to be largely determined by the matrix and the fiber/matrix interface.

Environmental Considerations

An important part of composite material evaluation for medical applications is the response of the material to the in vivo environment. In particular, fiber/matrix interfacial bond strength in some composite materials has been found to be significantly reduced by physiologic saline exposure [24], and creep resistance of some polymer matrices, such as polysulfone, has been found to be greatly reduced by exposure to lipids [39].

The rate of diffusion and the amount of swelling in environments simulating in vivo conditions are relevant environmental response properties which can be evaluated in composite materials. ASTM D 5229 provides a test method for measuring the through-the-thickness diffusion coefficient for moisture diffusion through thin composite plates based upon a weight-gain-versus-time method. Important parameters obtained from this test method are the percent maximum weight gain and the out-of-plane coefficient of diffusion. In this test method, plate width and length are specified to be very large compared to plate thickness to minimize errors caused by in-plane moisture diffusion via exposed edges of the plate. For specimens with thickness-to-width ratios greater than that specified in D 5229, weight gain studies are still meaningful for determining saturation weight gain levels, and specimen edges can be sealed with protective coatings (such as those used for moisture protection in strain gage applications) to minimize sample edge diffusion.

Because moisture diffusion can have a significant effect upon composite behavior, composite-based medical implant devices should be fully saturated prior to conducting performance tests of implant function. The ASTM provides a composite material environmental conditioning test method developed by the F04.14 Subcommittee on Composites (F 1634) which describes a weight-gain-versus-time method which should be followed to properly condition composite samples prior to mechanical performance evaluation.

FUTURE NEEDS FOR COMPOSITE MATERIALS EVALUATION

Composites possess great potential for the development of improved medical devices by providing materials with a much broader range of properties than can be obtained by homogeneous isotropic bulk polymers, metals, or ceramics. However, the heterogeneous, anisotropic nature of composite materials also makes the design of composite-based medical devices, and the prediction of their in vivo performance, very complex. While composite materials evaluation methods have been fairly well developed for the determination of basic materials characterization, much remains to be accomplished towards understanding and predicting actual composite-based medical device performance; this, therefore, represents one of the most important areas for the continued development of composite materials evaluation methods for medical applications.

PERTINENT ASTM TEST METHODS AND STANDARDS [11]

C 613. Test method for resin content of carbon and graphite prepregs by solvent extraction. Vol. 15.03.

D 638. Test method for tensile properties of plastics. Vol. 08.01.

D 695. Test method for compressive properties of rigid plastics. Vol. 08.01.

D 790. Test method for flexural properties of unreinforced and reinforced plastics and electrical insulating materials. Vol. 08.01.

D 792. Test method for specific gravity (relative density) and density of plastics by displacement. Vol. 08.01.

D 2343. Test method for tensile properties of glass fiber strands, yarns, and rovings used in reinforced plastics. Vol. 08.01.

D 2344. Test method for apparent interlaminar shear strength of parallel fiber composite by short-beam method. Vol. 15.03.

D 2584. Test method for ignition loss of cured reinforced resins. Vol. 08.02.

D 2734. Test method for void content of reinforced plastics. Vol. 08.02.

D 2990. Test method for tensile, compressive, and flexural creep and creep-rupture of plastics. Vol. 08.02.

D 3039. Test method for tensile properties of fiber-resin composites. Vol. 15.03.

D 3171. Standard test method for fiber content of resin-matrix composites by matrix digestion. Vol. 15.03.

D 3379. Test method for tensile strength and Young's modulus for high-modulus single-filament materials. Vol. 15.03.

D 3410. Test method for compressive properties of unidirectional or crossply fiber-resin composites. Vol. 15.03.

D 3479. Test method for tension-tension fatigue of oriented fiber, resin matrix composites. Vol. 15.03.

D 3518. Practice for inplane shear stress-strain response of unidirectional reinforced plastics. Vol. 15.03.

D 3529. Test method for resin-solids content of carbon fiber-epoxy prepreg. Vol. 15.03.

D 3544. Guide for reporting test methods and results on high modulus fibers. Vol. 15.03.

D 3800. Standard test method for density measurement of high-modulus fibers. Vol. 15.03.

D 3846. Test method for in-plane shear strength of reinforced plastics. Vol. 08.02.

D 4018. Test method for tensile properties of continuous filament carbon and graphite yarns, strands, rovings, and tows. Vol. 15.03.

D 4762. Standard guide for testing automotive/industrial composite materials. Vol. 15.03.

D 5229. Standard test method for moisture absorption properties and equilibrium conditioning of polymer matrix composite materials. Vol. 15.03.

D 5379. Test method for shear properties by V-notched beam test. Vol. 15.03.

F 1634. Standard practice for in vitro environmental conditioning of polymer matrix composite materials and implant devices. Vol. 13.01, 1996.

REFERENCES

1 Cheal EJ, Spector M, Hayes WC. Role of loads and prosthesis material properties on the mechanics of the proximal femur after total hip arthroplasty. *J Orthop Res*, 10 (1992), 405–422.

2 Magee FP, Weinstein AM, Longo JA, Koeneman JB, Yapp RA. A canine composite femoral stem: An in vivo study. *Clin Orthop*, 235 (1988), 237–252.

3 Chang F-K, Perez JL, Davidson JA. Stiffness and strength tailoring of a hip prosthesis made of advanced composite materials. *J Biomed Mater Res*, 24 (1990), 873–899.

4 Böstman OM. Current concepts review. Absorbable implants for the fixation of fractures. *J Bone and Joint Surg*, 73A (1991), 148–153.

5 Andriano KP, Daniels AU, Heller J. Biocompatibility and mechanical properties of a totally absorbable composite material for orthopaedic fixation devices. *J Applied Biomaterials*, 9 (1992), 197–206.

6 Smutz WP, Daniels AU, Andriano KP, France EP, Heller J. Mechanical test methodology for environmental exposure testing of biodegradable polymers. *J Applied Biomaterials*, 2 (1991), 13–22.

7   Topoleski LDT, Ducheyne P, Cuckler JM. The fracture toughness of titanium-fiber-reinforced bone cement. *J Biomed Mater Res*, 26 (1992) 1599–1617.

8   Pourdeyhimi B, Wagner HD. Elastic and ultimate properties of acrylic bone cement reinforced with ultra-high-molecular-weight polyethylene fibers. *J Biomed Mater Res*, 23 (1989), 63–80.

9   Gilbert JL, Ney DS, Lautenschlager EP. Self-reinforced composite poly(methyl methacrylate): Static and fatigue properties. *Biomaterials*, 16 (1995), 1043–1055.

10 Deng M. *Effects of Reinforcement and Irradiation on Thermal and Mechanical Properties of Ultrahigh Molecular Weight Polyethylene*, Doctoral dissertation, Clemson University, Clemson, SC, 1995.

11 *Annual Book of ASTM Standards*. West Conshohocken, PA: American Society for Testing and Materials, 1995.

12 *ASTM Standards and Literature References for Composite Materials*, 2nd ed. West Conshohocken, PA: American Society for Testing and Materials, 1990.

13 Evans FG. *Mechanical Properties of Bone*. Springfield, IL: Charles C. Thomas Publ., 1975.

14 Park JB, Lakes RS. *Biomaterials. An Introduction*. 2nd ed. New York: Plenum Press, 1992.

15 Black J. *Orthopaedic Biomaterials in Research and Practice*. New York: Churchill Livingstone, 1988.

16 UDEL P1700 polysulfone, *Design Engineering Data*, Amoco Performance Products, Inc., Marietta, OH, Amoco publication no. F-49959.

17 Polyetheretherketone, *Victrex PEEK*, ICI Advanced Materials, Wilmington, DE, publication no. VK2/0586.

18 Polyaryletherketone, *Ultrapek Properties Chart*, BASF Plastics, BASF publication no. F07e (8109) 5.90.

19 AS4 carbon fiber, *Hercules Graphite Fibers and Prepregs*, Hercules Advanced Materials and Systems Co., Magna, UT, publication no. 150-14 rev. 2-90 20M GTP.

20 E-glass fiber, *Glass Fiber Roving Property Data Sheet*, Owens Corning, Toledo, OH.

21 Kevlar 49 polyaramid fiber, *Kevlar 49 Aramid Fiber*, DuPont Inc., Wilmington, DE, publication no. E38532.

22 Spectra 1000 ultrahigh molecular weight polyethylene fiber, SPECTRA *High Performance Fibers for Reinforced Composites*, Allied Signal, Petersburg, VA, 1990.

23 AS4 carbon fiber reinforced APC2 polyetheretherketone thermoplastic, *Thermoplastic Composites Materials Handbook*, ICI Thermoplastic Composites, Laguna Hills, CA.

24 Latour RA, Jr., Black J. Fiber reinforced polymer composite biomaterials: Characterization of interfacial bond strength and environmental sensitivity. ASTM Symposium on *Biomaterials' Mechanical Properties*, ASTM STP 1173. Philadelphia, PA: American Society for Testing and Materials, 1994, 193–211.

25 Miller B, Muri P, Rebenfeld L. A microbond method for determination of the shear strength of a fiber/resin interface. *Composites Science and Technology*, 28 (1987), 17–32.

26 Drzal LT, Rich MJ. Effect of graphite fiber/epoxy matrix adhesion on composite fracture behavior. *Recent Advances in Composites in the United States and Japan*. ASTM STP 864. Philadelphia, PA: American Society for Testing and Materials, 1985, 16–26.

27 McDonough WG, Herrera-Franco PJ, Wu WL, Drzal LT, Hunston DL. Fiber-matrix bond tests in composite materials. *23rd Intl SAMPE Tech Conf*, 1991, 21–24.

28 Grande DH, Mandell JF, Hong KCC. Fibre-matrix bond strength studies of glass, ceramic, and metal matrix composites. *J Materials Science*, 23 (1988), 311–328.

29 Jamison RD, Gilbertson LN (Eds.). *Composite Materials for Implant Applications in the Human Body: Characterization and Testing*, ASTM STP 1178. Philadelphia, PA: American Society for Testing and Materials, 1993.

30 Kriz RD, Stinchcomb WW. Elastic moduli of transversely isotropic graphite fibers and their composites. *Experimental Mechanics*, 19 (1979), 41–50.

31 Zhang G. *Micromechanics of Compressive Behavior in Fiber Reinforced Polymer Composite Biomaterials*. Doctoral dissertation, Clemson University, Clemson, SC, 1994.

32 Zhang G, Latour RA, Jr., Kennedy JM, Schutte HD, Jr., Friedman RJ. Long-term compressive strength durability of CF/PEEK composite in physiologic saline. *Biomaterials*, 17 (1996), 781–789.

33 Hull D. Geometric aspects. *An Introduction to Composite Materials*. Chapter 4. New York: Cambridge University Press, 1981: 59–80.

34 Henneke EG, II. Destructive and nondestructive tests. *Composites, ASM Engineered Materials Handbook*, Vol. 1. Metals Park, OH: ASM International, 1987, 774–778.

35 Smith BW. Fractography for continuous fiber composites. *Composites, ASM Engineered Materials Handbook* Vol. 1. Metals Park, OH: ASM International, 1987, 786–793.

36 Atlas of Fractographs, Resin Matrix Composites. *Fractography, ASM Handbook*, Vol. 12. Metals Park, OH: ASM International, 1987, 474–478.

37 Sato N, Kurauchi T, Sato S, Kamigaito O. SEM observations of the initiation and propagation of cracks in a short fibre-reinforced thermoplastic composite under stress. *J Materials Science Letters*, 2 (1983), 188–190.

38 Robertson RE, Mindroiu VE. Discontinuous fiber composites. *Composites, ASM Engineered Materials Handbook*, Vol. 1. Metals Park, OH: ASM Intl., 1987, 794–797.

39 Asgian CM, Gilbertson LN, Blessing EE, Crowninshield RD. Environmentally induced fracture of polysulfone in lipids. *Trans Society for Biomaterials*, 12 (1989), 17.

ADDITIONAL READING

1 *ASM Engineered Materials Handbook, Composites*, Vol. 1. Metals Park, OH: ASM International, 1987.

2 Hull, D. *An Introduction to Composite Materials*. New York: Cambridge University Press, 1981.

3 Jones, RM. *Mechanics of Composite Materials*. New York: Hemisphere Publishing Co., 1975.

Chapter 4

Dental Materials

Robert G. Craig

The oral environment places special demands on materials used to replace hard tissues such as teeth and bone and soft tissues such as mucosa and skin. The oral cavity is a harsh region in which the materials come into contact with saliva, other body fluids, and many kinds of organisms (e.g. yeasts, bacteria, viruses). Another difference compared with other biomaterials is that dental materials are exposed to a wide range of temperatures, making the thermal properties particularly important. In addition to functioning and surviving in this environment the materials must be compatible with pulp, connective tissue, and/or bone.

Dental materials can be discussed as a unified topic because of special requirements such as esthetics and certain unique materials such as restorative composites and dental amalgam. A special requirement for a number of dental materials is that they match the optical properties of the tissues they are to replace. Dental materials are evaluated by a number of mechanical tests used for other biomaterials, but in addition special tests such as dynamic and creep compliance measurements are used to evaluate materials as different as maxillofacial elastometers and dental amalgam.

TYPES AND CLASSES OF DENTAL MATERIALS

Dental materials can be subdivided into types and classes of restorative and laboratory materials. The restorative materials are used to replace oral structures, and the laboratory materials are used to assist in the fabrication of restorations. The types and classes of materials and their principal uses are listed in Table 4-1. Detailed description of these classes and types are presented in dental materials textbooks [1].

Composition and Properties

The general compositions and properties of the restorative materials only are listed in Table 4-2. Additional information can be found in textbooks on dental materials [1, 2].

Methods of Forming

Amalgam   The alloy is mixed (triturated) with mercury (43–50%, depending on the alloy) in a mechanical mixer (amalgamator) in a plastic capsule (with or without a pestle, depending on the manufacturer's recommendations) for 6–20 sec. At these times, the mass has plastic qualities that enable it to be packed directly into cavity preparations.

Initial setting occurs within 10 min and the surface contour can be carved. Final polishing can be done at 10 min for high early-strength materials or at a later appointment for products that develop strength more slowly.

Table 4-1   Types, Classes, and Principal Application of Dental Materials

Type	Class	Principal application
Restorative Materials		
Amalgam	High copper	Posterior restoration of teeth
Resin composites	Microfilled	Anterior and posterior restoration of teeth
	Colloidal filled	Anterior and posterior restoration of teeth
	Hybrids	Anterior and posterior restoration of teeth
Noble alloy	Colloidal filled	Anterior and posterior restoration of teeth
Noble alloys	Gold-non-heat	Fixed bridges and crowns treatable
	Palladium silver	Restoration of single teeth
Base alloy	Nickel	Restoration of single and missing teeth, partial denture frameworks
	Cobalt	Partial denture framework and implants
	Iron	Orthodontic appliances and endodontic instruments
	Titanium	Implants, orthodontic wires, endodontic pins, posts, and files
Plastics	Poly(methylmethacrylate) (PMMA)	Dentures and artificial teeth
Ceramics	Feldspathic glasses	Single-crown restorations and denture teeth
	Alumina-reinforced glasses	Single-crown restorations and denture teeth
	Cast glass	Single-crown restorations
Cements	Zinc phosphate	Retain metallic restorations, thermal insulation
	Zinc oxide-eugenol	Temporary or permanent cement, pulp protection
	Zinc polyacrylate	Permanent cement
	Glass ionomer	Restorations and permanent cement
	Resin composite	Cement orthodontic brackets
Laboratory Materials		
Impression materials	Zinc oxide-eugenol	Edentulous mouths
	Agar	Dentulous patients
	Alginate	Dentulous patients
	Rubber (polysulfide, polyether, silicone)	Dentulous patients
Wax	Inlay	Patterns
	Base plate	Patterns
	Utility and miscellaneous	Maintaining position of parts
	Impression plaster	Mounting models
Gypsum	Model plaster	Models of patients' dentition
	Dental stone	Models of patients' dentition
	Improved stone	Models of patients' dentition
Casting investments	Gypsum bonded	Casting gold alloys and low melting base alloys
	Phosphate bonded	Casting high-melting base and gold alloys
	Silicate bonded	Casting high-melting base alloys

Table 4-2 Composition and Properties of Dental Restorative Materials

Material	Composition	Compressive strength, MPa @ 1 Hr 0.05 mm/min	Compressive strength, MPa @ 7 Days 0.2 mm/min	Tensile strength, MPa @ 15 min 0.5 mm/min	Tensile strength, MPa @ 7 days 0.5 mm/min	Creep, %	Dimensional change during setting, µm/cm
Amalgam High copper alloy	40–60% Ag, 22–30% Sn, 13–30% Cu, 0–5% In, 0–1% Pd	120–300	400–500	3–9	43–56	0.05–0.45	2–9

Material	Composition	Compressive strength (MPa) @ 24 hrs, 0.5 mm/min	Diametral Tensile strength (MPa) @ 24 hrs, 0.5 mm/min	Young's modulus, (GPa) @ 24 hrs	Linear coefficient of expansion $(10^{-6}/°C)$ @ 20–60°C	Water sorption mg/cm^2	Clinical wear µg/yr
Resin (BIS-GMA or UDMA) composites Microfilled	75–86 wt. % glass or quartz (51–76 vol. % glass or quartz) Balance	240–400	34–76	9–16	24–38	0.4–0.6	85–100
Colloidial filled	37–52 wt. % colloidal silica (22–36 vol. % colloidal silica) Balance diacrylate oligomers and momomers	270–330	28–33	3–6	45–70	1.2–2.2	25–60
Hybrids	Mostly microfiller with some colloidal filler plus oligomers and monomers	Properties intermediate to micro-filled and collodial-filled materials					

Table 4-2 Continued

Material	Composition	Yield strength MPa 0.2% offset		Tensile strength Mpa		Elongation %		Hardness, kg/mm²	
		Softened	Hardened	Softened	Hardened	Softened	Hardened	Softened	Hardened
Nobel Alloys									
Gold (non-heat-treatable)	76–78% Au, 1–3% Pd, 3–8% Ag, 8–12% Cu, 1% Zn maximum	160–180	160–180	315–375	315–375	26–35	26–35	95–100	95–100
Gold (heat-treatable)	73–75% Au, 2–4% Pd, 9–15% Ag, 12–18% Cu, 1% Zn maximum	200–240	290–310	400–450	510–550	30–40	12–22	120–150	150–170
Gold (heat-treatable)	50–62% Au, 1–3% Pd, 16–26% Ag, 8–11% Cu	400–450	790–830	550–590	860–900	15–20	3–4	170–200	260–300
Gold (heat-treatable)	35–50% Au, 3–10% Pd, 0–3% Pt, 13–30% Ag, 11–30% Cu	400–450	550–590	550–590	680–730	10–15	4–6	170–200	250–280
Palladium-silver	54–60% Pd, 28–38% Ag, 7–9% Sn	200–240	200–260	400–450	400–480	15–20	10–15	140–160	140–170

Material	Composition	Yield strength, MPA 2% offset, as cast	Tensile strength, MPa as cast	Elongation, % as cast	Hardness, kg/mm² as cast	Young's modulus, GPa as cast
Base Alloys						
Nickel	17% Cr, 5% Mo, 5% Al, 5% Mn, 0.5% Fe, 0.1% C	690	800	1.5–5	340	186
Cobalt	27–30% Cr, 0–13 % Ni, 4–5% Mo, 1–1.5% Fe, 0.2–0.5% C, 0.5%–0.6% Si, 0.5–0.7% Mn, 0–0.05% Ga, Balance Co	490–570	640–830	1.5–10.0	370–380	228
Iron	18% Cr, 8% Ni, 0.08–0.2% C, Minor % of Ti, Mn, Si, Mo, Balance Fe	Wrought 0.1% offset 1500–1700	Wrought 2000–2200	–	Wrought 520–540	Wrought — In Bending 122, In Torsion 134
Titanium	6% Al, 4% V, Bal. Ti	800–975	900–1025	12–15	–	In Bending 100, In Torsion 125

Table 4-2 Continued

Material	Composition	Proportional limit MPa	Tensile strength MPa	Elongation, %	Hardness, kgmm²	Young's modulus MPa
Plastics Poly(methyl-methacrylate)						
Powder	0.5–1.5% Benzoyl peroxide, 0.1–0.2% pigments (inorganic oxides), 0.1–0.5% opacifiers (TiO$_2$), balance PMMA	26	55	2	15–20	3800
Liquid	0.003–0.01% hydroquinone, 2–14% diacrylates, balance MMA; if processed at R.T., 0.5–1.5% N, N-dihydroxethyl-para-toluidine					

Material	Composition	Transverse strength, MPa	Shear strength, MPa	Diametral tensile strength, MPa	Hardness kg/mm²	Young's modulus GPa
Ceramics Feldspathic	75–85% feldspar, 12–22% quartz, 3–5% kaolin, 1% metallic oxide pigments and opacifiers includes Ti, Mn, Fe, Co, Cu, Ni, Sn, Zn, and rare earths	62–90	110	25–34	460	69
Alumina-reinforced	40–60% Al$_2$O$_3$ balance of above composition	138	145	37–42	–	36–96
Cast glass	Silica which after casting is ceramed to form mica	152	–	Comprressive strength 828	362	70

Table 4-2 *Continued*

Material	Composition	Compressive strength, MPA	Tensile strength, MPa	Young's modulus, GPa	Solubility in H_2O % in 24 hours
Cements					
Zinc Phosphate		62–117	4.8–6.2	12.1–13.7	0.2 maximum
Powder	90% ZnO, 8% MgO, 2% metal oxides of Si, Bi, Co, and Ba				
Liquid	38% H_3PO_4, 26% Zn and Al phosphate, balance H_2O				
Zinc oxide-eugenol					
Powder	69% ZnO, 29–30% rosin, 1–2% Zn acetate and sterate; modifications may contain 30% PMMA or 30% Al_2O_3				
Liquid	85% eugenol, 15% olive oil; modifications may contain 63% o-ethoxybenzoic acid	2–83	1.5–5.8	0.3–5.5	0.01–0.1
Zinc Polyacrylate					
Powder	90% ZnO, 10% MgO; some contain 15–18% polyacrylic acid	51–73	4.8–9.7	4.4	<0.05
Liquid	32–42% copolymer of mainly acrylic acid and some itaconic acid, 0.1–5% tartaric acid, balance water				
Glass Ionomer					
Powder	100% calcium fluoroalumino-silicate glass	117–135	3.5–5.5	5.6–9.5	0.4–1.5
Liquid	48% 2:1 copolymer of acrylic and itaconic acid, balance water				
Composite*					
Chemically Activated					
Paste #1	Diacryate oligomer and monomers 0.5–1% benzoyl peroxide	200	40	4.1–12	0.1
Paste #2	Diacrylate oligomers and monomers, 0.5–1% dihydroxyethyl-k-touluidine	270	50	9	0.1
Visible-light-activated (460 nm)					
Paste	Diacrylate oligomers and monomers, 0.2–1.0%; camphoroquinone 0.1–0.6% dimethylaminoethylmethacrylate				

*Note: Up to 85 wt % of filler present.

Resin Composites   Both chemical and visible light initiator systems are available. The chemical type is supplied as two pastes, and the visible as a single paste. For the former, equal volumes of the two pastes are mixed (spatulated) for about 20 sec; then the material is placed in a syringe and injected into the cavity preparation or the mixed material may be packed into the restoration. The material sets sufficiently in 5 min so that the excess may be removed and finishing done. Finishing is accomplished using fine abrasives followed by polishing compounds.

The visible-light-initiated types are formed by placing the single paste into the prepared cavity and then exposing it to high-intensity light of 460-nm wavelength (blue) for 30–60 sec. Finishing is the same as for the chemical-initiated type.

Noble and Base Alloys   The gold, palladium, nickel, and cobalt base alloys are processed by the lost-wax-casting method. Wax patterns are prepared and coated with a refractory investment. The investments contain various forms of silica and one of several binders, gypsum, phosphate, or silicate. After the investment sets, the wax is melted and burned out to form a mold, and the investment is heated to the appropriate temperature; the alloy is melted and then cast into the mold using a centrifugal casting machine.

The iron base alloys are used in the wrought condition and are supplied as drawn wires. Endodontic files and reamers are manufactured from these wires by grinding and twisting. Titanium and its alloys are supplied in the final cast or wrought form by the manufacturers and are rarely processed in a dental laboratory.

Plastics   Poly(methylmethacrylate) (PMMA) used in partial or complete dentures is processed by a dough-molding method. PMMA powder and methylmethacrylate (MMA) liquid are mixed in a ratio of 3:1 and solution is allowed to take place until the mix reaches a dough consistency. It is processed into a split mold produced by the lost-wax method. The investment in this instance is gypsum. The polymerization of the MMA is accomplished by free-radical initiation with benzoyl peroxide by heating to 74°C for 8 hr. If an amine accelerator is present, polymerization takes place at room temperature in 4 hr. Plastic teeth are manufactured by dough molding and heat using a variety of metal molds.

Ceramics   Ceramic restorations are prepared by painting a water slurry of the powder onto a die that has been covered with platinum foil. Excess water is removed by vibration and absorption of the water forming at the surface. After the correct contour has been built, the condensed ceramic is sintered, and final firing is done in a vacuum furnace. The final restoration is cemented to the tooth. Cast glass is fabricated using the lost-wax method. After casting it is surrounded by investment and ceramed to produce crystallinity.

Cements   Zinc phosphate, zinc oxide eugenol, zinc polyacrylate, and glass ionomer cements consist of a powder and a liquid in specific ratios mixed with a small spatula to the correct consistency. They are then used as cements for metallic restorations, as thermal insulation between the pulp and metallic restorative materials, or as temporary restorative materials.

Composite resin cements are generally supplied as two pastes mixed in equal quantities just before cementation. Their principal application is the cementation of orthodontic brackets to tooth enamel.

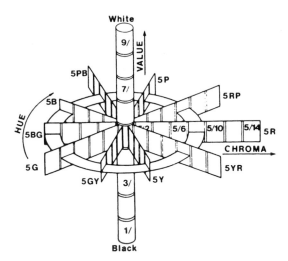

Figure 4-1 Munsell scales of hue, value, and chroma in color space. (Adapted from Powers JM, Capp JA, Koran A., *J Dent Res*, 56 (1977), 112.)

MEASUREMENT OF PHYSICAL PROPERTIES

Optical Properties

Color   The color of dental materials is evaluated using a visual method such as the Munsell Color System [3] or a spectrophotometric procedure for determining parameters called tristimulus values, which are computed relative to a standard source specified by the Commission Internationale de l'Eclairage (CIE) [4].

In the Munsell system, color is specified in three dimensions by value, hue, and chroma (Figure 4-1). The color is determined by visually comparing a sample of material with a large set of color tabs. The value from white 10/ to black 0/ is determined first, followed by matching the chroma (intensity) from achromatic/0 to saturated/18, and then the hue from 2.5 to 10 (in increments of 2.5) for 10 color families: red, R; yellow-red, YR; yellow, Y; green-yellow, GY; green, G; blue-green, BG; blue, B; purple-blue, PB; and red-purple, RP. Munsell notation for healthy human gingival tissue might be 5R 6/4, indicating a hue of 5 R, a value of 6, and a chroma of 4.

Color of materials before and after use can be compared in the Munsell Color System with a color difference formula [5]:

$$I = (C/5)(2\Delta H) + 6\Delta V + 3\Delta C$$

where C is the average chroma and ΔH, ΔV, and ΔC are differences in hue, value, and chroma. Differences in I of 5 can be detected by experienced observers.

In the tristimulus color system, spectral reflectance versus wavelength curves are obtained for a material in the visible region with a spectrophotometer. Tristimulus values (X, Y, Z) are calculated from the reflectance values relative to a particular light source and are related to the amounts of the three primary colors needed to match the color. The ratios of each tristimulus value to the sum are the chromaticity coordinates (x, y, z). The dominant wavelength (~hue) and excitation purity (~chroma) can be determined from a

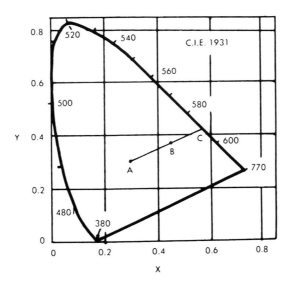

Figure 4-2 Chromaticity diagram according to the 1931 C.I.E. standard observer and coordinate system. Values of dominant wavelength determine the spectrum locus. The excitation purity is the ratio of the two lengths (AB/AC), where A refers to the standard light source and B the color being considered. Point C, the intersection of AB with the spectrum locus, is the dominant wavelength. From Craig RG (Ed.), *Restorative Dental Materials*, 10th ed., St. Louis: Mosby, 1997, 33.

chromaticity diagram (see Figure 4-2). The luminous reflectance z can then be calculated knowing x and y.

$$\Delta E(L^*, a^*, \text{and } b^*) = [(\Delta L^*)^2 + (\Delta a^*)^2 + (\Delta b^*)^2]^{1/2}$$

where L^*, a^*, and b^* depend on tristimulus values of a material and a perfectly white sample. Typical Munsell numbers and dominant wavelength, luminous reflectance, and excitation purity figures are listed in Table 4-3 for selected dental materials [6–10].

Color stability of dental materials has been evaluated using the CIE color notation by determining the color before and after aging in a Weather-Ometer, which permits exposure to ultraviolet light under controlled temperature and humidity [11, 12].

Opacity Opacity of dental materials has been judged qualitatively by comparing them with two opal glass standards. It is determined whether the opacity is between the standards by placing the wetted standards and a 1-mm-thick specimen on a striped black and white background, the latter having a daylight apparent reflectance of 70% relative to MgO.

The contrast ratio has also been used to measure the opacity by the ratio of the luminous reflectance with a black background to the luminous reflectance with a white background [6, 9, 11, 12]. Total transmittance measurements, which are six time times more sensitive to opacity, have been substituted for contrast ratios [13]. The optical infinite thickness is that thickness needed to produce a transmittance of 0 or a contrast of 1 and is useful in comparing opacity.

Dental materials used to replace human tooth structure are colored and cause a great deal of light scattering. The incident light decreases sharply with depth. The Kubelka-Munk equations [14, 15] describe the optical properties of such materials by two constants, K

Table 4-3   Color Notations for Various Dental Materials

| | | | Spectrophotometric Color | | |
| | | Dominant | Luminous | Excitation | Contrast |
Material	Munsel color	wavelength, nm	reflectance	purity	ratio
Denture acrylic (light pink) [89]	2.5R 5.5/6	611	23.8	0.31	0.92
Denture acrylic (blue-pink) [89]	10RP 5.5/6	631	21.5	0.24	0.93
Denture acrylic (purple) [89]	5RP 5.5/4	493	22.2	0.15	0.98
Tooth restorative composite (universal shade) [33]	2.5Y 7.5/3	579	59.4	0.27	0.68
Tooth restorative acrylic-unfilled (light yellow) [33]	7.5Y 8.0/2	576	64.7	0.23	0.80
Skin (Whites) [59]	–	591	30.9	0.29	
Skin (Blacks) [59]	–	588	21.9	0.36	
Maxillofacial silicone [127]	–	585	79.3	0.09	
Porcelain modifier (grey-green) [56]	–	552	15.3	0.12	
Porcelain modifier (grey-red) [56]	–	600	11.0	0.14	

and S, the absorption and scattering coefficients, which are functions of the wavelength of light. Kubelka then developed an equation for the reflectance R of a specimen in contact with a backing of known reflectance R_g, on sample thickness X as follows:

$$R = \frac{1 - Rg[a - b \operatorname{ctgh}(bSX)]}{a + b \operatorname{ctgh} bSX - Rg}$$

where

$$a = \frac{S + K}{S} \quad b = (a^2 - 1)^{1/2} \quad R = a - b$$

$$S = \frac{1}{bh} A R \operatorname{ctgh} 1 = \frac{a R_0}{b R_0} \quad K = S(a - 1)$$

where R_0 is the reflectance with an ideal black background.

These equations have been used to evaluate the optical properties of esthetic restorative dental materials [16–19]. Johnston modified the equation further to account for interfacial surface interactions as light enters and leaves the sample [20]. O'Brien et al. [21] showed that with these corrections, the Kubelka-Munk theory could predict reflectance of unpigmented ceramic over a pigmented substructure.

Surface Gloss   Major contributors to the appearance of esthetic dental restorations are surface gloss and the effect of roughness on gloss. Contrast gloss, the proportion of specular to diffuse reflection, has been measured with a goniophotometer [22]. An inverse linear relationship was found between contrast gloss and average surface roughness.

Fluorescence   Human teeth fluoresce in the blue region (450 nm) when exposed to ultraviolet light [23], and rare earths are usually added to esthetic dental restorative materials in order to reproduce the natural appearance.

A spectrophotofluorimeter has been used to obtain fluorescent spectra of various rare earth ions in a potassium feldspar glass [24]. These data permit formulation of ceramics with specific color qualities in ultraviolet light. Because of the possibility of energy transfer, the color cannot be predicted on the basis of the additive color-mixing method.

Thermal Properties

Thermal properties of special interest in dentistry are conductivity, diffusivity, and coefficient of thermal expansion.

Conductivity   The thermal conductivity of dental materials has been measured by a steady-state method using thermocouples [12, 25] and thermistors [26]. Values for selected dental materials are listed in Table 4-4. The conductivity of materials used to replace decayed portions of teeth is of interest, since thermal transfer to the living pulp is important. High thermal conductivity in materials can cause pain or even irreversible damage to the pulp.

Diffusivity   Thermal diffusivity is a measure of the transient heat flow and may be determined indirectly or directly. The diffusivity D may be calculated using the equation

$$\Delta = \frac{K}{C_\rho \times \rho}$$

Where K is the thermal conductivity, C_ρ, is the heat capacity at constant pressure (usually measured calorimetrically), and ρ is the density.

Values for some dental materials are listed in Table 4-4 [4, 27–31]. Since diffusivity is related to the rate of transfer of a thermal disturbance, it is interesting that dentin, which protects the pulp, has a lower value than enamel and that the values for cement more nearly match dentin while those for resin composite more nearly match enamel.

Table 4-4   Thermal Properties of Some Dental Materials

Material	Conductivity cal/sec/cm^2/°C/cm	Diffusivity mm^2/sec	Coefficient of expansion (/°C $\times$ 10^{-6})
Human enamel	0.0022	0.469	11.4
Human dentin	0.0015	0.183	8.3
Dental amalgam	0.055	–	25.0
Dental composite, microfilled	0.0026	0.675	26–40
Dental composite, colloidal filled	0.0014	0.211	55–68
Dental acrylic plastic	0.0005	0.123	76.0
Zinc phosphate cement	0.0028	0.290	–
Gold	0.710	–	14.4

Coefficient of Thermal Expansion   The thermal coefficients are usually measured with a dilatometer of some sort. The linear change with temperature has been measured with instruments ranging from a simple dial gauge to a cathetometer to a differential transformer [32, 34]. Values represent the change in length per unit length per degree change in temperature with units of per degrees Centigrade. Values for a selected number of dental materials are listed in Table 4-4.

The thermal expansion of restorative materials that replace a portion of a tooth should be close to the values for dentin and enamel in order to minimize the formation of crevices that permit the leakage of oral fluids during temperature changes. Also, porcelain (glass) fused to metal restorations must be made from ceramics and alloys with matching coefficients of thermal expansion in order to prevent cracking during fabrication.

Electrical Properties

Tarnish   Tarnish of dental alloys has been determined in a 2 percent sodium sulfide solution with a test developed by Nielsen and Tuccillo [35, 36]. Disk-shaped samples were mounted on the periphery of a rotating circular acrylic polymer plate, which was immersed in the sulfide solution half the time and exposed to air the remaining half. The extent of tarnish has been determined using a ranking system [35, 37], by photoreflection [37, 38], and by microprobe analysis [39]. Increases in gold or palladium in gold alloys decrease tarnish, with the latter being more effective. Increases in copper or silver increase the degree of tarnish. The interaction of these four elements on tarnish has been related to their concentrations and ratios. Below 55 percent noble content, microstructure strongly affected tarnish; therefore, alloy design and heat treatment are highly important in developing low nobility alloys with acceptable tarnish resistance.

Corrosion   Polarization measurements have been used to study the corrosion of dental amalgam [40–44]. It has been shown that the high-copper amalgams have better corrosion resistance than do the low-copper amalgams. Corrosion of amalgam is more severe in crevices and carved surfaces than in smooth and polished surfaces. Dental amalgam does show passive behavior, but the protective layer can be removed by abrasion and repassivation occurs slowly.

The corrosion of gold and silver-base casting alloys has also been studied by polarization measurements [45–48]. These studies established that alloying with palladium reduces corrosion in chloride solutions and tarnish of silver-base alloys in sulfide solutions. Palladium-rich compositions with silver show immunity or passivation over a wide range of potentials. Intermediate concentrations have a potential region of breakdown and subsequent passivation at higher anodic overpotentials than Pd-rich compositions. Finally, silver-rich compositions have little passivation tendency. Gold-rich alloys are immune at all potentials and intermediate gold alloys (>40 wt percent Au and >5 wt percent Pd) display passivity, depending on the other elements present. Copper enhances passivity, but the passivation current is relatively high. Silver-base alloy with 20 wt percent indium has low corrosion resistance at 100 mV noble to E_{corr}.

Ranking of the corrosion resistance of the gold- and silver-base alloys has been done based on $i_{crit.}/i_{pass.}$, $i_{corr.}$, and the relative positions of the anodic polarization profiles, with the latter generally being the most reliable. The rankings can be shifted, however, by wide ranges of corrosion potentials occurring in the mouth, as well as by variations in the casting procedure and heat treatment.

The corrosion of nickel-base dental casting alloys has also been reported using electrochemical methods including polarization curves, polarization resistance curves, and open circuit potentials [49] to rank alloys. Alloys containing more than 18–20 percent chromium may have their corrosion resistance altered by precipitation of an additional phase, alloys with high Mo or Mn content have better in vitro and in vivo corrosion resistance, and those without Mo or Mn are active and do not resist corrosion. Finally, Co or Ga improve the corrosion resistance of nickel-base alloys.

Nickel-chromium alloys for porcelain substrates have been examined electrochemically [50]. Anodic polarization curves and scratching at constant potentials in synthetic saliva showed that breakdown potentials were not affected by loss of passive films. Also, thermal treatment used in fabrication of the metal-ceramic restoration had no effect on corrosion. The corrosion resulted in dissolution of nickel-rich interdendritic regions.

A crevice cell configuration was developed [51] in an effort to study alloys for implants that would be reproducible and free from uncontrolled crevices and that would permit measurements within a short time.

Oral Galvanism   Measurements of currents and corrosion potentials of metallic restorations in the mouth have been reported [52–56]. Currents of 1–3 μA were observed, and values of 0.1–0.3 $\mu A/cm^2$ were measured with values increasing for the following couples: gold against gold, amalgam against amalgam, gold alloy or Co-Cr alloy and amalgam, and stainless steel and amalgam. Chewing by patients resulted in a twofold increase in current.

Chemical Properties

Corrosion Products   The analysis of phases in materials has been accomplished with x-ray diffraction, scanning electron microscopy, and microprobe; only a few examples are cited here [57–60]. Corrosion products from the interior of dental amalgams have been identified as $Sn_4(OH)_6Cl_2$ and SnO; Cu_2O and $CuCl_2 \cdot 3Cu(OH)_2$ were present in copper-rich amalgams. Corrosion products formed in copper-rich amalgams stored in Ringer's lactated solution consisted initially of $ZnSn(OH)_6$ in zinc-containing alloys and SnO_2 in most other alloys; Cu_2O formed next, followed by $CuCl_2 \cdot 3Cu(OH)_2$. When the amalgams were stored in 1 percent Na_2S, all brands produced HgS, while those placed in a mixture of 1 percent Na_2S and Ringer's lactated solution yielded first $CuSn(OH)_6$ and later Cu_2O. On the other hand, synthetic saliva caused a retardation of corrosion, and only small amounts of tin-rich products were observed even at 20 months.

Amalgams   Single-composition, high-copper amalgam alloys were found by microprobe analysis to be Ag_3Sn (γ), Cu_3Sn (ϵ) and in some cases Ag_4Sn (β). At higher Cu concentrations, more Cu was found in solution in γ and β. When reacted with mercury, mainly $Ag_{22}SnHg_{27}$ (γ_1) and Cu_6Sn_5 (η') were found with no Sn_8Hg (γ_2). If In is present, it is mainly in the γ and γ_1 phases, and when Pd is included it is mainly in ϵ, η', and γ_1 phases.

Polymers   The degree of polymerization of monomers or oligomers is important in denture prosthodontics where methyl methacrylate polymers are used and in bisphenol A-glycidyl methacrylate oligomers and other diacrylate monomers used in restorative dentistry. The degree of polymerization has a significant effect on the mechanical and biological properties of these products. The degree of polymerization is frequently estimated by the number of unreacted carbon-carbon double bonds. This number can be determined chemically by the addition of halogens to the double bond [61, 62], by standard multiple internal reflection infrared spectroscopy [63, 64], or by Fourier transform infrared analysis [65, 66].

Plaque   The interaction of dental plaque with restorative materials has been studied using Auger spectroscopy [67]. Adsorbed layers of plaque on gold alloy, dental amalgam, and composites formed in vivo were found to contain copper, tin, and silicon, respectively, indicating an interaction with the restorative materials.

Biological Properties

It is beyond the scope of this chapter to describe the various tests used to assess the biocompatibility of dental materials. A four-volume text has been published describing current knowledge of the biocompatibility of dental materials [68]. These volumes describe oral tissues and their response to preventive, restorative, and prosthodontic materials. Biocompatibility of dental materials is covered in Chapters VI-8, VIII-2, and VIII-4 of this handbook.

Of particular interest is the set of recommended tests for biological evaluation of dental materials that have been accepted by the American National Standards Institute and the American Dental Association [69]. Many tests are listed and not all are required for a given material. The particular tests required are based on the intended application of the material. Also, no tests for carcinogenesis are given; however, if the Ames or Styles test for mutagenic bacterial changes is positive, testing for carcinogenesis at an experienced laboratory is recommended. The document covers restorative, prosthetic, endodontic, periodontic, and orthodontic materials as well as the following miscellaneous products: investments, asbestos-containing products, low fusing metals, solders, fluxes, electroplating and polishing materials, die materials, and cleaning and polishing agents.

Initial tests on materials include cytotoxicity, hemolysis, Ames, Styles, dominant lethal, oral LD_{50}, IP-LD_{50}, and acute inhalation. Secondary tests are hamster's pouch mucous membrane irritation, dermal toxicity from repeated exposure, subcutaneous implantation in guinea pig, implantation in bone of guinea pig, and guinea pig sensitization. Finally, usage tests suggested are pulpal irritation, pulp capping, endodontic, and dental implant. Recently, in vitro quantitative tests have been developed for evaluating the cytotoxicity of alloys of dental interest [70].

Mechanical Properties

Standard text books [1, 2] on dental materials describe mechanical properties such as elastic modulus, proportional limit, yield strength, tensile and compressive strength, percentage elongation and compression, Poisson's ratio, fatigue strength, resilience, toughness, and hardness (Brinell, Rockwell, Knoop, and Vickers). The less common mechanical tests are reviewed in this section.

Diametral Tensile Strength (Brittle Materials)   This test is especially useful for brittle materials like cements and ceramics. The small size of some dental restorations has made the preparation of large, dumbbell-shaped tensile specimens impractical; also, clamping stresses during testing of small tensile specimens of plastics and ceramics frequently cause experimental problems. As a result, the tensile properties of these materials are usually estimated by the diametral tensile test [71, 72]. This test involves diametric compression of a disk with a thickness one-half its diameter between two plates until fracture occurs. The compressive force introduces tensile stresses normal to the diameter under load, and failure is tensile in character. The tensile strength is calculated as follows:

$$\text{Tensile strength} = \frac{2 \bullet \text{force}}{\pi \bullet \text{diameter} \bullet \text{thickness}}$$

In order for the test to be valid, fracture must occur along the diameter, and essentially no plastic deformation of the disk results where it contacts the two plates. Failure to respect these limitations has led to the publication of erroneous data; for example, PMMA materials exhibit too much contact deformation to be evaluated by this method. Materials whose properties are sensitive to the rate of strain should not be evaluated for tensile strength by this method. For brittle solids it is a useful test, since the preparation of small specimens is simplified and gripping problems are eliminated.

Shear Strength (Brittle Materials)   There is evidence that laminated structures such as porcelain fused to metals fracture in a shearing mode. Only limited data are available on shear in dental materials [73, 74] because of the practical difficulties of the test, e.g., producing true shear without introducing a bending moment.

A micropunch shear method was developed by Smith and Cooper [74] to eliminate bending, and a direct shear method was used by Johnston and O'Brien [73] to determine shear strength. The latter test demonstrated that the shearing tool must have low friction, the shearing edges must be sharp and hard, and the tool must induce failure with no significant bending or rotation of the sample. Shear strengths for feldspathic- and alumina-reinforced porcelain were approximately 128 and 165 MPa, respectively, substantially higher than the diametral tensile values (30 and 40 MPa) and somewhat higher than transverse strengths (88 and 108 MPa). In porcelain-metal systems where the bond strengths approximate the shear strengths, these data suggest failure in shear rather than tension.

In the micropunch shear test, the force required to push punches of 100-μm diameter through plane sections was determined. The shear strength was calculated as the force divided by the thickness times the circumference of the punch. This method permitted the determination of the shear strength of enamel (93 MPa) and dentin (118 MPa), as well as of materials such as dental amalgam (186 MPa) and acrylic polymers (128 MPa). The instrument consisted of a hydraulic loading device, a transducer load cell, and a binocular microscope to position the sample.

Bending and Torsional Properties (Orthodontic Wires and Endodontic Instruments)   The flexural properties of a number of dental materials are of greater importance than compressive, tensile, and shear qualities. Examples include stainless steel or other base metals used as wrought orthodontic wires [75] or stainless steel for endodontic files and reamers [76]. Bending and torsional moment versus the angle of bending or rotation, rather than stress-strain curves, are the parameters determined [77–79]. In addition, the number of 90° bends to failure and the number of rotational degrees to failure, both clockwise and counterclockwise, are measured.

The flexural properties of polymers used for denture bases is important since they are subjected to transverse bending during function. The flexural properties of a number of denture base polymers and the method used has been reported by Ruyter and Svendsen [80].

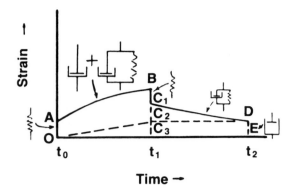

Figure 4-3 Creep and creep recovery curves for rubber impression material with mechanical models describing elastic (*OA* and *BC₁*), viscoelastic (*C₁,C₂*) and viscous strain (*DE*). Loading occurred at t_0 and release of loading at t_1. No further recovery of strain took place at t_2. The strain from *A* to *B* was viscoelastic plus viscous. Adapted from Craig RG (Ed.), *Restorative Dental Materials*, 10th ed., St. Louis: Mosby, 1997, 81.

Tear Properties (Elastomers)   The tear strength [81, 82] and energy [83] have been determined for elastomeric dental materials. Studies on hydrocolloid and rubber impression materials [84, 85] have shown the tear strength to be strain-rate sensitive, with higher values at higher rates of strain [84, 85]. As a result, compliance measurements provide useful data on these materials rather than stress-strain measurements.

Creep and Compliance (Elastomers, Restorative Polymers, and Amalgams)   Evaluation of materials whose properties are strain-rate sensitive is frequently done by determining creep strain at a fixed stress or by determining creep strain at a fixed stress combined with creep recovery. Stress decay at a fixed strain is also used [86–91]. Using the creep at a fixed stress combined with creep recovery, the strain can be subdivided into elastic, viscoelastic, and viscous creep as shown in Figure 4-3. A series of creep curves can be obtained at various stresses. These data can be converted to a compliance (strain/stress) versus time curve (see Figure 4-4). Again, this curve can provide an estimate of the elastic, viscoelastic, and viscous behavior; it is especially useful if the material is linearly viscoelastic (where

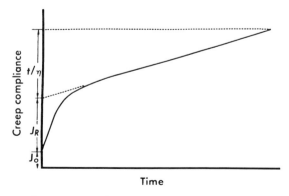

Figure 4-4 Creep compliance versus time for a soft denture lining material. J_0 is the elastic compliance, J_R is the viscoelastic compliance, and t/η is the viscous compliance. Adapted from Duran RL, Powers JM, Craig RG, *J Dent Res*, 58: (1979), 181.

the compliance is independent of the applied stress). A review of the use of short-term, time-dependent property data to predict long-term mechanical property behavior has been published by Smoluk [92].

In addition to static creep tests, Williams [93] has studied the cyclic creep of dental amalgam under conditions similar to those present in in vivo applications. Cyclic loading increased creep rates and reduced time to fracture dental amalgam.

Dynamic Properties (Soft Polymers) The evaluation of dynamic mechanical properties is frequently done with forced vibration methods [94]. The dynamic modulus, internal friction, and dynamic resilience were determined on maxillofacial materials over a temperature range of $-15°$ to $37°C$ using a Goodyear Vibrotester [94, 95]. Cylinders of the materials were vibrated at 60 cps at resonance under 8 percent compression and the properties measured. Plots of dynamic modulus versus temperature permit the determination of the second order transition point, which has been useful in selecting maxillofacial materials for clinical use.

Dynamic properties of materials used in the construction of athletic mouth protectors have been reported [96]. The dynamic modulus and resilience were determined at $23°$ and $37°C$ before and after use, and the values were used to select the most appropriate polymer for this application.

Fracture Toughness (Dental Restoratives and PMMA) Fracture toughness (K_{IC}), the critical stress intensity factor, is reported for selected materials in Table 4-5. Typical values are reported for micro and colloidal filled composites [97], and it can be seen that filler composition affects fracture toughness. The effects of oral temperatures and environment on fracture toughness are not significant, however, although the degree of conversion does increase the values. Storing composites in ethanol results in decreases in fracture toughness, probably as a result of softening of the polymer matrix. It has also been shown that fracture toughness values correlate with single-pass wear studies on composites.

The fracture toughness values of heat-cured denture base plastics are slightly greater than PMMA sheet material [98], but are three to five times less than those for high-impact denture base plastics.

The fracture toughness values for dental amalgams [99] show that composition and microstructure are important factors. The low-copper amalgams (<6 percent Cu) have

Table 4-5   Fracture Toughness of Dental Materials

Material	Fracture toughness, MN • m$^{-3/2}$
Dental composites	
>60 vol. % micro-filled	1.2–1.4
~40 vol. % colloidal-filled	0.8–0.9
PMMA	1.1
Denture base plastics—heat-cured	1.5
Denture base plastics—high impact	4–8
Dental amalgam	
Low-copper	1.5–1.6
High-copper	1.0–1.3
Dental ceramics—feldspathic	1.5–2.1

higher values of fracture toughness than do high-copper alloys ($\sim$13 percent Cu). The higher values for low-copper alloys are believed to be related to higher flow values resulting from the microstructure (i.e., the presence of a continuous γ_2 phase, Sn_{7-8} Hg). It should be noted that the fracture toughness of highly filled composites is intermediate between the low- and high-copper amalgams.

Denatal ceramics of the feldspathic type [100] have a fracture toughness of about 1.8 MN $\cdot$ m$^{-3/2}$ which is twice as great as that of human tooth enamel (0.9 MN $\cdot$ m$^{-3/2}$). Fracture toughness and acoustic emission behavior of dental composites has been reported [101].

Wear   Two- and three-body wear tests have been used to evaluate dental materials. Two-body tests have consisted of measurements of track width, depth, and type of failure from single and multiple passes of a diamond slider [102] and pin-on-disk or plate measurements [103–105]. The loss of volume on the pin as a function of sliding distance or the depth of the groove in the disk have been used to assess wear. The single- and multiple-pass sliding tests provide information about the wear process by examination of the wear tracks, while the pin-on-disk or plate methods provide some indication of the wear under service conditions.

The abrasiveness of dentrifrices on tooth structure represents a three-body wear system, and these tests are of particular interest in dentistry [106, 107]. Since toothpastes abrade enamel slowly, these tests use dentin as the wear surface to be evaluated under simulated *in vivo* conditions.

Clinical [108, 109] and simulated [110, 111] studies have also measured wear of restorative materials by periodically making dies from impressions of teeth containing restorations and using a variety of profile methods to determine the loss per time of service.

Bond Strength   The bond strength of restorative materials to tooth structure [112–116] or of ceramics to metals [117–121] is determined using tests that measure tensile or shear values. In the former tests, in vivo conditions have sometimes been simulated by storing the samples in body temperature fluids for various times before testing. In other studies, the stored samples have been temperature-cycled before testing to simulate oral conditions.

Filler-Matrix Interaction in Composites   Dielectric loss tangent and capacitance were measured [122] on a zirconia-silica filled UDMA composite which allowed the calculation of dielectric permittivities and real and imaginary electric moduli. Three relaxations α, β, and γ were observed where α was attributed to segmental motion of main chains, β to the motion of the free amide groups, and γ to local motion of $(CH_2)_n$. Adding filler had a pronounced effect on the thickness of the interfacial boundary layer. Increasing the filler concentration restricted the mobility of the main chains and decreased the thickness of the surface layer, while permitting more movement of the local chains in the loosely packed layer. The data showed that the optimum silane coverage of the filler was about three times the minimum uniform coverage and that higher amounts produced plasticizing effects. When the composite was treated with water, molecules of water were only found as fragments that formed non-freezing clusters. These clusters contained charges that were not stabilized by the hydrated amide groups. Water in silanated composites behaved much like the polymer at low temperatures, but increased plasticity at high temperatures. In non-silanated composites bulk water could exist at the interface; it can form disoriented structures of ice at low temperatures and can evaporate at high temperatures. Thus, dielectric measurements appear to be a good tool to detect phase transitions in composite systems and to investigate water-polymer interactions.

STRESS ANALYSIS OF DENTAL RESTORATIONS

Dental restorations are frequently very small and yet biting forces as high as 2000 N have been reported. As a result, materials with ultimate strengths of 1,000 MPa can fracture during use. Also, for brittle materials with low tensile or shear strengths, it is important to design restorations that will minimize these stresses during function.

Most of the current engineering methodsl [123] for stress analysis have been used to determine the optimum design of dental restorations [124–128]. A review of design analysis of fixed dental restorations was published in 1977 [129], and a review of the finite element method applied to dental problems including stress analysis and thermal gradients was done in 1984 [130]. Finally, an elementary review is presented in the undergraduate dental materials text, *Restorative Dental Materials* [1].

REFERENCES

1 Craig RG (ed.). *Restorative Dental Materials*, 9th ed. St. Louis: Mosby, 1993, 1–581.

2 Phillips RW. *Skinner's Science of Dental Materials*, 9th ed. Philadelphia: Saunders, 1991, 1–597.

3 *Specifying Color by the Munsell System*, ASTM D1535-1568, Part 20. Philadelphia: American Society for Testing and Materials, 1975, 383–404.

4 Civjan S, Barone JJ, Reinke PE, Selting WJ. Thermal properties of nonmetallic restorative materials. *J Dent Res*, 51 (1972), 1030–1037.

5 Nickerson D. The specification of color tolerances. *Textile Res*, 6 (1936), 509.

6 Dennison JB, Powers JM Koran A. Color of dental restorative resins. *J Dent Res*, 57 (1978), 557–562.

7 Johnston WM, O'Brien WJ. Color analysis of dental modifying porcelains. *J Dent Res*, 61 (1982), 484–488.

8 Koran A, Powers JM, Raptis CN, Yu R. Reflection spectrophotometry of facial skin. *J Dent Res*, 60 (1981), 979–982.

9 Powers JM, Koran A. Color of denture resins. *J Dent Res*, 56 (1977), 754–761.

10 Yu R, Koran A, Raptis CN, Craig RG. Cigarette staining and cleaning of a maxillofacial silicone. *J Dent Res*, 62 (1983), 853–855.

11 Craig RG, Koran A, Yu R, Spencer J. Color stability of elastomers for maxillofacial appliances. *J Dent Res*, 57 (1978), 866–871.

12 Powers JM, Dennison JB, Koran A. Color stability of restorative resins under accelerated aging. *J Dent Res*, 57 (1978), 964–970.

13 Hunter RS. *The Measurement of Appearance*. New York: Wiley, 1975, 1–348.

14 Kubelka P. New contributions to the optics of intensely light-scattering materials, Part I. *J Opt Soc Am*, 38 (1948), 448; Part II, Non-homogeneous layers, *J Opt Soc Am*, 44 (1954), 330.

15 Kubelka P, Munk F. Ein beltragzur optik der farbanstrochr. Zeit fur tech. *Physik*, 12 (1931), 593.

16 Miyagawa Y, Powers JM. Prediction of color of an esthetic restorative material. *J Dent Res*, 62 (1983), 581–584.

17 Miyagawa Y, Powers JM, O'Brien, WJ.: Optical properties of direct restorative materials. *J Dent Res*, 60 (1981), 890–894.

18 Colorimetry. Official recommendations of the 31st International Commission on Illumination (CIE), CIE Publication 15 (E-1.3.1), 1971, 124.

19 Yeh, CI, Miyagawa Y, Powers, JM. Optical properties of composites of selected shades. *Dent Res*, 61 (1982), 797–801.

20 Johnston WM. The color and translucency of feldspathic porcelain mixtures. Doctoral dissertation, University of Michigan, Ann Arbor, MI, 1983, 1–105.

21 O'Brien WJ, Johnston WM, Fanian F. Filtering effects of body porcelain on opaque color modifiers. IADR Paper No. 1369, Dental Materials Group Microfilm, 60th General Session, March 1982.

22 O'Brien WJ, Johnston WM, Fanian F, Lambert S. The surface roughness and gloss of composites. *J Dent Res* 63 (1984), 685–688.

23 Hall JB, Hefferren JJ, Olsen NH. Study of fluorescent characteristics of extracted human teeth by use of a clinical fluorometer. *J Dent Res*, 49 (1970), 1431.

24 Baran GR, O'Brien WJ, Tien TY. Color emission of rare earth ions in a potassium feldspar glass. *J Dent Res*, 56 (1977), 1323–1329.

25 Lisanti VF, Zander HA. Thermal conductivity of dentin. *J Dent Res*, 29 (1950), 493.

26 Soyenkoff BC, Okun JH. Thermal conductivity measurements on dental tissues with the aid of thermistors. *Am Dent Assoc J*, 57 (1958), 23.

27 Braden M. Thermal properties of dental composition. *J Dent Res*, 45 (1966), 1453–1457.

28 Brown WS, Dewey WA, Jacobs NR. Thermal properties of teeth. *J Dent Res*, 49 (1970), 752–755.

29 Powers J M. Tabulated values of physical and mechanical properties. In O'Brien WJ, Ryge G (eds.), *An Outline of Dental Materials and Their Selection*. Philadelphia: Saunders, 1978, 385–413.

30 Watts DC, Haywood CM, Smith R. Thermal diffusion through composite restorative materials. *Brit Dent J*, 154 (1983), 101.

31 Watts DC, Smith R. Thermal diffusivity in finite cylindrical specimens of dental cements. *J Dent Res*, 60 (1981), 1972.

32 Craig RG, Eick JD, Peyton FA. Properties of natural waxes used in dentistry. *J Dent Res*, 44 (1965), 1308–1316.

33 Fairhurst CW, Anusavice KJ, Hashinger DT, Ringle RD, Twiggs SW. Thermal expansion of dental alloys and porcelains. *J Biomed Mat Res*, 14 (1980), 435.

34 McLean JW, Hughes TH. The reinforcement of dental porcelain with ceramic oxides. *Brit Dent J*, 119 (1966), 251–267.

35 Lang BR, Bernier SH, Giday Z, Asgar K. Tarnish and corrosion of noble metal alloys. *J Prosthet Dent*, 48 (1982), 245–252.

36 Tuccillo JJ, Nielsen JP. Observations of onset of sulfide tarnish on gold-base alloys. *J Prosthet Dent*, 25 (1971), 629.

37 German RM, Wright DC, Gallant RF. In vitro tarnish measurements on fixed prosthodontic alloys. *J Prosthet Dent* 47 (1982), 399–406.

38 Lubovich RP, Kovarik RE, Kinser DL. A quantitative and subjective characterization of tarnishing in low-gold alloys. *J Prosthet Dent* 42 (1979), 534–538.

39 Tuccillo JJ, Nielsen JP. Microprobe analysis of in vivo discoloration. *J Prosthet Dent*, 31 (1974), 285.

40 Boyer DB, Chan KC, Svare CW, Bramson JB. The effect of finishing on the anodic polarization of high-copper amalgams. *J Oral Rehabil*, 5 (1978), 223–228.

41 Fairhurst CW, Marek M, Butts MB, Okabe, T. New information on high copper amalgam corrosion. *J Dent Res*, 57 (1978), 725.

42 Marek M. Acceleration of corrosion on dental amalgam by abrasion. *J Dent Res*, 63 (1984), 1010–1013.

43 Sarkar NK, Greener EH. Saline corrosion of conventional dental amalgams. *J Oral Rehabil*, 2 (1975), 49–62.

44 Tani G, Zucchi F. Electrochemical valuation of the corrosion resistance of commonly used metals in dental prostheses. *Minerva Stomatol*, 16 (1967), 710.

45 Johnson DL, Rinne VW, Bleich LL. Polarization-corrosion behavior of commercial gold- and silver-base casting alloys in Fusayama solution. *J Dent Res*, 62 (1983), 1221–1225.

46 Niemi L, Holland RI. Tarnish and corrosion of a commercial dental Ag-Pd-Cu-Au casting alloy. *J Dent Res*, 63 (1984), 1014–1048.

47 Sarkar NK, Fuys RA, Jr., Stanford JW. Application of electrochemical techniques to characterize the corrosion of dental alloys. In *Corrosion and Degradation of Implant Materials*, ASTM STP684. Philadelphia: American Society for Testing and Materials, 1978, 277–294.

48 Vaidyanathan TK, Prasad A. In vitro corrosion and tarnish analysis of the Ag-Pd binary system. *J Dent Res*, 60 (1981), 707–715.

49 Meyer JM, Wirthner JM, Barraud R, Susz CP, Nally JN. Corrosion studies on nickel-based casting alloys. In *Corrosion and Degradation of Implant Materials*, ASTM STP684. Philadelphia: American Society for Testing and Materials, 1979, 295–315.

50 DeMicheli, SM, Riesgo O. Electrochemical study of corrosion in Ni-Cr dental alloys. *Biomaterials*, 3 (1982), 209–212.

51 Sutow EJ, Jones DW. A crevice corrosion cell configuration. *J Dent Res*, 58 (1979), 1358–1363.

52 Arvidson K, Johansson EG. Galvanic series of some dental alloys. *Scand J Dent Res*, 85 (1977), 485–491.

53 Bergman M, Ginstrup O, Nilner K. Potential and polarization measurements in vivo of oral galvanism. *Scand J Dent Res*, 86 (1978), 135–145.

54 Gjerdet NR, Brune D. Measurements of currents between dissimilar alloys in the oral cavity. *Scand J Dent Res*, 85 (1977), 500–502.

55 Holland RI. Galvanic currents between gold and amalgam. *Scand J Dent Res*, 88 (1980), 269–272.

56 Nomoto S, Ano M, Onase H. Microprobe for measurement of corrosion potential of metallic restorations in mouth. *J Dent Res*, 58 (1979), 1688–1690.

57   Holland GA, Asgar K. Some effects on the phases of amalgam induced by corrosion. *J Dent Res*, 53 (1974), 1245–1254.

58   Lin JHC, Marshall GW, Jr., Marshall SJ. Corrosion product formation sequence on Cu-rich amalgams in various solutions. *J Biomed Mat Res*, 17 (1983), 913–920.

59   Mahler DB, Adey JD. Microprobe analysis of three high-copper amalgams. *J Dent Res*, 63 (1984), 921–925.

60   Marshall SJ, Lin JHC, Marshall GW, Jr. Cu_2O and $CuCl_2 \bullet 3Cu(OH)_2$ corrosion products on copper rich dental amalgams. *J Biomed Mat Res*, 16 (1982), 81–85.

61   Caul HJ, Schoonover LC. A method for determining the extent of polymerization of acrylic resins and its application for dentures. *Am Dent. Assoc J*, 39 (1949), 1–9.

62   Smith DC, Bains MED. The detection and estimation of residual monomer in polymethyl methacrylate. *J Dent Res*, 35 (1956), 16.

63   Ruyter IE, Svendsen SA. Remaining methacrylate groups in composite restorative materials. *Acta Odontol Scand*, 36 (1978), 75–82.

64   Vankerckhoven H, Lambrechts P, Van Beylen M, Davidson CL, Vanherle G. Unreacted methacrylate groups on the surface of composite resins. *J Dent Res*, 61(1982), 791–796.

65   Ferracane JL, Greener EH. Correlation between mechanical properties and conversion in unfilled Bis-GMA resins. IADR, Annual Session, March 1984, Dent Mat Gp Microfilm, Paper No. 544.

66   Koenig JL. Application of Fourier transform infrared spectroscopy to chemical systems. *Appl Spectroscopy*, 29 (1975), 293–309.

67   Skjorland KK. Auger analysis of integuments formed on different dental filling materials in vivo. *Acta Odontol Scand*, 40 (1982), 19–34.

68   Smith DC, Williams DF. *Biocompatibility of Dental Materials; Vol. I, Characteristics of Dental Tissues and Their Response to Dental Materials; Volume II, Biocompatibility of Preventive Dental Materials and Bonding Agents; Vol. III, Biocompatibility of Dental Restorative Materials, and Volume IV, Biocompatibility of Prosthodontic Materials*. Boca Raton, FL: CRC Press, 1982.

69   Council on Dental Materials and Devices. *Recommended Standard Practices for Biological Evaluation of Dental Materials*. American National Standards Institute/American Dental Association Document No. 41-1982. Chicago: American Dental Association, 1979.

70   Wataha JC, Craig RG, Hanks CT. Precision of, and new methods for testing *in vitro* alloy toxicity. *Dent Mat*, 8 (1992), 65.

71   Berenbaum R, Brodie J. Measurement of tensile strength of brittle materials. *Br J Appl Physics*, 10 (1959), 281.

72   Rudnick G, Hunter GR, Holden FC. An analysis of the diametral-compression test. *Mater Res Standards*, 3 (1963), 283.

73   Johnston WM, O'Brien, WJ. The shear strength of dental porcelain. *J Dent Res*, 59 (1980), 1409.

74   Smith DC, Cooper WEG. The determination of shear strength—a method using a micro-punch apparatus. *Br Dent J*, 130 (1971), 333.

75   Council on Dental Materials and Devices. New American Dental Association Specification No. 32 for Orthodontic Wire not Containing Precious Metals. *Am Dent Assoc J*, 95 (1977), 1169.

76   Council on Dental Materials and Devices. New American Dental Association Specification No. 28 for Endodontic Files and Reamers. *Am Dent Assoc J*, 93 (1976), 813.

77   Brantley WA, Augat WS, Myers CL, Winders RV. Bending deformation studies of orthodontic wires. *J Dent Res*, 57 (1978), 609.

78   Craig RG, McIlwain ED, Peyton FA. Bending and torsion properties of endodontic instruments. *Oral Surg, Oral Med, Oral Path*, 25 (1968), 239.

79   Dolan DW, Craig RG. Bending and torsion of endodontic files with rhombus cross sections. *J Endodont*, 8 (1982), 260.

80   Ruyter IE, Svendsen SA. Flexural properties of denture base polymers. *J Prosthet Dent*, 43 (1980), 95.

81   *Resistance to Tear Propagation in Plastic Film and Thin Sheeting by a Single-tear Method*. D1938–1967, ASTM Standards Part 27. Philadelphia: American Society for Testing and Materials, 1968, 669.

82   *Tear Resistance of Vulcanized Rubber*. D624–654, ASTM Standards, Part 28. Philadelphia: American Society for Testing and Materials, 1968, 341.

83   Webber RL, Ryge G. The determination of tear energy of extensible materials of dental interest. *J Biomed Mat Res*, 2 (1968), 231.

84   Herfort TW, Gerberick WW, Macosko CW, Goodkind RJ. Tear strength of elastomeric impression materials. *J Prosthet Dent*, 39 (1978), 59.

85   MacPherson GW, Craig RG, Peyton FA. Mechanical properties of hydrocolloid and rubber impression materials. *J Dent Res*, 46 (1967), 714.

86   Bertoletti RL, Moffa JP. Creep rate of porcelain-bonding alloys as a function of temperature. *J Dent Res*, 59 (1980), 2062.

87   Duran RL, Powers JM, Craig RG. Viscoelastic and dynamic properties of soft liners and tissue conditioners. *J Dent Res*, 58 (1979), 1801.

88   Goldberg AJ. Viscoelastic properties of silicone, polysulfide, and polyether impression materials. *J Dent Res*, 53 (1974), 1033.

89   Morris HF, Asgar K, Tillitson EW. Stress-relaxation testing, Part 1: A new approach to the testing of removable partial denture alloys, wrought wires, and clasp behavior. *J Prosthet Dent*, 46 (1981), 133.

90   Oglesby P. Viscoelastic behavior. In Dickson G, Cassel JM (Eds.), *National Bureau of Standards, Special Publ. 354*, July 1972, 127.

91   Ruyter IE, Espevik S. Compressive creep of denture base polymers. *Acta Odontol Scand*, 38 (1980), 169.

92   Smoluk GR. How to use time-dependent property data. *Modern Plastics*, Aug. 1964, 119.

93   Williams KR. Cyclic creep and fracture of dental amalgam. *Biomaterials*, 4 (1983), 255.

94   Gehman SD. Dynamic properties of elastomers. *Rubber Chem Tech*, 30 (1957), 1202.

95   Koran A, Craig RG. Dynamic mechanical properties of maxillofacial materials. *J Dental Res*, 54 (1975), 1216.

96   Godwin WC, Craig RG, Koran A, Lang BR, Powers JM. Mouth protectors in junior football players. *Physician and Sportsmedicine*, 10 (1982), 41.

97   Lloyd CH. The fracture toughness of dental composites. *J Oral Rehabil*, 9 (1982), 133.

98   Hill RG, Bates JF, Lewis TT, Rees N. Fracture toughness of acrylic denture base. *Biomat*, 4 (1983), 112.

99   Lloyd CH, Adamson M. The fracture toughness (K_{IC}) of amalgam. *J Oral Rehabil*, 12 (1985), 59.

100 Taira M, Nomwia Y, Wakasa K, Yamaki M, Matsui A. Studies on fracture toughness of dental ceramics. *J Oral Rehabil*, 17 (1990), 551.

101 Kim KH, Park JH, Imai Y, Kishi T. Fracture toughness and acoustic emission behavior of dental composite resins. *Engin Fract Mech*, 40 (1991), 811.

102 Craig RG, Powers JM. Wear of dental tissues and materials. *Internat Dent J*, 26 (1976), 121.

103 Powers JM, Allen LJ, Craig RG. Two-body abrasion of commercial and experimental restorative and coating resins and an amalgam. *Am Dent Assoc J*, 89 (1974), 1118.

104 Tillitson EW, Craig RG, Peyton FA. Friction and wear of restorative dental materials. *J Dent Res*, 50 (1971), 149.

105 Wu W, McKinley JE. Influence of chemicals on wear of dental composites. *J Dent Res*, 61 (1982), 1180.

106 American Dental Association Council on Dental Therapeutics. Abrasivity of current dentifrices. *Am Dent Assoc J*, 81 (1970), 1177.

107 Wright KHR, Stevenson JI. The measurement and interpretation of dentifrice abrasiveness. *J Soc Cosmetic Chem*, 18 (1967), 387.

108 Mitchem JC, Gronas DG. The continued *in vivo* evaluation of the wear of restorative resins. *Am Dent Assoc J*, 111 (1985), 961.

109 Wendt SL, Jr., Leinfelder KF. The chemical evaluation of heat-treated composite resin inlays. *Am J Dent*, 4 (1991), 10.

110 Pallav P, DeGee AJ, Davidson CL, Erickson RL, Glasspoole EA. The influence of admixing microfiller to small-particle composite resin on wear, tensile strength, hardness and surface roughness. *J Dent Res*, 68 (1989), 489.

111 DeLong R, Douglas WH. Development of an artificial oral environment for testing of dental restoratives: Bi-axial force and movement control. *J Dent Res*, 62 (1983), 32.

112 Bowen RL. Adhesive bonding of various materials to hard tooth tissues: 1. Method of determining bond strength. *J Dent Res*, 44 (1965), 690.

113 Bowen RL, Cobb EN. A method for bonding to dentin and enamel. *Am Dent Assoc J*, 107 (1983), 734.

114 Eden GT, Craig RG, Peyton FA. Evaluation of a tensile test for direct filling resins. *J Dent Res*, 49 (1970), 428.

115 Roydhouse RH, Rambosek GM. Pinhole test for adhesion. *J Dent Res*, 48 (1968), 1087.

116 Swartz ML, Phillips RW. A method of measuring adhesive characteristics of dental cements. *Am Dental Assoc J*, 50 (1955), 172.

117 Anthony DH, Burnett AP, Smith DL, Brooks MS. Shear test for measuring bonding in cast gold alloy-porcelain composites. *J Dent Res*, 49 (1970), 27.

118 Asgar K, Giday Z. Refinements on testing of porcelain to metal bond. *J Dent Res*, 57 (1978), 292.

119 Lubovich RP, Goodkind RJ. Bond strength studies of precious, semiprecious, and non-precious ceramic-metal alloys with two porcelains. *J Prosthet Dent*, 37 (1977), 288.

120   Malhotra ML, Maickel LB. Shear bond strength of porcelain-fused-to-alloys of varying noble metal contents. *J Prosthet Dent*, 44 (1980), 405.

121   Shell JS, Nielsen JP. Study of the bond between gold alloys and porcelain. *J Dent Res*, 41 (1962), 1424.

122   Mohsen NM. Physical, chemical and biological characterization of urethane dimethacrylate biomaterial composite. Doctoral dissertation, University of Michigan, Ann Arbor, MI, 1995, 288.

123   Tuppeny WH, Jr., Kobayashi AS. *Manual on Experimental Stress Analysis*, 2nd ed. Westport, CT, 1965, 1–67.

124   Craig RG, Peyton FA. Measurement of stresses in fixed-bridge restorations using a brittle coating technique. *J Dent Res*, 44 (1965), 756.

125   Craig RG, Peyton FA. Measurement of strains in fixed bridges with electronic strain gauges. *J Dent Res*, 46 (1967), 615.

126   Farah JW, Craig RG. Stress analysis of three marginal configurations of full posterior crowns by three-dimensional photoelasticity. *J Dent Res*, 53 (1974), 1219.

127   Farah JW, Craig RG, Sikarski DL. Photoelastic and finite element stress analysis of a restored axisymmetric first molar. *J Biomech*, 6 (1973), 511.

128   Nally JN, Farah JW, Craig RG. Experimental stress analysis of dental restorations, Part IX. Two-dimensional photoelastic stress analysis of porcelain bonded to gold crowns. *J Prosthet Dent*, 25 (1971), 307.

129   Craig RG, Farah JW. Stress analysis and design of single restorations and fixed bridges. *Oral Sci Rev*, 10 (1977), 45.

130   Craig RG. Dental mechanics. In Kardestuncer H, Norrie DH (Eds.), *Finite Element Handbook*. New York: McGraw-Hill, 1987, 3.330–3.334.

Chapter 5

Textiles

Roger W. Snyder
Robert Guidoin
Yves Marois

INTRODUCTION

Textiles are among the earliest of medical devices, having been used first as bandages, sutures, and ligatures and then as implants. Although there are many uses for textiles in medicine, such as bandages, cast material, drapes, sponges, and sutures, this chapter will concentrate on implants and tissue-contacting uses.

Textiles are assemblages of fibers [1]. These fibers may be a continuous monofilament, continuous multifilaments, or short lengths (staple). Filaments are solids with one dimension greater than the other two. They are usually circular in cross-section. Filaments can be natural or synthetic. Natural filaments occur as staple (e.g., wool, silk, and cotton); synthetic filaments are usually continuous. Most implantable textiles are fabricated of multifilament yarns. Synthetic filaments can be formed by any number of extrusion techniques, such as melt spinning, solvent spinning, or paste extrusion.

Vorhees et al. [2] first noted that a free suture end in the atrial wall became covered with "a glistening film, free of microscopic thrombi." This observation led to early trials with textiles as arterial replacements. A number of experimental materials and structures were tried [3]. Corrugations were added to prevent kinking [4]. Extensive experimental and clinical trials demonstrated the importance of porosity within the graft wall for the successful encapsulation of implanted textile prostheses [5–7].

Today, many woven and knit fabrications are available. The use of textiles has expanded to other areas of surgery. The basic theories have undergone little change, however [8].

TYPES OF FABRICATIONS

The earliest textile structures were woven. In weaving, one set of yarns is aligned lengthwise (warp) and a second yarn (filling or weft) is passed back and forth perpendicular to the warp (Figure 5-1A). Many patterns are possible and various surfaces, such as smooth, ribbed, and velour can be achieved.

Although braiding is done on different machinery, it is essentially a woven structure in which the yarns run at 45° to the axis of the fabrication. In triaxial weaving, there are two separate sets of warp yarns at ±60° to the weft yarn. This structure has not yet seen a medical application.

In knitting, either the warp yarn or the weft yarn is used to form the structure. The yarn is bent around a needle and looped around another yarn. Generally knit structures are not as strong as similar wovens and are more porous due to the more open fabrication. The advantage of knits is their flexibility.

In the simplest form of knitting, a single yarn travels in the weft direction, forming each row of stitches (Figure 5-1B). A second yarn can be used to form velour loops perpendicular

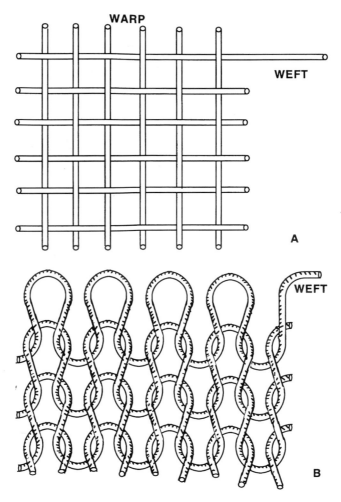

Figure 5-1 Typical textile fabrications: (A) simple weave pattern, (B) typical weft knit pattern, (C) typical warp knit pattern, (D) random felt pattern.

to the surface. This yarn travels with the body yarn. Warp knitting is more complex than weft. Yarns are assembled in the warp or machine direction similar to threading a weaving loom. A series of needles interact with these yarns to form the stitches (Figure 5-1C). Many implantable medical fabrics are warp knits.

The third class of fabrics is random (Figure 5-1D). These fabrics start out as a loose mat of staple yarns. Barbed needles are driven in and out of the mat, permanently entangling the fibers to form felt. In spun bonded material, the staple yarns are bonded to each other. Solvent welding, thermal welding or adhesives can be used. Because these materials do not rely on friction, they can be much thinner than felts. Some packaging materials, such as Tyvek® (E. I duPont de Nemours, Inc.), are made in this fashion and are impervious to microbes but porous to sterilizing media.

MATERIALS

Textiles can be fabricated from any fiber-forming material. Historically, experimental fabrics for implants have included such natural materials as silk and collagen and such

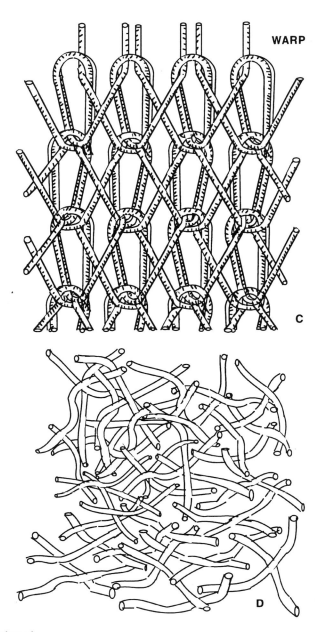

Figure 5-1 Continued.

manufactured materials as nylon, polyvinyl alcohol, polyethylene, and stainless steel. Currently three materials predominate: polyethylene terephthalate (PET), polytetrafluorethylene (PTFE), and polypropylene (PP) (see Chapter 2). These materials have demonstrated a good degree of bioendurance and biostability in the body, both as medical fabrics and as sutures.

The most widely used polymer in textiles today is PET. Until 1995, most of the PET used was duPont's Dacron® (E. I. duPont de Nemours, Inc.). However, Dacron® is no longer sold for use in implants (see Chapter 2). PET obtained from other manufacturers is currently being tested and used clinically outside the USA [9]. Because of the extensive clinical experience with Dacron®, careful testing of the substitute PETs will be required.

PET is available in different size filaments, filament counts, and cross-sectional shapes, as well as homopolymer and copolymer versions. It is also available with titanium dioxide and carbon fillers. PET is melt spun; that is, the polymer is melted and extruded to form filaments. Evidence suggests that PET shows an early 10–20 percent decrease in strength after implantation or in vitro cycling, but then stabilizes [10]. It is susceptible to fluid uptake, although no detrimental effect of this has been conclusively demonstrated. Successful implants in excess of 20 years have been reported.

Most PTFE textiles are felts. The only commercially available PTFE filament is duPont's Teflon® (E. I. duPont de Nemours, Inc.). However, Teflon® is no longer sold for use in implants (see Chapter 2). As of 1995, the Teflon® felts available for implant have been fabricated from stockpiled materials. It is unclear at the time of this writing whether or not there will be a replacement for PTFE felt.

PTFE is fabricated into filaments by mixing with cellulose-type fillers and solution spinning. The filaments are then oxidized, giving the filaments a dark chocolate color. The oxidized fillers are generally removed by using strong acid baths or long heat soaks. Implants approaching 20 years have been documented with little change noted [10]. In fact, evidence suggests a slight increase in strength that may be due to some crystalline changes.

The primary use of PP textiles was first as a mesh and soon after as a monofilament suture. PP filaments are generally thicker and stiffer than PET and PTFE. The resulting textile, even when knit in an open mesh, is inevitably very stiff. Stainless steel and tantalum meshes have also been used, but present the same stiffness problem.

A number of other fibers have been used in animal or clinical studies, including carbon, polyurethane (PU), and various bioresorbable suture materials. Carbon has been used in two forms: (1) carbonization of some other fabric such as rayon, and (2) direct fabrication with carbon filaments. This is difficult because of the brittleness of such filaments. Usually simple structures with few bends such as wovens and braids are used. It is also possible to coat these filaments in order to protect them during fabrication.

Two forms of PU textiles have been used experimentally. Lycra® (E. I. duPont de Nemours, Inc.), a filament form of segmented polyether polyurethane similar to Biomer®, has been knit or woven into vascular grafts to increase elasticity. PU can also be sprayed from solution directly onto a mandrel. The solvent evaporates as the material is being sprayed, forming filaments and bonding filaments to each other. This results in a material resembling a spun-bonded textile [11].

USES

The first use of implant textiles was as tissue buttresses. The more common use today is as arterial replacements; all textile vascular grafts are fabricated from PET. Woven grafts are used predominantly for the thoracic aorta and other locations in which bleeding would be critical. Knits are commercially available in simple and velour fabrications and are predominately used for smaller-diameter vessel replacements, such as femoral-popliteal bypasses. However, highly porous but efficiently preclotted fabrics can easily and safely be used in the thoracic aorta, and wovens have been used as femoral-popliteal bypasses. Both woven and knitted structures are used as aortoiliac bifurcations.

Defects created in arteries during endarterectomies, natural defects in ventricular walls, patent ducti, and transpositions are repaired using fabric patches. Woven and knit patches are used, depending upon the surgeon's preference. Some hernia repairs are reinforced with PET, PTFE, PP or bioresorbable meshes. Fabrics are also used in certain types of plastic surgical procedures, particularly in the repair of extensive damage due to tumor removal and injury.

Currently, one textile device is available for the repair of shoulder separations. This is a warp knit reinforced by seaming along the length. A number of textile structures have been designed and tested for ligament augmentation or replacement and tendon repair. Woven, warp-knit, and braided structures have been used. Materials include PET, PTFE, PP, PE and polyurethane-coated carbon [14].

One of the largest uses of medical textiles is as a constituent of multicomponent medical devices. Textiles have been used wherever a flexible structure is required or when ingrowth is desired, as in subcutaneous anchoring of skin penetration devices. Small squares of knit fabrics or felts are used as suture buttresses to prevent tissue tearing. Most heart valves have textile sewing rings. These are constructed of tubular or flat fabric and may be backed with felt. Both PET and PTFE materials are used. In addition, textiles may be used as strut covers if the design requires tissue ingrowth, in an attempt to limit fibrin formation. Textiles have been used experimentally as leaflets, but fatigue failure and other problems have not been overcome.

Textiles are also employed as filtering materials for arterial filters, cardiotomies, and oxygenators; PP, PET, and nylon materials have been used in these applications.

BIOLOGICAL RESPONSE

Textiles are porous and for the most part will exhibit a wick effect. In the initial stages of use, they will be filled with fluids such as plasma. The composition of these fluids depends primarily on the site of implantation and secondarily by the intramural characteristics and the dimensions of the fabrication. The natural fluids may also contain drugs, cells, and cellular elements and/or bacteria, any of which may affect subsequent events.

The healing response of textile vascular prostheses in animals has been well documented [12, 15, 16]. Barring toxic products introduced in processing, the tube is encapsulated according to a standard wound-healing mechanism. Most applications of textiles rely on this mechanism for permanent results. Encapsulation may be unstable because healing and viability of the inner capsule in contact with the blood stream depends on transmural blood supply as well as diffusion from the blood.

The microstructure of the encapsulation depends not only upon the structure of the textile, but also upon the material [12, 13]. For example, PET evokes a greater long-term tissue reaction than do bioresorbable lactide/glycolide copolymers [12]. Polyvinylidene fluoride (PVDF), a potential polymer candidate for numerous biomedical applications such as vascular prostheses and sutures [14], has recently been shown to generate low tissue reaction and better long-term biostability than those of the reference vascular suture, PP.

KEY CHARACTERISTICS

Textiles are available in a variety of patterns that can be modified by changing yarn content. Fabrics can be knit extremely thin, limited by the diameter of available filaments, or can be felted very thick, in excess of several inches. Ideal thickness for maximizing healing of vascular grafts is less than 0.75 mm [18], and the optimal filament diameter should range between 11–15 μm [9].

Surfaces can be smooth or ribbed or have a velour component. Each will affect the ingrowth and flow of blood differently. Textiles are porous unless coated or melted. Pore size can range from almost nonexistent, as in a thick felt, to the very large pores in a mesh. Pore size characterization is described in Chapter 2.

Textiles have different properties in the warp and weft directions. Because of the small cross-sectional area of filaments, the breaking strength is highly dependent on small changes in area as well as flaws and inclusions. Because of the random distribution of these flaws, the strength of the filaments and the fabric made from these fibers are statistical quantities. Three structural factors modify this strength: (1) the number of stitches per centimeter, (2) the radii of curvature introduced by the structure, and (3) any twisting of the yarns necessary for fabrication. Finally, the strength is decreased by any damage introduced during fabrication and processing.

When textiles are loaded uniaxially, four factors govern the resulting extension: (1) crimp or wrinkle deformation, (2) changes in bends in the yarn, (3) slippage between yarns, and (4) extension of filaments. The resulting load-deformation curves are complex. Any yarn slippage or plastic deformation of the filaments will result in a permanent deformation of the fabric. A structure that is loosely knit or woven may be subject to large permanent deformation without filament elongation.

Bending stiffness for a given fabrication is a function of yarn density, fabric thickness, and the stiffness of the polymer. Since most fabrics are very thin, filament stiffness dominates. Bending stiffness is further modified by the structure. Structures such as wovens, in which yarns must bend, are stiffer than knits, in which stitches may act as hinges.

Processing will affect both the biological response and the long-term fatigue life of a fabric. Many fabrics are heat treated to reduce porosity, stabilize the structure, and produce crimping. Excessive thermal exposure can degrade the polymer. Chemical cleaning (including using surfactants) or sterilization can leave residues that may be toxic or can modify the polymer surface. In addition, some polymers, such as PET, can trap certain fluids or ions into the molecular chain. These can leach out over time, with a microtoxic effect [19]. Chemical cleaning, such as scouring, can also damage the polymer if improperly controlled [20].

Various coatings have been proposed for vascular graft textiles. These coatings have three purposes: (1) to reduce the porosity, thus minimizing bleeding, (2) to promote tissue ingrowth, and (3) to improve blood and/or tissue compatibility. Commercially available grafts impregnated with crosslinked albumin or collagen have been extensively investigated and widely used. In a sense, the use of autologous blood (preclotting of vascular grafts during surgery) is also a coating technique. Silicone and both carbon- and plasma-deposited PTFE have been reported to improve the compatibility of vascular grafts.

TESTING

Yarn should be tested before fabrication. This includes not only identification of the polymer but any additives as well. In addition to the chemical characterization, the cross-sectional shape and dimension, number of filaments per yarn bundle, and any known lot numbers should be noted. The type of yarn processing, such as drawing, texturization, and number of twists per unit length should also be measured. The stitch pattern of the fabric and number of stitches per centimeter in both directions are also important.

One of the critical characteristics of a medical textile is its porosity. Three techniques have been used to characterize the porosity of these textiles: (1) physical dimensions, (2) air flow, and (3) water flow. Physical dimensions of pores are difficult to determine because of the flexibility of the structure and the pores. Air flow, characterized by pressure drop at fixed flow rates, was developed to characterize tight fabrics. This test is difficult to perform

Table 5-1   Typical Properties for Textile Vascular Prostheses

Structure type	Porosity $(cc/cm^2\text{-min})$	Radial Strength $(N/m \times 10^4)$	Handling
Woven	50–3800	2.8–3.5*	Difficult to suture* Little conformability*
Knit (weft)	1300–4000	0.7–1.5	Moderate to easy to suture; excellent conformability
Velour (warp)	1300–1800	0.7–1.8	Moderate to good suturability; good conformability
Typical artery	0	0.2–0.3	Excellent suturability and conformability when healthy

*For wovens with porosities of 50 to 200 cc/cm^2-min. Higher porosities have properties closer to those of knits.

on highly porous knit textiles such as those used in vascular grafts, but is frequently used for felts and tightly woven fabrics. Water porosity was developed [6, 7] as a more realistic test for grafts. Flow is measured at a fixed pressure (120 mm Hg) through a fixed area (1 cm^2). This measurement is related to the ease of tissue ingrowth through the wall of a healing vascular prosthesis but is not necessarily related to the difficulty expected in preclotting a graft. Preclotting efficiency can be modified by the fabrication and the wettability of the material. See Table 5-1 for typical values of porosity.

Multiple tests have been defined to measure strength of textiles. Uniaxial testing of dumbbell shapes is difficult, particularly if the structure frays easily. Uncut tubes and straight strips have been used and are preferable, particularly for applications requiring high uniaxial strengths. Uncut tubes can also be tested radially by using small pins inserted into the tube [21]. See Table 5-1 for typical values.

It is possible to pressurize tubes using liners provided that these liners are larger than the bursting diameter of the test sample. Relatively high pressures are required for woven tubes. Biaxial testing of flat samples is typically done with some variation of the Mullen burst test [22]. A sample is clamped between two rings and pressurized through a diaphragm. In addition to these tests, certain specialized strength tests, such as suture pullout tests, have been suggested.

There are currently no standard fatigue tests for medical textiles. Tests should simulate in-use conditions where possible. Cyclic pressurization of vascular prostheses using nonporous liners has been described [10]. Cyclic bending tests, designed to simulate grafts across flexion creases, have also been described. Cyclic tensile tests for ligament applications are recommended. All tests should be performed in fluids at body temperature.

Many textile tests, particularly for yarn characterization and fabric strength, have been standardized by the American Society for Testing and Materials (ASTM) [22]. These tests include methods for measuring of yarn properties such as tenacity, knot strength, and diameter; methods for measuring knit, woven and nonwoven fabrics such as air permeability, tenacity and elongation, stiffness, and seam strength; and methods for describing various types of test equipment. A standard also exists that describes further the specialized testing for vascular grafts [23]. At the time of this writing, standards for other medical products do not specifically address textiles.

It is important that the surface of the processed (as sterilized) polymer be thoroughly investigated. Particulate matter, stains, and low-molecular-weight polymer species could be present on the surface. These can be investigated using simple extraction techniques or SEM, IR, ESCA, and other instruments. These techniques are discussed in greater detail in Section 2. Physical damage to the filaments such as cracks, surface pits, and permanent deformation can be determined using microscopic techniques. Changes in crystalline content and molecular weight distribution, as well as basic polymer modification, may affect fatigue life and biological reactivity.

In addition to the standard toxicity and biocompatibility testing described in Sections III–VI, animal studies designed to simulate actual use should be performed. Vascular grafts have been implanted in a number of animals, with the canine and porcine preparations being the most common. Grafts designed for the aorta or its bifurcation can be studied experimentally as thoracoabdominal aortic bypasses, while small-diameter grafts can be studied as ilio-femoral or carotid bypasses or interpositional grafts. The calf model has been recommended for the study of heart valves. Ligaments can be studied in baboons and goats. For more details on implantology and postimplantation evaluation, see Sections VI, VII and VIII.

REFERENCES

1   Backer S. An engineering approach to textile structures. In Hearle JWS, Grosberg P, Backer S (Eds.), *Structural Mechanics of Fibers, Yarns, and Fabrics*. New York: Wiley; 1969.

2   Vorhees AB, Jaretski A, Blakemore AH. The use of tubes constructed from Vinyon-N cloth. I. Bridging arterial defects. *Ann Surg* 135 (1952), 332–336.

3   Deterling RA, Bhonslay SB. An evaluation of synthetic materials and fabrics suitable for blood vessel replacement. *Surgery*, 38 (1955), 71–89.

4   Edwards WS, Tapp JS. Chemically treated nylon tubes as arterial grafts. *Surgery*, 38 (1955), 61–70.

5   Harrison JH. Synthetic materials as vascular prostheses. *Am Jour Surg*, 95 (1958), 3–24.

6   Wesolowski SA, Fries CC, Karlson KE, DeBakey ME, Sawyer, PN. Porosity: Primary determinant of ultimate fate of synthetic vascular grafts. *Surgery*, 50 (1961), 91–96, 105–106.

7   Wesolowski SA. Evaluation of Tissue and Prosthetic Vascular Grafts. Springfield, IL: Charles C. Thomas, 1962.

8   Weslow A. Biologic behavior of tissue and prosthetic grafts. In Haimovici H (Ed.), *Vascular Surgery, Principles and Techniques*, 2nd ed. Norwalk, Appleton-Century-Crofts, 1984, 93–118.

9   King MW, Marois Y, Guidoin R, Ukpabi P, Deng X, Martin L, Paris E, Douville Y. Evaluating the Dialine® vascular prosthesis knitted from an alternative source of polyester yarns. *J Biomed Mater Res*, 29 (1995), 595–610.

10 Botzko K, Snyder R, Larkin J, Edwards WS. In vivo/in vitro life testing of vascular prostheses. In *Corrosion and Degradation of Implant Materials*, ASTM Special Publication 684. Philadelphia, PA: American Society for Testing and Materials, 1979, 76–88.

11 King MW, Zhang Z, Ukpab1 P, Murphy D, Guidoin R. Quantitative analysis of the surface morphology and textile structure of the polyurethane Vascugraft® arterial prosthesis using image and statistical analyses. *Biomaterials*, 15 (1994), 621–627.

12 Greisler HP. *New Biologic and Synthetic Vascular Prostheses*. Austin, TX: R.G. Landes Co., 1991.

13 Mallon WJ, Joyner WH, Seaber AV, Urbaniak JR. Vascular response to absorbable sutures in immature arteries. *Surg Forum*, 35 (1984), 527–529.

14 Cooperative retrieval program of explanted prostheses. Mechanisms of failure for anterior cruciate ligament prostheses implanted in humans. A retrospective analysis of 79 surgically excised explants. *Polymers and Polymer Composites*, 3 (1995), 79–97.

15 Weslowoski SA, Fries CC, Domingo RT, Fox LM, Sawyer PN. Fate of simple and compound arterial prostheses: Experimental and human observations. In Wesolowski SA, Dennis MD (Eds.), *Fundamentals of Vascular Grafting*, New York: McGraw-Hill, 1963.

16 Berger K, Sauvage LR, Rao AO, Wood SJ. Healing of arterial prostheses in man: Its incompleteness. *Ann Surg* 175 (1972), 118–127.

17 Laroche G, Marois Y, Guidoin R, King MW, Martin L, How T, Douville Y. Polyvinylidene fluoride (PVDF) as a biomaterial: From polymeric raw material to monofilament vascular suture. *J Biomed Mater Res*, 29 (1995), 1525–1536.

18 Sauvage LR, Berger K, Nakagawa Y, Mansfield PB. An external velour surface for porous arterial prostheses. *Surgery*, 70 (1971), 940–953.

19 Sawyer PN, Stanczewski B, Hoskin GP, Sophie Z, Stillman RM, Turner RJ, Hoffman HL, Jr. In vitro and in vivo evaluation of Dacron® velour and knit prostheses. *J Biomed Mater Res*, 13 (1979), 937–956.

20 Phaneuf MD, Quist WC, Bide MJ, LoGerfo FW. Modification of polyethylene terephthalate (Dacron®) via denier reduction: Effects on material tensile strength, weight, and protein binding capabilities. *J Appl Biomat*, 6 (1995), 289–299.

21 Snyder RW. Fabrication and testing of textile vascular prostheses. In Wright CB, Hobson RW, Hiratzka LF, Lynch TG (Eds.), *Vascular Grafting: Clinical Applications and Techniques*. Boston, MA: John Wright-PSG Inc., 1978, 12–22.

22 *Textiles—Yarns, Fabrics, General Test Methods*. American Society for Testing and Materials, Annual Book of Standards, 1984, Section 7.

23 *Standard for Vascular Graft Prostheses*, Association for the Advancement of Med Inst, ANSI/AAMI VP20-1994, August 1994.

Chapter 6

Absorbable Materials and Pertinent Devices

Karen J. L. Burg
Shalaby W. Shalaby

INTRODUCTION

Absorbable or biodegradable polymers have been used clinically for sutures and allied surgical augmentation devices to eliminate the need for a second surgery to remove functionally equivalent nonabsorbable devices [1, 2]. Although most of these devices were designed for repairing soft tissues, interest in using such transient devices, with or without biologically active components, in dental and orthopedic applications has grown significantly over the past few years [1, 3–9]. In addition, development of high performance microcomposites of high lactide/high glycolide copolymers to produce unique, absorbable surgical staples has been cited in the patent literature [10]. Due to the importance of surgical sutures, not only absorbable but also nonabsorbable types of sutures are addressed in this chapter.

TYPES OF ABSORBABLE POLYMERS AND THEIR COMPOSITES

Absorbable polymers have been the subject of a recent book [11], highlights of which are provided in this chapter. The most common types of absorbable polymers are polyesters that are made primarily of one or more of the following monomers: lactide, glycolide, e-caprolactone, p-dioxanone and trimethylene carbonate. Generally, degradation proceeds by hydrolytic scission of ester bonds in the polymer chain, releasing small chemical moieties as degradation products. Polyanhydrides have been explored primarily as matrices for controlled drug delivery. Other absorbable polymers have been investigated as candidates for biomedical devices and pharmaceutical formulations and include polyalkylene oxalates, polyester-amides, amino-acid-derived polymers, poly-2-hydroxyalkanoates (produced by fermentation) and biosynthetic polysaccharides.

APPLICATION OF ABSORBABLE AND RELATED NONABSORBABLE MATERIALS

Sutures and Other Wound Closure Devices

Sutures can be in two forms—monofilaments and twisted or braided multifilaments. They are utilized in incision closure, thereby reducing fluid loss, infection, and scarring while promoting rapid healing. Sutures fall into two categories, absorbable and nonabsorbable, examples of which are detailed in Tables 6-1 and 6-2. Generally, the absorbable sutures are used for shorter-term, internal closures while the nonabsorbables are used for longer-term, internal closures and accessible skin wounds. The suture specifications depend on the

Table 6-1 Properties of Absorbable Sutures

Class (chemical name)	Composition	Commercial name	Type	Break strength straight pull (MPa)	Break strength knot pull (MPa)	Elongation to break (%)	Young's modulus (GPa)	References
Polyesters								
Poly(p-dioxanone)	$[-O(CH_2)_2OCH_2CO-]$	PDS®	M	450–560	240–340	30–38	1.2–1.7	[57], [58]
Poly(glycolic acid)	$[-OCH_2CO_2CH_2CO-]$	Dexon®*	B	760–920	310–590	18–25	7–14	[59], [60], [61], [62], [63], [64]
Poly(glycolide-co-lactide)	$[OCH_2CO_2CH_2CO-]_{90}[OCH(CH_3)CO_2CH(CH_3)-CO]_{10}$	Vicryl®	B	570–910	300–400	18–25	7–14	[57], [65], [60]
Segmented glycolide trimethylene carbonate copolymer	$[-OCH_2CO-]_{67}[OCH_2CH_2CH_2OCO-]_{33}$	Maxon™	M	540–610	280–480	26–38	3.0–3.4	[66]
Segmented glycolide e-caprolactone copolymer	$[-OCH_2CO-]_{75}[-(CH_2)_5COO-]_{25}$	Monocryl®	M	628	315	39	0.8	[67]
Proteins								
Catgut (dry)	Protein		Tw	310–380	110–210	15–35	2.4	[57], [68], [63]
Regenerated collagen			M	<310	<110	15–35	<2.4	

*Monofilaments in fine sizes only.

Table 6-2 Properties of Nonabsorbable Sutures

Class (chemical name)	Composition	Commercial name	Type	Break strength straight pull (MPa)	Break strength knot pull (MPa)	Elongation to break (%)	Young's Modulus (GPa)	References
Cellulosics								
Cotton	Cellulose	Cotton	Tw	280–390	160–320	3–6	5.6–10.9	[59], [61], [62], [69]
Linen	Cellulose (Flax)	Linen	Tw					
Metals								
Stainless steel, 316L	17% Cr, 12% Ni, 2.5% Mo, 0.03% C, Bal. Fe	Flexon®	Tw	540–780	420–710	29–65	200	[59], [62], [64]
		Stainless Steel	M					
		Surgical Stainless Steel	M, Tw					
Polyamides								
Nylon 66	[—NH(CH$_2$)$_6$NHCO(CH$_2$)$_4$CO—]	Surgilon®	B	460–710	300–330	17–65	1.8–4.5	[66], [59], [60], [61], [62], [63], [64], [70], [69], [71]
		Dermalon®	M					
		Nurolon®	B					
Nylon 6	[—NH(CH$_2$)$_5$CO—]	Ethilon®	M					
		Supramid	S/C					
Polyesters								
Poly(butylene terephthalate)	[—O(CH$_2$)$_4$OCOC$_6$H$_4$CO—]	Miralene®	M	490–550	280–400	19–22	3.6–3.7	[71]
Poly(ethylene terephthalate)	[—O(CH$_2$)$_2$OCOC$_6$H$_4$CO—]	Dacron®	B	510–1060	300–390	8–42	1.2–6.5	[59], [60], [61], [62], [63], [64], [69]
		Ti.Cron®	B					
		Ethibond®*	B					
		Mersilene®	B					
		Ethiflex®	B					
		Polydek®	B					
		Tevdek®	B					
		Mirafil®	M					

Table 6-2 *Continued*

Class (chemical name)	Composition	Commercial name	Type	Break strength straight pull (MPa)	Break strength knot pull (MPa)	Elongation to break (%)	Young's Modulus (GPa)	References
Poly [Poly(tetramethylene ether)terephthalate-co-Tetramethylene Terephthalate]	$[-(OCH_2CH_2CH_2CH_2)_n$ $-OCO-C_6H_4CO]_{16}$ $[OCH_2CH_2CH_2CH_2$ $-OCOC_6H_4-CO]_{84}$	Novafil®	M	480–550	290–370	29–38	1.9–2.1	[58], [71]
Polyolefins								
Polypropylene	$[—CH_2CH(CH_3)—]$	Surgilene®	M	410–460	280–320	24–62	2.2–6.9	[66], [60], [61], [62], [63], [64], [71], [70], [72], [69]
		Prolene®	M					
		Polypro®	M					
Proteins								
Silk	Protein	Silk	B					[60], [61], [62], [63], [64], [69]
		Surgical Silk	B	370–570	240–290	9–31	8.4–12.9	
		Dermal®	Tw					
		Virgin Silk	Tw					

*Monofilaments in fine sizes only. Tw, twisted; M, monofilament; B, braided; S/C, sheathed or coated core.

tissue, implant location, size of wound, expected healing time, expected mechanical loads, and required suture configuration; therefore, there exist a series of mechanical tests with which to characterize the material. These include [12]: tensile testing to determine the modulus of elasticity, yield strength, yield elongation, ultimate elongation and breaking strength. In addition, knot tensile strength, knot security, and retention of required mechanical properties over the appropriate time period are assessed. The specific tests are detailed in the United States Pharmacopeia [13] as well as in the American Society for Testing and Materials (ASTM) standards (Specifications D3822, D4268).

Staples are alternate closure devices. They can be useful in closing larger surgical incisions, since the staples may be applied much faster than the sutures and provide equal resistance to infection. They are limited to locations which are not subject to large tensile loads and which do not have thicker or more sensitive tissue such as scar tissue or tissues with underlying bone, nerves, or vessels. Staples were originally developed in metallic materials [4], but now are being developed as absorbable devices [5, 6]. Tests employed to characterize staple functionality include progressive measurements of inflammatory response [16] as well as wound separation strength [15, 16].

Tissue adhesives are another application of absorbable materials to wound closure. The absorbable sutures and staples are ideal in tissues with moderate to high mechanical integrity; however, soft tissues such as liver, lung, and spleen are extremely difficult to repair with such devices. The tissue adhesives are considered more suitable for such applications; the butyl cyanoacrylates and fibrin-based glues have demonstrated sufficient strength and elasticity to be used in fragile tissue repair [7]. The fibrin-based glues, however, are not clinically approved in the United States and, although the butyl cyanoacrylates are readily available, they do not absorb in the body and therefore are potentially problematic. Ideally, the adhesive should be capable of rapid polymerization in a wet environment with minimal heat release, easy to apply, readily sterilizable, absorbable, and should not interfere with the normal healing process. A common test of tissue adhesive mechanical function is a tensile test to determine the adhesive strength of incised skin [17].

In a recent disclosure [7], a new composition of a cyanoacrylate tissue adhesive was described to consist of a water-miscible mixture of methoxypropyl cyanoacrylate. This composition polymerizes at a slower rate than the commonly known butyl cyanoacrylates upon contacting soft tissue, and the resulting polymers absorb in about one year. When used on soft tissues, the polymer forms a compliant film as compared to the hard crust known to form with the butyl cyanoacrylate polymer. Since the most important use of cyanoacrylates is in soft tissues, the latter property may be a distinct advantage of this new composition.

Cardiovascular Applications

Synthetic vascular grafts made of polyethylene terephthalate (Dacron®; E. I. duPont de Nemours and Co.) fabrics and expanded polytetrafluoroethylene (Teflon®; E. I. duPont de Nemours and Co.) have had great clinical success. However, device-induced infections which are associated with nonabsorbable implants including grafts evoked the need for developing fully or partially absorbable analogs, particularly those of PET. Thus, several attempts have been made to use absorbable textile constructions in the development of these grafts [9–22]. Such attempts entailed the use of poly-p-dioxanone, 10/90 poly-l-lactide-co-glycolide and polyglycolide fibers with or without PET fibers. However, to date, the success of these devices has been limited due to the relatively fast deterioration of the fabric mechanical properties before sufficient healing or regeneration of the biological tissues can occur.

Orthopedic Applications

Absorbable orthopedic applications include pins, plates, anchors, screws, and rods [10, 11, 12]. The pins are currently on the market, the plates and anchors are in clinical use, the screws are in trial stages, and the rods are still under development. The bioabsorbable polymers have found limited successful use in long bone fracture repair, as they have relatively low strength and stiffness. Attempts to remedy this problem include self-reinforcement, molecular orientation, and synthesis of new bioabsorbable materials.

A recent development is that of the absorbable suture anchor, traditionally a metallic device. This device consists of an anchor and suture; the anchor is embedded in the bone and the suture can then be utilized to reattach soft tissue to the bone [13, 15]. The important mechanical considerations for this device are the pushout, pullout, torsional, and suture strengths, as well as the retention of these properties over time.

Tissue Engineering

Most recently, absorbable materials have been incorporated into the growing field of tissue engineering as foams and scaffolds designed to support tissue growth. The absorbable material is used as a substrate upon which cells are seeded and cultured in vitro. Once the cells are suitably attached, the cell-polymer construct is implanted in vivo. The substrate may be shaped to best adapt to the target in vivo location; then, as the tissue forms and the absorbable material disappears, the newly formed tissue adopts the shape determined by the substrate. The selective use of parenchymal cells minimizes the amount of donor tissue required and, rather than implanting a large volume of avascular tissue which may not survive, the revascularization process occurs simultaneously with the tissue growth and material bioabsorption. The processing of an absorbable material allows a reproducible end product, and the use of tissue engineering concepts may eliminate both the cost and the risk of donor and recipient surgeries. Important processing factors include the spatial distribution of construct fibers, the dimensions of the implant, the wettability of the construct surface, the concentration of cells on the matrix, and the viscosity of the cell-bearing solution. Absorbable materials which have found use in tissue engineering include the synthetic polyesters, polyanhydrides, polyorthoesters, and polyetheresters, as well as the natural proteins and polysaccharides. Potential application sites include epidermis, dermis, ligament, tendon, bone, urothelium, vasculature, cartilage, nerve, liver, pancreas, cornea, trachea, esophagus, kidney, intestine, and heart [27–30].

MECHANISMS OF DEGRADATION AND SAFETY OF ABSORBABLE SYSTEMS

The degradation of absorbable polymers depends on many factors, among which are crystallinity, chain mobility, degradative medium, molecular orientation, weight-to-surface-area ratio, chemical composition, shape, molecular weight, molecular weight distribution, hydrophilicity/hydrophobicity, impurities, porosity, surface texture, and mass. Because the absorption process of synthetic biodegradable polymers is complex, it has motivated the development of several absorption models [31]. Degradability depends fundamentally on the presence of scissionable bonds in the polymer chain. As the material hydrolytically degrades, there are changes in the characteristics of the system, e.g., strength, viscosity, mass, overall molecular weight, and molecular weight distribution, until the polymer is solubilized directly or phagocytosed and solubilized. The internal structure of the polymer, its accessibility to the aqueous environment, and the transport of degradation products to the surrounding aqueous environment are key factors affecting the polymeric absorption profile.

It has been proposed [32–35] that "surface-center" differences may be an important factor in the degradation of aliphatic polyesters, inferring that the surface will degrade faster than the center initially, due to the early exposure to water. Once the water penetrates the internal structure of the implant and degradation products collect, the high concentration of carboxylic end groups lowers the pH and catalyzes the reaction further. In some cases a morphologically dissimilar outer layer of polymer forms an envelope or a crust, which appears to obstruct the escape of small internal degradation products to the surface. It is this delayed degradation phenomenon that is a safety concern, especially with the polyester biomaterials. During the early degradation stages, when the mass loss is minimal, there is generally minimal tissue reaction around the material. It is at a much later time, particularly with regard to the polylactide systems, that the exterior of the implant is finally breached and the interior pool of degraded, acidic material is released in high concentration into the surrounding environment. This is potentially detrimental to the local tissue and can result in swelling and sinus formation.

New materials have been specifically developed to exploit their aversion to water. The poly(orthoesters) (POE), for example, are a hydrophobic group which tend to erode by surface hydrolysis and thereby yield a more gradual degradation profile [36]. These materials, so far, have been determined to be nontoxic and may have great potential for biomedical use. They are, however, currently limited to low-load-bearing applications because of their low moduli and strength. The tyrosine-derived polycarbonates are a group of relatively hydrophobic polymers that have mechanical values comparable to the lactide systems and which, in preliminary investigations, exhibit favorable behavior in vivo [37]. The length of the alkyl ester pendent chain may be adjusted to vary the physicochemical and mechanical properties of the material to best suit the intended application. Hydrophobic anhydride copolymers also degrade in a manner characteristic of surface erosion. A variation of the relative amounts of monomeric precursors in this system will affect both the erosion duration and the crystallinity of the resultant copolymer [38]. The anhydrides were originally developed for drug delivery applications and as such have acquired Food and Drug Administration regulatory approval for use in clinical trials.

IN VITRO AND IN VIVO EVALUATION OF TYPICAL ABSORBABLE SYSTEMS

Although it is imperative to evaluate biomaterials in their final, functional form, preliminary assessment of basic material parameters and properties of intermediate forms can be equally significant. The basic testing of a biomaterial can pertain to its (a) chemical composition, and (b) inherent physical properties and (c) interaction with the biologic environment. An outline of common techniques used for the characterization and preliminary evaluation of the chemical, physical, and biological properties of biomaterials follows.

Chemical Properties

The first data to be acquired for a biomaterial should deal with chemical composition. The chemical structure and concentration of most or perhaps all of the components constituting a biomaterial system can be determined by testing, including tests based on

Table 6-3   Methods for Studying Basic Physical Properties

Property	Test methods	ASTM specifications
Thermal transitions e.g., melting (T_m), glass transition (T_g), and crystallization (T_c) temperatures	Differential scanning calorimetry (DSC), hot-stage optical microscopy, and thermal mechanical analysis	D3417, E537, E698, E794, E928, E967, E1269, E1356
Thermal stability	Thermogravimetric analysis (TGA)	E914, E1131, E1582, E1641
Molecular weight and/or molecular weight distribution	Gel-permeation chromatography, scattering membrane osmometry and solution viscosity	D2857, D3536, D3593, D3750, D4001
Surface bulk morphology	Optical microscopy, scanning electron microscopy (SEM), transmission electron microscopy (TEM), X-ray diffraction and birefringence	E20, E175, E858
Surface properties	Surface tension measurement and friction coefficient	D1894, D3028
Tensile properties	Stress-strain behavior using tensile tester	E1142
Dynamic mechanical properties	Dynamic mechanical analysis (DMA) and cyclic fatigue testing	E1142, E1640

Source: Based on material from [12].

(a) elemental analysis, (b) infrared spectroscopy (IR and ATR), (c) nuclear magnetic resonance (NMR) spectroscopy, (d) UV-visible spectroscopy, (e) gas and liquid chromatography, (f) mass spectroscopy, (g) electron spectroscopy for chemical analysis (ESCA), and (h) Auger electron spectroscopy (AES). To supplement some of these analytical methods, it is often necessary to subject the biomaterial to extraction, hydrolysis, and/or selected chemical modification. Details of the techniques are summarized in Chapter 2 of this handbook and are covered more completely in a number of reviews [39–41].

Physical Properties

For basic properties including a material's thermal, morphological, surface, and mechanical characteristics, a number of established test methods are available. A list of these testing techniques is given in Table 6-3. Details of the techniques described can be found in Chapter 2 and elsewhere [42–49].

Biological Properties

Evaluation of the basic biological properties of biomaterials in raw or intermediate forms develops qualitative and some quantitative data reflecting their interactions with the biological environment. This may assist investigators by providing some level of predictability as to the performance of the final system during use. Assessment of the biological properties is based, for the most part, on a series of in vitro, in vivo, and ex vivo test procedures (Table 6-4) used for evaluating the toxicological effects of biomaterials on viable cells (see Section III) and the compatibility of biomaterials with blood. The stability of biomaterials and the retention of their initial properties are discussed extensively in the literature [50–55] The material type is chosen in order to best modulate the absorption profile and the loss of mechanical properties and thus accommodate the healing tissue.

Table 6-4   Methods for Evaluating the Basic Biological Properties

Evaluation type	Test methods
Toxicological	
In vitro procedures	Tissue culture procedures
	Hemolysis assay
	Inhibition of cell growth or modification of cellular characteristic (in part for assessing mutagenicity)
In vivo procedures	Intradermal irritation test
	Systemic toxicity test
	Intramuscular implant test
	Carcinogenicity
	Teratologic
Blood Compatibility	
In vitro procedures	Kinetic clotting test
	Lindholm test
	Elliptical cell system
	Protein adsorption and platelet adhesion (steady uptake of plasma proteins, time-varying uptake of plasma proteins, time-varying platelet adhesion)
	Platelet retention with microbeads
	Shear-induced hemolysis
Ex vivo procedures	Stagnation point flow system
	Arteriovenous shunt system
In vivo procedures	Vena cava ring test
	Renal embolus test system
Retention of mechanical properties	Periodic monitoring of mechanical properties of suitable forms of biomaterials explanted from subcutaneous or intramuscular sites or immersed in a suitable buffered medium.

Source: Based on material from [12].

Following appropriate periods of residence, tissue reaction and cellular response to implanted bioabsorbable materials can be determined by several techniques. A semi-quantitative but rather subjective measure can be obtained through microscopic assessment of properly embedded and stained sections using a histologic grading and scoring scheme [14]. A more quantitative method involves staining of specially prepared tissue sections from around the implant where the intensity of staining is related to the level of enzyme activity in the cells. The intensity of staining can then be assessed in terms of the absorption of the transmitted light in the microscope using optical densitometry. Enzyme activity evaluated in this manner can be used as a quantitative index of cellular response. Finally, the thickness or area of the cellular reaction zone around the implanted bioabsorbable material can serve as a crude measure of the extent of reaction (see Sections VII and VIII).

REFERENCES

1   Schmitt EE. Controlled release of medicaments using polymers from glycolic acid. U.S. Patent (to American Cyanamid) 3,991,766 (1976).
2   Shalaby SW. In Swarbrick J, Boylan JC (Eds.), *Encyclopedia of Pharmaceutical Technology*, Vol. 1. New York: Marcel Dekker, 1988.
3   Bezwada RS, Arnold SC, Shalaby SW, Williams, BL. Liquid absorbable copolymers for parenteral applications. European Patent (to Ethicon, Inc.) 305,273 (1994).

4 Bhatia S, Shalaby SW, Powers DL, Lancaster RL, Ferguson RL. The effect of site of implantation and animal age on properties of polydioxanone pins. *J Biomater Sci, Polym Ed,* 6 (1994), 435.

5 Dunn RL, Ottenbrite RM (Eds.). *Polymeric Drugs and Drug Delivery Systems,* Vol. 467. ACS Symposium Series. Washington, DC: American Chemical Society, 1994.

6 Dunn RL, English JP, Cowsar DR, Vanderbilt DP. Biodegradable *In situ*-forming implants and methods of producing the same. U.S. Patent 4,938,763 (1990).

7 Damani NC. Sustained release compositions for treating periodontal disease. U.S. Patent (to Proctor & Gamble, Co.) 5,198,220 (1993).

8 Shalaby SW, Koelmel DF, Arnold S. Polyglycosalicylate. U.S. Patent (to Ethicon, Inc.) 5,082,925 (1992).

9 Wasserman D, Shalaby SW, Bousma OJ. Improved dental inserts for treatment of periodontal disease. U.S. Patent (to Ethicon, Inc.) 5,191,148 (1992).

10 Jamiolkowski DD, Gaterud MT, Newman HD, Jr., Shalaby SW. Surgical fastener made of glycolide-rich polymer blends. U.S. Patent (to Ethicon, Inc.) 4,889,119 (1989).

11 Shalaby SW (Ed.) *Biomedical Polymers: Designed-to-Degrade Systems.* New York: Hanser Publishers, 1994.

12 Shalaby, SW. In Lewin M, Preston J (Eds.), *High Technology Fibers.* Part A. New York: Marcel Dekker, 1985, 87.

13 *The United States Pharmacopeia. National Formulary.* Rockville, MD: United States Pharmacopeial Convention, 1994, 1475–1477; 1835–1836.

14 Steichen FM, Ravitch MM. Mechanical sutures in surgery. *Br J Surg,* 60 (1973), 60:191.

15 Shall LM, Cawley PW. Soft tissue reconstruction in the shoulder. Comparison of suture anchors, absorbable staples, and absorbable tacks. *Amer J Sports Med,* 22 (1994), 715.

16 Zachmann GC, Foresman PA, Bill TJ, Bentrem DJ, Rodeheaver GT, Edlich RF. Evaluation of a new absorbable Lactomer® subcuticular staple. *J Appl Biomater,* 5 (1994), 221.

17 Park JB, Lakes RS. *Biomaterials: An Introduction.* New York: Plenum Press, 1992.

18 Linden Jr. C, Shalaby SW. Absorbable Tissue Adhesives. U.S. Patent (to U.S. Army) 5,350,798 (1994).

19 Greisler HP. Arterial regeneration over absorbable prostheses. *Arch Surg,* 117 (1982), 1425.

20 Lommen E, Gogolewski S, Pennings AJ, Wildevuur CRH, Nieuwenhuis P. Development of a neoartery induced by a biodegradable polymeric vascular prosthesis. *ASAIO Trans,* 24 (1983), 255.

21 Niu S, Kurumatani H, Satoh S, Kanda K, Oka T, Watanabe K. Small diameter vascular prostheses with incorporated bioabsorbable matrices. A preliminary study. *ASAIO J,* 39 (1993), M750.

22 Lei BVD, Wildevuur CRH, Dijk F, Blaauw EH, Molenaar I, Nieuwenhuis P. Sequential studies of arterial wall regeneration in microporous, compliant, biodegradable small-caliber vascular grafts in rats. *J Thorac Cardiovasc Surg,* 93 (1987), 695.

23 Daniels AU, Chang MKO, Andriano KP, Heller J. Mechanical properties of biodegradable polymers and composites proposed for internal fixation of bone. *J Appl Biomater,* 1 (1990), 57.

24 Zhang X, Goosen MFA. Biodegradable polymers for orthopedic applications. *J Mater Sci Rev Macromol Chem Phys,* C33 (1993), 81.

25 Tunc DC. Orientruded polylactide-based body-absorbable osteosynthesis devices: A short review. *J Biomater Sci Polymer Edn,* 7 (1995), 375.

26 Nazre A, Krebs S, Lin S. Testing of a resorbable soft tissue anchor (RSTS) device. *Trans 21st Ann Mtg Soc Biomater,* 18 (1995), 434.

27 Langer R, Vacanti JP. Tissue engineering. *Science,* 260 (1993), 920.

28 Cima LG, Langer R. Engineering human tissue. *Chem Eng Progr,* 89 (1993), 46.

29 Hubbell JA, Langer R. Tissue engineering. *Chem Eng News,* 1995, 42.

30 Burg KJL, Shalaby SW. In Salamone JC (Ed.), *The Polymeric Materials Encyclopedia. Synthesis, Properties and Applications.* Boca Raton, FL: CRC Press, 1996.

31 Kronenthal RL. In Kronenthal RL, User Z, Martin E (Eds.). *Biodegradable Polymers in Medicine and Surgery.* New York: Plenum Press, 1974, 119.

32 Li SM, Garreau H, Vert M. Structure-property relationships in the case of the degradation of massive aliphatic poly-(-hydroxy acids) in aqueous media, Part 1: Poly(DL-lactic acid). *J Mater Sci Mater Med,* 1 (1990), 123.

33 Li SM, Garreau H, Vert M. Structure-property relationships in the case of the degradation of massive poly(-hydroxy acids) in aqueous media, Part 2: Degradation of lactide-glycolide copolymers: PLA37.5GA25 and PLA75GA25. *J Mater Sci Mater Med,* 1 (1990), 131.

34 Li SM, Garreau H, Vert M. Structure-property relationships in the case of the degradation of massive poly(-hydroxy acids) in aqueous media, Part 3: Influence of the morphology of poly(l-lactic acid). *J Mater Sci Mater Med,* 1 (1990), 198.

35 Ali SAM, Doherty PJ, Williams DF. Mechanisms of polymer degradation in implantable devices. 2. Poly(DL-lactic acid). *J Biomed Mater Res*, 27 (1993), 1409.
36 Daniels AU, Andriano KP, Smutz WP, Chang MKO, Heller J. Evaluation of absorbable poly(ortho esters) for use in surgical implants. *J Appl Biomater*, 5 (1994), 51.
37 Ertel SI, Kohn J. Evaluation of a series of tyrosine-derived polycarbonates as degradable biomaterials. *J Biomed Mater Res*, 28 (1994), 919–930.
38 Shieh L, Tamada J, Chen I, Pang J, Domb A, Langer R. Erosion of a new family of biodegradable polyanhydrides. *J Biomed Mater Res*, 28 (1994), 1465.
39 Haslam J, Willis HA. *Identification and Analysis of Plastics*. New York: Van Nostrand, 1965.
40 Schwarz JCP. *Physical Methods in Organic Chemistry*. London: Holden-Day, 1964.
41 Ke B, ed. *Newer Methods of Polymer Characterization*. New York: Wiley-Interscience, 1964.
42 Moncrieff RW. *Man-Made Fibers*, 6th ed. New York: Wiley, 1975.
43 Van Krevelen DW. *Properties of Polymers: Correlation with Chemical Structure*. New York: Elsevier, 1972.
44 Carter ME. *Essential Fiber Chemistry*. New York: Marcel Dekker, 1971.
45 Turi EA (Ed.). *Thermal Characterization of Polymeric Materials*. New York: Academic Press, 1981.
46 Carroll B (Ed.). *Physical Methods in Macromolecular Chemistry*. New York: Marcel Dekker, 1971.
47 Nielsen LE. *Mechanical Properties of Polymers and Composites*, Vol. 1 and 2. New York: Marcel Dekker, 1974.
48 Shalaby SW. In Turi EA (Ed.), *Thermal Characterization of Polymeric Materials*. New York: Academic Press, 1981.
49 Shalaby SW, Bair HE. In Turi EA (Ed.), *Thermal Characterization of Polymeric Materials*. New York: Academic Press, 1981.
50 Bruck SD. *Properties of Biomaterials in the Physiological Environment*. Boca Raton, FL: CRC Press, 1980.
51 Black J. *Biological Performance of Biomaterials: Fundamentals and Biocompatibility*. New York: Marcel Dekker, 1981.
52 Hastings CW, Williams DF (Eds.). *Evaluation of Biomaterials*. New York: Wiley; 1980.
53 Hastings CW, Williams DF (Eds.). *Mechanical Properties of Biomaterials*. New York: Wiley, 1980.
54 Williams DF (Ed.). *Biocompatibility of Clinical Implants*. Volume 2. Boca Raton, FL: CRC Press, 1980.
55 Bruck SD. Identification of biodegradation products of medical implants in adjacent tissues: An overview and recommendations. *J Long-Term Effects Med Implants*, 1 (1992), 357.
56 Gourlay SL, Rice RM, Hegyeli AF, Wade ZWR, Dillon JA, Jasse H, Kulkarni RK. *J Biomed Res*, 12 (1978), 219.
57 Doddi N, Versfelt CC, Wasserman D. Synthetic absorbable surgical devices of polydioxanone. US Patent (to Ethicon, Inc.) 4,052,988 (1977).
58 Ray JA, Doddi N, Regula D, Williams JA, Melveger A. Polydioxanone (PDS), a novel monofilament synthetic absorbable suture. *Surg Gynecol Obstet*, 153 (1981), 497.
59 Holmond DEW. Knot properties of surgical suture materials. *Europ Surg Res*, 6 (1974), 65.
60 Chu CC. Mechanical properties of suture materials: An important characterization. *Ann Surg*, 193 (1981), 365.
61 Herrmann JB. Tensile strength and knot security of surgical suture materials. *Am Surg*, 37 (1971), 209.
62 Holmlund DEW. Physical properties of surgical suture materials: Stress-strain relationship, stress relaxation and irreversible elongation. *Ann Surg*, 184 (1976), 189.
63 Marchant LH, Knap S, Braun H, Apter JT. Effect of elongation rate on the percentage elongation of surgical suture materials. *Surg Gynecol Obstet*, 139 (1974), 389.
64 Tera H, Aberg C. Tensile strengths of twelve types of knot employed in surgery using different suture materials. *Acta Chir Scand*, 142 (1976), 1.
65 Craig PH, Williams JA, Davis KW, Magoun AD, Levy AJ, Bogdansky S, Jones JP, Jr. A biological comparison of polyglycolic acid synthetic absorbable sutures. *Surg Gynecol Obstet*, 141 (1975), 1.
66 Katz AR, Mukherjee DP, Kaganov AL, Gordon S. Glycolide trimethylene carbonate (GTMC) copolymer: A new synthetic monofilament absorbable suture. *Surg Gynecol Obstet*, 161 (1985), 213.
67 Bezwada RS, Jamiolkowski DD, Lee I-Y, Agarwal V, Persivale J, Trenka-Benthin S, Erneta M, Suryadevara J, Yang A, Liu S. Monocryl® suture, a new ultra-pliable absorbable monofilament suture. *Biomater*, 16 (1995), 1141.
68 Conn J, Jr., Beal JM. Coated Vicryl synthetic absorbable sutures. *Surg Gynecol Obstet*, 150 (1980), 843.
69 Billmeyer FW, Jr. *Textbook of Polymer Science*, 3rd ed. New York: Wiley; 1984, 502.
70 Kaplan DS. Surgical sutures derived from segmented polyether-ester block copolymers. U.S. Patents (to American Cyanamid) 4,224,946 (1980), 4,246,904 (1981), 4,314,516 (1982).

71 *Proceedings of a Symposium on NOVAFIL Polybutester Suture*. Wayne, NJ: American Cyanamid, 1984.

72 Listner GJ. Polypropylene monofilament sutures. U.S. Patent (to Ethicon, Inc.), 3,630,205 (1971).

ADDITIONAL READING

1 Bronzino JD (Ed.). *The Biomedical Engineering Handbook*. Boca Raton, FL: CRC Press, 1995.

2 Dumitriu S (Ed.). *Polymeric Biomaterials*. New York: Marcel Dekker, 1994.

3 Göpferich A. Mechanisms of polymer degradation and erosion. *Biomat*, 17 (1996), 103.

4 Planck H, Dauner M, Renardy M (Eds.). *Degradation Phenomena on Polymeric Biomaterials*. Berlin: Springer-Verlag, 1992.

5 Shalaby SW, Hoffman AS, Ratner BD, Horbett TA (Eds.). *Polymers as Biomaterials*. New York: Plenum Press, 1984.

6 Shalaby SW, Ikada Y, Langer R, Williams J (Eds.). *Polymers of Biological and Biomedical Significance*. ACS Symposium Series, Vol. 520. Washington, DC: American Chemical Society, 1993.

7 Vert M, Feijen J, Albertson A, Scott G, Chiellini E (Eds.). Degradable Polymers and Plastics. Melksham: Redwood Press Ltd., 1992.

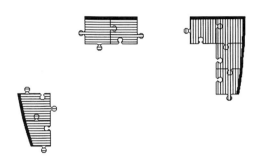
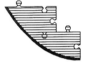
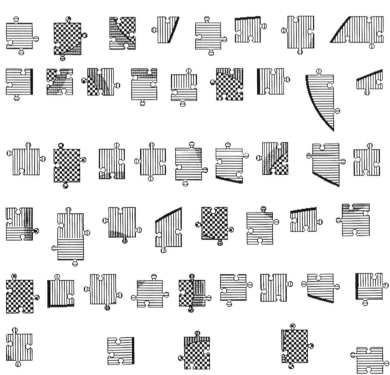

Section Two

Surface Characterization

Martine LaBerge

INTRODUCTION

The biomaterials literature has experienced an impressive burst of scientific publications in recent years that address biomaterial interactions with their biological host settings. More specifically, extensive studies have focused on the effect of the surface properties of materials and devices on cell and tissue responses. Initially, the performance of a medical device was primarily related to its design, material selection, and bulk material properties. It is now recognized that surface attributes, such as chemistry and topography, strongly dictate and influence the biological reactions to implants. On the other hand, the performance of a device can be greatly modified following a degradation of its surface, either chemical or mechanical, by the environment of the body and its selected sterilization process. The awareness of the materials community of the interactions between biomaterials surfaces and their hosts has been a driving force toward the establishment of experimental protocols aimed at fully understanding the effect of surface attributes on the performance and compatibility of biomaterials, and the effect of the environment on surface degradation. Surface degradation or change may occur due to chemical and mechanical processes such as corrosion, leaching, and mechanical wear, or be triggered by the selection of inappropriate sterilization processes such as oxidation and cross-linking of certain polymers by gamma irradiation. A thorough assessment of the pre-implantation surface properties of materials is an intrinsic part of the design process of implants. Besides fabrication processes, pre-implantation conditions include cleaning, handling, packaging, sterilization, storage, and any other procedures that an implant surface might encounter. Without this knowledge, implant designers cannot perform an accurate interpretation of failure or performance of implants.

Section II covers practical issues related to the evaluation and characterization of biomaterials surfaces. State-of-the art methodologies and standards available for the assessment of the chemical and physical properties of surfaces are described with an emphasis on their appropriate use and their limitations, as well as for the selection of reference materials introduced as an intrinsic part of a surface characterization protocol.

The following chapters are extremely valuable guides for planning experiments and selecting the most relevant techniques for surface characterization. Authors have discussed the most recent innovations in the field of surface science and engineering to help investigators answer their research goals and interpret their results. Topics of this section cover the applicability of techniques for chemical and physical surface analyses of materials such as surface infrared techniques, secondary ion mass spectroscopy, Auger electron microscopy, X-ray analysis, electron spectroscopy, atomic force microscopy, topography, contact angle measurement, surface charge analysis, and electron microscopy, among others. Protocols and new experimental techniques used to evaluate the surface degradation of metals and polymers due to the chemical and mechanical conditions in the body, such as corrosion and wear, are also discussed. A consequence of surface degradation is the production of particles or particulate matter that can trigger adverse body reactions. As discussed in this section, a thorough study and analysis of this particulate matter, including the understanding of its genesis, and the characterization of its physical and chemical attributes, is an important step toward evaluating and predicting implant performance.

Upon failure or inappropriate performance of implants and their surfaces, surface modification may be used to improve the biocompatibilty and biofunctionality of implants. Chemical treatments, surface alloying, molecular grafting, and self-assembling systems are popular design tools for the surface modification of polymers. Orthopaedic bearing surfaces can be used as an example of the relevance of surface modification in implant design. Aimed at enhancing their surface hardness, the surface modification of metallic components, most commonly utilizing plasma vapor deposition (PVD), ion implantation, and atmospheric controlled surface treatment, has been successful in reducing the wear rate of the components' surface wear on a short-term basis. Also, the surface modification of polyurethanes through the covalent incorporation of surface active side chains and the addition of oligomeric components is performed to improve their blood compatibility.

This section provides an understanding of the principles of surface characterization for a reader without relevant expertise in the field, and recommendations and suggestions for knowledgeable readers through a thorough review of new facts in this field.

Chapter 7

Biomaterial Surface Analysis

David W. Grainger
Kevin E. Healy

Widespread recognition that the surface of a biomaterial, employed either in a medical device or an assay, is a critical determinant of the biological response to the material has led to the use of an array of surface analytical methods aimed at biomaterials surface characterization. In addition, surface characterization can be an important component of the fabrication protocol, design process, and performance evaluation of materials and devices used in any industry that involves macromolecular or cell contact with synthetic materials. Elucidating specific surface properties of a material is important for a number of reasons. First, material surfaces interact with macromolecules (e.g., proteins, lipids, oligosaccharides) and cells in ways that influence subsequent biological responses. Secondly, because of interfacial thermodynamics, surface chemistry is distinct from that of its bulk material. Surfaces actively minimize their energy through continual processes of adsorption, restructuring, and chemical reactions, leading to a dynamic surface evolution through an array of physical and chemical features. Surfaces are challenging to understand fully because they change with their environment and are readily contaminated. Last is the issue of sensitivity: surfaces comprise a small fraction of a given material, limiting the amount of material interrogated by surface analytical methods. If a "typical" surface density is 10^{14} atoms cm^{-2} ($\sim$0.2 nmol cm^{-2}), then surface analytical methods must be able to resolve this relatively minute amount of material from signals emanating from the bulk material.

This chapter presents a concise introduction to the numerous strategies used to examine a material's surface as comprehensively as possible. It is beyond the scope of this chapter to provide even a fraction of the specific details for various methods: entire books and reviews are available to guide one further [1–10]. A wide range of surface-sensitive techniques are available to study the performance of materials and aid in problem-solving associated with devices fabricated from these materials. For example, polymeric, ceramic, and metallic components of devices can be characterized in terms of their surface chemistry or elemental composition with X-ray photoelectron spectroscopy (XPS or ESCA), Auger electron spectroscopy (AES), static and dynamic secondary ion mass spectrometry (SIMS), and attenuated total reflectance Fourier transform infrared spectroscopy (ATR-FTIR). Scanning force microscopy techniques such as atomic force microscopy (AFM) can be used to characterize the three-dimensional topography of a surface. Ellipsometry can give accurate information regarding the thickness of overlayers on reflective materials such as metal oxides. Figure 7-1 shows a flowchart outlining the various surface analytical methods currently available to the biomaterials researcher. While every technique is not commonly available at a single location, specialized surface analytical centers exist at industrial sites such as Physical Electonics, 3M, Kodak, Xerox, IBM, DuPont, Abbott Laboratories, Intel, Texas Instruments, ICI, Motorola, and Chevron; at academic institutions such as the University of Washington's NESAC/Bio, University of Lund, University of Toronto, SUNY Buffalo, University of Pittsburgh, University of Minnesota, and University of Münster; at

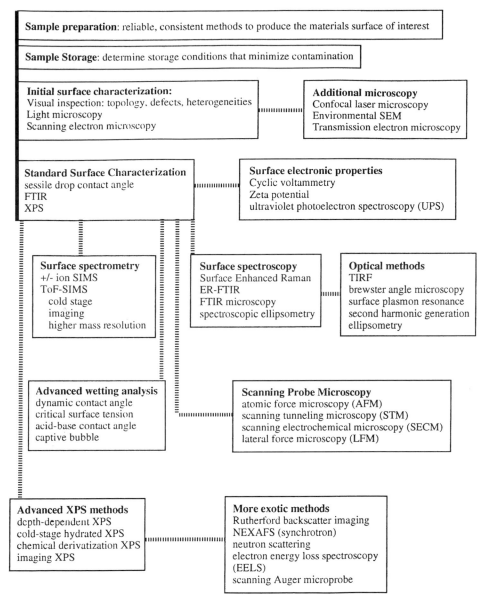

Figure 7-1 Flowchart of the various analytical methods currently available to the biomedical researcher and their respective analytical features.

government resources such as NIST, Brookhaven, and CSIRO; and at for-profit commercial analytical companies such as Charles Evans and Surface Science Labs that collectively contain most methods detailed in Figure 7-1. The flowchart begins with relatively common and inexpensive surface analytical methods and works down to more exotic, specialized, and expensive techniques that are not often readily available. To understand how one selects certain techniques and the order of progression from one technique to the next requires an appreciation of the surface physical chemistry of the material, knowledge of a specific question that could be addressed by surface analysis, and some idea of what level of resolution at which the surface should be examined. For example, characterization of surface modifications to improve device performance and identification of either contaminants or adsorbates require the use of surface analytical equipment capable of detecting changes in chemistry and elemental composition at the nanometer level (i.e., 10 Å), while a general, comparative approximation between materials might require only a few inexpensive routine analyses of lower surface resolution and informational content.

ASSESSING THE NEED FOR SURFACE ANALYSIS

A preliminary analytical approach is useful for all potential biomaterials surface characterization. A significant amount of effort (and money) can be spared by making a few careful choices from the beginning of any analysis. The decision of when to employ these techniques depends on the type of information desired and the depth into the material surface at which the information should be collected. It is rare that a single technique will provide adequate information for complete surface characterization of a material. Often, characterization of a material's surface requires the use of multiple techniques to generate a complete picture of the surface chemistry and structure.

What Is the Surface of Interest?

Table 7-1 shows that each surface analytical method considers the surface zone differently. This is shown schematically in Figure 7-2. Specifically, the depth of interrogation and the

Table 7-1 Surface Analytical Techniques Commonly Used for Biomaterials Characterization

Technique	Physical principle	Measured quantity	Depth of analysis	Analytical sensitivity
XPS (ESCA)	Photoelectron Effect: incident X-rays cause emission of electrons	Kinetic energy (or binding energy) of emitted core-level electrons	10–100 Å	0.1 at%
AES	Incident electrons cause emission of Auger electrons	Kinetic energy of Auger electrons	5–50 Å	0.1 at%
SIMS	Incident ions emit secondary ions of different mass	Mass/charge ratio of emitted ions	10 Å–1 μm	0.001 amu
ATR-FTIR	IR radiation is absorbed by molecules leading to unique vibrations of interatomic bonds	Absorbance as function of wave number	1–5 μm	1 mol %
AFM	Surface topography induced deflection of a cantilever is detected by reflected laser light and a photodiode	Quantitative three-dimensional images and surface physical properties	Depth or lateral resolution:1 Å	Atoms and molecules
Ellipsometry	Detects polarization change of coherent light reflected from a surface	Measures D and y that are then used to calculate overlayer thickness and surface coverage, adsorption kinetics, optical properties	Å to μm	2 Å pmol cm^{-2}

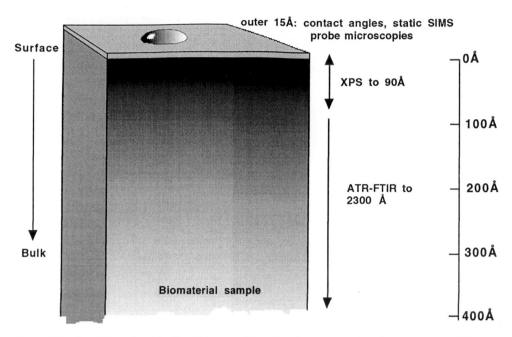

outer 15Å: contact angles, static SIMS
probe microscopies

Surface

XPS to 90Å

ATR-FTIR to
2300 Å

Bulk

Biomaterial sample

0Å

100Å

200Å

300Å

400Å

Figure 7-2   Depiction of an idealized biomaterial surface in cross section, demonstrating different analytical zones accessed by different surface analytical techniques.

type of analytical information returned must be considered when selecting given methods. The surface region for an ATR-FTIR experiment (up to ~2300 Å) is obviously not the surface zone analyzed by the atomic force microscope (top 10 Å) or a static SIMS experiment (top 10 Å). In addition, the type of information returned by each analysis is distinctly different. Regardless of surface depth resolution, the type of information required may dictate the sampling requirements (e.g., spectroscopic vs. surface energy vs. topology). Hence, one must decide the appropriate information to be gained from the surface analysis. To select surface analysis methods, the researcher should answer the following questions:

• "How deep is the relevant surface of my biomaterial of interest? What methods probe this surface zone?"
• "What type of surface information is required?" (e.g., compositional, energetic, dynamic, topological)
• "What analytical environment is appropriate?" (e.g., vacuum, ambient, or aqueous conditions)

In addition, quasi-stable surfaces (typically polymers) can exhibit lateral heterogeneities and depth-compositional gradients together with the structural dynamics to reorganize surface components either laterally or with the material's bulk. In these cases, methods that probe specifically at different zone depths or with different spatial resolution would be useful in order to rationalize these surface properties.

The protocol for analyzing a specific surface may be developed by formulating specific objectives for performing surface characterization. Relevant goals for a typical surface analysis are given in Table 7-2.

Table 7-2   Relevant Goals for Biomaterial Surface Characterization

Development of surface quality control criteria to monitor levels of
contamination and also provide a means to establish the true identity of a
biomaterial surface.

Monitoring for surface-active leachables contained within a sample bulk but
tending to collect on a biomaterial surface. Examples include plasticizers
and polymer fillers, oligomeric or unreacted chemical species, catalysts,
extrusion aids, mold-release agents, polishing compounds, and surfactant
processing agents.

Assess the impact of sterilization protocols on surface chemistry.

Evaluate surface oxidation, degradation, corrosion, or chemical reactions
over time in given environments.

Compare the effects of different biomaterial fabrication methods on surface
properties. Molding and casting surfaces of different chemistries (e.g.,
metal, glass-ceramic, glass, ambient air) are well known to produce distinct
surface properties in a given polymer film, metallic, or ceramic sample.

Correlate any given surface chemistry with biological response.
These responses include the activation of clotting factors, deposition of
proteins, inactivation of immobilized enzymes and antibodies, cell growth
and phenotypic expression, development of biofilms, activation of
macrophages, and growth of fibrous capsular tissue.

PREPARATION AND HANDLING OF SAMPLES
FOR SURFACE CHARACTERIZATION

Most biomedical devices should be fabricated to ensure reliability, consistency, and predictable performance. Quality control of the surface should be built into the sample analytical
routine. Surface analysis should be performed on samples identical (as much as possible)
to the actual device subject to the biological environment, implantation, or both. Once samples have been chosen, care should be taken to preserve the sample surface in its "original"
state. Since most biomaterials are fabricated and manipulated at atmospheric conditions,
certain levels of ubiquitous contamination (hydrocarbons, water vapor, siliceous species)
should be expected—even clean rooms will not eliminate these adsorbates. If sample preparation and handling are consistent protocols, then ambient contamination should remain at
relatively low and predictable levels. Common inadvertent contaminants include human
fingerprints (deposits of hydrocarbons and salts, typically sodium chloride), packaging materials (adhesive tape, paper or plastic wraps), and poor quality/contaminated solvents used
for surface rinsing/cleaning. For example, many envelopes and copy papers have surface
finishes (metal salts, clays) that will abrade away and deposit onto a sample surface if left
in contact. Plastic bags are often manufactured using highly surface-active silicone oils and
plasticizers (e.g., dioctyl phthalate) that readily transfer to any other sample surface. Therefore, sample storage or shipping protocols have the potential to substantially contaminate
the surfaces that are being carefully analyzed.

An important first step, then, is to determine the purity and reliability of all sample
preparation, handling and storage procedures/materials. The potential for the transfer of
contaminating materials to the sample surface must be ascertained, typically by a time-
dependent study of sample surface changes during storage or shipment. Commonly used
clean storage containers include Fluoroware® (Fluoroware, Inc., Chaska, MN) twist-top
single silicon wafer boats, acid-etched glass (borosilicate) dishes, cell-culture plastic ware
(polystyrene), and zip-lock-type electron microscopy polyethylene bags. However, quality
control and suppliers for these items are not guaranteed, and checks must be run periodically

to control for variability. Additionally, samples rinsed with alcohols or distilled water from common plastic laboratory squirt-bottles will often be contaminated by surface-active leachables found in the squirt-bottles from their manufacturing and thus also in the rinsing media.

SAMPLE ANALYSIS

A common rule applied by the seasoned surface analysis veteran is that conclusions regarding materials surface properties be drawn from as many different analytical methods as are financially and technically feasible. This means, of course, that surface analysis protocols be extensive as well as intensive: conclusions drawn from any single set of data are sure to be incomplete and hence misleading. Several principles govern the selection of a surface analytical protocol. First, the biological environment intended for the material is extremely heterogeneous and complex. Many surface analysis methods do not operate in conditions even close to biological complexity (e.g., UHV = *u*ltra*h*igh *v*acuum techniques including AES, XPS, dynamic or static SIMS). Nevertheless, information provided by UHV techniques are often extremely valuable and useful. The risk of artifacts is minimized by the rich informational content of UHV methods despite their apparent lack of direct correlation to a biological scenario.

The second guiding principle is that surface analysis data from many characterization techniques fit into a logical coherent and integrated picture for the biomaterials surface. Contradictory data among several methods should be suspect and subject to rigorous scrutiny to avoid misleading or erroneous conclusions. An integrated approach allows a system of checks. Poorly reproducible data should be carefully scrutinized and checked by at least two alternative methods.

A third guiding principle is that biomaterials surfaces need not be "perfect" to be successful. In fact, none of the vast amount of synthetic and fabrication expertise directed at biomaterials development to date has resulted in the ultimate biomaterial with ideal performance. More relevant, practical questions revolve around whether controlled levels of surface contamination present on all clinically used implant materials influence biological reactions, whether cells truly respond to surface microenvironments (heterogeneities) in controllable ways, and what types of surface properties influence biomedical device performance and consistency for a physician in a prescribed application over time.

A fourth important principle is that every surface analytical method has a potential to change the surface by its very process of interrogation. In short, surface analytical techniques can damage or alter samples being analyzed. Common examples are the loss of fluorine from fluorinated polymer samples exposed to X-rays under XPS analysis, and electron beam induced reduction of metal oxides during AES scanning Auger electron spectroscopy (SAM) analyses. Non-monochromatized X-ray sources can induce significant fluorine loss from the sample during a few minutes of XPS analysis. Even state-of-the-art XPS X-ray sources can remove fluorine from certain polymers in metal environments and induce oxidation of sulfur-containing compounds. Again, careful controls are needed to assess the potential for generating misleading data from fragile/labile surfaces.

SURFACE ANALYSIS METHODS

The following sections describe recommended methods and approaches to permit a thorough assessment of surface properties and judgment of suitable criteria for either acceptance or rejection. No effort is made in this chapter to correlate or speculate upon specific biomaterials' surface properties that promote or prevent certain biological responses. Indeed, such an understanding is still premature; generalizations are often scientifically unfounded and their implications are dangerous. It is generally acknowledged, nonetheless, that early surface events occurring rapidly upon implantation of a biomaterial into biological fluids determine subsequent responses reflecting "biocompatibility." These early events (occurring as fast as diffusional limitations dictate ~microseconds) involve adsorption of small organic molecules, then proteins, and ultimately cells to a biomaterial's surface. Certainly, surface parameters including surface composition, display of polar and apolar chemistry (surface energy), surface charge and topology are relevant to these critical events and have been the focus of many past efforts [1, 2, 4, 5, 8, 9].

Surface Wettability

Contact Angle and Surface Energy Measurements   While many surface analytical methods require sophisticated equipment and specialized operators, information on the outer few atomic layers of a material surface can be obtained with a relatively simple, inexpensive method called contact angles. Defined as the angle of the three-phase line between a solid surface, a liquid and a vapor in equilibrium, contact angle analysis is also known as "wetting" due to the convention of using liquids to probe solid surfaces in air. In combination with other techniques mentioned in this chapter, contact angles provide a readily accessible, valuable, first-line-of-analysis proven to be useful in virtually all areas of surface chemistry and engineering. Because of the interfacial nature of many biomaterials applications and the liquid-solid implant environment, contact angle analysis is a relevant and appropriate method. As simple as this method appears, it is one of the few in situ techniques to characterize the aqueous-biomaterial interface.

Contact angles lead the researcher to calculations of surface energies. Surface energy, in turn, is a reflection of the surface constitution–functional groups, polar or apolar species, and even acidic or basic chemistry–in the outer 2–10 Å. Because hydrophilicity and hydrophobicity remain two important classifications correlating biological interfacial behavior, wetting analyses, even in their crudest approximations, are valuable surface interrogation methods. Interpretation of contact angle data depends on the suitability of certain assumptions regarding the three-phase scenario: misleading data will result from misuse or ignorance of these assumptions. Classic sources of information on wetting, capillarity and surface tension are recommended reading to understand dynamics and thermodynamics of the three-phase line [1, 7, 11–13].

The basis for contact angle analysis lies most often on the interaction of a liquid with a solid surface in the presence of a vapor. A liquid drop placed on a solid surface (a sessile drop) often will not wet the surface (i.e., spread spontaneously) but, instead, will remain as a drop having a definite angle of contact on the surface. This situation is shown in Figure 7-3 as the idealized interface between an ideal non-deformable solid, an infinitely deformable liquid, and a vapor. The classic energy balance for this situation is provided by Young's equation:

$$\gamma_{SV} = \gamma_{LV} \, \cos\theta + \gamma_{SL} \tag{1}$$

where θ is the contact angle, and the interfacial free energies are given by γ_{SV} for the solid-vapor, γ_{SL} for the solid-liquid, and γ_{LV} for the liquid-vapor. Contact angles can be interpreted in terms of Young's equation directly if the following assumptions are valid [1]:

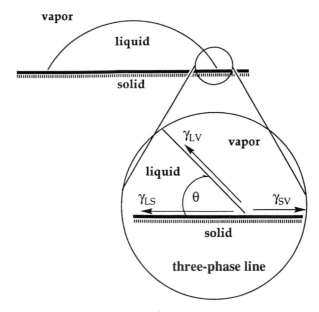

Figure 7-3 Ideal depiction of contact angle analysis, showing the liquid probe drop on a solid surface and the three-phase line with the interfacial energy balance.

• The solid surface is rigid and non-deformable (surface modulus of elasticity should exceed 3.5×10^5 dynes/cm^2).

• The solid surface is immobile and cannot re-orient in response to the liquid probe. Many polymer surfaces cannot fulfill this assumption.

• The solid surface is smooth ($\sim$0.1 mm RMS surface roughness regime): optically or visibly featureless is generally acceptable.

• The solid surface is homogeneous and uniform, lacking heterogeneous surface domains, patches or contaminants. Unclean surfaces most frequently violate this assumption.

• The liquid phase surface tension is known and remains constant. Transfer of surface contamination to the liquid surface from either the solid or vapor phases will change the liquid surface tension.

• The solid and liquid phases do not interact beyond the three-phase equilibrium (no surface swelling, extraction).

• The spreading pressure for the liquid on the solid is zero, meaning that the liquid vapor does not adsorb on the solid surface to change the solid surface-free energy.

Contact angle hysteresis and inaccurate wetting determinations result from situations where these assumptions are unfulfilled. True (reproducible, invariant) contact angle hysteresis can be a useful diagnostic tool, but must be distinguished from hysteresis related to sample non-adherence to the assumptions listed above.

Several different methods have been developed for contact angle measurements [1, 7, 12]:

• direct, microscopic measurements of the three-phase line for liquid drops or vapor bubbles against solid surfaces

• dimensional determinations for drops on surfaces, allowing contact angle determination from well-known trigonometric relationships

• capillary rise of a liquid of known surface tension

- DuNouy ring methods
- Wilhelmy plate methods

Many of these techniques are commercially available as turn-key instruments. The Wilhelmy plate method can be adapted to non-planar geometries, including cylindrical shapes relevant to catheters and tubing, fibers and discs [1, 14].

One note should be made to differences between so-called static and dynamic contact angle measurements. If the solid-liquid interface is in motion, the measurement is dynamic. Wilhelmy plate determinations are generally dynamic although low interfacial velocities approximate static measurements. Immersion of the solid surface into the probe liquid produces an *advancing* contact angle, θ_A while emersion of the solid from the liquid produces a *receding* contact angle, θ_R. The difference between advancing and receding angles, $\Delta\theta$, is termed the contact angle hysteresis. A solid-liquid pair fulfilling all the assumptions listed above should exhibit only one contact angle and, therefore, no hysteresis. However, because most real systems cannot fulfill all of these assumptions, hysteresis is commonly observed and is a useful diagnostic tool. A critical assessment must always be directed at the source of hysteresis, as two general types of hysteresis have been identified:

1 Thermodynamically stable hysteresis reproducible over many emersion-immersion cycles.
2 Kinetic hysteresis that changes with sample placement, time, cycling frequency.

Hysteresis interpretation must consider violation of the list of assumptions above and include effects of surface heterogeneity (contamination, domains), reactivity (i.e., polar/apolar interaction between probe liquids and the solid surface), metastable surface structures and chemistries (re-organization, reorientation), surface roughness (texture, particle adhesion, pinholes, pitting), solid surface swelling and liquid penetration, and surface deformation (mobility). Careful assessment of these interfacial factors in tandem with surface-sensitive knowledge from other analytical methods makes contact angle analysis a valuable surface characterization tool.

A popular extension of contact angle analysis is the determination of critical surface tension, γ_c, as originally described by Zisman's group [15]. This approach leads to an empirical determination of a surface energy related to the solid surface free energy. Experimentally, a series of pure liquids of varying surface tension are applied as drops to the sample solid surface. Contact angles are assessed for sessile drops for test liquids that span the non-wetting (contact angle $\theta > 90°$, $\cos\theta \sim 0°$) to wetting (contact angle $\theta \sim 0°$, $\cos\theta \sim 1.0$) regime. These data are plotted against the known surface tensions for the pure test liquids. The critical surface tension is defined by the x-intercept at $\cos\theta = 1$ (wetting) for the series of liquids. The method has proven useful for empirical correlations of solid surface energies with interfacial performance in various applications. Values of γ_c for various polymers are tabulated in the *Polymer Handbook* [16].

Surface Spectroscopy: Ambient Techniques

Surface-Sensitive Infrared Spectroscopy   Infrared (IR) absorption spectroscopy is a classical bulk characterization method providing chemical information on molecular structure of a material based on vibrational bands of bonded units. Nondestructive and applicable to wide varieties of materials, infrared interrogation of surfaces has been greatly enhanced by the use of Fourier methods to enhance signal-noise ratios and resolution. Nevertheless,

Fourier-transform infrared spectroscopy (FTIR) of surfaces still remains signal-limited in many cases. Where sufficient surface signal is obtained, the problem of resolving a given surface analytical zone from bulk-derived signal is difficult due to the depth of penetration (up to a micron).

As shown in Figure 7-4, several different FTIR surface-sensitive modes of analysis have been developed for obtaining representative surface IR spectra [17–20]. Several commercially available sampling "rigs" allow convenient access to spectroscopy from surfaces, of adsorbate reactions, and of events in aqueous media. Transparent films coated on reflecting metal mirrors are successfully analyzed by grazing incidence external reflection geometries with acceptable signal-to-noise ratios even for monolayers of material [21–23]. Films can be dip-coated or cast neatly onto metal substrates (evaporated gold mirrors) to produce these samples. Non-reflecting surfaces and powders can be analyzed in diffuse reflectance mode [19]. Attenuated total reflection (ATR-FTIR) methods have often been applied to biomaterials surfaces because hydrated and flow-cell samples in simplified aqueous solution can be analyzed using commercial components. An IR-transparent prism (typically germanium, ZnSe or silicon) is used as a waveguide to reflect the analytical IR signal multiple times internally as the beam traverses the prism. At each point of internal reflection a localized evanescent field is produced *external* to the prism, extending several microns into the external surroundings. External samples or media placed adjacent to the prism surface are sampled by this evanescent field, producing IR absorption/IR spectrum for all IR-active species within reach of the evanescent field. Acceptable signal-to-noise ratios often require physical compression (close contact) of the sample against the prism surface, a problem for rough or rigid irregular samples or parts. An ATR-FTIR circle cell (flow cell) has been used to study protein interactions in real time with thin films of biomaterials in ATR mode [24–26].

Surface Spectroscopy: Ultrahigh Vacuum Techniques

Electron Spectroscopy For Chemical Analysis (ESCA)   Also known by the synonym XPS (X-ray photoelectron spectroscopy), ESCA is the method of choice to provide high-resolution compositional information about biomaterials surfaces [1, 27, 28]. ESCA methods allow access to a rich variety of data summarized in Table 7-3.

Table 7-3   Information Possible from ESCA Studies of Biomaterials Interfaces

Identification of all elements except H and He present in the outer 100 Å of a surface at concentrations exceeding 0.1 atomic percent.

Determination of approximate surface composition (10%) semi-quantitatively.

Bonding information and molecular environments (oxidation states, bonding partners) in surface zone.

Identification of unsaturated and aromatic species from satellite ($p \to p$ *) transitions.

Further information on surface-exposed organic functional groups using derivatization methods.

Elemental depth profiles to 100 Å deep using angle-dependent ESCA analysis of different surface zones or photoelectrons with different depths.

Lateral resolution of surface domains/heterogeneities using models applied to angular-resolved data, or using small spot imaging methods (~ 20mm).

Identification of materials using valence bond spectra and bonding orbital information.

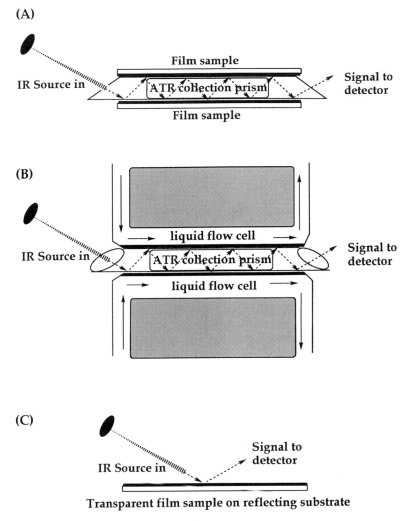

Figure 7-4 Modes of surface-sensitive measurement for infrared interrogation of biomaterials surfaces: (A) attenuated total reflection mode using a solid-phase IR collection prism and films pressed against each external prism face; (B) attenuated total reflection mode using a liquid flow cell with immersed collection prism (circle cell); (C) grazing incidence external reflection experiments using a single reflection off a reflecting substrate.

ESCA is based on photoemission of core-level electrons in an atom. Incident X-rays with energy ($h\nu$), usually monochromatic on modern systems, liberate core-level electrons with sufficient kinetic energy to escape from the material and pass through the vacuum chamber to the energy spectrum analyzer. Figure 7-5 schematically shows the photoemission process, the energy balance for the process described by Einstein in 1905, and a representative survey spectrum. Data are typically collected as survey spectra spanning the binding energy (B.E.) range of 10 to 1000 eV; subsequently high resolution spectra may be collected in a region of interest to examine the fine structure of specific core-level peaks (e.g., carbon $1s$, oxygen $1s$, titanium $2p$, etc.). The binding energy (B.E.) of the photoelectrons emitted depends on the atomic orbital from which they originated, the parent atom, and the chemical environment of the atom. A survey spectrum covering 0 to 1000 eV will contain

$$\text{B.E.} = h\nu - \text{K.E.} - (\phi + \delta)$$

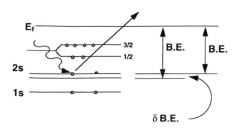

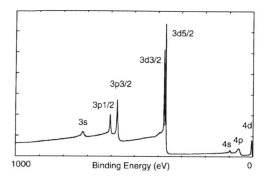

Figure 7-5 Schematic of the photoemission process and corresponding energy balance. An incident X-ray with energy (hn) liberates a core-level electron from the material with sufficient kinetic energy (K.E.) to be measured by the analyzer. The binding energy (B.E.) of the photoelectron is described by the energy balance, with knowledge of the work function of the spectrometer (ϕ). Changes in binding energy (δB.E.) for a particular photoelectron (i.e., 2s) occur when the chemical environment changes, possibly due to interatomic or intermolecular bonding. A model survey spectrum illustrates common photoelectrons detected with ESCA. (Adapted from figures provide by Dr. Patrick J. McKeown, Physical Electronics Incorporated, Eden Prairie, MN).

photoemission peaks from all elements (excluding H and He) present on a material surface up to 100 Å depth. Shifts in these ESCA peaks can be used to identify chemical state information for the outer atomic levels of a sample surface.

Innovations in ESCA sampling methods include angle-dependent capabilities for depth compositional mapping [29–31], cryogenic freezing of volatile or hydrated specimens for UHV analysis [32, 33], surface spatial mapping of chemistry [34–37], surface derivatization reactions to identify functional groups [38–41], and new X-ray sources [42]. While standard surface sample areas for a conventional ESCA instrument are circular spots approximately 150 mm across, newer "small-spot" instruments available commercially can analyze areas 1–10 mm across. Additionally, some instruments can raster the X-ray beam across selected spots. The primary benefit of these newer modifications is the capability of selecting smaller sample areas and "mapping" surface chemistry in these areas. Disadvantages include a greater risk of sample damage due to a higher flux of focused X-rays, a lower signal-to-noise ratio since smaller irradiated areas produce less photoelectrons, and significant charge neutralization problems on non-conducting samples. Sub-micron spatial resolution with ESCA is now possible using synchrotron radiation (e.g., at the Berkeley Advanced Light Source).

Together, these ESCA methods offer numerous advantages for biomedical materials surface analysis. Fragments of biomedical devices can be analyzed readily as retrieved, fabricated, or modified. Additionally, ESCA provides the capability to evaluate hydrated specimens; yields rich information on chemistries within a surface zone up to 100 Å deep; contributes relatively small sample destruction; establishes precedents for numerous data interpretation modes; allows rapid sampling and requires little sample preparation. Disadvantages include the requirement for eliminating sample outgassing into the UHV environment, access to specialized ESCA resources and operators with associated analytical costs, and the potential for sample damage if extended analysis times are required. The first disadvantage can be greatly reduced using cryogenic sampling methods mentioned above. The second disadvantage diminishes each year with the increased availability of these resources around the world.

Applications of ESCA to biomedical materials surface characterization and biocompatibility studies have been extensive. Studies of polymer surface dynamics [1, 43], protein adsorption to surfaces [44], and analysis of commercially available materials and medical devices have been performed [43–45]. Inorganic materials have also been studied using ESCA. Orthopaedic and dental applications include characterization of commonly prepared titanium implants [10, 46–48], contamination of dental implants from sterilization [49], failure analysis of ceramic-to-metal bonding [50], corrosion and oxidation of implant materials [51–54], and characterization of dental amalgams [55].

Secondary Ion Mass Spectrometry (SIMS)   SIMS is another UHV method that can supplement and augment surface analytical data available from ESCA [56–61]. Using a focused beam of ions (usually Xe^+ or Ga^+), this method produces a mass spectrum analogous to long-standing bulk mass-spectrum techniques of the outermost 10–15Å of a surface. Energy from the incident ion beam (3–5 keV) impacts the surface zone of a material, producing fragmentation of the outer atomic layers into neutral, anionic and cationic species. Conditions under which the flux of bombarding ions is low result in minimal surface etching and produce data consistent with the surface chemistry. These conditions are termed static SIMS [56, 57].

Recently developed time-of-flight SIMS (ToF-SIMS) is now a rapidly growing, commercially available SIMS method capable of high mass resolution [21, 62, 63]. The advantages of SIMS plus enhanced mass-measurement capabilities mean that synthetic polymer surfaces and high mass adsorbates (proteins, contaminants, genetic material) can be analyzed on surfaces with high precision. Complex fragmentation patterns presented by macromolecule mass spectroscopy data are often difficult to interpret unless simpler model studies are performed as a basis for understanding fragmentation. However, newer, multivariate statistical methods [64, 65] will attempt to improve analytical capabilities for polymer SIMS surface studies.

Information gained from SIMS analysis is shown in Table 7-4. This information is complementary in many respects to ESCA analysis and provides new, corroborative data from a different surface zone (see Figure 7-2). An example of SIMS analysis of poly(ethylene terephthalate) (PET), used frequently in commercial vascular grafts, is shown in Figure 7-6A. Positive ToF-SIMS survey (Figure 7-6B) and high resolution spectra (Figure 7-6C) demonstrate the ability to determine chemical species present at the surface with extremely high mass resolution. In addition to chemical information associated with the outermost materials surface chemistry, recent work has demonstrated that SIMS appears to be useful in identifying proteins adsorbed to interfaces [66].

Auger Electron Spectroscopy   Auger electron spectroscopy (AES) or scanning Auger electron spectroscopy (SAM) are versatile techniques capable of characterizing the top few molecular layers (0.5–5 nm), with detection limits on the order of 0.1 to 0.5 atomic percent.

Table 7-4   Surface Information Gained from SIMS Experiments

Surface zone restricted to top 10 Å of material (outermost 2 atomic layers).
Identification of hydrogen.
Molecular structure inferred from fragmentation patterns per mass spec.
Detection of high molecular weight fragments (polymers, biopolymers).
Useful for polymer, metal and ceramic samples.
Applicable to devices and samples with complex geometries (e.g.,
    powders, fibers, films, sponges, etc.).
Spatial resolution of composition in imaging mode.
High sensitivity to low surface concentrations.

In AES (SAM) the kinetic energy of electrons emitted from a parent atom are measured. All elements above He can be detected with either method. The strength of SAM is the excellent lateral resolution (~20 nm) capable with modern field emission electron sources. Due to this excellent spatial resolution, SAM is routinely coupled with scanning electron microscopy and has found wide acceptance in the fields of biomaterials, microelectronics, catalysis, corrosion science, tribology, metallurgy, adhesion science, and oxidation of metals. Depth profiling measurements are made by collecting Auger signal intensities while simultaneously using ion sputtering. The combination of surface sensitivity, excellent lateral resolution, and depth profiling capabilities allows SAM/AES to be used to investigate numerous phenomena associated with biomaterials fabrication, characterization, and performance testing. AES and SAM data are influenced by electron beam (incident electrons) interactions with the sample, so considerable care must be taken to minimize electron-beam-induced reduction or stimulated desorption of a sample, and, in the case of depth profiling, to prevent ion-dependent changes in peak shape and preferential sputtering of specific elements. The major drawback of these techniques is that they are limited in practice to the examination of inorganic materials, thin organic/inorganic coatings on base inorganic substrates, or inorganic coatings on organic materials. A comprehensive review of AES and SAM can be found elsewhere [2, 67].

AES and SAM both use electrons as the incident source and as the detected radiation. The underlying principle of both techniques is depicted in Figure 7-7, where an incident electron with sufficient energy elasticity scatters a core-level electron in an atom. The ionized atom may experience a number of different relaxation processes that emit either a photon or an electron. One potential mechanism is that an electron in a higher level fills the electron hole in the core energy level, which releases energy that appears either as a photon or is transmitted to a third electron which leaves both the atom and material surface with sufficient kinetic energy to be detected. The third electron in the process is called an Auger electron, which possesses kinetic energy that is governed by the atom and its chemical environment. The process of Auger electron emission leaves an atom in a doubly ionized final state. A thorough discussion of the nomenclature used to describe Auger emission, instrumentation, and spectral interpretation can be found in the literature [67, 68].

Standard AES analysis leads to data describing the elemental composition of the near surface region, and possibly the chemical state of a particular atom. Data are typically collected as a survey spectrum spanning the kinetic energy range of 10 to 1000 eV; subsequently, high resolution spectra may be collected in a region of interest to examine the fine structure of the Auger peaks. SAM studies combine AES analysis with scanning electron microscopy (SEM) to ascertain the spatial distribution of the elemental composition, or the

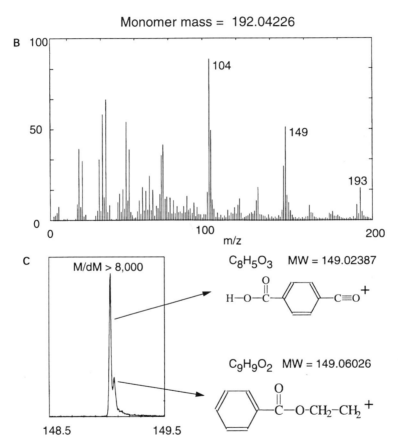

Figure 7-6 Positive ToF-SIMS spectra of a PET sample: (A) schematic of chemical structure of PET; (B) positive ToF-SIMS spectrum; (C) positive ToF-SIMS high resolution spectrum.

elemental composition at specific positions on a sample surface. Figure 7-8A shows an SEM micrograph indicating the points (1 and 2) where the AES measurements were made on a hydroxyapatite (HA) coated titanium sphere that was part of a porous coating on a Ti-6%Al-4%V alloy substrate. AES and SAM were used to identify the efficacy of the calcium phosphate coating on the beads (i.e., ceramic adhesion to the beads and interdiffusion of calcium or phosphorous into the titanium oxide). Figures 7-8B and 7-8C show the AES spectra for points 1 and 2 on the bead, respectively. These spectra display the data in the differentiated mode, $E \, dN(E)/dE$, where elements are identified by the kinetic energy of the minimum of the high energy negative excursion of the Auger peak. These figures emphasize the spatial resolution and the surface and chemical sensitivity of SAM.

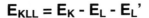

$$E_{KLL} = E_K - E_L - E_L'$$

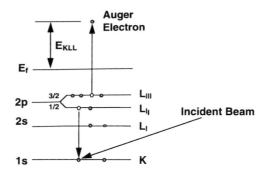

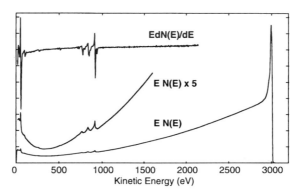

Figure 7-7 Schematic of the emission of Auger electrons from a parent atom, and the corresponding energy balance. The kinetic energy (E) of the emitted Auger electron depends on the specific Auger transition that occurs (i.e., KLL), and the chemical environment of the atom. A model AES survey spectrum illustrates the three common ways to represent collected data. (Adapted from figures provided by Dr. Patrick J. McKeown, Physical Electronics Incorporated, Eden Prairie, MN, originally published in reference [119] and used with permission.)

AES and SAM have also been used extensively to analyze the surface of orthopaedic and dental implants as a function of preparation [46, 69, 70], surface modifications or bioactive coatings [71, 72], oxidation and corrosion of biomaterials [53, 54, 73], implant failure [74], and bone response to the implant [75, 76].

AES depth profiling measurements are useful in analyzing the thickness and composition of metal oxides on implant materials [46, 53, 69, 76], surface modifications such as ion implantation or bioactive coatings on metal surfaces [72, 73], and composition gradients at either a surface or an interface. Quantitative depth profiling requires the use of a well-calibrated ion sputtering source to determine instrument parameters that minimize the interfacial depth resolution [77]. Furthermore, standards that model the actual sample are necessary to calibrate the ion sputtering rate. For example, an anodically oxidized titanium standard of known oxide thickness has been used to calibrate the sputter etch rate so that the oxide thickness of a titanium film exposed to a model biological environment could be measured [53, 54]. Thorough discussions addressing quantitative depth profiling are given in the literature [78, 79].

A

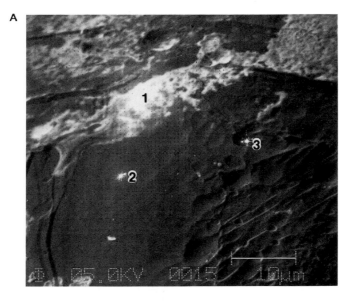

B

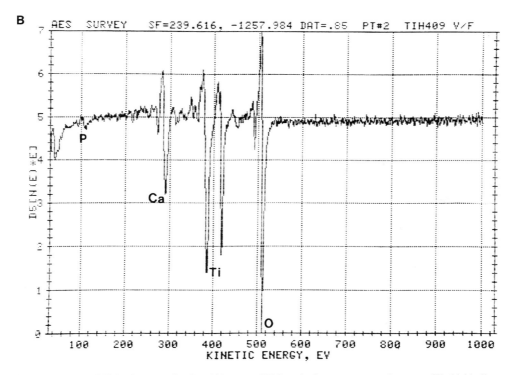

Figure 7-8 (A) SEM micrograph of an HA-coated Ti bead of a porous coating on a Ti_6Al_4V alloy substrate. Numbers indicate position of AES analysis in Figures 7-8B and C, points 1 and 2 respective; (B) AES survey spectrum in the differentiated mode taken at position 1; (C) AES survey spectrum in the differentiated mode taken at position 2. Consistent with a calcium phosphate (Ca-P) coating on titanium, calcium (Ca), phosphorous (P), oxygen (O), and titanium (Ti) were detected in these spectra. However, the P occurs in two distinct chemical states. At position 1 the P (120 eV) is incorporated into the oxide as a phosphide, and at point 2 the P exists as a phosphate, presumably as thin Ca-P coating (originally published in reference [73], used with permission).

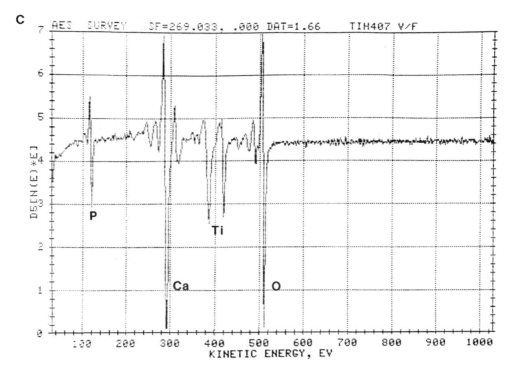

Figure 7-8 Continued.

Surface Sensitive Optical Techniques

Ellipsometry Ellipsometry is a valuable optical technique for determining the thickness and surface density of overlayers on reflective materials (e.g., SiO_2, titanium, gold, aluminum, platinum, etc.). Organic films and polymers can also be studied with ellipsometry if they are presented as a thin film on a reflective surface. The strength of ellipsometry lies in the technique's ability to accurately and non-destructively assess thickness and optical properties of either metal oxides, grafted organic molecules, or adsorbed proteins. Ellipsometry has found widespread use in the materials science community to determine the optical properties of unknown films and materials, assess dissolution and swelling of thin polymer films, and analyze oxidation and corrosion of metals and in situ kinetics of macromolecular adsorption to materials in aqueous environments [80–82]. Ellipsometry has not yet found extensive employment in the biomaterials community, possibly due to the fact that the optical models used to interpret data are considered too simplistic to accurately reflect the physical situation. However, advances in instrumentation and the wider availability of spectroscopic ellipsometry make this technique extremely valuable for surface engineering of materials and analysis of molecular adsorption to these materials.

Ellipsometry is based on the change in the polarization of polarized light (e.g., linear, elliptically) upon reflection at an interface. The ellipsometer actually measures the quantities "delta"(Δ) or psi (ψ), which are then used to calculate parameters of interest, such as index of refraction and thickness. The quantity Δ is the change in phase difference between the parallel component and perpendicular component of light that occurs upon reflection from either a surface or interface. (Parallel and perpendicular polarizations are defined with respect to the plane of incidence of the reflected light.) By definition, ψ is the angle whose tangent is the ratio of the magnitudes of the total reflection coefficients, r_p and r_s [83]. Both Δ and ψ are functions of wavelength (λ) or energy and are used in the fundamental equation of ellipsometry, given below,

$$\tan(\psi)e^{(i\Delta)} = r_p/r_s \qquad (2)$$

to calculate the total reflection coefficients, r_p and r_s. The total reflection coefficients are then used in conjunction with appropriate physical and mathematical models to calculate the parameter of interest, e.g., adsorbed protein layer thickness and surface density. The accuracy of the physical parameters calculated depends on the model used to make the estimate. Thus, materials properties and other physical parameters that are determined by ellipsometry are inherently dependent on the physical model assumed by the user and the mathematical treatment of that model. A more complete review of the practical issues of ellipsometry is given in reference [80], and the theoretical aspects are treated extensively in textbooks [83, 84].

The use of ellipsometry in biomaterials science and engineering has been somewhat limited to protein adsorption kinetics and isotherm measurements of proteins from media containing only a single protein [81, 82]. Recently, the scope of research employing ellipsometry has been broadened to include interactions of proteins with organic surfaces [85, 86], and the identification of the composition of proteins adsorbed to metals from human plasma [87], or organic surface modifications [88, 89]. The composition of proteins adsorbed to a surface were identified by using an indirect immuno-ellipsometry technique to measure the increase in thickness associated with the binding of antibodies directed toward specific proteins bound to the surface. A common problem associated with the measurement of overlayer thicknesses by ellipsometry is that the index of refraction ($N = n + ik$) of the layer and substrate need to be known a priori or determined simultaneously [90]. Accurate values of the index of refraction for proteins, thin polymer films, and organic layers are not usually available, so the researcher is left to estimate N. This problem is minimized by using a spectroscopic ellipsometer, where plots of Δ and ψ as a function of wavelength (or energy) are used to accurately determine the optical properties of the layer and calculate the parameter of interest. The accuracy of layer thicknesses and surface density in multilayer structures is also improved by making measurements with a spectroscopic ellipsometer [91].

Surface Plasmon Resonance (SPR) or Total Internal Reflection (TIR) Optical Sensing   Another surface analytical method that has emerged in the last five years with particular utility for biomaterials analysis is called either surface plasmon resonance (SPR) [92–96] or total internal reflection (TIR) optical sensing [97–99], depending on the optical configuration of the instrument. Both systems have been commercialized [100, 101] and perform virtually the same task of mass sensing of biomolecules in liquid milieu adsorbed or very near a biomaterial's interface. Both methods use an evanescent field to probe the area adjacent to the sensing interface (up to several hundred nanometers into the environment surrounding the surface) without the requirement for labeling or probes. Generation of the evanescent field is the major difference between the two general sensing strategies. The SPR system uses a thin metallic coating to generate a resonant coupling between incident probing light energy and surface plasmons (free electrons within the metallic film), producing a minimum in reflected light intensity. The incident angle at which this minimum occurs depends on the metal, but also more importantly upon the nature of the medium directly adjacent to the metal. Adsorption of molecules to this surface will change the angle at which the reflected light intensity minimum is detected, forming the basis for mass sensing. In the TIR sensor, a resonant mirror configuration is used to create an evanescent field external to the sensing element. Again, optical resonance conditions are established in the waveguide which are changed by the adsorption of molecules on the external surface of the sensing surface. Measurement is made in real-time using a flow cell configuration, and adsorption or ligand-receptor interactions can be observed conveniently and rapidly in any number of environments relevant to the biomaterials researcher. Additionally, sensing surfaces can be chemically and physically modified with a number of known conjugation chemistries to yield interfaces of relevant chemical features for the investigator.

Applications for these optical surface sensors are just beginning to be fully explored [96, 102, 103]. Sensing surfaces can be dip-coated, spin-coated, plasma-modified, chemically derivatized, and serially exchanged. Quantification of adsorbed amounts and binding and desorption kinetics are possible from both gas and liquid phases. New work [104, 105] indicates that apparent surface binding or adsorption kinetics must be carefully interpreted in terms of mass transfer limitations imposed by the immobilized surface layer or matrix where surface interactions occur. Tandem or synergistic surface-localized binding events can also be monitored. Recently, the SPR method has been developed into an imaging technique [106] by creating a surface plasmon microscope to map the surface topology. Lateral resolution of surface features of 20 μm and several Å in film thickness was obtained. More recent work has demonstrated the ability to use SPR to image protein monolayers on surfaces with applications to sandwich sensors and other protein-electrode-based devices [107].

Scanning Imaging Techniques

Atomic Force Microscopy (AFM)   AFM (or scanning force microscopy, SFM) and scanning tunneling microscopy (STM) are relatively new surface techniques, falling under the heading of "probe microscopies," that provide non-destructive quantitative topographical images of a surface with atomic-level resolution on rigid materials. Both techniques can be used in aqueous environments, but AFM has an enormous advantage for biomaterials research since it can image non-conducting materials under similar environmental conditions. Due to the inherent limitations of STM, AFM has become the instrument of choice for imaging synthetic biomaterials (commercial polymers, thin polymer films, metal oxides, etc.) and native biological materials (red blood cells, platelets, bone, dentin, etc.). Thus, this section focuses on AFM. In 1986 Binnig and co-workers published the first report describing the use of AFM [108]. Subsequently, Hansma and co-workers developed the technology for the current commercial instruments [109]. Current instruments ideally have lateral resolution better than 0.2 nm and vertical resolution near 0.1 nm. The potential impact of AFM in biomaterials research is substantial, since AFM both images with atomic resolution and measures frictional forces on the atomic scale (lateral force microscopy). Furthermore, it can be used to measure elastic and hardness properties of biomaterials on a nanometer scale.

An AFM operates by reflecting laser light off a microfabricated cantilever, with known spring constant $(0.1-1 \text{ Nm}^{-1})$, to a photodiode that records the deflection of the cantilever. The cantilever has a tip that comes to a point with near atomic dimensions that is scanned laterally over the surface (x and y directions). Constant force is maintained on the sample by using a feedback system that keeps the beam on the photodiode fixed [106]. This is accomplished by piezoelectric translators that adjust the z-axis of the sample while the sample is scanned laterally. This mode of operation is termed optical lever detection [108], and is used in most commercial instruments. Operating the AFM in a physiologically relevant medium such a water or buffered salt solutions is an advantage, since in air capillary forces tend to distort the precision of the applied force [108].

AFM has been used in numerous applications including the structural characterization of organic thin films [110], analysis of thin polymer films [111], nanoscale tribology of polymer films [112], protein adsorption to mica surfaces [113–115], measurement of elastic properties of biological materials such as bone [116], and monitoring of the effect of demineralizing conditioning agents on the structure of dentin [117]. AFM analyses on clinically available biomaterials include assessment of bone response to titanium implants with different morphology [75], and analysis of a solvent extraction process on the morphology of Biomer® [118]. The enormous potential of AFM in biomaterials research has been somewhat limited due either to artifacts associated with sample preparation methods or to limitations of the technique itself. An initial problem with AFM was that the tip shape influenced the images obtained, thus preventing accurate imaging of large structures or macromolecules. Recent advances in ultrasharp microfabricated Si_3N_4 tips have minimized the effect of tip shape on the images collected. Another limitation with AFM was the so called "sweeping" or "broom effect," where the high lateral forces generated by scanning the tip actually moved weakly adsorbed molecules or caused deformation of soft objects that were being imaged. This problem has also been minimized by using tapping mode AFM (TM-AFM) in liquids such as a buffered salt solution [114]. In TM-AFM, the cantilever is sinusoidally oscillated at a frequency (e.g., 15–35 kHz) which avoids generating lateral forces that can either move or distort objects [114]. The feedback control is different from that previously described for contact mode AFM. In tapping mode, the separation between the cantilever tip and the sample is controlled by the change in the amplitude of the sinusoidal wave that occurs upon approaching the surface. The change in the amplitude is corrected by the piezoelectric translators that adjust the z-axis to maintain constant amplitude. The instrument can be calibrated by using a sample with known height features in the range of the object to be imaged (e.g., for proteins a nm calibration standard would be used) [114]. In addition to TM-AFM one can minimize image artifacts by changing either the temperature or pH to increase the stiffness or strength of adsorption, respectively, of the object being imaged [114]. Furthermore, covalent coupling of the object of interest to the surface can significantly improve image quality. These recent advances in AFM instrumentation and sample preparation techniques should foster the use of AFM for analysis of clinically relevant biomaterials.

CONCLUSIONS

Surface characterization of biomaterials has enjoyed a renaissance of development and technological improvement with the recognition that the material interface plays a key role in mediating biological response and reactivity. New methods are continually evolving, improving the capabilities to probe materials surfaces and their interfaces with biological environments in many new and valuable ways. While a variety of surface analytical methods are now available to the biomaterial scientist, each case of surface characterization must be carefully evaluated to match desired analytical information with the method(s) and their respective capabilities. Few techniques actually are able to provide surface data of direct relevance to the biological implant environment; for example, few methods operate under water or in the presence of complex milieu such as serum. Instead, some of the more valuable methods (e.g., ESCA), operate often in high vacuum–of little relevance to biomaterials' applications. At best, only simulated environments approximating biological sites (for example, the evanescent wave biosensors, environmental SEM or hydrated ESCA or SIMS) are currently available from newer developments. Much of a biomaterial's surface description, therefore, must be inferred and extrapolated from the environment of the surface in the analytical scenario (e.g., UHV) to the material site of application (aqueous). Because surfaces of many biomaterials are synthetic polymers or proteins capable of metastable states of surface relaxation and restructuring, analytical methods must account for possible "chameleon-like" effects between vacuum, air, and water. The more complete the knowledge of the material and its possible surface composition and physical chemistry, the more confident the investigator may be regarding the surface's reactivity in a biological setting. The fullest impact of surface analysis in the biomaterials field will be realized by coupling surface characterization to a broader set of disciplines common to biomaterials development. The biomaterials specialist must become adept with a number of scientific concepts regarding surfaces and their behavior. Comprehensive understanding of the influence of materials interfacial chemistry in biological systems will be derived from an ability to direct diverse principles of surface physics, surface analysis, materials science and engineering, surface electrochemistry, synthetic chemistry, and cellular and molecular biology to the application of biomaterials in specific sites.

REFERENCES

1   Andrade JD. *Surface and Interfacial Aspects of Biomedical Polymers.* Volumes 1 and 2. New York: Plenum Press, 1985.

2   Briggs D, Seah MP (Eds.). *Practical Surface Analysis*, Volumes 1 and 2, 2nd ed. New York: John Wiley and Sons Ltd., 1990.

3   Ratner BD. Surface structure and properties. In Williams DF (Ed.), *Concise Encyclopedia of Medical and Dental Materials.* Oxford: Pergamon Press, 1990, 337–346.

4   Ratner BD. Characterization of biomaterial surfaces. In Ratner BD, Hoffman A, Lemons J, Schoen FJ (Eds.), *Biomaterials Science: An Introductory to Materials in Medicine.* San Diego: Academic Press, 1996.

5   Ratner BD. Contemporary methods for characterizing complex biomaterial surfaces. *Clin Mater*, 11 (1992), 25–36.

6   Somorjai GA. *Chemistry in Two Dimensions—Surfaces.* Ithaca, New York: Cornell University Press, 1981.

7   Adamson AW. *Physical Chemistry of Surfaces*, 4th ed. New York: Wiley-Interscience, 1990.

8   Horbett TA, Brash JD (Eds.). *Proteins at Interfaces.*, Volumes 1 and 2. Washington, DC: ACS Press, 1987, 1995.

9   Ratner BD (Ed.). *Progress in Biomedical Engineering, Vol. 6: Surface Characterization of Biomaterials.* Amsterdam: Elsevier, 1988.

10 Kasemo B, Lausmaa J. Surface science aspects on inorganic biomaterials. *In CRC Critical Reviews in Biocomptibility*, Boca Raton, FL: CRC Press, 1986, 335–80.

11 Aveyard R, Haydon DA. *Introduction to Principles of Surface Chemistry.* London: Cambridge Press, 1973.

12 Neumann AW. Contact angles. In Padday JF (Ed.), *Wetting, Spreading and Adhesion*, New York: Academic Press, 1978, 3–35.

13 Mittal KL (Ed.). *Contact Angle, Wettability and Adhesion.* Weinheim: VCP, 1993.

14 Pitt WL, Young, BR, Cooper SL. Measurment of advancing and receding contact angles inside polymer tubing. *Colloids Surf*, 27 (1987), 345–355.

15 Zisman W. Relation of equilibrium contact angle to liquid and solid constitution. In Fowkes FM (Ed.), *Contact Angle, Wettability and Adhesion. Adv. Chem. Ser. 43*, Washington: ACS Press, 1964, 1–51.

16 Brandup IJ, Immergut EH (Eds.). *Polymer Handbook*, 3rd ed. New York: Wiley & Sons, 1990.

17 Reichert WM. Evanescent detection of adsorbed films: Assessment of optical considerations for absorbance and fluorescence spectroscopy at the crystal/solution and polymer/solution interfaces. *Crit Rev Biocompat*, 5 (1989), 173–205.

18 Mirabella FM. Internal reflection spectroscopy. *Appl Spectrosc Rev*, 21 (1985), 145–78.

19 Urban M. *Vibrational Spectroscopy of Molecules and Macromolecules on Surfaces.* New York: Wiley-Interscience, 1993.

20 Knutson K, Lyman DJ. Surface infrared spectroscopy. In Andrade JD (Ed.), *Surface and Interfacial Aspects of Biomedical Polymers*, Volume 1. New York: Plenum Press, 1985, 197–247.

21 Wang W, Castner DG, Grainger DW. Ultrathin films of perfluoropolyether-grafted polysiloxanes chemisorbed via alkylthiolate anchors to gold surfaces. *Supramolec Sci*, 1996; in press.

22 Sun F, Castner DG, Mao G, Wang W, McKeown P, Grainger DW. Spontaneous polymer thin film assembly and organization using mutually immiscible side chains. *J Am Chem Soc*, 118 (1996), 856–866.

23 Porter MD. IR external reflection spectroscopy: A probe for chemically modified surfaces. *Anal Chem*, 60 (1988), 1143–54A.

24 Magnani A, Busi E, Barbucci R. In situ ATR/FTIR studies of protein adsorption on polymer materials: Effectiveness of surface heparinization. *J Mater Sci Mater Med*, 5 (1994), 839–847.

25 Lenk TJ, Ratner BD, Gendreau RM. IR spectral changes of bovine serum albumin upon surfaces. *J Biomed Mater Res*, 23 (1989), 549–557.

26 Cheng S-S, Chittur KK, Sukenik CN, Culp LA, Lewondowska K. The conformation of fibronectin on self-assembled monolayers of different surface compositions: An FTIR/ATR study. *J Colloid Interface Sci*, 162 (1994), 135–147.

27 Dilks A. X-ray photoelectron spectroscopy for the investigation of polymer surfaces. In Baker AO, Brudle CR (Eds.), *Electron Spectroscopy: Theory, Techniques and Applications*, London: Academic Press, 1981, 277–359.

28 Ratner BD, Castner DG. Electron spectroscopy for chemical analysis. In Vickerman JC, Read NM (Eds.), *Surface Analysis-Techniques and Applications*. Chichester, UK: John Wiley & Sons, 1995.

29 Fadley CS. Solid state and surface-analysis by means of angular-dependent X-ray photoelectron spectroscopy. *Prog Sol State Chem*, 11 (1976), 265–343.

30 Tyler BJ, Castner DG, Ratner BD. Regularization: A stable and accurate method for generating depth profiles from angle-dependent XPS data. *Surf Interface Anal*, 14 (1989), 443–450.

31 Ratner BD, Paynter RW. Polyurethane surfaces: The importance of molecular weight distribution, bulk chemistry and casting conditions. In Planck H, Engbers G, Syre I (Eds.), *Polyurethanes in Biomedical Engineering, Progress in Biomedical Engineering*, Vol. 1. Amsterdam: Elsevier Press, 1984, 41–68.

32 Ratner BD, Weathersby PK, Hoffman AS, Kelly MA, Scharpen LH. Radiation-grafted hydrogels for biomaterial applications as studied by the ESCA technique. *J Appl Polym Sci*, 22 (1978), 643–664.

33 Lewis KB, Ratner BD, Klumb LA, Ertel SI. Surface restructuring of biomedical polymers. *Trans Soc Biomat*, 14 (1991), 176.

34 Seah MP, Smith GC. Concept of an imaging XPS system. *Surf Interface Anal*, 11 (1988), 69–79.

35 Hoffmann DP, Proctor A, Hercules DM. Spatially resolved ESCA using Handamard masks. *Appl Spectrosc*, 43 (1989), 899–908.

36 Ebel H, Ebel MF, Mantler M, Barnegg-Golwig G, Svagera R, Gurker N. Imaging XPS with a hemispherical analyzer and multichannelplate detection. *Surf Sci*, 231 (1990), 233–239.

37 Briggs D. New developments in polymer surface analysis. *Polymer*, 25 (1985), 1379–1391.

38 Chilkoti A, Ratner BD, Briggs D. Plasma-deposited polymeric films prepared from carbonyl-containing volatile precursors: XPS chemical derivatization and static SIMS surface characterization. *Chem Mater*, 3 (1991), 51–61.

39 Chilkoti A, Ratner BD. An x-ray photoelectron spectroscopic investigation of the selectivity of hydroxyl derivatization reactions. *Surf Interface Anal*, 17 (1991), 567–574.

40 Batich, CD. Chemical derivatization and surface analysis. *Appl Surf Sci*, 32 (1988), 57–73.

41 Chilkoti A, Ratner BD. Chemical derivatization methods for enhancing the analytical capabilities of X-ray photoelectron spectroscopy and static secondary ion mass spectrometry. In Sabbatini L, Zambonin PG (Eds.), *Surface Characterization of Advanced Polymers*. Weinheim, Germany: VCH Verlag, 1993, 221–56.

42 Paynter RW. Surface analytical techniques in biomaterials development. In Williams DF (Ed.), *Techniques of Biocompatibility Testing*, Vol. 2. Boca Raton, FL: CRC Press, 1986, 49–80.

43 Mori H, Hirao A, Nakahama S, Senshu K. Synthesis and surface characterization of hydrophilic-hydrophobic block copolymers containing poly(2,3-dihydroxypropyl methacrylate). *Macromolecules*, 27 (1994), 4093–4100.

44 Paynter RW, Rantner BD. The study of interfacial proteins and biomolecules by X-ray photoelectron spectroscopy. In Andrade JD (Ed.), *Surface Interfac Asp Biomed Polym*, Vol. 2. New York: Plenum Press, 1985, 189–216.

45 Castner DG, Ratner BD, Hoffman AS. Surface characterization of a series of polyurethanes by X-ray photoelectron spectroscopy and contact angle methods. *J Biomater Sci Polym Edn*, 1 (1990), 191–206.

46 Lausmaa J, Kasemo B, Mattsson H. Surface spectroscopic characterization of titanium implant materials. *Appl Surface Sci*, 44 (1990), 133–146.

47 Klauber, C, Lenz LJ, Henry PJ. Oxide thickness and surface contamination of six endosseous dental implants determined by electron spectroscopy for chemical analysis: A preliminary report. *Int J Oral Maxilofac Implants*, 5 (1990), 264–271.

48 Healy KE, Ducheyne P. Hydration and preferential molecular adsorption on titanium *in vitro. Biomaterials*, 13 (1992), 553–561.

49 Lausmaa J, Kasemo B, Hansson S. Accelerated oxide growth on titanium implants during autoclaving caused by fluorine contamination. *Biomaterials*, 6 (1985), 23–27.

50 Anusavice KJ, Ringle RD, Fairhurst CW. Identification of fracture zones in porcelain-veneered-to-metal bond test specimens by ESCA analysis. *J Prosthetic Dentistry*, 42 (1979), 417–421.

51 Hofmann J, Michel R, Holm R, Zilkens J. Corrosion behaviour of stainless steel implants in biological media. *Surface Interface Anal*, 3 (1981), 110–117.

52 Ohnsorge J, Holm R. Surface investigations of oxide layers on cobalt-chromium-alloyed orthopaedic implants using ESCA technique. *Med Prog Technol*, 5 (1978), 171–177.

53 Healy KE, Ducheyne P. Oxidation kinetics of titanium thin films in model physiological environments. *J Colloid Interface Sci*, 150 (1992), 404–417.

54 Healy KE, Ducheyne P. The mechanisms of passive dissolution of titanium in a model physiological environment. *J Biomed Mater Res*, 26 (1992), 319–38.

55 Hanawa T, Takahashi H, Ota M, Pinizzotto RF, Ferracane JL, Okabe T. Surface characterization of amalgams using X-ray photoelectron spectroscopy. *J Dental Res*, 66 (1987), 1470–1478.

56 Castner DG, Ratner BD. Static secondary ion mass spectroscopy: A new technique for the characterization of biomedical polymer surfaces. In Ratner BD (Ed.), *Surface Characterization of Biomaterials, Progress in Biomedical Engineering*, Vol. 6. Amsterdam: Elsevier, 1988, 65–81.

57 Vickerman JC, Brown A, Reed NM. *Secondary Ion Mass Spectrometry, Principles and Applications*. Oxford, UK: Clarendon Press, 1989.

58 Pignataro S, Licciadello A. Static, imaging and dynamic SIMS in the study of surfaces and interfaces of materials. *Gazz Chim Ital*, 120 (1990), 351–363.

59 Katz W, Newman JG. Fundamentals of secondary ion mass spectrometry. *MRS Bulletin*, 7 (1987), 40–46.

60 Niehuis E. Secondary ion mass spectrometry of organic materials. In Benninghoven A, Huber AM, Werner HW (Eds.), *Proc Sixth Internatl Conf on Secondary Ion Mass Spectrometry (SIMS VI)*, Vol. 1. Chichester, UK: John Wiley & Sons, 1988, 591–598.

61 Davies MC, Lynn RAP. Static secondary ion mass spectrometry of polymeric biomaterials. *CRC Crit Rev Biocompat*, 5 (1990), 297–341.

62 Price D. The resurgence in time-of-flight mass spectrometry. *Trends Anal Chem*, 9 (1990), 21–25.

63 Sun F, Castner DG, Mao G, Wang W, McKeown P, Grainger DW. Spontaneous polymer thin film assembly and organization using mutually immiscible side chains. *J Am Chem Soc*, 118 (1996), 1856–1866.

64 Chilkoti A, Ratner BD, Briggs D. Developing multivariate statistical models of the surface chemistry of organic plasma deposited films based on the static SIMS spectra of model homopolymers. In Benninghoven A (Ed.), *SIMS VIII*. Chichester, UK: John Wiley & Sons, 1991.

65 Chilkoti A, Ratner BD, Briggs D. Static secondary ion mass spectrometric investigations of the surface chemistry of organic plasma-deposited films created from oxygen-containing precursors. 3. Multivariate statistical modeling. *Anal Chem*, 65 (1993), 1736–1745.

66 Mantus DS, Ratner BD, Carlson BA, Moulder JF. Static secondary ion mass spectrometry of adsorbed proteins. *Anal Chem*, 65 (1993), 1431–1437.

67 Hofmann S. High resolution auger electron spectroscopy for materials characterization. *Mikrochim Acta [Wein]*, 1 (1987), 321–345.

68 Briggs D, Rivière JC. Spectral interpretation. In Briggs D, Seah MP (Eds.), *Practical Surface Analysis: Vol. 1, Auger and X-ray Photoelectron Spectroscopy*, 2nd ed. New York: John Wiley & Sons, 1990, 85–141.

69 Binon PP, Weir DJ, Marshall SJ. Surface analysis of an original Brånemark implant and three related clones. *Int J Oral Maxillofac Implants*, 7 (1992), 168–75.

70 Lausmaa J, Kasemo B, Rolander U, Bjursten LM, Ericson LE, Rosander L, Thomsen P. Preparation, surface spectroscopic and electron microscopic characterization of titanium implant materials. In Ratner BD (Ed.), *Prog Biomed Eng Vol. 6: Surface Characterization of Biomaterials*, Amsterdam : Elsevier, 1988, 161–174.

71 Van Raemdonck W, Ducheyne P, De Meester P. Auger electron spectroscopic analysis of hydroxylapatite coatings on titanium. *J Am Ceram Soc,* 67 (1984), 381–384.

72 Kim CS, Ducheyne P. Compositional variations in the surface and interface of calcium phosphate ceramic coatings on Ti and Ti-6Al-4V due to sintering and immersion. *Biomaterials*, 12 (1991), 461–469.

73   Ducheyne P, Healy KE. The effect of plasma-sprayed calcium phosphate ceramic coatings on the metal ion release from porous titanium and cobalt-chromium alloys. *J Biomed Mater Res*, 22 (1988), 1137–1163.

74   Aparicio C, Olivé J. Comparative surface microanalysis of failed Brånemark implants. *Int J Oral Maxillofac Implants*, 7 (1992), 94–103.

75   Larsson C, Thomsen P, Lausmaa J, Rodahl M, Kasemo B, Ericson LE. Bone response to surface modified titanium implants: Studies on electropolished implants with different oxide thicknesses and morphology. *Biomaterials*, 15 (1994), 1062–1074.

76   Sundgren J-E, Bodö P, Lundström I. Auger electron spectroscopic studies of the interface between human tissue and implants of titanium and stainless steel. *J Colloid Interface Sci*, 110 (1992), 9–20.

77   Hunt CP, Seah MP. Characterization of a high depth-resolution tantalum pentoxide sputter profiling reference material. *Surface Interface Anal*, 6 (1984), 82–93.

78   Mathieu HJ, Datta M, Landolt. Thickness of natural oxide films determined by AES and XPS with/without sputtering. *J Vac Sci Technol A*, 3 (1985), 331–335.

79   Hofmann S. Depth profiling in AES and XPS. In Briggs D, Seah MP (Eds.), *Practical Surface Analysis: Vol. 1. Auger and X-ray Photoelectron Spectroscopy*, 2nd ed. New York: John Wiley & Sons, 1990, 143–199.

80   Tompkins, HG. *A User's Guide to Ellipsometry*. San Diego: Academic Press, 1993.

81   Cuypers PA, Corsel JW, Janssen MP, Kop JMM, Hermens WT, Hemker HC. The adsorption of prothrombin to phosphatidylserine multilayers quantitated by ellipsometry. *J Biol Chem*, 258 (1983), 2426–2431.

82   Ivarsson B, Lundström I. Physical characterization of protein adsorption on metal and metal oxide surfaces. *CRC Critical Reviews in Biocompatibility*, 2 (1986), 1–95.

83   Azzam RMA, Bashara NM. *Ellipsometry and Polarized Light*. Amsterdam: North-Holland Publishing, 1977.

84   Born M and Wolf E. *Principles of Optics: Electromagnetic Theory of Propagation Interference and Diffraction of Light*, 4th ed. New York: Pergamon Press, 1969.

85   Prime KL, Whitesides GM. Self-assembled organic monolayers: Model systems for studying adsorption of proteins at surfaces. *Science*, 252 (1991), 1164–1167.

86   Wahlgren MC, Paulsson MA, Arnebrant T. Adsorption of globular model proteins to silica and methylated silica surfaces and their elutability by dodecyltrimethylammonium bromide. *Colloids Surf*, A 70 (1993), 139–149.

87   Wälivaara B, Askendal A, Elwing H, Lundström I, Tengvall P. Antisera binding onto metals immersed in human plasma *in vitro. J Biomed Mater Res*, 26 (1992), 1205–1216.

88   Tengvall P, Lestelius M, Liedberg B, Lundström I. Plasma protein and antisera interactions with L-cysteine and 3-mercaptoproprionic acid monolayers on gold surfaces. *Langmuir*, 8 (1992), 1236–1238.

89   Lestelius M, Liedberg B, Lundström I, Tengvall P. In vitro plasma protein adsorption and kallikrein formation on 3-mercaptoproprionic acid, L-cysteine and glutathione immobilized onto gold. *J Biomed Mater Res*, 28 (1994), 871–880.

90   Arwin H. Optical properties of thin layers of bovine serum albumin, g-globulin, and hemoglobin. *Appl Spectrosc*, 40 (1986), 313–318.

91   Arwin H, Mårtensson J, Lundström I. Dielectric function of a protein monolayer at a gold/solution interface. *Appl Phys Commun*, 11 (1992), 41–48.

92   Kooyman RPH, Kolkman H, Van Gent J, Greve J. Surface plasmon resonance immunosensors: Sensitivity considerations. *Anal Chim Acta*, 213 (1988), 35–45.

93   Kooyman RPH, De Bruin HE, Eenik RG, Greve J. Surface plasmon resonance spectroscopy as a bioanalytical tool. *J Molec Struct*, 218 (1990), 345–50.

94   Jönsson U, Fägerstam L, Ivarsson B, Johnsson B, Karlsson R, Lundh K, Löfås S, Persson B, Roos H, Rönnberg I, Sjölander S, Stenberg E, Ståhlberg R, Urbaniczky C, Östlin H, Malmqvist M. Real-time biospecific interaction analysis using surface plasmon resonance and a sensor chip technology. *Biotechniques*, 11 (1991), 620–627.

95   Fägerstam L, Frostell-Karlsson A, Karlsson R, Persson B, Rönnberg I. Biospecific interaction analysis using surface plasmon resonance detection applied to kinetic, binding site and concentration analysis. *J Chromat*, 597 (1992), 397–410.

96   Davies J. Surface plasmon resonance: The technique and its applications to biomaterial processes. *Nanobiol*, 3 (1994), 5–16.

97   Cush R, Cronin JM, Stewart WJ, Maule CH, Molloy J, Goddard NJ. The resonance mirror: A novel optical biosensor for direct sensing of biomolecular interactions. Part I. Principle of operation and associated instrumentation. *Biosensors Bioelectron*, 8 (1993), 347–364.

98   Buckle PE, Davies RD, Kinning T, Yeung D, Edwards PR, Pollard-Knight D, Lowe CR. The resonance mirror: A novel optical biosensor for direct sensing of biomolecular interactions. Part II. Applications. *Biosensors Bioelectron*, 8 (1993), 365–370.

99   Davies RD, Edwards PR, Watts HJ, Lowe CR, Buckle PE, Yeung D, Kinning T, Pollard-Knight D. The resonance mirror: A tool for the study of biomolecular interactions. *Techniques Protein Chem*, 5 (1994), 285–292.

100 Davies RJ, Pollard-Knight D. An optical biosensor system for molecular interaction studies. *Am Biotech Lab*, July 1993, 52–54.

101 Malmqvist M. Biospecific interaction analysis using biosensor technology. *Nature*, 361 (1993), 186–187.

102 Malmqvist M. A surface plasmon resonance biosensor for characterization of biospecific interactions. In Hoch H, Jelinski L, Craighead H (Eds.), *Nanofabrication and Biosystems: Integrating Material Science, Engineering, and Biology.* Cambridge, UK: Cambridge University Press, 1996, 103–122.

103 O'Shannessy DJ. Determination of kinetic rate and equilibrium binding constants for macromolecular interactions: A critique of the surface plasmon literature. *Curr Opin Biotechnol*, 5 (1994), 65–71.

104 Schuck P, Minton AP. Analysis of mass transport-limited binding kinetics in evanescent wave biosensors. *Anal Biochem*, 240 (1996), in press.

105 Schuck P. Kinetics of ligand binding to receptor immobilized in a polymer matrix, as detected with an evanescent wave biosensor. I. A computer simulation of the influence of mass transport. *Biophys J*, 70 (1996), 1230–1249.

106 Yeatman EM, Ash EA. Surface plasmon scanning microscopy. *SPIE*, 897 (1988), 100–107.

107 Schmidt A, Spinke J, Bayerl T, Sackmann E, Knoll W. Streptavidin binding to biotinylated lipid layers on solid supports. *Biophys J*, 63 (1992), 1385–1392.

108 Binnig G, Quate CF, Gerber CH. Atomic force microscope. *Phys Rev Lett*, 56 (1986), 930.

109 Drake B, Prater CB, Weisenhorn AL, Gould SAC, Albrecht TR, Quate CF, Cannell DS, Hansma HG, Hansma PK. Imaging crystals, polymers, and processes in water with the atomic force microscope. *Science*, 243 (1989), 1586–1589.

110 Zasadzinski JA, Viswanathan R, Schwartz DK, Garnaes J, Madsen L, Chiruvolu S, Woodward JT, Longo ML. Applications of atomic force microscopy to structural characterization of organic thin films. *Colloids and Surfaces A: Physicochem Eng Aspects*, 93 (1994), 305–333.

111 Berquier J-M, Creuzet F, Grimal J-M. Atomic force microscopy images of polymer layers adsorbed on flat substrates of glass and silica. *Langmuir*, 12 (1996), 597–598.

112 Smithson RLW, Evans DF, Monfils JD, Guire PE. Ultrathin film characterization: Photoreactive polyacrylamide. *Colloids Surf B: Biointerfaces*, 1 (1993), 349–55.

113 Fritz M, Radmacher M, Cleveland JP, Allersma MW, Stewart RJ, Gieselmann R, Janmey P, Schmidt CF, Hansma PK. Imaging globular and filamentous proteins in physiological buffer solutions with tapping mode atomic force microscopy. *Langmuir*, 11 (1995), 3529–3535.

114 Marchant RE, Leas SA, Andrade JD, Bockenstedt PJ. Interactions of von Willebrand factor on mica studied by atomic force microscopy. *J Colloid Interface Sci*, 148 (1992), 261–272.

115 Taborelli M, Eng L, Descouts P, Ranieri JP, Bellamkonda R, Aebischer P. Bovine serum albumin conformation on methyl and amine functionalized surfaces compared by scanning force microscopy. *J Biomed Mater Res*, 29 (1995), 707–714.

116 Tao NJ, Lindsay SM, Lees S. Measuring the microelastic properties of biological material. *Biophysical J*, 63 (1992), 1165–1168.

117 Marshall GW, Balooch M, Kinney JH, Marshall SJ. Atomic force microscopy of conditioning agents on dentin. *J Biomed Mater Res*, 29 (1995), 1381–1387.

118 Nurdin N, Descourts P. Effect of toluene extraction on Biomer surface: II. An atomic force microscopy study. *J Biomat Sci, Polym Ed*, 7 (1995), 425–438.

119 Reichlmaier, S, Hammond JS, Hearn MJ, Briggs D. Analysis of polymer surfaces by SIMS. 17. An assessment of the accuracy of the mass assignment using a high mass resolution ToF-SIMS instrument, *Surface Interface Anal*, 21 (1994), 739–746.

ADDITIONAL READING

1   Andrade JD. *Surface and Interfacial Aspects of Biomedical Polymers.* Volumes 1 and 2. New York: Plenum Press, 1985.

2   Briggs D, Seah MP (Eds.). *Practical Surface Analysis*, Vols. 1 and 2, 2nd ed. New York: John Wiley and Sons Ltd., 1990.

3   Ratner BD. Surface structure and properties. In Williams DF (Ed.), *Concise Encyclopedia of Medical and Dental Materials*. Oxford, UK: Pergamon Press, 1990, 337–346.

4   Ratner BD. Characterization of biomaterial surfaces. In Ratner BD, Hoffman A, Lemons J, Schoen FJ (Eds.), *Biomaterials Science: An Introductory to Materials in Medicine*. San Diego: Academic Press, 1996.

5   Ratner BD. Contemporary methods for characterizing complex biomaterial surfaces. *Clin Mater*, 11 (1992), 25–36.

6   Somorjai, GA. *Chemistry in Two Dimensions–Surfaces*. Ithaca, New York: Cornell University Press, 1981.

7   Adamson, AW. *Physical Chemistry of Surfaces*, 4th ed. New York: Wiley- Interscience, 1990.

8   Horbett TA, Brash JD (Eds.). *Proteins at Interfaces*, Vol. 1. Washington, DC: ACS Press, 1987.

9   Horbett TA, Brash JD (Eds.). *Proteins at Interfaces*, Vol. 2. Washington, DC: ACS Press, 1995.

10 Ratner BD (Ed.). *Progress in Biomedical Engineering, Vol. 6: Surface Characterization of Biomaterials*. Amsterdam: Elsevier, 1988.

11 Kasemo B, Lausmaa J. Surface science aspects on inorganic biomaterials. *CRC Critical Reviews in Biocompatibility*, 4 (1986), 335–380.

Chapter 8

Ceramics and Glasses

William Lacefield
Alexis Clare

NEED AND RELEVANCE

Crystalline ceramics, amorphous ceramics and glass-ceramic materials represent an important group of materials used increasingly in implantology because of their unique properties. These materials range from high strength ceramics such as aluminum oxide to minimal-load-bearing materials such as the bioglasses. The biological response to these materials varies widely, resulting in the different types of ceramics being classified as anywhere from inert to bioactive. A full characterization of biomedical materials is needed in order to either predict their chance of success in a particular application or to correlate their performance to specific structural and chemical properties. Of primary importance from a biological standpoint is the nature of the surface of the implant that is presented to the surrounding tissues. For biomedical applications, the surface properties of the materials used are of greater importance than in practically any other application of materials; thus, full characterization of the surface becomes of critical importance. Properties and characteristics of the ceramic biomaterial's surface, such as chemistry, energy, rate of ion release, charge, texture and others have a profound influence on both the initial and long-term tissue response to the implant. Also, in some cases, the presence of organic species, foreign films and deposits, such as adsorbed proteins and contaminants on the surface of ceramic implant materials, are of primary interest and must be detected and identified.

Ceramic surfaces are becoming more a subject of surface analysis, although for the standard load bearing implant ceramics such as aluminum oxide and zirconium oxide, the surface composition is much closer to the bulk composition than is the case for metals and alloys. An example of a useful surface characterization would be the determination of what surface features and properties of single crystal aluminum oxide (sapphire) to explain why this material elicits a different response in the body as compared to the polycrystalline variety of the same composition. Another class of ceramic materials, the calcium phosphates, are widely used as particulate and for coating dental and medical implant devices. The primary starting material used for coatings is hydroxylapatite (HA), although the resulting coating may have a structure and properties quite different for dense, crystalline HA, and may vary from the outer to inner portion of the coating [1]. In this case, as in many other biomedical applications, a full characterization is indicated in order to correlate in vitro and in vivo properties.

FACTORS AFFECTING TESTS AND EVALUATION METHODS

As surface analysis is concerned with just the outer layers of materials and devices, proper handling and selection of the specimen to be analyzed is critical. It is desirable to analyze the actual implant specimens or other biomaterials in the same condition as they will be used in the body; for example, after sterilization procedures (see Chapter 15). If in vitro test specimens are being analyzed, it is important to prepare specimens so that replication of the actual implant surface is achieved. The surface should be processed in the same manner as the implant, with the same surface texture, heat treatment, and sterilization method (depending on which treatments are applicable). In some cases it may be necessary to subject the test specimen to a simulated physiologic solution at 37°C, at the correct pH and possibly containing proteins, if a relevant surface condition is desired. For retrieved in vivo specimens, proper handling is critical to preserve surface characteristics, especially when the goal of the analysis is to quantify adherence of molecules, detect contaminants, or observe fragments of the adjacent tissue layer.

During characterization of porous ceramic materials, such as those derived from the hydrothermal conversion of coral to hydroxylapatite, it is important to remember that surfaces exposed to the environment within the body and to bone or soft tissue typically extend to within the internal cavities of these types of implants. Another consideration is that the surface of the biomaterials may be changing with time, either as a result of the dissolution of material or the addition of materials from solution by reprecipitation or attachment of proteins or other biologic molecules. Factors which affect the attachment of proteins and other organic molecules to ceramic surfaces are the surface charge, zeta potential, specific energy, roughness and chemistry.

TESTS AND EVALUATION METHODOLOGIES

There are a number of characterization techniques which provide valuable information about the bulk (non-surface) condition of a material, and it may be useful to consider whether these techniques can also provide accurate surface information under certain conditions. For example, the structure and composition of a hydroxylapatite coating on a metal implant is commonly determined by a X-ray diffraction (XRD) and Fourier transform infrared analysis (FTIR) [2]. Even when providing compositional and structural information for these relatively thin coatings (typically 50 μm), XRD and FTIR in their common forms are considered to be bulk analysis techniques because the data obtained are from depths on the order of 1 μm below the true surface of the coating. Examples of bulk techniques which have been modified in order to make them useful for surface analysis are given in the following sections (see also Chapter 1). The rationale and techniques behind some of the surface analysis methods described in detail in Chapter 7 will not be discussed again in this chapter, but selected examples of the use of those methods in the analysis of ceramic materials will be provided.

X-ray Diffraction

X-ray diffraction (XRD), although not promoted for surface analysis, can provide some useful information about surface conditions when used in a glancing mode involving low incidence and refraction angles. In this technique a beam of X-rays of known wave length (for example, Cu Kα) is passed through the bulk or particles of the specimen, yielding a diffraction pattern characteristic of the material. The resulting pattern can be matched with a computer file catalog to confirm identity of the primary phase of the material. Extra peaks present in the material can then be noted and matched with suspected materials. The presence of amorphous material can be determined by the bulge in the baseline of the pattern. This technique has been shown to be valuable for determining the relative crystallinity of plasma sprayed hydroxylapatite coatings [3], the identification of secondary calcium phosphate phases in both powders and coatings [4], and the detection of apatite phases deposited on bioactive glass-ceramics [5]. Some peak shifting or broadening can be

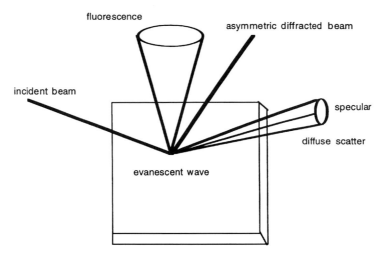

Figure 8-1 Summary of glancing angle X-ray methods (after Bowen and Wormington).

expected with specimens which are strained, thus giving information on the state of stress of the material. Limitations include the difficulty in distinguishing between amorphous, microcrystalline or poorly crystalline material.

Figure 8-1 provides a summary of methods in which XRD can be used for surface analysis [6]. The key point in all of these modifications to the basic technique is that the use of a "glancing angle" X-ray beam reflects from the specimen surface just in the way that a stone skims the surface of a pond. There are two basic ways of carrying this out, one of which is based on the fact that the refractive index of short wavelength (high energy) X-rays for most materials is slightly less than 1. In certain cases where X-rays are incoming at an angle below a "critical angle," total external reflection is observed which is entirely equivalent to total internal reflection. Generally the high refractive index medium is the air, whereas the low refractive index medium is the material. Under specific conditions there is an exponentially decaying electric field component dictated by the density and composition of the reflecting medium, and this variation can be used to provide surface data. As long as the wavelength of radiation used is far from the fluorescent absorption edge of all of the constituents in the material, one can determine the density at the surface by back-calculating the refractive index from measurement of the critical angle [7].

Most materials do not have simple, one-layer surfaces; they may have discreet surface layers, and, like light, X-rays reflected from the surfaces of two layers will interfere and can provide information regarding these layers and their composition. This can be achieved by examining the X-ray intensity at angles beyond the critical angle, without total external reflection, but actually penetrating the sample in a way that is determined by the absorption coefficient of the elements in the sample and hence composition-dependent. This technique is not limited to just one layer; it can be easily extended for up to five layers, and, in addition, the slope of the decay itself can be accessed to give information about surface roughness [7].

Infrared Analysis—Attenuated Total Reflectance

In the infrared (IR) analysis technique, compositional information is obtained by bombarding a specimen with an infrared beam and then monitoring the output of waves. Only the vibrational modes of atomic combination or molecules are determined using this technique. For example, when using Fourier transform infrared analysis (FTIR) on hydroxylapatite

—$(Ca_{10} PO_4)_6(OH)_2$—only the PO_4 and OH groups vibrate to produce the output that can be detected. FTIR is widely used to determine the degree of dehydroxylation of plasma sprayed hydroxylapatite coatings as a result of the high temperature coatings operation, since XRD is not able to provide this information [1]. IR techniques can also be used to determine the degree of HA crystallinity, when proper standards are available, by assessment of changes in phosphate adsorbtion in the 900–1200 cm^{-1} region of the IR spectrum [8].

The infrared technique utilizes the permanently polarized molecules (asymmetrical vibrational modes) of a specimen for determining composition, whereas a related technique, Raman analysis, measures changing polarization of molecules (symmetrical vibrational modes). Raman spectroscopy has been used to determine the surface reactions on bioactive glasses [9], the structure of calcium phosphate powders [10, 11] and the nature of coatings prepared by ion sputtering [12] and plasma spraying.

Standard FTIR gives information on phases present in a material, but generally provides data from a depth in excess of what would be considered the true surface layer. One form of FTIR known as attenuated total reflection (ATR) can provide information confined to the surfaces and interfaces of materials. This technique is used for characterization of ceramic and glass specimens which are difficult to analyze with standard IR spectroscopy, such as films, fibers, powders and pastes.

The principle behind ATR is that the incident infrared beam undergoes reflection as it passes the interface of two media possessing different densities (as described in Chapter 7). Total internal reflection can occur with specific materials of the proper geometry. ATR-FTIR has been used successfully for analyzing various ceramic surfaces such as thin sputtered coatings, with specific applications including the quantification of protein adsorption [13]. Samples can be analyzed in either liquid or air. Liquid samples can be studied using a liquid flow cell, while solids such as threads, fabric, fibers, paste powders, suspensions and collagen can be pressed against the surface of a substrate. In addition to being used in FTIR spectroscopy, the ATR technique has also been employed in conjunction with Raman spectroscopy and fluorescence spectroscopy [14].

Limitations of the ATR-FTIR technique include the very restricted specimen size and type in some cases. Ceramic materials can be studied by this method, but they usually must be deposited on the surface of a single crystal substrate. Quantitative information on protein attachment and confirmation can be obtained under only limited circumstances, usually requiring the necessity of using a substrate crystal of known parameters (e.g., germanium) with only a thin layer (usually well under 1 μm) of the surface of interest in order to get proper data collection [15]. For example, to determine protein attachment and conformation on a calcium phosphate surface using this technique, the material would have to be deposited (perhaps by sputtering) as a thin film (e.g., 25 nm) onto a single crystal [16]. In this example, it is not likely that the surface being tested would correspond exactly to an implant surface. Another problem is that heat treating or further processing in an attempt to create a surface more similar to that of a typical implant may result in damage to the germanium crystal.

Electron Spectroscopy for Chemical Analysis (ESCA)

One of the most valuable of the surface techniques is ESCA or electron spectroscopy for chemical analysis [17]. This technique is also known as X-ray photoelectron spectroscopy (XPS), another name for the same process of bombarding of a material specimen with X-rays and collecting and counting the electrons which are released.

Calcium phosphate powders and coatings can be characterized using ESCA in a nondestructive manner, and the surface composition can be related to bulk composition if a calibration curve is obtained [18].

Auger Electron Spectroscopy

Auger electron spectroscopy (AES) is a valuable tool for surface analysis of biomaterials. Data on surface composition is obtained by collection of the low-energy electrons released from the surface of a material as a result of bombardment of the specimen with electrons. This technique has been used to determine the nature of the surface on bioactive glasses and other calcium phosphate ceramics [19].

Secondary Ion Mass Spectrometry (SIMS)

A technique which is especially useful in identifying compounds and molecules from a surface is known as secondary mass spectrometry or SIMS. In this analysis method, only positive and negative ions are collected, thus providing important information about clusters of molecules rather than individual atoms. The beam which bombards the specimen surface in this technique consists of ions, not electrons or X-rays. These ions are usually generated from a source such as a liquid metal [20].

Advantages of the use of SIMS over other surface techniques is that all elements, including hydrogen, can be identified. Although SIMS is not generally used as often for determining the structure of ceramic materials as it is for polymers, this technique is especially useful for indentifying the composition of thin organic films, contaminants, adsorbed monolayer and adsorbed proteins on ceramics and glasses. Its advantages include a very rapid analysis time with high sensitivity and the capability of providing a semiquantitative determination of molecular structure.

Ellipsometry

Ellipsometry is a surface analysis technique which consists of the bombardment of a materials by polarized light followed by measurement of the resulting ellipse [21]. Some of the specific uses of ellipsometry for crystalline ceramics and glasses include the characterization of thin films on surfaces, including adsorbed gases, self-assembled monolayers and surfactants. As polarized light is used to bombard the specimen, there is no surface damage with this technique. The sensitivity is quite high for most of the applications for which this technique is typically used.

Scanning Tunneling Microscopy

As described in Chapter 7, a technique called scanning tunneling microscopy (STM) can be used to obtain compositional information on a very small (atomic size) scale [22]. An advantage of STM is that the specimens need not be in vacuum, as many analyses are conducted either in air or liquid. One limitation of STM for ceramic materials is that the surfaces need to be coated with a conducting material, as a current flow must develop between the probe and the surface.

Atomic Force Microscopy

The atomic force microscopy (AFM) technique is similar to STM and useful for surface imaging and wear studies of ceramic materials in addition to the metallic and polymeric analyses described in Chapter 7 [23]. AFM is based upon the principle of force detection since no electron flow is possible with non-conducting surfaces such as are characteristic of ceramic materials. This technique can be used equally well on either conductive or non-conductive surfaces, as it measures the repulsive/attractive forces associated with the surface under the probe. A major advantage of AFM is that it does not require high vacuum and use high energy beams like electron microscopy, and thus those materials that would be damaged under those circumstances are usually amenable to AFM. Care must be taken during specimen preparation and image processing to avoid misleading conclusions brought about by incorrect identification of artifacts.

Less Frequently Used Surface Composition Techniques

Optical spectroscopy to a certain extent can elucidate surface composition of ceramic materials. UV-visible reflectometry may reveal electronic structure and the presence of absorbing species such as rare earth and transition metals and is especially useful for strongly fluorescing species [24]. Diffuse reflectance infrared spectroscopy (DRIFTS) may provide some useful information, but generally probes too deeply into the structure to be considered a true surface analysis technique.

A combination of electron spectroscopy and vibrational techniques is used in EELS (electron energy loss spectroscopy), where electrons are reflected from the surface of the sample with altered energy profiles due to interactions with the surface of the sample; thus vibrational energy levels can be accessed [25]. This technique provides useful information on the composition and orientation of organic and other groups on surfaces.

A modification of the EXAFS (extended X-ray absorption fine structure) technique can be used for surface analysis by targeting a particular atomic type by focusing at the absorption edge for that atom [26]. Fine structure appears on the edge as a result of interference between the photoelectron ejected and the component of its wavefunction scattered from first neighbor atoms. These data may be Fourier transformed to obtain information regarding the pair distribution function of surface atoms. An alternative to this technique is low-energy electron diffraction or LEEDS [27]. LEEDS patterns give the surface order and the thickness of the surface layer, and can also be used to access defects in the surface such as steps or irregularities. However, data analysis and interpretation is somewhat difficult with this method.

Electron Microscopy

The widely used technique of scanning electron microscopy (SEM) has proven to be a valuable tool for determining surface morphology and texture of ceramic materials such as plasma sprayed coatings [28–30]. This technique utilizes a detector, photomultiplier, cathode ray tube and associated equipment to produce an image from the secondary electrons created by bombarding a specimen with a beam of electrons in vacuum [31–33]. Because of the large depth of field images characteristic of SEM, a topographical image of surface features can be readily obtained. SEM provides much more surface information than does another imaging method, light microscopy (LM), because of its better resolution, greater depth of field, and absence of light scattering on the surface. A modified LM technique, confocal microscopy, shows more promise than the conventional LM method for surface topographical analysis (see also Chapter 13). In this technique, high intensity light is reflected from the surface into a special detector which is usually hooked to an image processor [34]. Resolutions of up to 0.2 μm laterally and 0.4 μm vertically may be obtained, and specimens may be examined wet, dry or immersed in oil.

Compositional information of the actual surface of a specimen is generally not possible with the energy dispersive (EDS) or wave length dispersive (WDS) X-ray analysis systems which are commonly found on SEM. The penetrating nature of the X-rays means that information is collected to a depth that would be characteristic of the bulk material, not the true surface. In general, only if an Auger analysis system is used in conjunction with the SEM could the compositional information obtained be considered to be representative of the surface of the specimen only. However, an AES system is not typically found on an SEM because of the higher vacuum requirements of quantitative Auger analysis.

One problem associated with SEM is the damage to the biomaterial that may occur because of the energetic electrons and/or the high vacuum associated with the process [35]. Also, non-conducting biomaterials such as ceramics must be coated with a conducting layer to prevent charging by the electron beam; in certain cases this may alter somewhat the surface features of interest prior to observation.

Field emission microscopy (FEM) and its successor field ionization microscopy (FIM) have been reasonably well used as characterization tools for conductive biomaterial surfaces [36]. The former technique relies on a potential difference being applied between the sample, which has been etched to a sharp point, and a fluorescent screen. The emitted electrons hit the screen, causing the emission of light. The relative ease with which electrons are emitted depends upon the surface structure of the material. In FIM the potential is reversed between the sample and the screen; detection is secondary via the introduction of helium which is ionized by the protruding atoms on the irregular surface of the biomaterial. If the tip is cooled to $20°K$ resolution on an atomic scale can be achieved. In both cases these techniques require an inconvenient modification of the sample shape; there are now more advanced techniques in which his modification is not required.

Surface Profilometry

Another aspect of biomaterials which is of great importance in some applications is surface texture [37]. Texture in this usage implies a particular pattern of roughness which may or may not be consistent over the entire surface of the biomaterial (see Chapter 13). Information on the surface texture or surface roughness of a material is of importance in a number of biomedical devices. For example, the surface texture of an aluminum oxide implant may influence the interface with surrounding bone and degree of interlocking of bone and implant, the surface roughness of a hydroxylapatite coating may determine its push-out strength, and the plaque accumulation on a dental ceramic crown may be influenced by surface texture.

Other uses of a profilometer include the measure of the thickness of a surface film (such as a sputter deposited calcium phosphate coating) which has a discreet boundary with the remaining surface. In this instance, the stylus can be passed from the film onto the uncoated surface and the drop-off distance can be measured with the profilometer.

Surface Charge Measurement

The charge on an implant biomaterial may be an important factor in cases involving the attachment of proteins and organic molecules to the surface. There are various ways an implant can obtain a charged surface, such as by rubbing, contact with a charged material, or deposition of a charged species in vivo. Surface charge buildup on the surface is generally a factor for ceramic surfaces but not for metallic and carbon (graphite) surfaces which have the ability to dissipate charges. An example of a charged implant surface is a typical

HA coating on titanium, in which the negative charge on the ceramic surface apparently influences the type and quantity of proteins attracted to these surfaces.

The zeta potential of a surface is based on its charge, and can be calculated using measurements of the streaming potential obtained in a properly constructed in vitro experimental setup [38]. In a typical system, a sodium-chloride electrolyte is flowed past the surface of a specimen, and the streaming potential and pressure drop along short segments of the specimen are measured simultaneously. The zeta potential is influential in creating the double layer effect observed on some implant materials in solution, and can influence the type and adsorption rate of proteins on the surface.

Surface Energy Measurement

The energy of a crystalline ceramic or glass surface may be measured by looking at the way in which specific molecules adsorb [39]. For example the adsorption of a particular type of molecule can be determined by dividing the number of adsorption sites occupied by the number of sites available, and the rate at which adsorption or desorption took place can also be calculated. The latter may be monitored by the examination of gas flow rates in and out of a chamber containing the material, or alternatively a previously exposed sample may be heated instantaneously and the rise in pressure due to desorption noted; however, in the latter case care must be taken that the sample is not desorbing. The same effects may be observed in thermogravimetric analysis where the sample is monitored on a microbalance while thermal desorption occurs, but then again care must be taken not to compromise the sample. Lastly, these effects may also be accessed by radiotracing. Isotherm measurements may also give surface area information [40].

The most popular and the simplest way to estimate the surface energy is to measure the contact angle between the substrate and liquids of known surface tension with the equation:

$$\cos \phi_c = \{\gamma_{sg} - \gamma_{sl}\}\gamma_{lg}$$

where γ is the surface energy and the liquid gas interaction is known and the solid/gas interface is required [41]. A goniometer is typically used to measure the contact angle. Limitations of this approach are that this technique is subject to varying results due to differences in such factors as surface roughness, specimen curvature, operator ability, contaminants and progressive alterations of the test surface or liquid which occur during testing.

RECOMMENDATIONS AND CONCLUSIONS

Surface analysis is now recognized as an important aspect of the testing and evaluation for all types of inert and bioactive ceramic implant materials. The driving force behind the surface analysis of implant devices, in particular, is often a desire to obtain full characterization of a surface so that the information can be used to precisely correlate surface parameters to the observed in vivo performance, and thus provide the basis for better implant design and performance. The techniques for surface characterization and evaluation of ceramic materials referred to in this chapter are those most widely used at this time, but further advances and modifications of existing techniques are quite probable as the field of surface science continues to evolve. All of the current techniques have their limitations, which often necessitate the use of two or more analysis methods in order to obtain the desired characterization of the surface.

Important factors to consider in evaluation of biomaterials, as in any other type of analysis, include accuracy, speed and cost. There are low-cost methods, such as contact angle measurements, which can provide qualitative information about a surface and may be entirely satisfactory as quality control techniques requiring relatively low investment either in equipment purchases or in time. More quantitative techniques, such as Auger or ESCA, involve hundreds of thousand of dollars in basic equipment costs, and often require the services of a trained technician to operate. Their use, however, may be justified for research applications requiring precise compositional information, or where full characterization is needed for certification, quality control or other purposes.

There is often the temptation to use existing bulk techniques such as XRD and FTIR to obtain surface chemistry and structure if no true surface analysis techniques are readily available. As pointed out in this chapter, only with modifications of these techniques, usually requiring different or additional equipment, is it possible to obtain accurate surface information.

One of the best solutions for companies, universities and individuals wishing to overcome the high costs of some types of surface analysis is to investigate the possibility of shared equipment, often available with a user's fee which reflects such factors as maintenance and personnel costs. It is not unusual for universities, especially within the same state or region, to share usage of expensive equipment or even to plan purchases to avoid duplication of equipment within the region. Currently, researchers in the biomaterials field are fortunate to have a surface analysis resource established (by an NSF grant) at the University of Washington to provide a wide range of surface analysis techniques (ESCA, SIMS, ellipsometry, etc.). This is an option that should be considered for suitable biomaterials projects [42].

REFERENCES

1   Kim CS, Ducheyne P. Compositional variations in the surface and interface of calcium phosphate ceramic coating on Ti and Ti-6A1-4V due to sintering and immersion. *Biomaterials*, 12 (1991), 462–469.

2   Lacefield WR. Hydroxylapatite coatings. In Hench LL, Wilson J (Eds.), *Introduction to Bioceramics*. Singapore: World Scientific Publishing Company, 1993, 223–238.

3   Chen J, Wolke JGC, de Groot K. Microstructure and crystallinity in hydroxyapatite coatings. *Biomaterials*, 15 (1994), 396–399.

4   Ducheyne P, Van Raemdonck W, Heughebaert JC, Heughebaert M. Structural analysis of hydroxyapatite coatings on titanium. *Biomaterials*, 7 (1986), 97–103.

5   Kokubo T, Ito S, Huang ZT, HayashT, Sakka S, Kitsugi T, Yamamuro T. Ca, P-rich layer formed on high-strength bioactive glass-ceramic A-W. *J Biomed Mater Res*, 24 (1990), 331–343.

6   Bowen DK, Wormington M. In Gilfrich JV, Huang TC, Hubbard CR, James MR, Lachance GR, Smith DK, Predecki PK (Eds.), *Grazing Incidence X-Ray Characterization of Materials in Advances in X-Ray Analysis*. New York: Plenum Press, 1993, 171–184.

7   LaPuma PJ, Snyder RL, Zdzieszynski S, Bruckner R. Characterization of the Sn diffusion layer in the surface of float glass using grazing incidence X-ray reflectometry and fluorescence. In Schaeffer HA (Ed.), *Fundamentals of Glass Science and Technology, Proc Third Conf European Society of Glass Technology, Wurzburg, Germany, 1994*, 68.

8   Pleshko N, Boskey A, Mendelsohn R. Novel infrared spectroscopic method for the determination of crystallinity of hydroxyapatite minerals. *Biophysical Society*, 1991, 786–793.

9   Rehman I, Hench LL, Bonfield W, Smith R. Analysis of surface layers on bioactive glasses. *Biomaterials*, 15 (1994), 865–870.

10 Bertoluzza A, Simoni R, Tinti A, Morocutti M, Ottani V, Ruggeri A. Calcium phosphate materials containing alumina: Raman spectroscopical, histological, and ultrastructural study. *J Biomed Mater Res*, 25 (1991), 23–38.

11 Sauer GR, Zunic WB, Durig JR, Wuthier RE. Fourier transform Raman spectroscopy of synthetic and biological calcium phosphates. *Calcif Tissue Int*, 54 (1994), 414–420.

12 Chen TS, Lacefield WR. Crystallization of ion beam deposited calcium phosphate coatings. *J Mater Res*, 9 (1994), 565–574.

13 Skoog DA, Leary JJ. *Principles of Instrumental Analysis*. Fort Worth, TX: Saunders College Publishing, 1992, 252–295.

14 Mirabella FM, Harrick NJ. *Internal Reflection Spectroscopy: Review and Supplement*. Harrick Scientific Corporation, 1985.

15 Watkins RW, Robertson CR. A total internal reflection technique for the examination of protein adsorption. *J Biomed Mater Res*, 11 (1977), 915–938.

16 Zeng H, Chittur KK, Lacefield WR. Albumin adsorption on hard tissue replacement biomaterials. *Trans Fifth World Biomaterials Congress*, New York: John Wiley & Sons, 1996.

17 Ratner BD, Castner DR. In Vickerman JC, Reed NM (Eds.), *Electron Spectroscopy for Chemical Analysis in Surface Analysis—Techniques and Applications*. Chichester, UK: John Wiley and Sons, 1996.

18 Briggs D, Seah MP. *Practical Surface Analysis by Auger and X-ray Photoelectron Spectroscopy*. Chichester, UK: John Wiley & Sons; 1983, 41.

19 Ducheyne P, Healy KE. Surface spectroscopy of calcium phosphate ceramic and titanium implant materials. In Ratner BD (Ed.), *Surface Characterization of Biomaterials*. Amsterdam: Elsevier Scientific, 1988, 175–192.

20 Walls JM, Ionex VG. *Methods of Surface Analysis*. Cambridge, UK: Cambridge University Press, 1989, 13–14.

21 Tompkins HG. *A User's Guide to Ellipsometry*. New York: Academic Press, Inc., 1993.

22 Ito E, Takahashi T, Hama K, Yshioka T, Mizutani W, Shimizu H, Ono M. An approach to imaging of living cell surface topography by scanning tunneling microscopy. *Biochem Biphys Res Comm*, 177 (1991), 636–643.

23 Lal R, John SA. Biological applications of atomic force microscopy. *Am J of Phys*, 266 (1994), C1–21.

24 Good RJ, Stromberg RR, Patrick RL. In *Techniques of Surface and Colloidal Chemistry and Physics, Vol 1*. New York: Marcel Dekker, 1968.

25 Egerton RF. *Electron Energy Loss Spectroscopy*. New York: Plenum Press, 1986.

26 Strozier JA, Jepson, DW, Jona F. *Surface Physics of Materials, Vol 1*. New York: Academic Press, 1975, 56–73.

27 Murr, LE. *Electron Optical Applications in Material Science*. New York: McGraw-Hill, 1970, 267–272.

28 Maxian SH, Zawadsky JP, Dunn MG. *In vitro* evaluation of amorphous calcium phosphate and poorly crystallized hydroxyapatite coatings on titanium implants. *J Biomed Mater Res*, 27 (1993), 111–117.

29 Zyman Z, Weng J, Liu X, Zhang X, Ma Z. Amorphous phase and morphological structure of hydroxyapatite plasma coatings. *Biomaterials*, 14 (1993), 225–228.

30 Huaxia J, Marquis PM. Effect of heat treatment on the microstructure of plasma-sprayed hydroxyapatite coating. *Biomaterials*, 14 (1993), 64–68.

31 Goldstein JI, Newbury DE, Echlin P, Joy DC, Romig AD, Lyman CE, Fiori C, Lifshin E. *Scanning Electron Microscopy and X-ray Microanalysis*, 2nd ed. New York: Plenum Press, 1992.

32 Hayet MA. *Principles and Techniques of Electron Microscopy: Biological Applications*, 3rd ed. Boca Raton, FL: CRC Press, 1989, 377–378.

33 McCormack SM, Tormo FJ, Featherstone JD. A straightforward scanning electron microscopy technique for examining non-metal coated dental hard tissues. *Scanning Microsc*, 5 (1991), 269–272.

34 Danilatos GD. Bibliography of environmental scanning electron microscopy. *Microsc Res Tech*, 25 (1993), 529–534.

35 Wilson T, Sheppard C. Theory and Practice of Scanning Optical Microscopy. London: Academic Press, 1984, 1–4.

36 Morrison JR. *The Chemistry and Physics of Surfaces*. New York: Plenum Press, 1977.

37 Hutchings IM. *Tribology: Friction and Wear of Engineering Materials*. Boca Raton, FL: CRC Press, 1992, 4–7.

38 Ducheyne P, Kim CS, Pollach SR. The effect of phase differences on the time-dependent variation of the beta potential of hydroxyapatite. *J Biomed Mater Res* 26, 147–168.

39 Busscher HJ, Arends J. Determination of the surface forces γ^D and γ^P from contact angle measurements on polymers and dental enamel. *J Colloid Interface Sci*; 81 (1980), 75–79.

40 Andrade JD, Smith LM, Gregonis DE. The contact angle and interfacial energetics. In Andrade JD (Ed.), *Surface and Interfacial Aspects of Biomedical Polymers*. New York: Plenum Press, 1985, 249–292.

41 Zisman WA. Relation of the equilibrium contact angle to liquid and solid constitution. In Gould R (Ed.), *Contact Angle, Wettability, and Adhesion*. Washington, DC: American Chemical Society, 1964, 1–51.

42 University of Washington, Surface Analysis Recharge Center, Department of Chemical Engineering, Box 351750, Seattle, WA 98195.

ADDITIONAL READING

1   Kangasniemi IM, Vedel E, de Blick-Hogerworst J, Yli-Urpo AU, de Groot K. Dissolution and scanning electron microscopic studies of Ca,P particle-containing bioactive glasses. *J Biomed Mater Res*, 27 (1993), 1225–1233.

2   Filgueiras MR, La Torre G, Hench LL. Solution effects on the surface reactions of three bioactive glass compositions. *J Biomed Mater Res*, 27 (1993), 1485–1493.

3   Kieswetter K, Bauer TW, Brown SA, VanLente F, Merritt K. Characterization of calcium phosphate powders by ESCA and EDXA. *Biomaterials*, 15 (1994), 183–188.

4   Skoog DA, Leary JJ. *Principles of Instrumental Analysis*. Fort Worth, TX: Saunders College Publishing, 1992, 252–295.

5   Harrick NJ. *Internal Reflection Spectroscopy*. New York: Interscience Publishers, 1967.

6   Zyman Z, Weng J, Liu X, Li X, Zhang X. Phase and structural changes in hydroxyapatite coatings under heat treatment. *Biomaterials*, 15 (1994), 151–155.

7   Siegbahn K. Electron spectroscopy for atoms, molecules, and condensed matter. *Science*, 217 (1982), 111–121.

8   Berkowitz J. *Photoabsorption, Photoionization, and Photoelectron Spectroscopy*. New York: Academic Press, 1979.

9   Seah MP, Dench WA. Quantitative electron spectroscopy of surfaces: A standard data base for electron inelastic mean free paths in solids. *Surf Interface Anal*, 1 (1979), 2–11.

10 Ratner BD. The surface characterization of biomedical materials: How finely can we resolve surface structure? In Ratner BD (Ed.), *Surface Characterization of Biomaterials*. Amsterdam: Elsevier, 1988, 13–36.

11 Adamson AW. *Physical Chemistry of Surfaces*, 5th ed. New York: John Wiley & Sons, 1990, 330–337.

12 Toa N, Lindsay SM, Lee S. Measuring the microelastic properties of biological material. *Biophys J*, 63 (1992), 1165–1169.

13 Boland T, Ratner BD. Direct measurement by atomic force microscopy of hydrogen bonding in DNA nucleotide bases by atomic force microscopy. *Proc Natl. Acad. Sc. USA*, 92 (12) (1995), 5297–5301.

14 Eliades T, Lekka M, Eliades G, Brantley WA. Surface characterization of ceramic brackets: A multitechnique approach. *Am J Ortho & Dentofac Orthopedics*, 105 (1994), 8–10.

15 Ruse ND, Smith DC. Adhesion to bovine dentin—Surface characterization. *J Dent Res*, 70 (1991), 1002–1008.

Chapter 9

Corrosion and Biodegradation

Jack E. Lemons
Ramakrishna Venugopalan
Linda C. Lucas

NEED AND RELEVANCE

Over the past decades, quantitative analyses of basic biomaterial properties have been utilized to better optimize biocompatibility profiles for surgical implant devices. Correlations between results from preclinical and clinical investigations have provided critical comparisons of cause-effect relationships between the synthetic material properties and longer-term device function [1–10]. These activities have extended to materials-science-based investigations of the surfaces of explanted prostheses, specifically, the phenomena associated with biodegradation, the chemical and biochemical degradation of implant surfaces.

Since one of the primary goals of studies on biodegradation has been to improve the functional and longitudinal aspects of surgical implants, investigations have been extended to device-to-tissue interfaces and the overall host interactions. Biocompatibility has been described by Williams [11] as an appropriate response of a material intended for a specific application, and therefore research into biodegradation phenomena has been strongly influenced by clinical applications.

Many of the methodologies described in this chapter have evolved because of clinical applications in which multiple designs and materials are combined to achieve improved functional outcomes. Clearly, these outcomes have quite different bases, especially if one compares medical and dental reconstructive procedures. For load-bearing musculoskeletal devices, mechanical aspects necessitate stronger biomaterials. Therefore, most are metallic alloys with secondary utilizations of ceramic and polymeric components. Since corrosion is best understood with respect to metallic conductors, basic methodologies and interpretations for metallic biomaterials [12–13] will be presented in detail, while those for other classes of biomaterials will be summarized.

TEST METHODS

Metals and alloys proposed for implant systems can be evaluated using both *in vitro* direct current (DC) and alternating current (AC) or impedance electrochemical test methods.

DC Techniques

DC electrochemical techniques can be divided into pontentiostatic, potentiodynamic, galvanostatic and galvanodynamic methods. During an earlier era of non-automated test systems, common current-potential measurements like anodic polarization, polarization resistance and Tafel plots were obtained using potentiostatic techniques. Most modern electrochemical test systems can conduct these measurements using potentiodynamic (controlled potential) scanning techniques.

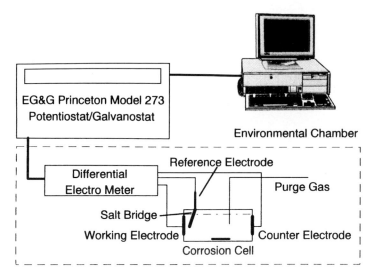

Figure 9-1 DC corrosion experimental configuration.

A schematic drawing of an automated potentiostat/galvanostat system is shown in Figure 9-1. The system consists of an IEEE 488.2 bus compatible potentiostat/galvanostat, a personal computer, a corrosion test cell chamber, electrodes (working/test, counter and reference), a Luggin probe/saltbridge, electrolyte solution, and atmosphere/temperature control systems. The system shown in Figure 9-1 has been standardized to ASTM [14]. Any changes to the components previously described necessitate re-standardization. Test specimens used for corrosion studies are prepared to appropriate surface finish.

Various electrolyte solutions (ranging from 0.9% saline solution to solutions containing other inorganic and organic additives) can be used to simulate a tissue fluid electrolyte solution [15–21]. The pH of the electrolyte solution varies based on electrolyte composition. The electrolyte solution can be oxygenated or deoxygenated by purging it with the appropriate gas. Tests are routinely conducted at $37 \pm 1°C$.

A schematic potentiodynamic polarization curve is shown in Figure 9-2 [22]. This curve is generated by scanning from cathodic potentials more active than the corrosion potential to anodic potentials more noble than the corrosion potential at a scan rate of 0.17 mV/sec [22]. The scan is then reversed and continued till the reverse scan crosses over the forward scan to generate a current-potential plot. Qualitatively, the current-potential plot can be divided into active, passive and transpassive regions [12, 23]. The active region is the region where corrosion increases with increasing applied potential. The passive region represents the state in which an alloy is deliberately passivated prior to surgical implantation. The transpassive region is that part of the plot where the applied potential is large enough to cause breakdown of the oxide/passivation layer.

In Figure 9-2, a linear region exists at a potential approximately 50 mV more active than the corrosion potential or more noble than the corrosion potential. In order to obtain the corrosion rate (I_{corr}) of this material, the linear region is extrapolated to the corrosion potential (E_{corr}). The accuracy of the Tafel method of extrapolation [24, 25] matches or exceeds the accuracy of conventional weight loss methods. However, to ensure accuracy of this method, the linear region must extend over a current range of at least one order of magnitude. For materials having more than one electroactive redox couple, the Stern-Geary [24, 26] current equation, which is a modified theory based on Tafel extrapolation, is used

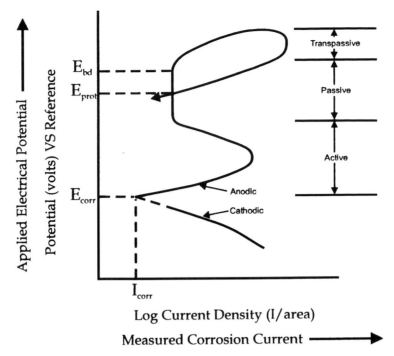

Figure 9-2 Schematic cyclic polarization curve.

to obtain the corrosion rate (I_{corr}). The Stern-Geary equation predicts that in a system with two electroactive redox couples,

$$I(E) = I_{corr}[10(E - E_{corr})/\beta a - 10(E_{corr} - E)/\beta c],$$

where E is the applied potential at any point in time and I is the measured current for E, β_a is the oxidation rate, and β_c is the reduction rate. The Stern-Geary equation also predicts that at potentials greater than E_{corr}, the anodic reaction predominates, while at potentials less than E_{corr}, the cathodic reaction predominates. On solving the equation one can observe that when $E = E_{corr}$, the value for I is zero. This does not mean that the system cannot actively corrode. It merely means that the anodic current exactly balances the cathodic current at E_{corr}. The I_{corr} is thus the magnitude of the current that flows in equal but opposite directions at E_{corr}.

The appearance of a knee shape [12, 23] in the cyclic cathodic and anodic polarization curve is used to determine the breakdown potential (E_{bd}) of the material. The E_{bd} is the least noble potential where pitting or crevice corrosion, or both, will initiate and propagate. This knee shape in Figure 9-2 means that for a small increment in applied potential there is a large increase in the measured current, signifying a breakdown of the surface oxide or the passivation layer. The potential at which the reverse scan crosses over the forward scan is called the protection potential (E_{prot}). The E_{prot} is the most noble potential where pitting or crevice corrosion will not propagate [22]. If the E_{bd} and the E_{prot} are the same, there will be no tendency to pit. If the E_{prot} is more noble than the E_{bd}, there will be no pitting. If the E_{prot} is more active than the E_{bd}, pitting may occur. Between the E_{prot} and the E_{bd}, pits already existing can propagate, but new pits cannot be formed. The area included in the loop formed by the scan between the E_{bd} and the E_{prot} is called the hysteresis. The size of

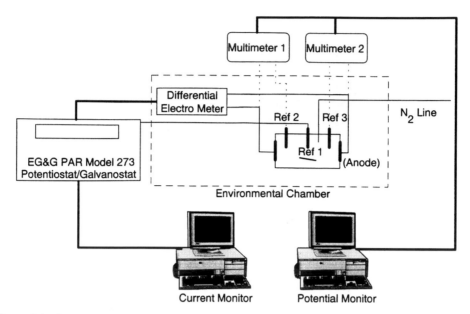

Figure 9-3 Experimental configuration for galvanic corrosion testing.

this hysteris is a rough indication of the susceptibility of a material to pitting corrosion. For specific details regarding such corrosion evaluations, the reader is referred to the citations of such work at the end of this chapter [27–42].

Various techniques have been developed for direct measurements of combinations (galvanic corrosion) of alloys [21, 27, 43–48]. These techniques are based on the theory of zero resistance ammetry. Most commercially available potentiostats/galvanostats can be modified to perform as zero resistance ammeters. The specific techniques for modification can be determined by discussion with the manufacturer. Figure 9-3 shows a corrosion test system for measuring the corrosion characteristics of an alloy couple [27].

Any alloy combination will have a cathode and an anode. The current flow ($I_{couple\ corr}$) between the anode and the cathode, because of galvanic (two metal) coupling, can be measured using the instrumentation shown in Figure 9-3. A schematic of the data generated for determining $I_{couple\ corr}$ is shown in Figure 9-4. The value for the $I_{couple\ corr}$ can be obtained

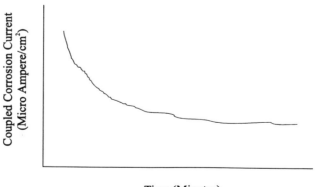

Figure 9-4 Schematic for coupled corrosion current measurement.

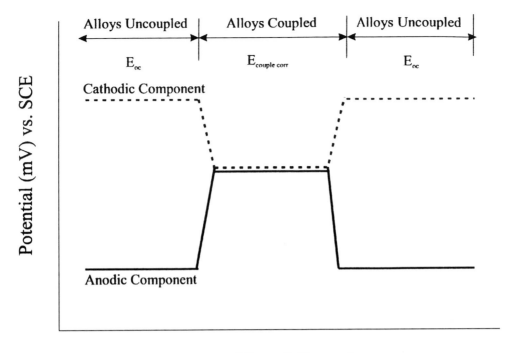

Figure 9-5 Schematic for coupled corrosion potential measurement.

by finding the y-intercept of the mid-point in the transition region of the current curve before it reaches negligible steady state values [27]. The current can also be integrated with respect to time to obtain the cumulated charge expressed during the test cycle [21].

Further additions to the galvanic corrosion measurement technique include continuous monitoring [27] of the open circuit potential ($E_{\text{o.c.}}$) of both components prior to coupling, the common coupled corrosion potential ($E_{\text{couple corr}}$) during coupling, and the $E_{\text{o.c.}}$ of both components after coupling. The coupled corrosion current ($I_{\text{couple corr}}$) as previously described is also monitored during coupling. A schematic illustrating the data acquired during such coupling experiments is shown in Figure 9-5.

No discussion of specific data obtained during such evaluations is included here for the sake of brevity. However, such techniques have been proposed and facilitate development of a profile for an acceptable couple combinations [21, 27, 43–48]. An example of such a profile is as follows: (1) the difference in $E_{\text{o.c.}}$ of the two materials and the coupled corrosion rate $I_{\text{couple corr}}$ should be as small as possible; (2) the $E_{\text{couple corr}}$ of the couple combination should be significantly lower than the E_{bd} of the anodic component; and (3) the repassivation properties of the anodic component of the couple should also be acceptable, defined as the absence of a large hysteresis.

DC techniques involving potentiostatic measurements are also used to determine diffusion coefficients of dissolved materials in solution, repassivation potentials, and repassivation rates. Galvanostatic (constant current) techniques are also used to determine passivation rates and to gauge thickness of passive films or electroplated layers [12, 23]. Galvanodynamic (controlled current) techniques can be used in place of their potentiodynamic counterparts. The galvanodynamic approach is required in systems which have a fluctuating, long-term, open circuit potential drift. A review of recent literature also reveals that a combination of the various techniques may be used to obtain specifically relevant results [49–53].

AC Techniques

Impedance electrochemical test systems can provide precise, error-free kinetic and mechanistic information [54–59] using a variety of techniques and output formats (Nyquist plots, Bode plots, Randles plots, etc.). This method can be used to make measurements in low conductivity solutions where DC techniques are subject to potential-control errors [60]. Furthermore, impedance systems can be used to determine the uncompensated resistance (R_Ω) of the electrochemical cell. Impedance techniques use waveforms of very small excitation voltage (5 to 10 mV peak-to-peak). Thus, the electrochemical test system is disturbed minimally because of the test technique [61, 62].

The primary advantage of impedance techniques is that a purely electronic circuit model can be used to represent an electrochemical system [59, 63–68]. Thus, an impedance (Z) plot obtained for an electrochemical system can be used to verify a mechanistic model or at least omit incorrect models. One can correlate physical or chemical properties with circuit elements and also extract deterministic values to the various components of the model by fitting the model to the data. Figure 9-6 shows a typical three-circuit element, Randles equivalent circuit. The simple three-circuit model is valid for a range of surface types involving titanium, Ti-6Al-4V, Co-Cr-Mo and 316L stainless steel [49, 55]. R_Ω is the uncompensated resistance of the electrolyte between the working and the reference electrodes, and R_p is the polarization or the charge transfer resistance at the working electrode/electrolyte interface. C_{dl} is the specific double-layer capacitance at the working electrode/electrolyte interface.

Nyquist Plot   A typical Nyquist (Cole-Cole) plot for the Randles cell is illustrated in Figure 9-7. The Nyquist plot is a plot of imaginary component of the impedance (Z'') against the real component of the impedance (Z'). The high frequency intercept, the uncompensated resistance (R_Ω), and the low frequency intercept, sum of R_Ω and R_p, can be used to determine R_p. The corrosion current density is obtained using the Stearn-Geary equation:

$$I_{corr} = (\beta_a \beta_c)/(2.3 R_p A_t (\beta_a + \beta_c)),$$

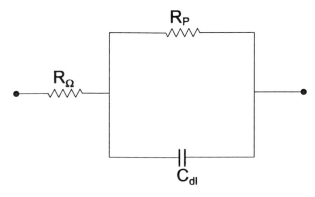

Figure 9-6   Schematic for three-element Randles equivalent circuit

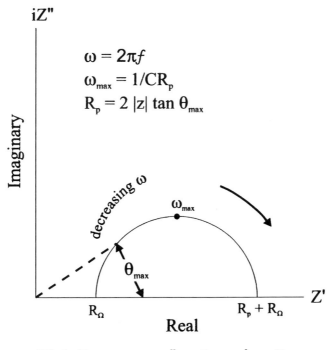

$$\omega = 2\pi f$$
$$\omega_{max} = 1/CR_p$$
$$R_p = 2\,|z|\,\tan\theta_{max}$$

High Frequency: $z'' \to 0 \Rightarrow z' \to R_\Omega$

Low Frequency: $z'' \to 0 \Rightarrow z' \to R_\Omega + R_p$

Figure 9-7 Nyquist plot for Randles equivalent circuit.

where β_a and β_c are the anodic and cathodic Tafel slopes, respectively, and A_t is the true electrode surface area. The angular frequency at the top of the Nyquist plot semicircle (ω_{max}) is used to determine the double-layer capacitance (C_{dl}). The primary advantage of using the Nyquist plot is that the effect of series circuit elements (like R_Ω) are explicitly illustrated. Furthermore, the shape of the Nyquist semicircle does not change with change in R_Ω. This is very advantageous when developing new corrosion cell configurations with limitations due to sample shape and size. The primary disadvantage of the Nyquist plot is that the frequency does not appear explicitly [60]. Consequently the C_{dl} can be calculated only after the frequency information is obtained. Also in electrochemical reactions having two rate-determining steps, i.e., two cell constants, the high impedance circuit signature will dwarf the low impedance circuit signature because of plot scaling (Figure 9-8) [60, 65, 66].

Bode Plot   The Bode plot ($\log|Z|$ vs. $\log\omega$ or Θ vs. $\log\omega$) illustrated in Figure 9-9 has several distinct advantages over the Nyquist plot. The primary advantage is that the frequency data appear on one axis, making it easy to understand the dependence of impedance on frequency. The Bode format is desirable when data scatter at the low frequency end prevents adequate fitting of the Nyquist semicircle. Also, in systems having two time constants, the Bode plot format (Figure 9-10) facilitates easy determination of the break points associated with the low impedance and high impedance circuits, thus overcoming the plot scaling problems associated with Nyquist plots [60, 65, 66]. However, the Nyquist plot obtained over the frequency range of 0.001 Hz to 10000 Hz provides a comprehensive first look at the behavior of most electrochemical systems.

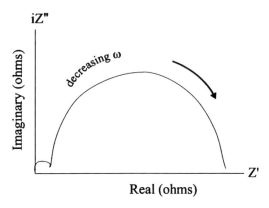

Figure 9-8   Nyquist plot for a cell with two time constants.

Other Plot Formats   Other useful plot formats are the plots of Z' vs. $\omega Z''$ and the capacitance plot (Y''/ω vs. Y'/ω). The admittance Y is the inverse of the Z. The Z' vs. $\omega Z''$ plot for a Randles cell allows for easy determination of the R_Ω, R_p and C_{dl} values using a straight line and slope intercepts on the y axis. The capacitance plot is used to emphasize electrochemical reactions with circuit elements in parallel. Various other plot formats are also used to analyze very specific aspects of impedance behavior of complex electrochemical systems [60, 69].

Equivalent Circuit Models   More complex circuit element models (than the one shown in Figure 9-7) can be used to model the material being tested [69, 70]. El-Basiouny and Mazhar [71] suggested a more complex model (Figure 9-11) for titanium, which is a

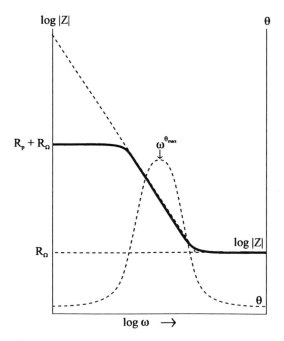

Figure 9-9   Bode plot (log Z vs. log ω or θ vs. log ω) format for Randles circuit.

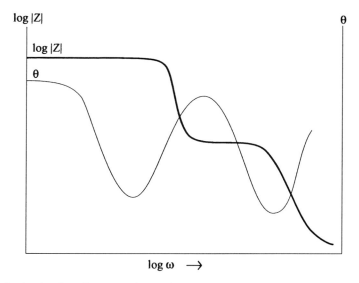

Figure 9-10 Bode plot (log Z vs. ω and Θ vs. log ω) for a two time-constant cell.

series combination of two parallel resistive-capacitive circuits representing two oxide coatings, an amorphous structure over a rutile (TiO_2) inner layer. Figure 9-12 is a representative equivalent circuit for a metal substrate coated with a porous, non-conductive film [63, 65, 67]. The additional circuit elements are the coating capacitance (C_c), the pore resistance (R_{po}), and the charge transfer resistance (R_{ct}).

The rate of any electrochemical reaction can be strongly influenced by diffusion of a reactant towards or a product away from the electrode surface. When such diffusion completely dominates the reaction mechanism, the impedance obtained is called a diffusion

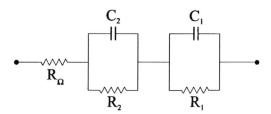

Figure 9-11 Equivalent circuit for titanium with its surface oxides.

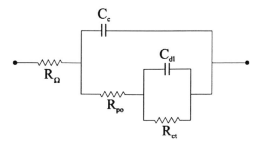

Figure 9-12 Equivalent circuit for metal substrate with porous non-conductive coating.

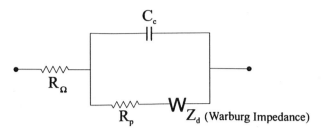

Figure 9-13 Equivalent circuit with Warburg diffusion element.

or Warburg impedance. Complex equivalent circuits [72, 73] can be constructed to explain such specific conditions that vary with the factors controlling corrosion. An example of this is the circuit illustrated in Figure 9-13 with the Warburg diffusion element (Z_d). A Nyquist plot manifesting charge transfer control and diffusion control is illustrated in Figure 9-14.

Impedance techniques are extremely versatile and can be used to determine changes in surface area and hence current density due to microscopic and macroscopic plastic deformation. Separating cause mechanisms for stress enhanced ion release (SEIR) phenomenon into passive film disruption and area changes caused by plastic deformation can also be accomplished using impedance techniques [49].

DEGRADATION OF CERAMICS AND POLYMERS

With regard to degradation of synthetic biomaterials, metals and graphite substrates differ from non-conductors such as high purity ceramics (aluminum and zirconium oxides, calcium phosphates and aluminates, and glasses and glass-ceramics) and high molecular weight polymers (polyethylene, polymethylmethacrylate, polydimethylsiloxane,

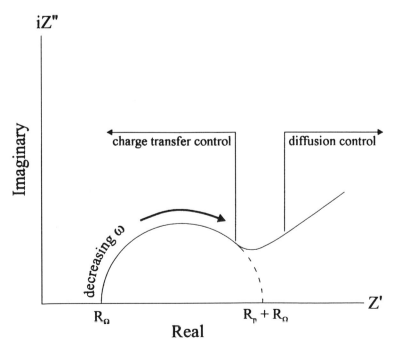

Figure 9-14 Nyquist plot manifesting charge transfer and diffusion control.

polytetrafluoroethylene and polyethyleneterephylate) [74–79]. The ceramics are crystalline and amorphous structures with predominately ionic bonds. Polymers are structures with primarily covalent atomic bonds. Therefore, environmental interactions within saline solutions can only be partially described by basic electrochemical theories. Physical-chemical properties and dissolution information must therefore be utilized to analyze the interactions between non-electrical conductors and tissues. Also, ceramics are brittle and exhibit no strain capacities beyond the elastic limit (rupture strength), while most of the polymeric biomaterials exhibit considerable plasticity (elongations) prior to mechanical fracture. Therefore, strain and residual stress characteristics are important considerations related to the biodegradation of metals and polymers, but are secondary for most ceramics [76–79].

Compared to other materials, the high density and purity ceramics such as aluminum and zirconium oxide are the most chemically stable of the biomaterials [80]. This inherent environmental characteristic is a result of the higher energy ionic bonds within the atomic structure plus the fact that these structures exist within a higher-order state of oxidation (e.g., Al_2O_3 and ZrO_2) [81]. In contrast, the calcium phosphates and aluminates are subject to chemical-biochemical dissolution, which is a strong function of local acidity [82]. Lower pH environmental conditions (e.g., in the presence of infection and inflammation) can result in active dissolution phenomena. On the more positive side, under normal physiological conditions, limited solubility has been directly associated with favorable aspects of bioactivity and biointegration [83, 84]. Glasses and glass ceramics exhibit similar properties, although the phosphate-rich surface zones have properties of a localized siliceous-gel reaction product [85]. Because of the complex nature of ceramic, glass, and glass-ceramic interactions with tissues and tissue fluids, chemical dissolution testing is normally accomplished through longer-term exposures within balanced and appropriately buffered simulated tissue fluids at $37 \pm 1°C$. Aliquots of solution are removed for elemental component analyses, and systems have now evolved to balance the solution chemistries (elements, temperature, flow) to better represent in vivo conditions. The in vitro analysis of environmental reactions of ceramics has evolved to a significant level, and a considerable literature exists that is specific to in vitro and in vivo analyses of bioceramic chemical properties [85].

Polymeric biomaterials usually have relatively lower biomechanical strengths and most exhibit substantial plasticity before fracture (100s of percent elongations) [86]. The average molecular weight and molecular weight distributions of polymerics have been shown to strongly influence biodegradation characteristics. This literature has expanded in recent years because of concerns about a combination of mechanical fretting (wear) and chemical interactions that have resulted in particulates (debris). The proceedings of a 1996 conference on polyethylene biomaterials provide detailed information on biodegradation phenomena [86]. Polymers, in general, are very stable under static biomechanical conditions, with most concerns about biodegradation focusing on lower molecular weight fractions as leachables. Also, there are possibilities of hydrolytic- and enzymatic-based degradations of regional polymer chain bonding sites. This has been a focus within the polydimethylsiloxane (silicone) polymers, especially with the prostheses that combine polymer and gel components. Once again, most emphasis has been on debris and particulates, plus the surface and bulk interactions between these forms and local and systemic tissue responses.

Analyses of polymers related to environmental degradation have been similar to those of the ceramic biomaterials, mostly depending on longer-term exposures within simulated tissue fluids at $37 \pm 1°C$. The degradation products from polymers in solution have been evaluated through mass and other spectrochemical analyses. Also critical to interpretations are the analyses of surface and bulk characteristics for pre- and post-environmental exposure specimens. To understand the environmental interactions, characterization of the biomaterials is necessary.

ANALYSES OF EXPLANTED DEVICES

A number of conferences, their associated proceedings, and now national and international standards have emphasized the value of analyses of explanted devices [10]. One area of emphasis has been corrosion of constructs, especially when device designs have utilized different alloys (galvanic interactions), combinations of alloys, ceramics and polymers, porous surfaces for tissue ingrowth, and surface modifications (ion implantation, anodizing, coatings, etc.; see Chapter 12) to enhance biomechanical and biochemical properties [87–89].

Investigations of devices, tissue, and tissue interfaces that have demonstrated unanticipated changes require special attention to assure specimen and sampling validity. These type specimens should not be pre-cleaned or pre-manipulated until examination is completed with a stereomicroscopic system (1–60x), coupled with sample collection for extended microscopy or spectroscopy studies as indicated. Available standards are specific in this regard and review is recommended prior to conducting studies on explanted devices [80]. Most importantly, preliminary stereomicroscopic examinations can lead to opinions about what might have caused the unanticipated features. However, confounding variables most often preclude quantitative analyses by observation alone, because of inadequate numbers of replicates, insufficient information about the conditions at the time of implantation, or incomplete records about function. More information is needed to establish cause-effect relationships. Therefore, investigators utilize these observations to develop hypotheses about what might have caused alterations in the devices. This normally leads to extended in vitro investigations, such as described previously, to determine the cause(s) (mechanisms) of the characteristics observed. Studies of explants, plus in situ specimens within cadavers that may represent successful applications, are very important to the assessment of the applicability of many in vitro methodologies. To further explain the interrelationships among several of these studies, the observations, tissue conditions, and clinical circumstances will be briefly reviewed.

Dental implants are often used as single or multiple site reconstructions and reconstructions are generally interconnected through an intraoral bridgework [90]. Different metals and alloys used for the implants, abutments, and bridgework necessitate mixed metal or galvanic corrosion evaluation [2, 3, 17, 18]. Clinical studies have shown preferential corrosion of stainless steel and carbon dental implant constructs with associated tissue reactions converting bone to granulation tissue, leading to their clinical loss [91]. In vitro investigations of these materials have demonstrated susceptibility to galvanic-type corrosion phenomena [2, 3, 17, 18, 92–94]. In general, analyses of explanted devices have shown minimal alterations (corrosion and biodegradation) for static combinations of titanium and titanium alloy, titanium and cobalt alloys, and titanium or cobalt systems when combined with carbon or intraoral bridges of noble gold or palladium alloys [2, 3, 90, 91]. Adverse observations have been associated with some stainless steel implants if combined with carbon, titanium and cobalt alloys, and some gold and palladium alloys [3, 91]. Similar circumstances were observed when nickel-chromium-beryllium crown and bridge alloys were placed in direct contact with titanium dental implant systems [17, 18, 28]. In selected circumstances, when the more active (anodic) components have been isolated from significant tissue fluid or saliva contact, enhanced corrosion has not been a significant observation or concern.

Most importantly, basic methodologies for evaluating corrosion or biodegradation phenomena have shown strong correlations with short- and long-term observations from investigations of clinical explants, tissues, and clinical outcomes. One of the advantages of combining in vitro laboratory investigations as an extension of questions raised from evaluations of explanted devices is the opportunity to better understand the value of retrospective analyses. These inputs therefore can be most important to establish more complete prospective protocols for extended in vitro and in vivo investigations.

RECOMMENDATIONS

A wide variety of in vitro methodologies currently exist to evaluate the corrosion and biodegradation of synthetic biomaterials. This type of information is required as one part of early investigations of safety and efficacy specific to surgical implant devices. Experience has shown that appropriate in vitro experiments can be predictors of longer-term interactions within a wide range of host (in vivo) environments. Importantly, the laboratory test series must include adequate simulations, so that the pre-clinical results will provide the basic data for eliminating inappropriate materials, combinations of materials within devices, or designs that may compromise the chemical-biochemical stability of any components.

When properly tested, synthetic biomaterials should minimally biodegrade and within host tolerance over the longer term. The goal should always be an appropriate lifetime of functional stability. Preclinical testing should assure, as best possible, no harm to the device and no harm to the host, which defines biocompatibility.

REFERENCES

1   Weinstein A, Gibbons D, Brown S, Ruff W (Eds.) *Implant Retrieval: Material and Biological Analysis*. NBS Special Pub. 601, Washington, DC: U.S. Printing Office, 1981.

2   Schnitman PA, Shulman LB (Eds.). *Dental Implants: Benefit and Risk*. PHS Pub. No. 81-1531, 1980.

3   Rizzo AA (Ed.) Proceedings of the 1988 Consensus Development Conference on Dental Implants. *J Dent Ed*, 52 (1988), 678–827.

4   Fraker AC, Griffin CD. *Corrosion and Degradation of Implant Materials: Second Symposium, ASTM STP 859*. Philadelphia, PA: American Society for Testing and Materials, 1985.

5   Syrett BC, Acharya A, (Eds.). *Corrosion and Degradation of Implant Materials, ASTM STP 684*. Philadelphia, PA: American Society for Testing and Materials, 1979.

6   Lemons JE. Device Retrieval and Analysis. Special Symposium on Orthopaedic Devices, AAOS Symposium, Atlanta, GA, 1984.

7   Lemons JE. Metallic corrosion and biodegradation in in vitro and in vivo environments. In Lin O, Chao E (Eds.), *Perspectives in Biomaterials*. Amsterdam: Elsevier, 1986, 245–253.

8   Retrieval and analysis of surgical implants and biomaterials. *Transactions, Society for Biomaterials Symposium*, Snowbird, UT, 1988.

9   Total Hip Replacement, NIH Consensus Conference. JAMA, 273, 1950–1956, 1995.

10 IDR[3] —Implant Data: Record, Report, *Review*, Society for Biomaterials Conference Proceedings, Buffalo, NY, 1996 (in press).

11 Williams DF (Ed.). An introduction to medical and dental materials. In *Concise Encyclopedia of Medical and Dental Materials*. Oxford: Permagon Press, 1991.

12 Fontana MG. *Corrosion Engineering*. New York: McGraw-Hill, Inc., 1986, 325–346.

13 Baboian R (Ed.). *Corrosion Tests and Standards: Application and Interpretation, Manual 20*. Philadelphia, PA: American Society for Testing and Materials, 1995.

14 Standard practice for conventions applicable to electrochemical measurements in corrosion testing. *In Annual Book of ASTM Standards: Metals, Test Methods and Analytical Procedures*, Vol 03.02. Philadelphia, PA: American Society for Testing and Materials, 1995, 30–37.

15 Bumgardner JD, Lucas LC. Surface analysis of nickel chromium dental casting alloys. *Dent Mat*, 9 (1993), 252–259.

16 Fusayama T, Katayori T, and Nomoto S. Corrosion of gold and amalgam placed in contact with each other. *J Dent Res*, 42 (1963), 1183–1197.

17 Johansson BI, Lemons JE, and Hao SQ. Corrosion of dental copper, nickel and gold alloys in artificial saliva and saline solutions. *Dent Mat*, 5 (1989), 324–328.

18 Johansson BI, Lucas LC, Lemons JE. Corrosion of copper, nickel, and gold dental casting alloys: An *in vitro* and *in vivo* study. *J Biomed Mater Res*, 23 (1989), 349–361.

19 Marek M. Measurement of metal ion release from biomedical implant alloys. Mechanical-Electrochemical interaction of passivating alloys used in medicine. In *Proc of the Symposium on Compatibility of Biomedical Implants, Vol. 94-15*. The Electrochemical Society, Inc., 1994, 73–84.

20 Meyer JM, Nally JN. Influence of artificial salivas on the corrosion of dental alloys. *J Dent Res*, 54 (1975), Abstract No. 76, 678.

21 Reclaru L, Meyer JM. Study of corrosion between titanium implant and dental alloys. *J Dent*, 22 (1994), 159–168.

22 Standard reference test method for making potentiostatic and potentiodynamic anodic polarization measurements. In *Annual Book of ASTM Standards: Metals, Test Methods and Analytical Procedures, Vol 03.02*. Philadelphia, PA: American Society for Testing and Materials, 1995, 48–58.

23 Shrier LL, Jarman RA, Burstein GT (Eds.). *Corrosion*. Oxford: Butterworth-Heinemann Ltd., 1995.

24 Stern M, Geary AL. Electrochemical polarization, I. A theoretical analysis of the shape of polarization curves. *J Electrochem Soc*, 104 (1957), 56–63.

25 Stern M. Electrochemical polarization, II. Ferrous-ferric electrode kinetics on stainless steel. *J Electrochem Soc*, 104 (1957), 559–563.

26 Stern M. Electrochemical polarization, III. Further aspects of the shape of polarization curves. *J Electrochem Soc*, 104 (1957), 645–650.

27 Venugopalan R. Development of test methods and instrumentation to measure galvanic corrosion in vitro. Master of Science thesis, University of Alabama at Birmingham, Birmingham, AL, 1995.

28 Lucas LC, Lemons JE. Biodegradation of restorative metallic systems. *Adv Dent Res*, 6 (1992), 32–37.

29 Williams DF. Titanium and titanium alloys. In Williams DF (Ed.), *Biocompatibility of Clinical Implant Materials, Vol. I.*, Boca Raton, FL: CRC Press, 1981, 11–42.

30 Ong JL, Lucas LC, Raikar GN, Gregory JC. Electrochemical corrosion analysis and characterization of surface-modified titanium. *App Sur Science* 72 (1993), 7–13.

31 Covington JS, McBride MA, Slagle WF, Disney AL. Beryllium localization in base metal dental castings. *J Biomed Mater Res*, 19 (1985), 747–750. .

32 Gregory DO. Nickel-chromium alloys in casting. *Miss Dent Assoc J*, 38 (1982), 18–20.

33 Ravhnholt G, Jensen J. Corrosion evaluations of two materials for implant supraconstructions coupled to a titanium implant. *Scand J Dent Res*, 99 (1991), 181–186.

34 Bundy KJ, Williams CJ, Leudemann RE. Stress-enhanced ion release: The effect of static loading. *Biomaterials*, 12 (1991), 627–639.

35 Gilbert JL, Samuel SM, Lautenschlager EP. Scanning electrochemical microscopy of biomaterials: Reaction rate and ion release modes. *J Biomed Mater Res*, 27 (1993), 1357–1366.

36 Tiara M, Lautenschlager EP. In-vitro corrosion fatique of 316L cold worked stainless steel. *J Biomed Mater Res*, 26 (1992), 1131–1139.

37 Gilbert JL, Buckley CA, Lautenschlager EP. Mechanical-electrochemical interaction of passivating alloys used in medicine. *Proc Symposium on Compatibility of Biomedical Implants, Vol. 94–15*. The Electrochemical Society, Inc., 1994, 319–330.

38 Buck BP. Impedance of thin and layered systems: Cells with even or odd number of interfaces. *Annals of Biomedical Engineering*, 20 (1992), 363–383.

39 Bundy KJ, Dillard J, Leudemann R. Use of AC impedance methods to study corrosion behavior of implant alloys. *Biomaterials*, 14 (1993), 529–536.

40 Lemaitre L, Moors M, Peteghem AP. A mechanistic study of the electrochemical corrosion of g_2 phase in dental amalgam, II. Introduction of a model. *J Oral Rehab*, 16 (1989), :543–548.

41 MacDonald DD. *Transient Techniques in Electrochemistry*. New York: Plenum Press, 1977.

42 MacDonald JR. Impedance spectroscopy. *Annals of Biomedical Engineering*, 20 (1992), 289–305.

43 Mansfeld F. Recording and analysis of AC impedance data for corrosion studies. *Corrosion, NACE 36* (1981), 301–307.

44 Technical Notes AC1-AC5. EG & G Princeton Applied Research. Electrochemistry Division, Princeton, NJ, 1989, 1990.

45 Franceschetti DR, Macdonald JR. Small-signal A-C response theory for electrochromic thin films. *J Electrochem Soc*, 129 (1982), 1754–1756.

46 Glarum SH, Marshall JH. An A-C admittance study of platinum/sulphuric acid interface. *J Electrochem Soc*, 126 (1977), 424–430.

47 Kendig M, Mansfeld F, Tsai S. Determination of the long-term corrosion behavior of coated steel with AC impedance measurements. *Corrosion Science*, 23 (1983), 317–329.

48 Lemaitre L, Moors M, Peteghem AP. A model for corrosion behavior of dental amalgams. *J Biomed Mater Res*, 23 (1989), 241–252.

49 Mansfeld F, Kendig MW, Tsai S. Evaluation of corrosion behavior of coated metals with AC impedance measurements. *Corrosion, NACE*, 38 (1982), 478–485.

50 Mansfeld F, Kendig MW, Tsai S. Recording and analysis of AC impedance data for corrosion studies, II. Experimental approach and results. *Corrosion, NACE*, 39 (1982), 570–586.

51 Mansfeld F, Kendig MW. Electrochemical impedance spectroscopy of protective coatings. *Werkstoffe und Korrosion*, 36 (1985), 473–483.

52 Sluyters JH. On the impedance of galvanic cells, I. Theory. *Recueil*, 79 (1960), 1092–1100.
53 El-Basiouny MS, Mazhar AA: Electrochemical behavior of passive layers on Ti. *Corrosion, NACE*, 38 (1982), 5.
54 De Levie R. The admittance of the interface between a metal electrode and an acqueous electrolte solution: some problems and pitfalls. *Annals of Biomedical Engineering*, 20 (1992), 337–347.
55 Mansfeld F, Lee CC, Kovacs P. Application of eletrochemical impedance spectroscopy (EIS) to the evaluation of corrosion behavior of implant materials. *Proc of the Symposium on Compatibility of Biomedical Implants, Vol. 94-15*. The Electrochemical Society, Inc., 1994, 59–72.
56 Vincenzini P (Ed.). *Ceramics in Surgery*. New York: Elsevier, 1983.
57 Oonishi H, Aoki H, Sawai K. *Bioceramics*. St. Louis: EuroAmerica, Inc., 1989.
58 Morrey BF (Ed.). *Biological, Material, and Mechanical Considerations of Joint Replacement, a Bristol-Myers Squibb/Zimmer Orthopaedic Symposium Series*. New York: Raven Press, Ltd., 1993.
59 Morrey BF (Ed.). *Total Joint Arthroplasty*. New York: Churchill Livingston, 1991.
60 Petty W (Ed.). *Total Joint Replacement*. Philadelphia: W. B. Saunders, 1991.
61 Cameron H (Ed.). *Bone Implant Interface*. St. Louis: Mosby, 1994.
62 *Annual Book of ASTM Standards, Emergency Medical Devices and Services, Vol. 13.01*. Philadelphia, PA: American Society for Testing and Materials, 1995.
63 Griss P, Krempien B, von Andrian-Werburg H, Heimke G, Fleine R, Diehm T. Experimental analysis of ceramic-tissue interactions. *J Biomed Mater Res*, 5 (1971), 39–48.
64 Ducheyne P, Lemons JE (Eds.). Bioceramics: Material characteristics versus in vivo behavior. *Annals of the New York Academy of Science*, Vol. 523, 1988.
65 Lacefield WR. Hydroxyapatite coatings. In Ducheyne P, Lemons JE (Eds.), Bioceramics: Material characteristics versus in vivo behavior. *Annals of the New York Academy of Science*, Vol. 523 (1988), 72–80.
66 deGroot K (Ed.) *Bioceramics of Calcium Phosphate*. Boca Raton, FL: CRC Press, 1983.
67 Yamamuro T, Hench L, Wilson J (Eds.). *Handbook of Bioactive Ceramics, I and II*. Boca Raton, FL: CRC Press, 1990.
68 Wright T, Goodman S (Eds.). Implant wear: The future of total joint replacement. *AAOS and NIH Symposium Proceedings*, Am Assoc of Orthop Surg Pub, Rosemont, IL, 1996.
69 Lemons JE (Ed.). *Quantitative Characterization and Performance of Porous Implants for Hard Tissue Applications, ASTM STP 953*. Philadelphia, PA: American Society for Testing and Materials, 1987.
70 Hockman R, Solnick-Legg H, Legg K. *Ion Implantation and Plasma Assisted Processes*. Metals Park, OH: ASM International, 1988.
71 Lucas LC, Lee JE, Lemons JE. In vitro corrosion investigations of TiN coated and nitrogen implanted Ti-6Al-4V alloy. *Orthopaedic Research Society Transactions*, 10 (1985), 323.
72 Misch CE (Ed.). *Contemporary Implant Dentistry*. St. Louis: CV Mosby, 1991.
73 Vitredent Root Replacement System, Product Information, Vitredent Corporation, Los Angeles, CA, 1973.
74 Thompson NG, Buchanan RA, Lemons JE. In vitro corrosion of Ti-6Al-4V and type 316L stainless steel when galvanically coupled with carbon. *J Biomed Mater Res*, 13 (1979), 35–44.
75 Buchanan RA, Lemons JE, Griffin CD, Thompson NG, Lucas LC. Effects of carbon coupling on the in vitro corrosion of cast surgical cobalt-base alloy. *J Biomed Mater Res*, 15 (1981), 611–614.
76 Lucas LC, Buchanan RA, Lemons JE. Investigations on the galvanic corrosion of multi-alloy total hip prosthesis. *J Biomed Mater Res*, 15 (1981), 731–747.

ADDITIONAL READING

1 Williams DF. *Concise Encyclopedia of Medical and Dental Materials*. Oxford: Pergamon Press, 1991.
2 Fontana MG. *Corrosion Engineering*. New York: McGraw-Hill, Inc., 1986.
3 Baboian R. *Corrosion Tests and Standards: Application and Interpretation, Manual 20*. Philadelphia, PA: American Society for Testing and Materials, 1995.
4 Technical Notes AC1–AC5. EG & G Princeton Applied Research, Electrochemistry Division, Princeton, NJ.
5 Shrier LL, Jarman RA, Burstein GT. *Corrosion*. Oxford: Butterworth-Heinemann Ltd., 1995.
6 Bard AJ, Faulkner LR. *Electrochemical Methods: Fundamentals and Applications*. New York: John Wiley and Sons, 1980.
7 MacDonald DD. *Transient Techniques in Electrochemistry*. New York: Plenum Press, 1977.
8 MacDonald JR. *Impedance Spectroscopy: Emphasizing Solid Material Systems*. New York: John Wiley and Sons, 1987.

Chapter 10

Friction and Wear

Martine LaBerge
John B. Medley
Jonette M. Rogers-Foy

INTRODUCTION

Investigators have been studying friction and wear phenomena for centuries. However, it was not until 1966 in a report published by the British Department of Education and Science that the studies of friction, lubrication and wear were officially integrated into a science, henceforth to be known as tribology [1]. Since this time, tribology has became a well established discipline in science and engineering and can be defined as the "science of interacting surfaces in relative motion including its related practices" [1]. Of the three interrelated phenomena, frictional behavior and wear resistance are the most commonly characterized parameters for biomaterials applications.

The study of friction involves the determination and characterization of static and kinetic coefficients of friction as well as frictional torque for a contact. The physical phenomena influencing friction include, but are not limited to, the direction and magnitude of relative motion between the surfaces in contact, the applied load, the environmental conditions such as type of lubricant and temperature, the topography of the surfaces (see Chapter 13), and the material properties of the contacting bodies.

While friction involves forces acting across a contact in the direction of sliding, wear involves how these forces act to remove material from the surfaces. Higher friction can give lower wear under some circumstances. For example, the separation of surfaces with lubricants of high viscosity often gives higher friction than dry contact while reducing wear significantly. The investigation of wear can include rate, mechanisms, transition between initial and steady-state wear, and generation and geometry of wear debris. Wear is influenced by the entire tribology of the contact, including, for example, the performance of lubricants. However, since ultimately wear is the removal of material from the surfaces, the properties of the materials are usually very important parameters in wear.

The tribological evaluation of biomaterials is a very broad subject. It could include detailed study of the many aspects of tribology such as applying theoretical models, laboratory investigations with devices of both simple and complex configuration, and in vivo studies with animals or humans. However, this chapter concentrates on laboratory studies using devices of simple configuration which can be used to isolate the tribological behavior of biomaterials. The more complex joint simulators are discussed because they are often used to compare biomaterial performance in implants.

CHARACTERIZATION OF
THE FRICTIONAL PROPERTIES

The clinical relevance of friction is applicable for different situations. In fact, the frictional behavior of polymeric biomaterials to be used for endoscopy or catheterization in urinary, tracheal, and cardiovascular tracts is assessed to predict mechanical injury of tissues and to minimize patient discomfort [2]. The characterization of the frictional properties of biomaterials is also assessed for the following applications:

- orthopaedic, especially for artificial joints [3, 4];
- dental, such as restorative materials [5, 6];
- cardiovascular, particularly for use in artificial vessels, valves, and stents [7]; and
- ophthalmological, for contact lenses and intraocular lenses [8–10].

Friction can be measured experimentally but only rarely predicted theoretically, with any accuracy. Friction tests can include the effect of motion of artificial materials on tissue response or tissue damage, the effect of coatings and chemical treatments of implant surface, and the evaluation of lubrication mechanisms.

Frictional Force

Friction is defined as the general resistance to motion experienced whenever a solid body slides over another [11, 12]. Friction is measured as a frictional force which can better be described as a resistive force parallel to the direction of motion. The frictional force (F) is normally proportional to the applied load (L) in a direction opposite to the sliding direction. However, if a surface has directional scratches, as are often observed on machined surfaces, the frictional force may vary from its assigned direction by a few degrees if the motion is at an angle to the direction of the scratches [13].

Two distinct frictional forces can be identified: the static or starting friction and the kinetic or dynamic friction. The static friction is the value of the tangential force required to initiate sliding, while the kinetic friction corresponds to the tangential force required to maintain sliding. Several parameters or variables will affect the frictional force of surfaces in tangential motion (Table 10-1). Each of these parameters must be taken into consideration

Table 10-1   Variables Potentially Affecting the Frictional Behavior of Materials

Variables potentially affecting the frictional behavior of materials [11, 13–15]

Physical Parameters:
    • Relative direction of motion
    • Relative velocity
    • Normal load
    • Contact geometry/area
    • Material properties
    • Interfacial temperature
    • Surface topography
    • Wear particle interaction
    • Atmosphere
Chemical Parameters:
    • Presence of surfactants/surface films
    • Presence of lubricants
    • Surface energy
    • Mutual solubility

when attempting to compare the frictional behavior of materials used in relative tangential motion. The frictional force also depends on the history of sliding, potentially indicating a time-dependent behavior for the kinetic friction [16]. Understanding the frictional behavior of materials is very important because it generally plays a complimentary role ultimately affecting the wear behavior [16].

Friction is a very broad description which can further be differentiated into a variety of types: dry, lubricated, sliding, rolling, hysteretic or viscous [15], just to name a few. Specific conditions applicable to dry friction are that the frictional force is independent of the contact area and sliding speed. This is known as Amontons' Law [17]. To briefly highlight the nature of dry friction, different models have been proposed. In 1987, Ludema summarized the current thoughts and models available for friction analysis in tribology [18]. These models have been derived from the pioneering work of Bowden and Tabor [19] and Rabinowicz [20] on the theory of adhesion, which implies that cold-welded junctions develop at individual asperity contacts due to high pressure and close surface proximity. These junctions are sheared by relative sliding, producing a friction force. Recent models describe the friction force as a combined effect of roughness, asperity deformation, adhesion at junctions and ploughing by asperities [21].

Coefficient of Friction

Typically, friction is described by a coefficient. The coefficient of friction (μ) is defined as the ratio of the tangential or frictional force (F) to the normal force (L)

$$\mu = F/L.$$

For sliding surfaces, the coefficient of friction is due to the combined effect of asperity deformation (μ_d), ploughing by hard surface asperities and/or wear particles (μ_p), and adhesion between the surfaces (μ_a) [16]. The parameters controlling the frictional behavior of materials as listed in Table 10-1 indicate that the coefficient of friction is not a material property. Consequently, friction should not be reported for a material pair without an accurate description of the test parameters. The static (μ_s) and kinetic (μ_k) coefficients of friction correspond to the static or starting frictional force and the kinetic or dynamic frictional force, respectively.

Friction Measurement

Often, the coefficient of friction is obtained by measuring the friction force between a stationary solid rubbing against a moving solid using transducers while applying a normal load with dead weights. Load cells [22] and strain gage arrangements have been used as force transducers [23–26]. Systems used to measure friction may also be used to evaluate the wear of materials.

The static coefficient of friction is calculated using the force required to initiate motion, whereas the kinetic coefficient of friction, which may vary during a test at a constant velocity, is often calculated from averaged force readings over the duration of the test. Frictional force should be acquired with a data acquisition system that allows for continuous recording at a very fast rate. American Society for Testing and Materials (ASTM) Standard G115-93 proposes a guide for "Measuring and Reporting Friction Coefficients" [27] designed to assist investigators in the selection of an appropriate method for measuring the frictional behavior of various materials.

In general, a large discrepancy, or, more precisely, an inconsistency, occurs when friction measurements taken under nominally identical conditions but from different laboratories are compared. This inconsistency occurs because unknown and thus uncontrolled parameters are acting in the friction testing. Therefore, all of the known parameters having any involvement in a particular tribosystem should be noted explicitly when reporting friction measurements in publications. In an attempt to better standardize methods for friction measurements, several standard procedures [27–36] for different materials have been issued by the ASTM.

CHARACTERIZATION OF WEAR PROPERTIES

Wear of biomaterials in implants has been shown to be detrimental to their long-term success, resulting in retrieval and revision. For example, wear of total joint replacements, as stated by Jacobs et al., has emerged as a central problem, limiting their long-term longevity [37]. Ultra high molecular weight polyethylene (UHMWPE) wear particles have been shown by many authors to trigger an osteolytic reaction which leads to implant loosening [38]. Wear of cardiovascular devices is also an important contributor to failure [39].

The wear of surfaces is a process resulting in the progressive loss of material mainly due to mechanical and/or chemical action. Wear involves many diverse mechanisms and phenomena which are often unpredictable. Unfortunately, surface deterioration or wear results from use and therefore cannot be avoided or eliminated, since wear is a direct consequence of two surfaces in relative motion interacting with each other.

Adhesive wear is characterized by the transfer of material from one surface to the other during relative motion. This type of wear is a consequence of adhesive forces acting at the junction of surface asperities. The transferred fragments may either be permanently or only temporarily attached to the other surface. Adhesive wear has been denoted as being the most commonly detected mechanism of wear; unfortunately, it is also the least preventable [40].

Abrasive wear is the result of a hard asperity damaging or ploughing the surface of a softer material. The presence of hard particles may be due to the original material properties of one of the surfaces or loose debris particles which have become entrapped between the two sliding surfaces and/or embedded into one of the surfaces, expediting abrasive wear. Generally, the resistance to abrasion can be related to the hardness of the material; however, this relationship is not directly proportional [11].

Fatigue wear is associated with cyclic stress variations, and the lifetime of the material is therefore dependent on the number of cycles. Cyclic deformation of the contacting surfaces leads to the initiation and propagation of microcracks [41]. Subsurface crack initiation generally occurs in the region of maximum shear stress which will depend upon the geometry of the materials. Both adhesive and abrasive wear can be considered to include fatigue phenomena, in that an individual wear particle may only be detached after repetitive frictional loading. However, the fatigue wear "mechanism" is usually reserved to describe subsurface microcracking leading to delamination, giving somewhat larger wear particles than typically found in adhesive or abrasive wear [42].

Corrosive wear is seen when the environment interacts chemically or electrochemically with one or both of the surfaces. Therefore, the wear rate is dependent on the environmental conditions affecting the chemical reactivity of the surfaces. This type of wear mechanism is important for biomaterials since they function in an extremely harsh environment, the human body.

Biomaterials used in the fabrication of orthopaedic, vascular, dental, and ocular implants are subject to mechanical and chemical constraints resulting in their wear. As such, wear mechanisms can be predominantly governed by the mechanical and/or chemical be-havior of the solids. More often than not, however, the wear processes listed above do not act independently. Realistically, a combination of two or more wear mechanisms may occur simultaneously and/or as a consequence of one another within the applied setting. Even though several mechanisms are involved in the materials wear process, one particular mechanism may be largely responsible for affecting their overall wear rate. The volume of material removed from the surface as a result of the wear processes has been described phenomenologically by different models.

Wear tests have been designed to predict the amount of material removal in specific conditions, compare the effect of different fabrication and sterilization processes, produce wear debris to be used in biocompatibility studies, or simply characterize the behavior of a new material destined for medical applications. To address each of these outcomes, tri-bosystems (pair of materials and their tribological environment and conditions) have to be carefully designed, monitored and evaluated for their applicability to different scenarios.

Wear Testing

The ultimate objective of any wear test is to obtain data on the performance and reliability of specific materials or devices in service conditions [43]. This performance is evaluated by measuring the wear rate of materials functioning in a particular tribosystem. According to Dowson [44], there are two main reasons for performing wear tests. The objective might be to ascertain the basic mechanisms of wear for a particular combination of materials, or to determine the more restrictive yet equally elusive rate of wear to facilitate the estimation of the useful life of the engineering components. Optimally, an experimental protocol aimed at investigating the wear properties of bearing materials must be designed to assess the effect of testing conditions on the materials.

As in friction testing, large differences in wear are reported by different laboratories for apparently identical test conditions. Once again, all possible influencing parameters must be recorded when performing wear tests. Also, ASTM standard protocols pertinent for the evaluation of wear performance of engineering materials are available [45–48]. However, only one ASTM standard procedure [36], entitled "Reciprocating Pin-on-Flat Evaluation of Friction and Wear Properties of Polymeric Materials for Use in Total Joint Prostheses," describes the testing protocol for characterizing the wear resistance of material combina-tions to be used in the design of artificial joints. (In the spring of 1996, a standard procedure was approved, in principle, by ASTM for simulator testing of hip implants and thus should appear eventually in the standards.) Several investigators have used modified or adapted versions of this standard to assess the wear resistance of bearing surfaces for orthopaedic applications [49–56]. The friction and wear behavior of other biomaterials for dental [57–67], cardiovascular [68–73], and ophthalmological [74] applications has also been assessed in the literature. Figure 10-1 summarizes the different steps involved in designing a wear testing protocol for materials. This rather extensive treatment can be modified to address specific research questions.

Selection of a Wear Test Apparatus

The ultimate goal of a wear test is to determine the wear rate (volumetric or linear) of materials in a tribological system which is part of an application of interest. As mentioned previously, it is notoriously difficult to obtain repeatable wear test results because the many

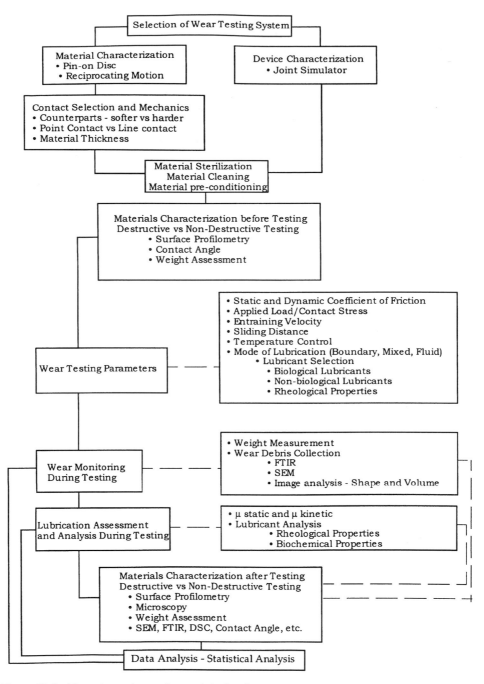

Figure 10-1   Flow chart of experimental design for wear measurement of biomaterials.

influencing variables are difficult to identify and/or control. Furthermore, it seems that there is an underlying random nature to the phenomena. At this point, a distinction must be made between fundamental studies and specific studies of actual components. Fundamental studies are commonly performed with geometrically simple and scaled-down specimen pairs in a kinematically simple apparatus. The general intent was to develop fundamental relationships to allow wear prediction of actual components in a variety of applications, in much the same manner as a tensile specimen allows yield stress to be determined so that the elastic-plastic transition of the same material in various engineering structures can be predicted. However, the many influencing parameters and the underlying random nature of wear prevent predictions of suitable accuracy in most tribological systems. Thus fundamental studies are generally only useful as screening tests which provide only the most approximate indications of actual component wear. Therefore, specific studies of actual components are performed using simulators which attempt to duplicate the conditions acting on a component in its in vivo service life. Although a simulator could be considered a type of wear test apparatus, it will be discussed separately in this chapter. Appropriate simulator conditions are difficult to establish, vary widely from investigator to investigator, and are expensive to apply. Thus the previously mentioned fundamental studies with a wear test apparatus are often performed first to narrow the scope of the investigation. Then, because even the validity of the simulator results cannot be established with certainty, animal models and clinical trials are also part of the tribological evaluations of biomaterials. A common line of investigation for a new tribological system (involving an innovative biomaterial) might be as follows:

- investigate fundamental behavior with a wear test apparatus
- test actual components in a simulator
- develop an animal model to provide a better simulation of the biological environment and to investigate the biomaterial's biological interactions
- perform clinical trials monitoring wear radiologically if possible and eventually study retrieved implants as they become available.

A somewhat similar list was presented by Clarke and McKellop [75].

When a new tribological system is proposed, assuming that it is appropriate to follow the above line of investigation, a wear test apparatus and associated test conditions must be chosen to initiate the study of fundamental behavior. The best test setup is one which loosely approximates the actual in situ conditions encountered during application. The following guidelines should be kept in mind when selecting (or designing) a wear system:

- equipment design must duplicate to some extent the biomechanical constraints observed in vivo.
- environmental conditions must be representative of conditions observed *in vivo*
- multivariable experimental designs should be carefully controlled and allow for multifactorial data analysis
- materials and bearing surfaces must be fully characterized before testing.

Even though the design of a wear system can be relatively complex, the apparatus for investigating the wear behavior (and frictional properties) of materials can be relatively simple. Several common arrangements are listed below:

- pin on disc (or flat)
- pin on cylinder
- cylinder on cylinder
- annular disk on annular disk
- two rotating discs

The relative motion of a sliding member on a stationary specimen can either be rotational or oscillatory as with the pin-on-disc, or linear reciprocating (back-and-forth) as with the

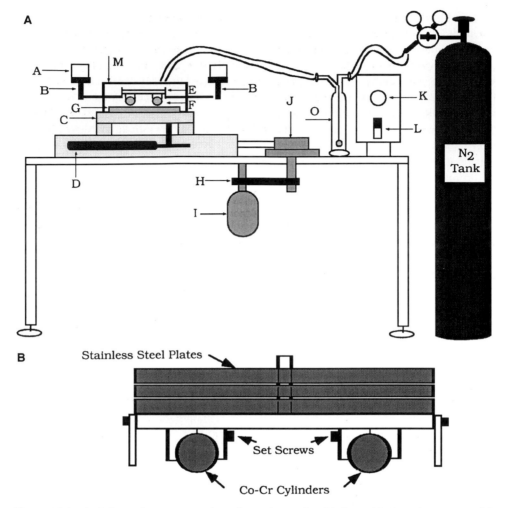

Figure 10-2 A. Schematic representation of a reciprocating friction table (not drawn to scale): (A) External support stand; (B) strain gages used as force transducers; (C) reciprocating platform; (D) linear voltage displacement transducer for distance monitoring; (E) specimen holder; (F) specimens (upper bearing material—stationary); (G) lower sliding bearing material; (H) belt; (I) motor; (J) Scotch yoke; (K) speed dial; (L) power switch; (M) environmental chamber box; (N) heating elements to control temperature of lower bearing material; (O) sparger filled with deionized water to produce moist, nitrogen-rich atmosphere.
B. A normal force is applied on the specimen holder using different weights such as stainless steel plates securely fastened.

pin-on-flat (Figure 10-2). For the linear reciprocating pin-on-flat apparatus, the pin can present a curved (cylindrical or spherical) or flat surface to the flat counterface.

Linear Reciprocating Pin-on-Flat Apparatus

In biomaterials evaluations, the linear reciprocating pin-on-disc apparatus is perhaps the most popular. The drive is reasonably simple (for example, a rotating shaft from an electric motor with a toothed belt to transfer motion to a scotch yoke which drives a flat table). By changing the counterface material or roughness, experiments can be designed to emphasize abrasive, adhesive, and/or fatigue wear mechanisms. The major advantages of conducting tests on a simplified model such as the pin-on-disc apparatus are as follows. First, major parameters influencing wear, such as load, ambient temperature, and velocity, can easily be controlled and monitored by the experimenter. Therefore, fundamental wear mechanisms can be studied. Second, the motion is preferred over the simpler constant rotary motion of a pin-on-disc apparatus because it is thought to better represent physiological motion. Third, costs of the materials and testing apparatus are considerably reduced in comparison to more sophisticated systems such as simulators.

The major disadvantage of the pin-on-disc apparatus is the inability to extrapolate the results obtained, with a reasonable expectation of accuracy, to predict the wear of actual components [76–80]. Even as a "screening" device to rank the wear behavior of material pairs, the apparatus may fail to predict in vivo results.

A linear reciprocating pin-on-flat apparatus can be used to obtain basic wear data for materials in a variety of biomedical applications. Specifically, polymers may be tested against metals or ceramics for potential use in total joint replacement [36]. Typically, when testing two materials in this particular configuration, a polymer pin is the stationary member, while a metal or ceramic flat surface is the moving member. However, there is no fixed convention regarding which material must serve as the stationary or the moving component, and different results in terms of wear mechanisms and wear rate can be expected with different arrangements [76–80]. If the flat material is a polymer and the pin is a metal, a track will be produced in the polymer as a result of both wear and creep. Also, edge effects may be present around the metal pin, specially for a line contact (cylinder-on-flat) and flat-on-flat configurations.

The stroke length can also influence wear. Under some circumstances, a large amount of a material transfer from a polymer pin to metal flat occurred when the stroke was long compared to the pin diameter [81]. The optimal choice of stroke length for testing joint replacement materials in a pin-on-flat configuration has not been established.

Another parameter which influences the wear is the heat generated by friction which is transferred to the surfaces and influences the wear mechanisms. The thermal properties of the materials transfer and the motion of the contacting surface relative to the frictional heat source influence the heat transfer. Davidson et al. [82] reported an increase of 5 to 10°C at the contacting surfaces of UHMWPE and metal in simulated hip joint conditions.

The selection of pin geometry is influenced by the desire to better approximate the in situ contact mechanics. Generally, the geometry of the pin will be one of the following types: spherical (point contact), cylindrical (line contact), or plane (often a truncated cone). For example, to imitate the contact pressure distribution experienced in the knee implant, line contact may be used, whereas a hip implant may be better represented by point contact. However, if the pin is to be considered a small representative section of a larger conforming contact in a joint replacement implant, a plane configuration with a reasonably constant pressure may be appropriate.

In using-plane ended polyurethane wear pins of a truncated cone configuration, Jin et al. [51] obtained a significantly lower coefficient of friction and wear rate with a small cone angle (30°) as compared to a larger cone angle (55°). Therefore, it is not just the choice of pin geometry but also fine details of the selected pin geometry that can be important to wear.

Hip Simulators

The wear in a linear reciprocating pin-on-flat apparatus can be influenced significantly by geometry, load and surface motion. It is difficult to establish appropriate values for these parameters to obtain wear that is related to that obtained by implants in vivo. Therefore simulator devices have been developed for tribological testing of biomaterials. Simulators have been used quite extensively in wear testing of heart valves and dental materials. In

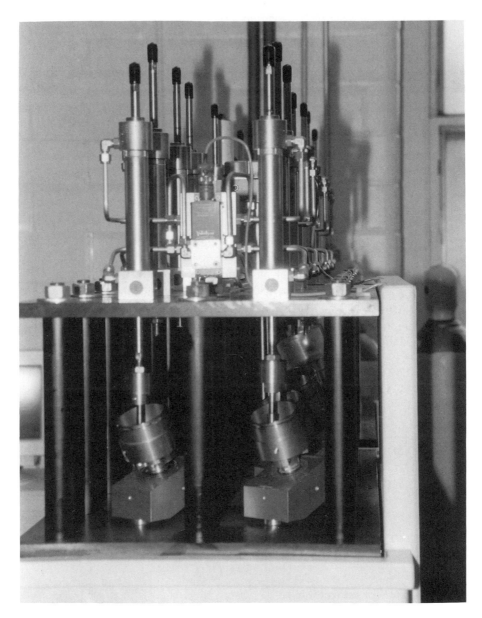

Figure 10-3 Photograph of a simulator apparatus (EW08 MMED made by MATCO, LaCanada, CA) with two banks of 8 channels where a channel is a mounting for an individual hip specimen.

orthopaedics, knee simulators have been developed, with perhaps the most promising efforts being made by Walker et al. [83]. However, in this chapter, hip simulators (Figure 10-3) are examined in some detail because they have been subject to quite intense research scrutiny for over 25 years [84]. Over the last years, hip simulator wear data have been presented by a number of groups (Table 10-2) and have involved testing of metal-polyethylene, ceramic-polyethylene, and metal-metal implants.

The central issue in hip simulator design is the extent to which the in vivo conditions are duplicated while having the capability to perform multiple tests simultaneously, main-

Table 10-2   Hip Simulators in the Recent Literature

Institution	Publication	Materials tested
Los Angeles Orthopaedic Hospital	[85]	metal-polyethylene ceramic-polyethylene
University of Leeds	[86]	metal-polyethylene ceramic-polyethylene
Helsinki University of Technology	[87]	metal-polyethylene ceramic-polyethylene
Sulzer Medical Technologies	[88]	metal-metal
Montreal General Hospital	[89]	metal-metal
New Jersey Institute of Technology	[90]	metal-polyethylene
Biomet, Inc.	[91]	metal-polyethylene
Loma Linda Medical Center	[92]	metal-polyethylene

taining a low cost of manufacture. The in vivo conditions that have been emphasized so far in the literature are essentially the choice of motions and loads transmitted. Usually, a representation [93] of an "average" walking cycle (Figure 10-4) is chosen to provide the angular positions of the femoral head over the cycle. The angular position of the acetabulum does not change significantly [94] and thus relative motions can be obtained from the femoral head positions. The joint force components [95] are also obtained from consideration of an average walking cycle (Figure 10-5). It is important to note that the resultant joint force vector changes in direction during walking, and thus the change in position of the peak contact pressure on the femoral head is not solely a function of the motion of

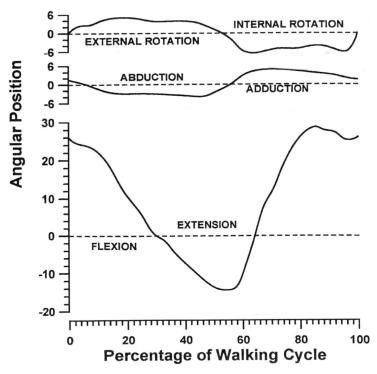

Figure 10-4   Angular position of the hip during walking after Johnston and Smidt [93] (a cubic spline interpolation of the data was used to obtain these curves).

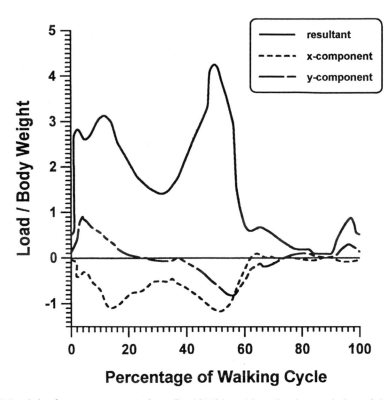

Figure 10-5 Joint force components from Paul [95] (a cubic spline interpolation of the data was used to obtain these curves). The origin of the Cartesian coordinate axes is located at the center of the femoral head of the left leg with x = horizontal in lateral direction, y = horizontal in the posterior direction, and z = vertical.

the femoral head [96]. Furthermore, the peak contact pressure moves on the acetabulum surface because of this shift in the direction of the joint force vector.

The only simulator that attempts to rigorously duplicate all kinematics (motions and loads) is one at the University of Leeds in which loads and angular displacements are input along the three coordinate axes. In addition, they place the implant specimens in the upright position rather than the upside-down position used in most simulators to avoid the risk of lubricant starvation. Other simulators, such the one shown in Figure 10-3, approximate the kinematics in order to simplify the apparatus, which improves reliability and reduces manufacturing costs. The details of the kinematics are important in developing a simulator, either in specifying an exact simulation or deciding on approximations. Therefore, discrete data used to construct spline interpolations giving the curves of Figures 10-4 and 10-5 and other existing determinations of the motion and loading of the hip joint during walking may be used as a basis for simulator design.

Having developed a simulator with a "good" kinematic representation of the hip in vivo, it might be thought that no further design considerations were required. However, a true simulation must deal with many other issues such as the extent to which thermal [97] and vibrational [98, 99] phenomena are represented. As yet, guidelines for thermal and vibrational simulation have not been developed. Finally, the biological environment must be considered in the simulation; this aspect is discussed in a subsequent section.

Given the complexity of simulator design, one may be tempted to use only more fundamental testing devices, such as the linear reciprocating pin-on-flat apparatus, and attempt to determine expressions to predict the wear in vivo. Unfortunately, such predictions are not accurate. Simulator studies have provided somewhat better predictions of actual component wear, despite the uncertainty in the extent to which the simulation must be performed. The key to simulator innovation is the continual comparison of wear results with those occurring in vivo [100, 101].

Specimen Cleaning and Sterilization

Prior to wear testing and evaluation, the metal, polymer or ceramic specimens must be cleaned. Rowland et al. described the importance of biomaterial cleaning for contaminant removal before physical assessment of the specimens [102]. Contaminants may include lubricating oils used during fabrication processes, or metal shavings, soaps, and fat as a result of handling. Oils and fats are excellent boundary lubricants [23] and in this respect might influence the resultant wear of the test materials. The Clemson Bioengineering Cleaning Protocol [102] has proven to be effective and has been used for cleaning wear specimens by investigators [24]. The ASTM standard procedure F 732 [36] suggests drying specimens with lint-free tissue followed by air drying for 30 minutes in a dust-free environment. Drying can also be performed under vacuum. Biomaterials tested for the fabrication of devices will eventually be sterilized before they are implanted. Therefore, wear specimens should be sterilized using a recommended method for that particular material prior to pre-conditioning or testing. It is important to ensure the cleanliness and sterility of test materials or devices since these will be the "operating" conditions at the time of implantation.

Pre-Conditioning of Wear Specimens (Soaking and Control)

Certain materials are susceptible to imbibing liquids from the environment [103]. In particular, polymeric materials can show a net increase in weight during a wear test due to fluid absorption [104].

For orthopaedic joint replacement, the ASTM standard protocol F-732-91 [36] recommends pre-conditioning polymeric specimens before testing in lubricated conditions. Obviously, it is important to consider this phenomenon in lubricated conditions; however, pre-conditioning of specimens should also be performed when there is the possibility of changes in the atmosphere (e.g., humidity) [104]. The goal of pre-conditioning is mainly to rule out artifacts in weight loss measurements of wear and minimize fluid absorption during the initial wear-in period.

During pre-soaking, polymer specimens are placed in the test lubricant and subjected to the same environment as the test specimens but are not subjected to wear. Specimens should be used for testing only after weight equilibrium has been attained. To account for the absorption of fluid by the polymer, Dowson et al. [44] exposed a pre-soaked control polymer pin to the same environmental conditions (temperature, static load, and lubricant) during the duration of the test. Any swelling or weight gain of the control polymer was then subtracted from the weight measurements of the test specimens to normalize the data.

Following F-732-91 [36], the specimens should be weighed on an analytical balance with an accuracy of at least ± 10 μg before testing and the same instrument is to be used for weight measurements during and after testing for gravimetric analysis. If this phenomenon is not taken into consideration, wear data may produce erroneous results because the polymer may actually gain weight instead of losing weight [103].

Selection of Lubricants

Wear tests can be conducted in dry or fluid environments. The former would be used if the sole purpose of the wear test were to compare the behavior of different materials. However, a dry environment is not representative of conditions found in the body. Therefore, the wear properties of biomaterials are normally characterized in a fluid environment. Even though different lubricants are used for wear testing, it is recommended to use a biological lubricant compatible with the clinical application. The type of lubricant used in wear tests will have a marked effect on the experimental wear rate. Table 10-3 lists lubricants used for the testing of biomaterials.

Fluids can be further classified as being Newtonian or non-Newtonian. The viscosity of Newtonian fluids is independent of the shear rate whereas for most biological fluids, including synovial fluid, viscosity is a function of shear rate and thus is non-Newtonian in nature. The viscosity of all liquid lubricants decreases as the temperature increases

Table 10-3   Lubricants Used for the Friction and Wear Testing of Biomaterials

Lubricant	Wear system	Remarks
Mineral oil [4, 105]	Rotating ring on a stationary conforming block (Journal bearing) Pendulum joint simulator	Selected following a comparative analysis between saline, plasma, synovial fluid, and mineral oil.
Distilled water [51, 53, 106–108]	Reciprocating pin-on-flat Rotating pin-on-flat Disk-on-flat	No viscosity effect or molecule transfer.
Saline solution [109–110]	Hip joint simulator Reciprocating pin-on-flat	Newtonian fluid, no boundary lubricant. Comparable to distilled water.
Bovine serum [50, 52, 111]	Hip joint simulator	0.1% sodium azide added to retard bacterial degradation.
Synovial fluid and synovial fluid aspirated from pathological joints [109]	Pendulum hip simulator	Difficult to obtain. Human fluids are considered a biohazard.
Phospholipid and hyaluronic acid solution [112]	Reciprocating pin-on-flat	Provides boundary lubrication of bearing surfaces.
Silicone fluid [113–114]	Hip joint simulator	Can be obtained in a whole range of viscosities and molecular weights. Being Newtonian, it eliminates the effects of velocity and film thickness on viscosity.
Synthetic lubricant (carboxymethyl cellulose) [115]	Hip joint simulator	Similar rheological properties to those of synovial fluid.
Glycerine and diluted glycerine [24]	Reciprocating pin-on-flat	Newtonian fluid that can be diluted to obtain a range of viscosities comparable to normal and degenerated synovial fluids.

[116]. Additionally, serum and synovial fluid contain proteins and lipids which may undergo conformational changes dependent on the temperature [117]. Healthy synovial fluid exhibits different rheological properties (viscosity vs shear rate) in comparison to degenerated synovial fluid [118–119]. The rheological properties may affect the lubrication mode and, consequently, the resultant wear processes of the surfaces. Because of the aforementioned phenomenon, the rheological properties of the lubricant should be characterized and monitored during testing, if possible.

Black [120] recommends using fresh serum for testing materials in contact with blood such as cardiovascular devices and a 50:50 mixture of serum and saline for soft tissue locations to approximate the intracellular fluid. Bovine serum seems to be the most widely used lubricant for orthopaedic bearing tests. As reported by Fisher and Dowson [55], bovine serum produces wear surfaces that closely resemble the wear surfaces found in retrieved orthopaedic UHMWPE components [53, 54]. Different dilute serum:saline solutions [49] are superior to pure saline but do not replace synovial fluid [120]. Filtered-sterilized serum is recommended since it contains less hemolyzed blood material, which has been shown to affect the lubricating properties of the serum [53]. However, biological fluids such as serum change in composition during testing, consequently affecting their viscosity and more importantly the wear process [55, 116]. Test parameters that will affect the composition of the lubricant are frictional heating [82], fluid degeneration [118], and calcium phosphorus precipitation in serum [52]. Temperature increases in the fluid can encourage evaporation as well as bacterial colonization. Evaporation of the lubricant or fluid environment can be prevented by enclosing the system or periodically (or continuously) replacing evaporated water with distilled water. Moreover, biological fluids used as lubricants are susceptible to degradation through bacterial colonization. To prevent this detrimental effect, antibiotics are frequently added to the solution. Antimicrobial agents such as sodium azide in very small concentrations (0.2% w/v) have also been used by investigators [50]. To prevent calcium precipitation on the bearing surfaces, decalcifiant agents such as EDTA (ethylene-diaminetetraacetic acid) have been added to serum at concentrations of 20 mM [52]. To preserve serum before its utilization in wear tests, it should be kept frozen.

Dumbleton [3] recommends changing the fluid at intervals of 24–48 hours to prevent the above changes in the tribosystem and keeping the temperature as constant as possible during testing by circulating the fluid. Ideally, a wear test should be conducted at body temperature (37°C) instead of room temperature (~25°C).

Selection of Operating Conditions for Simple Wear Testing Devices

Contact Stress and Applied Load   Loads giving a contact pressure representative of *in vivo* conditions should be selected. Different contact pressures for synovial joints have been reported in the literature (Table 10-4). Unfortunately, a static constant load typically used in simple wear testing devices is an over-simplification of the dynamic loading *in vivo*. In this respect, dynamic loading allows for fatigue wear and therefore is a better representation of clinical situations and clinical wear. However, in most pin-on-disc devices, at least one surface is subject to dynamic loading as the contact zone moves over it. Experiments have been conducted with critical contact pressures of up to 64 MPa [50] and 27 MPa [122] for orthopaedic applications (knee implants). For dental applications, a force of 1–2 N was used as a representative brushing force and 53 N was used for chewing force [58, 123].

Table 10-4   Joint Forces Observed During Common Activities

Activity/Joint	Hip [3, 121]	Knee (Patellofemoral joint) [3, 122]	Finger (Metacarpophalangeal joint) [121]	Shoulder (X BW) [121]
Level Walking	4.9–7.6 (X BW)	2.7–4.3 (X BW)	–	–
Up Stairs	7.2 (X BW)	4.4 (X BW)	–	–
Down Stairs	7.1 (X BW)	4.9 (X BW)	–	–
Up Ramp	5.9 (X BW)	3.7 (X BW)	–	–
Down Ramp	5.1 (X BW)	4.4 (X BW)	–	–
Lift arm	–	–	–	630 N
Abduction	–	–	–	2800 N
Pinch	–	–	9–380 N	–
Grasp	–	–	80–260 N	–

Sliding Velocity   Sliding velocity and type of motion (reciprocating, oscillating or rotating) will also affect the tribosystem. It is common practice to use a sliding velocity that corresponds to in vivo conditions. Further, the sliding velocity can be constant (e.g., rotating pin-on-disc apparatus) or sinusoidal (e.g., reciprocating apparatus). The velocity may be reported as an entrainment velocity, which is actually the average velocity of the lubricant into the contact. An increased velocity will often provide better conditions for lubrication.

Test Duration/Number of Cycles   The duration of a wear test should be determined based on the physiological cycling rate and on the clinical application. The failure of a cardiovascular device will possibly be catastrophic and therefore requires more attention in terms of number of cycles to failure.

A complete walking cycle is represented by two steps. One cycle on a reciprocating pin-on-flat system is obtained by two passes (return to starting point), while one cycle on a rotating pin-on-disc system corresponds to one turn. It is assumed that an average individual will make 2 million steps per year, while an active subject may make more than 10 million steps [124] at a maximum frequency of about 1 Hz. Therefore, the longer the test is performed, the closer to clinical applications the results may be. Frequency is the number of cycles/second and is dependent upon the sliding distance and velocity used for the tribosystem. Consequently, wear test duration can be specified as a frequency, cycle or distance per cycle (or stroke); total number of cycles or stroke; or total sliding distance [75]. In hip implant studies, investigators will normally assess wear resistance for one milion to five million cycles.

Wear and Material Characterization

An understanding of the wear process can only be obtained to the extent that valid data and information are available. There are three sources for information in a tribosystem: the worn surface, the subsurface, and the wear debris. Qualitative and quantitative assessments of these sources of data should be pursued before testing, during testing (if non-destructive), and after testing.

The amount of wear experienced within a tribosystem can be measured by the following techniques:

- weight loss
- dimensional changes
- comparison of the surface characteristics before and after testing
- characterization of wear debris [103].

A major disadvantage in the monitoring of wear and surface change during testing is associated with the fact that specimens must be removed to be characterized. Therefore, extreme caution must be taken to avoid weight or surface change resulting from repetitive mounting procedures. Additionally, care must be taken to avoid surface contamination since it would significantly influence the subsequent material wear behavior. By using a non-conforming contact geometry, such as the pin-on-disc, this effect can be minimized because wear debris can easily be removed from the test setup.

Some macroscopic, microscopic and profilometric techniques as well as weight measurements can be non-destructively applied to monitor wear.

Measurement of Wear   Changes in weight or dimensions may be used to give a quantitative measure of wear. Weight loss measurements can be very effective when small amounts of wear occur over large surface areas. However, difficulties with weight loss methods may arise if the weight loss occurs for reasons unrelated to wear. As mentioned previously, UHMWPE absorbs water and gains weight when immersed in an aqueous solution. Since wear testing of UHMWPE often occurs in an aqueous environment, weight loss methods of assessing wear must be adjusted to account for fluid absorption [36]. Linear and volumetric dimensional parameters can also be used to measure wear. The depth of wear tracks or material recession can be measured locally with precision calipers to measure loss of material. This method is typically performed by interrupting the wear test; however, the length of a specimen can also be monitored during testing by attaching transducers to the pin when using a pin-on-disc or pin-on-plate apparatus. Shortcomings with this method are that dimensional measurements must be corrected if materials are subject to surface creep during testing [3]. Additionally, increases in temperature as a result of friction may have an effect on the length of the pin. Wear volume can be extrapolated from linear dimensional changes and pin geometry. Subsequently, wear rates are calculated by dividing the wear volume by the sliding distance, allowing for a crude comparison of wear data.

In addition, a wear factor, K, can be used to characterize tribosystems. Wear coefficients are derived from wear models and therefore are dependent on wear mechanisms. The commonly used definition for wear factor is

$$K = V/LX,$$

where V is the volume of wear in mm^3, L is the applied load in Newtons, and X is the sliding distance. The wear factor may be influenced by other factors including sliding velocity, contact area, and lubrication.

Wear surfaces can also be characterized microscopically using optic or electron microscopy. However, it is difficult to separate surface changes associated with material removal (wear) from changes due to surface deformation (creep) and/or the transfer of counterpart material. In these cases, the use of elemental analysis as well provides a better assessment of surface wear. Profilometry techniques (stylus or non-contact), as described in Chapter 13, are commonly used to measure depth of wear with higher precision. Ultra-sounds have also been proposed as a non-destructive method to monitor material removal during reciprocation testing [125]. Scanning electron microscopy is also used to assess surface damage. However, the high voltage used in scanning electron microscopy can cause damage to polymeric surfaces such as ultra high molecular weight polyethylene. To account for this problem, authors have successfully used low voltage (1–2 kV compared to 15–25 kV) scanning electron microscopy to image UHMWPE [126].

Change in Surface Topography   Surface changes during tangential motion are observed by a deviation of the profile from initial measurements. Microtopographical parameters such as asperity numerical density, asperity spacing, asperity slope height, asperity tip radius, and curvature or error of form are also used as surface parameters and indicators of surface change. Precision and quality control assessment of surface microtopography is generally specified in terms of a single roughness parameter. However, the analysis of time-induced surface change in tribosystems requires a minimum of three parameters and a rigorous statistical treatment of experimental measurements [14]. Commonly used combinations of parameters to characterize a surface are:

- height, shape, and spacing of asperities
- size, spacing, and shape factors
- surface density, height distribution, and mean radius of asperities
- for a more general case, size, spacing, shape, height distribution of asperities, and micro-roughness of asperities which deform plastically under load.

Another surface parameter, the bearing area curve (BAC), indicates how much of the profile protrudes from a given height or depicts the area of an object cut by a plane at a specified height. The bearing area curve can be used in the modeling of rough bearing surfaces, their contact, surface deformation, surface change, and surface failure [127].

Roughness parameters are also used to determine the lubrication regimes of bearings. Experimental studies showed that when the lubricant film separating two contacting surfaces was thick enough to prevent their physical contact, the fatigue life and wear resistance of these surfaces was significantly increased. Optimum lubrication conditions and improved bearing life are achieved when both the film of fluid separating both contacting bodies is thick enough to provide full separation between the asperities at the contact, and the reduced surface roughness (σ) is much smaller than the fluid film generated between the contacting bodies.

The dimensionless film parameter, lambda (λ), is the ratio of the central lubricant film thickness (h_c) generated between the contact and the reduced surface roughness

$$\lambda = \frac{h_c}{\sqrt{\sigma_1^2 + \sigma_2^2}}$$

where σ_1 and σ_2 are the root-mean-square average of surface 1 and surface 2, respectively. The film parameter is used to define the lubrication mode such that full fluid film lubrication is achieved when $\lambda \geq 3$, mixed lubrication occurs when $1 \leq \lambda < 3$, and boundary lubrication occurs when $\lambda < 1$. These values provide a rough estimate of the magnitude of surface separation [127].

Wear Debris Analysis   Wear debris analysis is an important part of the diagnostic characterization of wear processes (see also Chapter 14). Particles of surface debris should develop characteristic shapes, sizes and features that relate to the wear mechanisms responsible for their production. Additionally, the production of wear debris may play a synergistic effect in the facilitation of other wear mechanisms. To accomplish the analysis, wear debris must be collected which is often a cumbersome and non-exact method. The end product may actually result in large inclusions of artifactual material and the potentiality for significant loss of wear debris particles during their extraction from the lubricant [128].

Debris collection and analysis is done by several methods. Ferrography is a popular method for isolating metallic debris involving the separation of debris from a fluid suspension on a microscope slide by a magnetic process [129, 130]. Additionally, wear particles can be extracted from a lubricant through filtration techniques and collected in a clean vial. Wear particles can be filtered from the lubricant using a gold filter with a very small pore size (order of magnitude below expected debris size) [24] and washed with an appropriate solvent to remove any lubricant residue. After complete drying, the debris can be weighed, observed with optical and scanning microscopy for image and contour analysis, and/or observed with infrared spectroscopy or other available techniques for elemental analysis.

Transfer films, such as UHMWPE, have been observed on metallic orthopaedic components [131, 132]. UHMWPE debris embedded in countersurfaces can be chemically analyzed by removing the film using a solvent and then analyzing the residue after solvent evaporation with infrared spectroscopy [133] as fully described in Chapter 14.

Statistical Relevance   Statistical analysis of compiled data is desirable. As emphasized previously, many parameters, both intrinsic and extrinsic to the tribosystem, can affect the outcome of wear measurements. Consequently, the probability of large variability between experiments is likely. Therefore, when performing wear tests, multiple samples should be tested to establish the statistical significance and/or repeatability of the material's or device's wear performance [75]. Additionally, appropriate controls and/or references should be tested in conjunction with experimental materials or devices to allow for accuracy, reliability and comparison between control and test materials.

Statistical methods can specifically be used for the determination of the following:

- wear rates
- distribution profiles of the wear rates, i.e., Gaussian, non-Gaussian, etc.
- effect of variables on the resultant wear rate
- wear rates for new materials in comparison to reference materials [134].

This list is certainly not all-inclusive; however, it provides one with the basis for the importance of statistics within the reporting of wear data.

Even though statistical methods may be applicable for more than one tribosystem, the results from one tribosystem may not be comparable to results from another tribosystem. For further explanation of the role of statistics in the evaluation of wear data, the reader is referred to Dumbleton [134] and Box et al. [135].

CONCLUSIONS

Before friction and wear testing, specimens should be cleaned and sterilized if applicable and characterized physically, mechanically, and chemically. Surface profilometry allows for the determination of roughness parameters. However, this surface characterization technique should be coupled with scanning electron microscopy or other visualization techniques. Samples and controls should be weighed before testing and pre-conditioned in the lubricant used for testing to measure weight changes due to absorption of the lubricant. Preferably tests should be conducted at body temperature (37°C) instead of room temperature (~25°C).

The lubricant should be selected to best represent the clinical conditions as well as loading magnitude (contact stress), loading mode (static or dynamic), and velocity. Wear testing can be conducted on different apparati with variation in time periods depending on the objective of the wear test. Normally, investigators attempt to obtain wear data for as long as possible to provide a better estimation of in vivo results and sometimes accelerated wear tests are proposed to optimize the time factor. The wear behavior for a test specimen should be assessed physically (surface characterization, contact angle, weight of specimen, dimension of specimens), chemically (Fourier transform infrared spectroscopy, etc.), and through the collection of wear debris and subsequent characterization. Lastly, it is crucial to conduct tests under stringent conditions and accurately report these criteria to ensure the proper assessment of results.

It has been demonstrated in this chapter that there are many parameters which need to be addressed to conduct scientifically valid friction or wear experiments. Wear is not a material property but instead a consequence of the entire contact tribology. As pointed out, the multitude of parameters which affect the results of wear tests are sometimes forgotten or deemed unimportant. Further research needs to be conducted on the parameters which truly affect wear.

REFERENCES

1   Department of Education and Science. *Lubrication (Tribology), Education and Research—A Report on the Present Position and Industry's Needs*. London: Her Majesty's Stationery Office, 1966.
2   Ikada Y, Ukama Y. *Lubricating Polymer Surfaces*. Lancaster, PA: Technomic Publishing Co., 1993, 55–71.
3   Dumbleton JH. *Tribology of Natural and Artificial Joints*. New York: Elsevier, 1981, 183–214.
4   Amstutz CH. Polymers as bearing materials for total hip replacement: A friction and wear analysis. *J Biomed Mat Res*, 3 (1968), 547–568.
5   Suzuki S, Suzuki SH, Cox CF. Evaluating the antagonistic wear of restorative materials. *JADA*, 127 (1996), 74–80.
6   Wassell RW, McCabe JF, Walls, AWG. A two-body frictional wear test. *J Dent Res*, 73 (1994), 1546–1553.
7   Woodell JE, Rogers JM, Childs D, Langan EM, Taylor S, LaBerge M. Effect of vascular stent geometry on porcine aorta damage: An *in vitro* model. *Proc Fifth World Biomaterials Congress*, Toronto, Ontario, Canada, May 29–June 2, 1996.
8   Kalachandra S, Shah DO. Polymers as ophthalmologic lubricating agents. *Mat Res Soc Symp Proc*, 110 (1989), 463–469.
9   Ichijima E, Kobayashi H, Ikada Y, Akita J, Ikeuchi K. An estimation method for the friction between a contact lens and corneal modes. *Japanese Soc Biomater Prep*, 1989, 95.
10 Reich S, Levy M, Meshorer A, Blumental M, Yalon J, Shetts W, Goldberg EP. Intra-ocular lens endothelial interface: Adhesive force measurements. *J Biomed Mat Res*, 18 (1984), 737–744.
11 Suh NP. *Tribophysics*. Englewood Cliffs, NJ: Prentice-Hall, Inc, 1986, 3–11.
12 Shigley JE, Mischke CR. *Bearings and Lubrication*. New York: McGraw-Hill Publishing Co., 1986.
13 Rabinowicz E. *Friction and Wear of Materials*. New York: John Wiley and Sons, Inc., 1965, 53–58.
14 Moore DF. *Principles and Applications of Tribology*. New York: Pergamon Press, 1975, 33–60.
15 Ludema KC. Friction. *CRC Handbook of Lubrication*. Boca Raton, FL: CRC Press, 1980, 31–48.
16 Suh NP, Sin HC. The genesis of friction. *Wear*, 69 (1981), 91–114.
17 Amontons G. On the resistance originating in machines. *Histoire de l'Academie Royale des Sciences avec les Memoires de Mathematique et de Physique*, 1699, 206–222.
18 Ludema KC. Friction, a study in the prevention of seizure. *ASTM Standardization News*, May 1987, 54–58.
19 Bowden FP, Tabor D. *The Friction and Lubrication of Solids*. Oxford: Clarendon Press, 1950.
20 Rabinowicz E. *Friction and Wear of Materials*. New York: John Wiley and Sons, Inc., 1965, 59–70.
21 Budinski KG. Friction in machine design. In Ludema KC, Bayer RG (Eds.), *Tribological Modeling for Mechanical Designers. ASTM STP 1105*. Philadelphia, PA: American Society for Testing and Materials, 1991, 89–126.
22 Hall HT, Powers DL, Bowman LS, LaBerge M. Effect of anti-inflammatory drugs on the properties of lapine articular cartilage. *Trans 42nd Annual Meeting Orthopaedic Research Society*, Atlanta, GA, February 18–22, 1996, 759.

23   Williams PF, Powell GL, LaBerge M. Sliding friction analysis of phosphatidylcholine as a boundary lubricant for articular cartilage. *J Eng Medicine (Inst Mech Eng)*, 207 (1993), 59–66.

24   Ruger LM, Love BJ, Drews MJ, Hutton WC, LaBerge M. Effect of antioxidant on the tribological properties of gamma sterilized ultra high molecular weight polyethylene. *Proc Fifth World Biomaterials Congress*, Toronto, Canada, May 29–June 2, 1996.

25   Rogers JM, Powell GL, Joseph PF, Pace TB, LaBerge M. Effect of phosphatidylcholine chain length on the friction of rigid bearing surfaces. *Proc Fifth World Biomaterials Congress*, Toronto, Canada, May 29–June 2, 1996.

26   Chow AB, Medley JB, LaBerge M. Mechanical and tribological analyses of elastomeric surface layers in load bearing implants. *Trans of 20th Annual Meeting of the Society for Biomaterials*, Boston, MA, 1994, 434.

27   Standard guide for measuring and reporting friction. *Annual Book of ASTM Standards*, G115-93. Philadelphia, PA: American Society for Testing and Materials, 1995, 13.01.

28   Test method for dynamic coefficient of friction and wear of sintered metal friction materials under dry conditions. *Annual Book of ASTM Standards*. Philadelphia, PA: American Society for Testing and Materials, 1989, 2.05.

29   Test method for frictional characteristics of sintered metal friction materials run in lubricants. *Annual Book of ASTM Standards*. Philadelphia, PA: American Society for Testing and Materials, 1989, 2.05.

30   Guidelines for reporting friction and wear test results of manufactured carbon and graphite bearing and seal materials. *Annual Book of ASTM Standards*. Philadelphia, PA: American Society for Testing and Materials, 1995, 13.01.

31   Test method for static and kinetic coefficients of friction of plastic film and sheeting. *Annual Book of ASTM Standards*. Philadelphia, PA: American Society for Testing and Materials, 1995, 8.01.

32   Test method for kinetic coefficient of friction of plastic solids. *Annual Book of ASTM Standards*. Philadelphia, PA: American Society for Testing and Materials, 1995, 8.02.

33   Test method for coefficient of friction, yarn to solid material. *Annual Book of ASTM Standards*. Philadelphia, PA: American Society for Testing and Materials, 1995, 7.01.

34   Method of testing fabrics woven from polyolefin monofilaments. *Annual Book of ASTM Standards*. Philadelphia, PA: American Society for Testing and Materials, 1988, 7.01.

35   Test method for coefficient of friction, yarn-to-yarn. *Annual Book of ASTM Standards*. Philadelphia, PA: American Society for Testing and Materials, 1995, 7.02.

36   Practice for reciprocating pin-on-flat evaluation of friction and wear properties of polymeric materials for use in total joint prosthesis. *Annual Book of ASTM Standards*. Philadelphia, PA: American Society for Testing and Materials, 1995, 13.01.

37   Jacobs JJ, Shanbhag A, Glant TT, Black J, Galante JO. Wear debris in total joint replacements. *J Am Acad Orthop Surg*, 2 (1994), 212–220.

38   Mittlmeier T, Walter A. The influence of prosthesis design on wear and loosening phenomena. *CRC Critical Reviews in Biocompatibility*, 3 (1987), 319–419.

39   Schoen FJ, Titus JL, Lawrie GM. Bioengineering aspects of heart valve replacement. *Annals of Biomed Eng*, 10 (1982), 97–128.

40   Dowson D. Basic tribology. In *An Introduction to the Bio-mechanics of Joints and Joint Replacement*. London: Mechanical Engineering Publications, Ltd., 1981, 49–60.

41   Rowe CN. Lubricated wear. In *CRC Handbook of Lubrication*. Boca Raton, FL: CRC Press, 1980, 209–225.

42   Stolarski TA. *Tribology in Machine Design*. Oxford: Heinemann Newnes, 1990, 13–30.

43   Evans DG, Lancaster JK. The wear of polymers. *Treatise on Materials Science and Technology*, 13 (1979), 85–140.

44   Dowson D, Atkinson JR, Brown KJ. Advances in polymer friction and wear. In Lee LH (Ed.), *Polymer Science and Technology Symposia Series*, Vol. 5B. New York: Plenum Press, 1974.

45   Terminology relating to wear and corrosion. *Annual Book of ASTM Standards*. Philadelphia, PA: American Society for Testing and Materials, 1995, 3.02.

46   Test method for ranking resistance of materials to sliding wear using block-on-ring wear test. *Annual Book of ASTM Standards*. Philadelphia, PA: American Society for Testing and Materials, 1995, 3.02.

47   Test method for wear testing with a crossed-cylinder apparatus. *Annual Book of ASTM Standards*. Philadelphia, PA: American Society for Testing and Materials, 1995, 3.02.

48   Test method for wear testing with a pin-on-disk apparatus. *Annual Book of ASTM Standards*. Philadelphia, PA: American Society for Testing and Materials, 1995, 3.02.

49   Streicher RM. Ceramic surfaces as wear partners for polyethylene. In Bonfield W, Hastings GW, Tanner KE (Eds.), *Bioceramics*, Vol 4. London: Butterworth-Heinemann Ltd., 1991, 9.

50   Schmidt MB, Lin M, Greer KW. Wear performance of UHWMPE articulated against ion implanted CoCr. *Trans 21st Annual Meeting of the Society for Biomaterials*, San Francisco, CA, 1995, 230.

51   Jin ZM, Dowson D, Fisher J. Wear and friction of medical grade polyurethane sliding on smooth metal counterfaces. *Wear*, 162–164 (1993), 627–630.

52   Medley JB, Krygier JJ, Bobyn JD, Chan FW, Tanzer M. Metal-metal bearing surfaces in the hip: Investigation of factors influencing wear. *Trans Orthop Res Soc*, 20 (1995), 765.

53   Brown KJ, Atkinson JR, Dowson D, Wright V. The wear of ultra high molecular weight polyethylene and a preliminary study of its relation to the in vivo behaviour of replacement hip joints. *Wear*, 40 (1976), 255–264.

54   Rose RM, Radin EL. Wear of polyethylene in total hip prostheses. *Clin Orthop Rel Res*, 170 (1982), 107–115.

55   Fisher J, Dowson D. Tribology of total artificial joints. *Proc Inst Mech Engrs*, 205 (1991), 73–79.

56   Dumbleton, JH. *Tribology of Natural and Artificial Joints*. New York: Elsevier, 1981, 94–103.

57   Wu W, McKinney JE. Influence of chemicals on wear of dental composites. *J Dent Res*, 67 (1982), 1180–1183.

58   Krejci I, Lutz F, Zedler C. Effect of contact area size on enamel and composite wear. *J Dent Res*, 71 (1992), 1413–1416.

59   Bloem TJ, McDowell GC, Lang BR, Powers JM. In vivo wear. Part II: Wear and abrasion of composite restorative materials. *J Pros Dent*, 60 (1988), 242–249.

60   McDowell GC, Bloem TJ, Lang BR, Asgar K. In vivo wear. Part I: The Michigan computer-graphic measuring system. *J Pros Dent*, 60 (1988), 112–120.

61   Dikson G. Physical and chemical properties and wear. *J Dent Res*, 58 (1979), 1535–1543.

62   Powers JM, Allen LJ, Craig RG. Two-body abrasion of commercial and experimental restorative and coating resins and an amalgam. *J Am Dent Assoc*, 89 (1974), 1118–1122.

63   Tillitson EW, Craig RG, Peyton FA. Friction and wear of restorative dental materials. *J Dent Res*, 50 (1971), 149–154.

64   Lugassy AA, Greener EH. An abrasion resistance study of some dental resins. *J Dent Res*, 51 (1972), 967–973.

65   Cordon M. Method for measuring the abrasion of dentin by dentifrices. *J Dent Res*, 50 (1981), 491–497.

66   Cornell JA, Jordan JS, Ellis S, Rose EE. A method of comparing the wear resistance of various materials used for artificial teeth. *J Am Dent Assoc*, 54 (1957), 608–614.

67   Pallav P, De Gee AJ, Werner A, Davidson, CL. Influence of shearing action of food on contact stress and subsequent wear of stress-bearing composites. *J Dent Res*, 72 (1993), 56–61.

68   Almond CH, Mayhan HG, Young RD, Simmons EM, Patterson BR, Biolsi ME, Davis SA, McClatchey BJ. A physiological approach to high-frequency testing of prosthetic ball valves. *J Thor Card Surg*, 67 (1974), 839–848.

69   Steinmetz GP, May KJ, Mueller V, Anderson HN, Merendino KA. An improved accelerated fatigue machine and pulse simulator for testing and developing prosthetic cardiac valves. *J Thor Card Surg*, 47 (1964), 186–198.

70   Koorajian S, Keller DP, Pierie WR, Starr A, Herr R. Criteria and systems for testing artificial heart valves in vitro. In *Prosthetic Heart Valves*. Springfield, IL: Charles C. Thomas, Publisher, 1969, 92–112.

71   Fettel BE, Johnston DR, Morris PE. Accelerated life testing of prosthetic heart valves. *Med Instrumentation*, 14 (1980), 161–164.

72   Noishiki Y, Yamane Y, Takahashi M, Kawanami O, Futami Y, Nihikawa T, Nogushi N, Nagaoka S, Mori Y. Prevention of thrombosis-related complications in cardiac catherization and angiography using a heparinized catheter. *Trans Am Soc Artif Org*, 33 (1987), 359–365.

73   Graiver D, Dural RL, Okada T. Surface morpholoy and friction coefficient of various types of Foley catheters. *Biomaterials*, 14 (1993), 465–469.

74   Sheets JW, Goldberg EP. Corneal endothelium damage with intraocular lenses: Contact adhesion between surgical materials and tissue. *Science*, 198 (1977), 525–527.

75   Clarke IC, McKellop HA. Wear testing. In *Handbook of Biomaterials Evaluation*. New York: Macmillan Publishing Co., 1986, 114–130.

76   Rigney DA. Introduction. In Rigney DA (Ed.), *Fundamentals of Friction and Wear of Materials*. Metals Park, Ohio: American Society for Metals, 1981, 1–12.

77   Hosseini SM, Stolarski TA. Morphology of polymer wear debris resulting from different contact conditions. *J Appl Poly Sci*, 45 (1992), 2021–2030.

78   Hosseini SM, Stolarski TA. Contact configuration effects on the dry and lubricated wear of polymers. *Surface Engineering*, 4 (1988), 322–326.

79   Weightman B. Friction, lubrication and wear. In *The Scientific Basis of Joint Replacement*. New York: John Wiley & Sons, Inc., 1977, 46–85.

80 Vaziri M, Spurr RT, Scott FH. An investigation of the wear of polymeric materials. *Wear*, 122 (1988), 329–342.

81 Dumbleton JH. *Tribology of Natural and Artificial Joints*. New York: Elsevier, 1981, 110–148.

82 Davidson JA, Scwartz G, Lynch G, Gir S. Wear creep and frictional heating of femoral implant articulating surfaces and the effect on long term performance. *J Biomed Mat Res*, 22A (1988), 69–91.

83 Walker PS, Blunn GW, Broome DR, Perry J, Watkins A, Sathasivam S, Dewar M, Paul JP. The kinematic conditions required for valid comparison of wear to total knees in a simulating machine. *Trans 42nd Annual Meeting of the Orthopaedic Research Society*, Atlanta, GA, February 18–22, 1996, 463.

84 Saikko, V. Tribology of total replacement hip joints studied with new hip joint simulators and a materials-screening apparatus. *Acta Polytechnica Scandinavia, Mechanical Engineering Series No. 110*, Helsinki, 1993, 1–44.

85 McKellop HA, Clarke IC. Evolution and evaluation of materials-screening machines and joint simulators in predicting in vivo wear phenomena. In Ducheyne P, Hastings GW (Eds), *Functional Behavior of Orthopaedic Biomaterials, Volume II: Applications*. Boca Raton, FL: CRC Press, 1984, 51–85.

86 Dowson D, Jobbins B. Design and development of a versatile hip joint simulator and a preliminary assessment of wear and creep in Charnely total replacement hip joints. *J Engrng in Med*, 17 (1988), 111–117.

87 Saikko V, Paavalainen P, Kleimola M, Slätis P. A five-station hip joint simulator for wear rate studies. *J Engrng in Med*, 21 (1992), 195–200.

88 Streicher RM, Schon R, Semlitsch M. Investigation of the tribological behaviour of metal-on-metal combinations for artificial hip joints. *Biomed Tech*, 35 (1990), 107–111.

89 Medley JB, Krygier JJ, Bobyn JD, Chan FW, Lippincott A, Tanzer M. Kinematics of the MATCO^{TM} hip simulator and issues related to wear testing of metal-metal implants. *J of Engrng in Med*, 25 (1996).

90 Pappas MJ, Makris G, Buechel FF. Titanium nitride film against polyethylene—a 48 million cycle wear test. *Clin Orthop*, 317 (1995), 64–70.

91 Shroeder DW, Pozorski KM. Hip simulator testing of isostatically molded UHMWPE: Effect of ETO and gamma irradiation. *Trans 42nd Annual Meeting of the Orthopaedic Research Society*, Atlanta, GA, February 18–22, 1996, 478.

92 Clark IC, Gustafson A, Jung H, Fujisawa A. Hip-simulator ranking of polyethylene wear—Comparisons between ceramic heads of different sizes. *Acta Orthop Scand*, 67 (1996), 128–132.

93 Johnston RC, Smidt GL. Measurement of hip-joint motion during walking: Evaluation of an electrogoniometric method. *J Bone Jt Surg*, 51A (1969), 1083–1094.

94 Murray MP, Drought AB, Kory RC. Walking patterns of normal men. *J Bone Jt Surg*, 46A (1964), 335–350.

95 Paul JP. Forces transmitted by joints in the human body. *Proc Instn Mech Engrs*, 181 (1966–67), 8–15.

96 Paul JP. Approaches to design—force actions transmitted by joints in the human body. *Proc R Soc Lond*, 192B (1976), 163–172.

97 Davidson JA, Schwartz G, Lynch G, Gir S. Wear creep and frictional heating of femoral implant articulating surfaces and the effect on long-term performance. Part II, friction, heating and torque. *J Biomed Mat Res*, 22A (1988), 69–91.

98 Skare T, Stahl JE. Static and dynamic friction processes under the influence of external vibrations. *Wear*, 154 (1992), 177–192.

99 Gee MG. Effect of test machine dynamics on the sliding wear of alumina. *Wear Testing of Advanced Materials, STP 1167*. Philadelphia, PA: American Society for Testing and Materials, 1992, 24–44.

100 McKellop HA, Campbell P, Park SH, Schmalzried TP, Grigoris P, Amstitz HC, Sarmiento A. The origin of submicron polyethylene wear debris in total hip arthroplasty. *Clin Orthop*, 311 (1995), 3–20.

101 Dowling JM, Atkinson JR, Dowson D, Charnely J. The characteristics of acetabular cups worn in the human body. *J Bone Jt Surg*, 60B (1978), 375–382.

102 Rowland SA, Shalaby SW, Latour Jr RA, von Recum AF. Effectiveness of cleaning surgical implants: Quantitative analysis of contaminant removal. *J Appl Biomat*, 6 (1995), 1–7.

103 Dowson D. Wear processes and test procedures. In *An Introduction to the Bio-mechanics of Joints and Joint Replacement*. London: Mechanical Engineering Publications, Ltd., 1981, 61–67.

104 Clarke IC, Starkebaum W, Hosseinian A, McGuire P, Okuda R, Salovey R, Young R. Fluid-sorption phenomena in sterilized polyethylene acetabular prostheses. *J Biomat*, 6 (1985).

105 Auger, DD, Dowson D, Fisher J, Jin MZ. Friction and lubrication in cushion form bearings for artificial hip joints. *Proc Instn Mech Engrs*, 207 (1993), 25–33.

106 Galante GO, Rostoker W. Wear in total hip prostheses: An experimental evaluation of candidate materials. *Acta Orthop Scand (Suppl.)*, 1973, 145.

107 Kang T, Rabinowicz E, Sector M. Distance-dependent mechanisms of wear of UHMWPE associated with reciprocating sliding. *Trans 19th Annual Meeting of the Society for Biomaterials*. Birmingham, AL, 1993, 13.

108   Saikko V, Paavolaien P, Kleimola M, Slätis P. A five-station hip joint simulator for wear rate studies. *Proc Instn Mech Engrs*, 206 (1992), 195–200.

109   O'Connor DO, Burke DW, Bragdon CR, Ramamurti BS, Harris WH. Dynamic frictional comparisons of different femoral head sizes and different lubricants. *Trans 21st Annual Meeting of the Society for Biomaterials*, San Francisco, CA, 1995, 230.

110   Agrawal CM, Micallef DM, Wirth MA, Lankford J, Dearnaley G, McCabe AR. The effects of diamond-like-carbon coatings on the friction and wear of enhanced UHMWPE-metal couples. *Trans 21st Annual Meeting of the Society for Biomaterials*, Birmingham, AL, 1993, 10.

111   McKellop HA, Röstlund TV. The wear behavior of ion-implanted Ti-6Al- 4V against UHMW polyethylene. *J Biomed Mat Res*, 24 (1990), 1413–1425.

112   Craig LE, LaBerge M. Effect of DPPC Concentration on the boundary lubrication of rigid bearings: An arthroplasty model. *15th Annual Conference of the Canadian Biomaterials Society*, Quebec City, July 1994, 33–34.

113   O'Kelly J, Unsworth A, Dowson D, Wright A. Pendulum and simulator studies of friction in hip joints. *Eng Med*, 8 (1979), 153–159.

114   Gore TA, Higginson GR, Kornberg RE. Some evidence of squeeze film lubrication in hip prostheses. *J Engrng in Med*, 10 (1981), 89–95.

115   Unsworth A, Pearcy MJ, White EFT, White G. Frictional properties of artificial joints. *Eng Med*, 17 (1988), 101–104.

116   Alexander AL. The viscosity of lubricants. *Lubrication*, 78 (1992), 1–16.

117   Huang C, Li S, Wang Z, Lin H. Dependence of the bilayer phase transition temperatures on the structural parameters of phosphatidylcholines. *Lipids*, 28 (1993), 364–370.

118   Ly DP, Bellet D, Boyer P, Roques C. Rheological behavior of synovial fluids. *Biorheology*, 17 (1980), 321–329.

119   Cooke AF, Dowson D, Wright V. The rheology of synovial fluid and some potential synthetic lubricants for degenerate synovial joints. *IMechE: Eng Med*, 7 (1978), 66–72.

120   Black J. Friction and wear. In *Biological Performance of Materials*. New York: Marcel Dekker, 1992, 92–109.

121   An KN, Chao, EYS, Kaufman KR. Analysis of muscle and joint loads. In Mow VC, Hayes WC (Eds.), *Basic Orthopaedic Biomechanics*. New York: Raven Press, 1991, 1–50.

122   Greer KW, Jones DE. The importance of standardization of wear test parameters in the simulation of knee wear mechanisms. *Trans of 20th Annual Meeting of the Society for Biomaterials*, Boston, MA, 1994, 408.

123   McConnell D, Conroy C. Comparison of abrasion produced by a simulated manual versus a mechanical toothbrush. *J Dent Res*, 46 (1967), 1022–1027.

124   Dumbleton JH. *Tribology of Natural and Artificial Joints*. New York: Elsevier, 1981, 74–109.

125   Long M, Rack HJ. Ultrasonic method for *in situ* continuous wear measurements of orthopaedic titanium alloys. *Proc Fifth World Biomaterials Congress*, Toronto, Canada, May 29–June 2, 1996.

126   Pienkowski D, Jacob R, Hoglin D, Saum K, Kaufer H, Nicholls PJ. Low-voltage scanning electron microscopic imaging of ultrahigh-molecular-weight polyethylene. *J Biomed Mat Res*, 29 (1995), 1167–1174.

127   Hamrock BJ. *Fundamentals of Fluid Film Lubrication*. New York: McGraw-Hill, Inc., 1994.

128   Ruff AW, Ives LK, Glaeser WA. Characterization of wear surfaces and wear debris. In Rigney DA (Ed.), *Fundamentals of Friction and Wear of Materials*. Metals Park, Ohio: American Society for Metals, 1981, 235–290.

129   Scott D. Debris examination: A prognostic approach to failure prevention. *Wear*, 34 (1975), 15–22.

130   Barnwell FT. The use of temper colors in ferrography. *Wear*, 44 (1977), 163–171.

131   Briscoe BJ, Tabor D. Friction and wear of polymers: The role of mechanical properties. *Brit Poly J*, 10 (1978), 74–78.

132   Briscoe BJ, Stolarski TA. Transfer wear of polymers during combined linear motion and load axis spin. *Wear*, 104 (1985), 121–137.

133   McGovern TE, Black J, Jacobs JJ, Graham RM, LaBerge M. In vivo wear of Ti6Al4V femoral heads: A retrieval study. *J Biomed Mat Res*, 1996.

134   Dumbleton JH. *Tribology of Natural and Artificial Joints*. New York: Elsevier, 1981, 149–182.

135   Box GEP, Hunter WC, Hunter JS. *Statistics for Experimentors*. New York: John Wiley & Sons Inc., 1978.

Chapter 11

Reference Materials

Anne E. Meyer

THE NEED FOR AND RELEVANCE
OF REFERENCE MATERIALS

The need for standard reference materials in research and testing is widely recognized. Generally we can place the use of these materials in one of two categories: a check on analytical accuracy and precision from laboratory to laboratory, given the application of the same analytical procedure or set of procedures, or a means toward understanding how the results of a variety of experimental techniques interrelate and describe the system studied. The first category is most common in analytical laboratories (chemical, biological, and physical testing). Regulatory agencies, such as the United States Environmental Protection Agency and most health administrations, frequently require the inclusion of primary reference material characterization in the routine workload of service and research laboratories. Often the reference materials are included in round-robin testing. As testing procedures become more standardized in biomaterials research, reference materials play a key role in identifying any systematic errors that may creep into a laboratory's techniques.

The second category is fundamental to the development of new biomaterials and biomedical devices. One characteristic of this type of research is that new experimental methods frequently are introduced to the field: methods for in vitro, ex vivo, or in vivo testing. Reference materials are used to develop and calibrate a new method, thus defining the capability of the new technique. The results from using reference materials with a new or modified technique also help to bring that technique into use in ongoing biomaterials research, in which correlation of results from a wide variety of material tests is crucial to understanding short- and long-term consequences of material use.

The reference material, in a given system, should produce a consistent and quantifiable "response" or interaction with system components. Depending on the reference material used, the response can be either "good" or "bad." The results must be reproducible, however, to ensure that the experimental method and conditions are consistent. The reference material need not be the same material intended for use in fabricating a biomedical device. An investigator may choose to use two reference materials: one that is similar to the material of device construction and one that is likely to elicit the opposite response. It must be stressed, however, that a test protocol should not be revised to accommodate a particular reference material. For instance, if the temperature range of a test system will degrade one type of reference material, the temperature should not be adjusted to accommodate the reference material; rather, a reference material that will not be temperature-sensitive should be selected.

A wide variety of reference materials are currently available. Many have been developed with the objective of providing known bulk material chemical and/or mechanical characteristics. An example is the reference grade polyethylene available from the National Institute of Standards and Technology (NIST), formerly the National Bureau of Standards [1]. NIST has created an inventory of a large number of "reference materials" and *standard* reference materials." Standard Reference Materials (SRMs) are much more thoroughly characterized and controlled as to composition and reproducibility [2]. Designation of a material as an SRM by NIST is a lengthy and costly process. The cost for a laboratory to acquire SRM samples from NIST, therefore, is much greater than if only reference-material-grade samples are required. Individual researchers also can develop their own "laboratory reference" materials for more frequent use in experiments. Lab reference materials are discussed in greater detail below.

The remainder of this chapter will focus on reference materials for surface-specific studies, such as the interaction of proteins or cells with materials.

SOURCES AND SELECTION OF REFERENCE MATERIALS

Both NIST and the National Institutes of Health (NIH), particularly, the National Heart, Lung, and Blood Institute (NHLBI) have been sources of reference materials and standard reference materials (NHLBI referred to the latter as "primary reference materials") for the biomaterials research community.

In 1977, NHLBI reviewed its progress in biomaterials development and determined that significant gaps existed in the understanding of blood-material interactions, and that reliable approaches to the study of biomaterials and their interactions with blood needed to be defined (although NHLBI focused on blood-material interactions, the results of their efforts also apply to soft tissue-material and hard tissue-material systems). Two expert panels were formed by NHLBI, the working group on physicochemical characterization of biomaterials and the working group on blood-material interactions. By 1980, both panels published their recommendations for standardized methods and materials [3, 4]. The reports later were published as a single volume in the second edition [5]. The physicochemical characterization panel made specific recommendations for the production of particular reference materials, including polyethylene, fluorinated ethylene propylene, filler-free polydimethylsiloxane, graphitic carbon, and "natural" reference materials. The panel emphasized the need for materials that were consistent from sample to sample, requiring extensive characterization, including molecular weight distribution; glass transition temperature; degree of tacticity; polymerization conditions; residual monomer and catalyst levels; refractive index at common wavelengths; ultraviolet, visible, and infrared spectra; swelling and solubility information; solubility parameter; hardness; stress-strain relations; elastic modulus; surface energy parameters; surface composition; degree of roughness; and toxicity. Obviously, many of the characteristics concern bulk properties of a material, but are of interest because inconsistency within the bulk often results in changes at the surface of a material, especially if the test material is subjected to mechanical stress during an experiment.

Three materials were selected by NHLBI for immediate attention: low-density polyethylene (LDPE), polydimethylsiloxane (PDMS), and fluorinated ethylene propylene (FEP). Beginning in 1979, NIH funded projects for the production and thorough characterization of these "primary reference materials." As of 1984, LDPE and PDMS were available for general use by the biomaterials research and testing community. Shortage in supplies delayed the large-scale production of the primary reference fluoropolymer, leading individual researchers to select commercially available film stock of conventional tetrafluoroethylene/ethylene (TFE) as a useful substitute. Different textures and/or surface chemistries on the two sides of the PDMS primary reference and TFE lab standard materials, however, are a cause of confusion in test results, if researchers are not careful to keep track of sample "sidedness" during experiments and analyses [6]; this has not been a problem with the

LDPE primary reference material, as its two sides are very similar. Work to develop a polyurethane primary reference material is in progress.

Recent discussions were held regarding the transfer of the NHLBI inventory of primary reference materials to NIST, indicating an increasing commitment by NIST to biomaterials. NIH, however, continues to support development of new reference materials that are relevant to cardiovascular devices, hard- and soft-tissue implants, and other biomedical devices.

In selecting a reference material (of any grade), each test director must consider the following questions: How has the material previously been characterized? Are the descriptors that are key to one's own work defined? If only bulk characteristics are given in the specification of the material, then it is unlikely that the surface quality of the material has been defined or carefully controlled; there are likely to be contaminants on the surface of the material. If surface characteristics of a reference material are not provided and there is no other suitable material available, researchers should consider performing their own series of "quality control" tests on a number of samples to determine the consistency of the sample surfaces. Another approach is to acquire an inventory of commercially available material (enough to fill the researcher's needs for 5–10 years) for development as a "lab reference material."

At first glance, selection and qualification of one's own reference material appears to be relatively straightforward and inexpensive: purchase the material, clean, characterize, and use. Commercially available polymers, for instance, generally contain stabilizers and processing aids. Metal and ceramics acquire contaminants from processing, packaging, storage, and handling. These contaminants will not often affect the bulk characteristics of a material, but definitely will alter its surface qualities. Subsequent treatments, such as sterilization by autoclaving or ethylene oxide, are also known to seriously compromise the initial surface properties of even originally clean materials [7, 8]. The following stages in development of lab reference materials must be considered, each contributing to sample reproducibility: anticipated inventory requirement, cleaning procedures, surface spatial consistency and "sidedness," sterilization technique, storage modality, and shelf-life. The stability of packaging materials also is very important. In the case of hard materials (e.g., metals, alloys, ceramics), means to recycle lab reference materials, restoring them to their original condition, should be evaluated if a great deal of effort is required to acquire a stock of known bulk composition or to prepare specimens of specific dimensions. Characterization of the clean, sterile, packaged lab reference samples by a higher level of analysis than is generally performed by the laboratory is recommended to avoid future surprises. For instance, comprehensive contact angle analyses and X-ray photoelectron spectroscopy (or scanning Auger microprobe analyses or secondary ion mass spectrometry) should be undertaken to highlight the nature of the outermost aspects of the prepared reference material. If surface texture is a key aspect of the laboratory's research, analysis of reference materials should include atomic force microscopy as well as scanning electron microscopy. A detailed, written protocol of preparation and analysis methods and results should be prepared, checked for accuracy by all those involved in development of the lab reference material, and revised until the document is a reliable handbook for future consultation.

Once a reference material (of any grade) is deemed suitable for an experimental program, the researcher must then be extremely alert to the manner in which the material is treated when it is removed from inventory. Have the materials been treated carelessly? What is the potential for contamination by handling? Are the reference materials prepared for exposure in the same manner as other test samples? If not, are the differences consistent and documented? Are the post-exposure procedures consistent and documented? A short, written description of reference material properties and handling tips (e.g., to avoid confusion with sample sidedness) is recommended when sharing reference materials with new colleagues in one's own lab, and essential when sharing materials with collaborators from other laboratories.

In summary, the investigator must not only be sensitive to the quality of the reference material that is selected, but also must be watchful of how the material is handled and treated before, during, and after exposure to the test system.

CHARACTERIZATION METHODS

In addition to bulk characteristics that may affect material performance, a number of material surface properties can greatly influence the outcome of exposure to biological systems. Key surface characteristics include chemical composition, reactivity, surface energy, surface charge, and texture. Methods recommended for determining these properties are included in this volume and elsewhere [10–16].

OTHER RECOMMENDED REFERENCE MATERIALS

Most of the reference materials currently available to the biomaterials research and testing community are polymers. Other commonly used biomaterials include metals, ceramics, and stabilized tissue; still others incorporate specialized coatings such as collagen and heparin. Additional progress in the field of tissue engineering may require an entirely new class of reference materials. The remainder of this chapter highlights a few suggestions for metal, ceramic, and tissue reference materials. Different commercial sources of the materials are available; none has been qualified to the extent necessary for NIST Standard Reference Materials.

Pyrolytic Carbon

This material is available in two versions: low temperature isotropic (LTI) and a similar material alloyed with silicon (to improve wear properties). The recommendation for a standard, or primary, reference material is the LTI (pure carbon) version, polished to a smooth surface finish with 0.25-micron diamond dust.

Pure Metals and Metal Alloys

Metal and metal alloys are discussed at great length in other sections of this book, particularly bulk properties and corrosion tendencies. In the selection of a metal reference material for surface evaluation, a number of factors come into play: control of texture, surface composition, and reproducible preparation methods. Polishing residues can be particularly troublesome. A large number of metals could serve well as reference materials, for instance, the more corrosion-resistant stainless steels (iron/chromium alloys), the cobalt/chromium alloys, and titanium.

Ceramics

Ceramics also have been addressed elsewhere in this book; these materials are most frequently used to replace or encourage growth of bony tissues. Calcium hydroxyapatite is an obvious choice as a reference material. Commercial sources of dense crystalline hydroxyapatite in block form are available, but, like most of the materials suggested here, are not produced as reference materials and, therefore, should be prepared for testing in individual laboratories by each laboratory's own standardized and documented protocol. Like clean metals and metal alloys, clean ceramics are easily contaminated.

Stabilized Tissue

The need for a reference stabilized tissue material is great. While the NIH panels discussed earlier in this chapter recommended such a reference material, efforts to produce polymeric materials took priority.

Ideally, like the other reference materials already discussed, the tissue should be processed and its properties thoroughly documented under strict quality control requirements. It would seem that tissue materials used in medical devices currently marketed in the U.S. (note that the U.S. Food and Drug Administration does not "approve" materials) would fill the need for reference materials until a standard tissue reference is developed. Stabilized tissue materials include pericardium, porcine valves, bovine heterografts, and human umbilical cord vein grafts marketed by cardiovascular device companies.

REFERENCES

1   U.S. Department of Commerce, National Institute of Standards and Technology. *Standard Reference Materials Catalog*. Gaithersburg, MD. Published on a regular basis.

2   Mears TW and Young DS. Measurement and standard reference materials in clinical chemistry. *Am J Clin Pathol*, 50 (1968), 411–421.

3   *Guidelines for Blood-Material Interactions*. Report of the National Heart, Lung, and Blood Institute Working Group, NIH Publ. No. 80-2185, NIH, Washington, DC, 1980.

4   *Guidelines for Physicochemical Characterization of Biomaterials*. Report of the National Heart, Lung, and Blood Institute Working Group, NIH Publ. No. 80-2186, NIH, Washington, DC, 1980.

5   *Guidelines for Blood-Material Interactions*. Report of the National Heart, Lung, and Blood Institute Working Group, NIH Publ. No. 85-2185, NIH, Washington, DC, 1985.

6   Schmidt JA, von Recum AF. On the use of primary reference grade polydimethylsiloxane. *J Applied Biomaterials*, 4 (1993), 73–76.

7   Baier RE, Meyer AE, Akers CK, Natiella JR, Meenaghan MA, and Carter JM. Degradative effects of conventional steam sterilization on biomaterial surfaces. *Biomaterials*, 3 (1982), 241–245.

8   Baier RE, Meyer AE. Surface energetics and biological adhesion. In Mittal KL (Ed.), *Physicochemical Aspects of Polymer Surfaces*, Vol. 2. New York: Plenum Press, 1983, 895–909.

9   Keller JC, Draughn RA, Wightman JP, Dougherty WJ, Meletiou SD. *Intl J Oral & Maxillofac Implants*, 5 (1990), 360–367.

10 Zisman WA. Relation of the equilibrium contact angle to liquid and solid constitution. In Contact Angle: *Wettability and Adhesion*. Advances in Chemistry Series, Vol. 43. Washington, DC: American Chemical Society, 1964, 1–64.

11 Ratner BD (Ed.). *Surface Characterization of Biomaterials: Progress in Biomedical Engineering*, Vol. 6. Amsterdam: Elsevier, 1988.

12 *Surface Measurement and Characterization*. Proc of SPIE, the International Society for Optical Engineering, Bellingham, WA, Vol. 1009, 1989.

13 Silage DA, Baran GR. Morphometric assessment of surface conformation as an estimate of roughness. *J Microscopy*, 173 (1994), 239–243.

14 Vesenka J, Mosher C, Schaus S, Ambrosio L, Henderson E. Combining optical and atomic force microscopy for life science research. *Biotechniques*, 19 (1995), 240–248.

15 Firtel M, Beveridge TJ. Scanning probe microscopy in microbiology. *Micron*, 26 (1995), 347–362.

16 Stemmer A. A hybrid scanning force and light microscope for surface imaging and three-dimensional optical sectioning in differential interference contrast. *J Microscopy*, 178 (1995), 28–36.

Chapter 12

Property Modification

Jennifer A. Neff
Karin D. Caldwell

INTRODUCTION

A biomedical material selection process typically begins with the identification of those bulk physical and mechanical properties which are required for a device to accomplish a desired task. Such characteristics as flexibility or rigidity, porosity or impermeability, electrical insulation or ability to pass current are but a few examples of properties that may dictate the choice of material for a given application. However, a *biomaterial* by definition will be required to function in a biological environment, where it will come in contact with living tissues or chemically complex body fluids, such as blood and tears. Over the years it has become clear that compatibility with this environment is first and foremost regulated by the material's surface and, as a result, an extraordinary effort has been made to develop methods for tailor-making desired surfaces on a vast number of different bulk materials. It is beyond the scope of the present chapter to provide an exhaustive account of this large research effort; instead, the following text will attempt to give a brief, and by necessity selective, summary of some recent developments and concerns in the area of biomaterials surface modification.

General Approaches to Surface Activation

Two major strategies present themselves for the biocompatibilization of a surface, namely its transformation to become either bioactive or bioinert. The former includes surfaces that are modified to present active functionalities which range in size and complexity from small ionic groups to large extracellular matrix proteins and which, therefore, bind key proteins, e.g. in the complement or coagulation cascades of blood or those functioning as integrin receptors on the membranes of cells. The latter is designed to minimize all interactions — favorable as well as adverse. Even though the final result of a surface modification procedure may be a "stealth" coating, the attachment of this coating may well proceed via an active intermediate. It may therefore be of some use to begin by taking a general look at the arsenal of methods now available to modify surfaces of the more commonly used classes of materials.

Plasma Modification   When a rarefied gas is exposed to an energy input in the form of high power radio frequency, highly reactive ions and radicals are formed. Due to the low concentration of neighbors in the gas phase, numerous radicals avoid recombination and survive until they hit some object in their way with which they can combine. The result of this combination is typically the formation of a covalent bond with the surface of the object and, hence, the plasma technique is well suited to introduce a large variety of groups on surfaces of virtually any chemical composition [141, 195, 197]. Materials ranging from metals [183, 186] to polymers [105] have been surface-modified in this manner to display amine groups (ammonia plasma) [21, 43, 107], alcoholic hydroxides (hydroxyethyl methacrylate) [108, 127], carbonyl and carboxylic acid functionalities (oxygen plasma)

[152)], as well as sulphonate groups (sulphur dioxide plasma) [105]. These functional groups lend themselves well to further derivatization, as will be discussed below. In addition, more complex plasmas, produced with larger molecules and applied for longer periods of time, lead to the build-up of polymeric films on the exposed surface [50, 196].

Although these techniques have great versatility, they are somewhat difficult to control. Factors such as energy and angle at collision will affect the nature of the bond created with the surface; hence a variety of chemistries may result from the impact. The sensitivity to impact energy, in turn, makes it difficult to treat an object of complex geometry in a fully reproducible manner, and a pattern of chemically distinct shadows may well result in the absence of meticulous care in the reactor design. One further complication of particular concern for polymeric substrates above their glass transition temperature is associated with the dynamic nature of such matrices. In an effort to minimize its energy, a newly modified system will undergo more or less rapid molecular rearrangements that may ultimately cause a burial of the introduced reactive groups in the interior of the matrix. Storage of plasma modified polymer products can therefore be a problem.

Silanization   The modification of silica surfaces with organic phases has been well developed since the pioneering work of Plueddeman [147]. The modification most commonly involves reacting an amphoteric or weakly acidic oxide (or hydroxylated) surface with a tri-alkoxy silane of the general formula $(R_1-O)_3-Si-R_2$ to form a siloxane linkage between the two. Those alkoxide groups which fail to bond to the surface are generally induced to link laterally by a combined hydrolysis/condensation reaction. The R_1-groups of the tri-alkoxy silane are for the most part of methyl- or ethyl-type, while R_2 contains the functional group to be implanted on the surface. A variety of silanes are commercially available today, so that the researcher has a large latitude in selecting a surface chemistry which matches the chemical nature of the ligand to be covalently attached. Most commonly, the R_2-groups are of the end-substituted propyl variety, with amino-, 3-glycidoxy-, and mercapto-groups as representative examples of useful reactivities for work with proteins, nucleic acids, and carbohydrates [53, 82, 116, 150, 187].

Direct Chemical Activation   Many polymeric biomaterials are susceptible to hydrolysis under extreme conditions of pH. This is, for instance, true for the frequently used polyesters, which opens an avenue for modification of polycarbonate (PC), polyethylene terepthalate (PET), polymethylmethacrylate (PMMA), polylactic acid (PLA), and polylactic glycolic acid (PLGA) polymers, among others, by creating surface hydroxyls and carboxylic groups that are suitable for further ligand attachment, e.g. by chemistries outlined in Figure 12-1. In addition to a hydrolytic chain scission, a hydrazinolytic reaction [15] may sometimes be desirable, as it introduces amine groups which, unlike the primary amines whose pK lies around 9.5–10, are deprotonated and hence reactive even at low pH [167]. A chemical cleavage of the polyurethane backbone can be accomplished by an exchange reaction involving a second isocyanate, e.g. hexamethylenediisocyanate [55] which, in turn, enables subsequent functionalization; the otherwise highly stable polysulphones are easily aminated in two-step reactions involving either a chloromethylation or a chlorosulphonation step, followed by reaction with a diamine [148]. Polystyrene, in turn, is amenable to derivatization, e.g. through the introduction of alcohols, carboxyls, or sulfhydryl groups [124]. In this case, the substituents are affixed to the pendant aromatic rings in a reaction that does not primarily involve chain cleavage.

As no general rules can be stated regarding the choice of reactants and reaction conditions, specific examples of such chemical polymer activation are given below. Although

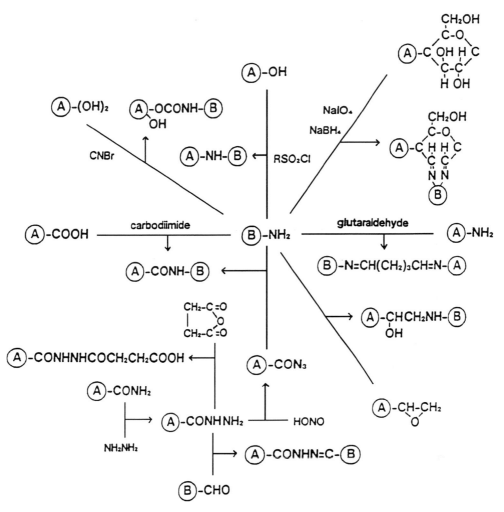

Figure 12-1 Reaction strategies available for covalent linking of two moieties, A and B. Reproduced from Reference 80 with permission.

often practical tools for providing chemical access to a surface, these modification techniques are by their very nature somewhat destructive and may change both surface morphology as well as a material's ability to withstand future degradation.

Physisorption A general listing of the means available for surface modification would not be complete without a mentioning of those processes which rely on adsorption. Like the previous category, these methods are materials specific, both with regard to the substrate and the adsorbing entity.

A material whose cohesive energy differs significantly from that of the liquid in which it is immersed will tend to accumulate surface active species at the solid/liquid interface in order to reduce the existing interfacial tension. In aqueous environments, non-polar materials such as polyethylene (PE), or the hard segment, e.g. the methyl diphenyl isocyanate (MDI) domains in certain biomedical polyurethanes (PU), give rise to large interfacial tensions, while the opposite holds for such polar polymers as polyvinyl pyrrolidone (PVP) or cellulose. In an aqueous environment, amphipathic molecules are therefore likely to adsorb strongly to non-polar surfaces, while such adsorption is less likely to occur on hydrophilic sufaces. Since most proteins have surface active properties even in their native form, and since these properties typically become more pronounced as the protein is forced to unfold at the interface, it stands to reason that the proteins of plasma, tears, and other biological fluids have a tendency to accumulate and bind to hydrophobic materials with which they come in contact.

Specific examples of adsorption-based biosurface modification will be addressed below. In the present context it is sufficient to recall that the adsorption of a surface active polymer, whether natural or synthetic, is likely to result in a multi-point attachment to the substrate. This fact accounts for the virtually irreversible immobilization which is often seen when macromolecular surfactants and proteins come in contact with a surface. The adsorption-based surface modification can, therefore, act as a stepping stone for one or more subsequent modification reactions, as will be demonstrated below.

Chemical Linking to Functional Surface Groups

Once functionalized as described above, the surface is ready for the attachment of a desired ligand or modifier. For several decades, protein chemists have been actively developing bifunctional reagents for immobilization, crosslinking, and labelling of biomolecules, and excellent monographs exist [192] which detail these reactions. Furthermore, both homo- and hetero-bifunctional reagents with high specificity are now commercially available, making the modification process ever more tractable. Although activated biomaterials will include functional groups of a large variety, the most common linking reactions will be those involving amines, alcohols, aldehydes, and carboxylic acids. Figure 12-1 [79] summarizes several useful reactions for accomplishing such linking. Among these, the conversion of alcoholic -OH groups into reactive esters by treatment with sulfonyl halides, e.g. tosyl-, tresyl- or fosyl chlorides [133)], or by succinimidyl- [125] or p-nitrophenyl-[103] chloroformates in non-aqueous solvents, provide powerful means for subsequent coupling of amines or thiols under mild aqueous conditions. Figure 12-1 also outlines a useful method for coupling carbohydrates to any amine-containing compound. This approach is based on the periodate-mediated oxidation of the sugar into an aldehyde and the subsequent Schiff's base formation with the deprotonated amine or hydrazine, followed by a reduction with $NaBH_4$ [63]. Schiff's base formation is the basis also for coupling by means of the homo-bifunctional glutaraldehyde, a commonly used cross-linking reagent for proteins which, in this context, serves as a linker between amine-containing entities. Carboxylic acid groups, in turn, whether originally present on a surface or produced by ester hydrolysis, are most commonly coupled to amines or alcohols following carbodiimide activation [29]. This coupling occurs in aqueous milieu, and is therefore suitable for use even with fragile biomolecules.

Lastly, among reactions suitable for activation of products resulting from hydrazinolysis is the treatment with nitrite to form an azide (low center in Figure 12-1). This compound is photoactivable and provides a means for spatially precise coupling of a variety of polymers, including peptides, carbohydrates, and polyurethanes. In the arsenal of commercially available hetero-bifunctional reagents, those containing azides (e.g. in the form of azido-phenyl groups) [2] are steadily gaining in popularity.

While the surface attachment of a given protein may effectively proceed via any of a number of exposed primary amines, the linking process can in some cases chemically involve or sterically impact that portion of the molecule which is responsible for its biological activity. This is frequently the case in the important bioanalytical process of antibody immobilization, in which the N-terminal antigen binding sites should ideally be protected from involvement in the surface linking. Strategies for attachment should then consider directional immobilization via groups known to be removed from the active site, in this case an activated thiol or carbohydrate group in the hinge region [63, 136]. In order to reduce the steric hindrance to biological activity presented by the surface, the bioactive ligand may often be productively attached via a non-interactive tether, e.g. of polyethylene glycol (PEG).

A more detailed and extensively referenced account of reaction conditions used for practical ligand attachment is given by Drumheller and Hubbell [35].

BIOINERT SURFACES

Steric exclusion mechanisms have long been invoked to stabilize colloidal suspensions [131]. Since the 1960s biochemists have been aware that the addition of small quantities of certain water-soluble polymers to dilute solutions of proteins can accomplish their concentration, and ultimately precipitation, with full retention of biological activity. Rather than stemming from a bonded interaction between the two components, this effect was found to result primarily from a preferential hydration of the polymer with the resultant steric exclusion of protein from its hydration sphere. Of the many highly water-soluble polymers that possess this steric exclusion property there were only a few, most notably PEG, dextran, and PVP, that appeared to leave the proteins in their native conformation without a tendency to form complexes of significant stability [72]. Later findings by Abukowski et al. [1] indicated that PEG had the power to confer non-immunogenicity to proteins to which it had been grafted. This opened the possiblity of protecting not only proteins but also tissues and synthetic materials from adverse reactions by a host organism in which they had been implanted. Encouraging results obtained in the early 1980s [122, 130] have resulted in a significant biomaterials research effort directed towards surface modification with hydrogels and other compounds with minimal tissue interaction.

Immobilization of Synthetic Polymers

Covalent Attachment   The early work by Nagaoka et al. [130] investigated the effect of chain length of end-grafted polyethylene oxide (PEO) on the adsorption of plasma protein as well as on the activation of platelets and found a significant reduction in both upon increasing the number of EO units in the chain until it contained about 50 monomer units. This finding is fully consistent with observations of excluded volume phenomenon in protein solutions that indicate a diminishing effect on the exclusion for polymer chains larger than about 5,000 Da (or just under 115 EO units per chain) [67]. In recent years, PEO has been successfully grafted to biomedical-grade polyurethanes with clearly demonstrable effects related to reduced protein uptake and the activation of platelets [14, 55]. PET has likewise been successfully PEO-grafted, in this case by means of a plasma polymerization procedure [48]. Surfaces that are hydrophobic by nature [162] or have been made hydrophobic, e.g. by silanization [4, 179)], can be induced to adsorb PEO-containing block copolymers via their hydrophobic blocks. Following adsorption, these blocks are then affixed to the surface by plasma treatment or g-irradiation [4, 105)], leaving the PEO chains in a mobile and highly hydrated state, serving as effective protein shields and suppressors of thrombogenicity.

An alternative route to PEO-based surface protection involves photochemical attachment, which has been successfully implemented on synthetic surfaces [180)]. Recently, the ability to accomplish photo-induced surface attachment of PEO has been extended also to living tissues, whose protection after trauma is hoped to lead to reduced thrombosis and suppression of restenosis [58, 110, 166, 189]. The approach involves a series of steps of which the first is an adsorption of the dye Eosin Y to the tissue to be protected. After flushing to remove the excess dye, the polymerizable PEO derivative (e.g., acrylic-terminated oligolactide-modified PEO) is introduced together with triethanolamine (TEOA), which serves as an initiator. A short pulse (20 seconds) of visible laser light (488–514 nm) is delivered to the reaction site by means of an optical fiber. This energy input excites the dye, leading in turn to radical formation by the TEOA and a subsequent polymerization of the PEO derivative. The technique has been successfully applied to stented arteries whose load of adherent platelets was reduced to 1/30 of the load seen in the absence of treatment [166]. By careful control of illumination time, intensity, and polymer concentration, it has been possible to control the thickness (5–100 μm) of the gel barrier which forms on the vessel surface [110].

To judge from the solution behavior of protein-polymer mixtures, the type of surface protection afforded by PEO and its derivatives should also result from treatment with dextran or PVP. Although not as commonly used, these polymers have nevertheless proven to have similar protective qualities. Thus, a recent study by Österberg et al. [138] compared the fibrinogen rejection by surfaces covered on the one hand by side-on or end-on immobilized dextran, and on the other by end-on polymerized PEG. Although there is no information on the relative surface concentrations of these polymer-coated products, the study clearly shows that comparable protein rejections can be generated by dextran and PEO, although, unlike the situation for PEO, the mode of attaching the dextran coating is crucial for its efficiency.

The attachment of PVP to polyurethane catheters [44] has similarly been seen to result in decreased fibrinogen and fibronectin adsorption, as well as in suppressed adhesion of both *Staphylococcus aureus* and *S. epidermidis*.

Besides dextran, there is a host of mucopolysaccharides thought to act as surface protectants in a manner similar to PEO. In a recent development, photocurable films were produced from hyaluronic acid and chondroitin sulfate, both highly water-swellable biopolymers [120], and implanted in test animals to cover injuries caused to the peritoneum. One week after implantation, the films had attached to the injured tissue, but their back-sides remained free from any attachment. This is in contrast to similarly injured control animals that were shown to develop adherent tissue consisting of fibroblasts and collagen fibers between the peritoneal defect and the omentum. These films, which were photocurable through the substitution of nontoxic dimerizable chromophors, such as cinnamate or thymine, were biodegradable with a minimum of inflammatory response.

Although the creation of "cilia-like" [5] high entropy surfaces through the attachment of PEO, PVP, polysaccharides, and other hydrophilic polymers may be the most commonly used approach to achieving bioinertness, the plasma deposition of many small molecules has proven highly effective in suppressing fibrinogen deposition and platelet activation. Ulubayram and Hasirci [181] found polyurethane surfaces modified with either hydroxyethylmethacrylate (HEMA) (contact angle 55°) or hexamethyldisiloxane (HMDSO) (contact angle 90°) to adsorb fewer platelets than did the untreated polymer (contact angle 70°). This is somewhat surprising in view of the large differences in hydrophobicity between the three materials. Kiaei et al. [83] did likewise observe reduced platelet adhesion to HMDSO-modified Dacron® (E. I DuPont de Nemours & Co., Inc., Wilmington, DE) vascular grafts. By contrast, work by Lin and Cooper [104] indicated no differences in hemocompatibility between untreated low density polyethylene (LDPE) and LDPE surfaces that had been plasma-modified with either HMDS alone, or in mixture with SO_2.

Other hydrophobic surface modifiers include the fluorocarbons, which have been uti-lized by several groups [10,45,54,85,146] with positive results. Despite a satisfactory hemocompatibility, the surface treatment described by Pizzoferrato et al. [146] had the draw back of increasing bacterial adhesion.

Given that protein adsorption is implicated in such adverse reactions to a material as thrombus formation, neutrophil activation, inflammatory response and capsule formation, the relationship between biocompatibility and surface hydrophobicity, which is known to correlate with protein uptake, clearly needs to be better understood. Recent work by Silver et al. [164] involved the production of a series of self-assembled alkyl siloxane monolayers on plasma-oxidized polydimethyl siloxane (PDMS) surfaces. Here, the C-(9-11) alkyl chains were terminated by groups that varied widely in hydrophobicity. Among the hydrophilic end groups were an acetate group, an OH-terminated trioxyethylene to simulate PEO, and an acetate analogue of this compound, while the hydrophobic specimens included underiva-tized siloxane (Silastic®, Dow Corning Corp., Midland, MI) and a PE sample, in addition to the methyl- and trifluoromethyl-terminated alkanes. In contrast to the hydrophilic sur-faces, all of which were found to be highly thrombogenic, the hydrophobic surfaces showed lower platelet adhesion and fibrinogen deposition. This led the authors to conclude that the most hydrophobic surfaces are the most hemocompatible. A similar study [114] on monolayer-covered silica and glass concluded that alkane chains terminated by methyl- or fluoromethyl groups were much less prone to protein uptake and epithelial cell adhesion than those terminated by an acetate or a methanolic group. It should be noted that the overall protein adsorption on these surfaces is high, with reported fibrinogen uptakes of $17 \ pmol/cm^2$ and above, which is about two orders of magnitude higher than what is found on Pluronic[TM] (Wyandott Chemical Corp., Wyandott, MI) F108 coated PS surfaces dis-cussed below [102]. A definitive answer to the biocompatibility question is therefore not at hand and will require more extensive model studies.

Adsorption of Synthetic Amphiphiles   The voluminous evidence of a lack of ad-verse biological response to surfaces grafted with PEO and similar hydrophilic polymers has led to a search for alternative and convenient ways to attach these polymers to potential biomaterials. For example, although PEO shows a slight tendency to adsorb to hydrophobic surfaces in an aqueous environment, the interaction is very weak, and the polymer is easily displaced by more strongly adsorbing species, such as plasma proteins. Hubbell and his group [32, 34] have devised a novel method for providing a permanent surface protection of common biomaterials, e.g. PET, PU, and PMMA. This method, which does not involve a plasma treatment or other incorporation of reactive chemical groups that might create problems if left on the surface after a grafting reaction, is built on the formation of inter-penetrating networks at the biomaterial surface. By swelling the base polymer in a solvent which is also capable of dissolving PEO, it is possible to accomplish diffusive mixing at the interface between the solid polymer and the PEO solution. After some time, the device is quenched by immersion in water, which is a solvent for PEO but a non-solvent for the base polymer. The molecular weight of the trapped PEO was found to affect its ability to provide surface protection for all base polymers studied, with an optimum in platelet and protein rejection being caused by the 18.5 kDa polymer.

From a practical standpoint, the simplest form of PEO-based surface protection is obtained through direct adsorption of a block copolymer, which is designed to contain hy-drophobic blocks for anchoring the molecule on a hydrophobic surface, and pendant PEO blocks to reduce interfacial tension and provide the desired steric shield. This form of sur-face modification, while inherently less durable than that provided by covalent attachment, has the clear advantage of being easily applicable to devices of any geometry without the introduction of chemical linkage groups that themselves may be the source of unwanted cell or protein adhesion if left unprotected. Most commonly used in this regard are the triblocks consisting of two PEO-chains surrounding a polypropylene oxide PPO center block, although diblocks consisting of PEG-esterified fatty acids [113] have recently shown promise as protein repellents. A set of more complex constructs with excellent protein repelling qualities were recently synthesized by Kopecek and coworkers [99].

The PEO/PPO/PEO triblocks are commercially available as poloxamers or Pluronic^{TM} surfactants, and can be obtained with a variety of block lengths; they have been demonstrated by several authors to effectively reduce protein uptake [3, 62, 97, 102, 135] and cell adhesion. Coated surfaces have also shown suppressed bacterial adhesion, with reductions of nearly two orders of magnitude observed for three different strains of *S. epidermidis* on PS [13].

In an effort to identify biocompatible carriers for controlled drug release, Illum and coworkers realized that a reduced uptake by macrophages of PS latex particles could be obtained by simple coating with several of the poloxamers [65]. The efficiency of this reduction was clearly increased with increasing PEO block length. Similar findings were made by Müller [155] who also gave convincing evidence of the importance of the PPO block length for good surfactant adhesion, and thereby effective cellular repulsion. By using a poloxamer with 98 EO units in the flanking blocks and 67 PO units in the central anchoring block, these workers found an almost complete suppression of the phagocytosis of 3.2 μm PS particles by freshly isolated human granulocytes. The study was carried out in protein-free medium, and it could well be argued [49] that the surface protection afforded by the adsorbed surfactant might vanish in a highly protein-rich medium, in which displacement of the surfactant could easily take place. Yet, when injected intravenously in rats, adsorption coated nanoparticles (75 nm PS colloids coated with Pluronic^{TM} F108) were found to remain considerably longer in circulation than their uncoated counterparts, with half-lives for clearance amounting to 13 hours and 30 minutes, respectively [171].

The tenacity of the complex formed between Pluronic^{TM} F108 and a hydrophobic (polypropylene (PP)) membrane was demonstrated by Schroën et al. [160] who found protein repulsion by the coated membrane to be unimpaired by 10 days of continuous operation in a bioreactor. Despite these encouraging findings, it must be recognized that, depending on the nature of the interacting components, surface-surfactant complexes might be more or less stable and may well require the formation of covalent bonds in order to withstand disruption by competing adsorbates. This can be accomplished by radiation treatments of various kinds, as discussed above [4, 105].

Surface Protection with Biological Materials

Proteins   The most abundant protein in plasma is serum albumin (HSA); because of its high concentration in combination with a relatively high diffusivity, this protein will be the first to populate any surface in contact with blood [60]. On hydrophilic surfaces, HSA is easily displaced by other less abundant, but more tenaciously binding proteins, including fibrinogen (HFB), in a displacement train commonly referred to as the "Vroman Effect" [191]. On hydrophobic surfaces, this displacement is less pronounced [39, 134, 145]. Surface "passivation" with serum albumin has long been known to reduce thrombogenicity and discourage platelet and phagocyte adherence [61, 87]. Also bacterial adhesion is suppressed by surface protection with albumin, as shown in recent work with titanium plates given a carbodiimide cross-linked and highly hydrolysis-resistant surface coating with albumin [168]. The securing of an albumin coating on blood-contacting materials has therefore been the focus of much attention [51, 94, 144)].

One problem with the pre-albumination of implants is the finite life-time of the protective molecule in the plasma environment. A logical goal for surface modification is, therefore, to ensure that the biomaterial is kept in a constantly albuminated state. The approach taken by Cooper et al. [144] is to provide the surface with long-chain alkyl groups, to which albumin has a specific affinity, while Eaton et al. are accomplishing a highly specific albumin attachment to the dye cibachron blue, tethered to surfaces of blood-contacting Pellethane[TM] (Dow Chemical Co., Midland, MI) via a dextran spacer arm [80].

Adsorbed fibrinogen has long been implicated in the thrombogenicity of a blood-contacting material [199]. More recently, it has also been suggested that adsorbed fibrinogen binds and activates phagocytic cells, and hence actively participates in the production of an inflammatory material response [174]. A general goal in designing biocompatible materials has, therefore, until recently been to reduce the uptake of fibrinogen to the greatest possible degree. However, in the late 1980s two articles emerged that laid the foundation for a slight shift in this approach [106, 159]. These authors demonstrated the absence of a direct correlation between platelet activation and the surface concentration of fibrinogen adsorbed on a series of methacrylate polymers. By probing the adsorbed fibrinogen with an ^{125}I-labeled anti-fibrinogen antibody, they noted instead that such a correlation existed with the amount of recognizable antigen on the surface. Based on these findings they concluded that excessively surface-denatured fibrinogen was inconsequential as a cause of thrombus formation. Rather, those molecules that had suffered only minor conformational changes, and were still recognizable by the polyclonal anti-fibrinogen, were the culprits responsible for platelet activation. Recently, Kiaei et al. [84] produced some strong supporting evidence for this conclusion in an investigation of glow-discharge tetrafluoroethylene treated surfaces. The low surface free energy of their fluorocarbon materials would give rise to a particularly high interfacial tension when immersed in an aqueous solution of fibrinogen, and as a result, the highly surface active fibrinogen would adsorb and spread on the polymer surface. The spreading, measured as reduced elutability with the surfactant sodium dodecyl sulfate, was found to increase with residence time [20] while the platelet activation showed a time-dependent decrease. Of the surfaces produced, those with the lowest surface energy displayed the highest fibrinogen uptake and the lowest platelet adhesion, in good agreement with the original suggestion by Salzman et al.. In a similar vein, Brash and coworkers [193] compared the platelet activation by a variety of different adsorption complexes between PE and fibrinogen. While the regularly adsorbed fibrinogen led to significant platelet adhesion/activation, a companion sample that had been heat-denatured at 70°C for 15 minutes showed no greater platelet activation than the neat PE in a PBS/albumin buffer. A heat treatment or other fibrinogen denaturation scheme could, therefore, offer a new approach to hemocompatibilization. The validity of such speculations will have to be tested in a whole blood environment.

Phospholipids   The search for an ideal biomimetic surface coating has also led to investigations of phospholipid polymers as model cell membranes and therefore potentially biocompatible materials [57]. Recent studies have produced some very encouraging results with phospholipid-derivatized surfaces that merit a closer look. Thus, Ishihara et al. [68, 70, 71] performed a cerium ammonium nitrate initiated attachment of 2-methacryloyloxyethyl phosphorylcholine onto celluose membranes, to be used in hemodialysis. While the un-treated membrane showed significant platelet adhesion and aggregation within 30 minutes of contact, the grafted product failed to show any adherent cells, even after 180 minutes. In addition, the grafting treatment resulted in a strong reduction in complement activation. More recently, the same group was able to accomplish a similarly successful derivatization of a segmented PU [69].

In a separate approach, phosphatidylcholine (PC) moieties were covalently attached via one of their fatty acid chains to a modified glass surface [91]. Even this construct showed very low adhesion of platelets, with less than 0.4% of the surface covered, compared to the 25.3% seen on underivatized glass, and cell spreading that was ten times larger on the neat glass than on the PC film. No albumin was detected on the derivatized surface, indicating the presence of a protection mechanism that differs significantly from that seen on C-18-grafted surfaces [144]. The lack of a strong interaction of either albumin or fibrinogen with PC-containing model surfaces is also borne out by a recent total internal reflection fluorescence (TIRF) study on hydrophobized silica to which the phospholipid had been merely adsorbed [112]. Similar surfaces covered with phosphatidic acid (PA) showed drastically different behavior, with strong adsorption of both proteins. While PA may not hold particular promise, it is clear that PC grafting has a prominent future as a surface modification strategy for biomaterials.

MODEL SURFACES

It is clear from the above survey that designing an ideal surface for a particular biomaterial application can be a most complex problem, given the many components with which a surface as a rule will have to react, and the many different functional groups that are known to influence such reactions. In order to answer basic questions about the interactions be-tween a surface, on the one hand, and proteins or cells on the other, model studies must be designed that allow comparisons between surfaces of different compositions recorded under as close to identical conditions as possible. The need for such studies has led to the design of patterned surfaces that offer a systematic variation in composition within a limited area. Substrates of this kind allow the simultaneous testing of multiple chemistries or morphologies under one and the same set of environmental conditions.

A breakthrough in the analysis of protein adsorption to surfaces with gradually vary-ing chemistries was made by Elwing et al. [40] with their design of gradient surfaces, in which a hydrophobic silane was allowed to diffuse across a liquid-liquid phase boundary and thereby create a concentration gradient which was imprinted on a glass slide immersed in the two-phase system. The gradient could easily be characterized in terms of contact angle/position pairs of data. By immersing the whole surface in one and the same pro-tein solution, the relative depositions on the different substrate chemistries could easily be determined. This informative technique has since been refined in a number of ways. For instance, by mounting the gradient surfaces in a flow cell where they could be exposed to protein solutions of varying concentrations, and observing the cell by total internal reflec-tion fluorescence (TIRF) using a charge coupled device (CCD) camera, Hlady was able to observe not only the adsorption end-points, but also the rates of protein adsorption to the different surface compositions [59]. In recent years, wettability gradients have been produced also by other means, e.g. by plasma discharge in an oxygen atmosphere and a gradual exposure of a hydrophobic substrate (polydimethylsiloxane) which became hy-drophilized in the process [47]. Plasma discharge was also used to gradually activate PE film for graft co-polymerization of PEG-monomethacrylates. The result was a gradient surface

consisting of comb-like PEO-PMMA constructs of increasing length. This surface modification resulted in a strongly position dependent platelet adhesion, with uptakes being the
highest at the untreated end and gradually reducing to near-zero at the end with the longest
exposure time [98].

While the ability to gradually modify a surface is extremely useful in creating a general
understanding of interactions with a particular chemistry, the specific understanding that
comes from knowing the exact spatial distribution of functional groups on a given surface
can only be offered by the self-assembled monolayer (SAM) chemistry, primarily developed
by Whitesides and his group [129]. By adsorbing alkane thiols with different end-group
chemistries onto gold substrates, one can assume to produce defect-free surface coatings
with known distances between the surface groups.

With these tools, our basic understanding of the relationship between surface composition, protein adhesion, and the attachment/activation and growth of cells in surface contact
is likely to grow at an increasingly rapid rate.

BIOACTIVE MATERIALS

Cell adhesion to artificial materials is influenced by chemical structure, interfacial forces,
and surface topography, all of which influence the nature and extent of protein adsorption.
Therefore, interfacial properties may influence cell adhesion either directly by cell-surface
interactions, or indirectly by modulating protein adsorption and, subsequently, protein-
mediated cell adhesion. Biologically specific signals can also mediate cell-material interactions. Various types of biochemical signals such as compatible crystal structure and
adhesive ligands for cell receptor interactions have been incorporated at the surface of
synthetic biomaterials in order to improve their biocompatibility.

The first part of this section looks at modifications of surface physical, chemical,
and topographical properties used to study and enhance biocompatability. The second part
of this section deals with biomimetic materials and provides a brief review of materials
endowed with ligands for cell surface receptors and approaches used to pattern substrates
with these ligands. Finally, surface modifications used to enhance hard tissue bonding are
covered.

Physical and Chemical Properties

Surface hydrophobicity, or wettability is an important determinant of cell adhesion. It is
related to surface free energy and is typically evaluated by water contact angle. Smaller water
contact angles correspond to more hydrophilic surfaces and higher surface free energies. In
general, more hydrophilic substrates support cell adhesion and spreading to a greater extent
than hydrophobic materials which have low surface free energies [7, 96].

The wettability of a material and related affinity for cells can be increased by incorporation of polar groups at the surface as discussed above [28, 42]. PS substrates modified by
radiofrequency plasma discharge to produce surface hydroxyl and carboxyl groups display
impoved cell adhesion when compared to untreated PS substrates [41, 100, 184].

Differences in cell interactions with wettable and nonwettable substrates may be due in
part to differences in composition, density, and/or conformation of adsorbed proteins. Cell
binding to extracellular matrix (ECM) adhesion proteins such as fibronectin or vitronectin
is mediated by cell surface receptors called integrins, which bind to relatively small domains on their protein ligands [194]. Variations in surface orientation, conformation, or

packing density of these or other adhesion proteins may result in differences in the accessibility or binding affinity of integrin recognition domains which, in turn, may affect the nature of cell-surface interactions. For the purpose of studying the effect of wettability on cell-substrate and cell-protein interactions, it is desirable to use a single substrate with a range of wettabilities as discussed under model surfaces above. Specifically, work with wettability gradient surfaces has shown that protein adsorption occurs to a greater extent on hydrophobic substrata than on hydrophilic substrata, that exchange of a preadsorbed protein by another protein occurs more readily on hydrophilic substrata than on hydrophobic substrata, that adsorption-induced conformational changes are greater on hydrophobic substrates than on hydrophilic substrates, and that cell adhesion reaches a maximum on moderately hydrophilic substrates which have a contact angles around 60 degrees [96]. Conformation and biological activities of adsorbed adhesion proteins such a fibronectin (FN) and vitronectin (VN) have been studied in relation to substrate chemical and physical properties [7, 74, 101, 142, 182]. In order to study the cellular response to plasma fibronectin (pFN) adsorbed to substrates of different surface chemistries, Lewandowska et al. derivatized glass substrates with self assembled monolayers of aliphatic chains having specific chemical endgroups [101]. The chemical groups studied, [CH_3], [SH], [$SCOCH_3$], [NH_2], [SO_3H], and [SiOH], yielded surfaces with wettabilities that ranged from advancing and receding contact angles of 30° and <10° to 82° and 77°, respectively. The amounts of pFN bound and the attachments of either 3T3 fibroblast or neuroblastoma cells were found to be similar for all surface chemistries with the exception of [NH_2], which promoted greater fibroblast attachment. There were, however, considerable variations in the degree of cell spreading and differentiation observed for the different substrates. Spreading and microfilament bundle reorganization on [SH], [$SCOCH_3$], and [SO_3H], substrates could be completely inhibited by the presence of the well known adhesion peptide, GRGDS [194] which is a competitive inhibitor of cell binding to FN. On [CH_3] substrates, however, GRGDS had less of an inhibitory effect on these responses, and on [NH_2] substrates, no effect whatsoever was observed. In the case of neuroblastoma cells, the pattern of neurite outgrowh was also found to vary with surface chemistry. Long neurites formed on [SO_3H], and [SiOH] surfaces, shorter neurites formed on [SH] and [$SCOCH_3$] surfaces, and few neurites formed on [CH_3] and [NH_2] surfaces. On the [NH_2] surface, neural cells displayed pseudopodial spreading. The most striking responses by either cell type were observed on [CH_3] and [NH_2] surfaces. These responses were similar for each cell type on the two chemistries but differed from the general response observed on the remainder of the test substrates. [CH_3] substrates are hydrophobic, whereas [NH_2] substrates are hydrophilic. Differences in cellular responses to test substrates, therefore, cannot be attributed primarily to differences in their degree of hydrophilicity, but instead are likely due to differences in the nature of FN interaction with specific chemistries. Overall, the results of this research and other similar studies indicate that FN adsorption onto a surface results in conformational changes in the protein. The nature of these changes depends on both surface chemical and physical properties. Different conformational changes result in differences in the accessibility, avidity, and proximity of cell and heparin binding domains which in turn affect the cellular response to materials precoated with adhesion proteins [7, 74, 101, 142, 182].

Surface Topography

In addition to chemical and physical surface properties, surface topography has an important effect on the tissue response to an implant, as discussed in Chapter 13. The nature of cell contacts at the tissue/material interface can effect the anchorage of an implant and, subsequently, the amount of friction that can occur between the implant material and surrounding tissues. In the case of soft tissue implants, this factor may be particularly important as it has been hypothesized that friction at the material/tissue interface may contribute to a sustained inflammatory response [185]. Model surfaces having well defined microgroves have been prepared using photolithographic techniques and used to study the effect of surface texture on cell/material contacts and cell alignment. [22, 30, 123]. Meyle et al. demonstrated that surface grooves of 1 μm pitch and 1 μm depth lead to intense fibroblast contact with the surface as evidenced by the extension of cellular processes into the grooves [123]. den Braber et al. produced similar surfaces which had grooves 0.5 μm in depth and 2, 5, or 10 μm in width [30]. On surfaces having 2 μm-size grooves, fibroblasts were found to elongate and align parallel to the grooves. This phenomenon was also observed on 5 μm-size grooves, but to a lesser extent, while no such effect was seen on 10 μm-size grooves. Together, the results of these studies suggest that surface features between 1 and 5 μm may have the greatest effect on cell contact and guidance. Techniques used to alter surface topographies of hard tissue replacement materials such as titanium are described later in this section.

Biomimetic Materials

Cell behavior on synthetic materials is commonly enhanced by immobilization of ECM adhesion proteins by either adsorption or covalent coupling [11, 52, 75, 81, 90, 126, 151, 161, 190, 198]. It is clear from the above discussion, however, that protein adsorption is a complex process which is difficult to control. Depending on the method of conjugation, covalently immobilized proteins may undergo surface-induced conformational changes similar to those described for adsorbed proteins. In addition, protein layers are susceptible to denaturation and proteolytic degradation and may, therefore, not be suitable for long-term applications. As mentioned above, cell surface receptors recognize and bind to relatively small domains on their protein ligands. These binding domains often contain the Arg-Gly-Asp (RGD) amino acid sequence and can be reproduced as synthetic peptides [194]. Because of the difficulties associated with protein adsorption, many researchers have sought to replace the function of adhesion proteins with short synthetic peptides corresponding to their cell binding domains.

Cell Adhesion Peptides   Cell adhesion peptides have been immobilized on surfaces by both adsorption and covalent coupling. Chemistries for ligand conjugation and immobilization are reviewed above. Important parameters to consider when assessing the usefulness of various immobilization methods are the ability to control, vary, and quantify the number of active ligand sites, the cell adhesive properties of the base material and its tendency toward nonspecific protein adsorption, and its mechanical properties, in order to assess its suitability for various implant or biodevice applications.

The most widely studied cell adhesion motif is the RGD tripeptide, which comprises the cell binding domain of fibronectin and is common to several other ECM adhesion proteins [194]. While the intact ECM proteins are frequently attached to substrates by means of adsorption, this avenue is not directly available for immobilization of the small model peptides. The efficiency of protein adsorption is proportional to molecular size, and proteins with molecular weights below about 10,000 do not coat plastic efficiently. Adhesion peptides typically have molecular weights below 2000, and must, therefore, be conjugated to larger proteins or other carrier molecules to enhance their coating efficiency. Tashiro et al. coupled an RGD-containing peptide corresponding to the RGD site of laminin to a larger protein, Keyhold Limpet Hemocyanin (KLH) [175]. Both the protein-conjugated peptide and its underivatized analog were adsorbed onto tissue culture dishes, where promotion of neurite outgrowth was found only in the dishes containing the larger RGD-KLH conjugate. Ruoslahti and Pieschbacher used a similar but simplified approach whereby they prepared a RGD-containing oligopeptide corresponding to the RGD site of fibronectin which had a hydrophobic tail consisting of leucine residues [156]. The peptide was found to support adhesion of numerous cell types onto a number of different polymeric and inorganic substrates. Although adsorption is an attractive approach to peptide immobilization because of its simplicity, it is not optimal. While coating densities may be readily determined on such surfaces, these densities do not necessarily reflect peptides active for cell adhesion. In addition, nonspecific protein adsorption is likely to occur on any surface that would support peptide- or protein-conjugated peptide adhesion. This problem may be minimized, however, by use of a postmodification treatment with albumin.

Massia and Hubbell used silane-modified glass as a base material to immobilize a RGD peptide through the N-terminus of a glycine spacer residue. It was found that fibroblast attachment was supported by a surface RGD density of 0.1 fmol/cm^2, while spreading and focal contact formation required a surface density of 10 fmol/cm^2 or greater [118]. Although this study provided valuable information regarding appropriate ligand densities for biomaterials design, the system used was limited to service as a research tool due to the undesirable mechanical properties of glass. This same group has coupled RGD to both PET and polytetrafluoroethylene (PTFE) which are more practical materials for bioapplications [115]. Indeed, in protein-free medium there was a clear difference between derivatized and underivatized surfaces in terms of cell adhesion. However, in serum-containing medium, the difference observed was somewhat less spectacular, which suggests that non-specific protein adsorption may have contributed to the degree of cell adhesion. Kondoh et al. and Matsuda et al. have both coupled RGD-containing peptides to polyvinyl alcohol (PVA) films [93, 119] although with different chemical techniques. While Kondoh achieved coupling through isocyanation of surface hydroxyl groups followed by conversion to an activated ester and RGD conjugation, Matsuda used carbonyl diimidazole to activate surface hydroxyls and acomplish RGD attachment. Using either of these methods, the number of peptides incorporated could be varied by altering the reaction conditions. Derivatized PVA films were found to support endothelial cell (EC) adhesion and growth, whereas PVA alone did not. Imanishi et al. linked RGDS peptides to amino groups created on silicon rubber [66], and were able to show that fibroblast cell attachment to the RGD-immobilized silicon increased with increasing concentration of peptides linked to the surface. In a different approach, Sugawara and Matsuda derivatized GGGRGDSP at its N-terminal with 4-azidobenzoyloxysuccinimide [169]. The derivatized peptide was covalently immobilized on PVA films or tissue culture polystyrene precoated with poly(N, N dimethylacrylamide-co-3-azidostyrene) by adsorption followed by UV irradiation and found to enhance cell adhesion.

Nearly all of the RGD-modified materials described thus far will support protein adsorption to some extent. Consequently, the grafted peptides might not constitute the only cell adhesion signal on such surfaces. In order to fully control the cell adhesive properties of a surface, it is necessary for the base material to resist protein adsorption. PEO has been shown to inhibit protein adsorption [49]. Drumheller and Hubbell have designed semi-interpenetrating polymer networks of PEO and acrylate polymers that enable peptide conjugation yet resist any nonspecific protein adsorption [33]. This group was able to show that in the absence of peptide, yet in the presence of serum, no cell adhesion occurred on the polymer networks. When peptides were grafted to the surface at a density of 475 pmol/cm^2, fibroblast adhesion was well supported. In this case, peptides were grafted to exposed carboxylic acid moieties of the incorporated acrylic acid. It might be possible to vary the number of active sites for peptide immobilization by varying the molar ratio of acrylic acid to PEO incorporated in the polymer networks. Varying this ratio, however, may affect the protein resistant properties of the base material.

An alternative approach to preparing protein resistant surfaces conjugated with RGD is to use PEO molecules as spacer arms for peptide coupling. This can be accomplished using PEO-PPO-PEO triblocks that are immobilized to hydrophobic substrates through simple adsorption. End groups of the PEO arms can be derivatized with pyridyl disulfide structures and serve as coupling sites for thiolated peptides [103]. By mixing underivatized triblocks with derivatized triblocks prior to adsorption, the surface density of peptides can be readily varied. This approach should prove promising for enhancing cell adhesion and growth in a wide variety of bioapplications because it is theoretically applicable to any material having suitable hydrophobicity [132]. In addition, this type of peptide grafting chemistry could provide a useful tool for evaluating the concentration effects of specific ECM components on cellular function.

Heparin Binding Domains   Another type of cell adhesive domain present in adhesion proteins is a heparin binding domain. These domains consist of short stretches of positively charged amino acids such as arginine and glycine. Cells bind to these domains through electrostatic interactions with cell surface proteoglycans containing negatively charged chondroitin sulfate and/or heparin sulfate groups. In this same way, amine-rich oligopeptides are capable of promoting cell adhesion when immobilized to a substrate. Massia and Hubbell covalently grafted N, N-dimethylaminoethyl-amine (NNDMAEA), arginine, and lysine to sulfonyl chloride activated glass and demonstrated that the presence of these groups on the surface promoted cell adhesion [117].

Glycoconjugate-Mediated Cell Adhesion   Cell surface glycoproteins recognize and bind to simple sugars. This type of interaction has been the focus of efforts to engineer biomaterials which selectively promote adhesion of a specific cell type. Hepatocytes interact with monosaccharides via the hepatocyte asialoglycoprotein receptor. Kobayashi et al. developed a lactose-carrying styrene homopolymer which when coated onto PS culture dishes promoted selective adhesion of hepatocytes [89, 90], while Lopina et al. created galactose-modified PEO star gels which sustained both long-term culture and differentiated function of hepatocytes [109]. Surface glycoconjugates of vascular endothelial cells display high affinity for the lectin Ulex Europaeus I (UEA I), which led Ozaki et al. to bind this lectin to Dacron™ using the 1-ethyl-3-(dimethylaminopropyl) carbodiimide hydrochloride cross-linking agent [139]. The UEA I/Dacron™ surfaces supported a 100-fold increase in endothelial cell attachment compared to unmodified Dacron™, yet did not support adhesion of monocytes, smooth muscle cells, or fibroblast.

Growth Factors   Immobilization of growth factors is yet another strategy which has been used to improve cell growth and differentiated function at the cell-material interface. Liu et al. covalently immobilized insulin and collagen on PU to enhance endothelial cell growth for application to vascular grafts [107]. The proteins were immobilized by use of a plasma treatment in the presence of ammonia gas to create amino groups on the polymer surface followed by protein coupling to these groups using dimethyl suberimidate. Long-term growth, normal endothelial cell cobblestone morphology, and prostacyclin secretion were supported by the modified graft material. In an effort to enhance bone ingrowth into orthopedic materials, Arm et al. modified porous hydroxyapatite (HA) implants with platelet-derived growth factor (PDGF) [6]. This growth factor is osteogenic and functions in bone growth and fracture healing. Porous ceramic implants were adsorption-coated with a mixture of PDGF and albumin which permitted sustained release of the growth factor in an active form. PDGF-modified HA showed a trend toward increased interfacial shear strength and bone ingrowth compared to untreated HA [165].

Patterned Substrates Substrates have been patterned in two dimensions with biospecific signals for the purpose of manipulating cell attachment, morphology, growth, and function. Patterned substrates are typically prepared using photolithographic techniques, often in combination with either silane chemistry or photoreactive compounds. Kleinfeld et al. patterned cell adhesive amines and non-adhesive alkyl chains on silcon-based substrates using a silane coupling agent and lithographic processing [88]. With these substrates, it was possible to direct high-resolution adhesion and growth of dissociated neurons. Similar procedures have been applied to the patterning of substrates for localized protein adsorption, and as such used to direct the attachment and/or differentiated function, of neural, epithelial, and hepatocyte cells [9, 153, 165]. Photoimmobilization in conjunction with masking techniques have enabled patterning of adhesion peptides to a variety of materials [23, 169]. Sugawara et al. derivatized a RGD-containing peptide with a photoreactive moiety, phenyl azide, and immobilized it to a nonionic, hydrophilic polymer by UV irradiation as discussed earlier [169]. By using a photomask during UV irradiation, it was possible to create two-dimensional patterns of endothelial cell adhesion with feature sizes on the order of microns. Clemence et al. used a maleimide-containing diazirine photo-cross-linker to immobilize a YIGSR cell adhesion peptide to hydroxylated fluorinated ethylene propylene [23]. Neuroblastoma x glioma cells were found to attach and differentiate well on peptide-modified areas, whereas very little adhesion occurred on unmodified areas.

Numerous applications exist for substrates patterned with bioactive moieties. By enabling control of neural cell attachment and neurite outgrowth, patterned substrates will provide a valuable tool for scientists to study and model the development and mechanisms of information processing in neural systems. Such substrates may also have potential use in biosensor application. Micropatterning technology should also prove particularly valuable in the development of biohybrid artificial organs, where it is crucial not only to maintain cells in a stable differentiated state, but also to grow adequate numbers of them in a small volume while allowing for efficient mass transport.

TISSUE BONDING MATERIALS

Metals

The long-term success of many orthopedic and dental implants is dependent on their ability to become well integrated with bone. Ti, Ti-Al-V alloy and Co-Cr-Mo alloy are popular materials for hard tissue implants due to their excellent mechanical properties; however, their surface properties are not well suited for bonding to bone. Modifications of both surface topography and surface chemistry have led to significant improvements in the integration of such materials with bone.

Surface Topography Surface texture at the microscopic level has been shown to be an important determinant of the cellular response to an implant and, subsequently, the degree of tissue integration [95, 143, 188]. Rough surfaces display higher levels of osteoblast attachment when compared to smooth surfaces [12]. For this reason, metal implants are routinely treated by rough polishing, grit, or sand blasting to improve their interactions with cells. The result of such treatments is an osseoconductive surface or one which permits osseointegration.

Surface texture at the macroscopic level is an important feature of implants designed for cementless fixation. Porous surfaces with pore sizes in the range of 100 to 350 microns have proven optimal for osseointegration and implant fixation [18]. Surfaces with these types of rougosity are most commonly produced, either through plasma spraying of titanium powder, or by sintering titanium beads or a wire mesh onto the implant surface [128].

Surface Chemistry   Because the crystal structures of some bioceramics are compatible with those of hydroxyapatite (HA) found in bone, they are osseoinductive or active for promoting bone formation. Coating metallic implants with bioceramics may enhance bone formation at the implant surface, result in more rapid increases in interfacial strength between the implant and bone, and allow for cementless fixation [8, 17, 24, 31, 46, 56, 73, 77, 111, 137, 157, 158, 176]. In addition, ceramic coatings may protect against metallic ion release [36]. HA and calcium phosphate ceramics are the most widely used bioceramics for coating metallic implants. Such bioceramics are commonly deposited onto metals by the plasma spray method [8, 24, 25, 27, 31, 46, 77, 137]. Coatings produced by vacuum plasma spray have been found to display better adhesion properties than do coatings produced by air plasma spray [16]. Other methods for producing bioceramic coatings include sintering [170], pulsed laser deposition [177], radiofrequency magnetron sputtering [64], electrolytic deposition [154], electrodeposition [26], and the biomimetic method [92]. Redepenning et al. coated stainless steel implants with HA in a two-step process, beginning by electrolytic deposition of brushit onto the metal, followed by conversion of the formed brushit layer into HA through a high-temperature, high-pH treatment [154]. Similarly, Dasarathy et al. produced HA-metal composite coatings on titanium by electrodeposition [26]. This process makes use of an electrolytic bath to codeposite a metal with another metal, nonmetal, or ceramic onto a substrate. Using this method, the HA particles are mechanically fixed within the metal matrix at the surface.

In an alternate approach, Kokubo et al. have produced apatite layers on ceramics, metals, and polymers using the biomimetic method [92]. This two-step method consists of a nucleation step which occurs in simulated body fluid containing glass powders and a growth step which takes place in simulated body fluid alone. Here, apatite layer thickness is readily controlled by varying the time allowed for the growth step. An advantage of the latter three methods is that they employ non-line-of-sight procedures and can, therefore, be applied to irregularly shaped implants.

Although bioceramic coatings have proved beneficial for promoting bone in growth, their brittle nature makes them susceptible to failure both within the coating and at the coating/implant interface. For this reason, it is not clear whether or not they actually improve long-term implant function. HA/metal composite coatings similar to those prepared by Dasarathy et al. and described above are likely to be less prone to such failures and may, thus, increase implant lifetimes [26].

Polymers

Repair of some soft tissues such as ligaments or tendons require tough flexible materials that are also capable of bonding to bone. Apatite-coated polymers are well suited for such applications. Tretinnikov and Ikada have produced high density polyethylene materials having a firmly bonded carbonated HA layer by surface graft polymerization of a phosphate-containing monomer followed by immersion in simulated physiologic solution [178]. Tanahashi et al. have used a biomimetic process similar to that described above [92] to produce apatite coatings on a variety of polymeric materials including PET, PMMA, polyamide 6, and polyethersulfone [172, 173].

THERAPEUTIC MATERIALS

In addition to providing mechanical function, biomaterials often serve as delivery systems for pharmacological agents. The entirety of Chapter 27 is dedicated to drug delivery implants. Here, we will only briefly discuss the surface modification of biomaterials with pharmacological agents for the purpose of improving implant function and prolonging implant lifetime.

One of the greatest challenges in biomaterials engineering is the development of blood-compatible materials. In vivo, events that lead to thrombus formation are regulated by endothelial cells. Approaches used to improve endothelial cell adhesion and growth on bio-materials for blood-contacting devices were described above. However, the production of stable endothelial linings on synthetic materials has not yet been achieved. An alternative strategy to preventing thrombus formation is to modify the surface of biomaterials such that they have anticoagulant activity. Heparin is a well known natural anticoagulant and has been immobilized onto material surfaces by a variety of methods, as reviewed by Kim and Feijen [86]. Some examples include adsorption in the form of an albumin conjugate, covalent immobilization directly onto the surface, and covalent immobilization via spacer arms [38, 76, 86, 140]. Park et al. immobilized heparin onto polyurethaneurea surfaces using hydrophilic, PEO spacer arms [140]. This group demonstrated that the use of PEO tethers leads to decreased platelet adsorption compared to unmodified surfaces and surfaces containing heparin immobilized by alkyl spacer arms. In addition, in shunt experiments under low flow and low shear, PEO-immobilized heparin was found to have greater activity than did alkyl-immobilized heparin as evidenced by longer occlusion times. Another approach to rendering material surfaces resistant to thrombus formation is by incorporating charged moieties which to some extent mimic the anticoagulant effects of heparin. Thus, antithrombic effects have been achieved using sulfonated dextrans and PS [19, 78, 121]. Similarly, Silver et al. have prepared sulfonated PU and demonstrated that surface sulfonate groups provide an anticoagulant effect by interacting with thrombin, plasma proteases, and fibrinogen [163].

A major concern for the success of orthopedic implants, particularly those used in fracture fixation, is prevention of infection. Optimal antimicrobial treatment after surgery requires an administration technique that yields a high, localized concentration of antibiotic. To achieve this, antibiotics have been incorporated at implant surfaces. Dunn et al. used electrophorectic migration of ciprofloxacin ions and ciprofloxacin HCl particles to deposit the antibiotic salt onto positively biased, porous titanium substrates [37]. The modified substrates were shown to deliver antibiotics for up to 5 days. Price et al. used a biodegradable copolymer, polylactic-co-glycolic acid, as a carrier for gentamicin antibiotic [149]. Stainless steel fracture plates coated with the gentamicin-containing polymer displayed sustained antibiotic delivery for more than 15 days.

ACKNOWLEDGMENTS

J. A. N. gratefully acknowledges fellowship support from the Whitaker Foundation under the Biobased Engineering Program at the Department of Bioengineering, University of Utah.

REFERENCES

1   Abuchowski A, van Es T, Palczuk NC, Davis FF. Alteration of immunological properties of bovine serum albumin by covalent attachment of polyethylene glycol. *J Biol.Chem*, 252 (1977), 3578–3586.

2   Aldenhoff YBJ, Koole LH. Studies on a new strategy for surface modification of polymeric biomaterials. *J Biomed Mat Res*, 29 (1995), 917–928.

3   Amiji M, Park K. Prevention of protein adsorption and platelet adhesion on surfaces by PEO/PPO/PEO triblock copolymers. *Biomaterials*, 13 (1992), 682–692.

4   Amiji M, Park K. Surface modification by radiation-induced grafting of PEO/PPO/PEO triblock copolymers. *J Coll Interface Sci*, 155 (1993), 251–255.

5   Andrade JD, Nagaoka S, Cooper SL, Okano T, Kim SW. Surfaces and blood compatibility: Current hypotheses. *ASAIO J*, 10 (1987), 75–84.

6   Arm DM, Tencer AF, Bain SD, and Celino D. Effect of controlled release of platelet derived growth factor from a porous hydroxyapaptite implant on bone ingrowth. *Biomaterials*, 17 (1996), 703–709.

7   Atankov G, Grinnell F, and Groth T. Studies on the biocompatibility of materials: Fibroblast reorganization of substratum-bound fibronectin on surfaces varying in wettability. *J Biomedical Materials Research*, 30 (1996), 385–391.

8   Augat P, Claes L, Hanselmann KF, Suger G, Fleischmann W. Increase of stability in external fracture fixation by hydroxyapatite-coated bone screws. *J Applied Biomaterials*, 6 (1995), 99–104.

9   Bhatia SN, Toner M, Tompkins RG, Yarmush ML. Selective adhesion of hepatocytes on patterned surfaces. *Annals New York Academy of Sciences*, 745 (1994), 187–209.

10 Bohnert JL, Fowler BC, Horbett TA, Hoffman AS. Plasma gas discharge deposited fluorocarbon polymers exhibited reduced elutability of adsorbed albumin and fibrinogen. *J Biomat Sci, Polym Ed*, 1 (1990), 279–297.

11 Bonzon N, Lefebvre F, Ferre N, Daculsi G, Rabaud M. New bioactivation mode for vascular prostheses made of Dacron^{TM} polyester. *Biomaterials*, 16 (1995), 747–751.

12 Bowers KT, Keller JC, Michaels CM. Optimization of surface micromorphology for enhanced osteoblast responses in vitro. *Int J Oral Maxillofac Implants*, 7 (1992), 302–310.

13 Bridgett MJ, Davies MC, Denyer SP. Control of staphylococcal adhesion to polystyrene surfaces by polymer surface modification with surfactants. *Biomaterials*, 13 (1992), 411–416.

14 Brinkman E, Poot L, Does VD, Bantjes A. Platelet deposition studies on copolyether urethanes modified with poly(ethylene oxide). *Biomaterials*, 11 (1990), 200–205.

15 Bronzon N, Lefebvre F, Ferre N, Daculsi G, Rabaud M. New bioactivation mode for vascular prostheses made of Dacron$^{®}$ polyester. *Biomaterials*,16 (1995), 747–751.

16 Brossa F, Cigada A, Chiesa R, Paracchini L, and Consonni C. Adhesion properties of plasma sprayed hydroxylapatite coatings for orthopedic prostheses. *Biomed Mater Eng*, 3 (1993), 127–136.

17 Burr DB, Mori S, Boyd RD, Sun TC, Blaha JD, Lane L, Parr J. Histomorphometric assessment of the mechanisms for rapid ingrowth of bone to HA/TCP coated implants. *J Biomed Mater Res*, 27 (1993), 645–653.

18 Cameron HU. The implant bone interface: Porous metals. In Hurley R (Ed.), *Bone Implant Interface*. St. Louis: Mosby, 1994, 145–168.

19 Charef S, Tapon-Bretaudiere J, Fischer A, Pfluger F, Jozefowicz M, Labarre D. Heparin-like functionalized polymer surfaces: Discrimination between catalytic and adsorption processes during the course of thrombin inhibition. *Biomaterials*, 17 (1996), 903–912.

20 Chinn JA, Posso SE, Horbett TA, Ratner BD. Postadsorptive transitions in fibrinogen adsorbed to Biomer: Changes in baboon platelet adhesion, antibody binding, and sodium dodecyl sulfate elutability. *J Biomed Mat Res*, 25 (1991), 535–555.

21 Chu T-J, Caldwell KD, Weiss RB, Gesteland RF, Pitt WG. Low fluorescence background electroblotting membrane for DNA sequencing. *Electrophoresis*, 13 (1992), 105–114.

22 Clark P, Connolly P, Curtis ASG, Dow JAT, Wilkinson CDW. Topographical control of cell behavior: II. Multiple grooved substrata. *Development*, 108 (1990), 634–635.

23 Clemence JF, Ranieri JP, Aebischer P, Sigrist H. Photo-immobilization of a bioactive laminin fragment and pattern-guided selective neuronal cell attachment. *Bioconjugate Chem* 6 (1995), 411–417.

24 Cook SD, Thomas KA, Kay JF, Jarcho M. Hydroxyapaptite-coated porous titanium for use as an orthopedic biologic attachment system. *Clin Orthop* 230 (1988), 303–312.

25 D'Antonio JA, Capello WN, Crothers OD, Jaffe WL, Manley MT. Early clinical experience with hydroxyapatite-coated femoral implants. *J Bone Joint Surg*, 74 (1992), 995–1008.

26 Dasarathy H, Riley C, Coble HD, Lacefield WR, Maybee G. Hydroxyapaptite/metal composite coatings formed by electrodeposition. *J Biomed Mater Res*, 31 (1996), 81–89.

27   de Groot K, Geesink R, Klein CP, Serekian P. Plasma sprayed coatings of hydroxylapatite. *J Biomed Mater Res*, 21 (1987), 1375–1381.

28   Dekker A, Reitsma K, Beugeling T, Bantjes A, Feijen J, van Aken WG. Adhesion of endothelial cells and adsorption of serum proteins on gas plasma-treated polytetrafluoroethylene. *Biomaterials*, 12 (1991), 130–138.

29   Delden CJ, Engbers GHM, Feijen J. Interaction of antithrombin III with surface-immobilized albumin-heparin conjugates. *J Biomed Mat Res*, 29 (1995), 1317–1329.

30   den Braber ET, de Ruijter JE, Smits HTJ, Ginsel LA, von Recum AF, Jansen JA. Quantitative analysis of cell proliferation and orientation on substrata with uniform parallel surface micro-grooves. *Biomaterials*, 17 (1996), 1093–1099.

31   Denissen HW, Kalk W, de Nieuport HM, Mkaltha JC, van de Hooff A. Mandibular bone response to plasma-sprayed coatings of hydroxyapatite. *Int J Prosthodont*, 3 (1990), 53–58.

32   Desai NP, Hubbell JA. Solution technique to incorporate polyethylene oxide and other water-soluble polymers into surfaces of polymeric biomaterials. *Biomaterials*, 12 (1991), 144–153.

33   Drumheller PD, Elbert DL, Hubbell JA. Multifunctional poly(ethylene glycol) semi-interpenetrating networks as highly selective adhesive substrates for bioadhesive peptide grafting. *Biotechnology and Bioengineering*, 43 (1994), 772–780.

34   Drumheller PD, Hubbell J. Semi-interpenetrating polymer networks of PEG copolymers as biospecific cell adhesive substrates. *Trans Soc Biomaterials*, 17 (1994), 60.

35   Drumheller PD, Hubbell JA. Surface immobilization of adhesive ligands for investigations of cell-substrate interactions. In Bronzino JD (Ed.), *The Biomedical Engineering Handbook*. Boca Raton, FL: CRC Press, Inc., 1995, 1583–1596.

36   Ducheyne P, Healy KE. The effect of plasma-sprayed calcium phosphate ceramic coatings on the metal ion release from porous titanium and cobalt-chromium alloys. *J Biomed Mater Res*, 22 (1988), 1137–1163.

37   Dunn DS, Raghavan S, Volz RG. Ciprofloxacin attachment to porous-coated titanium surfaces. *J Applied Biomaterials*, 5 (1994), 325–331.

38   Ebert CD, Kim SW. Immobilized heparin spacer arm effect on biological interactions. *Thromb Res*, 26 (1982), 43–57.

39   Elgersma AV, Zsom RIJ, Lyklema J, Norde W. Adsorption competition between albumin and monoclonal immuno-gama-globulins on polystyrene lattices. *J Coll Interface Sci*, 152 (1990), 410–428.

40   Elwing H, Welin S, Askendahl A, Nilson U, Lundström I. A wettability gradient method for studies of macromolecular interactions at the solid/liquid interface. *J Coll Interface Sci*, 119 (1987), 203–210.

41   Ertel SI, Chilkoti A, Horbett TA, Ratner BD. Endothelial cell growth on oxygen-containing films deposited by radio-frequency plasmas: The role of surface carbonyl groups. *Biomaterials*, 12 (1991), 443–448.

42   Ertel SI, Ratner BD, Horbett TA. Radiofrequency plasma deposition of oxygen-containing films on polystyrene and poly(ethylene terephthalate). *J Biomed Mater Res*, 24 (1990), 1637–1659.

43   Fischer AB, Bizios R, Sheu MS, Loh IH. Plasma-modified surfaces for enhanced endothelialization. *Trans Soc Biomat*, 17 (1994), 21.

44   Franscois P, Vaudaux P, Nurdin N, Mathieu HJ, Descouts P, Lew DP. Physical and biological effects of a surface coating procedure on polyurethane catheters. *Biomaterials*, 17 (1996), 667–678.

45   Garfinkle AM, Hoffman AS, Ratner BD, Reynolds LO, Hanson SR. Effects of tetrafluoroethylene glow discharge on patency of small diameter Dacron® vascular grafts. *Trans ASAIO*, 30 (1984), 432–439.

46   Geesink RG, de Groot K, Klein CP. Bonding of bone to apatite-coated implants. *J Bone Joint Surg*, 70 (1988), 17–22.

47   Gölander CG, Pitt WG. Characterization of hydrophobicity gradients prepared by means of radio frequency plasma discharge. *Biomaterials*, 11 (1990), 32–35, 1990.

48   Gombotz WR, Guanghui W, Hoffman AS. Immobilization of poly(ethylene oxide) on poly(ethylene terephthalate) using a plasma polymerization process. *J Appl Polymer Sci*, 37, 1989.

49   Gombotz WR, Guanghui W, Horbett TA, Hoffman AS. Protein adsorption to poly(ethylene oxide) surfaces. *J Biomed Mat Res*, 25 (1991), 1547–1562.

50   Gombotz WR, Hoffman AS. Gas-discharge techniques for biomaterial modification. *CRC Critical Reviews in Biocompatibility*. Boca Raton, FL: CRC Press, 1987, 1–42.

51   Guidoin RA. Albumin coating of a knitted polyester arterial prosthesis: An alternative to preclotting. *Ann Thorac Surg*, 37 (1984), 457–465.

52   Haegerstrand A, Bengtsson L, Grillis C. Serum proteins provide a matrix for cultured endothelial cells on expanded polytetraflourocthylene vascular grafts. *Scand J Thoracic*, 27 (1993), 21–26.

53   Halling PJ, Dunnill P. Improved nonporous magnetic supports for immobilized enzymes. *Biotech Bioeng*, 21 (1979), 393–416.

54   Han DK, Jeong SY, Kim YH, Min BG. Surface characteristics and blood compatibility of polyurethanes grafted by perfluoroalkyl chains. *J Biomater Sci Polym*, 3 (1992), 229–241.

55 Han DK, Park KD, Ryu GH, Kim UY, Min BG, Kim YH. Plasma protein adsorption to sulfonated poly (ethylene oxide)-grafted polyurethane surface. *J Biomed Mat Res*, 30 (1996), 23–30.

56 Hayashi K, Uenoyama K, Matsuguchi N, Sugioka Y. Quantitative analysis of in vivo tissue responses to titanium-oxide- and hydroxyapatite-coated titanium alloy. *J Biomed Mater Res*, 25 (1991), 515–523.

57 Hayward J, Chapman D. Biomembrane surfaces as models for polymer design: The potential for hemocompatibility. *Biomaterials*, 5 (1984), 135–142.

58 Hill-West JL, Chowdhury SM, Slepian MJ, Hubbell JA. Inhibition of thrombosis and intimal thickening by in situ photopolymerization of thin hydrogel barriers. *Proc Natl Acad Sci*, 91 (1994), 5967–5971.

59 Hlady V. Spatially-resolved adsorption kinetics of immunoglobulin G onto the wettability gradient surface. *Applied Spectroscopy*, 45 (1991), 246–252.

60 Hlady V, Andrade JD. Plasma protein adsorption: The big twelve. *Ann NY Acad Sci*, 516 (1987), 158–172.

61 Horbett T. Plasma adsorption on biomaterials. In Cooper SL, Peppas NA (Eds.), *Biomaterials: Interfacial Phenomena and Applications*. Washington, DC: ACS, 1982, 233–244.

62 Horbett TA, Weathersby RK. Adsorption of proteins from plasma to a series of hydrophilic-hydrophobic copolymers. I. Analysis with the in situ radio-iodination technique. *J Biomed Mat Res*, 15 (1981), 403–423.

63 Huang S-C, Caldwell KD, Lin J-N, Wang H-K, Herron JN. Site-specific immobilization of monoclonal antibodies using spacer-mediated antibody attachment. *Langmuir*, in press.

64 Hulshoff JE, van Dijk K, van der Waerden JP, Wolke JG, Ginsel LA, Jansen JA. Biological evaluation of the effect of magnetron sputtered Ca/P coatings on osteoblast-like cells in vitro. *J Biomed Mater Res*, 29 (1995), 967–975.

65 Illum L, Jacobsen LO, Müller RH, Mak E, Davis SS. Surface characteristics and the interaction of colloidal particles with mouse peritoneal macrophages. *Biomaterials*, 8 (1987), 113–117.

66 Imanishi Y, Ito Y, Liu L, and Kajihara M. Design and synthesis of biocompatible polymeric materials. *J Macromol Sci-Chem*, A25 (1988), 555–570.

67 Ingham KC. Precipitation of proteins with polyethylene glycol: characterization of albumin. *Archives of Biochemistry and Biophysics*, 186 (1978), 106–113.

68 Ishihara K, Aragaki R, Ueda T, Watanabe A, Nakabayashi N. Reduced thrombogenicity of polymers having phospholipid polar groups. *J Biomed Mat Res*, 20 (1990), 1069–1077.

69 Ishihara K, Hanyuda H, Nakabayashi N. Phospholipid polymers having a urethane bond in the side chain as coating material on segmented polyurethane. *Trans Soc Biomat*, 18 (1995), 83.

70 Ishihara K, Nakabyashi N, Fukumoto K, Aoki J. Improvement of blood compatibility on cellulose dialysis membrane: 1. Grafting of 2-methacryloyloxyethyl phosphoryl choline on to a cellulose membrane surface. *Biomaterials*, 13 (1992), 145–149.

71 Ishihara K, Takayama R, Nakabayashi N, Fukumoto K, Aoki J. Improvement of blood compatibility on cellulose dialysis membrane: 2. Blood compatibility of phospholipid polymer grafted cellulose membrane. *Biomaterials*, 13 (1992), 235–239.

72 Iverius PH, Laurent TC. Precipitation of some plasma proteins by the addition of dextran or poly-ethylene glycol. *Biochim Biophys Acta*, 133 (1967), 371–373.

73 Jansen JA, van de Waerden JP, Wolke JG, de Groot K. Histologic evaluation of the osseous adaptation to titanium and hydroxyapatite-coated titanium implants. *J Biomed Mater Res*, 25 (1991), 973–989.

74 Juliano DJ, Saaedra SS, Truskey GA. Effect of the conformation and orientation of adsorbed fibronectin on endothelial cell spreading and the strength of adhesion. *J Biomed Mater Res*, 27 (1993), 1103–1113.

75 Kaeler J, Zilla P, Fasol R, Deutsch M, Kadlets M. Precoating substrate and surface configuration determine adherence and spreading of seeded endothelial cells on polytetrafluoroethylene grafts. *J Vasc Surg*, 9 (1989), 535–541.

76 Kang IK, Kwon OH, Lee YM, Sung YK. Preparation and surface characterization of functional group-grafted and heparin-immobilized polyurethanes by plasma glow discharge. *Biomaterials*, 17 (1996), 841–847.

77 Kangasniemi IM, Verheyen CC, van der Velde EA, and de Groot K. In vivo tensile testing of flourapatite and hydroxylapatite plasma-sprayed coatings. *J Biomed Mater Res*, 28 (1994), 563–572.

78 Kanmangne FM, Labarre D, Serne H, and Jozefowicz M. Heparin-like activity of insoluble sulphonated polystyrene resins. Part I. Influence of the surface density, nature and binding of substituted anionic groups. *Biomaterials*, 6 (1985), 297–302.

79 Kawaguchi H. Polymer materials for bioanalysis and bioseparation. In Tsuruta T, Hayashi T, Kataoka K, Ishihara K, Kimura Y (Eds.), *Biomedical Applications of Polymeric Materials*. Boca Raton, FL: CRC Press, 1993, 299–324.

80 Keogh JR, Velander FF, and E JW. Albumin binding surfaces for implantable devices. *J Biomed Mat Res*, 26, 1992.

81   Kesler KA, Herring MB, Arnold MP, Glover JL, Park HM, Helmus MN, Bendick PJ. Enhanced strength of endothelial attachment on polyester fibronectin substrate. *J Vasc Surg*, 3 (1986), 58–64.

82   Khamlichio S, Serres A, Muller D, Jozefonvicz J, Brash JL. Interaction of IgG and albumin with functionalized silicas. *Coll Surf B: Biointerfaces*, 4 (1995), 165–172.

83   Kiaei D, Hoffman AS, Hanson SR. Ex vivo and in vitro platelet adhesion on RFGD deposited polymers. *J Biomed Mater Res*, 26 (1992), 357–372.

84   Kiaei D, Hoffman AS, Horbett TA, Lew KR. Platelet and monoclonal antibody binding to fibrinogen adsorbed on glow-discharge-deposited polymers. *J Biomed Mat Res*, 29 (1995), 729–739.

85   Kiaei D, Hoffman AS, Ratner BD, Horbett TA. Interaction of blood with gas discharge treated vascular grafts. *J Appl Polym Sci. Appl Polym Symp* 42 (1988), 269–283.

86   Kim SW, Feijen J. Surface modification of polymers for improved blood compatibility. *CRC Critical Reviews in Biocompatibility*, 1 (1985), 229–260.

87   Kim SW, Lee R, Oster H, Coleman D, Andrade JD, Lentz D, Olsen D. Platelet adhesion to polymer surfaces. *Trans Am Soc Art Int Org*, 20 (1974), 449–455.

88   Kleinfeld D, Kahler H, Hockberger PE. Controlled outgrowth of dissociated neurons on patterned substrates. *The Journal of Neuroscience*, 8 (1988), 4098–4120.

89   Kobayashi A, Kobayashi K, Akaike T. Control of adhesion and detachment of parenchymal liver cells using lactose-carrying polystyrene as substratum. *J Biomat Sci, Polym Ed*, 3 (1992), 499–508.

90   Kobayashi K, Kobayashi A, Akaike T. Culturing hepatocytes on lactose-carrying polystyrene layer via asialoglycoprotein receptor-mediated interactions. *Meth Enzymol*, 247 (1994), 409–418.

91   Köhler AS, Mooradian DL, Parks PJ, Rao G, Furcht LT. Grafting of modified phospholipids to glass: Evaluation of platelet interaction and analysis of surface morphology. *Trans Soc Biomat*, 18 (1995), 18.

92   Kokubo T, Hata K, Nakamura T, Yamamuro T. Apatite formation on ceramics, metals, and polymers induced by a CaO-SiO$_2$-based glass in a simulated body fluid. In Bonfield W, Hasting GW, Turner KE (Eds.), *Bioceramics*. London: Butterworth-Heinemann, 1991, 113–120.

93   Kondo A, Makino K, Matsuda T. Two-dimensional artificial extracellular matrix: bioadhesive peptide-immobilized surface design. *J Applied Polymer Science*, 47 (1993), 1983–1988.

94   Kottke-Marchant K, Anderson JM, Umemura Y, Marchant RE. Effect of albumin coating on the in vitro blood compatibility of Dacron™ arterial prostheses. *Biomaterials*, 10 (1989), 147–155.

95   Larsson C, Thomsen P, Aronsson BO, Rodahl M, Lausmaa J, Kasemo B, Ericson LE. Bone response to surface-modified titanium implants: Studies on the early tissue response to machined and electropolished implants with different oxide thicknesses. *Biomaterials*, 17 (1996), 605–616.

96   Lee HB, Lee JH. Biocompatibility of solid substrates based on surface wettability. In Wise DL, Trantolo DJ, Altobelli DE, Yaszemski MJ, Gresser JD, Schwartz ER (Eds.), *Encyclopedic Handbook of Biomaterials and Bioengineering. Part A: Materials*. New York: Marcel Dekker, Inc, 1995.

97   Lee J, Martic PA, Tan JS. Protein adsorption on pluronic copolymer-coated polystyrene particles. *J Coll Interf Sci*, 131 (1989), 252–266.

98   Lee JH, Jeong BJ, Khang GS, Lee HB. Plasma protein adsorption and platelet adhesion onto comb-like PEO gradient surfaces. *Trans Soc Biomat*, 18 (1995), 146.

99   Lee JH, Kopeckova P, Kopecek J, Andrade JD. Surface properties of copolymers of alkyl methacrylates with methoxy(polyethylene oxide)methacrylates and their application as protein-resistant coatings. *Biomaterials*, 11 (1990), 455–463.

100 Lee JH, Kopeckova P, Kopecek J, Andrade JD. Surface properties of copolymers of alkyl methacrylates and their application as protein-resistant coatings. *Biomaterials*, 11 (1990), 169–177.

101 Lewandowska KE, Pergament, Sukenik N, Culp LA. Cell-type-specific adhesion mechanisms mediated by fibronectin adsorbed to chemically derivatized substrata. *J Biomed Mater Res*, 26 (1992), 1343–1363.

102 Li JT, Caldwell KD. Plasma interactions with Pluronic™-treated colloids. *Colloids and Surfaces B: Biointerfaces*, 1996.

103 Li JT, Carlsson J, Lin J-N, and Caldwell KD. Chemical modification of surface active poly(ethylene oxide)-poly(propylene oxide) triblock copolymers. *Bioconjugate Chemistry*, in press.

104 Lin JC, Cooper SL. Surface characterization and ex vivo blood compatibility study of plasma modified small diameter tubing: Effect of sulfur dioxide and hexamethyldisiloxane plasmas. *Biomaterials*, 16 (1995), 1017–1023.

105 Lin JC, Cooper SL. Surface characterization and ex vivo blood compatibility study of plasma modified small diameter tubing: Effect of sulfur dioxide and hexamethyl-disiloxane plasmas. *Biomaterials*, 16 (1995), 1017–1023

106 Lindon JN, McManama G, Kushner L, Merrill EW, Salzman EW. Does the conformation of adsorbed fibrinogen dictate platelet interactions with artificial surfaces? *Blood*, 68 (1986), 355–362.

107 Liu SQ, Ito Y, Imanishi Y. Cell growth on immobilized cell growth factor. 9. Covalent immobilization of insulin, transferrin, and collagen to enhance growth of bovine endothelial cells. *J Biomed Mater Res*, 27 (1993), 909–915.

108 Lopez GP, Ratner BD, Rapoza RJ, Horbett TA. Plasma deposition of ultrathin films of poly(2-hydroxyethyl methacrylate): Surface analysis and protein adsorption measurements. *Macromolecules*, 26 (1993), 3247–3251.

109 Lopina ST, Edward GW, Merrill W, Griffith-Cima L. Hepatocyte culture on carbohydrate modified star polyethylene oxide hydrogels. *Biomaterials*, 17 (1996), 559–569.

110 Lyman MD, Melanson D, Sawhney AS. Characterization of the formation of interfacially photopolymerized thin hydrogel in contact with arterial tissue. *Biomaterials*, 17 (1996), 359–364.

111 Maistrelli GL, Mahomed N, Fornasier V, Antonelli L, Li Y, Binnington A. Functional osseointegration of hydroxyapatite-coated implants in a weight-bearing canine model. *J Arthroplasty*, 8 (1993), 549–554.

112 Malmsten M, Lassen B. Competitive protein adsorption at phospholipid surfaces. *Colloids and Surfaces B: Biointerfaces*, 4 (1995), 173–184.

113 Malmsten M, van Alstine JM. Adsorption of poly(ethylene glycol) amphiphiles to form coatings which inhibit protein adsorption. *J Coll Interface Sci*, 177 (1996), 502–512.

114 Margel S, Vogler EA, Firment L, Watt T, Haynie S, Sogah DY. Peptide, protein, and cellular interactions with self-assembled monolayer model surfaces. *J Biomed Mat Res*, 27 (1993), 1463–1476.

115 Massia SP, Hubbell JA. Human endothelial cell interactions with surface-coupled adhesion peptides on a nonadhesive glass substrate and two polymeric biomaterials. *J Biomed Mat Res*, 25 (1991), 223–242.

116 Massia SP, Hubbell JA. Immobilized amines and basic amino acids as mimetic heparin-binding domains for cell surface proteoglycan-mediated adhesion. *J Biological Chemistry*, 267 (1992), 10133–10141.

117 Massia SP, Hubbell JA. An RGD spacing of 440 nm is sufficient for $a_v b_3$ integrin-mediated fibroblast spreading and 140 nm for focal contact and stress fiber formation. *J Cell Biology*, 114: 1089–1100, 1991.

118 Matsuda T, Kondo A, Makinl K, Akutsu T. Development of a novel artificial matrix with cell adhesion peptides for cell culture and artificial and hybrid organs. *ASAIO Transactions*, 35 (1989), 677–679.

119 Matsuda T, Miwa H, Moghaddam ML, Iida F. Newly designed tissue adhesion prevention technology based photocurable mucopolysaccharides. *ASAIO J*, 39 (1993), M327–M331.

120 Mauzac M, Aubert N, Jozefonvicz J. Antithrombic activity of some polysaccharide resins. *Biomaterials*, 3 (1982), 221–224.

121 Merrill EW, Salzman EW. Polyethylene oxide as a biomaterial. *J Am Soc Artif Intern Organs*, 6 (1983), 60–72.

122 Meyle J, Gultig H, Wolburg N, von Recum AF. Fibroblast anchorage to microtextured surfaces. *J Biomed Mat Res*, 27 (1993), 1553–1557.

123 Migonney V, Fougnot C, Jozefowicz M. Heparin-like tubings. I. Preparation, characterization, and biological in vitro activity assessment. *Biomaterials*, 9 (1988), 145–149.

124 Miron T, Wilchek M. A simplified method for the preparation of succinimidyl carbonate polyethylene glycol for coupling to proteins. *Bioconjugate Chemistry*, 4 (1993), 568–569.

125 Mooney D, Hansen L, Vacanti J, Langer R, Farmer S, Ingber D. Switching from differentiation to growth in hepatocytes: Control by extracellular matrix. *J Cellular Physiology*, 151 (1992), 497–505.

126 Morra M, Occhiello E, Garbassi F. The effect of power discharge on the acid-base properties of thin films deposited from hydroxyethylmethacrylate. *J Colloid Interface Sci*, 164 (1994), 325–332.

127 Morscher EW. The current status to acetabular fixation in primary total hip arthroplasty. *Clin Orthop*, 274 (1992), 172–193.

128 Mrksich M, Whitesides GM. Using self-assembled monolayers to understand the interactions of man-made surfaces with proteins and cells. *Ann Rev Biophys Biomol Struct*, 25 (1996), 55–78.

129 Nagaoka S, Mori Y, Takiuchi H, Yokota K, Tanzawa H, Nishiumi S. Interaction between blood components and hydrogels with poly(oxyethylene) chains. In Shalaby SW, Hoffman AS, Ratner BD, Horbett TA, *Polymers as Biomaterials*. New York: Plenum Press, 1984, 361–374.

130 Napper DH. *Polymeric Stabilization of Colloidal Dispersions*. San Diego, CA: Academic Press Inc., 1983.

131 Neff JA, Caldwell KD, Tresco PA. Use of PEO-containing surfactants for immobilization of cell adhesion peptides. I. Control of surface peptide density. Manuscript in preparation.

132 Nilsson K, Mosbach K. Immobilization of ligands with organic sulfonyl chlorides. *Meth Enzymol*, 104 (1984), 56–69.

133 Norde W. Adsorption of proteins from solution at the solid-liquid interface. *Adv Colloid Interface Sci*, 25 (1986), 267–340.

134 Norman ME, Williams P, Illum L. In vivo evaluation of protein adsorption to sterically stabilized colloidal carriers. *J Biomed Mat Res*, 27 (1993), 861–866.

135 O'Shannessy DJ. Hydrazido-derivatized supports in affinity chromatography. *J Chromatogr*, 590 (1990), 13–21.

136 Oonishi H, Yamamoto M, Ishimaru H, Tsuji E, Kushitani S, Aono M, Ukon Y. The effect of hydroxyapatite coating on bone growth into porous titanium alloy implants. *J Bone Joint Surg*, 71 (1989), 213–216.

137 Osterberg E, Bergstrom K, Holmberg K, Schuman TP, Riggs JA, Burns NL, Alstine JM, Harris JM. Protein-rejecting ability of surface-bound dextran in end-on and side-on configurations: Comparisons to PEG. *J Biomed Mat Res*, 29 (1995), 741–747.

138 Ozaki KC, Phaneuf MD, Hong SL, Quist WC, LoGerfo FW. Glycoconjugate mediated endothelial cell adhesion to dacron polyester film. *J Vasc Surg*, 18 (1993), 486–494.

139 Park KD, Okano T, Nojiri H, Kim SW. Heparin immobilization onto segmented polyurethaneurea surfaces—Effect of hydrophilic spacers. *J Biomed Mater Res*, 22 (1988), 977–992.

140 Parker JL, Cho DL, Claesson PM. Plasma modification of mica: Forces between fluorocarbon surfaces in water and a nonpolar liquid. *J Phys Chem*, 93 (1989), 6121–6125.

141 Pettit DK, Hoffman AS, Horbett TA. Correlation between corneal epithelial cell outgrowth and monoclonal antibody binding to the cell binding domain of adsorbed fibronectin. *J Biomed Mat Res*, 28 (1994), 685–691.

142 Piattellli A, Scarano A, Piatelli M, Calabrese L. Direct bone formation on sand-blasted titanium implants: an experimental study. *Biomaterials*, 17 (1996), 1015–1018.

143 Pitt WG, Cooper SL. Albumin adsorption on alkyl chain derivatized polyurethanes: I. The effect of C-18 alkylation. *J Biomed Mat Res*, 22 (1988), 359–382.

144 Pitt WG, Park K, Cooper SL. Sequential protein adsorption and thrombus deposition on polymeric biomaterials. *J Coll Interface Sci*, 111 (1986), 343–362.

145 Pizzoferrato A, Arciola CR, Cenni E, Ciapetti G, Sassi S. In vitro biocompatibility of a polyurethane catheter after deposition of fluorinated film. *Biomaterials*, 16 (1995), 361–367.

146 Plueddeman EP, Clark HA, Nelson LE, Hoffman KR. New silane coupling agents for reinforced plastics. *Mod Plastics*, 39 (1962), 135–146, 187–195.

147 Pozniak G, Krajewska B, Trochimczuk W. Urease immobilized on modified polysulphone membrane: Preparation and properties. *Biomaterials*, 16 (1995), 129–134.

148 Price JS, Tencer AF, Arm DM, Bohach GA. Controlled release of antibiotics from coated orthopedic implants. *J Biomed Mater Res*, 30 (1996), 281–286.

149 Puleo DA. Activity of enzyme immobilized on silanized Co-Cr-Mo. *J Biomed Mat Res*, 29 (1995), 951–957.

150 Ramalanjaona G, Kempczinski RF, Rosenman JE, Douville EC. The effect of fibronectin coating on endothelial cell kinetics in polytetraflouroethylene grafts. *J Vasc Surg*, 3 (1986), 264–272.

151 Ramsey WS, Hertel W, Nowlan ED, Binkowski NJ. Surface treatments and cell attachment. *In Vitro*, 20 (1984), 802–808.

152 Ranieri JP, Bellamkinda R, Jacob J, Vargo TG, Gardella JA, Aebischer P. Selective neuronal cell attachment to a covalently patterned monoamine on fluorinated ethylene propylene films. *J Biomed Mater Res*, 27 (1993), 917–925.

153 Redepenning J, Schelessinger T, Burnham S, Lippiello L, Miyano J. Characterization of electrolytically prepared brushite and hydroxyapatite coating on orthopedic alloys. *J Biomed Mater Res*, 30 (1996), 287–294.

154 Rudt S, Müller RH. In vitro phagocytosis assay of nano- and microparticles by chemiluminescence. II. Effect of surface modification by coating of particles with poloxamer on the phagocytic uptake. *J Controlled Release*, 25 (1993), 51–59.

155 Ruoslhati E, Pierschbacher M. Tetrapeptides useful in surgery and therapeutic reconstruction and treatment of injuries. U. S. Patent, 1986.

156 Siballe K. Hydroxyapatite ceramic coating for bone implant fixation. mechanical and histological studies in dogs. *Acta Orthop Scand Suppl*, 255 (1993), 1–58.

157 Siballe K, Hansen ES, Brockstedt-Rasmussen H, Hjortdal VE, Juhl GI, Pedersen CM, Hvid I, Bunger C. Gap healing enhanced by hydroxyapatite coating in dogs. *Clin Orthop*, 272 (1991), 300–307.

158 Salzman EW, Lindon J, McManama G, Ware JA. Role of fibrinogen in activation of platelets. *NY Acad Sci*, 516 (1987), 184–195.

159 Schroen CGPH, Wijers MC, Cohen-Stuart MA, van der Padt A, van't Riet K. Membrane modification to avoid wettability changes due to protein adsorption in an emulsion/membrane bioreactor. *J Membrane Sci*, 80 (1993), 265–274.

160 Seeger IM, Klingman N. Improved In vivo endothelialization of prosthetic grafts by surface modification with fibronectin. *J Vasc Surg*, 8 (1988), 467–482.

161 Shue M-S, Hoffman AS, Feijen J, Harris JM. Glow discharge immobilization of PEO surfactants for non-fouling biomaterial surfaces: A mechanism study. *Trans Soc Biomaterials*, 17 (1994), 138.

162 Silver JH, Hart AP, Williams EC, Cooper SL. Anticoagulant effects of sulfonated polyurethanes. *Biomaterials*, 13 (1992), 339–344.

163 Silver JH, Hergenrother RW, Lin J-C, Lim F, Lin H-B, Okada T, Chaudhury MK, and Cooper ST. Surface and blood-contacting properties of alkylsiloxane monolayers supported on silicone rubber. *J Biomed Mat Res*, 29 (1995), 535–548.

164 Singhvi R, Kumar A, Lopez GP, Stephanopoulos GN, Wang DIC, Whitesides GM, Ingber DE. Engineering cell shape and function. *Science*, 264 (1994), 696–698.

165 Slepian M, Massia S, Kieras M, Dehdashti B, Khosravi F. Endovascular photopolymerized gel paving of stented porcine femoral arteries, acute in-vivo efficacy. *Trans Soc Biomaterials*, 18 (1995), 32.

166 Smith PAS. *Derivatives of Hydrazine and Other Hydronitrogens Having N-N Bonds*. Boston: Benjamin/Cummings, 1983.

167 Stuart GW, McDowell SJ, McDaniel SE, An YH, Friedman RJ. Cross-linked albumin-coated surfaces to prevent bacterial adhesion onto titanium plates. *Trans Soc Biomat*, 19 (1995), 414.

168 Sugawara T, Matsuda T. Photochemical surface derivatization of a peptide containing Arg-Gly-Asp (RGD). *J Biomed Mater Res*, 29 (1995), 1047–1052.

169 Takatsuka K, Yamamuro T, Kitsugi T, Nakamura T, Shibuya T, Goto T. A new bioactive glass-ceramic as a coating material on titanium alloy. *J Applied Biomater*, 4 (1993), 317–329.

170 Tan JS, Butterfield DE, Voycheck CL, Caldwell KD, Li JT. Surface modification of nanoparticles by PEO/PPO block copolymers to minimize interactions with blood components and prolong circulation in rats. *Biomaterials* 14: 823–833, 1993.

171 Tanahashi M, Yao T, Kokubo T, Minod M, Miyamoto T, Nakamura T, Yamamuro T. Apatite coated on organic polymers by biomimetic process: improvement in its adhesion to substrate by glow discharge treatment. *J Biomed Mater Res*, 29 (1995), 349–357.

172 Tanahashi M, Yao T, Kokubo T, Minod M, Miyamoto T, Nakamura T, Yamamuro T. Apatite coated on organic polymers by biomimetic process: Improvement in its adhesion to substrate by NaOH treatment. *J Applied Biomaterials*, 5 (1994), 339–347.

173 Tang L, Eaton JW. Adsorbed fibrinogen mediates acute inflammatory responses to biomaterials. *J Exper Med*, 178 (1993), 2147–2156.

174 Tashiro K, Sephel GC, Greatored D, Sasaki M, Shirashi N, Martin GR, Martin HK, Kleinman HK, Yamada Y. The RGD containing site of the mouse laminin A chain is active for cell attachment, spreading, migration, and neurite outgrowth. *J Cellular Physiology*, 146 (1991), 452–459.

175 Thomas KA, Kay JF, Cook SD, Jarcho M. The effect of surface macrotexture and hydroylapatite coating on the mechanical strengths and histologic profiles of titanium implant materials. *J Biomed Mater Res*, 21 (1987), 1395–1414.

176 Torrisi L. Micron-size particles emission from bioceramics induced by pulsed lazer deposition. *Biomed Mater Eng*, 3 (1993), 43–49.

177 Tretinnikov ON, Ikada KK. In vitro hydroxyapaptite deposition onto a film surface-grafted with organophophate polymer. *J Biomed Mater Res*, 28 (1994), 1365–1373.

178 Tseng Y-C, McPherson T, Yuan CS, Park K. Grafting of ethylene glycol-butadiene block copolymers onto dimethyl-dichlorosilane-coated glass by g-irradiation. *Biomaterials*, 1995, 963–972.

179 Tseng Y-C, Park KJ. Synthesis of photoreactive poly(ethylene glycol) and its application to the prevention of surface-induced platelet activation. *Biomed Mater Res*, 26 (1992), 373–391.

180 Ulubayram K, Hasirci N. Properties of plasma-modified polyurethane surfaces. *Coll and Surf B: Biointerf*, 1 (1993), 261–269.

181 Underwood PA, Steele JG, Dalton BA. Effects of polystyrene surface chemistry and the biological activity of solid phase fibronectin and vitronectin, analyzed with monoclonal antibodies. *J Cell Science*, 104 (1993), 793–803.

182 van Ooij WJ, Surman D, Yasuda HK. Plasma-polymerized coatings of trimethylsilane deposited on cold-rolled steel substrates: Part 2. Effect of deposition conditions on corrosion performance. *Progr Organic Coatings* 25 (1995), 319–337.

183 van Wachem PB, Hogt AH, Beugeling T, Feijen J, Bantjes A, Detmers JP, van Aken WG. Adhesion of cultured human endothelial cells onto methacrylate polymers with varying surface wettability and charge. *Biomaterials*, 8 (1987), 323–328.

184 von Recum AF. New aspects of biocompatibility: Motion at the interface. In Heimke G, Soltze U, Lee AJC (Eds.), *Clinical Implant Materials*. Amsterdam: Elsevier, 1990, 297–302.

185 Wang TF, Yasuda HK. Modification of wettability of a stainless steel plate by cathodic plasma polymerization of trimethylsilane-oxygen mixtures. *J Appl Polymer Sci*, 55 (1995), 903–909.

186 Weetall HH. Covalent coupling methods for inorganic support materials. *Methods Enzymol*, 44 (1976), 134–148.

187 Wennerberg A, Albrektsson T, Johansson C, Anderson B. Experimental study of turned and grit-blasted screw-shaped implants with special emphasis on effects of blasting material and surface topography. *Biomaterials*, 17 (1996), 15–22.

188 West JL, Hubbell JA. Comparison of covalently and physically cross-linked polyethylene glycol-based hydrogels for the prevention of postoperative adhesions in a rat model. *Biomaterials*, 16 (1995), 1153–1156.

189 Williams SK, Jarrell BE, Friend L, Radomski JS, Carabasi RA, Koolpe E, Mueller SN, Thornton SC, Marinucci T, Levine E. Adult human endothelial cell compatibility with prosthetic graft material. *J Surg Res*, 38 (1985), 618–629, 1985.

190 Wojciechowski PW, Brash JL. Fibrinogen and albumin adsorption from human blood plasma and from buffer onto chemically functionalized silica substrates. *Colloids and Surfaces B*, 1 (1993), 107–117.

191 Wong SS. *Chemistry of Protein Conjugation and Cross-Linking*. Boca Raton, FL: CRC Press, 1991.

192 Woodhouse KA, Skarja GA, Bishop P, Brash JL. Platelet interactions with cross-linked fibrin and thermally denatured fibrinogen surfaces. *Trans Soc Biomat*, 18 (1995), 33.

193 Yamada K. Adhesive recognition sequences. *J Biological Chemistry*, 266 (1991), 12809–12812.

194 Yasuda H. *Plasma Polymerization*. New York: Academic Press, 1985.

195 Yasuda H. Plasma polymerization and plasma modification of polymer surfaces. In Ebdon G (Ed.), *New Methods of Polymer Synthesis 6* London: Blackie Academic, 1995, 161–196.

196 Yeh YS, Iriyama Y, Matsusawa Y, Hanson SR, Yasuda H. Blood compatibility of surfaces modified by plasma polymerization. *J Biomed Mater Res*, 27 (1988), 795–818.

197 Zilla P, Fasol R, Preiss P, Kadletz M, Deutsch M, Schima H, Tsangaris S, Groscurth P. Use of fibrin glue as a substrate for in vitro endothelialization of PTFE vascular grafts. *Surgery*, 105 (1989), 515–522.

198 Zucker MB, Vroman L. Platelet adhesion induced by fibrinogen adsorbed onto glass. *Proc Soc Exper Biol Med*, 131 (1969), 318–320.

Chapter 13
Surface Topography

Andreas F. von Recum
Carolyn E. Brown
Clare E. Shannon
Martine LaBerge

NEED AND RELEVANCE

This chapter focuses on surface topography as a known modifier of histo-compatibility. It presents the tissue/surface interactions related to topography and describes topographic characterization methods used for the assessment of surface texture and their limitations.

The effect of implant surface roughness on the surrounding tissue has been observed by a number of investigators (see also Chapters 7, 8, and 12). Powell and Gibbons [1] reported a notable difference between breast capsules of smooth versus textured implant material. The textured sac (texture consisted of 75 μm square pillars with heights of 150 μm) had greater cellularity, particularly giant cells, and lower collagen density as compared to smooth implants surrounded by inactive fibrocytes. From their findings it would appear that the texture dimensions of Powell and Gibbons maintained a stimulus for chronic inflammation. Pollock [2] conducted a retrospective study of nearly 200 patients and found that silicone implants with textured surfaces had less capsular contracture as compared with smooth-surface silicone implants. Smahel et al. [3] concluded that textured polymeric surfaces prevented compact capsule development, as compared to smooth polymeric implants, in rats. It is important to note that neither Pollock nor Smahel and associates reported on textural details (size, shape, distribution). Schmidt and von Recum [4] reviewed published histological responses attributed to the NIH reference material polydimethylsiloxane. Curious about the reported large histological variance, they then characterized the surface profile of the top and the bottom of the NIH test material specimens and found significant differences between both sides, probably related to the manufacturing process. Since the specimen sites were not identified in the literature, the histological variance might be due solely to the topographic differences.

It is not yet entirely understood how implant surface topography affects the tissue response, but a number of investigators point to a direct relationship between capsule thickness and tissue/implant interfacial motion. Kupp et al. [5] reported that surface roughness of intra-muscular implants related to capsule thickness where the degree of interfacial motion was speculated to be the etiological factor. Picha and Drake [6] found that capsule thickness can be reduced by up to a magnitude when fixed by sutures, indicating that the reduction of motion between the implant and the tissue can significantly change the tissue response. Since surface roughness can serve as a means for tissue interdigitation or anchorage, it was tested by many as a means to reduce interfacial motion. Indeed Vaughan et al. [7] reported that fibroblasts actually anchor in surface pores of 1 μm. Campbell and von Recum [8] additionally observed that fibroblasts produced collagen strands penetrating into such pores for distances of up to 150 μm. Salthouse and Matlaga [9] found that the shape of the cross section of suture materials had a significant influence on the degree of inflammatory response. von Recum [10] reported on a reverse correlation between tissue attachment to the implant surface and responding chronic inflammation. He speculated that mechanical forces (friction and motion) at the interface play a causative role in maintaining chronic inflammation. In summary, it appears that micro-motion at the tissue/implant interface must be considered a cause of chronic inflammation, capsule thickening, and contracture [11] and therefore needs to be factored into the design of implants.

Campbell and von Recum [12] have experimentally demonstrated that the dimensions of the textural configurations (in their experiments pores within polymeric filters) have a profound modifying effect on biocompatibility and that average pore sizes between 1 and 2 μm diameter elicited the mildest overall tissue response. Smaller (0.5 μm) and larger pore diameters (3, 5, and 10 μm) had more pronounced inflammatory responses, capsule formation, and signs of contracture.

It has been well reviewed by a number of authorities [13–15] that individual cells and bacteria can recognize certain surface topographical configurations, including infinite grooves and ridges, and finite pillars and wells, if these configurations are within certain size ranges which appear to be below the size of the average tissue cell. According to these findings cells preferably attach, elongate, migrate, and reproduce along suitable events textured onto cell culture substrata. The advent of photolithography as a surface-texturing technique has enabled us to design surface configurations down to sub-micron sizes and study the cellular responses to such textured substrates [14]. Schmidt et al. [15] demonstrated that macrophages cultured on textured silicone substrates (with textural configurations including wells, hills, ridges, and grooves in the size range from 1 to 10 μm) had different metabolic and morphological responses to various configuration dimensions and configuration densities. Green et al. [16], using the same substrata, demonstrated that fibroblasts were able to differentiate hills from wells and ridges from grooves even though their three-dimensional dimensions, either into or out of the surface, were the same (see Figure 13-1).

The cues that are the signals to which cells (macrophages or fibroblasts) and granulation tissue appear to respond are not yet clearly identified but must be associated with certain elements of the topographic configurations and must be within or below cellular size ranges. Wu [17] deduced from his implantation experiments that sharp configuration contours and edges seem to contain the stimulating signals. For a detailed review of this subject see von Recum and van Kooten [18].

In summary, surface topography has been shown to affect biocompatibility and often indirectly influence the designed performance of surgical implants in several ways. Motion at the interface between bone and bone implants impairs bone healing and actually promotes bony tissue lysis. Bone tissue interdigitation with appropriate surface topological configurations has effectively reduced interfacial motion, improved long-term fixation of the implant in its bony implantation site, and promoted direct bone healing at the implant interface and across the bone defect.

Motion at the interface between soft tissues and their implants has been shown to increase tissue capsule thickness and capsule contraction. Soft tissue implants, especially those with motion or mobility inherent in their function such as blood pumps, vascular grafts, and breast implants, have been impaired by the contracting tissue capsule, which increasingly restricts their free mobility and actions, reduces their effective volume, or destroys their desired cosmetic contouring effect. The provision of tissue interdigitating means on the implant surface has greatly reduced the described detrimental effects, but has not necessarily reduced the overall inflammatory response to the implant.

Surface texturing within a micrometer range of topological configuration sizes has been shown to influence the tissue response to the implant on a cellular level by reducing the number of inflammatory cells at the interface and reducing the thickness of the tissue

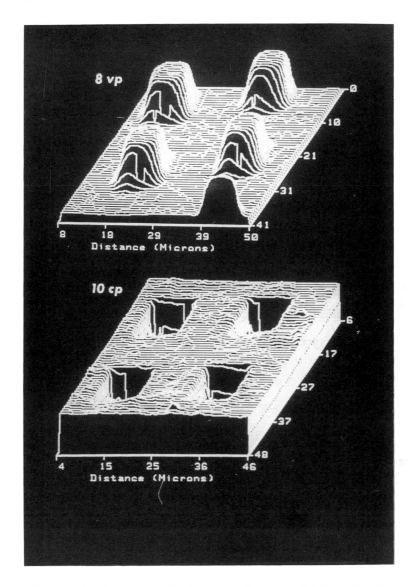

Figure 13-1 Topographical evaluation of an implant surface using light beam interferometry. The z-direction of the surface phenomena clearly show protuberances (top) or indentations (bottom).

capsule. It is speculated that the reduction of interfacial motion on a cellular level is, to a large degree, responsible for chronic inflammation and capsular contraction.

From all of this evidence it becomes clear that surface topography is an important variable of implant performance. Therefore, surface topography of implants needs to be characterized and controlled. In the following text we propose topographic assessment methods and discuss their diagnostic value and technical limitations.

DEFINITIONS OF TOPOGRAPHY

Topography may be defined as the morphology or configuration of a surface. A differentiation can be made between two different topographic characteristics: roughness and texture. These are briefly defined below. In addition, Table 13-1 lists some frequently used terms.

Table 13-1 Definition of Surface-Related Terms

Term	Definition
Discontinuity	a change in the direction from one surface plane into another as produced by hills, pits, valleys, grooves, or ridges extending out of or into the main plane; the edge where two or more planes meet
Configuration	a purposefully created topographic detail in a plane like a groove, ridge, hill, or well
Macro	details that can (almost) be detected with the naked eye and are somewhere above 20 μm in dimension
Macro-Textured Surfaces	coarse surface textures produced by beads or wires attached to the surface of a metallic implant, or by the textile fibers (also comprising the bulk material) of a vascular graft
Micro	details that are smaller than 20 microns and are not detectable with the unaided eye
Micro-Textured Surfaces	designed surfaces with configurations of regular size and density including grooves, wells, ridges, and hills, the dimensions of which are smaller than 20 μm
Roughness	a surface with multiple, randomly-sized and distributed discontinuities, as they are generated by natural formation or surface-finishing methods; some of the parameters characterizing roughness are listed below:
Ra	Roughness average (Ra) or Center-Line Average (CLA) or Arithmetic Average (AA). Arithmetic mean of the vertical deviation from the mean. $$R_a = \frac{1}{n}\sum_{i=1}^{n}|z_i|$$ z_i are measured from the center-line defined as the line which divides the profile with a net deviation of 0
RMS	Root Mean Square of the roughness average value corresponding to Ra. Standard deviation of the profile for a Gaussian height distribution. $$R_a = \sqrt{\frac{1}{n}\sum_{i=1}^{n}z_i^2}$$
PV	Peak to Valley: vertical distance between maximum peak and maximum valley within the scan length $$R_t = \max(z_i) - \min(z_i)$$
Probability Density Function (Ψ)	$$\int_{-\infty}^{\infty}\Psi(z)\,dz = 1$$ Probability that surface heights lie between z and dz. $\Psi(z)$ may be Gaussian for some surfaces and non-Gaussian for others.
Skewness (s)	$$s = \frac{1}{R_q^3}\int z^3\Psi(z)\,dz$$ Measure of the departure of the probability density function from symmetry.
Autocorrelation function r(l)	$$r(l) = \frac{1}{R_q^2}<z(x).z(x+l)>$$ Reveal surface periodicities inherent to production or finishing.
Wa	Waviness Average: average deviation of waviness height from the mean line.
WMS	Root Mean Square of waviness average value corresponding to Wa.
Texture	A surface topography comprised of purposefully-designed surface configurations with controlled dimensions and surface distribution.
Topography	The configuration of a surface including its relief and the position of its natural and/or man-made configurations.

All surfaces contain irregularities or asperities that can be divided into three main categories: roughness, waviness, and error of form. Roughness includes closely spaced irregularities and surface textures inherent in the fabrication process. At the microscopic level, roughness concerns the horizontal spacing of the surface features. Roughness is created by hills and valleys of varying amplitude and spacing larger than molecular dimensions. Surface waviness consists of surface irregularities of greater spacing than roughness while error of form is a gross deviation from a nominal shape. Surface irregularities may be the cumulative result of the crystal structure of the material, the fabrication processes, or purposeful surface finish including etching, grinding or sandblasting. Surface roughness can be described and quantitated by topographic methods and expressed as measurements of the surface profile.

Texture, in our terminology, is represented by any deliberate array of configurations including but not limited to grooves, ridges, hills, or pores. They are designed into a substrate surface, created by machining, sintering, or etching, and resulting in purposeful, regular surface topography with defined dimensions and surface distribution. Currently used in orthopedic applications, they have typical configuration diameters (of pores, beads, or wires) larger than 50 μm. Textured surfaces cannot be adequately characterized by measuring a linear profile. Additional parameters including dimensions of the textural configurations and their distribution over the surface will also have to be described [19].

Porosity can be considered a special case of texture. It can consist of individual surface pores or interconnecting pores throughout the bulk material. It has been used for tissue anchorage to vascular grafts having effective pore diameters above 20 μm and usually below 60 μm (see also Chapters 1, 5 and 43). For bone ingrowth the typically recommended pore entry size lies between 75 and 250 μm [19]. Porosity has been created by sintering, etching, casting, leaching, foaming, or textile manufacturing methods using fibers.

Micro-texture must be considered a special case of texture where the textural configurations are sized in cellular and sub-cellular dimension. Such surfaces have been created by micro-machining, photo-lithography, or ion beam etching, and their carefully controlled surface configurations have dimensions ranging from a few hundred nanometers to less than 10 μm.

Particulate matter is often found around implants in situ because of material disintegration due to chemical decomposition and/or mechanical wear. Particulate matter is sometimes purposefully implanted as a bone substitute or contour generating filler. The particles, predominately through their size and topography, have become a great medical concern since they can stimulate especially severe inflammatory responses that are not explainable through their bulk or surface chemistry (for more details see Chapter 14).

TESTS AND EVALUATION METHODOLOGIES

Surface Cleanliness

Characterizations should be performed on clean implant surfaces to avoid erroneous results from loose surface contaminants. Therefore the implants are cleaned thoroughly to remove loose debris and organic contaminants. We recommend the Clemson Implant Cleaning Protocol [20], according to which each implant is placed in a porous plastic cassette (as they are used for histological specimen embedding) to avoid direct contact with unclean surfaces. In addition, a pair of Teflon® (E. I. DuPont de Nemours & Co., Inc., Wilmington, DE)-coated forceps is also cleaned along with the implants to be used in subsequent implant handling. The cleaning procedure includes successive ultrasonic submersion of the implant cassette and Teflon®-coated forceps into 75% acetone in ultra pure de-ionized water and 1% detergent solution (Liquinox, Alconox Inc., New York, NY) for 20 minutes each, followed by three 15-minute ultrasonic rinses in ultra pure de-ionized water. Using the cleaned forceps, the cassette including the implant is transferred to a vacuum desiccator to dry. The dried implant is removed from the cassette and transferred to the surface characterization stage. The researcher must beware of contamination with dust and avoid handling the implant either with bare or gloved hands (glove powder will contaminate the implant surface). Optimally the surface characterization procedure is performed on a clean bench with laminar airflow.

Surface Electron Microscopy

The surface of an implant should be evaluated first with a scanning electron microscope (SEM) to obtain an overview of the surface topography, its uniformity, its approximate range of roughness, the spatial arrangement of textural configurations, and the presence of gross artifacts, defects, or contaminants. The surface of the specimen must be electrically conductive in order to achieve an SEM image. If the surface is not conductive, a thin metallic coating is applied to the surface; typical coating materials are gold or carbon. Then a fine probe of electrons scans the surface; each pixel signal is detected in sequence of the specimen-electron interaction. In this serial detection method the reflected (or back-scattered) beam of electrons is amplified and used to modulate the intensity of a TV-like image tube, which is scanned at the same rate as the electron probe [21]. SEM gives a direct image of the textured surface (see Figure 13-2). At low magnifications, this process allows for an overall evaluation of topographic configurations, configuration regularity, and a qualitative range of surface roughness. At higher magnifications, a quantitative method for evaluation of the configuration size and distribution can be developed with the aid of ASTM standards E 82-91, E 112, and E 1181, which are methods for the determination and characterization of the average grain size, grain size distribution, and crystal orientation of metallic materials [22–24]. These ASTM standards can be directly applied for the evaluation of topographic configuration size and distribution. ASTM E1181 recommends the use of a parallel array of test lines spaced 5.0 mm apart. Measurements from five randomly selected fields are taken to acquire a representation of the surface configuration size and distribution of a given sample within a 95% confidence limit. When the sample is visibly anisotropic and principal directions are not obvious, measurements from four equally spaced angular positions of the grid (for example, at 0, 45, 90, and 135 degrees) are recommended for each field. Selection of the photographic magnification of each field under evaluation is dependent upon the number of configurations visible in a particular field; ASTM recommends that each field should contain a minimum of 50 configurations and a maximum of 150 configurations in the field to be counted. Statistical determination of the spacing between each surface configuration can be conducted by measuring the distance (pitch) between configurations along a given length. For a given photographic field, a polar chart is placed in the center of the photograph in which the distance between each configuration is measured along the lengths of the 60-degree projection lines to determine the average spacing between each configuration (ASTM E 82-91). These measurement procedures can be conducted by hand (a time-consuming method) or by an automated image analysis system.

The disadvantages of SEM analysis are the lack of immediate configuration quantification, the insufficient depth analysis, and the need for sputtered coatings of non-conductive surfaces, thus preventing the scanning of surfaces that are subsequently used for implantation. Also, the high voltage used in scanning electron microscopy can cause damage of polymeric surfaces such as ultra high molecular weight polyethylene. To account for this

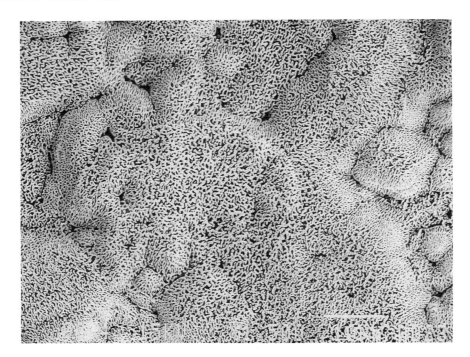

Figure 13-2 Scanning electron micrograph (magnification 1500X) showing a titanium surface treated with ion beam etching methodology (courtesy of NASA Lewis Research Center, Cleveland). The texture on the depicted surface is composed of configurations in two size ranges. The larger configurations represent titanium grain size and orientation, the smaller configurations represent etched ridges and grooves in a size range around one micron. SEM provides excellent qualitative, visual representation of the surface morphology but offers little direct quantitative information, especially in the z-axis.

problem, authors have successfully used low voltage (1–2 kV compared to 15–25 kV) scanning electron microscopy to image polymers [23].

Profilometry

Surface profilometry is commonly characterized along the vertical direction by height (amplitude) parameters and along the horizontal direction by spatial (wavelength) parameters. A surface is characterized in terms of surface parameters which commonly include arithmetic average roughness (R_a), root-mean-square roughness (RMS or R_q), and maximum peak-to-valley height (R_t or PV) (Table 13-1). In general, $R_a \leq R_q \leq R_t$. The roughness average is an ambiguous parameter. There is no indication whether the R_a value is the mean of many small deviations from the mean value or a few larger ones. Since different surface profiles can demonstrate the same R_a values, these data are not a direct representation of surface change resulting from tangential motion. Moreover, R_a, R_q, and R_t do not fully reflect the shape of the surface since they depend only on the profile height, rather than on the spacing between heights. Hence, these parameters do not carry any information about the size of asperities, slopes, and frequency of their occurrence. They are useful only when comparing surfaces produced with the same technique. Therefore, more informative surface parameters can be used. Moore [24] reviews surface parameters highlighting the slopes of the asperities, the degree of sharpness at asperity peaks, and the direction of asperities.

Table 13-2   Advantages and Limitations on Contacting and Non-contacting Profilometry

Technique	Function	Advantages	Disadvantages
Stylus Profilometry [30]	A diamond stylus is dragged across the specimen surface and the vertical motion the stylus is of transformed into an electrical analog voltage. The motion of the stylus replicates the topography of the specimen.	• Convenient to use • Wide dynamic range is available • Can cover distances from tens of microns to tens of millimeters • Vertical sensitivity can be better than 10 nm	• Can cause surface damage • Lateral resolution limited by tip radius • Two-dimensional representation of surface • Does not accommodate curved surfaces (e.g. acetabular cups)
Interferometry (Bushman) [31,32]	Interferometer measures surface topography by combining a path of light reflecting off the surface with a path of light reflecting off a reference surface. When the two paths become equal and combine, the light waves interfere to produce a pattern of fringes in a series of phase shift. The optical path of these data is used to determine surface height differences.	• Non-contact technique • Excellent vertical resolution • 3D or 2D surface representation • Attractive for soft surfaces	• Size of scanned area depends on objective magnification • Moderate reflectivity of the surface required • Not suitable for very rough surfaces • Incident light can penetrate the surface and be reflected necessitating correction

Likewise, similar measurements can be made on the waviness data. Definitions for some of the more important parameters are provided in Table 13-1. Non-contacting and contacting profilometers are available to quantify the microroughness of surfaces and their advantages and limitations are compared in Table 13-2 [25–27].

Light Beam Interferometry   Topographical surface evaluation can be conducted with a non-contacting white light interferometer which provides projection measurements of the surface profile through digital phase shifting interferometry (see Figure 13-3). Optical measurements are collected by the interferometer's magnification head. The optical measurements formulate a detailed map of the sample surface by combining the path of light reflecting off the surface with the light reflected off the magnification head reference surface. Then a computer image of the surface with its corresponding dimensions is generated. The resolution of this method is dependent on the light source implemented, which is in the nanometer range. Two-dimensional and three-dimensional surface profiles can be obtained. Line scan analysis from two-dimensional profilometers can give misleading topographical results because the periodicity of configuration events is dependent upon the

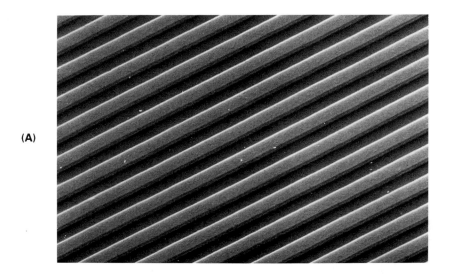

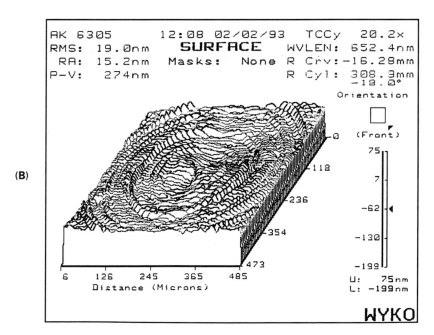

Figure 13-3 **(A)** Posterior surface of a commercially available intraocular lens machined out of PMMA sheets. **(B)** Machining marks are seen and quantifiable as shown in the 3-D scan using a non-contacting white light interferometry. Distances in the z-axis are represented by color changes which can be read from the color code on the right side of the 3-D reproduction.

location of the scan. The use of three-dimensional profilometers will determine more accurately the periodicity of surface configurations of a given area. The use of non-contacting topographical profilometers require that the material being observed is reflective. Therefore some polymeric materials must be coated like those prepared for SEM. Non-contact surface profilometry allows for the evaluation of softer materials like polymers and biologicals and offers distinct advantages over more destructive modes of topographical measurements discussed in this chapter.

One main disadvantage of interferometry is the small area (cut-off area) characterized, necessitating several scans of the surface to obtain a representative surface roughness. A typical cut-off area would be 500 μm × 500 μm (Linnik 20X magnification head, TOPO-3D, Wyko Corp., Tucson, AZ). Additionally, one should be concerned with the lateral and vertical resolution of the equipment since asperities larger than 1 μm in height cannot necessarily be detected by all non-contact profilometers. This limiting factor could provide inaccurate data regarding the surface profile. Hence, one should have some basic knowledge regarding the expectations of the surface roughness for accurate interpretation of data.

Mechanical Stylus Profilometry   Mechanical surface profilometers assess the surface profile by measuring the pole-tip displacement of a stylus which directly traces across the surface. The primary advantages of mechanical stylus profilometry are the generation of direct, reproducible, quantitative data.

Profile data are collected as the stylus traces the surface of the implant. As for the non-contacting profilometers, several scans of the same implant in equally distributed locations are recommended. Depending on the instrument used, the profile data are separated into low frequency waviness data and high frequency roughness data by selecting a cut-off filter appropriate for the implant tested. Stylus profilometry can be applied to a variety of materials from metals to biological tissue such as articular cartilage. Unfortunately, this method can actually damage highly polished or soft surfaces. In contacting profilometry, the stylus is normally made of diamond and a typical tip radius of approximately 2 μm with an applied static load of less than 7×10^{-4} N. Consequently, if the size of the stylus tip is larger than the asperities, this technique does not allow for a true representation of the surface roughness. Because of contact between the stylus and the surface, the surface profile can be distorted resulting in narrowed peaks and broadened valleys. Benabdallah and Chalifoux proposed a model to predict the extent of surface damage in contact profilometry, especially for soft materials, as a function of indenter shape and asperity angle [26]. Also, the textures of some biomaterial surfaces are highly anisotropic, resulting in different profiles for different scanning directions [27]. Stylus measurement will be magnified in both vertical and horizontal directions with a ratio of 50:1 [28]. It is therefore important to take this difference in magnification into consideration. Therefore, care must be taken in selecting the appropriate surface profilometer in order to obtain the best possible representation of the surface analyzed.

Figure 13-4 represents a black and white reproduction of a color graph generated by a contact profilometer (DEKTAK™ Profilometer, Sloan Technology, Santa Barbara, CA) showing the profile of a 5 mm trace on a cylindrical titanium implant. The three lines (shown in three different colors in the original) represent the actual trace of the stylus and the data separated into high frequency roughness data and low frequency waviness data. Calculated Ra, RMS, PV, Wa, WMS parameters are shown on the left side .

In summary (see Table 13-2), advantages of the mechanical stylus method are its direct measurement with a stylus on the original, non-coated implant surface as it will be implanted. It allows a much larger range of focal depth because the light beam interferometry and measurements can be made on a surface with curvature. A disadvantage is that the stylus scratches the surface and the test specimen can therefore not be used for further evaluations

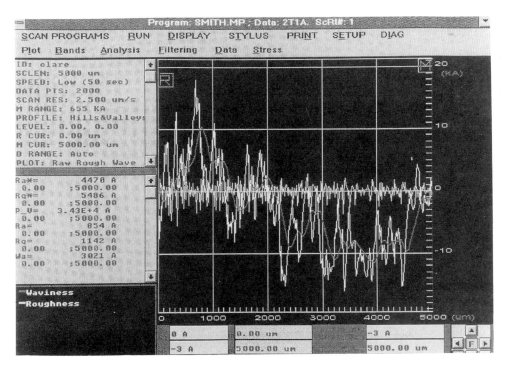

Figure 13-4 Roughness data of the machined surface of a titanium cylinder implant that was used in a biocompatibility study [38]. The surface is scanned with a mechanical stylus profilometer. The scans are shown on the right; the calculated roughness parameters are shown on the left.

or implantations. Also this method is limited to use on surface details larger than the stylus tip diameter.

Combining the quantitative data of profilometry with the three-dimensional visual information of SEM is commonly recommended to provide a complete picture of surface topography [29].

Laser Scanning Confocal Microscopy   When topographic configurations are of submicron dimensions, the resolution of white light beam interferometry and mechanical stylus profilometry is insufficient for accurate measurements, especially in the z-axis. Laser scanning confocal microscopy (LSCM) offers a higher resolution in the z-axis (700 nm). Optical sections in the z-axis can be taken at 0.2 μm intervals. We use a BioRad MRC1000 confocal setup linked to a Zeiss Axiophot microscope equipped with all necessary optics, including a Krypton-Argon laser, and image analysis software and hardware. A scanning of a silicon surface with photo-etched parallel grooves of one 1 μm depth and 1 μm width is shown in Figure 13-5. The native surface can be scanned, but only very small sections (field size of 60 μm) can be scanned at one observation time. LSCM is not cost-effective for routine surface characterization procedures but excellent for research purposes where it offers great opportunities to study in three dimensions the spatial interactions of cells on micro-textured surfaces.

CRITICAL PROBLEMS AND DIRECTIONS FOR FUTURE EVALUATIONS AND RESEARCH

Since the cause/effect relationships between surface topographic profile and biological response are not clear, general surface profiles for implants cannot be recommended at this

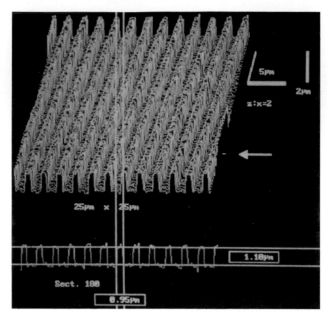

Figure 13-5 Laser scanning confocal light microscopic reproduction of a silicon wafer surface with photo-etched, parallel grooves of 1 μm width, 1 μm depth and 1 μm distance (courtesy of J. Meyle, University of Tübingen, unpublished data).

time. More research will have to clarify what topographic surface cues are recognized by what cell types and lead to what biological responses. It may well turn out that certain surface profiles stimulate metabolic, production, or reproductive activities of some cells but not others. Certain surface profiles might alter the competitive race for the implant surface in favor of either bacteria, connective tissue or inflammatory cells, respectively. It is already clear that textured dental implants not only promote bony anchorage but also favor plaque adherence.

A relationship between surface topography and histocompatibility has, however, been clearly documented. More research will be an excellent investment in the improvement of histocompatibility of currently available materials. For example it will be possible to select materials for their best mechanical, thermal, or chemical fit. Their biocompatibility can then be corrected with topographic designs. Until then, we can keep the histocompatibility performance of an implant constant by controlling its topographic profile.

SPECIFICATIONS/STANDARDS

1   ASTM, E 89-91: Standard test method for determining the orientation of a metal crystal. In *1995 Annual Book of Standards*, v03.01. Philadelphia, PA: American Society for Testing and Materials, 1995, 228–252.

2   ASTM, E112: Standard test methods for determining average grain size. In *1995 Annual Book of Standards.*, v03.01. Philadelphia, PA: American Society for Testing and Materials, 1995, 228–252.

3   ASTM, E1181: Standard test method for characterizing duplex grain sizes. In *1995 Annual Book of Standards.*, v03.01. Philadelphia, PA: American Society for Testing and Materials, 1995, 777–790.

REFERENCES

1   Powell E, Gibbons DF. Effect of implant compliance and surface texture on fibrous capsule morphology and myofibroblast population. *Biol Eng Soc*, (1982), 21–33.

2   Pollock H. Breast capsular contracture: A retrospective study of textured versus smooth silicone implants. *Plastic and Reconstructive Surg*, 92 (1993), 404–407.

3   Smahel J, Hurwitz PJ, Hurwitz N. Soft tissue response to textured silicone implants in an animal experiment. *Plastic and Reconstructive Surg*, 92 (1993), 474–479.

4   Schmidt JA, von Recum AF. On the use of primary reference grade polydimethylsiloxane. *J Appl Biomaterials*, 4 (1993), 73–76.

5   Kupp T, Hochman P, Hale J, Black J. Effect of motion on polymer implant capsule formation in muscle. In Winter GD, Gibbons DF, Plenk H (Eds.), *Biomaterials*. New York: John Wiley and Sons, 1982.

6   Picha GJ, Drake R. The effect of pillar surface microstructure and implant micro-environment on the soft tissue response. Abstract, *16th Annual Meeting Transactions*, Society for Biomaterials, Charleston, SC, USA, May 20–23, 1990.

7   Vaughan FL, Bernstein IS, Freed P, Kantrowitz A. The use of biological process in the development of a long-term percutaneous energy transmission system. In Schycher M (Ed.), *Biocompatible Polymers, Metals, and Composites*, Chapter 27. Lancaster: Technomic Publishing Comp. Inc., 1983.

8   Campbell CE, von Recum AF. Microtopography and soft tissue response. *J Invest Surg*, 2 (1989), 51–74.

9   Salthouse TN, Matlaga BF. Some cellular effects related to implant shape and surface. In Rubin LR (Ed.), *Biomaterials in Reconstructive Surgery*. St. Louis: Mosby, 1983, 40–45.

10   von Recum AF. New aspects of biocompatibility: Motion at the interface. In Heimke G, Soltesz U, Lee AJC (Eds.), *Clinical Implant Materials*. Amsterdam: Elsevier, 1990.

11   von Recum AF. Effects of implant surface microtexture on histological tissue response. In Kogel HC (Ed.), *The Prosthetic Substitution of Blood Vessels: Actual State and Future Development*. Munich, Germany: Quintessenz, 1991, 297–302.

12   Campbell CE, von Recum AF. Microtopography and soft tissue response. *J Invest Surg*, 2 (1989), 51–74.

13   Jauregui HO. Cell adhesion to biomaterials. *ASAIO*, 33 (1987), 66–74.

14   Curtis ASG, Clark P. The effects of topographic and mechanical properties of materials on cell behavior. *Critical Reviews in Biocompatibility*, 5 (1990), 343–362.

15   Meyle J, Wolburg H, von Recum AF. Surface micromorphology and cellular interactions. *J Biomat Appl*, 7 (1993), 362–374.

16   Schmidt JA, von Recum AF. Texturing of polymer surfaces at the cellular level. *Biomaterials*, 12 (1991), 385–389.

17   Schmidt JA, von Recum AF. The macrophage response to microtextured silicone. *Biomaterials*, 13 (1992) 1095–1069.

18   Green AM, Jansen JA, von Recum AF. The fibroblast response to microtextured silicone surfaces: Texture orientation into or out of the surface. *J Biomed Mat Res*, 28 (1994), 647–653.

19   Wu EY. Surface texture versus material type (titanium, hydroxyapatite and silicone): A biocompatibility study in rabbits. Master of Science thesis, Clemson University, Clemson, SC, 1991.

20   von Recum AF, Van Kooten T. The influence of micro-topography on cellular response and the implications for silicone implants. *J Biomaterials Science, Polymer Edition*, 7 (1995), 181–198.

21   Schmidt JA, von Recum AF. Surface characterization of microtextured silicone. *Biomaterials*, 13 (1992), 675–681.

22   Pilliar RM. Porous-surfaced metallic implants for orthopaedic applications. *J Biomedical Materials Research*, 21 (1987), 1–33.

23   Rowland SA, Shalaby WS, Latour Jr. RA, von Recum AF. Effectiveness of the Clemson bioengineering cleaning (CBC) protocol for implants: Quantitative analysis of contaminant removal. *J Appl Biomat*, 6 (1995), 1–7.

24   O'Conner DJ, Sexton BA, Smart RStC. *Surface Analysis in Materials Science*. Berlin, Germany: Springer-Verlag, 1992.

25   Standard test method for determining the orientation of a metal crystal. In *1995 Annual Book of Standards.*, v03.01. Philadelphia, PA: American Society for Testing and Materials, 1995, 228–252.

26   Standard test methods for determining average grain size. In *1995 Annual Book of Standards.*, v03.01. Philadelphia, PA: American Society for Testing and Materials, 1995, 228–252.

27   Standard test method for characterizing duplex grain sizes. In *1995 Annual Book of Standards.*, v03.01. Philadelphia, PA: American Society for Testing and Materials, 1995, 777–790.

28   Pienkowski D, Jacob R, Hoglin D, Saum K, Kaufer H, Nicholls PJ. Low-voltage scanning electron microscopic imaging of ultrahigh-molecular-weight polyethylene. *J Biomed Mat Res,*, 29 (1995), 1167–1174.

29   Moore DF. *Principles and Applications of Tribology*. New York: Pergamon Press, 1975, 33–60.

30   Sherrington I, Smith EH. Modern measurement techniques in surface metrology: Part I. Stylus instruments, electron microscopy and non-optical comparators. *Wear*, 125 (1988), 271–288.

31 Sherrington I, Smith EH. Modern measurement techniques in surface metrology: Part II. Optical instruments. *Wear*, 125 (1988), 289–310.

32 Bhusan B, Wyant JC, Meiling J. A new three-dimensional non-contact digital optical profilometer. *Wear*, 122 (1988), 301–312.

33 Benabdallah SMH, Chalifoux JP. Ploughing of soft asperities by a hemisperical indenter. *Tribology International*, 22 (1989) 383–388.

34 Schmidt JA, Black J. Determination of three-dimensional morphometry of adherent cells by surface profilometry. *Biomaterials.*, 13 (1992), 483–487.

35 Hamrock BJ. *Fundamentals of Fluid Film Lubrication*. New York: McGraw Hill, Inc., 1994.

36 Ungersböck A, Rahn B. Methods to characterize the surface roughness of metallic implants. *J Mater Sci Mater in Med*, 5 (1994), 434–440.

37 Cannon CE. Microsurface texturing: An industrial approach for soft tissue implants. Master of Science thesis, Clemson University, Clemson, SC, 1996.

38 Shannon CE. Types I and III collagen in the tissue capsules of titanium and stainless steel implants. Master of Science thesis, Clemson University, 1995.

ADDITIONAL READING

1 von Recum AF, Van Kooten T. The influence of micro-topography on cellular response and the implications for silicone implants. *J Biomater Sci, Polymer Edition*, 7 (1995), 181–198.

2 O'Conner DJ, Sexton BA, Smart RStC. *Surface Analysis in Materials Science*. Heidelberg, Germany: Springer-Verlag, 1992.

Chapter 14

Particulate Material

Laurie C. Carter

EFFECTS OF PARTICULATE MATTER

Contemporary biomaterials, whether polymeric, ceramic or metallic, are well accepted by the biologic milieu in their bulk forms, yet their particulate breakdown products often generate aggressive inflammatory, granulomatous and/or osteolytic responses [1]. This concept is illustrated by lessons learned from experience with total joint replacements. In the nearly four decades since Sir John Charnley revolutionized treatment of the osteoarthritic hip with cemented total hip arthroplasty, prosthesis loosening has been the most frequent long-term complication necessitating revision. Even in the absence of frank loosening, focal aseptic osteolysis has been described around cemented femoral stems [2]. In 1977, Willert and Semlitsch first implicated the macrophagic response to particulate wear debris as the etiologic cause of the observed osteolysis, which was eventually described as "Willert's phenomenon" [3]. The standard progression begins with the generation of wear debris which stimulates development of a synovial-like granulomatous membrane containing histiocytes, fibroblasts, foreign body giant cells and particulate debris [4]. Macrophage recruitment and proliferation is followed by phagocytosis of debris, activating macrophages to release such cellular mediators of osteolysis as interleukins IL-1 and IL-6 and the prostaglandin PGE_2 which signal cells in the local environment to resorb bone [5]. Recently, Horowitz and Purdon offered a revision of this paradigm by demonstrating in vitro that macrophage phagocytosis of polymethylmethacrylate (PMMA) particles activates elaboration of tumor necrosis factor (TNF) but not IL-1 or PGE_2, but that when the macrophage died and released its contents, osteoblasts then secreted the PGE_2 which led to bone resorption [6].

Peri-prosthetic osteolysis was first associated with particulate PMMA in cemented devices, a phenomenon which came to be known simply as "cement disease" [7]. However, development of cementless techniques for implant fixation revealed that similar periprosthetic osteolysis and loosening occur in the absence of PMMA, suggesting a role for other wear debris particles found in tissues at revision [8]. PMMA was formerly blamed for all the ills of cemented joint arthroplasties to the extent that the terms aseptic loosening and "cement disease" became synonymous [9]. Histopathologic analysis of tissues adjacent to successful cemented and failed cementless joint replacements have revealed that PMMA, as a component per se, cannot be held accountable for implant loosening. Retrieved tissues from stable cemented prostheses display a paucity of cement particles, few macrophages, minimal fibrous tissue and few foci of bone resorption [4, 10]. Boss and associates described healthy tissue reactions to stable cemented components in contrast to granulomatous interfacial membranes studded with prosthetic detritus apposed to loose cementless components [1]. Since the pathosis is independent of PMMA cementation but dependent on the interfacial accumulation of diverse wear particles, the term "small particle disease" is a more accurate descriptor.

Hypersensitivity reactions to PMMA have been well documented [11], but attention has only recently been turned to non-allergic ramifications of cement-induced activation of the immune system. T lymphocyte products may lead to bone resorption by monocyte/macrophage activation and by the release of TNF-α or β, IL-1 and TGF-β [12].

For many years, medical grade silicone rubber was considered to be an inert, well-tolerated biomaterial, but during the 1980s and early 1990s many reports of pathosis subsequent to local or distant effects of silicone degradation particles were published [13, 14]. Leong, Disney and Gove blamed the severe inflammation and fibrosis of the liver in patients undergoing hemodialysis on spallation of silicone particles from blood pump tubing [15]. Pierce and Boretos report that custom fit of polymeric implants involving cutting or modification at the surgical site can elaborate a host of particles which are held by electrostatic forces to the device, later to be liberated within the vascular tree [16]. Carter (Hartman) and colleagues examined tissues surrounding failed Silastic® (Dow Corning Corp., Midlan, MI) TMJ interpositional implants and described inflammatory polykaryon formation containing numerous particles of silicone debris of two basic morphologic forms [17]. Solitary, irregularly shaped homogeneous fragments averaging 175–250 μm were viewed, although the bulk of the specimen was replete with small, coarse, refractile granules averaging 50 μm. These specimens were further characterized by synovitis, dystrophic calcification, fibrocartilaginous metaplasia, hyalinization and scarring. Energy dispersive X-ray microanalysis (EDX) revealed prominent peaks for silicone in both the pseudocapsular and regional lymph nodal tissues. This represented the first genuine documentation of silicone migration from Silastic implants; prior reports had inferred the presence of silicone on morphologic criteria alone.

Despite the fact that Charnley abandoned the use of PTFE acetabular cups in 1962 because particulate wear produced a severe foreign body reaction, resulting in the production of granulomatous tissue and osseous erosion, a variety of PTFE-based composites containing either carbon, aluminum or hydroxyapatite (termed Proplast I, Proplast II and Proplast-HA, respectively) were used for facial augmentation purposes as well as TMJ interpositional implants [18, 19]. Examination of Proplast specimens removed because of return of severe pain or functional impairment revealed that the implant was surrounded by a thick fibrocollagenous capsule characterized by intensive and extensive granulomatous inflammation (Figure 14-1). The exciting agent for this inflammatory response was the diffuse bimodal presence of highly refractile, yellow-brown filaments and coarse granules or large, irregularly shaped, clear, smooth, refractile chunks of implant material (Figure 14-2). Severe host reactions to particulate Proplast debris led to erosion of facial bones or destruction of the condyle/fossa/base of the skull complex, with perforation into the middle cranial fossa with dural violation accompanied by CSF leakage [20, 21].

In 1955, Oppenheimer and associates had difficulty in comprehending the carcinogenic activity of plastics inasmuch as they are insoluble in aqueous systems and chemically rather inert, causing speculation that some physico-chemical interaction between polymeric degradation products and the tissues resulted in neoplasia [22]. Specifically, it was hypothesized that the degradation products were carcinogenic via the effects of free radical depolymerization of nucleic acids. A great deal more work needs to be done in assessing the relationship between wear debris and the long-term induction of neoplasia truly caused by the presence of the particulate detritus and its effects. Perhaps a mechanistic factor can be identified relating particulate detritus to genetic changes in cells.

Titanium is widely regarded as the quintessentially biocompatible metal for use in biomedical devices, a reputation based on the metal's excellent corrosion resistance and "biological indifference." Misadventures with titanium have arisen from the poor tribological properties of the metal and its alloys. Lalor and associates demonstrated by immunocytochemistry that deposition of titanium particles in tissues obtained at revision surgery were

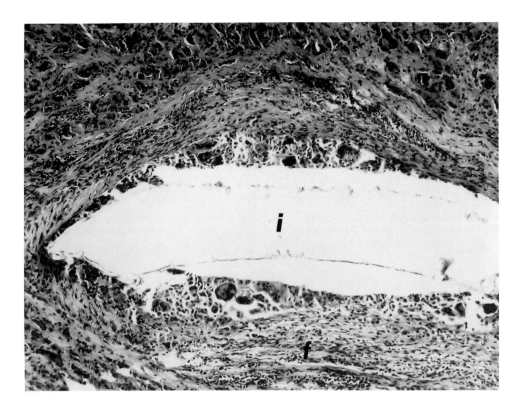

Figure 14-1 Large chunk of implant material (i) rimmed by non-cohesive giant cells and macrophages, with a peripheral zone of fibroendothelial proliferation (f). Hematoxylin and eosin, original magnification ×100.

present in macrophages and associated with T lymphocytes in the absence of B lymphocytes and plasma cells, suggesting a Type IV contact sensitivity and potential for titanium immunogenicity [23]. Haynes and co-workers (1993) reported on the release of inflammatory mediators by macrophages stimulated by particulate titanium [24].

Moreover, release of particulate titanium wear debris has been reported to eventuate in hepatic and splenic dissemination of wear particles and structural nodal changes including necrosis and fibrosis in association with particulate metallic debris, the concentration of which was greater if the prosthesis was loose. Macrophages in the peri-implant interfacial membrane become damaged with excessive accumulation of cytolysosomes, blurring of the cell membrane and nuclear pyknosis, a response which varies directly with particulate load and is most severe in association with wear particles from Co-Cr alloy [25]. Particulate cobalt has been shown to reduce cell viability in very small doses [26]. The self-perpetuating nature of the pathologic response to metallic debris is exemplified by the separation of frankly necrotic nodal tissue from apparently healthy tissues by a "tideline" of macrophages containing abundant metallic debris [27]. This intimates a cyclic cascade of cytokine activity leading to tissue necrosis with recruitment of living macrophages to zones of effete macrophages and rephagocytosis of wear debris.

Although titanium is generally regarded as non-toxic, the long-term clinical implications of elevated serum titanium levels are unknown at present. Examples of titanium-derived pathosis and vanadium toxicity have been reported [28]. Implants of biomaterials into young patients and those with pathoses causing reduced tolerance of environmental disturbances

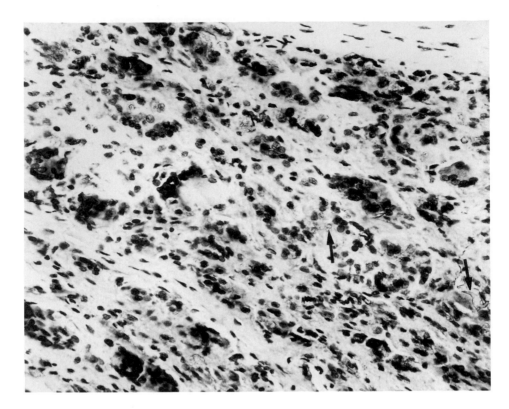

Figure 14-2 Proplast TMJ interpositional implant retrieval specimen shows a multiplicity of small, irregular, filamentous and coarse granular foreign material within a matrix of granulomatous inflammation. Hematoxylin and eosin, original magnification ×250.

(i.e., renal insufficiency) arc of some concern, especially when the site of implantation precludes employment of such biologic safety nets as the selective permeability of the gut and implant degradation products are permitted intimate contact with body fluids [29].

Although reports of local malignancy adjacent to implants are scant, two independent epidemiologic studies have reported a threefold increased risk of leukemia and lymphoma ten years after joint replacement [30,31]. It is of interest that the levels of particulate cobalt in the deep lymph nodes in the study reported by Case and colleagues [27] were similar to those reported in foundry workers who developed lung cancers after chromium exposure [32].

James and co-workers (1995) used confocal differential interference contrast (DIC) microscopy to examine the reaction of a patient's blood monocyte/macrophage population to particulate titanium alloy debris from that individual's failed total hip replacement [33]. After fifteen minutes, filamentous membranous extensions came in contact with particles and membrane perturbations were viewed. At one hour, partial particulate ingestion was observed; by six hours most cells were replete with particles. Over the 24–48 hour period, cytoplasmic swelling increased.

Relationship of Particle Morphology to Response to Particulates

Boss and co-workers (1995) stated that standard definitions of biocompatibility do injustice to the factual in vivo situation inasmuch as they ascribe behavioral traits based on chemical composition and presume solid state bulk form [1]. However, failures involving implants composed of supposed biocompatible materials have taught that the size, shape, surface area, density and surface topography of both the native implant and its breakdown products, in addition to their chemistry, account for the unwanted exuberant tissue reactions which, if severe, can result in catastrophic implant failure. The material composition of the particulate debris [25, 36], its rate of production [35], size [36], shape [37] and surface characteristics [38] all affect the biological response. Examples of aggressive responses to particulate debris of a variety of biomaterials which demonstrate biotolerant behavior in their bulk form will serve to illustrate this point.

Interfacial membranes and areas of osteolysis in cemented and uncemented arthroplasties have been found to contain wear particles from PMMA (in cemented prostheses), polyethylene and metal. Glant and associates (1993) found that particulates (titanium, polystyrene and PMMA) in the nonphagocytosable size range ($>5\,\mu$m) have very little or no effect on elaboration of IL-1 or PGE_2 by peritoneal macrophages [39]. Furthermore, conditioned media from cultures with nonphagocytosable particles did not stimulate ^{45}Ca release from calvarial bones. On the other hand, phagocytosis of submicron particles of Ti, PS or PMMA stimulated peritoneal macrophages to secrete IL-1 and PGE_2 in a dose- and time-dependent method, while only Ti particles exhibited enhanced bone resorptive activity, as measured by ^{45}Ca release. The quantity of the deposited PMMA particulates is thought to play a role in the extent and intensity of the inflammatory reaction [1].

In total joint replacement, only when polyethylene wear debris is in the form of small, irregularly shaped particles with well-defined edges does an aggressive granulomatous response arise as a prequel to aseptic loosening of the joint [1]. The aggressive inflammatory response to small and angular polymeric debris is adverse because of macrophage secretion of inflammatory mediators which potentiate significant tissue destruction. This reaction is inappropriate and renders polyethylene bioincompatible under the circumstances. The chemical composition of polyethylene, a biotolerant material, does not endow it with an all-inclusive biocompatible nature. The physical properties of size, shape and surface topography predict the response to the material. Using tissue digestion and isolation techniques followed by scanning electron microscopy (SEM) examination of polyethylene (PE) wear debris, Campbell and associates (1995) determined that the majority of particles were submicron in size and that individual particles were either rounded or elongated [40].

In an analysis of tissues from failed titanium alloy total hip replacements, Shanbhag and associates (1994) found that the majority of particulates were polyethylene, with a mean size of $0.53 \pm 0.3\,\mu$m, similar in size to particles seen in virgin base resin used to make acetabular components [41]. The fact that some retrieved particles were smaller in size than those in the base resin they ascribed to attrition and oxidative degradation after the particles' release into the joint space.

Experiments exploring cellular response to ultra-high molecular weight polyethylene (UHMWPE) have been hindered by the difficulty in obtaining adequate quantities of debris in sizes simulating that found in wear debris adjacent to arthroplasties [42]. Investigators have generally used primary UHMWPE grain as fabricated (20–$200\,\mu$m) or dental bur reduction of solid UHMWPE which yields a smallest size fraction of approximately $16\,\mu$m. Leigh and colleagues (1992) point out that as the upper size limit for macrophage phagocytosis is about 3–$7\,\mu$m and most of the PE wear debris in the interfacial membrane around failed total hip replacement is submicron in size, the challenge particles typically used are too large in mean diameter by a factor of 10–100 [42]. Cryogenic attrition using liquid nitrogen in a freezer mill followed by sieving provides a very satisfactory method for obtaining particles of desired size range for most polymeric, ceramic and osseous materials

[42, 43]. SEM micrographs reveal that as-received grain consists of both a dense highly crystalline phase and an amorphous phase. Inasmuch as both types of particle may be released during in vivo wear, biological activity studies of UHMWPE may need to address both particle size and crystallinity of PE challenge materials.

Differences in the articulating surface conformity between total hip replacement (THR) and total knee replacement (TKR) have profound effects on the wear mechanisms involved and hence the physical nature of the PE wear particles generated [44]. Increased contact stresses which exceed the yield strength of PE occur in TKR which are characterized by minimal conformity of the bearing surfaces. This results in subsurface delamination, pitting and fatigue cracking with release of PE particles averaging 2–20 μm in size. Despite voluminous PE wear, aggressive inflammatory osteolysis is not problematic in TKR, where the large PE particles are associated with a foreign body polykaryon response.

The conformity of the bearing surfaces in THR results in wear mechanisms involving adhesion and abrasion with generation of an extensive population of submicron particles. Histologic examination of peri-implant interfacial membranes reveals sheets of plump histiocytic macrophages and a paucity of giant cells, associated with painful osteolysis and implant loosening. Macrophage activation is related not only to particulate size but also particle number. Kabo and associates (1993) determined that volumetric wear of a conventional PE acetabular component averages over 1 cm^3 over ten years, which assuming an average particle size of <1 μm^3 equates to trillions of particles [45]. Since macrophage activation is related to the number of particles ingested, "small particles disease" appears to be especially problematic in THR due to the tremendous numbers of wear particles leading to significant osteolysis.

The effect of sterilization methods, oxidative degradation and mechanical stress on bulk UHMWPE and its wear particles represent another area needing further study. Rimnac and associates (1994) reported that oxidative degradation initiated by gamma radiation sterilization continues to occur in storage in distilled water prior to implantation, as discerned by an increase in carbonyl peaks [46]. Further oxidative degradation then occurs in vivo upon exposure to oxidizing agents in synovial fluid such as hydrogen peroxide and superoxide and hydroxyl radicals [47]. Moreover, chain scission in PE due to mechanical loading results in the creation of additional free radicals [48]. Clearly, investigation of the effects of oxidative degradation and mechanical stress, taken alone and together, on polymers in vivo needs further investigation.

Using atomic force microscopy, James and co-workers (1995) found that particulate titanium alloy debris from a failed total hip replacement was mostly submicron in size and either globular or elongated in shape [33]. Elongated particles showed an extremely smooth surface with fine grain boundaries and sharp/jagged edges.

Both metal wear particles and metal reaction products (ions, metal-protein complexes) are present in interfacial membranes adjacent to loose joint replacement prostheses. While metal wear particles result in macrophage migration and proliferation and bone resorption, metal reaction products may seriously inhibit the formation of hydroxyapatite [49]. Conventional recovery techniques for retrieving metal from tissues involved dissolving blocks of tissue in acids. However, this technique dissolved wear particles into ions and rendered quantitation of the separate concentrations of ions and wear particles impossible. Blumenthal and co-workers (1994) described a procedure for freezing harvested tissues with subsequent tissue degradation in sodium hypochlorite and chloroform-methanol solution [49]. Separation of ions from wear particles via centrifugation enabled measurement of the concentration of each metal species by atomic absorption spectroscopy. This procedure should permit elucidation of the separate contributions of metal debris and metal reaction products to implant loosening.

In response to stimulation with small sized titanium particles ($<3\ \mu$m), Yao and colleagues (1995) demonstrated marked up-regulation of fibroblastic metalloproteinases at both the mRNA and protein levels and a discoordinately small elevation of tissue inhibitor of metalloproteinase (TIMP) [50]. Moreover, conditioned media from titanium particle-stimulated fibroblasts significantly inhibited expression of collagen genes in osteoblast-like cells. Shanbhag and associates (1994) showed that titanium particles stimulate fibroblast, release bone-resorbing metalloproteinases, proliferate more aggressively, and form an interfacial membrane which provides access for wear debris particles to enter the effective joint space where they may further suppress osteoblastic function and contribute to progressive osteolysis [5]. While the predominant mechanism for peri-prosthetic osteolysis has been considered to be macrophage recruitment and phagocytosis of debris followed by the release of osteolytic agents, these data indicate that fibroblasts may also play a key role in the pathogenesis of osteolysis, rather than merely passively filling in the voids left by resorption of bone [50].

Boss and colleagues (1995) write that the attribute of biocompatibility is subject to neither an all-or-none law nor subordinate to unique chemical constituencies [1]. They contend that biocompatibility depends on the circumstances under which a biomaterial confronts the tissues at the interface, thus rendering biocompatibility a relativistic rather than an absolute concept. Williams (1994) points out that interfacial reactions involving biocompatibility are often autocatalytic, a circumstance creating thresholds below which failure cannot be predicted but above which it is rapid and catastrophic [51]. Pierce and Boretos suggested that perhaps the "questions most germane to the sequelae of the unintentional clinical administration of particles are: What size constitutes a particle? What are the safe limits of size and quantity? What are the biological risks?" [16].

Relevance

• The increasing array of biomaterials available for long-term implantation in humans begs biocompatibility testing not just of the bulk material but of the material and its breakdown products following short-, intermediate-, and long-term implantation or simulation conditions.

• Not only the chemical composition of the bulk material but also the mechanisms of physical and chemical degradation in a given in vivo situation as well as the size, shape, surface topography, number, density and surface area of the wear particles need to be accounted for when designing experiments to test for situational biocompatibility both in vitro and in vivo.

• While IL-1 and PGE_2 have been implicated in periprosthetic osteolysis, other cytokines, including IL-6, IL-8, PDGF, TNF-α and TGF-β, may also play a role in particulate-mediated pathways of tissue repair, inflammation and tissue catabolism, possibly involving activation of the cyclooxygenase and leukotriene pathways. Investigation of the effects of various particles on these cytokines is essential to elucidate the complex stimulatory, secretory and signalling mechanisms involved in the local milieu leading to interfacial membrane formation and implant loosening.

• The association between disseminated implant-generated wear debris and the development of subsequent pathosis such as alteration in immune surveillance and neoplasia remains to be explored.

TESTING METHODS FOR PARTICULATES

Detection methods for the quantitation, measurement and morphological analysis of particulates largely depends on both the size and the chemical composition of the particles in question. For larger particles (the λ of visible light being 0.4–0.7 μm), conventional light microscopy allows a reasonable assessment of the gross morphologic size and shape of particulates. Many native and biomaterial particulates may appear refractile; however, transmitted light microscopy alone is incapable of revealing true birefringency. A quarter wave plate is used for bidirectional light polarization which will reveal the truly birefringent nature of certain particulate materials such as bone, collagen, amyloid, crystals of uric acid or calcium pyrophosphate, UHMWPE or PMMA. There are no specific stains which can identify the exact nature of particulate debris in tissues. Oil Red O is a stain with high sensitivity but not 100% specificity for polyethylene [52].

Energy Dispersive X-Ray Microanalysis (EDX)

Currently available microanalytic instrumentation provides a simple, thrifty and speedy method for the precise elemental composition of many particles in peri-implant tissues. In the case of finely dispersed particulate debris in the oral tissues, Carter (Hartman) and associates (1986) demonstrated that EDX identified elemental compositions related to amalgam tattoo or gold impregnation, allowing separation of these materials from melanin pigmentation, hemosiderin deposition or "lead lines" from heavy metal ingestion [53]. Inasmuch as the appropriate management of patient cases depends on accurate diagnosis, and the morphologic features between the items on the differential diagnosis were confounding, the definitive diagnosis rested on the ability to determine the specific elemental composition of the foreign material. Likewise, Carter (Hartman) and colleagues (1988) made the diagnosis of silicone in tissues surrounding Silastic™ TMJ implants and regional lymph nodes by EDX [17]. Formerly, silicone in tissues was "identified" on a presumptive, inferential basis. Although EDX alone cannot make the separate identification of debris from polymers with similar chemical composition (i.e., polymers containing C, H and O, albeit in different concentrations and arrangements), it has the capability of precisely identifying metal debris and those polymer particles with a distinctive elemental composition (such as silicone rubber).

In EDX, unstained 10 μm paraffin sections are mounted directly on carbon stubs, exposed to radiofrequency glow discharge treatment for ten minutes to vaporize all superficial organic contaminants and sputter-coated with gold to reduce charging. Specimens are then placed in a SEM equipped with an energy dispersive X-ray microanalysis system. An exciting voltage of 30 kV at 100–120 μA is recommended, with magnifications dependent on the size of the particulate in question and counting times of approximately 100–300 sec/specimen. Collected spectra are background subtracted after initial peak identification, and full scale vertical counts depend on the amount of a given element present in the tissues. Inductively-coupled argon plasma (ICAP) analysis offers a somewhat more sophisticated form of elemental microanalysis in biologic samples, including tissues as well as fluids.

Ultrastructural Examination

For submicron particles, ultrastructural analysis is required. Techniques such as scanning electron microscopy (SEM), transmission electron microscopy (TEM), atomic force microscopy (AFM) and confocal differential interference microscopy (DIC) allow for exquisitely sensitive analysis of the particle number, size, shape, surface area, surface topology and other morphologic features of the particles themselves and of the cellular components which react to them. Ultrastructural examination of wear particles by conventional

TEM methods is limited because the size of the wear particles often exceeds the section thickness and debris is torn out of the specimen during ultramicrotomy.

Particle Isolation Methods

An alternative method facilitating morphologic and quantitative evaluation of particles involves isolation of the particles from the tissues and subsequent SEM evaluation. Several methods of tissue digestion using NaOCl or papain digests have been proposed for the recovery of metallic or bone cement particles [54, 55]. The high density of these particles facilitates their isolation from tissues because centrifugation readily results in pelleting. On the other hand, particles such as polyethylene, with a density lighter than water (0.93–0.94 g/cm^3), require an alternative isolation technique based on sodium hydroxide tissue digestion and ultracentrifugation over a sucrose gradient [40]. Fourier transform infrared spectroscopy (FTIR) and differential scanning calorimetry (DSC) can then verify the nature of the recovered polymer, and samples of the particles can then be spread onto a stub and examined by SEM.

In Vivo Examination of the Cellular Response to Particulate Biomaterials

The chick egg chorioallantoic membrane (CAM) model represents a reliable and inexpensive system for the induction of a cellular response to implanted particulate native and biomaterials [43]. This model differs from cell culture methods in that it is an in vivo, dynamic system. Although the embryonic chick immune system is somewhat immature, both eosinophils and osteoclast precursors have been demonstrated in the circulation of embryonic chickens [56]. In this method, particles are prepared by cryogenic milling and sieving to the desired particle size range. Two mg samples are sterilized by gamma radiation and stored in the dark. Embryonated white Leghorn chicken eggs are windowed according to the method of Krukowski and Kahn [57]. After an additional 4 days, the CAMs are implanted with one of the particulate samples (Figure 14-3). After 9 days of implantation, induced cell plaques are harvested and analyzed by a battery of histochemical, immuno-

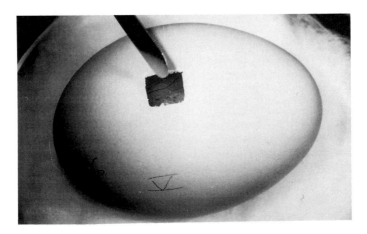

Figure 14-3 Two mg sterile particulate 75–150 mm PMMA being implanted onto the vascular CAM.

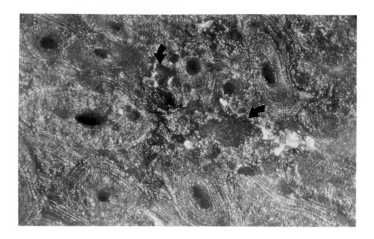

Figure 14-4   Reflected light microscopy of bone wafer cultured with particulate Proplast-HA on chick CAM reveals the presence of numerous lacunar excavations (arrows).

cytochemical, ultrastructural and tissue culture assays [43]. In a variation on this model, bovine cortical bone wafer may be placed on the developing CAM cell plaque to assay for the presence of resorption pits (Figure 14-4).

REFERENCES

1   Boss JH, Shajrawi I, Aunullah J, Mendes DG. The relativity of biocompatibility: A critique of the concept of biocompatibility. *Isr J Med Sci*, 31 (1995), 203–209.

2   Harris WH, Schiller AL, Scholler JM, Freiberg RA, Scott R. Extensive localised bone resorption in the femur following total hip replacement. *J Bone Joint Surg*, 58A (1976), 612–618.

3   Willert HG, Semlitsch M. Reactions of the articular capsule to wear products of artificial joint prostheses. *J Biomed Mater Res*, 11 (1977), 157–164.

4   Goldring SR, Schiller AL, Roelke M, Rourke CM, O'Neill DA. The synovial-like membrane at the bone-cement interface in loose total hip replacements and its proposed role in bone lysis. *J Bone Joint Surg*, 64A (1983), 575–580.

5   Shanbhag AS, Jacobs JJ, Black J, Galante JO, Glant TT. Macrophage/particle interactions: Effect of size, composition and surface area. *J Biomed Mater Res*, 28 (1994), 81–90.

6   Horowitz SM, Purdon MA. Mediator interactions in macrophage/particulate bone resorption. *J Biomed Mater Res*, 29 (1995), 477–484.

7   Jones LC, Hungerford DS. Cement disease. *Clin Orthop*, 225 (1987), 192–206.

8   Maloney WJ, Jasty M, Harris WH, Galante JO, Callaghan JJ. Endosteal erosion in association with stable uncemented femoral components. *J Bone Joint Surg*, 72A (1990), 1025–1034.

9   St. John K (Ed.). *Particulate Debris from Medical Implants: Mechanisms of Formation and Biological Consequences*. Philadelphia, PA: American Society for Testing and Materials, 1992, 90–108.

10 Horowitz SM, Doty SB, Lane JM, Burstein AH. Studies of the mechanism by which the mechanical failure of polymethylmethacrylate leads to bone resorption. *J Bone Joint Surg*, 75A (1993), 802–813.

11 Fries IB, Fisher AA, Salvati EA. Contact dermatitis in surgeons from methylmethacrylate bone cement. *J Bone Joint Surg*, 57A (1975), 547–549.

12 Herman JH, Solder WG, Anderson D, Appel AM and Hopson CN. Polymethylmethacrylate-induced release of bone-resorbing factors. *J Bone Joint Surg*, 71A (1989), 1530–1541.

13 Garrido L, Pfleiderer B, Papisov J, Ackerman L. In vivo degradation of silicones. *Magn Reson Med*, 29 (1993), 839–843.

14 Derlin C. Silicone breast implants and breast feeding. *Pediatrics*, 94 (1994), 547.

15 Leong AS, Disney AP, Gove DW. Spallation and migration of silicone from blood pump tubing in patients on hemodialysis. *N Engl J Med*, 206 (1982), 135–140.

16   Pierce WS, Boretos JW. The dilemma of patient exposure to ubiquitous foreign particles. *J Biomed Mater Res*, 17 (1983), 389–391.

17   Carter (Hartman) L, Bessette R, Baier R, Meyer A, Wirth J. Silicone rubber temporomandibular joint (TMJ) meniscal replacements: Postimplant histopathologic and material evaluation. *J Biomed Mater Res*, 22 (1988), 475–484.

18   Charnley J. An artificial bearing in the hip joint: Implications of lubricating. *Fed Proc* 25 (1962), 1079–1080.

19   Homsy C. Biocompatibility of perfluorinated polymers and composites of these polymers. In Williams DF (Ed.), *Biocompatibility of Clinical Implant Materials*. Boca Raton, FL: CRC Press, Inc., 1982, 59–77.

20   Berarducci J, Thompson D, Scheffer R. Perforation into middle cranial fossa as a sequel to use of a Proplast-Teflon implant for temporomandibular reconstruction. *J Oral Maxillofac Surg*, 48 (1990), 496–498.

21   Chuong R, Piper M. Cerebrospinal fluid leak associated with Proplast implant removal from the temporomandibular joint. *Oral Surg, Oral Med, Oral Pathol*, 74 (1992), 422–425.

22   Oppenheimer BS, Oppenheimer ET, Danishefsky I, Stout AP, Eirich F. Further studies of polymers as carcinogenic agents in animals. *Cancer Res*, 15 (1955), 333–340.

23   Lalor PA, Revell PA, Gray AB, Wright S, Railton GT, Freeman MA. Sensitivity to titanium: A cause of implant failure? *J Bone Joint Surg*, 73B (1991), 25–28.

24   Haynes DR, Rogers SD, Hay S. The differences in toxicity and release of bone-resorbing mediators induced by titanium and cobalt-chromium alloy wear particles. *J Bone Joint Surg*, 75A (1993), 825–834.

25   Howie DW. Tissue response in relation to type of wear particles around failed hip arthroplasties. *J Arthroplasty*, 5 (1990), 337–348.

26   Maloney W, Lane Smith R, Castro F, Schurman D. Fibroblast response to metallic debris in vitro. *J Bone Joint Surg*, 75A (1993), 835–844.

27   Case P, Langkamer VG, James C, Palmer MR, Kemp AJ, Heap PF, Solomon L. Widespread dissemination of metal debris from implants. *J Bone Joint Surg*, 76B (1994), 701–712.

28   Jacobs JJ, Skipor AK, Black J, Urban RM, Galante JO. Release and excretion of metal in patients who have a total hip replacement component made of titanium-base alloy. *J Bone Joint Surg*, 73A (1991), 1475–1486.

29   Callen BW, Lowenberg BF, Lugowski S, Sodhi RN, Davies JE. Nitric acid passivation of Ti6Al4V reduces thickness of surface oxide layer and increases trace element release. *J Biomed Mater Res*, 29 (1995), 279–290.

30   Gillespie WJ, Frampton CM, Henderson RJ, Ryan PM. The incidence of cancer following total hip replacement. *J Bone Joint Surg*, 70B (1988), 539–542.

31   Visuri T, Koskenvuo M. Cancer risk after Mckee-Farrar total hip replacement. *Orthopedics*, 14 (1991), 137–142.

32   Hyodo K, Suzuki S, Furuya N, Meshizuka K. An analysis of chromium, copper and zinc in organs of a chromate worker. *Int Arch Occup Environ Health*, 46 (1980), 141–150.

33   James RE, Maloney WJ, Braunstein D, Smith RL. Surface topology of retrieved TiAlV particulate debris and its effect on the human macrophage cellular membrane. *Trans Soc Biomat*, 18 (1995), 116.

34   Escalas F, Galante J, Rostoker W. Biocompatibility of materials for total joint replacement. *J Biomed Mater Res*, 10 (1976), 175–195.

35   Johanson NA, Bullough PG, Wilson PD Jr, Salvati EA, Ranawat CS. The microscopic anatomy of the bone-cement interface in failed total hip arthroplasties. *Clin Orthop*, 218 (1987), 123–135.

36   Cohen J. Assay of foreign-body reaction. *J Bone Joint Surg*, 41A (1959), 152–166.

37   Matlaga BF, Yasenchak LP, Salthouse TN. Tissue response to implanted polymers: The significance of sample shape. *J Biomed Mater Res*, 10 (1976), 391–397.

38   Salthouse TN. Some aspects of macrophage behavior at the implant interface. *J Biomed Mater Res*, 18 (1984), 395–401.

39   Glant TT, Jacobs JJ, Molnar G, Shanbhag AS, Valyon M, Galante JO. Bone resorption activity of particle-stimulated macrophages. *J Bone Miner Res*, 8 (1993), 1071–1079.

40   Campbell P, Ma S, Yeom B, McKellop H, Schmalzried TP, Amstutz HC. Isolation of predominantly submicron-sized UHMWPE particles from periprosthetic tissues. *J Biomed Mater Res*, 29 (1995), 127–131.

41   Shanbhag AS, Jacobs JJ, Glant TT, Gilbert JL, Black J, Galante JO. Composition and morphology of wear debris in failed uncemented total hip replacement. *J Bone Joint Surg*, 76B (1994), 60–67.

42   Leigh HD, Taylor P, Swaney A and Black J. Research and development: Production of fine particulate ultra high molecular weight poly(ethylene) for biological response studies. *J Appl Biomat*, 3 (1992), 77–80.

43   Carter L. Analysis of the cellular healing response of the chick chorioallantoic membrane to implanted poly (glycolic acid). Doctoral dissertation, State University of New York at Buffalo, Buffalo, NY, 1993.

44   Schmalzried T, Jasty M, Rosenberg A, Harris W. Polyethylene wear debris and tissue reactions in knee as compared to hip replacement prosthesis. *J Appl Biomat*, 5 (1994), 185–190.

45 Kabo JM, Gebhard JS, Loren G, Amstutz HC. In vivo wear of polyethylene acetabular components. *J Bone Joint Surg*, 75B (1993), 254–258.

46 Rimnac CM, Burstein AH, Carr JM, Klein RW, Wright TM, Betts F. Clinical and mechanical degradation of UHMWPE: Report of the development of an in vitro test. *J Appl Biomat*, 5 (1994), 17–21.

47 Hooper C. Free radicals: Research on biochemical bad boys comes of age. *J NIH Res*, 1 (1989), 101–106.

48 Franconi BM, DeVries KL, Smith RH. Free radicals and new end groups resulting from chain scission: II. Mechanical degradation of polyethylene. *Polymer*, 23 (1982), 1027–1033.

49 Blumenthal NC, Cosma V, Jaffe N, Stuchin S. A new technique for the quantitation of metal particles and metal reaction products in tissues near implants. *J Appl Biomat*, 5 (1994), 191–193.

50 Yao J, Glant TT, Lark M, Mikecz K, Jacobs J, Hutchinson N, Hoerrner L, Keutnner K, Galante J. The potential role of fibroblasts in periprosthetic osteolysis: Fibroblast response to titanium particle. *J Bone Miner Res*, 10 (1995), 1417–1427.

51 Williams DF. Titanium: Epitome of biocompatibility or cause for concern? *J Bone Joint Surg*, 76B (1994), 348–349.

52 Guttmann D, Schmalzried T, Jasty M and Harris W. Light microscopic identification of submicron polyethylene wear debris. *J Appl Biomat* 4 (1993), 303–307.

53 Carter (Hartman) L, Natiella J, Meenaghan M. The use of elemental microanalysis in verification of the composition of presumptive amalgam tattoo. *J Oral Maxillofac Surg*, 44 (1986), 628–633.

54 Emmanual J, Yapp R, Hedley A. Recovery of biomaterial wear debris from membranes of failed joints for characterization. *Trans Soc Biomat*, 13 (1990), 254.

55 Lee J-M, Salvati E, Betts F, DiCarlo EF, Doty S, Bullough PG. Size of metallic and polyethylene debris particles in failed cemented total hip replacements. *J Bone Joint Surg*, 74B (1992), 380–384.

56 Kahn A, Simmons D, Krukowski M. Osteoclast precursor cells are present in the blood of preossification chick embryos. *Dev Biol*, 84 (1981), 230–234.

57 Krukowski M, Kahn A. Inductive specificity of mineralized bone matrix in ectopic osteoclast differentiation. *Calcif Tissue Int*, 34 (1982), 474–479.

ADDITIONAL READING

1 Coleman DL. Particulate contamination and characterization. In *Guidelines for Physico-Chemical Characterization of Biomaterials*. NIH Publication 80-2186, Devices and Technology Branch, NHLBI 1980, 91–93.

2 Glant TT, Jacobs JJ. Response of three murine macrophage populations to particulate debris: Bone resorption in organ cultures. *J Orthop Res*, 12 (1994), 720–731.

3 Goldring MB, Goldring SR. Skeletal tissue response to cytokines. *Clin Orthop Rel Res*, 258 (1990), 245–278.

4 Kirchen ME, Campbell PA, Cindrick RS. Transmission electron microscopy of macrophages containing polyethylene wear debris. *Trans Soc Biomat*, 18 (1995), 170.

5 Murray DW, Rushton N. Macrophages stimulate bone resorption when they phagocytose particles. *J Bone Joint Surg*, 72B (1990), 988–992.

6 Peters MS, Schroeter AL, van Hale HM and Broadbent JC. Pacemaker contact sensitivity. *Contact Dermatitis*, 11 (1984), 214–218.

7 Shinto Y, Uchida A, Yoshikawa H. Inguinal lymphadenopathy due to metal release from a prosthesis: A case report. *J Bone Joint Surg*, 75B (1993), 266–269.

Chapter 15

Sterilization Effects

Virginia C. Chamberlain
Byron Lambert
Fuh-Wei Tang

The purpose of medical product sterilization is to render the product free of microbial contamination. In practice, this involves designing a reliable sterilization process.

Sterilization processes are validated by investigating their lethality to either the natural product bioburden or to a worst case challenge, e.g., standardized microorganisms exhibiting high resistance to the mode of sterilization. International standards regarding traditional device sterilization methods and associated topics have been developed recently and can be obtained through the Association for the Advancement of Medical Instrumentation in Arlington, Virginia [1].

There are a variety of sterilization methods using physical and/or chemical agents which can be considered for sterilization of a particular device. Agents to be reviewed in this chapter are ethylene oxide (EtO) gas, radiation (gamma or electron beam), steam, liquid chemical (e.g., aldehydes or oxidizing agents), plasma, and gases other than ethylene oxide (e.g., ozone, hydrogen peroxide and chlorine dioxide). These agents interact with microbial components, thereby killing the microorganisms.

Sterilization agents, of course, interact with the biomaterials as well as the microorganisms. Therefore, in addition to assuring adequate sterilization of a device, the sterilization process must be compatible with the device and container or packaging materials so that the functionality of the device and the microbial barrier properties of the primary package are not significantly compromised during processing or afterward. Chemical residues from the sterilization process must be considered in terms of their impact on the efficacy of implant applications and in terms of safety for the patient from a toxicological perspective. Many devices and their packaging consist of polymeric materials unstable at high temperatures and therefore unsuitable for heat sterilization. For these devices, ethylene oxide and radiation sterilization have been the most prevalent means of industrial device sterilization. Traditionally, health care facilities have used heat, ethylene oxide, and liquid chemicals for sterilization and reprocessing of reusable devices between patients. Recently, because of environmental concerns regarding ethylene oxide gas mixtures, newer sterilization methods have been developed and are increasingly used, particularly in healthcare facilities.

Some heat labile devices, such as enzyme-containing contact lens solutions, are not terminally sterilized but are aseptically filled. This process is outside the scope of the chapter but a few comments are appropriate. Containers, equipment, and some solution components are usually sterilized prior to aseptic fill; heat labile components are usually filter sterilized prior to the aseptic fill. The container, equipment, and filter materials must be compatible with the product and not impart undesirable residues to the product.

Damage may occur during sterilization if device materials are not adequately evaluated. Package seals and adhesives must be able to withstand the physical and chemical conditions of sterilization. Embrittlement of plastic packaging can result in cracking and crazing, compromising the microbial barrier. Packaging must be strong enough to withstand normal handling including shipping of the device.

DESIGNING A DEVICE INTENDED TO BE STERILIZED

Materials scientists should be involved from the beginning of device design. If the intended use of a device necessitates that it be sterilized prior to patient use, then this must be considered during the initial material design phase for the device. Stresses accumulated within materials in configuring the device can increase the potential for adverse effects of sterilizing conditions. Exposure of devices to the extremes of sterilization conditions must be assessed. For example, for radiation sterilization, the materials effects of the maximum dose, including that from initial sterilization and any resterilization allowed, must be considered. If the device is intended to be reused, then materials must be selected which can withstand repeated reprocessing. Nonsterilizable parts of a device, such as electrical components, must be adequately encapsulated by materials to protect them and the patient. Design validation testing is required to verify these aspects. These requirements can be found in IOS (International Organization for Standardization) quality and sterilization standards and in the proposed revision of the FDA regulation, Good Manufacturing Practice (GMP) for Devices.

Packaging materials including seals and adhesives must be selected which allow for penetration of the sterilizing agent, fit the configuration of the device without being punctured by the device, and can withstand sterilizing conditions such as temperature, relative humidity, pressure, and chemical concentration. An ISO standard for medical device packaging has been approved. When devices are used soon after sterilization, some sterilization processes conducted in health care facilities do not utilize packaging.

BIOMATERIAL STABILITY OVER TIME

Sterilization effects need to be considered both immediately after sterilization and over time after sterilization. The latter is of particular concern when the sterilization process initiates reactive species that propagate over time and result in the associated degradation of material properties over time. Device material selection and sterilization selection should, therefore, include consideration of the biomaterial's stability over the projected and/or labeled service lifetime. This includes consideration of wear testing (see Chapter 10) as well as aging over time. For example, a heart valve may be able to cycle two billion times in a "time zero" wear test, equivalent to a 20-year survivorship. However, due to aging over time, it may not be able to cycle another one billion times after 10 years of use or after 10 years of real time aging on a shelf.

Elevated temperature is often used to accelerate (i.e., simulate) the aging of polymeric materials based on an Arrhenius type of logic in which the rate of degradation mechanisms increases in conjunction with increased temperature. For example, a common and conservative assumption is that the rate of aging increases by a factor of 2 for every 10-degree increase in temperature. By using this model, one month of aging at 57°C can simulate 4 months of aging *in vivo* at 37°C.

ETHYLENE OXIDE

The sterilizing ability of ethylene oxide gas was investigated during World War II by the Army's biological warfare laboratory [2]. Ethylene oxide is a very reactive epoxide and

Table 15-1 EtO Sterilization

Material class	Effects of EtO sterilization on bulk properties of biomaterials
Polymers [5]	Compatible with most polymeric materials —Residues may be toxic; often requires degassing process. —Some materials (for example, certain hydrophilic coatings) are sensitive to the humidity of the ETO process. —Certain extremely temperature sensitive materials are not compatible, even with the moderate prolonged heat of the process.
Metals/Alloys	Compatible; corrosive effects need to be considered.
Ceramics	Compatible; porous materials may retain EtO residues.
Electronics	Compatible; sparking must be avoided; corrosive effects need to be considered.
Biologicals	—May be sensitive to the temperature of the process or to the effects of the EtO as an alkylating agent. —Residues may be toxic; requires degassing process.

alkylating agent which can react with carboxyl, amino, sulfhydryl, hydroxyl, or phenolic radicals in proteins and DNA [3]. This compromises the metabolism and reproduction of bacterial cells.

As mentioned above, ethylene oxide sterilization permits sterilization of most heat- and/or moisture-sensitive materials such as plastics. The efficacy of EtO sterilization depends on the process pressure, temperature, humidification, gas concentration, and exposure time [4]. The typical EtO sterilization process consists of a vacuum phase to remove air, a humidification phase with steam, gas exposure, and air removal. EtO sterilization efficiency requires at least 30% relative humidity, 400 mg/L EtO, and 125–130°F.

Pure EtO is flammable and explosive. For sterilization, it has traditionally been diluted with inert gases such as chlorofluorocarbon (CFC) or carbon dioxide to reduce flammability; pure EtO can be employed with the appropriate explosion-proof equipment. Anticipation of the banning of CFC manufacturing in January 1996 stimulated increased use of 100% EtO or radiation sterilization by industry, the development of HCFC substitutes for CFCs, and the emergence of new sterilization techniques for use in healthcare facilities not equipped for use of the explosive 100% EtO.

Due to the low temperatures used, EtO sterilization does not impact the bulk properties of most biomaterials. EtO is an alkylating agent and may impact the physical properties of some materials (see Table 15-1). Packaging materials must allow air removal and penetration of moisture and EtO gas without damage to the packaging or its seals during vacuum and pressure excursions. In addition, device residues including EtO, ethylene glycol and ethylene chlorohydrin must be within safe levels. These and other inert process residues resulting in films or spots should be considered (see Table 15-2). Some materials (e.g., polyurethanes) have a greater affinity to absorb and retain EtO residues than other materials. This necessitates storing the device post-sterilization, often at elevated temperatures, in order to degas the toxic residues.

RADIATION

Radiation sterilization involves either exposure to gamma rays from Cobalt-60 or accelerated high energy electrons. X-ray sterilization is under development, but is not extensively

Table 15-2   Sterilization Effects on Surface Properties [6]

Sterilization method	Effects on surface properties
Plasma —Increases reactivity of surface (surface free energy) —Leaves no residue —Cleans organic and inorganic films from surfaces —Increases bioadhesion	—Positive impact on implant applications —Negative impact on applications such as heart valves
EtO, Steam, Other Gases —Possible toxic residues (EtO & liquid chemical); —Corrosion products (steam) —Decreases reactivity of surface (surface free energy) —Inorganic and organic films and spots —Decreases bioadhesion	—Negative impact on implant application —Positive impact on applications such as heart valves
Radiation —Leaves no residue —No cleaning effect —Negligible effect on surface reactivity or bioadhesion	—Negligible effect

used. Because of the extensive shielding requirements, radiation sterilization is mainly used by industry, but some health care facilities contract for this service.

The effects of radiation on microbes have been attributed to direct impingement of radiation on cellular molecules, probably resulting in disruption of molecular bonds within DNA. In addition, cell destruction has been attributed to the formation of free radicals and other moieties such as peroxides [3].

In the early years of radiation sterilization, a dose of 25 kGy was considered adequate for device sterilization. The need for use of lower doses compatible with many more materials led to the development of dose-setting methods demonstrating the lethality of radiation to natural product bioburden rather than to a more resistant microbial challenge. If product bioburden can be controlled to a low level, then lower sterilization doses can be validated and more materials are compatible with the process. On the other hand, dose-setting studies have led to the necessity of doses higher than 25 kGy to kill some device bioburdens.

The primary interaction with matter of both gamma rays and accelerated high energy electrons ultimately results from low energy (approximately 100 eV) secondary electrons generated from primary electrons. They produce charged species, free radicals and excited molecules in close proximity to the point of origination. These high energy species return to lower energy states with the final effect of molecular crosslinking and chain scission. The observable physical and chemical property changes are a product of the resulting crosslinked molecular networks, broken molecular chains and gaseous (e.g., H_2) and low molecular weight scission products. In addition, free radicals are often sufficiently stable to survive past the initial irradiation event and can continue to significantly impact the ongoing radiation chemistry and resulting physical properties depending on their half life, the oxygen environment and the material thickness. The radicals are more troublesome if they persist over time. Residual free radicals are susceptible to interactions with oxygen, resulting in highly reactive peroxide radicals and further molecular chain scission and degradation of physical properties over time.

The source of secondary electrons is high energy primary electrons. The primary electrons in the case of electron beam sterilization are generated directly by the accelerator. In gamma sterilization, the gamma rays produce the primary electrons through an energy deposition process called Compton Scattering. It is interesting to note that despite the differences in origination, the interactive agent, the low energy secondary electron, is identical for electron beam and gamma sterilization. The observed differences in material effects between the two sterilization methods result, therefore, strictly from differences in the rate at which these species are introduced; 25 kGy in seconds with electron beam and in hours with gamma sterilization. Indeed, this is one of the main differences between gamma radiation and electron beam radiation. The oxidative degradation of the electron beam system is limited because oxygen within the material is consumed rapidly and cannot be replaced through oxygen diffusion during the time frame of irradiation, whereas there is sufficient time during gamma irradiations. This makes some materials such as polypropylene radiation compatible with electron beam while they are not acceptable with gamma radiation in certain applications. In addition, different levels of oxidative degradation can be observed between surface and bulk area of materials because of the differences in availability (concentration differences) of oxygen.

The effect of radiation on materials is mainly determined by their chemical composition, conformation and morphology. The variation of these factors can lead to different levels of crosslinking and chain scission; the ratio of these two defines the final material effect. In general, crosslinking can increase tensile strength and toughness for most polymeric materials while chain scission causes degradation such as loss of strength and embrittlement of materials.

At radiation sterilization dose levels (typically up to 50 kGy, depending on the dose required to kill the device bioburden) the effect on the bulk properties of most biomaterials is small (see Table 15-3). Due to the dose rate effects discussed above, materials effects including discoloration and embrittlement are more severe with gamma radiation sterilization rather than with electron beam exposures. Due to ongoing radical reactions with oxygen in certain polymers, material degradation may persist over time after sterilization. This has been observed in ultra high molecular weight polyethylene hip implants sterilized with gamma radiation [7].

One advantage of radiation sterilization is that it typically does not result in significant levels of toxic or non-toxic residues (see Table 15-2).

STEAM

Of all the sterilization methods, steam sterilization has been used the longest. The mechanism of heat sterilization is associated with denaturation of microbial proteins. Pure saturated steam is a very efficient means of sterilization, typically operating at elevated pressures between temperatures of 121°C and 133°C. The process can involve air removal with vacuum or by gravity displacement.

Due to the high temperatures involved, its use for device sterilization is limited to metallic or other heat resistant materials including some textiles and polymers [5]. Boiler water additives are commonly used to decrease the corrosive nature of the steam to the sterilizing vessel or to metallic devices. The FDA has established limits for boiler water additives for food sterilization and considers those levels also safe for device sterilization (21CFR 173.).

Table 15-3   Radiation Sterilization

Material class	Effects of radiation sterilization on bulk properties of biomaterials
Polymers [8]	—Compatible with most polymeric materials at sterilization dose range up to 50 kGy. —Some materials (e.g., acetal, unstabilized polypropylene and polytetrafluoroethylene—PTFE) need to be carefully evaluated.
Metals/Alloys	—Compatible —Temperature increase caused by radiation needs to be carefully monitored to avoid damage on coating or bonding materials.
Ceramics	Compatible
Electronics [9]	—Not compatible with active components (ICs, semiconductors) —Acceptable with most passive components (resistors, capacitors)
Biologicals	Acceptable in some applications

Steam sterilization has found long-term use for sterilization of metallic surgical instruments, but may be of concern for implant materials. Deposition of hydrophobic organics and hygroscopic salts on implant materials such as Germanium and Vitallium has been indicated during steam sterilization (see Table 15-2). These surface contaminants may adversely influence adhesion to implant surfaces in the body.

LIQUID CHEMICAL

Liquid chemical sterilants usually consist of formulations utilizing one or more sporicidal agents, the "active ingredients," and one or more "inert" ingredients such as buffers, anti-corrosive agents, and detergents. The inert ingredients can influence the sporicidal activity of the active ingredients. Aldehydes such as glutaraldehye and oxidizing agents such as hydrogen peroxide and peracetic acid are common active ingredients of liquid chemical sterilants.

Liquid chemical sterilization involves the immersion of a device in a solution at a particular temperature for a period of time. This type of sterilization does not provide for the extensive process monitoring commonly used in terminal processes such as those above for which microbial or physical/chemical monitoring systems are available. It is employed industrially mainly for sterilization of devices made from animal or human tissues which cannot be subjected to other means of terminal sterilization. The devices may then be packaged in a container with the sterilant which is intended to be rinsed off prior to use.

In healthcare facilities, devices are exposed to liquid chemical sterilants for a shorter time than required for sterilization, but adequate to kill microorganisms such as mycobacterium tuberculosis. This process, called high-level disinfection, permits the reuse of expensive devices within a shorter time than required for terminal sterilization methods. These devices are not packaged and are subject to contamination after removal from the process.

Glutaraldehyde has the potential to cross-link with unsaturated structures; hydrogen peroxide and peracetic acid can be corrosive. In addition, leaching of device materials additives such as plasticizers can occur. For reused devices, the effects of repeated liquid chemical exposures on device materials must be evaluated.

PLASMA

Radiofrequency gas plasma (glow discharge) was initially researched for surface cleaning of biomaterials [10]. Subsequently, it was adapted for device sterilization [11]. The process used hydrogen peroxide gas excited by radiofrequency discharge and enhanced by vacuum and ultraviolet radiation effects.

One commercially available plasma process uses hydrogen-peroxide-seeded gas plasma. It operates at less than 50°C. Reaction products, oxygen and water, are non-toxic. Sterilization of lumens with diameters below 6 mm and longer than 31 cm was contraindicated. It is compatible with metallic and polymeric devices, but not with cellulosics, linens, and liquids.

Another commercially available system uses gaseous peracetic acid and plasma [12]. It also operates at low temperatures and there are no toxic residues produced. It was approved initially for use on stainless steel instruments without hinges. Use on devices with lumens, implantable devices, or bone tissue was contraindicated. It is compatible with Tyvek® (E. I. DuPont de Nemours & Co., Inc., Wilmington, DE) and Tyvek® mylar packaging.

OTHER GASES

Gaseous sterilization systems employing gases other than ethylene oxide are emerging due to the environmental concerns. These include systems using ozone, hydrogen peroxide, and chlorine dioxide.

Vaporized Hydrogen Peroxide

One system is based on the use of vaporized hydrogen peroxide with steam at atmospheric pressure. The main application for this technology is barrier isolators. Lethality is due to protein oxidation. Surface contaminants such as oils, salts, and residues will inhibit or stop penetration to surfaces. Materials degradation and binding with hydrogen peroxide are of concern with this sterilizing agent [12].

Chlorine Dioxide

Chlorine dioxide is an oxidizing agent which is nonflammable at sterilizing concentrations and non-ozone-depleting. The gas must be generated as needed, not stored in cylinders as is EtO. At the time this chapter was written, this process had been approved in Canada, with U.S. approval pending. For this process a porous package is required for gas penetration. The process is compatible with coated and uncoated Tyvek® packaging, but is not compatible with cellulosics due to chlorine dioxide binding [12].

Ozone

Ozone previously used for treatment of drinking water, has been developed for device sterilization. It can be generated from air with electricity. It decomposes to oxygen, leaving no toxic residues.

Table 15-4   Typical Effects of Sterilizing Agents on Materials

	Bulk material effects	Surface material effects	
		Applications requiring STRONG bioadhesion (e.g., implants)	Applications requiring WEAK bioadhesion (e.g., heart valves)
Ethylene Oxide	—Effects are typically negligible. —Hydrophilic materials may not be compatible. —Residues are toxic.	Negative impact	Positive impact
Radiation	—Effects small for most polymers at doses less than 50 kGy. —Effects can be significant, e.g., in acetal, unstabilized propylenes and PTFE. —Not compatible with active electronics.	Negligible impact	Negligible impact
Steam	—Applicable only to heat-resistant materials —Corrosive effects need to be considered with metals —Not compatible with most biologicals	Negative impact	Positive impact
Liquid Chemical	Applicable only to biologicals	n/a	n/a
Plasma	Effects are typically small	Positive impact	Negative impact
Other Gases	Dependent on the nature of the gas; see text	Negative impact	Positive impact

CONCLUSION

Generally observed effects of sterilizing agents on materials are summarized in Table 15-4. With the current level of interest in developmnet of new sterilization technologies for use on medical devices, there will be a continuing need for testing of materials effects of these physical and chemical agents.

REFERENCES

1   Association for the Advancement of Medical Instrumentation, 3330 Washington Boulevard, Suite 400, Arlington, VA 22201-4598.
2   Phillips CR, Kaye S. The sterilizing action of ethylene oxide. I. Review. *Am J Hyg*, 50 (1949), 270–279.
3   DeRisio R. Sterilization concepts and methods of sterilization employed by the hospital and industry. In Gaughran ERL, Morrissey RF, and Wang Y, (Eds.), *Sterilization of Medical Products*, Vol. IV. 1986, 17–31.
4   Loshbaugh C. *Microbiological Considerations for EtO Sterilization*. MDDI, 1980.
5   *The Effects of Sterilization Methods on Plastics and Elastomers*. New York: Plastics Design Library, 1994.
6   Baier RE, Meyer AE. Implant Surface Preparation. *International J Oral & Maxillofacial Implants*, 3 (1998), 9
7   Baier RE , Meyer AE, Natiella JR. Implant surface physics and chemistry: Improvements and impediments to bioadhesion. *Proc Second International Congress on Tissue Integration in Oral, Orthopedic, and Maxillofacial Reconstruction*, Minneapolis, MN, September, 1990, 240.

8   Baier RE. Conditioning surfaces to suit the biomedical environment. *J Biochemical Engineering*, 104 (1982), 257.

9   Sutula LC. Impact of gamma sterilization on clinical performance of polyethylene in the hip. *Clinical Orthopaedics and Related Research*, 319 (1995), 28.

10 Morrissey CJ. NASA/JPL Report No. NPO16424/5904.

11 Morrissey CJ. NASA Tech Brief, 9 (1985), #107.

12 Skeins WE, Williams JL. Ionizing radiation's effect on selected biomedical polymers. In Szycher M (Ed.), *Biocompatible Polymers, Metals, and Composites*, Chapter 44. Society of Plastics Engineers, 1978.

ADDITIONAL READING

1   Ley FJ. The effect of irradiation on packaging materials. *J Society of Cosmetic Chemists*, 27 (1976), 483–489.

2   Holmes-Siedle A, Adams L. *Handbook of Radiation Effects*. New York: Oxford University Press, 1993.

3   Philips CR, Kaye S. The sterilizing action of gaseous ethylene oxide. *Am J Hyg*, 50 (1949), 280–306.

4   Baier RE, Carter JM, Sorensen SE, Meyer AE, McGowan BD, Kasprzak, SA. Radiofrequency gas plasma (glow discharge) disinfection of dental operative instruments, including handpieces. *J Oral Implant*, 18 (1992), 236–245.

5   Kowalski JB. Presentation at Fundamentals of Medical Device Sterilization, HIMA, Baltimore, MD, 1996.

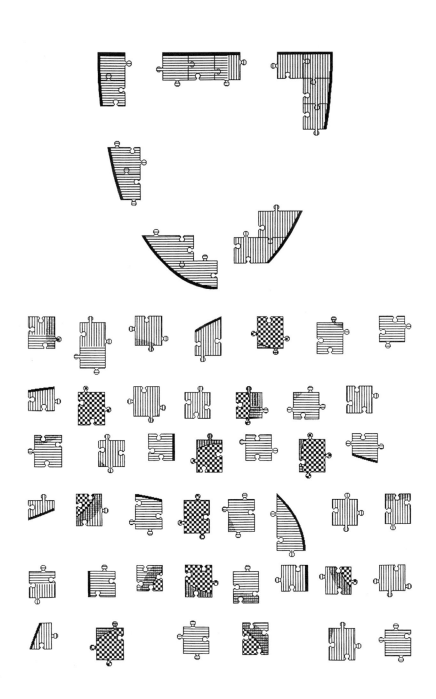

Section Three

Toxicological Evaluations

W. Homer Lawrence

INTRODUCTION

Biomedical devices are employed to strengthen or replace a compromised physiological function. These are usually composed of one or more synthetic materials (biomaterials) fabricated into a functional device. It is important that such devices do not create new (toxicological) problems for the patient, or aggravate existing physiological problems.

Critical evaluation of any material intended for biomedical applications is essential prior to, or early during device development. The scope of such tests should be quite broad and dictated only in part by the intended application of the material. It is generally important that the material is compatible with biological systems with which it comes into contact, and that these biological systems should not adversely affect the material. Additionally, toxicological evaluations of the intact device are important to help ensure that the material has not been significantly altered, or that toxic leachables were not introduced, during its manufacture and sterilization, and to ensure its safety for the intended use. Functionality of the device is primarily in another domain except as it may be altered by the biological system during use to adversely affect its function.

In essence, toxicological tests should ensure, as much as possible, the safety of the material when used in humans. Since, in general, safety may be viewed as inversely related to toxicity—as toxicity increases, safety tends to decrease and vice versa—these tests may be considered either "toxicity tests" or "safety tests" based upon the approaches and goals.

In this section, Chapter 16 places into perspective some of the problems that may be encountered in the biomedical applications of plastics and other materials and discusses how these may contribute to the toxicity or unacceptability of a biomaterial or device. Approaches are also presented for the prevention of certain types of biomaterial toxicity. This chapter also considers the appropriateness of various testing procedures and the importance of understanding the results and relevance of toxicity tests.

Chapter 17 discusses preclinical safety-toxicity evaluation of biomaterials from the perspective of an industrial testing laboratory. Both in vivo and in vitro tests are considered with some of these being conducted upon the material per se, while others utilize extracts of the material. Included are recommended tests and guidelines or protocols prepared by certain professional or regulatory organizations.

The problem of hypersensitivity of the patient to biomaterials or devices, particularly implanted devices, is considered in Chapter 18. The immune system and types of hypersensitivity reactions are briefly reviewed, as well as the mechanisms involved in these reactions.

Recommendations are presented for evaluating the potential for biomaterials (devices) to induce hypersensitivity reactions.

Material-induced carcinogenicity continues to be of concern, especially in connection with long-term implants, although scientific opinion differs with regard to the phenomenon in humans. Chapter 19 reviews the background and theories for material-induced tumors. Experimental evaluation of biomaterials for their tumorigenic potential is discussed along with interpretation of results obtained from such tests. Certain in vivo/in vitro, or in vitro/in vivo, techniques were developed in the early to mid-80s which offered promise as more rapid means of evaluating materials for solid-state carcinogenic potential. Unfortunately, however, this promise has not yet been realized.

The satisfactory culmination of safety-toxicity testing for a biomaterial leads to the development of a medical device and its in vivo testing. Chapter 20 focuses upon these final stages of biomaterial evaluation, when the materials have been constructed into device configuration. Some of the "in-use" and additional supporting tests are discussed; these are used to detect and quantify, if possible, the tendency for the material to induce problems when it is employed in a specific biomedical application.

Chapter 16

Perspectives

W. Homer Lawrence

The ever-increasing uses of biomaterials for patient implants and as components of various medical devices that have intimate contact with blood, tissues, or drug solutions make it imperative that they be properly evaluated for safety/toxicity prior to introduction into patients. Biomaterials are most useful in medicine, surgery, and health care when they are shaped, formed, or constructed into specific configurations, termed devices, for particular applications. Undoubtedly biomedical devices have produced significant, even life-saving, benefits to numerous patients. It is not clear, however, how many patients may have suffered adverse effects, including death or serious disability, from such devices. While adverse effects from devices have been documented for some patients, there is a much larger group in which it is not clear whether some of the patients' problems were due solely to the underlying disease or pathological state, or whether device usage was responsible for, or a contributing factor to, the problems.

Biomedical materials and/or devices are intended to benefit patients who generally have an anatomical, biochemical, or physiological disorder or defect, and therefore use of the material or device should not impose any unnecessary adverse or toxic stress upon the patient. Consequently, any toxic potential of a candidate biomaterial should be determined, and appropriate steps should be taken to minimize any adverse effect to the patient. Thus, when considering benefits versus risks from such devices, it is not adequate simply to consider them in terms of whether the risks to the patient are greater if the device is or is not used, but rather in terms of whether or not, in the context of current knowledge and technology, the device produces the *maximum benefit* to the patient with a *minimum of risk*.

TOXICITY TESTING OF POTENTIAL BIOMATERIALS

Reasons for Testing

When a new material is being considered for use in a biomedical area, it is important to know a number of things about the candidate material. Generally it is the material's physical properties that first suggest it may be suitable for the application. This may be followed by consideration of its suitability to be formed or shaped into the desired configuration during the manufacturing process and then sterilization of the finished product. Sometimes consideration of the material's potential toxicity or biological incompatibility is largely ignored in the early phases of planning or development, which could be very expensive and result in considerable lost time for the developer.

Toxicological evaluation of biomaterials, or candidate materials, is an extremely important part of their development for biomedical applications. Although selected screening tests may be employed to obtain a preliminary assessment, this is best accomplished by determining the *toxicological profile* of a new biomaterial or device, just as it is for a new drug, in order to assess intelligently its safety. In this respect, biomaterials show a kinship to drugs because there is no single, quick, and simple test that will provide all of the information needed for safety-toxicity assessment. The toxicological profile may also help to delineate conditions and limits for safe applications for the material.

The process of obtaining the toxicity-safety profile for a biomaterial and/or device may require various modifications to standard or classic toxicity testing procedures as well as utilizing new and innovative approaches. There are times when a standard test, or the standard conditions for the test, should be modified to evaluate a particular material. Thus, rigid adherence to a particular protocol, without incorporating reasonable modifications, may not provide the best or most relevant toxicity data for the material.

Unlike drugs, whose purpose is to produce a dose-related physiological change during use, most biomaterials ideally should not interact with blood, tissues, or biochemical systems in the patient even during prolonged contact or use, and therefore should not exhibit a quantity-related effect. Thus, toxicological evaluations of biomaterials are intended to ensure, as much as possible, compatibility of the biomaterials with the environment in which they are used.

It is also important to recognize that a biomaterial may be suitable for a particular biomedical application, but may be unsuitable for a different use. Therefore, in evaluating the suitability of a material one must look not only at the total toxicity data, but must also specifically consider data that are most appropriate to the intended use of the material when fabricated into its device.

The nonuniformity of generic materials is another reason to conduct toxicity tests. Often one hears that a particular material is suitable for a specific purpose because another material of the same generic class has been successfully used for that purpose. Such assumptions are unjustified and may subsequently lead to serious problems. One cannot take toxicological data from one biomaterial and safely extrapolate that data to other materials of the same generic class. For example, there are many different formulations that may be used to produce a polyvinyl chloride (PVC), polyurethane, or silicone polymer, and these, coupled with various manufacturing processes, not only yield polymers with different physical properties, but all too often with different toxicological characteristics. Even when one is considering a particular brand name polymer, it is necessary to be sure there have not been any changes in formulation, source of ingredients, or manufacture of the polymer since it was evaluated for toxicity-safety.

Scheduling of Testing

A new potential biomaterial, or one whose toxicological profile is unknown, should be evaluated for toxicity and/or biocompatibility at an early stage in its consideration for a biomedical application. If the material exhibits significant evidence of toxicity, it should be examined closely to determine whether or not it is feasible to make it suitably biocompatible *before* proceeding with design and development of the device. If the undesirable effects of the material cannot be eliminated or corrected, an alternate material should be considered. It is important to start development with suitable materials to avoid wasting time and money in designing and fabricating an item that must be discarded because of unacceptable compatibility properties.

Using materials with physical and toxicological properties that make them suitable, the design and fabrication of a biomedical item may proceed. Once the item is in its finished form, it should again be subjected to toxicological evaluation to ensure that the procedures involved in its fabrication, sterilization, etc., have not introduced substances or modified the material(s) in such a way that the biocompatibility of the original material(s) have not been altered.

USUAL CAUSES OF TOXICOLOGICAL PROBLEMS FROM BIOMATERIALS

The usual causes for biological incompatibility of materials are (a) biologically active leachable substances; (b) physical contact of the material, particularly with regard to thrombosis and cancer induction; and (c) biodegradation of the material, which alters its physical or compatibility properties and/or produces free bioactive molecules.

Most instances of acute biological incompatibility of a material, as detected in primary screening tests, appear to be due to the release of one or more substances (called "leachables") to the biological system. In some cases, this form of incompatibility may be resolved by identifying the offending substance and its source and then taking steps to eliminate it from the material.

Toxic leachables may also be due to sterilant residues (e.g., liquid or gaseous sterilants), or to degradation products produced by excessive heat or radiation of some materials, as discussed below in the section on leaching.

DETOXIFYING POTENTIAL BIOMATERIALS

Sometimes a candidate biomaterial exhibits evidence of significant toxicity in initial screening toxicity tests. Toxic leachables are most often responsible for adverse effects noted in short-term screening tests; therefore, it may be possible to "clean up" the material to eliminate this aspect of toxicity.

The first step is to identify the leachable and/or its source and then to prevent its occurrence in or remove it from the material. Depending upon the leachable and its source, it may be necessary to use more highly purified starting materials, modify the formulation, employ better stoichiometric synthesis, or prevent extraneous contamination during the manufacturing process. If the toxic leachable is a sterilant residue or degradation product resulting from sterilization of the material and/or device, it may be necessary to change sterilization methods or modify the sterilization or poststerilization conditions.

Occasionally, it may be possible to "clean up" the polymer by aeration or applied vacuum, extensive washing, or selective extraction to remove the leachable substances.

CAUSATIVE MECHANISMS OF ADVERSE EFFECTS

Leaching

As previously indicated, the presence of biologically active substances, both within or upon a polymer, that are capable of being solubilized by biological fluids or contacting media (leachables) are the most frequent cause for a material's acute incompatibility with biological systems (excluding thrombosis). Leaching is a surface phenomenon; however, many substances contained in the matrix of a polymer may migrate to the surface where leaching occurs (see also Chapter 2). In these cases, the substance contained in the polymer may act as a reservoir to provide long-term migration to the surface where leaching may occur. The rate-limiting step in this process may be either the rate of migration or rate of leaching from the surface, depending upon the substance involved, the polymer, and the extracting medium. The presence of a plasticizer may facilitate migration of other substances within the polymer.

Sources of Leachables

Leachables may be intentional or unintentional additives, or both. Intentional additives are those substances deliberately added to the formulation for a particular purpose, such as plasticizers, stabilizers, colorants, radiopaques, ultraviolet (UV) absorbants, or added but unintentionally present, such as residual monomers, incompletely polymerized molecules (low molecular weight polymers), and polymerization initiators. Unintentional additives would include contaminants from impure starting materials, sterilant residues, and products of polymer degradation. The designations of "intentional" and "unintentional" relate to those substances knowingly and unknowingly added; none of these substances are intended to be leachables (excluding the use of polymers as drug delivery systems).

Partial degradation of the polymer may result from (a) heat and/or radiation during the manufacturing or sterilization process or (b) biological degradation. The former should be detectable from acute screening tests, whereas the latter would be apparent only after prolonged contact with the biological system. It should also be noted that both types of polymer degradation tend to change the physical properties of the material as well as to provide potentially toxic leachables.

Sterilization

Sterility of most biomedical devices is of prime importance, but the choice of sterilization methods is often limited by material characteristics (for more details see Chapter 15).

Steam and dry heat are advantageous methods because they do not leave a toxic residue, but many polymeric materials cannot withstand the heat and/or humidity without deforming or degrading. Also, in the device configuration, there may be areas in which steam does not readily penetrate. Chemical sterilants, particularly ethylene oxide (EtO), have been quite widely used. With EtO, freshly sterilized materials may contain significant quantities of EtO, which require thorough degassing before they are suitable for use. Ethylene oxide is very reactive, and in the presence of chloride it may form the very toxic 2-chloroethanol (ethylene chlorohydrin), as well as ethylene glycol and other products; such reaction products may remain in the device after EtO degassing. Recent evidence of the carcinogenicity of EtO has imposed greater restrictions upon its usage. Like EtO, liquid chemical sterilants, such as formaldehyde and glutaraldehyde solutions, do not require high temperatures, but it is sometimes difficult to remove the sterilant completely by flushing, particularly in low-flow areas of a device, and from sorption onto or into some polymers. Radiation sterilization has achieved considerable popularity for a number of reasons (including ease, reliability, cost, and convenience). However, different polymers exhibit varying degrees of instability to radiation, resulting in additional cross-linking or breakage of polymer chains. As a consequence, there may be a change in the appearance and physical properties of the polymeric material, while polymer degradation may produce toxic leachable substances.

Selection of an appropriate sterilization method (see Chapter 15) is of prime importance. If an inappropriate method is used, or if it is improperly used, a biologically compatible device may be transformed into one that is physically or biologically unacceptable. This is one reason why a finished device should be evaluated for toxicity even if previous tests had indicated that all of its component materials were suitable.

Drug-Plastic Interactions

Permeation and sorption (absorption and adsorption) are phenomena that are often considered together because they have certain characteristics in common; however, they also exhibit certain differences. Either or both of these processes may be observed with many polymeric materials. Sorption tends to remove substances from the contacting medium, either onto its contacting surface or into the matrix of the polymer. Permeation is the process of a substance migrating through the polymer; it is bidirectional, concentration-dependent, and preceded by absorption.

Selective permeability of a polymer to specific molecular species may be a highly desirable characteristic and serve as the basis for certain biomedical applications, such as hemodialyzers and oxygenators. On the other hand, permeation (and sorption) may have a detrimental effect upon a diagnostic or therapeutic product. Generally, this problem tends to be most acute when the material is used as a container. For example, oxygen permeating into the container may oxidize and destroy a sensitive drug or diagnostic product, or carbon dioxide permeation might alter the pH of the solution and create a formulation incompatibility. On the other hand, if the solvent permeates without the active ingredient, the preparation may become excessively potent or precipitate.

Sorption may create problems when very potent drugs or diagnostic agents, which are present in low concentrations, are involved. Such losses from the formulations may result in a lack of therapeutic effect and false negative tests, respectively. In a similar fashion, sorption or permeation of an antimicrobial additive may compromise the expected sterility of a product during its use.

While sorption and permeation may not be true toxic phenomena *per se*, they may nevertheless lead to undesirable or toxic consequences.

Biodegradation and/or Biotransformation

Prolonged contact of a biomaterial with biological systems often results in alterations of the chemical and physical properties of the biomaterial. There are, of course, a few biomedical applications (such as absorbable sutures or some controlled drug release systems), in which biodegradation of the material is a desirable characteristic, but it is undesirable for most applications.

Biodegradation and/or biotransformation may take the form of biological molecules attaching to, or penetrating into, the polymer, or of biological reactions altering the polymeric structure of the material. In this last case, the result may be an increase or decrease in cross-linking, degradation, or fragmentation of polymer chains with a concomitant change in physical, mechanical, and biocompatibility characteristics.

These degradation products may initiate or participate in local or systemic toxic reactions, hypersensitivity reactions or other adverse effects. The possible relationship of polymer biodegradation to carcinogenic phenomena is discussed in Chapter 19.

Sometimes prolonged contact with a biological environment alters the biomaterial to such an extent that the device fails to perform its intended function. As an illustration, consider the ball and cage heart valves in which the silicone balls sometimes became deformed or chipped, resulting in failure of the heart valve. Because this type of problem involves an interaction of the biological environment with the material, in vitro tests are of little value in predicting a problem of this nature, other than assurance that the original (unchanged) material will perform satisfactorily for the anticipated duration of its use.

Physical Contact

Most biomaterials exhibit relatively good compatibility during short-term contact with tissues, excluding blood (see Chapters 22, 23, 34, and 43), unless toxic leachables are involved. However, after a biomaterial is placed into the body (biological system), the body's defense systems attack it in an attempt to destroy or isolate it. Most implanted biomaterials are biodegraded rather slowly, and thus it is common for the body to attempt to isolate it by enclosing it in a fibrous capsule (see Chapter 38). Anatomic location of the implant affects the type and efficiency of the encapsulation process, with subcutaneous or muscle sites demonstrating this phenomenon quite readily.

The long-term effects of a biomaterial in contact with tissues are less clear. Physical properties of the implanted material may be altered by leaching, biodegradation, calcification, encapsulation, etc., which may impair its function or make it aesthetically less acceptable for cosmetic purposes. In addition, there is the question of tumorigenesis associated with long-term implantation of materials (see Chapter 19).

APPROPRIATE TOXICITY TESTING

The appropriateness of a particular toxicity test will depend upon a number of factors. Among these are the stage of testing (preliminary, toxicological profile, relevant to use, or in-use) and the purpose of the test. A new material may merely be subjected to a few preliminary screening tests to ascertain if it has a marked tendency to induce acute reactions. This screens out grossly undesirable materials before they undergo more expensive and time-consuming evaluations. This procedure may also be employed as a first approximation to determine how effectively a reactive biomaterial candidate was detoxified in the cleanup process before proceeding to more extensive testing.

Before a new material is seriously considered for biomedical applications, it should be evaluated in an appropriate battery of tests (toxicological profile) to determine and delineate its probable scope of safe application. These tests should be of a broad nature and not limited or targeted to use of the material; in fact, some potential uses of and limitations for the material may be suggested from the results of these tests.

Once a probable application for the material has been targeted, based upon results of the toxicological profile, the physical properties of the material, and the designer's and/or manufacturer's needs or desires, the material should be considered in terms of results from relevant tests. This may include tests from the toxicological profile that are relevant to the intended use as well as additional tests targeted to the intended application. This phase of evaluation should provide significant safety data on the material for this purpose and indicate what type of adverse (or toxic) reactions, if any, might be expected from the material during its use for this purpose.

The last preclinical phase involves preparing the material into its device configuration and evaluating it for toxicity and/or safety in animal models that mimic, as much as possible, the clinical application of the device (see Chapter 20). For those items that normally would remain in the patient for extended periods of time, it would also be desirable to evaluate the physical properties (elasticity, tensile strength, etc.) of the material before and after use in animals to see if there are any indications of biodegradation or biotransformation from prolonged contact with the biologic system (see Sections I and II). Significant changes in physical properties of a material from in vivo exposure should alert one to the likelihood of subsequent device failure.

UNDERSTANDING THE RESULTS AND RELEVANCE
OF TOXICITY TESTS

Some people view the results from toxicity tests on a material as branding the material "toxic" or "nontoxic," with little consideration given to the tests or their meaning. Others rely strictly on a numerical system which assigns a numerical value to each test result. If the total (or average) value from all tests exceeds a specified value the material is unsuitable, whereas if the test value is less than the specified value, the material is acceptable. I would like to warn against a dogmatic approach to both of these positions, and instead, recommend consideration of (a) the purpose of the test, (b) the degree of response produced in the test, and (c) the relevance of these factors to the intended use of the material.

Most preclinical tests are designed to evaluate a particular aspect of a material's compatibility with the living system. Since the majority of short-term compatibility tests are concerned with detecting biologically active ("toxic") leachables from the material, one should consider the test itself, the conditions under which it was performed, the sensitivity of the test, and the type of response produced. For example, should one have the same level of concern about a material whose extract produces only a slight retardation in growth of cells in culture as about a material whose extract kills 50% or more of the mice to which it is administered?

Most toxicological evaluations of a biomaterial include a number of tests, measuring different end-points, whose individual sensitivities (concentration and/or quantity required to reach detection threshold) cover a relatively broad range. One should keep in mind that, when discussing in vivo, ex vivo, or in vitro biological tests' sensitivities, we are referring to biological activity of the test substance (or leachable); this is a combination of quantity and activity. Thus, a small quantity of a very active substance may produce the same or greater response than a larger quantity of a less active substance. Furthermore, the final response may be markedly affected by the ability of the test system to metabolize, partition (distribute), and excrete the bioactive component.

What does the test measure? One should consider the results in terms of what the test is designed to detect. Various tests may be employed to detect such parameters as primary irritation, hypersensitivity induction, cellular death, inhibition of cellular growth, alterations of isolated heart contractions, evidence of overt toxicity, and even death. All of these, whether qualitative or quantitative, indicate the presence of a biologically active substance, although the end-points are not always death of the cell or animal; if there is sufficient activity present, one could anticipate subtle or overt toxic changes in vivo.

The sensitivity of the particular test should also be considered. Some tests will detect a bioactive leachable at levels considerably lower than that needed to detect the same bioactive leachable in other tests. For example, a toxicant will generally show a cytotoxic response to cells in culture (agar overlay tissue culture test) at a lower concentration than is needed to elicit a detectable response in the rabbit intradermal or dermal irritation test or the systemic toxicity test in mice. On the other hand, other tests (e.g., inhibition of cell growth and isolated perfused rabbit heart) tend to detect the presence of bioactive compounds at concentrations below those required for a cytotoxic response in the agar overlay tissue culture test. Nevertheless, a positive response from these more sensitive tests is an indication of the presence of a bioactive leachable or contaminant.

Quantitative test responses are desirable end-points; however, one should not be misled by the numbers. Some tests lend themselves readily to quantitation of results, whereas others are inherently qualitative tests. In an attempt to quantitate some test data, a number of arbitrary classifications may be established for responses (a simple example would be "mild," "moderate," and "severe") to which numerical values may be assigned. Objective criteria are established, insofar as possible, for classifying the response, but subjective factors are often involved in the evaluation process. Data of this type may be viewed as semiquantitative (or pseudoquantitative). The training and experience of the evaluator is often critical. For instance, in the histological evaluation of rabbit muscle's response to a 7-day implant, one would expect to see some tissue damage from the implantation process even in the absence of a toxic reaction to the implant. Thus, it is necessary to evaluate the site carefully to distinguish between those abnormalities that are associated with physical insertion of the sample versus those that result from the release of a cytotoxic substance from the implant.

The range of detectable responses from a particular test may pose interpretative problems when comparing data from a series of tests. Sometimes the more sensitive tests may reach their response maxima at bioactivity levels that may be below threshold levels for the less sensitive tests. The various tests tend to measure different parameters or biological activities and, therefore, due to mechanistic differences, there is no constant quantitative relationship between the relative sensitivities of the tests. Although general guides or approximations can be developed for relative sensitivities of various test systems, any specific quantitative relationship developed for a test substance may be different for a different test substance. This phenomenon provides additional justification for the use of a battery of tests to evaluate a biomaterial, rather than any single test.

Most properly conducted tests used for the acute evaluation of a biomaterial indicate if there is a bioactive substance leaching from the material. To assess the possible toxic hazard from this unwanted contaminant (or adulterant), additional studies are needed to identify and quantitate the substance. Unless the substance can be removed from the material, as discussed earlier, dose–response studies on this substance should be performed in animals to provide a basis for assessing the potential hazard of the leachable to the patient. It is often difficult to assess the toxic hazard from a device leachable when in use in a patient because of the difficulty of distinguishing between adverse effects of the underlying disease process or the leachable.

Thus, in summary, one should understand the tests employed, what they measure, the kind of response produced (if any), the significance of this response in man (or determined in animals and extrapolated to man), and the possible consequences of the leachable to the diseased patient. This is not to imply the presence of any leachable is desirable, but rather, if it cannot be eliminated, an informed decision may be made concerning its potential toxic hazard if appropriate information is available.

ADDITIONAL READING

1 ASTM Committee F-4 on Surgical Implant Materials. *Plastics in Surgical Implants*. ASTM Special Technical Publication No. 386. Philadelphia, PA: American Society for Testing and Materials, 1965.
2 Autian J. Plastics in pharmaceutical practice and related fields, Part 1. *J Pharm Sci*, 52 (1963), 1–23; Part II, 105–122.
3 Autian J. Toxicity, untoward reactions, and related considerations in the medical use of plastics. *J Pharm Sci*, 53 (1964), 1289–1301.
4 Autian J. Interaction between medicaments and plastics. *J Mond Pharm* 4 (1966), 316–341.
5 Autian J. Problems in the use of polymeric materials in medical and biomedical applications. *Ann NY Acad Sci*, 146 (1968), 251–261.
6 Autian J. Toxicological problems and untoward effects from plastic devices used in medical applications. *Essays Toxicol*, 6 (1975), 1–33.
7 Bischoff F. Organic polymer biocompatibility and toxicology. *Clin Chem*, 18 (1972), 869–894.

8 Bruck SD. *Blood Compatible Synthetic Polymers—An Introduction*. Springfield, IL: Charles C. Thomas Publ., 1974.

9 Bruck SD (Ed.). *Controlled Drug Delivery. Vol. I, Basic Concepts; Vol. II, Clinical Applications*. Boca Raton, FL: CRC Press, 1983.

10 Cooper J. *Plastic Containers for Pharmaceuticals Testing and Control*. Geneva: World Health Organization, 1974.

11 Dillingham EO, Webb N, Lawrence WH, et al. Biological evaluation of polymers, I. Poly (methyl methacrylate). *J Biomed Mater Res*, 9 (1975), 569–596.

12 Doull J, Klaassen CD, Amdur MO (Eds.). *Casarett and Doull's Toxicology, The Basic Science of Poisons*, 2nd ed. New York: Macmillan, 1980.

13 Eckardt RE, Hindin R. The health hazards of plastics. *J Occup Med*, 15 (1973), 808–819.

14 Guess WL, Autian J. Biological testing of plastics to be used in medical practice. *Am J Hosp Pharm*, 21 (1964), 260–267.

15 Gunther DA. Absorption and desorption of ethylene oxide. *Am J Hosp Pharm*, 26 (1969), 45–49.

16 Harrison JH. Synthetic materials as vascular prostheses, II. A comparative study of nylon, Dacron, Orlon, Ivalon Sponge and Teflon in large blood vessels with tensile strength studies. *Amer J Surg*, 95 (1958), 16–24.

17 Hayes AW. *Principles and Methods of Toxicology*. New York: Raven Press, 1982.

18 Klein E, Villarroel F. *Evaluation of Hemodialyzers and Dialysis Membranes*, Pub. No. 77-1294. Washington, DC: U.S. Dept. of Health, Education and Welfare, 1977.

19 Lawrence WH. Phthalate esters: The question of safety. *Clin Toxicol*, 13 (1978), 89–139. An Update. *Clin Toxicol*, 15 (1979), 447–466.

20 Lawrence WH. Phthalate esters: The question of safety. *Clin Toxicol*, 15 (1979), 447–466.

21 Lawrence WH, Beyer SA, Raje, RR, et al. The isolated perfused rabbit heart test for detecting leachables in biomedical devices. In G Li Plaa, Duncan WAM (Eds.), *Proc First International Congress on Toxicology: Toxicology as a Predictive Science*. New York: Academic Press, 1978, 652–653.

22 Leininger RI. Changes in properties of plastics during implantation. *Plastics in Surgical Implants*. ASTM Special Technical Publication No. 386. Philadelphia, PA: American Society for Testing and Materials, 1965, 71–76.

23 Leininger RI, Mirkovitch V, Peters A, et al. Changes in properties of plastics during implantation. *Trans Am Soc Artif Intern Org*, 10 (1964), 320–321.

24 Marcus E, Kim HK, Autian J. Binding of drugs by plastics, I: Interaction of bacteriostatic agents with plastic syringes. *J Am Pharm Assoc, Sci Ed*, 48 (1959), 457–462.

25 McHenry MM, Smeloff EA, Fong WY, et al. Critical obstruction of prosthetic heart valves due to lipid absorption by Silastic. *J Thorac Cardiovasc Surg*, 59 (1970), 413–425.

26 NHLBI Working Group. *Guidelines for Blood-Material Interactions*. Pub. No. 80-2185. Washington, DC: U.S. Department of Health, Education and Welfare, 1980.

27 Pelling D, Sharratt M, Hardy J. The safety testing of medical plastics. I. An assessment of methods. *Food Cosmet Toxicol*, 11 (1973), 69–83.

28 Roberts WC, Morrow AG. Fatal degeneration of the silicone rubber ball of the Starr-Edwards prosthetic aortic valve. *Am J Cardiol*, 22 (1968), 614–620.

29 Rubin LR, Bromberg BE, Walden RH. Long-term human reaction to synthetic plastics. *Surg Gynecol Obst*, 132 (1971), 603–608.

30 Turner JE, Lawrence WH, Autian J. Subacute toxicity testing of biomaterials using histopathologic evaluation of rabbit muscle tissue. *J Biomed Mater Res*, 7 (1973), 39–58.

31 Williams DF. The properties and medical uses of materials. *Biomed Eng*, 6 (1971), 62–69, 106–113, 152–156, 205–208, 260–265, 300–307.

32 Williams DF. Future prospects for biomaterials. *Biomed Eng*, 10 (1975), 207–212, 218.

33 Winter GD, Leray JL, de Groot K (Eds.). *Evaluation of Biomaterials*. New York: Wiley, 1980.

Chapter 17

Testing

Paul Upman

The trend toward global standardization of measurement systems has affected the medical device industry. It is now possible to conduct and assemble one set of safety evaluation data to satisfy most major markets in the world. That is to say, the same biocompatibility data should now be sufficient to satisfy reviewers or regulators in all major countries. Careful thought must go into the interpretation of the international requirements and the development of testing protocols that permit developing universally relevant data in support of device biocompatibility. This chapter will address the industrial toxicology testing methods most often used to evaluate biocompatibility of materials and devices. Emphasis will be placed on the rationale for test selections to insure that good science wins out over the "fill-in-the-blank" approach. For details of the methods discussed, the reader should consult the numerous references that exist for most of the procedures.

HISTORICAL PERSPECTIVE
ON BIOCOMPATIBILITY REQUIREMENTS

The current systematic approach to evaluating biocompatibility of materials and devices evolved over many years and was influenced by many industry leaders and published information [1–3]. The most profound influence on testing schemes, however, occurred with the announcement of the Tripartite Biocompatibility Guidance in early 1987 [4]. This guidance was simultaneously issued as a "draft" document by the U.K., Canada, and the U.S. The Tripartite document was never finalized, but most device manufacturers accepted the guidance as a regulation and followed it almost to the letter. Regulatory personnel likewise used the document to insure that the manufacturer addressed all the concerns as suggested by the Tripartite guidance. Although the Tripartite matrix was interpreted as a list of testing that must be done, there was never a requirement as such to do so. The option was always present to use published information, resin or component part vendor data, and clinical experience to satisfy some or all of the biocompatibility questions. Today's requirements are similar in this regard.

Shortly after the widespread introduction of the Tripartite guidance, the International Organization for Standardization (ISO), a world-wide federation of national standards bodies, developed a similar guidance document [5] eventually known as ISO 10993-1, and formally titled the "Biological Evaluation of Medical Devices-Part 1: Guidance on Selection of Tests." This standard greatly resembled the Tripartite in style, content and format.

For a short period of time (1993–1995), manufacturers had to deal with both the Tripartite guidance for FDA submissions and the ISO guidance for the European community. Fortunately, in mid-1995, the FDA agreed to embrace the ISO 10993-1 document, but with minor modifications. This was done by way of a General Program Memorandum, GP#95-1, issued in May and effective July 1, 1995 [6]. The testing scheme matrix, standardized by ISO and modified by the FDA for device submissions in the U.S., has been reproduced in this chapter (Table 17-1). The reader is directed to the original and complete ISO 10993-1 document, as it contains a significant amount of information that is not apparent by viewing the matrix alone.

The information presented in this chapter will follow the major test headings indicated by the testing scheme matrix. The options that may be exercised in a given situation will be discussed. For the most part, this chapter deals with the in vivo biological methods used to demonstrate biocompatibility. Reference will be made to other chapters in this Handbook that describe relevant in vitro methods or specialized procedures needed to satisfy required testing.

What to Test: Components or Device

Before embarking on a discussion of testing methods, it is important to decide what the test article really is. Which part of the device to test becomes a significant issue whenever there is more than one component part to a device. Even a single material device (e.g., rubber urinary catheter) can present a question as to whether or not the device should be cut or not cut during the preparation or actual testing, because the cut surface may present opportunities for the leaching of toxic or irritant chemicals that might not be available from the intact surface alone.

Ideally, one would develop a biocompatibility profile for each component available for use in a device. Then, one would restrict the components used in devices to those that have been shown to be acceptable for the intended use. In fact, many major device manufacturers do just that. Such files are maintained on each acceptable material and this information is made available to engineers charged with creating and modifying devices. Having this individual information does not preclude final product testing, but it certainly can minimize the amount of testing, money and time needed to evaluate the final device.

There are many who believe that a device should be evaluated as a complete, final product. Those responsible for reviewing safety data accept results of testing conducted on the entire final product, or on a composite of the parts used in the final device. Whether intentional or not, both the Tripartite and ISO guidelines use the term "device" when discussing testing, implying that it is acceptable to evaluate the entire device by the methods indicated. The ISO document (Section 4.3) does state: "This guide is concerned with the tests to be carried out on materials and/or the final product." Evaluations of the entire final product or composite sampling of the product become possible when one considers that many of the test methods are accomplished by using extracts and not the material of the device itself. In the case of implantation studies, however, testing multiple components at the same time may not be practical unless the entire device is implanted as in the clinical setting. For a better understanding of extraction principles and methods, the reader is directed to the U.S. Pharmacopeia [7], and to the international guidance on sample preparation [8]. (See also Table 17-2.)

To show biocompatibility, one must demonstrate a lack of irritant and toxic leachables (or degradation products) available from the device to the patient. Most investigators agree that in general it is important to use both an aqueous and a nonaqueous extraction vehicle in order to detect leachables that are soluble at both ends of the chemical polarity spectrum. Thus, the extract preparation will mimic potential actions of the aqueous and lipid constituents of tissue, bone and blood.

Unless a device is filled or completely covered with the extraction fluid, the guidance given in Table 17-2 should be followed. This allows for at least some standardization of this critical variable. It is important that all extraction tests conducted on a given device

Table 17-1   Material Biocompatibility (Per FDA and ISO Guidance) Phase II Involves Advanced Biocompatibility Testing Appropriate to the Intended Use of the Component Material. These Tests are Designed to Challenge Various Biological Models with the Test Material or a Suitable Extract. Specific Safety Evaluation Programs are Designed in Accordance with FDA Guidance (May 1, 1995) and ISO (International Organization for Standardization) 10993 Standards

Device categories		Contact duration A=Limited (≤24 Hours) B=Prolonged (24 Hours-30 Days) C=Permanent (>30 days)	Cytotoxicity	Sensitization	Irritation/intracutaneous reactivity	Acute systemic toxicity	Subchronic toxicity	Genotoxicity	Implantation	Hemocompatibility	Chronic toxicity	Carcinogenicity	Reproductive/developmental	Biodegradation
Body contact														
Surface devices	Skin	A	X	X	X									
		B	X	X	X									
		C	X	X	X									
	Mucosal membrane	A	X	X	X									
		B	X	X	X	O	O		O					
		C	X	X	X	O	X	X	O		O			
	Breached or compromised surfaces	A	X	X	X	O								
		B	X	X	X	O	O		O					
		C	X	X	X	O	X	X	O		O			
Externally communicating devices	Blood path, indirect	A	X	X	X	X				X				
		B	X	X	X	X	O			X				
		C	X	X	O	X	X	X	O	X	X	X		
	Tissue/bone/dentin communicating[1]	A	X	X	X	O								
		B	X	X	O	O	O	X	X					
		C	X	X	O	O	O	X	X		O	X		
	Circulating blood	A	X	X	X	X		O²		X				
		B	X	X	X	X	O	X	O	X				
		C	X	X	X	X	X	X	O	X	X	X		
Implant devices	Tissue/bone	A	X	X	X	O								
		B	X	X	O	O	O	X	X					
		C	X	X	O	O	O	X	X		X	X		
	Blood	A	X	X	X	X			X	X				
		B	X	X	X	X	O	X	X	X				
		C	X	X	X	X	X	X	X	X	X	X	X	X

Source: Table Based Upon FDA Blue Book Memorandum #G95-1.
X = tests per ISO 10993-1
O = additional tests, which may be applicable in the U.S.
Note[1] = tissue includes tissue fluids and subcutaneous spaces.
Note[2] = for all devices used in extracorporeal circuits.

Table 17-2   Surface Area of Specimen to be Used (7)

Form of Material	Thickness	Amount of sample for each 20 mL of extracting medium	Subdivided into
Film or sheet	<0.5 mm	Equivalent of 120 cm^2 total surface area (both sides combined)	Strips of about 5 × 0.3 cm
	0.5 to 1 mm	Equivalent of 60 cm^2 total surface area (both sides combined)	
Tubing	<0.5 mm (wall)	Length (in cm) = 120 cm^2/ (sum of ID and OD) circumferences)	Sections of about 5 × 0.3 cm
	0.5 to 1 mm (wall)	Length (in cm) = 60 cm^2/ (sum of ID and OD) circumferences)	
Slabs, tubing, and molded items	>1 mm	Equivalent of 60 cm^2 total surface area (all exposed surfaces combined)	Pieces up to about 5 × 0.3 cm
Elastomers	>1 mm	Equivalent of 25 cm^2 total surface area (all exposed surfaces combined)	Do not subdivide[2]

[1]When surface area cannot be determined due to the configuration of the specimen, use 0.1 g of elastomer or 0.2 g of plastic or other polymers for every 1 mL of extracting fluid.
[2]Molded elastomeric closures are tested intact.

at the same time should be prepared in the same way. Specifications should be set and followed in all future testing that may be required when there are significant changes to the device or a component in the device (ISO 10993-1, Section 4.6). Whenever discrepancies exist for like testing of the same material or device, whether at the same facility or between facilities, the differences can usually be traced to variations in preparation methods.

When confronted with the question of what to test, the investigator must determine the best approach that will demonstrate the biocompatibility of the device for the intended use. Thus, an intravenous bag with tubing set, spike and filter may best be studied by filling and extracting the device with the intended extraction fluid. An implantable drug delivery device that has exposure to subcutaneous tissue and a conduit to the vascular system requires a different approach. If the number of component parts in a device becomes too large, one must consider that a single component that is toxic may be "diluted out" or masked and not manifest itself as a problem. This is possible because most extraction ratios (weight or area to given volume) remain constant as volumes of fluid are adjusted up or down, depending upon total area or weight of the device or parts cut out for extraction.

Regardless of whether the components or final product is being tested, the component part or device should have been exposed to all the manufacturing steps, including appropriate sterilization. There is some evidence that the method of sterilization or cycle used may influence the outcome of biocompatibility tests due to ethylene oxide residuals remaining or polymer degradation following exposure to radiation [9]. Testing final product or simulated final components takes into account any processing steps or adhesives used during the final stages of manufacture that might otherwise be overlooked.

TEST METHODS FREQUENTLY USED

Cytotoxicity

Many, if not all, existing guidance documents call for in vitro cytotoxicity data. Various methods are described in the literature [10], in the U.S. Pharmacopeia [11], and in ISO 10993-5: Tests for cytotoxicity: in vitro methods [12]. One or more of the methods described (direct contact, agar overlay, elution) can be used to screen materials, to investigate post-marketing anomalies, or to qualify materials initially and following minor changes. Cytotoxicity methods are known to be sensitive, economical and quick to conduct. While most device materials are noncytotoxic, biomaterials that show cytotoxicity should not be abandoned until the cause is known. In some cases the materials used may, as a generic class, typically show cytotoxicity. Some materials known to be cytotoxic have found useful niches as devices that are acceptable for certain uses, for example, natural or synthetic rubber products, certain adhesives, electrode gels, etc. [13]. Materials or extracts that show cytotoxicity by the usual methods of preparation should be titrated out to a nontoxic dilution, or the sample preparation modified to yield a nontoxic dose. This does not make the problem go away but provides a test method and baseline data that may be usable in the future to clear up questions or problems that may occur. In other words, if the "nontoxic" dose can be defined at the same time that all the remaining biocompatibility work is done, then a useful in vitro method exists to monitor future lots of the same product without resorting to time-consuming in vivo studies to troubleshoot problems. As an example, some latex surgical glove and condom manufacturers establish a dilution at 1:16 as the maximum nontoxic titer they wish to have. Latex rubber devices at this level of "non-cytotoxicity" generally show acceptable results in other testing and in clinical use.

A complete description of relevant cytotoxicity methods can be found in Chapter 21.

Sensitization

Proof needs to be provided that the device or biomaterial has minimal likelihood to cause an allergic response following exposure to the patient. This is especially critical for invasive or implantable devices because, unlike topical products, they cannot be easily retrieved.

In some cases there may, in fact, be ample literature available to demonstrate that the device or materials in question are, or are not, acceptable for repeat or long-term contact with humans. As an example, much information exists in literature with regard to the safe use and implantation of certain "medical grade" stainless steel and titanium metal alloys, particularly those manufactured to ASTM (American Society for Testing and Materials) specifications. Some of the typical reactions noted in the literature are skin rashes to eye glass frames containing nickel, patient and user reactions to rubber gloves, and anaphylactic reactions to latex balloons on barium enema catheters [14].

In those cases where the material is not well known or may indeed have a different formulation than that used in the past, sensitization studies will need to be performed in animals (or humans). Although much effort has gone into the development of in vitro methods [15], nothing has surfaced that concerned scientists and regulatory bodies will accept as an alternative to the classical "guinea pig" methods [16].

The device community tends to rely on the standard Magnuson-Kligman Maximization test [17] for the evaluation of nearly all kinds of devices. Also used are the repeated patching methods published by Buehler. Both the nine-patch [18] and three-patch [19] induction methods are appropriate for many topically used devices.

Maximization Method   In the Maximization test, both aqueous (saline) and nonaqueous (vegetable oil) extractions can be prepared of entire devices or individual components according to methods previously described [7, 8]. The shape and size of the part is not a critical concern when using extracts. Thus any implantable device, blood contact device or topical product may lend itself to extractions, whereas only materials with a flat surface can be tested via the repeated patch methods.

The aqueous and nonaqueous extracts are initially combined with Freund's complete adjuvant and dosed intradermally in the scapular region. Separate injections of the test material extract and Freund's adjuvant are also given. As a minimum, 10 animals should be dosed with each extract. At least five untreated control animals are maintained. A week later, the same site is pretreated with a surfactant (sodium lauryl sulphate) *to eliminate any skin barrier* to a topical patch of the material extract to be applied to this same site on the following day. Two weeks after this second induction, the same test animals, as well as the control group for each extractant, are challenged with a topical patch of the appropriate extract to the flank. If the material is "patchable," then the opposite flank can be used as an exposure site to the material itself. The data assessment is the same as for chemicals; any reaction at the test site not noted at the control sites could be indicative of a sensitization reaction. As with chemicals, a rechallenge is recommended if the results are equivocal.

Repeated Patch Method   In the case of the repeated patch test method, the material to be evaluated is cut to a 2.5 cm by 2.5 cm size for each patching. Liquids, gels and pastes are applied as a 0.5 ml or 0.5 g dose. A group of 10 animals is patched either three times one week or once a week for three weeks. Treatments each consist of a six-hour occluded patching. After a two-week recovery, all test and control animals are challenged by topical patching. Any response seen in the test animals and not seen in the control animals may indicate that a delayed dermal sensitization has occurred. For relatively inert materials (fabrics, polymers, rubber), it is recommended that the full nine-patch series be done so that the strongest challenge can be demonstrated as not producing an allergic response. For raw materials (polymer resin compounds) and components (gels or pastes) that are more chemical in nature, the abbreviated three-patch induction procedure is acceptable.

While these classical methods have been documented well in the literature as capable of screening out sensitizing cosmetics, drugs, and industrial chemicals, there is little proof that they can detect sensitizers in extractables from devices. However, we have seen subtle reactions to certain polymers that could be related to high monomer content (unpublished data). It is widely known, for example, that latex gloves that "pass" a sensitization test in guinea pigs can indeed "find" a nurse or doctor or patient somewhere who will develop a serious dermal allergy. Nonetheless, the guinea pig has been established as the best screening model to identify potential sensitizing materials. In recent years, some attempts have been made to replace these classical methods with the mouse ear swelling assay (MESA) or the mouse local lymph node assay (MLNA), which rely on a reaction in the ear or an evaluation of lymph nodes at the base of the ear, respectively [20]. These methods bear watching, but widespread acceptance has not yet surfaced. Unlike the "grandfathered" guinea pig assays, any new methodology will have to stand up to closer validation before a switch can be made.

Routine protocols for both the maximization and repeated patch tests call for dose determinations prior to the actual assay. Unlike chemicals or cosmetics, there is rarely a need to pretreat a group of animals with devices or extracts to establish a nonirritant dose for the induction treatments in these two assays. Nearly all extracts of devices, polymers, fabrics, metals, and other "chemical-like" gels and pastes generally are nonirritating under these circumstances. This, in effect, saves two to six guinea pigs for each assay conducted. Extracts and materials are tested at full strength as often as possible.

Likewise, for laboratories conducting these tests on a regular basis, using trained personnel and written standard procedures, there is no need to conduct studies of positive control materials with every assay. There are in fact no reliable polymers or device material positive controls. Typically, laboratories use chemical sensitizers to demonstrate that the model works. In reality, the rare delayed sensitization responses seen as a result of biomaterial allergy are quite subtle and may even require scoring in natural lighting, unlike chemical allergens that often produce a rather dramatic response. In lieu of frequent positive control testing of chemicals, most laboratories conduct quarterly assays to validate the model (animals, methods, personnel) on a periodic basis. This seems adequate to validate the model for use throughout the year, providing no significant changes are made in any of the variables.

Antigenicity Assay A third type of study often used to evaluate potential allergenicity, particularly with biologically derived device materials (e.g., natural ligaments, skin, collagen) is an antigenicity assay. No specific models for devices have been formally validated, but various published approaches can be modified to include biomaterials or extracts of biomaterials [21, 22]. Again the guinea pig is used, but the induction phase takes the form of large-volume intraperitoneal dosings over a two-week period. After a two-week recovery, the test and control animals are challenged by intravenous injection. If the animals have become sensitized (developed antibodies), the test animals will react rather dramatically. Reactions range from repetitive face pawing to convulsions and death, as is the case with anaphylactic shock.

Irritation or Intracutaneous Injection

The nature of the device's exposure to the body dictates the type of irritation method used to show compatibility. The test matrix very wisely indicates "irritation or intracutaneous" so as not to imply that any one method with the term "irritation" in its title will suffice. ISO 10993 Part 10: Tests for Irritation and Sensitization [23] provides a wealth of guidance as to the methods available for detecting irritation. The investigator is responsible for selecting the appropriate method.

Primary Skin Irritation This study, familiar to most toxicologists and based on methods published many years ago [24], has value for the evaluation of topically used devices. Such devices as electrodes, bandages used on superficial wounds, surgical drapes, gowns, and surgical gloves (for user protection) are examples. On occasion, as in the case of irregular-shaped objects, extracts may be prepared and patched, but for the most part, this test should be used for materials "as is." If it is necessary to work with extracts, the intracutaneous injection test described later in this chapter should be employed.

The basic primary skin irritation study design calls for six rabbits to be patched on fur-clipped skin. However, for most topically used devices, three rabbits consistently showing little or no response is adequate proof that dermal irritation is not a potential hazard [25]. If the results are equivocal, the three additional rabbits can be added to produce a larger sampling for analysis.

Current thinking among toxicologists is that abraded skin sites, as used in the past, do not show any different response than intact sites. However, this work was performed on

Table 17-3 Primary Irritation Response Categories in Rabbits

Response category	Mean score (PII)[1]
Negligible	0 to 0.4
Slight	0.5 to 1.9
Moderate	2 to 4.9
Severe	5 to 8

[1] The Primary Irritation Index (PII) is determined by adding the Primary Irritation Score for each animal and dividing the total score by the number of animals.

chemicals and it is not known that the information applies to solid materials used in devices. The occluded patches should stay in place a minimum of four hours. Many laboratories leave the patches in place for the full 24 hours, as in the original study design, again because the changes are likely to be subtle. It is suggested that the treated site be observed for erythema and edema at 1, 24, 48 and 72 hours after patch removal. A Primary Irritation Index is calculated by adding all the scores and dividing by the number of dosed sites (Table 17-3). An index of less than 2 would be expected for adhesive electrodes and gels, and less than 0.5 for solid materials. Serious consideration of replacement materials would have to be given if the material proves to be dermally irritating.

When patching adhesive-backed products, there is a tendency to cause mechanical damage to the animal skin. In such cases, nonirritating solvents (alcohol, mineral oil) may be used to help remove the patches. While such mechanical irritation may indeed occur clinically, it is important to separate irritation caused by leachable components vs. mechanical damage.

Mucosal Irritation   These models should be used for materials in contact with parts of the body lined with similar tissue. Everyone can see the need to evaluate ocular products (lenses, solutions) in the various ocular models available [26], but many investigators fail to carry this thinking over to products used in the oral, vaginal and rectal cavities, or in the urethra and/or bladder. Direct contact and extract dosing methods exist for vaginal devices [27, 28, 29] that can readily be adapted to dosing the rectal cavity or the urinary bladder. ISO 10993-10 also provides guidance in this regard. Primary skin irritation methods are simply not adequate to evaluate the irritation potential of devices in contact with mucosal tissue.

Dental materials, which are considered medical devices and subjected to the same international guidelines, present some unique challenges. However, ample methods exist that permit the painting of liquids on rat or hamster cheeks [30], the application of solid pieces of material in cheeks or pouches of hamsters [31], or actual oral implants to mimic clinical situations [32].

Intracutaneous Injection   These test models have been widely used and described in the U.S. Pharmacopeia [7]. For most materials, extracts need to be prepared using saline and cottonseed or sesame oil according to the previously referenced standard methods. Five intradermal injections of 0.2 ml each are given to the fur-clipped skin of a minimum of two rabbits. Each day for up to three days, the injected sites are subjectively scored for erythema and edema, and a comparison is made with a vehicle-only "extract" which is commonly called a "blank." For the most part, all injected sites on each animal tend to react very similarly, and there seems to be no need to individually score injected sites or to manipulate data for individual sites. Conclusions can easily be made on mean scores collected over three days and compared to the control response similarly scored. Care must be taken in selecting a vegetable oil that is low in background irritation. Subtle reactions can be masked if the oil control extract alone produces a score greater than 2 erythema or edema.

The intracutaneous method has a good track record for detecting the presence of irritant or biologically active leachables present in the device. It is by far the irritation screening test of choice for most biomaterials or devices. At times this same method can be modified to dose implantable device materials neat or as used clinically (viscoelastics, biological adhesives, collagens). Small volume doses such as 0.1 ml are given intradermally to rabbit backs, at multiple sites. The smaller volume helps to eliminate pressure necrosis that can occur when larger volumes are forced into the tight intradermal space. Reactions are scored as above. Care must be taken that a "bleb" in the tissue that is caused by sample residue at the site is not scored as "edema." Experienced personnel can distinguish the difference by palpation of the sites.

Acute Systemic Toxicity

As noted in the test requirement matrix (Table 17-1), many devices should be subjected to an acute systemic toxicity screen.

Mouse Injection Test   In many cases, the simple mouse injection test as provided in several Pharmacopeias [7] will suffice. These models were developed for dosing extracts made from polymers used to construct injection vials. They have long been used to evaluate biomaterials used in devices. In most cases, five mice dosed intravenously with a saline extract or dosed intraperitoneally with a vegetable oil extract will provide ample evidence that no significant level of acutely toxic leachables have come from the material. Adverse reactions generally appear within the first 24 hours after dosing. Animals are observed for a minimum of three days. Clinical signs such as lethargy, hyperactivity, convulsions, body weight loss and death are critical parameters monitored and compared to a vehicle control group of mice.

Oral and Dermal Tests   The injection test is quite a severe challenge as the animals are parenterally dosed with an extract prepared under exaggerated conditions and at the highest volume tolerated (50 ml/kg). Care should be taken when considering the acute toxicity potential of materials that are not clinically exposed to mucosal tissue or blood, or that are not injected or implanted. There may indeed be better ways to approach the question. For example, a dental device may be better evaluated by a single oral dose of extracts (aqueous, nonaqueous), or a suspension of pulverized hardened or reacted materials [32]. An electrode gel may better be evaluated by the classical dermal toxicity model as published for cosmetics and household products [24] where a single large g/kg body weight dose is applied to the fur-clipped skin of rabbits or rats. It is important that the acute systemic evaluation have some relevance to the end use of the device.

Pyrogen Test   In recent years, much attention has been given to the material-mediated rabbit pyrogen test. Some believe that there is a potential for chemical leachables from a device to cause a febrile (pyrogenic) reaction in patients. This reaction would be similar to that seen when patients experience intravenous exposure to an endotoxin-contaminated solution. However, the causative agent would be of chemical origin. Therefore, it has become customary to screen new devices intended for blood contact or implantation for material-mediated pyrogenic leachables. Because existing in vitro methods such as the limulus amebocyte lysate gel clot method are specific for the detection of surface endotoxin contamination from gram negative bacteria the in vitro methods cannot be used for this purpose. Only the rabbit pyrogen test as described in various pharmacopeias is considered effective at detecting material-mediated pyrogens. The sample must be extracted in saline according to preparation ratios and temperatures as indicated in Table 17-2, and not subjected only to surface rinsing, as one might do for lot-to-lot release of a final product.

Subchronic Toxicity

These tests determine the effects of constant tissue exposure or repeated treatment to an animal model for a period of time up to 10 per cent of the animal's life span. Such a study would be necessary for any device in contact with the patient for more then 1 day (and up to 30 days). The route of exposure and actual expected length of exposure dictates the animal model to use. Also included in this category of testing would be a device that has very limited exposure to the patient, but with repeated episodes over a period of time, such as periodic treatment over any period of time. Examples are a syringe used to dose a desensitizing solution and instruments and supplies used during in vitro fertilization where the contact may be repeated but not long-term. In contrast, dialysis devices used several times a week for a prolonged period of time would require more extensive evaluation as discussed below.

For the most part, no standard protocols exist for the subchronic evaluation of devices. ISO 10993 Part 11: Tests for Systemic Toxicity [33] does little to help in this regard. The approach taken by this guidance document is to reference numerous classical toxicology methods previously established for the safety evaluation of drugs and industrial chemicals. The investigator must select a protocol that closely resembles what needs to be done, and then must create the modifications necessary to render it applicable to devices. For example, there is rarely a need for multiple concentrations or levels to be given of an extract or implant. Therefore, most device subchronic studies can be conducted with one test and one control level. The referenced protocols are best used for number and type animal to be used, length of time to run the exposure, type of blood studies to conduct and the extent of histopathology and statistical analysis needed. Device toxicologists are challenged to use common sense in adapting referenced protocols to biocompatibility evaluations. The key elements to keep in mind: treatment or implant should mimic end use of the device; constant or repeated exposure must be part of the design; and systemic evaluations must be made. Thus, simple implant studies that have both test and control materials in the same animals, and use local irritant findings to evaluate the device, regardless of the length of time of the implantation, are not acceptable as true "subchronic" evaluations of a device.

Genotoxicity

With the advent (or explosion) of in vitro methods validated for the detection of mutagenic changes, medical devices must undergo genotoxic evaluations with increasing frequency. Prior to this time, there were no reliable methods to evaluate devices. Except in rare cases [34], the methods in widespread use for drugs and industrial chemicals have not been shown to detect mutagenic changes induced by a biomaterial. This is true primarily because device materials have a very low potential to do such harm. However, biologically active leachables from device materials should be fair game for evaluation by any of the in vitro models validated for chemical screening.

According to the previously cited guidance matrix (Table 17-1), devices that contact the body for over 30 days, contact with circulating blood, or are implantable would require

Table 17-4 Implantation Test in Rabbits: Microscopic Evaluation

	Test article	USP negative control	
Inflammation			
Polymorphonuclear	____	____	
Lymphocytes	____	____	
Plasma cells	____	____	
Macrophages	____	____	
Giant cells	____	____	
Necrosis	____	____	
Subtotal (x2)[a]	____	____	
Fibroplasia	____	____	
Fibrosis	____	____	
Fatty infiltrate	____	____	
Subtotal[b]	____	____	
Total[c]	____	____	= ____

Parameters scored on a 0–4 basis. Irritant score key: ≤ 02, nonirritant, 3–8 slight irritant, 9–15 moderate irritant, >15 severe irritant.
[a]Inflammatory response weighted (x2).
[b]Recovery response, not weighted.
[c]Test (−) Control = Irritant Score.

a mutagenicity screen. The most common test is the Ames salmonella bacteria reverse mutation assay. In moving from chemicals or drugs to solid polymers and materials used in devices, one must prepare aqueous (saline) and nonaqueous (DMSO) extracts in the standard fashion (Table 17-2), then subject the extracts to the assay. In the event DMSO degrades the device during extraction, isopropyl alcohol may be used as the medium for extracting the lipid soluble components that may become available to the patient.

In addition to the Ames test which evaluates primarily gene mutations in a bacterial model, there is now a requirement to evaluate DNA and chromosomal effects on mammalian cells [35]. This can be accomplished by established in vitro methods or by means of animal models. The in vitro approach is suggested as the first step. With many of the in vitro methods an extraction of the device can be prepared directly in tissue culture media. A detailed presentation of typical in vitro assays is presented in Chapter 24.

Implantation

As expected, virtually any implantable devices will require an evaluation following implantation in an animal model. Most of the implant methods employed found their basis in the original Pharmacopeia rabbit muscle implant procedures [7]. These procedures have remained essentially unchanged over the years, though there has been some refinement, including the development of histological scoring systems to augment the basic macroscopic observations (see Table 17-4).

While the original implant studies lasted only three to five days, the implant tests used to study the effects of various device materials may be conducted for any length of time, up to the lifespan of the animal, in order to parallel human exposure. The most relevant guidance may be found in ISO 10993 Part 6: Tests for Local Effects Following Implantation [36].

There are several issues to keep in mind when using implant studies to evaluate biomaterials. First, most reviewers (European Notified Body) and regulators (U.S. FDA) are accustomed to seeing a simple muscle implant test on materials that have prolonged or permanent contact with mucosal tissue, blood, or bone, as well as subcutaneous, brain or muscle tissue. A significant body of data and experience exists, and very good reference materials are readily available as negative and positive controls [36]. Much can be understood about a material following a simple screening study such as a two-week implant test in rabbit muscle. Beyond this simple short screen, it is suggested that the implant site and animal model be varied as necessary to mimic the actual clinical implant or exposure site. Animals smaller than the rabbit may be possible for peritoneal and subcutaneous studies, while a larger animal may be better for bone [37] and brain work.

Second, unless implant studies are set up purposely to examine systemic changes in the host (clinical blood studies, remote organ pathology) they are essentially an examination of local reactions at the site of the implant. Such information is very valuable, but regardless of the length of time of implantation, one cannot expect to gather adequate information to meet subchronic and chronic biocompatibility needs. The techniques, animal models, and intervals as discussed by ISO 10993-6 can, however, be helpful in designing such a systemic study.

Thirdly, for devices in contact with the body for more than two weeks, it is important to set the implant intervals to bracket the time of human exposure or to show that the reaction to the implant has stabilized. Thus, a device in contact for two months should be examined at one week and eight weeks. For a biomaterial expected to degrade or absorb over two to three months, sampling intervals should be set during this time of change, such as one, four and twelve weeks. Histopathology should always be a final part of any implant study as much can be learned by microscopic analysis (see Table 17-4, Microscopic Scoring System). Considerably more information can be found about implantology in Sections VI through VIII of this handbook.

Hemocompatibility

Traditionally, toxicologists used red blood cell hemolysis and thrombogenicity as measures of blood compatibility. A more thorough evaluation of hemocompatibility was left to those investigators actually doing efficacy-like studies, or to clinical trials. The reason for this was that standard methods did not exist that would allow for blood compatibility study on materials and devices, and that would predict the performance in clinical use. The myriad of methods found in the literature bears witness to the challenges faced in designing models that can reliably predict blood compatibility.

The guidance document published as ISO 10993 Part 4: Selection of Tests for Interactions with Blood [38] presents the challenge well. This document approaches the issue from the clinician's perspective. The concerns are detailed: thrombosis, coagulation, effects on platelets, effects on hematology, and effects on immunology (complement activation) of the blood. The reader is directed to Chapters 22 and 23 for a better understanding of blood compatibility and a discussion of the frequently used methods available to date.

Chronic Toxicity

Ready-made protocols for systemic toxicity tests do not exist. Guidance can be found in ISO 10993 Part 11: Tests for Systemic Toxicity [33], but there are no protocols described or referenced. For doing systemic toxicity work, one needs to conduct studies similar to those described above, but for longer periods of time. Chronic evaluations, defined as greater than 10 per cent of the animal lifespan (and up until death), are required for all materials in contact with the body for more than 30 days, regardless of the exposure site (see Table 17-1). Common sense dictates that the length of the study need only slightly exaggerate the human exposure time; in the case of a device that is in permanent contact, the study should be conducted for no longer than the average lifespan of the animal model employed. For example, an orthopedic device in the body for two months may be adequately studied over a three-month period in a relevant implant model. An artificial joint expected to remain in place for the lifetime of the host may require study for up to two years in a rat that has a typical life expectancy of 18 to 30 months. In some cases, the length of time may be shortened if the reaction to the material is expected to stabilize, or the material becomes encapsulated, absorbed, or replaced by natural bone or tissue. Very few chronic systemic studies (except for carcinogenicity) may need to go beyond one year in the typical rabbit and rodent models.

Carcinogenicity/Reproductive Toxicity

Biocompatibility studies that address the tumorigenic and teratogenic potential of implantable devices are rarely conducted. At this time, there is heavy reliance on a battery of genotoxicity studies to rule out potential carcinogenicity, as there is evidence of a high correlation between these in vitro assays and lifetime tumorigenic studies in rodents [39].

There is also a sparsity of studies on reproductive effects. This is probably a testament to the clean and relatively safe history of medical devices. Before the need arises to undertake such complex and costly studies, materials that would have the potential to effect changes of these types are generally cast aside in favor of more compatible materials. For example, permanent implants require full characterization of potential leachables and/or degradation products. Should suspicious leachables be detected that may indicate a concern, then such testing would be required. ISO 10993 Part 3: Test for Genotoxicity, Carcinogenicity and Reproductive Effects [35] describes three areas that might require such study:

    (a)   resorbable materials and devices, unless there are significant and adequate data on human use or exposure;
    (b)   materials and devices where positive results have been obtained in genetic toxicity testing on mammalian cells;
    (c)   materials and devices introduced into the body and/or its cavities with a permanent or cumulative contact of 30 days or longer, except when significant and adequate human-use history is available.

In the event carcinogenicity work is needed, there is some guidance available. One such protocol is ASTM F-1439-92 [39], which takes into account that implants are to be studied. A second is OECD Guidelines 451 [40] that provide general guidance but do not address implantables. Typically these lifetime studies are conducted in rodents. Among all the usual arguments surrounding the use of rodents to predict human experience is that of the solid state tumor effect that often manifests itself in animals, due to shape and size of the implant alone [41, 42]. Alternative methods for implanting [43] or repeated dosing of extracts may be attempted, but to date no methods have been accepted as reliable predictors.

Anyone planning carcinogenicity work in laboratory animals should complete a series of in vitro mutagenicity assays, discuss the need with the regulatory body in the country of intended marketing, and then draft a protocol that is scientifically sound and based on published guidance. Care must be taken in the selection of species and strain for the study, the number of animals to implant with the test article, and what (if anything) can be used as negative or positive controls.

As discussed above, none of the traditional methods for the study of reproductive effects have been widely used on devices. Protocols exist for multigenerational study, teratogenicity, and mutagenicity study [44], but are used primarily for drugs and industrial chemicals. It has not been established whether device exposure should be by implantation or repeated dosing with extractions of the device. The extract dosing approach for teratogenicity would be acceptable to pregnant animals during the critical middle phase of gestation (as opposed to implanting and explanting a device). The alternative would be to implant the animals for the entire length of gestation, which would not be consistent with validated methods available to the drug and chemical industries. Multigenerational studies could, on the other hand, be conducted following implantation of the animals. The size (or gram per kilogram body weight) and location of the treatment should mimic and/or exaggerate clinical use of the device. At the present time, there are no defined requirements for the reproductive evaluation of devices. One can surmise that implants placed in younger populations of child-bearing age may be likely candidates for such study, particularly if the device is not considered life-saving or is optional to current treatment.

CONCLUSION

The toxicity test methods presented here, along with the literature citations, provide substantial information to those responsible for evaluating the biocompatibility of medical devices and materials. This scientific field is continuously evolving, and additional in vitro and in vivo models will be needed to better evaluate new generations of biomaterials and devices.

REFERENCES

1   Selecting generic biological test methods for materials and devices, Designation F 748-91. *ASTM Standards Book*, Volume 13. Philadelphia, PA: American Society for Testing and Materials, 198–203.
2   Guidelines for the Preclinical Safety Evaluation of Materials Used in Medical Devices, HIMA Report 85-1.
3   Autian J. The new field of plastics toxicology methods and results. *CRC Critical Reviews—Toxicology*, 2 (1973), 1–40.
4   *Tripartite Biocompatibility Guidance*, GPM#87-1. Washington, DC: DHHS, 1987.
5   Guidance on selection of tests. *Biological Evaluation of Medical Devices*, Part 1. ANSI/AAMI, 1994, 10993–1.
6   Evaluation and testing. *Use of ISO 10993*, Part I. Washington, DC: DHHS, ODE, GPM#95-1, 1995.
7   Biological reactivity tests, *in vivo*. U.S. Pharmacopeia 23, (1995), 1699–1702.
8   Sample preparation and reference materials. *Biological Evaluation of Medical Devices*, Part 12. Draft International Standard (ISO/DIS 10993-12), 1994.
9   Shintani H. The relative safety of gamma-ray, autoclave and ethylene oxide gas sterilization of thermosetting polymers. *Biomedical Instrumentation and Technology*, 29 (1995), 513–519.
10 Wilsnack RE, Meyer FJ, Smith JG. Human cell culture toxicity testing of medical devices and correlation to animal tests. *Biomaterials, Medical Devices and Artificial Organs*, 1, 545–562.
11 Biological reactivity tests, *in vitro*. U.S. Pharmacopeia, 23 (1995), 1697–1699.
12 Tests for cytotoxicity: *In vitro* methods. *Biological Evaluation of Medical Devices*, Part 5. ANSI/AAMI, 1993, 10993–10995.
13 Guess WL. Natural rubber closures: A need for further research. *P&MC Industry*, Mar/Apr 1983, 30–31.
14 Allergic reactions to latex-containing medical devices. FDA Medical Alert, MDA91-1. Washington, DC: DHHS, Mar. 29, 1991.
15 Cosmides G, et al. Alternatives to the use of live vertebrates in biomedical research and testing: An annoted bibliography. *ILAR News*. Washington, DC: National Academy Press, 1952, 34.
16 Skin sensitization testing. Monograph No 14 *European Chemical Industry Ecology and Toxicology*, Mar. 1990.
17 Magnusson B, Klihman AM. The identification of contact allergens by animal assay. The guinea pig maximization test. *J Invest Dermatol*, 52, (1969), 268.

18 Buehler EV. Delayed contact hypersensitivity in the guinea pig. *Arch Dermatol*, 91 (1965), 171.

19 Buehler EV, Griffith JF. Experimental skin sensitisation in the guinea pig and man. In Maibach HI (Ed.) *Animal Models in Dermatology*. London: Churchill Livingstone, 1975, 56.

20 Kimber I, Dearman R. Approaches to the identification and classification of chemical allergens in mice. *J Pharm Tox Methods*, 1 (1993), 11–16.

21 Kabst EA, Mayer M. *Anaphylaxis and Allergy. Experimental Immunology*, 2nd ed. Springfield, IL: Charles C. Thomas, 1961, 268–325.

22 Protein hydrolysiate injection. *U.S. Pharmacopeia*, 23 (1995), 1337–1338.

23 Tests for irritation and sensitization. *Biological Evaluation of Medical Devices*, Part 10. ISO 10993–10, 1995.

24 Federal Hazardous Substances Act Regulations, Code of Federal Regulations Title 16, Consumer Product Safety Communication Part 1500, 1973, 38.

25 Derelanko M, et al. Reliability of using fewer rabbits to evaluate dermal irritation potential. *Fund Applied Tox*, 21 (1993), 159–163.

26 Guidance Document for Class III Contact Lenses. Div. Ophthalmic Devices, ODE/CDRH U. S. FDA, 1988.

27 Auletta C. Vaginal and rectal administration. *J Am Colleqe of Tox*, 1994.

28 Eckstein P, et al. Comparison of vaginal tolerance tests of spermicidal preparations in rabbits and monkeys. *J Reprod Fert*, 20 (1969), 85–93.

29 Chvap LM, et al. Reaction of vaginal tissue of rabbits to inserted sponges of various materials. *J Biomed Mat Res*, 13 (1979), 1–13.

30 Bourrinet P, et al. Interlaboratory study for assessment of potential irritative properties of hygiene products on hamster cheek pouch. *Laboratory Animal Science*, 45 (1995), 36–40.

31 Wilson J, Francis A. The hamster cheek pouch as a model for testing biomaterials. *Evaluation of Biomaterials*. New York: John Wiley & Sons, 1980, 325–332.

32 Secondary tests for biological evaluation of dental materials. *Toxicity Testinq of Dental Materials*. Boca Raton, FL: CRC Press, Inc., 1985, 55–85.

33 Tests for systemic toxicity. *Biological Evaluation of Medical Devices*, Part 11. ANSI/AAMI, 11 (1993), 10993.

34 Schweikl H. Mutagenicity of denture bonding agents. *J Biomed Mat Res*, 28 (1994), 1061–1067.

35 Tests for genotoxicity, carcinogenicity and reproductive effects. *Biological Evaluation of Medical Devices*, Part 3. ANSI/AAMI 3 (1993), 10993.

36 Tests for local effects following implantation. *Biological Evaluation of Medical Devices*, Part 6. ANSI/AAMI, 6 (1995), 10993.

37 Practice for assessment of compatibility of biomaterials for surgical implants, Designation F98183. *ASTM Standards Book*, Volume 13. Philadelphia, PA : American Society for Testing and Materials, 306–310.

38 Selection of tests for interactions with blood. *Biological Evaluation of Medical Devices*, Part 4. ANSI/AAMI, 4 (1993) 10993.

39 Performance of lifetime bioassay for the tumorigenic potential of implant materials, Designation F1439-92. *ASTM Standards Book*, Volume 13. Philadelphia, PA : American Society for Testing and Materials, 761–765.

40 Carcinogenicity studies. OECD Guidelines for Testing Chemicals, No. 451. Paris, France: OECD, 1981.

41 Brand L, Brand K. Testing implant materials for foreign body carcinogenesis. *Biomaterials* (1980), 819.

42 Memol V, et al. Malignant neoplasms associated with orthopedic implant materials in rats. *J Orthoped Res*, 4 (1986), 346–355.

43 Ternant R, et al. Predictions of chemical carcinogenicity in rodents from *in vitro* genetic toxicity. Science, (198), 933–941.

44 *Guideline for the Assessment of Drug and Medical Device Safety in Animals*. Pharmaceutical Manufacturers Assoc., Feb. 1977.

Chapter 18

Hypersensitivity Induction

Katharine Merritt

THE PROBLEM OF HYPERSENSITIVITY REACTIONS TO BIOMATERIALS

Hypersensitivity reactions to biomaterials are of concern since the symptoms they cause in the patient may be of sufficient magnitude to necessitate removal of the device which is otherwise functioning well. These reactions can occur to a variety of devices, ranging from surface-contacting materials to major implants such as total joint replacements. Hypersensitivity reactions are the consequence of the immune system's recognizing components of the biomaterial as foreign and responding in special ways. With increasing knowledge about the mechanisms of the immune response as well as about the components and mechanisms of degradation of the material, the number of these reactions is decreasing. However, these reactions still occur in some individuals and are particularly disturbing since they tend to be unpredictable.

There is abundant literature on the reactions of patients to devices and compilations of the literature are occasionally presented [1–4]. Although the issue of sensitivity to materials was under consideration in the 50s and 60s, it was the reactions to metal-metal total hip joint prostheses necessitating removal of these devices that prompted a closer look at the problem [5–7]. The consequences of an immune reaction to a biomaterial's components vary and range from mild fleeting symptoms to severe compromise of host or device function.

This chapter will discuss the immunological principles behind the reactions and methods to evaluate a material's potential for causing sensitivity reactions. In addition there is a brief discussion on the immune response's role in evaluating materials.

TYPES OF HYPERSENSITIVITY REACTIONS

Hypersensitivity reactions are manifestations of the interaction of the immune system with substances called antigens. The overall mechanisms and manifestations were described in the early 1970s and the framework has not changed significantly [8]. There is deeper understanding of the intercellular communications and the signaling molecules, but the basic concepts remain unaltered.

The generally accepted definition of an antigen is a substance that stimulates the immune response to respond; the immune response in turn reacts specifically to this antigen. It is the extreme specificity of this response which makes it so useful. There is some confusion in this definition of the term "antigen"; the fully correct usage would define a substance that stimulates the immune response as an immunogen or as immunogenic, whereas an antigen reacts with immune response produced. However, "antigen" is the term generally used and some care must be taken to determine if it is immunogenic. This will be explained in more detail later.

What Makes a Substance Immunogenic?

The purpose of the immune response is to protect the body against harmful substances such as bacteria, viruses, toxins, and cancer cells. Thus it must be remembered that the immune response is in general a beneficial response.

Foreign Origin   The first rule of the immune system is that it does not react with self tissue. Thus an immunogenic substance is usually of foreign origin such as the harmful substances listed above. The greater the difference between the substance and our own components, the more likely it will elicit an immune response. This also must be considered when extrapolating animal test results to the human situation. The human may respond to substances in a way that a particular animal species does not, and the reverse also may be true. This is especially a problem in hypersensitivity responses. Animal testing may not detect all substances which can cause sensitivity in humans.

Size   The antigen is processed through a complex series of cellular interactions and therefore it must be of sufficient size. The usual estimate of size cutoff is 5,000 daltons. Substances smaller than that are generally poor immunogens. However, small molecular weight substances may bind to cells or proteins and be presented as a large antigen with only the small substance recognized as foreign. These small substances are called haptens. Haptens are antigenic in that they react with the immune system, but they are not immunogenic until combined with larger carriers.

Chemistry   Proteins are highly immunogenic and thus are also good carriers for haptens. Carbohydrates are often immunogenic, and lipids and nucleic acids are generally non-immunogenic.

Processing   In order for a substance to be immunogenic, it must be processed by the immune system. The exact method of processing is unknown, but in general the immunogens are internalized by macrophages or cells resembling macrophages. These cells are collectively referred to as antigen processing cells (APCs). The substance is degraded by the APCs and presented to the immune system in conjunction with the appropriate human major histocompatibility complex (HLA marker).

The presentation in conjunction with an HLA marker is an important topic in immunology and cannot be treated here with the detail it deserves. The presentation with an HLA marker helps in defining self from nonself, and helps prevent damage to the host [9, 10].

The concept of processing also includes the subject of route of administration. All animals eat things that are foreign and would stimulate an immune response if contacted directly in the bloodstream or tissue. The gastro-intestinal tract is lined with APCs and clusters of lymphocytes which will react with and neutralize antigens. The skin contains dendritic cells called Langerhans Cells [11, 12] which process and present the antigenic message to lymphocytes. There may be similar cells in the buccal mucosa. The brain seems also to have some antigen-processing capacity [13].

Another issue of processing concerns foreign substances that cannot be processed by the APCs. This is often the important issue with biomaterials since the material must be processed by an APC for an immune response to occur. Thus immune responses and hypersensitivity response are not to the material but to degradation products. If the material is not degradable, then one of two things usually happens: (a) the material is biocompatible and the inflammatory system accepts it and walls it off with a fibrous capsule, or (b) the macrophage finds the material not biocompatible and continues to try to phagocytize and digest it. This results in the accumulation of activated or "angry" phagocytic cells and in a chronic inflammatory response with the formation of a large tissue mass. Figure 18-1 depicts the cellular reaction occurring in the peri-implant tissue with polyethylene debris from a total joint replacement.

TYPES OF IMMUNE RESPONSES

The immune response has two separate components, both of which involve lymphocytes. This chapter will not replace a good knowledge of immunology and there are several good textbooks [8, 10, 14]. The hallmark of the immune system is the small lymphocyte. Lymphocytes are part of the group of cells called white cells which circulate in the blood and are present in tissue of specialized organs such as the spleen or lymph nodes. Accumulations may also be seen at the site of an immune reaction. Lymphocytes are classified as T cells, B cells, or null cells. These are identified by markers to be discussed shortly. The antigen is processed by the APC and then in most cases is presented to a particular T cell called a T helper cell. This cell reacts with the HLA signal and the antigen fragment and presents it to either a B cell or a T cell. How this choice of B or T cell is made is still an immunologic mystery. However, it is now recognized that there are two types of T helper cells, Th1 and Th2, and elucidation of their responses may answer this question.

B Cell Responses

The B cell is the initiating cell of the arm of the immune response called humoral immunity. The B cell possesses on its surface small amounts of antibody which will react with the antigen. This reaction leads to B cell differentiation into plasma cells. Plasma cells are protein factories and produce the protein antibody that is specific for the antigenic stimulus; this antibody will react specifically with this particular antigen in the body or in the test tube. By definition, antibodies react with antigens, and all antibodies are immunoglobulins. Immunoglobulin (Ig), the generic term for these proteins, can be of any of five classes. IgM is produced first and is also, along with IgD, one of the immunoglobulins on the surface of the B cell recognizing the antigen. IgG, produced later in the immune response, is in higher concentration; IgA is produced at surfaces—notably the GI tract; IgE is produced in small quantities but is responsible for one type of hypersensitivity reaction. These five types of antibodies circulate in the blood and may be found in tissue fluid. B cells and plasma cells may be found in the tissue at the site of the antigen.

T Cell Responses

If the helper T cell presents the antigen to another T cell, which is usually called the cytotoxic T cell, then the resultant immune reactions are called cell-mediated immunity. This immune response involves the accumulation of lymphocytes at the site of the antigen.

Identification of B Cells and T Cells

These cells are all small lymphocytes and thus morphologically they are identical. They can, however, be specifically identified on the basis of surface markers. The B cell as indicated above has IgM and IgD on the surface. Thus procedures identifying these molecules will

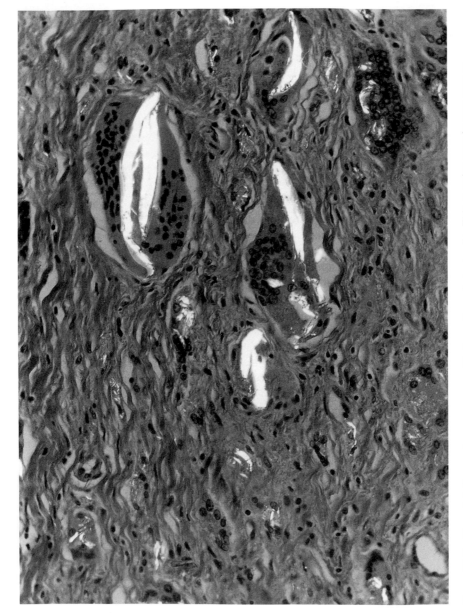

Figure 18-1 Chronic inflammatory response with formation of giant cells. This reaction was in response to polyethylene particles.

identify which lymphocytes are B cells. T cells do not contain immunoglobulins. However they do have special markers in the group called cluster differentiation antigens (CD markers). All T cells express the marker CD3 and most also express CD2. Thus these are pan T cell markers and will give a total count of T cells. The T helper cell expresses CD4 in addition to CD3, and testing for CD4 will identify T helper cells. The T cytotoxic cells express CD3 and CD8 but not CD4. Thus in doing an immunologic work-up, a blood sample can be obtained and aliquoted for four tests: a total white cell count, a total lymphocyte count, the per cent expressing immunoglobulins, and the per cent expressing CD3. This will indicate the general health of the immune response since about 20 per cent of the white cells should be lymphocytes. The number of T cells should be about twice that of the B cells. Then additional tests can be done with CD4 and CD8 markers to determine the number of T helper and T cytotoxic cells. The number of CD4 expressing cells should be greater than those expressing CD8. Alteration in these values will indicate an immunological problem [14].

Null Cells

These are small lymphocytes lacking the CD3 markers or immunoglobulins on their surfaces and therefore are not identified as T or B cells. Whether these null cells have temporarily lost their identifying surface markers, have yet to express them, or are a separate subset of small lymphocytes remains to be determined.

CLASSIFICATION OF HYPERSENSITIVITY REACTIONS

Hypersensitivity is most simply defined as the inadvertent damage to the host as a result of an immune reaction. What was supposed to be a beneficial response eliminating foreign substances, instead harms the host. Allergy, sensitivity, and hypersensitivity are generally used synonomously. Hypersensitivity reactions fall into several classifications; the one this chapter will use is the classification of Type I, II, III, and IV [8, 10, 14]. Types I–III are mediated by the humoral system (antibody), whereas Type IV is mediated by T cells.

Type I Hypersensitivity

This reaction is mediated by the reaction of IgE antibody with antigen. Ragweed allergy (hay fever) is the most common of these. The reaction of the IgE antibody, which is usually attached to the surface of specialized cells in the tissue, with antigen results in the release of vasoactive amines, including histamine, from these specialized cells. These vasoactive amines cause the runny nose, watery itching eyes, itching and swelling in the skin. Severe reactions in the bloodstream lead to anaphylactic shock and are life-threatening. These reactions occur within minutes of contact with the antigen. This type of hypersensitivity is the most feared of all the reactions, and materials are usually carefully screened for their ability to stimulate IgE responses. However, animal models for human IgE responses are not adequate. Despite screening tests, this hypersensitivity reaction is occurring to latex products, such as examining gloves, and has been observed to occur to collagen products.

Type II Hypersensitivity

Type II Hypersensitivity reactions are similar in end result to that of Type I but the mechanism is different. In this case, instead of the IgE antibody being on the surface of cells with the vasoactive amines, the antigen is on the surface. Antibody of the IgG or IgM class will then react with the antigen and cause permutations of the cell membrane and the release of these vasoactive amines. This rarely occurs with biomaterials. It is much more of a concern with drugs that bind to platelets. However, any small substance can cause Type II reactions, and it may be a special problem with the biomaterial-based drug delivery systems.

Type III Hypersensitivity

Type III hypersensitivity is rarely seen. This results from the precipitation of antigen-antibody complexes in the small blood vessels blocking blood flow. The symptoms are apparent from specialized organs with small blood vessels as important components and are most commonly expressed in lung, kidney, and joints. For this sensitivity reaction to occur, the antigen and antibody must both be present at the same time, in the correct proportions. This is rare with biomaterials and again is most likely to occur in slow release or slow degradation materials with constant antigenic stimulation of the system.

Type IV Hypersensitivity

Type IV hypersensitivity results from the reaction of cell-mediated immunity. The cytotoxic T cells and macrophages accumulate at the site of the antigen and cause a reaction which ranges from swelling to massive tissue destruction. The most recognized of these reactions is contact dermatitis, of which poison ivy is a common example. Many chemicals cause a contact dermatitis. This hypersensitivity is of concern in the use of biomaterials, and the reaction may be local to the skin, local in the deep tissue, or systemic, depending on the location of contact. Most of the reactions to the biomaterials are due to the fact that the chemicals used to make these materials are used commonly in the activities of daily living. Metal salts, corroding metals, jewelry, cookware, and flatware all can cause sensitivity reactions, with nickel, cobalt, and chromium being common causes of contact dermatitis. These metals are components of stainless steel or cobalt-chromium alloys used in implants. Thus reactions can occur in previously sensitized individuals. These Type IV reactions have been observed to occur to various other materials, including collagen products, latex, and acrylics.

CYTOKINES

It has been recognized in the last two decades that intercellular communication in the immune response involves soluble mediators called cytokines [8, 10, 14]. These are substances that are produced by one cell and influence another cell which may or may not be of the same type. Some of these cytokines are produced by macrophages and some by lymphocytes. Again, this is a complex subject and the reader desiring more information is referred to other sources [15–17].

Many of these cytokines fall into the category of interleukins (IL). The best studied to date are IL-1, which seems to be important in responses to cardiovascular materials; IL-1's subset IL-1b, which stimulates bone-resorbing cells; IL-2, which promotes the growth of lymphocytes; IL-4, which is important in the development of B and mast cells and in the responses of certain T cells; IL-6, which is important in macrophage lymphocyte interaction and also a factor in bone resorption; IL-10, which affects the production of a number of other interleukins and cytokines; and IL-12, which also seems to control the immune response and is less well studied.

Among the cytokines not classified as interleukins but important in the biological reaction to implants are the interferons, tumor necrosis factor alpha (TNFa), and the simple molecule nitric oxide (NO) [19, 20]. These are proinflammatory molecules and have a major impact in controlling inflammatory and immune responses. Prostaglandin E2 (PGE2) also plays a major role in responses to biomaterials since it interacts with other cells and seems to have a role in bone resorption. Although the impact of these simple molecules on the biological response remains to be elucidated, the reader needs to be aware of their existence so as to understand this rapidly developing area.

EVALUATING BIOMATERIALS FOR IMMUNE AND HYPERSENSITIVITY RESPONSES

Testing for biocompatibility of materials is generally done under the categories described by ISO 10993 (21) and ASTM 748 [22]. Extracts and degradation products of the material must be included in the testing. The immunological testing described in these documents specifies only testing for dermal sensitivity in animals. The ISO document also suggests testing for IL-1 release with blood-contacting materials. Other aspects of the immune response which are important in evaluation of biocompatibility may be covered in future documents.

Immunotoxicity

Immunotoxicity covers the testing of whether or not a substance alters the general immune system. It does not address the issue of whether it is immunogenic. The test parameters include total lymphocyte counts, the identification of T and B cells, responses of T cells to mitogens, and total immunoglobulins produced. Again these are not markers of immune responses or hypersensitivity, but determine aspects of toxicity to the immune system.

Testing for Specific Immune Responses and Sensitivity

These are important tests to be done on substances that are intended to be implanted in the body and that may be immunogenic. Testing should be done with the intact biomaterial and with the extracts and degradation products.

Choice of Animal   Since the immune responses are under genetic control in the animals, there are responders and non-responders. Ideally the biomaterial is tested in the species in which the product will be used. However, screening tests are often done in experimental animals. Because the immune responses of the guinea pig most closely resemble human responses, preliminary tests are generally done in this species. Rabbits, mice, hamsters, and rats are sometimes used for special aspects. However, clinical testing is generally needed, and the patients receiving the device are followed for specific and nonspecific immune responses.

In Vivo **Responses**   The skin test is generally the only in vivo test done. Extracts or degradation products are injected just under the skin or placed onto the skin. The site is observed at 15 minutes, 30 minutes, 24 hours and 48 hours. Hypersensitivity reactions of Type I (IgE mediated), with redness and swelling from fluid accumulation, will occur in 15–30 minutes. This test needs to be done carefully by trained personnel, since the procedure can produce life-threatening Type I responses in highly sensitive patients. Type IV reactions occur in 24–48 hours and are marked by redness and swelling from a hard tissue mass of accumulated cells. Most of the tests for humoral immune responses and some for the cell-mediated responses are done in vitro using blood obtained from the patient.

In Vitro Testing   Testing procedures for the specific immune response to substances are well defined. Protocols are available in immunologic methods books [23, 24] and only briefly reviewed here.

Most of the tests for responses of the humoral immune system are done using solid phase assays and based on enzyme markers (ELISA or EIA tests) or radio-isotope markers (RIA). These test protocols are defined to either measure antibody or antigen. Since in the biocompatibility tests we are usually interested in determining whether a patient has produced an immune response to a substance and what type of antibody is produced, we will use a protocol to measure antibody. The procedure is simple and involves multiple washings to remove unbound material after each step. The first step is to attach the antigen to a solid surface such as polystyrene tubes or wells. Many substances will adhere by themselves at a neutral to high pH. Some substances will bind to proteins, such as albumin, already coating the plate [25, 26]. The patient's serum is then allowed to interact with the solid surface. Then antisera directed against the human IgG, IgM, or IgE antibodies are reacted with the complex. These antisera are tagged with an enzyme or a radio-isotope. The amount of enzyme or radio-isotope reacting is then measured and the magnitude of the immune response determined. These well-documented, simply performed tests require only small amounts of serum and clearly identify the production of immune responses directed specifically against the antigen.

The tests for cell-mediated immunity use white cells obtained in the blood sample. These tests have several drawbacks: the cells must be alive when the tests are done, strict aseptic technique is required, and the procedures are lengthy and relatively difficult. The tests are based on the knowledge that T cells responding to an antigen will produce soluble factors. The cytokines then cause other T cells and perhaps B cells to divide. Thus the number of cells increases. This can be detected by doing cell counts or by using a radio-labeled substance such as tritiated thymidine or I-125 or I-131 labeled uridine which will be taken up by dividing cells. The magnitude of increase in cell count at 5–7 days is indicative of the immune response to the substance added. Some substances are pan T cell stimulants and therefore control populations need to be included in the test to distinguish an immunogen from a pan T cell stimulant. This test is commonly called the lymphocyte transformation test (LTT).

Another factor that is produced is called migration inhibition factor. This factor is produced by lymphocytes and prevents the amoeboid movement of cells such as polymorphonuclear leukocytes and macrophages. These tests are simple to perform.

Much of the work on biological responses to particulate debris is based on detecting the release of cytokines following macrophage-particle interactions. The most commonly tested are IL-1, Il-6, TNFa, PGE2, and NO in murine cells [27, 28]. Commercial test kits or simple reagents are available for these assays. In some circumstances the production of these substances following lymphocyte interaction with antigens is being assessed. This is a rapidly growing area of research and evaluation.

EFFECTS ON THE SPECIFIC IMMUNE RESPONSE

In addition to determining a substance's ability to influence the immune system, to stimulate specific humoral responses, or to stimulate specific cell-mediated responses, it is important to determine the effect of the material on immune responses to other antigens. Tests to determine if the material suppresses or enhances specific immune responses to unrelated antigens may be needed. Substances to boost the immune system have been sought for years and there are many substances bought over the counter, including vitamins and natural products, that are touted to boost resistance to disease and cancer. In addition, there are substances sold as adjuvants that are designed to boost the immune response in animals being used to raise immunologic reagents, or added to vaccines to boost the immune response in domestic and farm animals as well as humans. The actual mechanism by which the adjuvants work is often obscure, but basically they either stimulate the lymphocytes directly to grow and divide or they provide a slow release of antigen for a continual stimulation over several days. Oily substances, gels, and colloidal suspensions are known to serve as adjuvants and materials falling into these categories should be evaluated. Unfortunately, we may not know what to do with the answer since substances that enhance the immune system are believed to be advantageous, as long as they don't stimulate undesirable responses.

CONCLUSIONS

With the increasing development of biomaterials, including materials of animal origin, genetically engineered products, or implantation of cell systems, it is critical to understand the problems that can result from specific immune responses and hypersensitivity responses to the material and from immunotoxicity of the device.

Although procedures for evaluating materials and responses are already available, immunological tests must be carefully performed with extracts and degradation products to prove the safety of those materials. Some specified tests are designed for biocompatibility testing in animal systems, some are designed for testing patients in clinical trials, and some can be used for diagnosis of specific problems.

Since immune reactions, especially hypersensitivity reactions, are under genetic control, animal testing is not a final step and clinical evaluations are needed. Even with clinical evaluations, the percentage of patients with the propensity to develop such sensitivity reactions may be so small that the responses do not occur in the test populations. We cannot assure that no patient will respond; however, we can keep the responses to a minimum with adequate testing.

REFERENCES

1   Menne T, Maibach HI. Systemic contact allergy reactions. *Immunol Allergy Clinic N.A.*, 9 (1989), 507–522.
2   Merritt K. Biochemistry/hypersensitvity/clinical reaction. In Lang BR, Morris HF, Razzoog ME (Eds.), *International Workshop on Biocompatibility, Toxicity, and Hypersensitivity to Alloy Systems Used in Dentistry.* Ann Arbor, MI: The University of Michigan Press, 1986, 195-s 223.
3   Gawkrodger DJ. Nickel sensitivity and the implantation of orthopaedic prostheses. *Contact Dermatitis,* 28 (1994), 257–259.
4   Merritt K, Brown SA. Effects of metal particles and ions on the biological system. *Techniques in Orthopaedics,* 8 (1993), 228–236.
5   Evans EM, Freeman MAR, Miller AJ, Vernon-Roberts B. Metal sensitivity as a cause of bone necrosis and loosening of the prosthesis in total joint replacement. *J Bone Joint Surg,* 56B (1974), 626–642.
6   Benson MKD, Goodwin PG, Brostoff J. Metal sensitivity in patients with joint replacement arthroplasties. *Brit Med J,* 4 (1975), 374–375.
7   Elves MW, Wilson JN, Kemp HBS. Incidence of metal sensitivity in patients with total joint replacements. *Brit Med J,* 4 (1975), 376–378.
8   Roitt I. *Essential Immunology.* London: Blackwell Scientific Publications, 1971.
9   Chicz RM, Urban RG. Analysis of MHC presented peptides: Applications in autoimmunity and vaccine development. *Immunology Today,* 15 (1994), 155–160.
10 Benjamin E, Leskowitz S. *Immunology. A Short Course.* New York: Wiley-Liss, 1991.
11 Kimber EA. Epidermal cytokines in contact hypersensitivity: Immunological roles and practical applications. *Toxicology in vitro,* 7 (1993), 295–298.

12   Choi KL, Sauner DN. The role of Langerhans cells and keratinocytes in epidermal immunity. *J Leuk Biol*, 39 (1986), 343–358.

13   Streit WJ, Kincaid-Colton CA. The brain's immune system. *Scientific American*, 273 (1995), 54–61.

14   Golub ES, Green DR. *Immunology, A Synthesis*, 2nd ed. Sunderland, MA: Sinauer Assoc., 1992.

15   Julius M, Maroun CR, Haughn L. Overview of functions of CD4 and CD8. *Immunology Today*, 4 (1993), 177–182.

16   Mizel SB. The interleukins. *The FASEB J*, 3 (1989), 2379–2388.

17   Miyajima A, Kitamura T, Harada N, Yokota T, Arai K-I. Cytokine receptors and signal transduction. *Annual Review of Immunology*, 10 (1992), 295–331.

18   Goldring SR, Goldring MB. Cytokines and skeletal physiology. *Clin Orthop Rel Res*, 324 (1996), 13–23.

19   James SI. Role of nitric oxide in parasitic infections. *Microbiol Rev*, 59 (1995), 533–547.

20   Oppenheim JJ. Summary of the fifth conference on the molecular mechanisms and physiological activities of cytokines. *J Leuk Biol*, 56 (1994), 687–691.

21   *AAMI Standards and Recommended Practices in Biological Evaluation of Medical Devices*, Vol 4. Arlington, VA: AAMI, 1995.

22   *ASTM Book of Standards*, Vol 13. Philadelphia, PA: American Society for Testing and Materials, 1995.

23   Rose NR, Friedman H. *Manual of Clinical Immunology*. Washington, DC: American Society for Microbiology, 1992.

24   Coligan JE, Kruisbeek AM, Margulies DH, Shevach EM, Strober W. *Current Protocols in Immunology*. New York: John Wiley, 1992.

25   Yang J, Merritt K. Detection of antibodies against corrosion products in patients after Co-Cr total joint replacements. *J Biomed Mater Res*, 28 (1994), 1249–1258.

26   Wolf LE, Lappe M, Peterson RD, Ezrailson EG. Human immune response to polydimethylsiloxane (silicone) screening studies in a breast implant population. *FASEB J* & (1993), 1265–1268.

27   Shanbhag AS, Jacobs JJ, Black J, Galante JO, Glant TT. Human monocyte response to particulate biomaterials generated in vivo and in vitro. *J Orthop Res*, 13 (1995), 792–801.

28   Horowitz SM, Purdon MA. Mediator interactions in macrophage/particulate bone resorption. *J Biomed Mater Res*, 29 (1995), 477–484.

Chapter 19

Tumor Induction

W. Homer Lawrence
James T. Dalton

REASONS FOR CONCERN

Observations of malignant tumors in association with implanted synthetic polymers and other foreign materials have been reported in both humans and experimental animals for a number of years. The question of whether or not there is a causal relationship between implanted materials and tumor development in humans is still not resolved. However, continued clinical reports of tumor occurrence, coupled with demonstrated production of tumors by implanted materials in animals, has created concern that implanted biomaterials and/or devices may induce malignant tumor formation in humans. A number of clinical reports of tumors in humans, in association with implanted materials, is summarized in Table 19-1.

Material-induced malignant tumors have been well documented in experimental animals, particularly in rodents. Experimentally, tumors (principally sarcomas) have been produced by almost all solid materials tested, including various synthetic polymers, glass, and metal films. Clinically, tumors have been reported in association with implanted synthetic polymers and metals as well as with asbestos, unremoved bullets, and shrapnel. Various terms have been applied to this phenomenon, such as a solid-state, foreign-body (FB), smooth-surface, or material-induced carcinogenesis. In this chapter, we will focus on tumor induction by synthetic polymers that may find use as, or in, biomedical devices.

BACKGROUND

Recognition of material-induced carcinogenesis is often attributed to Turner [1], who in 1941 reported a sarcoma around a bakelite disk implanted subcutaneously (sc) in the rat. Oppenheimer et al. [2] reported sarcomas in rats after wrapping one kidney in cellophane; their intention was to produce hypertensive rats. This was followed by sc implants that also produced sarcomas. During the next decade or so, Oppenheimer and associates investigated various aspects of material-induced tumors, such as material specificity, latent periods, precancerous stages, and importance of physical forms of the material [3–8].

In 1959, Alexander and Horning [9] reported the results of studies to determine a "critical size" necessary to produce solid-state carcinogenicity, a term suggested by Bischoff and Bryson in 1964 [10] Goldhaber [11, 12] and Dukes and Mitchley [13] presented data that support the earlier observations of Oppenheimer et al. [5] concerning the importance of impermeability of the implanted material. Bates and Klein [14] found a higher incidence of tumors from a smooth film than from the same film roughened prior to implantation.

From these early investigations, one can derive a number of characteristics for the phenomenon termed "solid-state carcinogenesis." Some of the major ones are:

1 Composition of the material per se appears to be of little importance (unless it contains leachable carcinogens) because a wide variety of materials elicit a similar response.

Table 19-1   Some Material-Associated Tumors in Humans

Material	Application	Reported tumors	References
Medical device and polymethylmeth-acrylate	Total hip arthroplasty	Malignant fibrous histocytoma	Bago-Granell, et al.[57]
Metal grenade fragments	War wound	Angiosarcoma	Hayman and Huygens[58]
Mandibular staple bone plate	Repair mandible	Squamos cell carcinoma	Friedman and Vernon[59]
Dacron, woven	Repair abdominal aortic aneurysm	Angiosarcoma	Fehrenbacher et al.[60]
Silicone prostheses	Metacarpophalangeal joints of both hands	Malignant lymphoma	Digby and Wells[61]
Dacron, woven	Repair abdominal aortic aneurysm	Primary malignant fibrous histocytoma	Weinberg and Maini[62]
Vitatron pacemaker	Cardiac pacemaker	"Breast cancer," 2 cases	Dalal et al.[63]
Vitallium	Sherman plate and screws	Ewing's sarcoma	Tayton[64]
Medtronic model 5942 pacemaker	Cardiac pacemaker	Carcinoma of breast, 2 cases	Biran et al.[65]
Silicone gel-filled prosthesis	Augmentation mammaplasty	Infiltrating duct cell adenocarcinoma	Hausner et al.[66]
Dacron, woven prosthesis	Arterial graft	Sarcoma	O'Connell et al.[67]
Vitatron pacemakers	Cardiac pacemaker	Carcinoma, 2 cases	Zafiracopoulos and Rouskas[68]
Teflon—Dacron, woven	Prosthetic, femoral artery	Fibrosarcoma	Herrmann et al.[69]
Polymethylmeth-acrylate (Lucite)	Extrapleural plombage	Chondrosarcoma extraskeletal	Thompson and Entin[70]
Silicone sponge (Silastic, RTV 53G2)	Augmentation mammaplasty	Carcinoma	Hoopes et al.[71]
Polyurethane (Etheron)	Augmentation mammaplasty	Carcinoma	Hoopes et al.[71]
Polyvinyl alcohol (Ivalon)	Augmentation mammaplasty	Carcinoma, 2 cases	Hoopes et al.[71]

2   A continuous, impermeable surface is important since perforations, weaves, or powders tend to reduce or abolish tumorigenicity of the material.

3   The implant must be of at least a minimum ("critical") size.

4   The implant must remain in situ for a minimum period of time. The studies of Oppenheimer et al. [6] found the presarcomatous changes occurred when the material was in place for about 6 months, although tumors may not appear for many more months.

With this very brief background, we now consider some of the theories that have evolved for this phenomenon.

THEORIES FOR MATERIAL-INDUCED CARCINOGENICITY

Theories for material-induced carcinogenicity can be separated into five broad categories: (a) chemical leachables, (b) biodegradation products, (c) physical contact of the material,

(d) facilitation of maturation for existing preneoplastic cell(s), or (e) a combination of two or more of these.

Chemical Leachables

Some chemicals with demonstrated (or suspected) carcinogenic potential are employed in polymer synthesis and device production. Consequently, there may be carcinogenic substances (residues from synthesis or fabrication, contaminants, sterilization residues or degradation products, etc.) in the material and/or device that are released to the tissues following implantation or contact. While this may account for some cases of carcinogenicity, accumulated data indicate that it does not adequately explain most cases of material-induced tumors.

Biodegradation

Although synthetic polymeric materials were once thought to be inert to the biological environment and immune to degradation by the biologic system, we now know this is generally not the case. Ample evidence has been presented to show that synthetic polymeric materials can be altered or degraded by prolonged exposure to the biological system. Harrison [15], Leininger et al. [16], and Leininger [17] found that many polymeric materials showed a decrease in tensile strength and/or percent elongation after being implanted in dogs for a few months to 3 years. Mirkovitch et al. [18] found polyurethane strips lost 77% of their tensile strength when implanted for 8 months in the abdominal wall of dogs, and that polyurethane aortic grafts became distorted, stiff, and brittle during 3-year implantations in dogs. Harrison [15] reported, along with other adverse effects, the complete breakdown of the nylon fabric in an aortic graft after 21 months in a dog, resulting in a dissecting aneurysm that ruptured. Oppenheimer et al. [5] and Sherman and Lyons [18], using ^{14}C-labeled polymers, reported biodegradation of implanted polystyrene, polyethylene, polymethyl methacrylate [5], and polyurethane [19].

Hueper [20] suggested that tumors he found after implanting a polyurethane foam or powder, but not disks, in rats resulted from biodegradation products of the polyurethane. In this study, Hueper found carcinomas more frequently than sarcomas; this is in contrast to most studies of "solid-state" tumorigenesis in which sarcomas predominated. Autian et al. [21], using particles below the "critical size," implanted a group of 17 chemically different polyurethanes and one polyethylene in rats for a 2-year study to see if they could correlate tumorigenicity with chemical structure of the polymers. (If the polyurethanes are biodegraded to carcinogenic substances, one might expect to find that the tumorigenic potential varied with chemical structure of the polymers, unless the primary carcinogen was a common feature of all the polyurethanes.) They found tumorigenic incidence varied with the implanted material, but did not find a consistent correlation with chemical structure; the polyethylene also produced a significant incidence of tumors. In a follow-up study [22] this group, using the most tumorigenic polyurethane from the previous study, found a positive relationship between incidence of tumors and quantity of polymer implanted, and an inverse relationship between time for detection of tumors and quantity implanted.

Earlier studies by Oppenheimer et al. [6] produced sarcomas in rats implanted sc with a nylon film, but not when the nylon was powdered prior to implantation. Since the nylon powder would expose a much greater surface area, and hence should be more susceptible to biodegradation, this would imply the carcinogenic activity of nylon was not due to biodegradation of the polymer. In 1953, Fitzhugh [23] suggested that free radicals from the polymers might be responsible for tumor initiation, a concept that was not supported by Oppenheimer et al. [24].

Physical Contact

Physical contact induces tumors by causing the formation of reactive centers on the polymer and blocking metabolism of adjacent cells. Oppenheimer et al. [5] suggested the possibility of "creation of reactive centers in the polymer as a result of degradation" (biodegradation) to which proteins or other basic tissue constituents might bind. This concept of biological molecules reacting with or binding to synthetic polymers in vivo and speculation about the forces involved were supported by Kordan [25] and Ecanow et al. [26]. Molecular/cellular binding to the foreign polymer may create physiochemical changes that alter adjacent cellular metabolism, thereby promoting tumor initiation [5, 26].

On the other hand, Brand et al. [27] concluded that "preneoplastic cells have acquired their neoplastic determination at a site distant from the implanted foreign body (FB) and independent of direct physical or chemical reaction with it." They exclude the FB as the direct inducer of "cellular neoplastic potential and determination," a theory that is compatible with sarcoma production by various implanted materials.

Facilitation of Maturation for Existing Preneoplastic Cells

In 1959, Alexander and Horning [9] suggested the mode of action for material-induced tumors might be that "the film alters the normal environment of the neighboring cells in such a way as to favor the induction (or selection) of discontinuous variations leading to malignancy." Furthermore, they suggested that the action of the carcinogenic implant "might be to create an environment which provides a favourable condition for the establishment of the spontaneously mutated cell."

This concept for solid-state (or FB) carcinogenesis is described in detail by Brand et al. [27]. Briefly, the implanted polymeric material induces cellular proliferation and its encapsulation. Cells with neoplastic determination may be present in normal tissue. The capsule around the implanted material must undergo a series of sequential changes to provide the necessary environment for the cells with neoplastic determination to undergo preneoplastic development and provide the FB surface for preneoplastic cells to mature. Various aspects of this process have been described by Brand, Buoen and associates [27–42].

Several years earlier, Oppenheimer et al. [6] studied the presarcomatous stage and latent periods of tumor formation in rats following implantation of a polystyrene film. They found that removal of the film [while leaving the pockets (capsules) in place] within 6 months did not result in subsequent tumor formation at the implant sites, but if the films were in place for more than 6 months before removal, tumors may still form at the sites. However, if both the films and pockets were removed within 12 months after implantation, tumors were not subsequently produced at the implant sites. Furthermore, they reported that tumors seemed to originate in the inner layer of the capsule adjacent to the implanted material, a finding that is in general agreement with that of Brand et al. [27].

Combined Effects

There is also the possibility that two or more of these mechanisms may be involved in some cases of tumorigenesis. For example, a chemical leachable or biodegradation product may induce neoplastic change in adjacent cell(s), and the capsular environment permits it to develop, mature, and express itself as a tumor.

FACTORS WHICH MODIFY TUMORIGENICITY

Implant Size

The implant must be of sufficient size to induce solid-state tumors. In the sc site of rats, Alexander and Horning [9] determined the "critical size" to be approximately 0.5×0.5 cm, with larger implants exhibiting greater tumor-inducing activity. The critical or threshold size for humans is not known, but if the rat data were extrapolated to humans, based upon body size, it would require a very large implant. However, Bischoff and Bryson [10] point out that this phenomenon has a functional relationship to adjacent cells, and a weight comparison is not applicable: "the quantitative factors are not only animal *versus* implant size, but also the number of cells in contact with the unbroken smooth surface (threshold size)."

Surface

Maximum tumorigenesis is present when the material has a smooth, continuous surface. Tumorigenic incidence is reduced if the surface is roughened [14], contains perforations [6, 11–13], or is woven [6], or if the material is powdered [6].

Irritation

Mechanical irritation per se from implanted materials does not seem to induce tumor formation [3, 6]. This concept is supported by Northdurft [43], who found that the original nodule of a solid-state tumor did not develop at a sharp edge or corner of an implant where the greatest mechanical irritation should occur, and Salyamon [44] who concluded that nonspecific inflammation has an anticarcinogenic effect, whereas "carcinogenesis is a result of inhibition of inflammation."

Rigidity of Implant

Variations in flexibility or rigidity of an implant appear to have little or no influence upon tumorigenicity [6], unless (a) the flexible implant becomes folded or displaced, or (b) the rigid implant becomes broken or produces continual irritation. In both of these cases (a and b) the tumorigenicity tends to be reduced or abolished.

Duration

The implant must remain in situ for a sufficient period of time to induce tumors via the solid-state mechanism; short-term contact appears to be ineffective. In the rat, the latent period was determined to be about 6 months, with appearance of tumors after approximately 300 days or more [6]. Comparable periods have not been established in man, although Druckrey [45] has suggested that the latent period may be as much as 50 to 60 years in some cases.

Species and Strains

There are marked differences between species with regard to induction of solid–state (FB) tumorigenesis. Rats and mice appear to be particularly susceptible, hamsters and dogs less susceptible, while chickens and guinea pigs are especially resistant [46]. Material-induced tumors have been produced in many strains of rats and mice, although there appears to be some quantitative differences in incidences and/or latent periods.

Age and Sex

Most studies on material-induced tumors are initiated in young animals to provide for long-term observation. However, data from Oppenheimer et al. [6] and Brand et al. [46] indicate that age of the animal at implantation does not significantly affect tumor formation. The length of the latent period for solid-state carcinogenesis is not determined by the age of the animal, "but according to the time necessary for certain changes to occur" [6]. Both male and female animals have been used to demonstrate tumor formations. In some cases, there appears to be little or no difference between males and females, whereas in other cases there may be slight differences in latent periods and/or incidence of tumors.

EXPERIMENTAL EVALUATION OF BIOMATERIAL TUMORIGENICITY

Evaluating a potential biomaterial for solid-state, smooth-surface, FB, or materialinduced carcinogenicity raises some very basic questions: "What is one looking for?" "What action is to be evaluated?" "Is it relevant to humans?"

There are indications that this phenomenon is real and reproducible in rodents. A number of material-associated tumors in humans have been reported, although a causal relationship has not been demonstrated. Some believe materials implanted in humans pose a significant risk for tumor induction. On the other hand, there are those who contend the solid-state (FB or smooth-surface) mechanism of carcinogenesis does not operate in humans, and the low incidence of reported material-associated tumors in humans is simply coincidental and not induced by the material.

Rationale

Experimental induction of tumors in rodents by implanted materials is a generally recognized phenomenon; however, there is considerable controversy concerning its applicability to implanted biomaterials and devices in humans. Consequently, until more definitive data are available, it would be prudent to evaluate new biomaterials, intended for long-term implantation, to ensure that they do not exhibit undue tumor-inducing activity. It would appear, at this time, that the most suitable test would involve long-term implantations in the rat.

Previous studies of material-induced tumorigenesis in rodents generally reveal that only a portion of the implanted animals produce demonstrable tumors during the observation periods (for example, see Refs. 6 and 21). A time difference between implantation of the material and appearance of tumors has also been observed. Thus, an in vivo evaluation of a candidate biomaterial in the rat should be designed to determine the *relative incidence* of tumor production and the *relative rapidity* of tumor formation as compared to a material that has been clinically satisfactory for a long time, if possible, when used for the same purpose or in a very similar manner.

Tumorigenic Evaluation in the Rat

The experiment is designed for 2 years or more; thus young rats of 6 to 8 weeks of age are selected as the experimental animals. If only one sex is employed, male rats would be recommended. However, the phenomenon has been observed in many experiments using both male and female rats and mice. A sufficient number of rats should be used in each group to permit statistical evaluation of the results for up to 2 years postimplantation. There should be three or more groups of rats of equal numbers: (1) one or more to be implanted with the biomaterial(s) under evaluation; (2) one with a "reference material" (a clinically satisfactory material that has a long history of usage, if possible, and that is used in the same or very similar manner to that for the proposed use of the biomaterial under investigation); and (3) a sham-operated group in which the implantation procedure is performed but without the actual implantation of any material. All animals should be of approximately the same age and weight, and the operative procedures should be the same for all groups.

All implants (biomaterial being evaluated and reference material) should be the same with regard to size, shape, and surface finish. In general, the subcutaneous site is preferred because it has been more thoroughly investigated, although other sites have also been used. One may opt to focus upon the possibility of biodegradation and tumorigenesis by implanting the solid material in one side of the animals and the material in its powdered form on the other side, as Oppenheimer et al. did with nylon [6].

After recovery from the implantation procedure, the animals should be checked for general health and weighed weekly. About 6 to 8 months postimplantation, the implant sites should receive close attention in order to detect tumor formations as early as possible. Care should be exercised, however, to avoid physical damage to the tissue or implanted material. Dead or moribund animals should be necropsied and examined carefully for the presence of tumors. If suspicious lesions are found, they should be examined histologically for confirmation.

Data records should include information on (a) the number of animals in each group that developed tumors at the implant sites, and which sites, especially if more than one form of material is used; (b) the number of tumors that develop at implant sites and remote sites, as well as the histologically determined type of tumor; (c) unusual weight gain or loss; and (d) the number of non-tumor-related deaths in each group.

Evaluation of test results should include, for each group including nonimplanted ("sham") controls, (a) the number of animals at risk for the observation period (i.e., original number of animals in the group corrected for non-tumor-related deaths [47]); (b) the incidence of tumors (percent of animals at risk that developed tumors); and (c) the approximate latent period (mean and range) for tumor detection. Data from the biomaterial(s) under evaluation are compared to that from the reference material; the nonimplanted ("sham") controls provide an estimate for the incidence of spontaneous tumors, if any.

Alternative Methods of Evaluation

In vivo studies in rats remain the "gold standard" for evaluation of material-induced tumorigenesis. However, the duration and costs associated with such studies are formidable, and emphasize the need for development of alternative methods to evaluate potential biomaterials for carcinogenicity.

The Ames test [48, 49] is a widely recognized in vitro method for evaluation of mutagenic potential, and is commonly used as a screening tool for chemical carcinogens. It is relatively inexpensive to perform and provides results in a timely fashion (i.e., days to weeks for completion as compared to up two years for completion of in vivo testing). The Ames test employs genetically altered bacteria which return to the normal nutrient requirements of the original strain when grown in the presence of a mutagenic substance. The rate of reversion to the normal nutrient requirements is related to the mutagenicity of the compound.

Despite its widespread use, the Ames test is only useful for detecting mutagenic leach-ables present in the material and/or device. It is not designed to evaluate material-induced tumorigenesis, which according to prevailing theories [27] requires cellular proliferation and encapsulation of the material, and is not likely to be amenable to adaptation for these purposes.

In the late seventies and early 1980s, several in vivo-in vitro methods were evaluated for their potential to identify material-induced tumorigenesis. Buoen et al. [34] examined the development and origin of plastic film-induced preneoplastic cells in mice using a combination of in vivo transplant and in vitro cell culture techniques. These studies showed that preneoplastic cells, from which tumors would eventually arise months later, can be grown and characterized in vitro. A portion of this work (namely, the implantation of plastic sample, in vivo maturation, removal of implant tissues, with subsequent in vitro growth of maturing preneoplastic cells) would appear to offer promise as a screening test for material-induced tumorigenicity of a biomaterial.

In contrast to the studies by Buoen et al. using in vivo exposure and subsequent in vitro growth, Boone et al. [50] presented a method in which normal subcutaneous connective tissue cells were removed from mice, cultured in vitro on polycarbonate plastic plates, and then re-implanted for tumorigenicity testing. Thus, normal connective tissue cells were first grown on the plastic surface in vitro, and when these plastic plates were covered with cultured connective tissue cells, they were implanted subcutaneously in mice to observe for sarcoma formation. Boone et al. reported a tumorigenic incidence up to 78 percent and a latent period of 24–79 weeks with this method. They noted that the frequency of tumor production correlated directly with the time the cells spent in culture prior to implantation in mice and that there was an inverse correlation between the time the cells spent in culture and the latent period before appearance of sarcomas in mice after implantation of cells attached to the plastic plates. They obtained the highest incidence of tumor production (78 percent) and the shortest latent periods (24–40 weeks) in an experiment in which the cells were cultured 130 days (18.6 weeks) prior to implanting the plastic plates with attached cells. However, it is important to note that the total time required for this method, including in vitro culture and in vivo follow-up (about one year), approaches the amount of time required for conventional in vivo tumorigenic evaluation.

Another approach, as presented by Ziche and Gullino [51], involved the sequential use of mice and rabbits and targeted angiogenesis as a predictive indicator for plastic-induced sarcoma formation. These investigators implanted plastic coverslips subcutaneously in mice, and removed the coverslips along with adhering cells one to sixteen weeks after im-plantation. The coverslips were then cut into small pieces ($\sim$1 mm^2) and implanted in the cornea of rabbits. Corneal implants were observed daily with a slit lamp stereomicroscope for evidence of angiogenesis. A positive response was characterized by sprouting of cap-illaries from the limbal vessels within 6 to 8 days. By 10 to 12 days, an extensive network of capillaries enveloped the plastic sample. They found the highest incidence (56 percent) of positive reactions occurred (a) with larger coverslips, and (b) when they remained in mice 2 to 3 weeks before removal for corneal implantation. Thus, these data are in accord with various previous studies in rats in which larger implants produced a higher incidence of tumors and shorter latent periods. The primary advantage of this method was that it required only about 4 to 5 weeks for completion, as compared to 2 years or more for the classical animal carcinogenicity test.

To varying degrees, each of the aforementioned methods (those of Buoen, Boone, Ziche and Guillino) could conceivably save time and money if used for routine evaluation of material-induced tumorigenesis. Several more recent examples of such procedures can be found. Okada et al. [53, 54] used a spontaneously regressing mouse fibrosarcoma cell line to show that foreign bodies can promote tumor growth in normal mice, using a procedure similar to that reported by Boone et al. [50]. These investigators also showed that response of host inflammatory cells to the foreign body is a critical step in progression to the malignant phenotype during material-induced tumorigenesis. Langer and coworkers [55, 56] advocated the use of rabbit corneal implants as a means to visualize and quantitate in vivo angiogenesis and inflammatory response to biomaterials. These results suggest the possibility of utilizing such methods for a more rapid and inexpensive assessment of solid-state carcinogenicity. For example, if positive responses during corneal implantation in the rabbit could be sufficiently correlated with tumor development in intact animals or humans, one could reduce the time required for testing from two years to approximately one to two months. However, validation of such a model would require extensive studies correlating the results from numerous different types of biomaterials in both the test system and classic animal carcinogenic tests. Thus, the commitment of time and resources required to validate such models has hampered their further development, despite their original description nearly two decades ago.

Interpretation of Results

It is much easier to interpret the results of the tests discussed than to answer the more central question: "What is the significance of these results to the human in whom a biomaterial or device is implanted?" Opinions differ widely concerning the carcinogenic risk from implanting a biomaterial andor device in humans. Brand and Brand [52], based upon tests with human tissues and clinical reports of material-associated tumors in man, concluded that implantation of polymeric materials (biomaterials and/or devices) poses little or no carcinogenic risk to the recipient. Although the incidence is low, material-associated tumors continue to be reported in the literature. Whether there is some causal relationship or whether the occurrences are purely coincidental is still a matter of debate.

Studies from rodents have shown that all solid materials with a smooth surface which are implanted for a sufficient period of time will produce tumors. Usually tumors were not observed in all implanted animals, and the time of tumor detection (latent period) also varied. Because of differences in species and strains of animals, composition and purity of implanted polymers, size and surface characteristics of the implants, and procedures and operator techniques, it is not feasible to make quantitative comparisons of tumorigenic incidence and latent periods for various polymeric materials. However, it appears that differences do exist. The rationale for use of the subcutaneously implanted rat test described earlier is to evaluate the candidate biomaterial by comparing its tumor-inducing activity (relative tumorigenicity) with that of a relevant, clinically satisfactory reference material. Results, then, would be presented in terms of whether the test material was more, less, or equivalent to the reference material in regard to its tumorigenic potential, as opposed to testing to see whether or not it will produce tumors.

A variety of more rapid and inexpensive testing methods has been reported. However, before any of these alternative methods is accepted as a means to evaluate material-induced tumorigenesis, in lieu of classic animal studies, proper validation is necessary. This would include correlations between various materials, types of materials, incidences of tumors, latent periods, etc. Nonetheless, it would be valuable if more rapid and less expensive methods for evaluation of material-induced tumorigenesis were developed. Technologies that use tissue culture and other noninvasive methods may eventually be developed that could substitute for extensive animal or human tests.

REFERENCES

1   Turner FC. Sarcomas at sites of subcutaneously implanted Bakelite disks in rats. *J Natl Cancer Inst*, 2 (1941), 81–83.

2   Oppenheimer BS, Oppenheimer ET, Stout AP. Sarcomas induced in rats by implanting cellophane. *Proc Soc Expt Biol Med*, 67 (1948), 33–34.

3   Oppenheimer BS, Oppenheimer ET, Stout AP. Sarcomas induced in rodents by imbedding various plastic films. *Proc Soc Expt Biol Med*, 79 (1952), 366–369.

4   Oppenheimer BS, Oppenheimer ET, Stout AP, et al. Malignant tumors resulting from embedding plastics in rodents. *Science*, 118 (1953), 305–306.

5   Oppenheimer BS, Oppenheimer ET, Danishefsky I, et al. Further studies of polymers as carcinogenic agents in animals. *Cancer Res*, 15 (1955), 333–340.

6   Oppenheimer BS, Oppenheimer ET, Stout AP, et al. The latent period in carcinogenesis by plastic in rats and its relation to the presarcomatous stage. *Cancer*, 11 (1958), 204–213.

7   Oppenheimer ET, Willhite M, Danishefsky I, et al. Observations on the effects of powdered polymer in the carcinogenic process. *Cancer Res*, 21 (1961), 132–136.

8   Oppenheimer ET, Willhite M, Stout AP, et al. A comparative study of the effects of imbedding cellophane and polystyrene films in rats. *Cancer Res*, 24 (1964), 379–387.

9   Alexander P, Horning, ES. Observations on the Oppenheimer method of inducing tumors by subcutaneous implantation of plastic films. In Wolstenholme GEW, O'Connor M (Eds.), *Ciba Foundation Symposium on Carcinogenesis. Mechanisms of Action*. Boston, MA: Little, Brown & Co., 1959, 12–25.

10 Bischoff F, Bryson G. Carcinogenesis through solid state surfaces. *Progr Exp Tumor* Res, 5 (1964), 85–113.

11 Goldhaber P. The influence of pore size on carcinogenicity of subcutaneously implanted Millipore filters. *Proc Am Assoc Cancer Res*, 3 (1961), 228.

12 Goldhaber P. Further observations concerning the carcinogenicity of Millipore filters. *Proc Am Assoc Cancer Res*, 3 (1962), 323.

13 Dukes CE, Mitchley BCV. Polyvinyl sponge implants: Experimental and clinical observations. *Brit J Plast Surg*, 15 (1962), 225–235.

14 Bates RR, Klein M. Importance of a smooth surface in carcinogenesis by plastic film. *J Natl Cancer Inst*, 37 (1966), 145–151.

15 Harrison JH. Synthetic materials as vascular prostheses. *Amer J Surg*, 95 (1958), 16–24.

16 Leininger RI, Mirkovitch V, Peters A, et al. Change in properties of plastics during implantation. *Trans Amer Soc Artif Int Organs*, 10 (1964), 320–321.

17 Leininger RI. Change in properties of plastics during implantation. *Plastics in Surgical Implants*, ASTM Technical Publication No. 386. Philadelphia, PA: American Society for Testing and Materials, 1965, 71–76.

18 Sherman RT, Lyons H. The biological fate of implanted rigid polyurethane foams. *J Surg Res*, 9 (1969), 167–171.

19 Mirkovitch V, Akutsu T, Kolff WJ. Polyurethane aortas in dogs. Three-year results. *Trans Amer Soc Artif Int Organs*, 8 (1962), 79–84.

20 Hueper WC. Experimental production of cancer by means of implanted polyurethane plastic. *Am J Clin Path*, 34 (1960), 328–333.

21 Autian J, Singh AR, Turner JE, et al. Carcinogenesis from polyurethanes. *Cancer Res*, 35 (1975), 1591–1596.

22 Autian J, Singh AR, Turner JE, et al. Carcinogenic activity of a chlorinated polyether polyurethane. *Cancer Res*, 36 (1976), 3973–3977.

23 Fitzhugh AF. Malignant tumors and high polymers. *Science*, 118 (1953), 783.

24 Oppenheimer BS, Oppenheimer ET, Stout AP, et al. Reply to malignant tumors and high polymers. *Science*, 118 (1953), 783–784.

25 Kordan A. Localized interfacial forces resulting from implanted plastics as possible physical factors involved in tumor formation. *J Theoret Biol*, 17 (1967), 1–11.

26 Ecanow B, Gold BH, Sadove M. The role of inert foreign bodies in the pathogenesis of cancer. *Brit J Cancer*, 36 (1977), 397.

27 Brand KG, Buoen LC, Johnson KH, et al. Etiological factors, stages, and role of the foreign body in foreign body tumorigenesis. A review. *Cancer Res*, 35 (1975), 279–286.

28 Brand KG, Buoen LC, Brand I. Foreign body tumorigenesis: Timing and location of preneoplastic events. *J Natl Cancer Inst*, 47 (1971), 829–836.

29 Karp RD, Johnson KH, Buoen LC, et al. Foreign-body tumorigenesis. No requirement for tissue anoxia. *J Natl Cancer Inst*, 50 (1973), 1403–1405.

30 Brand KG, Buoen C, Brand I. Foreign-body tumorigenesis in mice: Most probable number of originator cells. *J Natl Cancer Inst*, 51 (1973), 1071–1074.

31 Johnson KH, Ghobrial HK, Buoen LC, et al. Nonfibroblastic origin of foreign body sarcomas implicated by histological and electron microscopic studies. *Cancer Res*, 33 (1973), 3139–3154.

32 Thomassen MJ, Buoen LC, Brand KC. Foreign-body tumorigenesis: Number, distribution and cell density of preneoplastic clones. *J Natl Cancer Inst*, 54 (1975), 203–207.

33 Brand KG, Buoen LC, Brand I. Foreign-body tumorigenesis induced by glass and smooth and rough plastic. Comparative study of preneoplastic events. *J Natl Cancer Inst*, 55 (1975), 319–322.

34 Buoen LC, Brand I, Brand KG. Foreign-body tumorigenesis: In vitro isolation and expansion of preneoplastic clonal cell populations. *J Natl Cancer Inst*, 55 (1975), 721–723.

35 Brand KG, Buoen LC, Brand I. Foreign-body tumorigenesis by vinyl chloride vinyl acetate copolymer: No evidence for chemical cocarcinogenesis. *Natl Cancer Inst*, 54 (1975), 1259–1262.

36 Brand KG. Diversity and complexity of carcinogenic processes: Conceptual inferences from foreign-body tumorigenesis. *J Natl Cancer Inst*, 57 (1976), 973–976.

37 Brand KG, Buoen LC, Brand I. Multiphasic incidence of foreign-body-induced sarcomas. *Cancer Res*, 36 (1976), 3681–3683.

38 Michelich VJ, Buoen LC, Brand KG. Immunosuppression studies in foreign-body tumorigenesis: No evidence of tumor-specific antigenicity. *J Natl Cancer Inst*, 58 (1977), 757–761.

39 Johnson KH, Buoen LC, Brand I, et al. Light-microscopic morphology of cell types cultured during preneoplasia from foreign-body-reactive tissues and films. *Cancer Res*, 37 (1977), 3228–3237.

40 Thomassen MJ, Buoen LC, Brand I, et al. Foreign-body tumorigenesis in mice: DNA synthesis in surface-attached cells during preneoplasia. *J Natl Cancer Inst*, 61 (1978), 359–363.

41 Michelich VJ, Brand KG. Effects of gonadectomy on foreign-body tumorigenesis in CBA/H mice. *J Natl Cancer Inst*, 64 (1980), 807–808.

42 Johnson KH, Ghobrial HKG, Buoen LC, et al. Ultrastructure of cell types cultured during preneoplasia from implant surfaces and foreign-body-reactive tissues in mice. *J Natl Cancer Inst*, 64 (1980), 1383–1392.

43 Nothdurft H. Tumorerzeugung durch Fremdkor perimplantation. *Abh Deut Akad Wiss Berlin, Kl Med*, 3 (1960), 80.

44 Salyamon LS. The role of inflammation in the mechanism of carcinogenic, co-carcinogenic and certain anti-carcinogenic effects. *Probl Oncol*, 7 (1961), 44–50.

45 Druckrey H. Berliner Symposium uber Fragen der Carcinogenese. *Abhandl Dtsch Akad Wiss Berlin, Kl Med*, 3 (1960), 98–112.

46 Brand KC, Johnson KH, Buoen, LC. Foreign body tumorigenesis. *CRC Crit Rev Toxicol*, 4 (1976), 353–394.

47 Pilgrim HI, Dowd JE. Correcting for extraneous death in the evaluation of morbidity or mortality from tumor. *Cancer Res*, 23 (1963), 45–48.

48 Ames BN. The detection of chemical mutagens with enteric bacteria. In Hollaender A (Ed.), Chemical Mutagens: *Principles and Methods for Their Detection*, Vol. 1. New York: Plenum Press, 1971, 267–282.

49 Ames BN, McCann J, Yamasaki E. Methods for detecting carcinogens and mutagens with the salmonella/mammalian microsome mutagenicity test. *Mutation Res*, 31 (1975), 347–364.

50 Boone CW, Takeichi N, Eaton SA, et al. Spontaneous neoplastic transformation in vitro: A form of foreign body (smooth surface) tumorigenesis. *Science*, 204 (1979), 177–179.

51 Ziche M, Gullino PM. Angiogenesis and prediction of sarcoma formation by plastic. *Cancer Res*, 41 (1981), 5060–5063.

52 Brand KG, Brand I. Risk assessment of carcinogenesis at implantation sites. *Plast Reconstr Surg*, 66 (1980), 591–595.

53 Okada F, Hosokawa M, Hamada J-I, Hasegawa J, Kato M, Mizutani M, Ren J, Takeichi N, Kobayashi H. Malignant progression of a mouse fibrosarcoma by host cells reactive to a foreign body (gelatin sponge). *Br J Cancer*, 66 (1992), 635–639.

54 Okada F, Hosokawa M, Hamada J.-I, Hasegawa J, Mizutani M, Takeichi N, Kobayashi H. Progression of a weakly tumorigenic fibrosarcoma at the site of early phase of inflammation caused by plastic plates. *Jpn J Cancer Res*, 84 (1993), 1230–1236.

55 Langer R, Brem H, Tapper D. Biocompatibility of polymeric delivery systems for macromolecules. *J Biomed Mater Res*, 15 (1981), 267–277.

56 Peppas NA, Langer R. New challenges in biomaterials. *Science*, 263 (1994), 1715–1720.

57 Bago-Granell J, Aguirre-Canyadell M, Nardi J, et al. Malignant fibrous histiocytoma of bone at site of total hip arthroplasty: A case report. *J Bone Joint Surg*, 66 (1984), 30–40.

58 Hayman J, Huygens H. Angiosarcoma developing around a foreign body. *J Clin Pathol*, 36, (1983), 515–518.

59 Friedman KE, Vernon SE. Squamous cell carcinoma developing in conjunction with a mandibular staple bone plate. *J Oral Maxillofac Surg*, 41, (1983), 265–266.

60 Fehrenbacher JW, Bowers W, Strate R, et al. Angiosarcoma of the aorta associated with a dacron graft, *Ann Thorac Surg*, 32, (1981), 297–301.

61 Digby JM, Wells AL. Malignant lymphoma with intranodal refractile particles after insertion of silicone prostheses. *Lancet*, 2(8246), (Sept. 12, 1981), 580.

62 Weinberg DS, Maini BS. Primary sarcoma of the aorta associated with a vascular prosthesis: A case report. *Cancer*, 46, (1980), 398–401.

63 Dalal JJ, Winterbottam T, West RR, et al. Implanted pacemakers and breast cancer. *Lancet*, 2(8189), (Aug. 9, 1980), 311.

64 Tayton KJJ. Ewing's sarcoma at the site of a metal plate. *Cancer*, 45, (1980), 413–415.

65 Biran S, Keren A, Farkas T, et al. Development of carcinoma of breast at the site of an implanted pacemaker in two patients. *J Surg Oncol*, 11, (1979), 7–11.

66 Hausner RJ, Schoen FJ, Pierson KK. Foreign-body reaction to silicone gel in axillary lymph nodes after an augmentation mammaplasty. *Plast Reconstr Surg*, 62, (1978), 381–384.

67 O'Connell TX, Fee HJ, Golding A. Sarcoma associated with dacron prosthetic material: Case report and review of the literature. *J Thorac Cardiovasc Surg*, 72, (1976), 94–96.

68 Zafiracopoulos P, Rouskas A. Breast cancer at site of implantation of pacemaker generator. *Lancet*, 1(7866), (June 1, 1974), 1114.

69 Herrmann JB, Kanhouwa S, Kelley RJ, et al. Fibrosarcoma of the thigh associated with a prosthetic vascular graft. *N Engl J Med*, 248, (1971), 91. Also reported in: Burns WA, Kanhouwa S, Tillman L, et al. Fibrosarcoma occurring at the site of plastic vascular graft. *Cancer*, 29, (1972), 66–72.

70 Thompson JR, Entin SD. Primary extraskeletal chondrosarcoma: Report of a case arising in conjunction with extrapleural lucite ball plombage. *Cancer*, 23, (1969), 936–939.

71 Hoopes JE, Edgerton MT, Jr., Shelley W. Organic synthetics for augmentation mammaplasty: Their relation to breast cancer. *Plast Reconstr Surg*, 39, (1967), 263–270.

Chapter 20

In-Use Testing of Biomaterials in Biomedical Devices

John A. Thomas

REASONS FOR IN VIVO TESTING OF BIOMATERIALS IN END-USE CONFIGURATION

Over 50 implanted devices have been made from more than 40 different materials or their combination (Table 20-1) [1]. Prior chapters have addressed specific toxicological reactions between a particular biomaterial and living tissue. Therefore, and for purposes of discussing in vivo testing within the context of this chapter, no references will be made to either biomaterial-evoked immune reactions or carcinogenesis. While both of these phenomena are important for assessing the compatibility of usefulness of a particular biomaterial, in vivo or in-use testing within the definitions of this chapter will focus upon nonimmunogenic and noncarcinogenic evaluations (see Table 20-2). Current discussions will address the major physiological systems and the extent to which a particular biomaterial or a device itself will alter such functions by precipitation of toxicological reactions. Emphasis will be placed upon alterations that occur while the material or the device is in use.

The functionality of the biomedical device must be physiologically acceptable. Perhaps the most significant toxicological concern continues to be thrombogenesis. Unfortunately, despite intensive and ongoing research, the mechanisms of interaction between blood and polymeric surfaces remains largely unknown. When the cardiovascular system is involved, toxicological evaluations necessitate a thorough knowledge of blood coagulation and platelet aggregation. A battery of blood clotting assays is often required to assess fully the biomaterial's ability to affect adversely hemodynamics and thrombogenicity. Adhesion of blood platelets to polymeric surfaces continues to be a major concern in the design of any new medical device (see also Chapters 22 and 23).

Interfacial problems may involve thrombogenicity in the short term (and sometimes carcinogenicity in the long term), yet in-use toxicological testing may also be concerned with on-site chemical breakdown of the biomaterial. Chemical breakdown and/or leachables may need to be assessed from an in vivo toxicological standpoint, depending upon the characteristics of the particular biomaterial. Any chemical breakdown of a biomaterial that leads to a significant increase in a metal or metals would likely require in-use toxicological assessment focusing on renal function. A chemical breakdown into any particularly toxic organic intermediate substance would indicate evaluation of both hepatic and renal function. A potential intermediate chemical breakdown product that affected the excretory system might also have an adverse effect on other physiological areas, such as the musculoskeletal, neural, endocrine, and/or reproductive systems. Whether the particular breakdown chemical(s) is lipophilic and undergoes bioaccumulation or is readily detoxified to a polar metabolite and is quickly excreted will, in large measure, dictate the toxicological approach to the safety evaluation of the biomaterial.

Table 20-1   Selected Implant Devices and Examples of Biomaterials Used*

Biomedical devices	Biomaterials
Corneal prosthesis	PMMA (polymethylmethacrylate)
Intraocular lens	PMMA; Nylon; polypropylene; silicone rubber
Eustachian tube	Silicone rubber; Teflon
Middle ear prosthesis	PMMA; Proplast; glasses; ceramics
Chronic catheters	Polyethylene; hydrophilic coatings; silicone rubber
Heart valves	Co-Cr alloys; Ti alloys
Vascular prostheses	Segmented polyurethanes; Nylon; PTFA; PET
Joints	Stainless Steel; Co-Cr alloys; Ti alloy; Ti-Al-V alloy; silicone rubber
Vertebral spacers	Al_2O_3
Dental prostheses	Stainless steel; Co-Cr-Mo alloys; Ti and Ti alloys; Proplast
Artificial cartilage	Crystallized hydrogel-PVA (polyvinyl acetate); polyurethane polymers
Artificial ureter & bladder	Teflon; Nylon-polyurethane
Artificial skin	Processed collagen; PCA (polycaprolactone) foam
Sutures	Stainless steel; silk; nylon; Dacron; catgut; polypropylene
Drug delivery systems	Silicone rubber; hydrogels; ethylene-vinyl acetate copolymer
Infusion pumps	Titanium; epoxy

*Modified from Hench.[1]

Table 20-2   Suggested General Toxicological Evaluation of Medical Devices in Relation to Their Function

Biomedical device	CVS[†]	Excretory[‡] and metabolic	Neurological[§] function	Reproductive[‖] system	Respiratory system	Other[#]
Heart valves and vascular prosthesis	+	±	−	−	±	
Intraoccular lens	−	±	−	−	−	+
Catheters (CVS)	+	±	−	−	−	
Catheters (G-U)	−	±	−	+	−	±
Orthopedic devices	−	±	+	−	−	+
Drug delivery system	+	+	−	±	±	+

Physiological systems

Note: +, Toxicological assessment recommended; ±, depends upon specific biomaterial.
*To be monitored by appropriate testing methods and to what extent there is device-induced changes from normal.
[†]Thrombogenesis: blood coagulation, platelet adhesion/function, etc.
[‡]Renal and hepatic function tests; pulmonary elimination also involves respiratory system.
[§]Includes both peripheral nervous system and central nervous system.
[‖]May include teratory studies in female, include genitourinary system.
[#]Depending upon biomaterial characteristics, test may involve dermal toxicity, special senses, ototoxicity, ocular defects, microbiological/immunological assessment, hematopoietic, etc.

Renal plasma flow is commonly assessed by infusing *p*-aminohippuric acid (PAH) or iodopyracet (Diodrast) and measuring urine and plasma concentrations. Glomerular filtration rate (GFR) can be measured by such methods as the inulin clearance test. Dyes such as phenol red and sulfonphthalein can be employed as an index of renal tubular secretion. Chemically induced changes in renal function parameters, such as PAH, GFR and inulin clearance, can be readily assessed in experimental animals.

PHYSIOLOGICAL SYSTEMS AND IN-USE TESTING

Cardiovascular System

Consideration of biomaterials for blood-contacting applications should take into account blood-biomaterial interactions [3] (see also Chapters 35 and 44). Blood coagulation is generally considered in terms of contributions from factors such as platelet activation; intrinsic, extrinsic and common pathways; and control systems participating in thrombus inhibition and fibrinolysis [4] (for in vitro examinations see Chapters 22 and 23).

Assuming the biomedical device that involves the cardiovascular system achieves its functionality, the greatest in vivo toxicological concern is thrombogenicity of the biomaterial. Several approaches have been devised to reduce thrombogenicity, including modifying the chemistry of the polymer, changing the flow pattern and the physical properties of the surface, precoating with human protein, and incorporating antithrombotic agents into the biomaterial [3, 4].

Several toxicological tests have been devised that assess the thrombogenicity of such artificial surfaces as those found on vascular grafts, dialysis membranes, cardiopulmonary bypasses and oxygenators, blood pumps, and vascular catheters. Although a number of in vitro tests are available, none can be directly applied to the in vivo or the clinical situations. Table 20-3 summarizes a series of thrombogenicity assays that can be carried out in vivo, in vitro, and ex vivo.

Many modifications of in vivo testing for thrombogenicity of devices have been reported. Platelet labeling with ^{111}In-oxine and in vivo imaging with a gamma camera represents a noninvasive radioisotopic technique for the detection of platelet deposition [5]. Similarly, the accumulation of ^{111}In-labeled platelets in human femoropopliteal bypass grafts have been employed to evaluate thrombogenicity in vivo [6]. The thrombogenicity

Table 20-3   Toxicological Assessment of Thrombogenicity*

Platelet tests	Blood coagulation tests	General tests
Total count	Partial thromboplastin time	Scanning electron microscopy
Release of constituents (BTG, acid phosphatase, 5HT, TXB_3 PF4	Fibrinogen and degradation products	Test cells constructed of materials under test
	Assays of factors XII, XI, and V	Artificial circulations
Survival of platelets	Fibrinopeptide A (FPA)	Arteriovenous anastomoses of materials to be tested
Adhesion, platelets	Fibrinogen turnover	Estimation of platelet—fibrin emboli
Aggregation, platelet [111]Indium-labeled platelets	Immunofluorescent staining for fibrinogen	

*Source: Modified from Forbes [4].

of different suture materials has been assessed using the scanning electron microscope (SEM) [7]. Hanson el al. [8] have described an in vivo evaluation of artificial surfaces, using a nonhuman primate (baboon) arteriovenous (A-V) shunt model. An ex vivo A-V shunt model using dogs and SEM techniques to determine the type and amount of blood cells adhering has been employed successfully to test hydrogel/silicone rubber composite material [9]. Some ex vivo blood compatibility tests have used human arm veins [10]. Catheters can be inserted into several anatomical sites and can be used to deliver drugs by the intravenous route or the peritoneal route.

Endocrine System

The pancreas and the uterus have been sites for the use of biomedical devices in the endocrine system. A hybrid artificial pancreas for experimental animals, comprised of microporous hydrogel membranes, has been described [11, 12]. A special microporous semipermeable membrane and diffusion chamber made of polymerized 2-hydroxyethylmethacrylate (pHEMA) synthesized to encapsulate pancreatic beta cells has been evaluated in diabetic rats. Insulin permeability can be used to assess the transfer of hormone across these artificial membranes. Histological evaluation of the membrane's compatibility may also be included in the battery of toxicological tests.

Artificial insulin infusion devices currently represent a more clinically useful approach to the control of diabetes mellitus [13]. Many of these insulin infusion pumps are still externalized, yet totally implantable devices represent a more adaptable method for long-term ambulatory use in the diabetic patient. Both blood glucose levels and circulating blood insulin concentrations represent physiological monitors for the infusion pump's effectiveness in maintaining euglycemia. Miniaturization of the infusion pump, whether for insulin or for some other drug or hormone, aids in patient acceptance of these medical devices.

Blackshear et al. [14] have described a totally implantable insulin delivery system. This device requires vascular access and consists of two chambers, the inner one containing insulin and the outer one a fluorocarbon liquid. The fluorocarbon exerts a vapor pressure that propels the insulin through the system and, via a silicone rubber cannula, into the venous circulation. Blood incompatibility remains a toxicological problem with this approach.

Biomaterials and/or devices can be implanted into the uterine lining. Intrauterine devices (IUDs) are available in both an unmedicated form (i.e., biological inert biomaterial) or a medicated form (i.e., copper-containing or progesterone-containing biomaterial) [15]. The toxicological concern of such devices involves inflammatory reactions (pelvic inflammatory disease or PID), and the risk of infection (e.g., gonococcal and nongonococcal organisms). The use of a copper-containing IUD enhances leukocytic infiltration into the uterus. Blood levels of copper are not usually affected and, hence, pose no particular toxicological problem. Other IUDs may contain progesterone or mestranol.

Several bioerodible polymers have been used in contraceptive drug delivery systems [16, 17]. Polyhydropyrans have been used to encapsulate various progesterones and estrogens for their subsequent release, leading to inhibition of ovulation. Patient acceptance of uterine implants for controlling fertility has not been as widespread as either oral contraceptives or IUDs. In-use toxicological assessment, aside from infection and inflammatory reactions, may involve monitoring blood levels of estrogens and progesterone, as well as serum gonadotropins [18].

Biomaterials, including polyurethane-related polymers, have been used for penile prostheses and breast implants. Polyurethane-related polymers are stronger and more resilient than silicone polymers. Fibrous capsular contracture remains the most common complication following augmentation mammoplasty. Using a rabbit model, silicone implant capsules can be deliberately seeded with *Staphylococcus epidermidis*, causing an increased hardness and thickness of the capsules along with an inflammatory response [19].

Skeletomuscular System

Biomaterials may be utilized in a variety of ways within the skeletomuscular system. Specifically, biomaterials have been used in artificial joints, bone bonding, percutaneous leads, catheters, absorbable sutures, dental materials, and so-called synthetic skin. The mechanical requirements of arthroplasty most often call for the use of stainless steel and a variety of alloys, including nickel and cobalt (for specifics, see Section I). Ceramic and plastic materials have also been used in certain bone and joint replacements. Some artificial finger joints have been made with high performance silicone elastomers. Various bioglass formulations possess specific surface activities, to the extent that they can be used to insure bonding with living tissues. Wilson et al. [20] have described a series of in vivo toxicological tests that aid in determing the biocompatibility of bioglass. A convenient animal model for testing bone substitute materials uses the cranial vault of the rabbit and allows for radiological and histological assessment of implant resorption and ingrowth of new bone [21].

A number of composite resins and other biomaterials have been employed in restorative dentistry [22, 23, 24] (see also Chapters 3, 4, and 37). Polymethylmethacrylate is, perhaps, one of the most commonly used dental bases. A large number of chromium-cobalt partial denture frameworks are also used clinically. Casting alloys, particularly gold, have traditionally been utilized for permanent crown and bridge materials. Some gold solders contain cadmium, which may pose a toxicological consideration. Some porcelains contain uranium oxide, but there is no evidence of toxicological damage. Temporary cements characteristically contain zinc oxide, but not to the extent that they pose a toxicological concern. Polymers used in restorative dentistry as well as maxillo-facial reconstruction surgery contain many toxic ingredients (Table 20-4) [25]. These chemicals may have been ingredients inherent in a formulation, contaminants, sterilants, solvents or degradation products.

Marion et al. have described an in vivo implant technique to assess dental biomaterials [26] (see also Chapter 37). Likewise, McClugage et al. [27] have employed an in vivo model for evaluating the response of dental pulp to various biomaterials. This rat model allows sequential microscopic observations of the microvascular system of dental pulp before and after application of pulp-capping agents, cementing agents, or cavity liners.

Table 20-4   Identified Toxic Ingredients in Polymers*

Aluminum	Ethylene oxide
Acrylonitrile monomer	Formaldehyde
Arsenic	Lead
Benzene	Mercaptobenzothiazole
Benzoic peroxide	Methylene dianiline
Bisphenol A	Nickel
Cadmium	Pyrene
Carbon tetrachloride	Tricresyl phosphate
Dibutyl tin	Triphenyl phosphate
Ethylene dichloride	Vinyl chloride monomer

*Source: Northup [25].

Synthetic materials for covering burn wounds have been developed. So-called synthetic skins are utilized for a short-term dressing material and as a longer-term skin substitute [28, 29]. These skin substitutes consist of preformed films (e.g., PVC, polymerized methacrylate, polyurethane, acrylonitrile, animal collagen and fibrin), and spray-on films (e.g., acrylic caprolactone, polyvinyl alcohol, and Silastic). In general, the in vivo toxicological assessment of skin substitutes encompasses their ability to provide a barrier against bacterial invasion and immunogenicity in the instance of animal collagens and related films.

Genitourinary (G-U) System

Medical devices are used to maintain the patency of functionality of the G-U system (Table 20-5). Some of these devices (e.g., catheters) may come into direct contact with tissues in the G-U tract; other devices may simply be used to measure urine flow and, hence, do not necessarily come into contact with epithelial lining. The use of indwelling catheters may be followed by urethritis, cystitis, formation of vesicle calculi, vesicoureteral reflux, and penoscrotal junction fistulas. The in vivo testing of catheters, assuming biocompatibility, usually involves microbiological assessment and examination for local tissue irritation due to increased in situ residence time. Tissue irritation is exceedingly difficult to quantify, although local inflammatory reactions can be assessed semiquantitatively by histological methods (see Sections VII and VIII).

The use of artificial kidneys and membrane oxygenators presents some specific toxicological problems that need to be assessed. Therapeutic hemodialysis may employ a hollow fiber dialyzer or a parallel flow (plate) dialyzer. In the former, blood passes through hollow fibers lying in dialysis fluid (dialysate). In the latter, blood flows along one side and dialysate along the other side of a membrane. The evaluation of dialyzers entails assessment of residual blood volume, the in vivo clearance of substances with a low molecular weight,

Table 20-5   Genitourinary Tract and Dialysis Medical Devices

Device	General use
Urologic instruments	biopsy
Urodynamics system	diagnosis
Urine flow/volume system	diagnostic
Enuresis alarm	monitoring
Penile implant	prosthesis
Fiberoptic light, urethral catheter	surgical device
Urology evacuator	surgical device
Ureteral stent	surgical device
Water jet renal stone dislodger	surgical device
Ureteral stone dislodger	surgical device
Urethrotome	surgical device
Urologic table	surgical device
Suprapubic catheter	therapeutic device
Urological catheter	therapeutic device
Urine collector	therapeutic device
Implanted urinary continence device	therapeutic device
Non-implanted urinary continence device	therapeutic device
Ureteral dilator	therapeutic device
Hemodialysis system	therapeutic device
Peritoneal dialysis system	therapeutic device
Isolated kidney perfusion system	therapeutic device

and the in vitro clearance of substances with a higher molecular weight [30]. The National Institute of Arthritis, Metabolic Disease and Diabetes (NIAMDD) has established criteria for evaluating the toxicity potentials of dialyzers [31]. One toxicological consideration involving allergic reactions is known as "cuprophan hypersensitivity." Cuprophan hypersensitivity, a blood-material interaction, occurs in such extracorporeal circuits as artificial kidneys or membrane oxygenators. Sheep are a particularly useful and sensitive animal model to evaluate such membrane-related problems as hypersensitivity [32]. The sheep reproducibly develops acute cardiopulmonary reactions after receiving blood previously in contact with cuprophan and certain other dialyzer fibers. Other toxicological assessments may involve the release of trace metals (e.g., zinc) from disposable coils during hemodialysis. Dialysis dementia syndrome reportedly occurs during chronic hemodialysis and is sometimes characterized by elevated brain levels of aluminum [33]. Aluminum-containing antacids or elevated municipal water levels of aluminum are contributing etiological factors.

Many of the same toxicological evaluations employed for hemodialysis need to be addressed in peritoneal dialysis. Peritoneal dialysis is often preferred over that of extracorporeal dialysis. Ray et al. [34] have described an evaluation of biocompatibility of polymers for the development of peritoneal dialysis catheters. A technique is available that examines the morphology of bacterial colonies adhering to peritoneal dialysis catheters by scanning and transmission electron microscopy [35].

REFERENCES

1   Hench LL. Biomaterials. *Science*, 208 (1980), 826–831.
2   National Institutes of Health. Clinical applications of biomaterials-consensus conference. *JAMA*, 249 (1983), 1050–1054.
3   Courtney JM, Lamba NMK, Sundaram S, Forbes CD. Biomaterials for blood-contacting applications. *Biomat*, 15: 737–744, 1994.
4   Forbes CD, Prentice CRM. Thrombus formation and artificial surfaces. *Brit Med Bull*, 34 (1978), 201–207.
5   Dewanjee MK, Kaye MP, Fuster V, et al. Noninvasive radioisotopic technique for detection of platelet deposition in mitral valve prosthesis and renal microembolism in dogs. *Trans Am Soc Artif Intern Organs*, 36 (1980), 475–480.
6   Goldman M, Norcott HC, Hawker RJ, et al. Femoropopliteal bypass grafts—An isotope technique allowing in vivo comparison of thrombogenicity. *Brit J Surg*, 69 (1982), 380–382.
7   Dahlke H, Dociu N, Thurau K. Thrombogenicity of different suture materials as revealed by scanning electron microscopy. *J Biomed Mater Res*, 14 (1980), 251–268.
8   Hanson SR, Harker LA, Ratner BD, et al. In vivo evaluation of artificial surfaces with a nonhuman primate model of arterial thrombosis. *J Lab Clin Med*, 95 (1980), 289–304.
9   Vale BH, and Greer RT. Ex vivo shunt testing of hydrogel-silicone rubber composite materials. *J Biomed Mater Res*, 16 (1982), 471–500.
10   Fischer JP, Fuhge P, Burge K, et al. Methods for the production and characterization of polymers with improved blood compatibility. *Angew: Makromoleuk Chem*, 105 (1982), 131–165.
11   Klomp GF, Hashiguchi H, Ursell PC, et al. Macroporous hydrogel membranes for a hybrid artificial pancreas. II. Biocompatibility. *J Biomed Res*, 17 (1983), 865–871.
12   Ronel SH, D'Andrea MJ, Hashiguchi H, et al. Macroporous hydrogel membranes for a hybrid artificial pancreas. 1. Synthesis and chamber fabrication. *J Biomed Mater Res*, 17 (1983), 855–864.
13   Bruck SD. The role of biomaterials in insulin delivery systems. *Int J Artif Organs*, 3 (1980), 299–304.
14   Blackshear PJ, Rohde TG, Grotting JC, et al. Control of blood glucose in experimental diabetes by means of a totally implantable insulin infusion device. *Diabetes*, 28 (1979), 634.
15   Chien YW. Medicated intrauterine devices: Development considerations and clinical uses. *Parenteral Drug Assoc*, 34 (1980), 295.
16   Buckles RG. Biomaterials for drug delivery systems. *J Biomed Mater Res*, 17 (1983), 109–128.
17   Langer R, Brem H, Tapper D. Biocompatibility of polymeric delivery systems for macromolecules. *J Biomed Mater Res*, 15 (1981), 267–277.
18   Thomas JA, Bell JH. Endocrine toxicology. In Hayes AW, Jr. (Ed.), *Methods in Toxicology*. New York: Raven Press, 1982.

19 Shah F, Lehman JA, Tan J. Does infection play a role in breast capsular contracture? *Plast Reconstr Surg*, 68 (1981), 34–38.

20 Wilson J, Pigott GH, Schoen FJ, et al. Toxicology and biocompatibility of bioglasses. *J Biomed Mater Res*, 15 (1981), 805–817.

21 Frame JW. A convenient animal model for testing bone substitute materials. *J Oral Surg*, 38 (1980), 176–180.

22 Heys RJ. Biologic considerations of composite resins. *Dent Clin North Am*, 25 (1981), 257–270.

23 Brown RM, Tyas MJ. Biological testing of dental restorative materials *in vitro*. *J Oral Rehabil*, 6 (1979), 365–374.

24 Caputo AA. Biological implications of dental materials. *Dent Clin North Am*, 24 (1980), 331–341.

25 Northup SJ. Current problems associated with toxicity evaluation of medical device materials and future research needs. *Fund & Appl Toxicol*, 13 (1989), 196–204.

26 Marion L, Haugen E, Major, IA. Methodological assessments of subcutaneous implantation techniques. *J Biomed Mater Res*, 14 (1980), 343–357.

27 McClugage SG, Jr., Holmstedt JOV, Malloy RB. An in vivo model for evaluating the response of pulp to various biomaterials, *J Biomed Mater Res*, 14 (1980), 631–638.

28 Davies JWL. Synthetic materials for covering burn wounds: Progress towards perfection. Part 1. Short-term dressing materials, *Burns*, 10 (1983), 94–103.

29 Davies JWL. Synthetic materials for covering burn wounds: Progress towards perfection. Part 2. Longer-term substitutes for skin. *Burns*, 10 (1983), 104–108.

30 Gorgels J, Tan BH, Go IH. An evaluation of the performance of current dialyzers in routine use and in vitro. *Dialysis Transplant*, Oct./Nov. 1976, 68–76.

31 Klein E, Autian J, Bower JD, et al. *Evaluation of Hemodialyzers and Dialysis Membranes*, DHEW Publication No. (NIH) 77-1294. Washington, DC: NIH, 1977.

32 Walker JF, Lindsay RM, Peters SD, et al. A sheep model to examine the cardiopulmonary manifestations of blood-dialyzer interactions. *ASAIO J*, 6 (1983), 123–129.

33 Bogden JD, Zadzielski E, Weiner B, et al. Release of some trace metals from disposable coils during dialysis. *Amer J Clin Nutrit*, 36 (1982), 403–409.

34 Ray AR, Verma K, Chaudhry VP. Evaluation of biocompatibility of polymers for the development of peritoneal dialysis catheter. *Ind J Med Res*, 74 (1981), 308–311.

35 Marrie TJ, Noble MA, Corterton JW. Examination of the morphology of bacteria adhering to peritoneal dialysis catheters by scanning and transmission electron microscopy, *J Clin Microbi*, 118 (1983), 1388–1398.

ADDITIONAL READING

1   Bou-Abboud NN, Patat JL, Guillemin G, Issahakian S, Forest N, Ouhayoun JP. Evaluation of the osteogenic potential of biomaterials implanted in the palatal connective tissue of miniature pigs using undecalcified sections. *Biomaterials*, 15 (1994), 201.

2   Ciapetti G, Stea S, Cenni E, Sudanese A, Marraro D, Toni A, Pizzoferrato A. Toxicity of cyanoacrylates in vitro using extract dilution assay on cell cultures. *Biomaterials*, 15 (1994), 92.

3   Henderson LW. Immunotoxicity of blood-synthetic membrane interactions. *Fund & Appl Tox*, 13 (1989), 228–234.

4   Hunt JA, Williams DF. Quantifying the soft tissue response to implanted materials. *Biomaterials*, 16 (1995), 167–170.

5   Ikada Y. Surface modification of polymers for medical applications. *Biomaterials*, 15 (1994), 725–736.

6   Laing PG. World standards for surgical implants: An American perspective. *Biomaterials*, 15 (1994), 403–407.

7   Marchant RE. The cage implant system for determining in vivo biocompatibility of medical device materials. *Fund & Appl Tox*, 13 (1989), 217–227.

8   Meyer U, Szulczewski DH, Barckhaus RH, Atkinson M, Jones DB. Biological evaluation of an ionomeric bone cement by osteoblast cell culture methods. *Biomaterials*, 14 (1993), 917–923.

9   Richardson RR, Miller JA, Reichert WM. Polyimides as biomaterials: Preliminary biocompatibility testing. *Biomaterials*, 14 (1993), 627–634.

10 Sunderman FW, Jr. Carcinogenicity of metal alloys in orthopedic prostheses: Clinical and experimental studies. *Fund & Appl Tox*, 13 (1989), 205–216.

11 Van Sliedregt A, van Loon JA, van der Brink J, de Groot K, van Blitterswijk CA. Evaluation of polylactide monomers in an in vitro biocompatibility assay. *Biomaterials*, 15 (1994), 251.

12 Wening JV, Marquardt H, Katzer A, Jungbluth KH, Marquardt H. Cytotoxicity and mutagenicity of Kevlar®: An in vitro evaluation. *Biomaterials*, 116 (1995), 337–340.

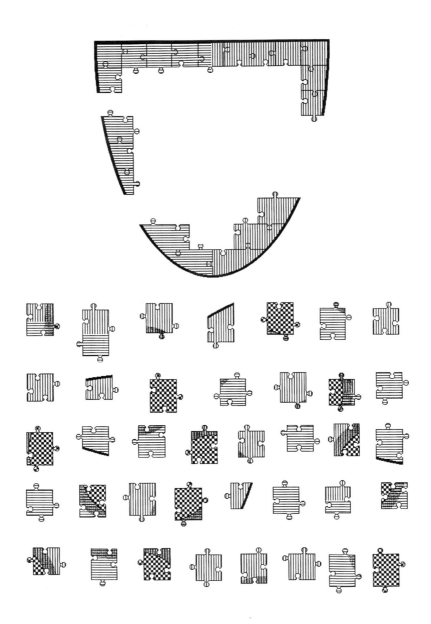

Section Four

In Vitro Assessment of Safety

Richard F. Wallin

INTRODUCTION

There are many in vitro methods that can be used to great advantage to evaluate the potential toxicity of biomaterials. Nevertheless, until relatively recent times, cytotoxicity and hemolysis testing were synonymous with in vitro biomaterial testing.

The Tripartite Guidance issued in 1987, the ISO 10993 standards still under development, and the FDA G95-1 Blue Book Memorandum effective July, 1995 all describe the range of biologic effects that may be caused by the chemicals present in or on medical device materials. These documents provide systematic approaches for testing materials for their various toxicologic properties. Careful review of these documents indicates that there are numerous potential biologic effects of materials that are subject to direct investigation using in vitro techniques. Some of these have now been developed into test procedures that have become as routine as cytotoxicity and hemolysis tests. For other biologic effects, standard methods have not yet been developed. In some cases, in vitro methods may never completely provide the necessary answers to specific questions about materials.

In addition to cytotoxicity and hemolysis, complement activation, bacterial endotoxin tests, and a variety of genotoxicity tests such as the Ames reverse mutation, sister chromatid exchange, and chromosomal aberration tests are now frequently used to test biomaterials. ISO 10993 standards describe a series of hemocompatibility issues that are excellent candidates for in vitro test methods: effects on thrombosis, coagulation, platelets, hematology, and immunology. For the most part, however, standard tests that address these five categories of effects remain to be developed. In principle, sensitization is another effect that should be detectable in vitro but for which in vitro methods have not yet been developed.

By their nature, in vitro models tend to be sensitive and specific. They are generally based upon exposure of a biological or physiological "test system" to a "test article," to use Good Laboratory Practice (GLP) language, in an isolated environment unlike that which exists in the intact mammalian body. Thus effects are likely to be either exaggerated, due to concentration effects and the absence of protective mechanisms present in the intact animal, or unobservable, due to a lack of target elements in the biological system used. For example, one could rather easily design alternative in vitro test methods that would address the effects of a material on the coagulation of blood; however, it would be difficult to imagine single in vitro methods capable of detecting acute or chronic, systemic toxicity.

It remains for laboratories around the world to identify which of the potential toxicologic effects of biomaterials can best be addressed by sensitive, specific in vitro methods. These must then be developed and validated to show that they are capable of being reproduced, that they adequately separate active from inactive control materials, and ideally, that they are relevant to the clinical situation in which a patient is exposed to a biomaterial.

Because they are so sensitive, in vitro test methods sometimes indicate false positive results, that is, results that show toxicity without clinical relevance. There are numerous examples of biomaterials that fail various of the common in vitro tests such as cytotoxicity and complement activation and yet are in routine clinical use. Generally, this is because further in vivo and clinical testing have shown the suitability of the biomaterial for its intended use. Likewise, because they are so specific, in vitro tests that show negative or acceptable results must be viewed carefully because in vitro tests usually detect only the effects they were designed to detect. Thus a negative cytotoxicity test result offers little information about the suitability of a material for long-term implantation during which the material may undergo biodegradation with release of toxic breakdown products.

The importance of characterizing biomaterials under toxicologic investigation has often been overlooked. Without some level of characterization, investigators cannot be sure about the identity of the biomaterials they have studied. With information about the physical and chemical properties of biomaterial test articles, it may be possible to minimize or even eliminate the need for further testing in vitro or in vivo because of the minute quantity or inocuous nature of the extractables present. Physicochemical data also form the basis for materials specifications that allow manufacturers to assure that every lot of material used in their products is the same in ways that are toxicologically important.

Chapter 21

Mammalian Cell
Culture Models

Sharon J. Northup
John N. Cammack

INTRODUCTION

Mammalian cell culture techniques have been applied to the field of biomaterials research and development for more than two decades. Cytotoxicity tests are the first in a sequenced program of tests for biocompatibility. The earliest procedures were based on morphological measures of cell viability or death. These procedures were adapted by many laboratories and have achieved widespread use and have become internationally recognized standards. Protein assays have become the most frequently used functional assay and are exemplified in the inhibition of cell growth assay. Biochemical methods can measure such cell functions as deoxyribonucleic acid (DNA) synthesis, protein synthesis and adenosine triphosphate (ATP) levels. Cell function tests such as adhesion and phagocytosis are highly sensitive but have low toxicity-ranking agreement and reproducibility [1].

RELEVANCE OF *IN VITRO* ASSAYS

Darby [2] described the cell culture assays as in vitro correlates of the in vivo local tissue toxicity assays such as irritation and implantation assays. The rationale for the use of cultured mammalian cells for analysis of toxicity rests on the fact that actions of chemicals that produce disease and death in the animal or human are ultimately exerted at the cellular level. Thus, investigation of cellular response is the cornerstone for establishing biological response to foreign materials.

Frazier [3] described three interfaces between in vitro methodology and animal toxicology: screening, mechanistic studies and considerations for risk assessment. Screening tests are the most developed and are likely to remain the major focus of in vitro toxicology. However, mechanistic studies probably will become increasingly more important, both in toxicological evaluations and for risk assessment.

Toxicity as a term for cellular responses reflecting chemical injury is used loosely. The term generally includes any chemically induced change in structure and function of affected cells, ranging from cell death to a transient and reversible aberration in a single enzymatic reaction. Regardless of the end point measured, the production of a toxic response in a cell appears to involve the interactions of virtually all subcellular processes—nucleic acid function, membrane transport and permeability, energy production, chemical metabolism and much more—as the cell attempts to maintain its functional integrity while disposing of the exogenous chemical. The ultimate toxic response made by the cell to an exogenous chemical represents a summation at the cellular level of the extent of perturbation of many subcellular processes. The variation in the quality of the toxic response with dose also suggests that more cellular processes are perturbed as the chemical dose is increased [4].

Except in a very few instances, it appears reasonable to suggest that cellular toxic responses often may not result from the modification of single macromolecules or the perturbation of single cellular processes [5].

Cells from different tissues and species appear to give very similar results when all other assay variables are identical, indicating that it may not be that important to match cell culture type with the target tissue for local toxicity tests. However, there are exceptions when testing pure chemicals which have specific mechanisms of action such as interference with mitotic spindle formation, inhibition of discrete metabolic pathways or inhibition of synthesis of a macromolecule which is the measured endpoint [6]. In comparing cells with animals, one pitfall often exists: the method of measuring dose. For proper comparison, the dosage should be expressed as a standard unit such as "moles per cell" [7]. That is, toxicity measures may be expected to vary with changes in the dose of the agent per cell or when cells are affected by the added stress of growth.

CELL CULTURE TECHNIQUES

Cell Selection

Several types of cell culture systems are available routinely for toxicity studies in vitro (Table 21-1). A *primary culture* is a fresh isolate of cells or tissue that is cultured in vitro. Primary cell cultures may be obtained from fragments of tissue or from a suspension of individual cells obtained by treatment of the tissue with proteolytic enzymes. The monolayer of cells that grow out from a tissue explant usually contains a variety of cell types representative of that tissue. After a few days in culture, one cell type will become predominant. Primary cells will grow until the culture becomes confluent. Further growth is obtained by subculturing in fresh nutrient media and culture dishes. As the primary culture ages, growth becomes slower with the culture eventually dying.

Continuous *cell lines* are derived from primary cultures that have become adapted to grow in vitro. Cell lines are propagable cultures of cells that usually may be passaged for a limited number of times in vitro. Continuous cell strains, unlike primary cells, can be cultured indefinitely. Often the cell strain is cloned from a single cell so that every cell has an identical genetic origin. Consequently, cell strains represent more uniform cell populations than do cell lines. Continuous cell strains are obtainable from biological supply houses and individual investigators. These cultures are usually carefully tested to determine whether the culture is free from contaminating microorganisms, such as mycoplasmas, bacteria, fungi, and cytopathic viruses. Information on history, genealogy (species origin, sex, age, and tissue), karyotype, morphology, and culture techniques may be supplied with each continuous cell strain.

The availability of characterized cell strains provides significant advantages: (a) the investigator can obtain "clean" standard cells at the same passage level over the years for

Table 21-1   Characteristics of cell cultures

Parameter	Primaries	Cell lines	Cell strains
Culture life	Hours to days	Months to immortal	Often immortal
Function	Excellent	Variable	Limited
Proliferation	None to very limited	Usually limited	Often unlimited
Karyotype	Diploid	Diploid or aneuploid	Often aneuploid

systematic experimentation; (b) the origin, history, and characteristics of the cells have been described and documented; (c) there are a large variety of cell types available; (d) time-consuming and costly long-term serial subcultivation of cells is not necessary; and (e) there is "insurance" against the total loss of valuable cells through contamination, alteration, or accident. Of additional importance are the advantages to be gained by efforts to improve and standardize procedures and culture media.

The adherent cell strains L-929 and WI-38 are used most frequently for testing medical devices and materials. Other frequently used adherent cell strains include MRC-5, 3T3, IMR-90, HR-218, HFS-15, and HeLa. Most of these are fibroblast-like cells, which are relatively easy to maintain in vitro. Fibroblastic cell strains are limited in that they lack the differentiated morphology, metabolism, and function of specialized tissues of the body.

Culture Media

A crucial parameter for successful culturing of cells is the provision of proper nutrients. The minimal nutritional requirements for cultured cells were first defined in a classic paper by Eagle [8]. Twenty-seven factors, defined as essential for growth, formed the basis of a medium known as "Basal Medium, Eagle" or BME. The defined medium consisted of a mixture of essential amino acids, vitamins, electrolytes, and carbohydrates, supplemented with serum. This basal medium, which required frequent replenishment for the cells to continue growing, was replaced by Eagle's minimum essential medium (MEM) in which the concentrations of the various components were increased to enable cells to continue growing in culture for several days between medium changes. Medium 199 is a more complex medium containing over 60 ingredients.

The media or components are commercially available as dry powders or in various concentrations from 1X to 100X. The concentrated media are diluted with sterile water, followed by addition of balanced salt solution, L-glutamine (if not included), serum, bicarbonate, and antimicrobials, if required. Many investigators prefer to add L-glutamine as a separate component because it is not stable in solution.

Balanced salt solutions (BSS) supply essential electrolytes and contribute to the maintenance of osmotic balance for cultured cells. The solutions are supplied separate from the nutrient media components because of solubility characteristics. Eagle's and Hank's BSS are those in common use today. These contain sodium, potassium, magnesium, phosphate, and calcium salts which are essential for viability.

Correct pH of culture media is generally achieved with a bicarbonate/CO_2 buffer system. Phenol red indicator, which is often included in the medium, imparts a light red color to the medium at the optimal cellular pH range of 7.2 to 7.5. Zwitterionic buffers, such as HEPES and TRICINE, have also been used in cell culture medium. An atmosphere of 5 per cent CO_2 in air is not required when the zwitterionic buffers are used. An exception to this is for cloning cells, where bicarbonate is essential for cell function.

Serum is a very complex, natural additive to the majority of culture media. Serum contains a wide variety of macro- and micronutrients that are not present in commonly used culture media. These include proteins, hormones and growth stimulators. The age and species of the donor are important variables in selecting sera for cell cultures. Commercially available sera have been sterile filtered and assayed for possible bacterial, mycoplasmal, viral and endotoxin contamination. Additional tests are performed to ensure that each batch of serum will support the growth of cells in culture. When necessary, an investigator may request serum from a specific batch to support the growth of a given cell culture.

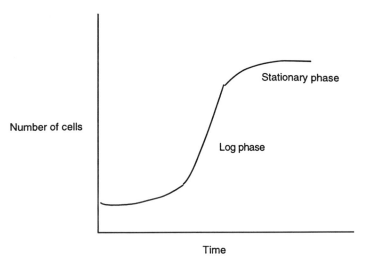

Figure 21-1 Growth phases of cells in vitro.

Antimicrobials and Antibiotics

All culture media provide an excellent environment for the growth of microbial contaminants. The usual cell culture procedures, which involve frequent opening of culture vessels, provide ample opportunities for contamination. In the absence of antimicrobials, stringent precautions are necessary to ensure that contamination does not occur. Inclusion of antimicrobial agents in stock cultures is discouraged because the antimicrobial is potentially cytotoxic and because selection of antimicrobial-resistant strains of microorganisms in long-term cultures must be avoided. Penicillin is frequently used to control gram-positive bacterial contamination. Streptomycin sulfate or the more stable dihydrostreptomycin sulfate may be used to control gram-negative bacterial contamination.

Under optimal environmental conditions, cultured cells usually display logarithmic growth patterns that are population-dependent (Figure 21-1). At very low cell concentrations, growth may be very slow because there is dilution of cellular micronutrients in the culture medium. At high cell concentrations, growth ceases as a result of cell contact inhibition. The selection of culture growth phases can be a source of variation when comparing different assays. For example, cellular proliferation requires log-phase cells, whereas biochemical modifications can be measured in either log or stationary phase cells.

Sample Preparation

The International Organization for Standardization (ISO) standard recommends standard methods for sample preparation (ISO 10993-12. Biological evaluation of medical devices— Part 12: Sample preparation and reference materials; see Table 21-2). Samples for cytotoxicity testing should be adequately cleaned to prevent misleading results or contamination of the test system. Nonsterile samples may be tested in cultures containing antibiotics in the media.

Several of the cytotoxicity assays described below are suitable for testing solid samples. The standard size of 1 cm^2 projected surface area was initially derived from the surface-area-to-volume ratio from the U.S. Pharmacopeia biological tests for plastics (Chapter 88, Biological Tests In Vivo) and proportioned to the volume of culture medium in the direct contact assay.

Table 21-2   Recommended surface-to-volume ratios for preparation of extracts

Example of materials	Thickness (mm)	Extraction ratio (surface area/volume)
Metal, synthetic polymer, ceramic or composite film, sheet and tubing wall	≤ 0.5	6 cm^2/mL
Metal, synthetic polymer, ceramic and composite tubing wall, slab and molded items	> 0.5	3 cm^2/mL
Natural elastomer	≤ 1.0	3 cm^2/mL
Natural elastomer	> 1.0	1.25 cm^2/mL
Pellets	irregular	0.1 to 0.2 g/mL 6 cm^2/mL

Some cell culture methods use an extract of the material for cytotoxicity testing. Extract solvents include culture medium with or without serum, saline, vegetable oil, dimethyl sulfoxide, etc. The extract solvent should be compatible with the cell culture and not be adversely affected by the extraction temperature. Extracts are often prepared at the highest extraction temperature compatible with the physical characteristics of the extract solvent and sample (i.e., without softening or causing other physical changes in the material). In the case of plastic samples, the extraction temperature should not exceed the glass transition temperature (the temperature at which a plastic's crystalline structure changes to the amorphous state) or cause hydrolysis of covalent bonds. Groth et al. [9] note that care should be taken to adopt the extraction conditions appropriate to the clinical application because different extraction media may result in different cytotoxic potentials of the extract. Because of these variables, the conditions for preparing extracts of biomaterials have been carefully standardized to improve the reproducibility of the data.

Endpoints

Perhaps the most fundamental manifestation of cellular toxicity is cell death. Cell death is generally divided into two broad categories: necrosis or cytotoxic-induced cell death and apoptosis or programmed cell death [10]. Although some degree of overlap exists between these two modes of cell death, the segregation of the two responses by morphology as well as by time of appearance, tissue location and type and strength of stimulus suggests that necrosis and apoptosis are quite discrete processes. Cellular necrosis is associated with disruption of ionic pumps of the plasma membrane, leading to cytoskeletal disorder, cellular and organelle swelling, cell shape changes, and blebbing (i.e., formation of fluid-filled vesicles) of the cell membrane. An intracellular calcium overload leads to irreversible mitochondrial dysfunction. In fact, gross swelling of mitochondria is in general considered to indicate irreversibility. Finally, rupture of nuclei, organelles, and plasma membrane takes place as well as loss of chromatin from disintegrating nuclei (karyolysis). Vacuolation, a response which has historically been considered a sign of cytotoxicity, is a reversible process that is believed to result from uptake by lysosomes and ensuing entrapment of materials with basic properties [11]. Lysosomal vacuolation is produced by the uptake of water and swelling due to osmotic demand. Apoptosis is the result of an active cellular process under genetic control. The reaper gene, which was originally found in drosophila, encodes a small peptide that leads to programmed cell death in that species. The reaper gene, or one similar, may be responsible for mammalian cell apoptosis. Apoptosis is characterized by condensation, basophilic staining of chromatin, nuclear disintegration, and a shrinkage of cell volume with a concomitant increase in the cell density [12].

Cytotoxicity may be determined microscopically or macroscopically through the use of vital stains. Vital stains are used to discriminate between live and dead or injured cells on the basis of membrane permeability. Vital stains, such as neutral red, are taken up by the lysosomes of healthy viable cells. Dead or injured cells do not retain neutral red and remain colorless. Trypan blue, on the other hand, is taken up by dead or injured cells but does not stain live cells. Microscopic determinations require discrimination between live cells and those that may be fixed by leachable substances from the test sample. For example, the formaldehyde released from some polymeric adhesives during the curing process can fix cultured cells, causing them to appear normal.

Reference Controls

Polymeric materials, which may be used as positive and negative controls for cytotoxicity assays to confirm the performance of the test method, are available from the U.S. Pharmacopeial Convention, Inc., Rockville, MD. Other reference control materials and suppliers are listed in ISO 10993-12.

MAMMALIAN CELL CULTURE STANDARDS

The following sections summarize ISO procedures for cytotoxicity testing (ISO 10993-5. Biological evaluation of medical devices—Part 5: Tests for cytotoxicity: in vitro methods). ISO 10993-5 recommends testing a sample portion of a finished device, a portion of one of its components or an extract thereof. This standard has also been adopted by national standards organizations in the U.S., Europe, Asia and Latin American countries which participated in development of the standard. These standards are recommended and accepted internationally by the health authorities who regulate approval of medical devices.

Other cell culture assays for unique products are listed in the product standards of ISO, American Society for Testing Materials, American Dental Association, etc. For example, the Australian Ministry of Health has published cell culture assays for urinary catheters and blood containers; Japan has a colony-forming cytotoxicity assay for contact lenses [13]. Most standards and guidelines are revised periodically to reflect changes in standard practices. The interested reader should contact the respective association for the current edition of these standards.

Agar Diffusion Assay

This assay, which derives from work by Guess et al. [14] and Dulbecco [15], employs a monolayer of cells with a semi-solid agar overlay on which the test article is placed. This assay is based on the migration or diffusion of toxic substances from the test article through the agar to the cellular monolayer. The slow diffusion of leachable substances through the agar results in a concentration gradient around the test article and a zone of dead cells if the leachable substances are toxic. The agar overlay also protects the cells from physical damage by certain kinds of test articles, such as materials that may float or move about in a liquid culture medium or high-density samples that would traumatize the cells by direct contact. In addition, liquid samples absorbed on filter disks or powders may be tested by this assay. The assay is also useful for small samples, which provide a limited amount of material for extraction, and for samples which have different surfaces (e.g., surface finish or adhesive).

In the standard assay (Figure 21-2), a suspension of adherent cells is pipetted into a culture dish and incubated until the cells attach to the surface of the dish. The cells are

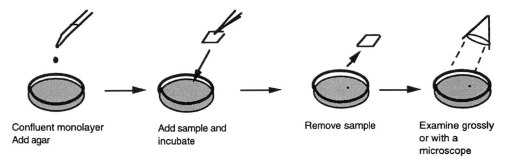

Confluent monolayer   Add sample and   Remove sample   Examine grossly
Add agar   incubate   or with a
                                                                 microscope

Figure 21-2 Schematic of agar diffusion assay.

incubated until a near-confluent monolayer of cells is formed. Thus, differences in cell type and size of culture dish affect the number of cells seeded and incubation period prior to use. After the monolayer is established, the culture medium is removed and the cells are rinsed with phosphate buffered saline. Culture medium containing 1 percent agar and serum is then added to the culture dishes. To avoid heat denaturation of serum proteins, the agar is melted and cooled to approximately 45°C before being added to the culture medium. The test articles are then placed on the semi-solid agar surface and the prepared cultures incubated for 24–72 hours. If desired, a vital stain, such as neutral red, may be added before or after incubation with the test article. Cytotoxicity may be measured objectively or estimated subjectively using descriptive terms (e.g., none, slight, moderate or severe) or semi-quantitative numeric terms (e.g., 0, 1, 2, etc.) (See Table 21-3).

The type of agar is a critical factor for this assay. Agar is a natural product derived from red algae and is available in a variety of grades, molecular weight ranges, and gel temperatures. The preferred type for the agar diffusion assay is Bacto-agar or agarose. Wilsnack et al. [16] noted that agarose, which gels at 32°C, prevents the thermal shock associated with preparation of agar overlays at 40°–45°C. They also found that Sudan black and Giemsa stains placed on filter disks showed greater diffusion in agarose than in agar. These differences were attributed to the presence of charged groups that are integral to agar and impede the diffusion of both acidic and basic substances. Agarose does not significantly alter the diffusion rate of charged compounds because it lacks agaropectin. The increased diffusion rate with agarose must be weighed against the potential for decreased concentration of the diffusable chemicals. That is, diffusion of a very low concentration of a toxic chemical may be too rapid to effect a toxic cellular concentration.

The agar diffusion assay has been validated for dose response (content validity), correlation with the direct contact assay (concurrent validity) and the intramuscular implantation assay in rabbits (construct and predictive validity) [17, 18]. Guess et al. [14], who tested

Table 21-3 Reactivity Grades for Agar Diffusion Test and Direct Contact Test

Grade	Reactivity	Description of reactivity zone
0	None	No detectable zone around or under sample
1	Slight	Some malformed or degenerated cells under sample
2	Mild	Zone limited to area under sample
3	Moderate	Zone extends 0.5 to 1.0 cm beyond sample
4	Severe	Zone extends greater than 1.0 cm beyond sample but does not involve entire dish

100 different plastic samples, found the agar diffusion assay using L-929 cells gave results identical to those obtained with the direct contact assay for 94 percent of the samples. The remaining 6 percent gave negative responses in the agar diffusion assay, responses attributed to the low concentration of chemicals diffusing through the agar overlay.

Wilsnack et al. [16] modified the agar diffusion assay by overlaying the agarose with an additional 4 mL of culture medium. This method was not as sensitive as the Extract Dilution assay in detecting cytotoxicity with rubber, polyvinyl chloride, polypropylene, polyethylene, silicone rubber, an unidentified copolymer, and paper materials.

Brown et al. [19] compared the standard agar diffusion assay with a modification wherein the cells were suspended in an agar media matrix free of vital stains or indicators. The agar media suspension modification allowed for more cell growth and replication than the confluent monolayer. This test design increased the sensitivity of the assay, as was shown by a lower toxicity detection level for benzalkonium chloride. This modification also makes it possible to increase the assay exposure period to 7 days from the conventional 1 day.

Imai et al. [20] used the agar diffusion assay to evaluate the biological effects of dental materials. By varying the thickness of the agar overlay between 1 and 5.5 mm, they demonstrated "thickness dependent" or diffusion-dependent cytotoxicity. Varying the amount of serum in the agar overlay from 10 to 50 percent demonstrated interaction or binding of toxicants with serum proteins.

Direct Contact Assay

This assay, which derives from work of Rosenbluth et al. [21], employs a monolayer of cells on which the test article is placed in direct contact with the cells. The biological response is usually determined after 24 hours exposure although in some instances the exposure period may be extended to 48 hours. Like the agar diffusion assay, this assay is based on the diffusion or migration of substances into the culture medium.

In the standard assay (Figure 21-3), 2 mL of a suspension of cells in culture medium is added to a 35 mm culture dish. The cultures are incubated for 24 hours at 37°C, allowing the cells to attach to the base of the dish. The concentration of cells in the innoculum and cellular replication rate determines the time required for establishment of a monolayer. Individual culture dishes ensure there is no chemical interaction among extractives of different test articles. The volume of culture medium is reduced before adding the test article to minimize any physical movement of the test article. Movement of the test article has the potential for traumatizing the cellular monolayer and could inadvertently be misinterpreted

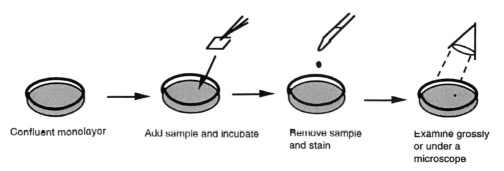

Confluent monolayor   Add sample and incubate   Remove sample   Examine grossly
                                                               and stain   or under a
                                                                                       microscope

Figure 21-3   Schematic of direct contact assay.

as a cytotoxic response. The cultures are then incubated for 24–48 hours and the amount of cytotoxicity determined by observation either using a phase contrast microscope or following histochemical staining. Subjective-descriptive terms (i.e., none, slight, moderate or severe) or numeric terms (i.e., 0, 1, 2, etc.) are given in Table 21-3.

The direct contact assay has been applied to a wide variety of materials used in medical devices. The assay has content, concurrent, construct and predictive validity as described for the agar diffusion assay. Rosenbluth et al. [21] tested 112 plastic samples obtained from administration devices, containers, catheters, and other medical devices. He found that the direct contact assay had greater sensitivity for detecting toxic plastic samples than the intramuscular implantation assay.

Extract Dilution Assay

In this assay, a serially diluted extract of a material is evaluated for cytotoxicity. An exception would be the situation in which the culture medium is the extractant and, hence, dilution may or may not occur. Standard surface-to-volume ratios for preparing extracts are summarized in Table 21-2.

In the standard assay, a suspension of cells is added to a culture dish. The cultures are incubated for 24 hrs at 37°C, allowing the cells to attach to the base of the dish. The culture medium is removed and replaced with fresh medium containing the sample extract. Concentrated culture medium is recommended for use in diluting aqueous extracts to retain optimal culture media osmolality for the cells. The cultures are incubated for an appropriate interval, usually 24 to 72 hours. Any toxic substances in the extract will be evenly distributed in the culture medium, resulting in changes in monolayer density rather than yielding zones of toxic and normal cells. Cytotoxicity is commonly evaluated after histochemical staining. Malformed or degenerated cells may be observed if they were not lost prior to fixation. Assay interpretation is usually based on a subjective evaluation of the decrease in monolayer density and the extent of affected cells (Table 21-4). One modification of this assay involves removing and liquefying the stained cells and then quantifying the color with a spectrophotometer. Alternatively, live cells may be observed by phase microscopy and scored at 24-hour intervals.

The Extract Dilution Assay has content, construct, concurrent and predictive validity as described for the agar diffusion assay. Wilsnack et al. [16] compared the sensitivity with the agar diffusion assay, systemic injection in mice, intracutaneous irritation in rabbits, and intramuscular implantation in rabbits (viz., U.S. Pharmacopeia 88, Biological Reactivity in

Table 21-4   Reactivity Grades for Elution Test

Grade	Reactivity	Conditions of all cultures
0	None	Discrete intracytoplasmic granules; no cell lysis
1	Slight	Not more than 20% of the cells are round, loosely attached, and without intracytoplasmic granules; occasional lysed cells are present
2	Mild	Not more than 50% of the cells are round and devoid of intracytoplasmic granules; extensive cell lysis and empty areas between cells
3	Moderate	Not more than 70% of the cell layers contain rounded cells and/or are lysed
4	Severe	Nearly complete destruction of the cell layers

Vivo). Using WI-38 cells, they observed toxic cell culture responses from 7 of 18 different polyvinyl chloride (PVC) extracts prepared with culture medium. No responses were observed using saline or cottonseed oil extracts sorbed into disks in a modified agarose overlay assay or when the plastic samples were placed on the surface of the agarose and in turn overlaid with culture medium. All PVC samples were nontoxic in the standard animal bioassays. Tests with rubber materials showed greater toxicity when tested using culture medium extracts in vitro than when tested using cottonseed oil extracts in vivo in the intracutaneous rabbit test. However, in vitro and in vivo assays frequently yielded different results with rubber samples. The rationale for differing results may be due to the type of chemicals extracted by different solvents as well as the detection limit of the biological assay.

CELL FUNCTION ASSAYS

Cell function assays are used in evaluating the compatibility of materials used in medical devices in order to obtain objective measures. A comprehensive comparison of cell function assays was reported by Johnson et al. [1]. In this study, ten materials were tested in assays measuring proteins, nucleic acids, glucose, ATP, phagocytosis, and cellular adhesion. Primary cells and established cell strains were evaluated. Results with biochemical methods demonstrated good agreement in toxicity ranking of materials, regardless of which cell culture was used. Methods that measured phagocytosis and adhesion were highly sensitive but had low toxicity ranking agreement and reproducibility. Furthermore, assays using established cell lines were more reproducible than assays using primary cell types (i.e., lymphocytes, mixed white blood cells, peritoneal macrophages, and mouse embryo cells).

Biochemical methods can measure such cell functions as DNA synthesis, protein synthesis, or metabolic rate as measured by glucose or ATP concentration. The most widely accepted cell function assay is the inhibition of cell growth assay [22]. Cell growth is determined by protein analysis after exposure to an aqueous extract of the material. The authors have recommended preparing multiple extracts of different masses of material in order to correct for diffusion of extractable chemicals. Other investigators have used varying dilutions of a single extract. In either case, the objective is to determine whether the extract affects cell growth and to note the mass of material or concentration of extract where this occurs. The data are compared with that from a database of other materials similarly tested. The MTT [3-(4,5-dimethylthiazol-2-yl)2,5-diphenyl tetrazolium bromide] assay is a colorimetric method of determining cell viability based on reduction of the yellow tetrazolium salt MTT to a purple formazan dye by mitochondrial succinnic dehydrogenase in viable cells. Osborne et al. [23] found that MTT produced higher incorporation in untreated control cultures but lower background staining following treatment with maximally cytotoxic concentrations of surfactant over a linear range of absorbencies. Assessment of membrane integrity forms the basis of assays measuring ^{51}Cr release [24, 25] or lysosomal enzymes such as lactic dehydrogenase [26]. These assays have not been used extensively for assessment of medical device/material biocompatibility.

MATERIALS EVALUATION

Each biomedical material or formulation component must be tested for biocompatibility because there is extensive variation in their physical and chemical properties. For example, it is widely known that low molecular weight organotin stabilizers (6 carbons or less) may leach from a flexible polymer, resulting in toxicity in a biological assay (see also Chapters 2, 16, and 17). This effect is related to the aqueous solubility and comparatively high toxicity of these chemicals which have also been used as pesticides. The higher molecular weight organotin compounds are insoluble (less than 1 part per 10,000 parts) in aqueous media and have been used as stabilizers in plastic formulations that are radiation sterilized. Plastisols may give toxic responses if they contain high amounts of selected plasticizers or if residual solvents released during curing are present at high levels at the time of assay. Residual solvents frequently contribute to the biological response to adhesive materials. Heavy metal ions or residual monomers may inhibit the activity of cellular enzymes. Synthetic elastomers may release acetic acid or formaldehyde if improperly cured. Latex and natural rubber materials contain a variety of potentially toxic, leachable chemicals as mercaptobenzothiazoles and thiocarbamates [27, 28]. In addition, sterilization methods may affect the biocompatibility of materials (see also Chapter 15). The toxicity of residual ethylene oxide is widely recognized. Materials are differentially sensitive to radiation and may form free radical reaction products of an antioxidant or other chemical additive.

CURRENT ISSUES

Standardization of cell culture methods is one of the most important current issues for the evaluation of biocompatibility of medical devices. In general, the best standards are based on methods which have become widely accepted by a variety of investigators and/or industrial firms. The next stage of standards development is interlaboratory testing to ensure reproducibility and reliability among different laboratories.

Progress toward standardization has been achieved by interlaboratory testing using the same methods and materials and by voluntary development of detailed assay procedures. The reliability of the test method is based upon obtaining consistent results between laboratories using the same test or in the same laboratory over time. For example, Turner, Spyratou and Schmidt [29] emphasized variation in test results which were attributable to frequency of changing the culture medium, the initial cell number and the surface area available for growth of an adherent cell strain.

Bultitude and Boocock [17] reported an interlaboratory trial of the direct contact, agar overlay, and extract dilution assays. This report is very useful in describing the variables affecting these assays. The test samples consisted of a low-density polyethylene; polyvinyl chlorides with either calcium zinc, dibutyl tin dilaurate (3000 ppm), dioctyl tin thioglycolate (1300 ppm) or two unidentified tin stabilizers (1400 and 60 ppm); silicone rubber; natural rubber; and di-n-butyl phthalate. In the direct contact assay, there was considerable variability among the laboratories in demonstrating the amount of toxicity. However, the relative ranking of the samples was very similar. The agar overlay and extract procedures were carried out using a wide variety of conditions and were not comparable. The most favored method was that with which the laboratory was most familiar.

The University of Tennessee [22] conducted an interlaboratory study of the agar overlay and inhibition of cell growth assays along with in vivo and hemolysis assays. Five independent, replicate assays were conducted on each of four materials (clear vinyl, gum rubber, black neoprene, and polyurethane). All laboratories ranked the materials in the same order of toxicity; however, the magnitude of the differences in toxicity rating varied among the laboratories due to individual subjective judgment.

Travenol Laboratories, Inc. [30] reported an interlaboratory study of six assays on six materials. The assays were low cell density with L-929 or citrullinemia cells, confluent cell density (protein analysis) with L-929, ^{3}H-uridine uptake by mixed human lymphocytes, phagocytosis by mouse macrophages, and DNA synthesis in mouse embryo cells. The low cell density is an extract dilution assay using a low cell population such that individual clones of cells are formed whereas the confluent cell density assay uses an established monolayer of cells. All of these assays yielded objective numerical data rather than the qualitative data characteristic of the previous interlaboratory studies. The test materials were polyethylene, stainless steel 316, polyurethane, silver, and unstabilized and dibutyl tin dilaurate stabilized polyvinyl chlorides. These materials covered the range of nonreactive to highly toxic samples. The toxicity classifications of the materials were differentiated by all assays. However, there was greater variation in the data for those assays that required more complex technical skills. The low cell density method with L-929 cells and macrophage phagocytosis assays exhibited the best repeatability, reproducibility, and relative merit.

A second major issue is the use of cytotoxicity data for risk characterization. Risk characterization involves integration of information from hazard identification, dose-response assessment and exposure assessment to develop a qualitative or quantitative estimate of the likelihood that any hazards associated with the material will be realized in exposed humans [31]. The standardized methods described in this chapter have been validated as screening tests but not for the purpose of interpreting the results for extended clinical use of a medical device nor for unique types of medical devices. That is, the assays were established on the basis of correlative results with some measure of in vivo toxicity in animals rather than a mechanistic basis of the response of the test system to in vivo pathology in humans. As described by Frazier [3], the information obtained from in vitro test systems is based on the concentration of chemical which produces a given cellular effect. For risk characterization, the chemical concentration in vitro needs to be compared with the target tissue dosage which results from an exposure to the chemical in vivo. That is, the concentration in vitro can be related to in vivo effects through physiologically based toxicokinetic models of exposure dosages.

True risk characterization is not currently attainable because the composition of the medical device frequently turns out to be too complex to identify and quantify all potentially extractable species. The inability to define and prepare precise dosages precludes a thorough dose-response assessment, i.e., the quantitative relationship between the dose and the toxic response. On the assumption that extraction occurs from or close to the surface of the device, the amount of chemical(s) extracted will be proportional to the exposed surface area. Dose concentration is therefore often determined by interfacial area per unit volume of solvent at extraction. However, more extensive studies by Till et al. [32] have shown that the migration of chemicals from a solid plastic material into liquid solvents is controlled by diffusional resistance within the solid, chemical concentration, time, temperature, mass transfer resistance on the solvent side, fluid turbulence at the solid-solvent interface and the partition coefficient of the chemical in the solvent. The diffusion-controlled release of extractable chemicals is illustrated in Figure 21-4 which shows that the available extractable pool of low molecular weight chemicals may be less than the total pool. This explains in part why different extraction media may result in different cytotoxic potentials [9, 20].

Complete dissolution of a medical device or material is an alternative approach for *in vitro* testing. Its main limitation is that it does not simulate the intended clinical application, or it may create degradation products that do not occur in the clinical application. Therefore, the actual clinical dosage or agent exposed to the cells in toxicokinetic terms may be overexaggerated because the rate of diffusion from the intact material or medical device may be very slow or different from complete dissolution.

One could cite many reported examples of materials that have performed well in animals and yet have "failed" cell culture tests [33]. Whether this observation is related to

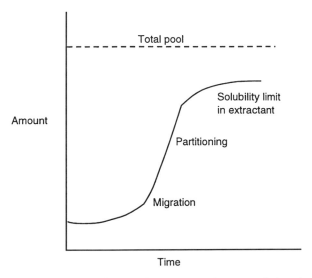

Figure 21-4 Schematic of factors affecting the amount of extracted chemicals from a plastic material.

dose-response effects in vitro, metabolism in vivo or other factors has not been determined. As the field of new material development progresses, it is important that toxic materials be detected early in the development process—but care must be taken not to discard materials with potential. Since nearly all cell culture studies employ relatively short periods of exposure to the materials, the extrapolation is limited to studies of comparable duration in animals or humans. A variety of reports have shown very good correlation of toxicity between in vitro and in vivo acute biocompatibility studies (14, 16, 21, 34). Extension of cell culture tests to measure selected aspects of cellular function (e.g., protein synthesis and glucose metabolism) and the use of greater exposure periods will provide additional dimensions to biocompatibility assessment.

LIST OF SPECIFICATIONS AND STANDARDS

1   Guidance on selection of tests. *Biological Evaluation of Medical Devices*, Part 1. Geneva: International Organization for Standardization, 1994.

2   Tests for cytotoxicity: in vitro methods. *Biological Evaluation of Medical Devices*, Part 5. Geneva: International Organization for Standardization, 1993.

3   Sample preparation and reference materials. *Biological Evaluation of Medical Devices*, Part 12. Geneva: International Organization for Standardization, 1993.

4   *F-813 Standard Practice for Direct Contact Cell Culture Evaluation of Materials for Medical Devices*. West Choshocken, PA: American Society for Testing and Materials, 1992.

5   *F-895 Standard Practice for Agar Diffusion Cell Culture Screening for Cytotoxicity*. West Choshocken, PA: American Society for Testing and Materials, 1990.

6   *Recommended Standard Practices for the Biological Evaluation of Dental Materials*. Chicago: American Dental Association, 1982.

7   *Biocompatibility Testing of Device Materials in Canada*. Ottawa, Ontario: Environmental Health Directorate, Health Canada, 1994.

8   *Medical Equipment—Single Use Urethral Catheters (Sterile) for General Medical Use*. North Sydney, NSW: Standards Australia, 1989.

9   Cytotoxicity test (Colony Assay). *Guidelines for Basic Biological Tests of Medical Materials and Devices (Japan)*, Part I. Tokyo: National Institute of Health Science, 1995.

REFERENCES

1   Johnson HJ, Northup SJ, Seagraves PA, et al. Biocompatibility test procedures for materials evaluation in vitro. I. Comparative test system sensitivity. *J Biomed Mater Res*, 17 (1983), 571–586.
2   Darby TD. Safety evaluation of polymer materials. *Ann Rev Pharmacol Toxicol*, 27 (1987), 157–167.
3   Frazier JM. Validation of in vitro models. *J Am Coll Toxicol*, 9 (1990), 355–359.
4   Seibert H, Gülden M, Voss J-U. Comparative cell toxicology: The basis for in vitro toxicity testing. *ALTA*, 22 (1994), 168–174.
5   Grisham JW, Smith GJ. Predictive and mechanistic evaluation of toxic responses in mammalian cell culture systems. *Pharmacol Rev*, 36 (1984), 151S–171S.
6   Riddell RJ, Panacer DS, Wilde SM, Clothier RH, Balls M. The importance of exposure period and cell type in in vitro cytotoxicity tests. *ALTA*, 14 (1986), 86–92.
7   Tardiff RG. In vitro methods of toxicity evaluation. *Ann Rev Pharmacol Toxicol*, 18 (1978), 357–369.
8   Eagle H. Nutritional needs of mammalian cells in culture. *Science*, 122 (1955), 501–504.
9   Groth T, Falck P, Miethke R-R. Cytotoxicity of biomaterials—basic mechanisms and in vitro test methods: A review. *ALTA*, 23 (1995), 790–799.
10 Majno G, Joris I. Apoptosis, oncosis and necrosis: An overview of cell death. *Am J Pathol*, 146 (1995), 3–15.
11 Valtolina M, Forster R. Induction of cytoplasmic vacuolation by two alkyl-diamine compounds. *ALTA*, 19 (1991), 30–38.
12 Arends MJ, Morris RG, Wyllie AH. Apoptosis: The role of endonuclease. *Am J Pathol*, 136 (1990), 593–608.
13 Tsuchiya T, Arai T, Ohhashi J, Imai K, Kojima H, et al. Rabbit eye irritation caused by wearing toxic contact lenses and their cytotoxicities: In vivo/in vitro correlation study using standard reference materials. *J Biomed Mater Res*, 27 (1993), 885–893.
14 Guess WL, Rosenbluth SA, Schmidt B, et al. Agar diffusion method for toxicity screening of plastics on cultured cell monolayers. *J Pharm Sci*, 54 (1965), 1545–1547.
15 Dulbecco R. Production of plaques in monolayer tissue cultures by single particles of an animal virus. *Proc Natl Acad Sci (USA)*, 38 (1952), 747–752.
16 Wilsnack RE, Meyer FJ, Smith JG. Human cell culture toxicity testing of medical devices and correlation to animal tests. *Biomat Med Dev Art Org*, 1 (1973), 543–562.
17 Bultitude FW, Boocock G. *Interlaboratory Trial of Cell Culture Methods for BSI Technical Committee SGS/26-Toxicity Tests for Medical Rubber and Plastics*. London: Ministry of Defense, AWRE Chemistry Division. 1977.
18 Johnson HJ, Northup SJ, Seagraves PA, et al. Biocompatibility test procedures for materials evaluation in vitro. II. Objective methods of toxicity assessment. *J Biomed Mater Res*, 19 (1985), 489–508.
19 Brown IM, Kaplan MM, Szabocsik JM. An improved in vitro screening method for cytotoxicity. *Dev Biol Stand*, 19 (1977), 299–307.
20 Imai Y, Watanabe A, Chang P-I, et al. Evaluation of the biological effects of dental materials using a new cell culture technique. *J Dental Res*, 61 (1982), 1024–1027.
21 Rosenbluth SA, Weddington GR, Guess WL, et al. Tissue culture method for screening toxicity of plastic materials to be used in medical practice. *J Pharm Sci*, 54 (1965), 156–159.
22 University of Tennessee, Materials Science Toxicology Laboratories. *Determination of Levels of Chemical Purity for Biomaterials Used as Surgical Implants*. Quarterly Report No. 15-16: Part II. Contract No. FDA 223-73-5231. Washington, DC: National Technical Information Service, 1978.
23 Osborne R, Perkins MA, Roberts DA. Development and interlaboratory evaluation of an in vitro human cell-based test to aid ocular irritancy assessments. *Fund Appl Toxicol*, 28 (1995), 139–153.
24 Ulreich JB, Chvapil M. In vitro toxicity testing: A quantitative microassay. In Brown SA (Ed.), *Cell-Culture Test Methods ASTM STP 810*. Philadelphia, PA: American Society for Testing and Materials, 1983, 102–113.
25 Ulreich JB, Chvapil M. A quantitative microassay for in vitro toxicity testing of biomaterials. *J Biomed Mater Res*, 15 (1981), 913–922.
26 Grasso P, Gaydon J, Hendy RJ. The safety testing of medical plastics. II. An assessment of lysosomal changes as an index of toxicity in cell cultures. *Fd Cosmet Toxicol*, 11 (1973), 255–263.
27 Wood RT. Validation of elastomeric closures for parenteral use: An overview. *J Parenteral Drug Assoc*, 34 (1980), 286–294.
28 Nakamura A, Ikarashi Y, Tsuchiya T, Kaniwa M-A, Sato M, Toyoda K, et al. Correlations among chemical constituents, cytotoxicities and tissue responses: In the case of natural rubber latex materials. *Biomat*, 11 (1990), 92–94.
29 Turner TD, Spyratou O, Schmidt RJ. Biocompatibility of wound management products: Standardization of and determination of cell growth rate in L929 fibroblast cultures. *J Pharm Pharmacol*, 41 (1989), 775–780.

30 Travenol Laboratories, Inc. *Development of test procedures for the evaluation of implantable biomedical materials in vitro. Round robin tissue culture program.* FDA Contract 223-77-503. Washington: U.S. Department of Health, Education and Welfare, 1979.

31 *Science and Judgment in Risk Assessment.* Washington, DC: National Academy Press, 1994.

32 Till DE, Reid RC, Schwartz PS, et al. Plasticizer migration from polyvinyl chloride film to solvents and foods. *Fd Chem Toxicol*, 20 (1982), 95–104.

33 Brown S. Developing biocompatibility test methods: ASTM Committee F-4. *Med Device Diag Ind*, 1 (1979), 25–32.

34 Johnson HJ, Northup SJ. Tissue-culture biocompatibility testing program. In Brown SA (Ed.), *Cell-Culture Test Methods ASTM STP 810.* Philadelphia, PA: American Society for Testing and Materials, 1983, 25–34.

Chapter 22

Hemocompatibility: Effects on Cellular Elements

Patrick J. Parks

INTRODUCTION

When biomaterials interact with blood, formed elements cause thrombosis, embolism, and inflammation. This chapter provides an overview of the mechanisms involved in the reactions of formed elements of blood to materials and measurements that monitor these events.

The interaction of the formed elements of blood with biomaterials reflect a sequence of events that includes both humoral and cellular components. The initial phases of blood-material interactions are well known (Figure 22-1). Following exposure of a material to blood, there is a rapid, almost immediate, coating of the biomaterial by a protein layer. The proteins comprising the adsorbed layer can and do undergo exchange, and the composition of the protein layer varies over the time of blood exposure. It still is not possible to predict the *a priori* relationship between any characteristic of a material or device and the composition of the proteins in the adsorbed layer. The complexities of blood flow and the intrinsic variability among patients [1] contribute to the inability to predict concisely. However, certain general principles are known. Fibrinogen preferentially adsorbs [2–9] and can displace proteins such as albumin. Similarly, elements of the contact activation phase of coagulation including Factor XII and High Molecular Weight Kininogen also adsorb. Together, these and a series of other proteins that include the complement sequence contribute to and in many cases determine the cellular reaction to a biomaterial. The reactions of the cellular elements of blood to a biomaterial are bound inextricably with the humoral response to the material.

WHOLE BODY INFLAMMATORY RESPONSE

The "Total Body Inflammatory Reaction" or "Whole Body Inflammatory Response" is a collection of physical and chemical changes that are associated with blood exposure to a biomaterial. The findings include [10, 11] bleeding, thrombosis with its attendant complications, massive fluid shifts, and activation of cellular and humoral defense mechanisms. The term implies both inflammatory and hemostatic abnormalities, and reflects the interaction between these systems. The inflammatory and hemostatic components of the Whole Body Inflammatory Response will be considered separately.

The inflammatory response includes cytokines [12, 13], activated neutrophils [14, 15] and activated complement sequence proteins (Figure 22-2). Complement forms one of several humoral defense mechanisms, is an example of a cascade, and, as a humoral mediator, has been considered and described in detail elsewhere [16–18]. Small amounts of initiator from one of two pathways lead to the formation of C3 convertase. This enzyme produces biologically active compounds of the complement system which include the frequently measured components, C3a and C5a [12, 19, 20]. The products of complement system activation induce changes on circulating neutrophils via receptors for these components [21–25].

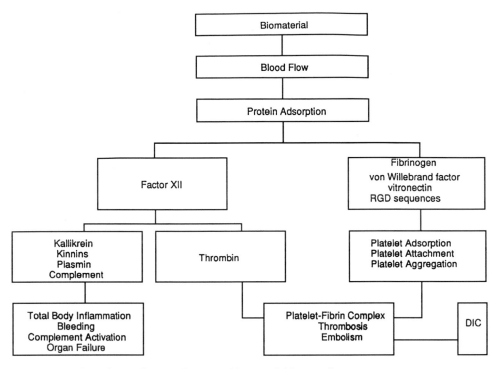

Figure 22-1   Flowsheet of events in blood–biomaterial interactions.

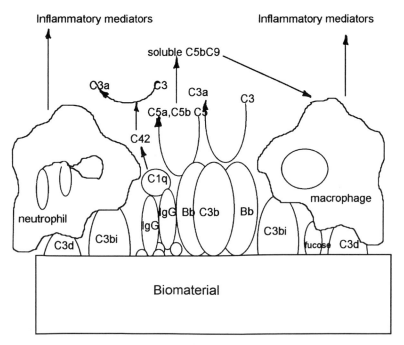

Figure 22-2   Schematic representation of major interactions involving formed elements of blood with complement and biomaterials.

Neutrophils adhere to the surface of a material as a result of binding to the available receptors. The complement components can be both ligands and chemoattractants; for example, C5a induces neutrophil chemotaxis in addition to binding to the neutrophil membrane.

The attachment, activation and partial or complete degradation of the third component of complement, C3, is critical to the cellular activation process [25]. Intact C3b, and the breakdown product C3bi form the ligands for binding to CR1 and CD11b/CD18 receptors, respectively, with neutrophils. Regulation of the CD11b receptor also occurs with cardiopulmonary bypass [23]. Attachment of the neutrophils to the complement receptor will lead to the formation of oxidative metabolites capable of inducing injury to local endothelium [24, 26]. Additional mediators include elastase and myeloperoxidase from azurophilic granules as well as lactoferrin from specific granules following surface-induced activation [23]. Attachment of neutrophils also can produce local concentrations of leukotriene B4 or platetet activating factor [26] which can contribute to thrombus formation at the point of adherence of the neutrophils. However, even in the absence of serum, mononuclear cells in contact with Cuprophan can be activated [27, 28] and are capable of producing inflammatory mediators. The pathway is L-fucose dependent [29] and has been observed with Cuprophan dialysis membranes. However, this pathway also shows sensitivity to the complement system. Amplification of the cell pathway occurs following exposure to the Terminal Complement Complex, or Membrane Attack Complex, composed of the last portions of the complement sequence, C5–C9 [29].

The systemic findings with blood-contacting devices are not unique to biomaterials; similar findings have been observed in massively injured trauma patients [30]. Intravascular leukostasis, especially involving the lungs [31], hypotension, and hypoxemia can be found both in trauma patients and in patients with blood-contacting devices [32]. The multi-organ failure syndrome that is encountered with trauma patients includes edema and eventual failure of organs distal from the original site of injury; this syndrome reflects the systemic effects of complement [30]. Through a similar mechanism, neutropenia occurs as a result of reversible leukostasis and leukocyte aggregate formation within the first fifteen minutes of dialysis [25], cardiopulmonary bypass [33] and apheresis [31], although to varying degrees. Leukopenia is the direct result of complement activation and release, leading to neutrophil aggregates [14, 22, 23, 25, 34]. While complement activation can occur as a result of the type of surgery [35], the contact of blood with a material is the more significant source of complement activation. The local and systemic presence of activated complement components allows neutrophils to adhere to endothelial cells throughout the body [14] as well as at the anastamotic junctions of vascular grafts [24]. Given neutropenia as an outcome of cellular activation, measurement of the neutrophil count before and after exposure to a biomaterial can serve as one indicator of interaction. Monocytes attach to surfaces in a manner similar to the way in which neutrophils attach. However, the monocyte number in the circulation is an order of magnitude lower than the neutrophil count, and cell differential counts will be relatively insensitive in measuring changes in monocyte counts. Direct measurement of monocyte count using current cell counting devices may be more accurate, but the measurement of the products of stimulated monocytes (e.g., IL-1) forms a more useful marker of cellular activation [23, 25, 27].

A variety of experimental [1, 14, 21, 36–38] and/or recommended test methods useful in predicting the potential of a biomaterial for inducing leukocyte activation and subsequent inflammatory reactions are available [39]. The cost-to-benefit ratio for a particular test or set of tests and the required specificity of results makes practical test selection more difficult. Serum or plasma markers that predict the ability of a material to activate complement form one potential method for predicting, in part, the inflammatory potential of a material

[25, 40–43]. Complicating the general utility of such a method is the clinical setting; alternative pathway activation is responsible to a great extent or completely responsible for complement activation on synthetic biomaterials [14, 16–18, 25, 41, 44–46]. By comparison, the use of protamine during cardiopulmonary bypass produces complement activation via the classical pathway to an extent greater than that caused by the biomaterial [47], making clinical interpretation of material-induced complement activation difficult. The adsorption of various complement components [20, 33, 44, 46, 48–50] limits predictive value of blood levels for most components of the complement system with the exception of the soluble form of the terminal complement complex, sC5bC9 (51). Intuitively, low levels of complement activation by a biomaterial would suggest low levels of cellular activation since they are related. The measurement of sC5bC9 acts as a fluid phase "surrogate" for cellular activation, although interpretation of the measured levels are dependent on the clinical condition. Further, the magnitude of change of a given parameter does not necessarily correlate with the clinical outcome, and parameters may change over a period of time, making an isolated measurement of limited significance [1]. For example, the long-term sequela of amyloidosis in chronic hemodialysis patients is related to beta 2 microglobulin production and release [14]. In this context, measurement of beta 2 microglobulin production as a result of biomaterial exposure would appear useful. Complement-mediated granulocyte elastase release also is a significant marker [1], having utility in cardiopulmonary bypass and dialysis since elastase augments beta 2 microglobulin expression [25] in addition to having direct effects.

In addition to the classical cellular elements of the inflammatory response—neutrophils, lymphocytes and monocytes—the inflammatory response affects endothelial cells. Independent of the application, endothelial cells will be activated to varying degrees. No direct measure of such a diverse population of cells exists. Vascular grafts in humans involving large vessels such as the aorta function in the absence of an endothelial layer [24, 52]. The in vitro attachment of cellular elements to form a new endothelial layer aims at enhancing the survival of vascular grafts of all diameters [53–56] and measurements that imply biocompatibility include cell migration [53], cell adhesion [53, 55, 56], and cell products [53]. Until methods that lead to successful re-endothelialization in vitro prior to implantation or to sufficient re-endothelialization in vivo after implantation are devised, the surface of any permanent vascular device will be subject to the same potentially adverse reactions as those seen with temporary blood-contacting devices and will require an identical approach to analysis and management [57].

Secreted products from endothelial cells serve as markers that integrate over the entire body's surface of the endothelium [23, 54]. Radioactive isotopic markers can isolate those portions of the endothelium that are involved with adhesion or aggregation of other formed elements [1, 58]. However, a practical marker of endothelial status at a given site remains to be developed. The measurement of endothelial reactions to a biomaterial will continue to be derived from analysis of secreted products that reflect varying contributions to the whole body inflammatory response [23].

HEMOSTATIC ABNORMALITIES

Coagulation

The humoral aspects of blood coagulation are considered in detail elsewhere (see Chapters 23 and 44). The coagulation sequence is the result of a series of proteins acting in sequence; the entire series behaves as an enzyme amplification system, beginning with extremely low levels of activator (e.g., Factor XII) and ending with a thrombus or clot. As is common with biochemical pathways associated with homeostasis, there is more than one initiating pathway [23]. Thrombin production is the most significant result of activation of the coagulation sequence. Thrombin has a range of effects on the formed elements involved in the interaction of blood with biomaterials, predominantly encouraging thrombosis. The local concentration of thrombin is critical to the formation of thrombus or thromboembolism on a biomaterial surface [59]. If success is defined as the absence of clinically significant thrombosis or thromboembolism, then a successfully designed material aims at the reduction or abrogation of local surface-induced thrombin formation [36, 60, 61] and/or control of the amount of thrombin in the circulation as a result of contacting a biomaterial surface [23]. To date, success has been limited at best [60, 62].

Disseminated Intravascular Coagulation

The model used for the hemostatic component of the response of the formed elements of blood to a biomaterial is the condition of disseminated intravascular coagulation (DIC). There is a voluminous literature on disseminated intravascular coagulation, and the literature reflects the broad range of etiologies and the equally broad spectrum of reactivity. Fulminant DIC occurs infrequently in the context of devices or biomaterials [4], and the type of blood activation customarily observed with materials exposure may be so mild as to have no clinical effect on outcome [63]. The diagnosis of DIC requires evidence for four separate events: procoagulant activation, fibrinolytic activation, inhibitor consumption, and end-organ damage or failure.

Procoagulant activation is measured conveniently by fibrinopeptide A, and the activation fragment of prothrombin, PF1.2 [4]. Similarly, fibrinolysis can be measured most specifically by D-dimer [4], a specific product of fibrin breakdown, or less specifically by fibrinogen degradation products which reflect both fibrinogen and fibrin breakdown [4]. The major inhibitor of thrombosis is antithrombin, previously antithrombin III, which combines stoichiometrically with thrombin and prevents thrombin's procoagulant effects. The level of thrombin anti-thrombin complexes, measured immunologically, serves as direct evidence of both procoagulant activation and inhibitor consumption [4]. End organ damage or failure results from thromboemboli [23, 57]. All of the findings necessary to document the existence of disseminated intravascular coagulation can be found with the devices and materials used for blood contact [4, 57]. These findings also imply that the measurement of the humoral components associated with disseminated intravascular coagulation will be pertinent and potentially predictive in the understanding of the influence of a biomaterial on the hemostatic system.

Measurement of fluid phase coagulation-related parameters can reflect the formed element contribution to hemostatic abnormalities. Endothelial cells form a variety of biologically reactive molecules. Thrombin induces endothelial cells to produce tissue plasminogen activator in excess, leading to a hyperfibrinolytic state [23, 64]. Hyperfibrinolysis leads to excess bleeding [63], commonly requiring therapy [65]. While the contribution of the endothelial cell cannot be measured directly, the measurements that define hyperfibrinolysis act as a substitute.

The circulating formed elements that contribute to the hemostatic abnormalities seen with biomaterials interactions include the neutrophil, monocyte, erythrocyte and platelet. The neutrophil effects include platelet-neutrophil aggregates. Monocytes can also form aggregates with platelets, and can form tissue factor [23, 25], contributing to the activation of coagulation factors. Erythrocytes contribute to the hemostatic abnormalities as a result of hemolysis [4, 15, 64]. Long-term devices, e.g., prosthetic cardiac valves or vascular grafts, may be accompanied by compensated hemolytic processes. The degree of compensation in chronic hemolysis is reflected in the reticulocyte count. However, the confounding variables that can arise over extended time of contact make the measurement of limited value. The degree of hemolysis is sensitive to parameters other than the biomaterial surface; blood flow [1] and complement activation [4] are among these. There are no guidelines available a priori for the measurement of a satisfactory or clinically safe level of hemolysis. Intravascular hemolysis of any degree theoretically can be sufficient to begin fulminant DIC [4]. Since the erythrocyte does not have secreted products, the measurement of the erythrocytic contribution to biomaterial interaction continues to be free plasma hemoglobin [15, 62].

It is observed empirically that the adsorbed protein layer on a biomaterial—in particular, adsorbed complement proteins—are prime determinants of the formed element response. Similarly, the contribution of platelets to the hemostatic portion of the response is in large part determined by the presence of fibrinogen on the surface of the biomaterial. While proteins having the arginine-glycine-aspartate, or RGD, sequence have the capacity to bind to platelets [8], the platelet receptors GPIIbIIIa and GPIb-IX preferentially bind to fibrinogen and von Willebrand factor, respectively [9]. Platelets are anucleate cell fragments with a collection of bioactive compounds stored within specific granules [7, 66, 67]. The alpha granules contain platelet factor 4 (PF4), von Willebrand factor, platelet derived growth factor, and fibrinogen and factor V among others [66]. The dense granules contain adenosine diphosphate (ADP), serotonin, calcium and phosphate [66].

The attachment of platelets to the surface of a biomaterial is receptor-mediated, in a fashion analogous to neutrophil attachment (Figure 22-3). Unactivated platelets can bind to fibrinogen adsorbed onto surfaces via GPIc-IIa receptors [9]. The ability of platelets to bind without activation suggests that the enumeration of platelets on a surface of a biomaterial will have limited utility in predicting thrombotic potential. Small amounts of thrombin formed through the coagulation sequence are sufficient to activate platelets [4, 68]. With platelet activation, the receptor for fibrinogen, GPIIb IIIa, is exposed and the conversion of the platelet to the activated state can be monitored with monoclonal antibody to GPIIb IIIa [67].

The further conversion of prothrombin to thrombin accelerates platelet activation and can lead to platelet secretion. The surface of the activated platelet is the preferred surface for prothrombinase assembly and conversion of prothrombin to thrombin. Secretion of the contents of the alpha granules accelerates thrombin formation. The secretion of factor V from the alpha granules further accelerates the response [69, 70]. Secretion from the alpha granules need not be coupled to the secretion from the dense granules, and the sequential activation of platelets can be monitored by the molecules released from the alpha and dense granules. Secreted products from the alpha granules, for example beta thromboglobulin and platelet factor 4, can be used to monitor platelet activation with secretion [7, 15, 66, 67, 71, 72]. Similarly, ATP release can be measured in functional assays of platelets [68, 73]. The secretion of alpha granules is accompanied by the exposure of membrane markers that are otherwise unavailable for binding; specifically, granule membrane protein-140 (GMP-140), also designated CD62 or PADGEM (platelet activation dependent granule external membrane protein) [22] and cell sorting methods can detect the presence of GMP-140 on the surface of circulating platelets.

Activation and aggregation of platelets will proceed as a result of ADP and serotonin, released from the dense granules. The ability of platelets to adhere to one another in the process of aggregation is strictly dependent on the IIb3 integrin [5], which is the GPIIb IIIa receptor. Therefore, aggregation requires activation [5] as does platelet spreading since it involves the same receptor. With platelet aggregation and shape change, membrane-bound arachidonic acid is released and forms thromboxane A2 [66]. Thromboxane A2 or

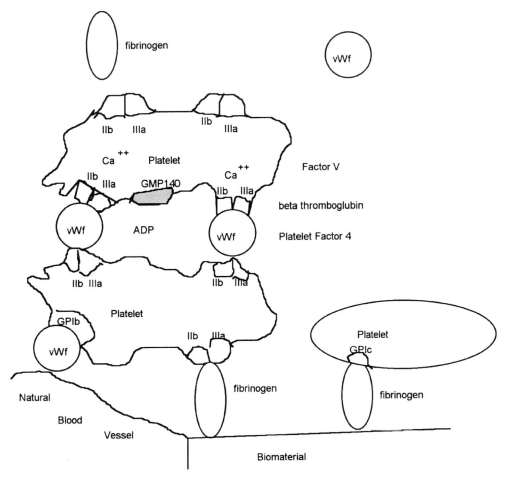

Figure 22-3 Schematic of platelet surface interactions.

its stable metabolite, thromboxane B2, forms additional measures of platelet activation [68]. Thrombin is a sufficiently strong agonist that up to 90% of the contents of both the alpha granules and dense bodies may be secreted in a thromboxane A2 independent fashion, implying that inhibition of the arachidonic acid pathway pharamacologically will not influence platelet function on biomaterials. Since platelet attachment to a surface and to other platelets is the major role for platelets, it is anticipated and has been verified that exposure of platelets to a material will result in a decrease in platelet number. Measurement of platelet number and platelet size through the mean platelet volume gives an index of activation that can illustrate time-dependent changes in hemostasis [4, 68].

The process of platelet adhesion is redundant with respect to both ligand and receptor [5]. It is possible for platelets to adhere to surfaces containing ligands such as von Willebrand factor via the GPIb receptor [5, 9]. The process of attachment of platelets to biomaterials follows the sequence of platelet activation, exposure of the GPIIb IIIa receptor, and binding to fibrinogen or other adsorbed protein on the surface. Attachment of one platelet to the other following adsorption to a biomaterial is dependent on von Willebrand factor [58]. The attachment and subsequent aggregation of platelets is acccompanied by a change in markers that involve primarily GPIb and GPIIb IIIa. These same markers can be used to monitor the embolic potential in using flow cytometric methods [74, 75]. Fragmentation of the platelets into highly reactive microparticles capable of producing thrombin leads to GPIb positive elements with characteristic light scatter profiles [67], although the potential for biologically active microparticles of platelets that are GPIb negative remains as a result of the shedding of GPIb from the surface of activated platelets [76]. Emboli commonly involve platelets complexed with monocytes [22] and measurement of the activation marker CD11b serves as a marker for both monocyte activation and platelet-cell aggregates [22].

SUMMARY

The recommended tests for screening a biomaterial should include the measurement of C3 convertase and platelet dependent prothrombinase, neither of which is practical at present. The proper set of measurements is that which predicts clinical behavior for a given condition. The long-term sequelae of renal dialysis and vascular grafts differ, implying a different set of measurements. The evolution of tests from morphology to cell sorting carries with it the potential to measure the molecular events involved in interaction of the formed elements of blood with biomaterials. However, caveats exist for many of the molecular markers. Monoclonal antibodies characteristically react less well across species lines than polyclonal antibodies; a monoclonal antibody with utility in human studies may not react in preclinical studies depending on the species chosen for preclinical testing. The antibodies have the potential to lead to contradictory results by reacting to subtly different antigenic determinants and by reacting under differing experimental conditions. Refinement of the methods and the extension to animal models, however, carries the greatest potential for analysis. While it is not possible to provide a definitive recommended list for the formed elements, a minimum set of measurements for analyzing the interaction of blood with biomaterials can be described. The measurements should include the number density of the formed element where this can be performed unambiguously, a surface marker that indicates the degree of activation, and a soluble marker that correlates with the activation state, preferably at multiple time points over the course of the interaction of the blood with the biomaterial.

REFERENCES

1   Sundaram S, Courtney JM, Taggart DP, Tweddel AC, Martin W, McQuiston AM, et al. Biocompatibility of cardiopulmonary bypass: Influence on blood compatibility of device type, mode of blood flow and duration of application. *Int J Artificial Organs*, 17 (1994), 118–128.

2   Janvier G, Caix J, Bordenave L, Revel P, Baquey C, Ducassou D. An ex vivo original test using radiotracers for evaluating hemocompatibility of tubular biomaterials. *Appl Radiat Isot*, 45 (1994), 207–218.

3   Panichi V, Casarosa L, Gattai V, Bianchi AM, Andreini B, Migliori M, et al. Protein layer on hemodialysis membranes: A new immunohistochemistry technique. *Int J Art Org*, 18 (1995), 305–308.

4   Bick RL. Disseminated intravascular coagulation: Objective criteria for diagnosis and management. *Med Clin N Amer*, 78 (1994), 511–543.

5   Shattil SJ. Regulation of platelet anchorage and signaling by integrin $a_{IIb}b_3$. *Thromb Haemost*, 70 (1993), 224–228.

6   Garrett KO, Pautler SV, Johnson PC. The inability of low-molecular-weight dextran, aspirin, and prostaglanding E1 to inhibit monolayer platelet adhesion to polyethylene. *J Lab Clin Med*, 121 (1933), 141–148.

7   Groth T, Mihanetzis G, Missirlis Y, Wolf H. The interrelationship between platelet adhesiveness and released platelet factors during standardized in vitro blood/biomaterial contact. *Adv Biomat*, 10 (1992), 247–251

8   Elam J-H, Nygren H. Adsorption of coagulation proteins from whole blood onto polymer materials: relation to platelet activation. Biomaterials, 13 (1992), 3–8.

9   Goodman SL, Cooper SL, Albrecht RM. Integrin receptors and platelet adhesion to synthetic surfaces. *J Biomed Mater Res*, 27 (1993), 683–695.

10 Loisance D. Les biomateriaux cardiovasculaires. *Bull Acad Nat Med*, 179 (1995), 537–546.

11 Downing SW, Edmunds LH. Release of vasoactive substances during cardiopulmonary bypass. *Ann Thorac Surg*, 54 (1992), 1236–1243.

12 Hirano T. The biology of interleukin-6. In Kishimoto T (Ed.), *Interleukins: Molecular Biology and Immunology*. Basel: Karger, 1992, 153–180.

13 Zellweger R, Ayala A, Zhu X-L, Holme KR, DeMaso CM, Chaudry IH. A novel anticoagulant heparin improves splenocyte and peritoneal macrophage function after trauma-hemorrhage and resuscitation. *J Surg Res*, 59 (1995), 211–218.

14 Schulman G. A review of the concept of biocompatibility. *Kidney Int*, 43 (1993), S209–S212.

15 de Haan J, Boonstra PW, Tabuchi N, van Oeveren W, Ebels T. Retransfusion of thoracic wound blood during heart surgery obscures biocompatibility of the extracorporeal circuit. *J Thorac Cardiovasc Surg*, 111 (1996), 272–275.

16 Hakim RM. Complement activation by biomaterials. *Cardiovasc Pathol*, 2 (1993), 187S–197S.

17 Kazatchkine MD, Nydegger UE. The human alternative pathway. Biology and immunopathology of activation and regulation. *Prog Allergy*, 30 (1982), 193–234.

18 Kazatchkine MD, Carreno MP. Activation of the complement system at the interface between blood and artificial surfaces. *Biomaterials*, 9 (1988), 30–34.

19 Kazatchkine MD, Fearon DT, Metcalfe DD, Rosenberg RD, Austen KF. Structural determinants of the capacity of heparin to inhibit the formation of the human amplification C3 convertase. *J Clin Invest*, 67 (1981), 223–228.

20 Nilsson UR, Storm KE, Elwing H, Nilsson B. Conformational epitopes of C3 reflecting its mode of binding to an artificial polymer surface. *Molecular Immunol*, 30 (1993), 211–219.

21 Parsson H, Nassberger L, Thorne J, Norgren L. Metabolic response of granulocytes and platelets to synthetic vascular grafts: Preliminary results with an in vitro technique. *J Biomed Mater Res*, 29 (1995), 519–525.

22 Rinder CS, Bonan JL, Rinder HM, Mathew J, Hines R, Smith BR. Cardiopulmonary bypass induces leukocyte platelet adhesion. *Blood*, 79 (1992), 1201–1205.

23 Edmunds LH. Why cardiopulmonary bypass makes patients sick: Strategies to control the blood-synthetic surface interface. *Adv Cardiac Surg*, 6 (1995), 131–167.

24 Greisler HP. Interactions at the blood/material interface. *Ann Vasc Surg*, 4 (1990), 98–103.

25 Jahns G, Haeffner-Cavaillon N, Nydegger UE, Kazatchkine MD. Complement activation and cytokine production as consequences of immunological bioincompatibility of extracorporeal circuits. *Clin Matl*, 14 (1993), 303–336.

26 Matsuda T, Itoh S, Anderson JM. Endothelial injury during extracorporeal circulation: Neutrophil endothelium interaction induced by complement activation. *J Biomed Mater Res*, 28 (1994), 1387–1395.

27 Betz M, Hansch GM, Rauterberg EW, Bommer J, Ritz E. Cuprammonium membranes stimulate interleukin 1 release and arachidonic acid metabolism in monocytes in the absence of complement. *Kidney Int*, 34 (1988), 67–73.

28 Jahn B, Beta M, Deppisch R, Janssen O, Hansch GM, Ritz E. Stimulation of beta 2 microglobulin synthesis in lymphocytes after exposure to cuprophan dialyzer membranes. *Kidney Int*, 40 (1991), 285–290.

29 Deppisch R, Ritz E, Hansch GM, Schols M, Rauterber EW. Bioincompatibility: Perspectives in 1993. *Kidney Int*, 45 (1994), S77–S84.

30 Nuytinck HK, Offermans XJ, Kubat K, Goris RJ. Whole body inflammation in trauma patients; an autopsy study. *Prog Clin Biol Res*, 236 (1987), A55–A61.

31 Hammerschmidt DE, Craddock PR, McCullough J, Kronenber RS, Dalmasso AP, Jacob HS. Complement activation and pulmonary leucostasis during nylon fiber filtration leucapheresis. *Blood*, 51 (1978), 721.

32 Hakim RM. Clinical sequelae of complement activation in hemodialysis. *Clin Nephrol*, 26 (1986), S9–S12.

33 Liu L, Elwing H. Complement activation on solid surfaces as determined by C3 deposition and hemolytic consumption. *J Biomed Mater Res*, 28 (1994), 767–773.

34 van Oeveren W. Leukocyte and platelet activation during extracorporeal circulation. *Cells Matl*, 4 (1994), 187–195.

35 Garred P, Fosse E, Fagerhol MK, Videm V, Molines TE. Calprotectin and complement activation during major operations with or without cardiopulmonary bypass. *Ann Thorac Surg*, 55 (1993), 694–699.

36 Wendel HP, Heller W, Gallimore MJ, Hoffmeister H-E. Heparin-coated oxygenators significantly reduce contact system activation in an in vitro cardiopulmonary bypass model. *Blood Coag Fibrinolysis*, 5 (1994), 673–678.

37 Combe C, Pourtein M, de Precigout V, Baquey A, Morel D, Potaux L, et al. Granulocyte activation and adhesion molecules during hemodialysis with cuprophane and a high-flux biocompatible membrane. *Am J Kidney Dis*, 24 (1994), 437–442.

38 Kaplan SS, Basford RE, Jeong MH, Simmons RL. Mechanisms of biomaterial-induced superoxide release by neutrophils. *J Biomed Mater Res*, 28 (1994), 377–386.

39 *Biological Evaluation of Medical Devices. AAMI Standards and Recommended Practices*, Volume 4. Arlington, Virginia: Association for the Advancement of Medical Instrumentation, 1995.

40 Chenoweth DE, Henderson LW. Complement activation during hemodialysis: Laboratory evaluation of hemodialyzers. *Art Org*, 11 (1987), 155.

41 Cheung AK. Biocompatibility of hemodialysis membranes. *J Am Soc Nephrol*, 1 (1990), 150–161.

42 Hakim RM. Complement activation by biomaterials. *Cardiovasc Pathology*, 2 (1993), 187S–197S.

43 Janatova J, Cheung AK, Parker CJ. Biomedical polymers differ in their capacity to activate complement. *Compl Inflam*, 8 (1991), 61–69.

44 Fukumara H, Yoshikawa S, Miya M, Hayashi H. In vitro activation and adsorption of complement components by hollow fibers for plasma separation. *J Jap Soc Biomat*, 6 (1988), 23–28.

45 Gutierrez A, Alvestrand A, Bergstrom J, Beving H, Lantz B, Henderson LW. Biocompatibility of hemodialysis membranes: A study in healthy subjects. *Blood Purif*, 12 (1994), 95–105.

46 Pascual M, Plastre O, Montdargent B, Labarre D, Schifferli JA. Specific interactions of polystyrene biomaterials with factor D of human complement. *Biomaterials*, 14 (1993), 665–670.

47 Moorman RM, Zapol WM, Lowenstein E. Neutralization of heparin anticoagulation. In Gravlee GP, Davis RF, Utley JR (Eds.), *Cardiopulmonary Bypass: Principles and Practice*. Baltimore: Williams & Wilkins, 1993, 381–406.

48 Montdargent B, Toufik J, Carreno MP, Labarre D, Jozefowicz M. Complement activation and adsorption of protein fragments by functionalized polymer surfaces in human serum. *Biomaterials*, 13 (1992), 571–576.

49 Vogt W, Luhmann B, Hesse D. "Inactivated" third component of complement (C3b-Like C3; C3i) acquires C5 binding capacity and supports C5 activation upon covalent fixation to a solid surface. *Complement*, 1 (1984), 87–96.

50 Pascual M, Schifferli JA. Adsorption of complement factor D by polyacrylonitrile dialysis membranes. *Kidney Int*, 43 (1993), 903–911.

51 Berger M, Broxup B, Sefton MV. Using ELISA to evaluate complement activation by reference biomaterials. *J Matl Sci Matls Med*, 5 (1994), 622–627.

52 Guidoin R, Chakfe N, Maurel S, How T, Batt M, Marois M, et al. Expanded polytetrafluoroethylene arterial prostheses in humans: Histopathological study of 298 surgically excised grafts. *Biomaterials*, 14 (1993), 678–693.

53 Pronk A, Hoynck van Papendrecht AA, Leguit P, Verbrugh HA, Verkooyen RP, van Vroonhoven TJ. Mesothelial cell adherence to vascular prostheses and their subsequent growth in vitro. *Cell Transpl*, 3 (1994), 41–48.

54 Zhang JC, Wojta J, Binder BR. Growth and fibrinolytic parameters of human umbilical vein endothelial cells seeded onto cardiovascular grafts. *J Thorac Cardiovasc Surgery*, 109 (1995), 1059–1065.

55 Zilla P, Preiss P, Groscurth P, Rosemeier F, Deutsch M, Odell J, et al. In vitro lined endothelium: Initial integrity and survival. *Surgery*, 116 (1994), 524–534.

56 Hirabayashi K, Saitoh E, Ijima H, Takenawa T, Kodama M, Hori M. Influence of fibril length upon ePTFE graft healing and host modification of the implant. *J Biomed Mater Res*, 26 (1992), 1433–1447.

57 Schoen FJ, Clagett GP, Hill JD, Chenoweth DE, Anderson JM, Eberhart RC. The biocompatibility of artificial organs. *ASAIO Transactions*, 33 (1987), 824–833.

58 Sheppeck RA, Garrett KO, Bentz ML, Johnson PC. Platelet deposition on polyethylene: Dependence of second layer platelet attachment on von Willebrand's disease plasma. *ASAIO Transactions*, 37, (1991), M260–M261.

59 Wagner WR, Hubbell JA. Local thrombin synthesis and fibrin formation in an in vitro thrombosis model result in platelet recruitment and thrombus stabilization on collagen in heparinized blood. *J Lab Clin Med*, 116 (1990), 636–650.

60 Lindhout T, Blezer R, Schoen P, Willems GM, Fouache B, Verhoeven M, et al. Antithrombin activity of surface-bound heparin studied under flow conditions. *J Biomed Mater Res*, 29 (1995), 1255–1266.

61 Ericson DG, Parks PJ. Heparin-coated cardiopulmonary bypass and platelet preservation. *IBC Biocomp Blood Interact Matls*, June 26, 1995, 185.

62 Gorman RC, Ziats N, Rao AK, Gikakis N, Sun L, Khan MM, et al. Surface-bound heparin fails to reduce thrombin formation during clinical cardiopulmonary bypass. *J Thorac Cardiovasc Surg*, 111 (1996), 1–11.

63 Kesten S, de Hoyas A, Chaparro C, Westney G, Winton T, Maurer JR. Aprotinin reduces blood loss in lung transplant recipients. *Ann Thoracic Surgery*, 59 (1995), 877–879.

64 de Haan J, Boonstra PW, Monnink SHJ, Ebels T, van Oeveren W. Retransfusion of suctioned blood during cardiopulmonary bypass impairs hemostasis. *Ann Thorac Surg*, 59 (1995), 901–907.

65 Verstraete M. Clinical application of inhibitors of fibrinolysis. *Drugs*, 29 (1985), 236–261.

66 Mruk JS, Chesebro JH, Webster MWI. Platelet aggregation and interaction with the coagulation system: Implications for antithrombotic therapy in arterial thrombosis. *Coronary Art Dis*, 1 (1990), 149–158.

67 Abrams CS, Ellison N, Budzynski AZ, Shattil SJ. Direct detection of activated platelets and platelet-derived microparticles in humans. *Blood*, 75 (1990), 128–138.

68 Bick RL. Platelet function defects associated with hemorrhage or thrombosis. *Med Clin N Amer*, 78 (1994), 577–607.

69 Swords NA, Mann KG. The assembly of the prothrombinase complex on adherent platelets. *Arterioscler Thromb*, 13 (1993), 1602–1612.

70 Tracy PB, Nesheim ME, Mann KG. Platelet factor Xa receptor. *Meth Enzymol*, 215 (1992), 329–360.

71 Orchard MA, Goodchild CS, Prentice CRM, Davies JA, Benoit SE, Creighton-Kemsford LJ, et al. Aprotinin reduces cardiopulmonary bypass induced blood loss and inhibits fibrinolysis without influencing platelets. *Br J Haem*, 85 (1993), 533–541.

72 Weiss HJ, Lages B. Evidence of tissue factor-dependent activation of the classic extrinsic coagulation mechanism in blood obtained from bleeding time wounds. *Blood*, 71 (1988), 629.

73 Owen WG, Bichler J, Ericson DG, Wysokinski W. Gating of thrombin in platelet aggregates by PO_2 linked lowering of extracellular calcium concentration. *Biochemistry*, 34 (1995), 9277–9281.

74 Gemmell CH, Sefton MV, Yeo EL. Platelet-derived microparticle formation involves glycoprotein IIb IIIa. Inhibition by RGDS and a Glanzmann's thrombasthenia defect. *J Biol Chem*, 268 (1993), 14586–14589.

75 Gemmell CH, Ramirez SM, Yeo EL, Sefton MV. Platelet activation in whole blood by artificial surfaces: Identification of platelet derived microparticles and activated platelet binding to leukocytes as material induced activation events. *J Lab Clin Med*, 125 (1995), 276–287.

76 Fox JEB. Shedding of adhesion receptors from the surface of activated platelets. *Blood Coag Fibrinolysis*, 5 (1994), 291–304.

Chapter 23

Hemocompatibility: Effects on Humoral Elements

Suneeti Sapatnekar
James M. Anderson

INTRODUCTION

The widespread use of biomaterials in blood-contacting applications is a feature of modern clinical practice. Contact of blood with a biomaterial surface activates plasma enzyme cascades, and may result in potentially serious consequences for the patient with an implanted biomaterial. For example, surface thrombosis due to activation of the coagulation cascade can occlude a small-diameter vascular graft, necessitating its removal and replacement. However, the potential for activation of the plasma enzyme cascades would depend upon the chemical composition, physical form and site of implantation of the biomaterial. Biomaterial-induced activation of plasma enzyme cascades contributes significantly to blood incompatibility of the surface; in order to improve blood compatibility, it is necessary to design biomaterial surfaces that do not activate the plasma enzymes to an appreciable extent. The purpose of this chapter is to present an overview of biomaterial-induced activation of four major plasma enzyme systems (the coagulation, fibrinolytic, kinin and complement systems) and the approaches to detecting and preventing their activation.

When blood contacts a biomaterial, the first event is the adsorption of plasma proteins upon the surface of the biomaterial. The layer of adsorbed protein directs the course of subsequent events at the blood-biomaterial interface, and may ultimately determine the fate of the biomaterial. The composition of the layer of adsorbed plasma proteins depends upon the surface properties of the material and changes over time. Generally, the first proteins to be adsorbed are the relatively abundant plasma proteins, such as albumin, fibrinogen and fibronectin, but these are soon replaced by trace proteins, including factor XII and high molecular weight kininogen (HMWK) [1]. Adsorption of factor XII, followed by contact activation, is a critical event in the process of activation of the plasma enzyme cascades at the blood-material interface. Activated factor XII is the key enzyme in initiating the coagulation, fibrinolysis and kinin cascades (Figure 23-1). Depending upon the extent of activation of coagulation/fibrinolysis, the outcome could range from a subtle activation of platelets to a major thrombo-embolic complication, or an episode of abnormal bleeding. If activation of the kinin cascade is prominent, the result could be relatively localized leukocyte activation or a systemic inflammatory reaction. Activated factor XII fragments can potentially induce activation of the classical pathway of complement. However, activation of the alternative pathway is the more commonly described mode of complement activation on artificial surfaces. As in the case of activation of the coagulation/fibrinolytic systems, products of activated complement are potential activators of leukocytes and platelets.

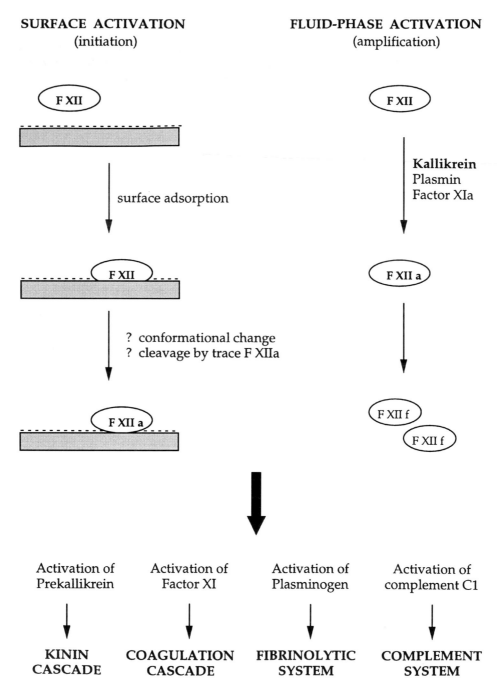

Figure 23-1 Mechanism of factor XII activation on biomaterial surfaces.

ACTIVATION OF THE CONTACT SYSTEM

The potential for contact activation depends upon the surface properties of the biomaterial. Surface defects tend to promote coagulation by disrupting the flow of blood at the blood-biomaterial interface. Similarly, textured surfaces tend to be more thrombogenic than smooth surfaces. However, fibrin formation on textured surfaces may promote tissue ingrowth, thus decreasing the reactivity of the surface over time, whereas a smooth surface continues to remain reactive [2].

Negatively charged surfaces have traditionally been considered to be good activators of factor XII, but it now appears that the optimal spacing of negative charges, rather than the absolute negative charge, is probably more important [3]. Contact activation of factor XII occurs in two steps. Following adsorption on an appropriate surface, the factor XII molecule undergoes auto-activation. This process is also known as solid-phase activation. The mechanism of factor XII auto-activation may involve a conformational change in the molecule that exposes an active site or a site for proteolytic cleavage. Alternatively, trace amounts of activated factor XII (factor XIIa) present in the blood could induce proteolytic activation of surface-adsorbed factor XII.

Factor XII adsorption on the surface is generally associated with adsorption of its substrates, factor XI and prekallikrein. Factor XI and prekallikrein are complexed to the cofactor protein, HMWK, which mediates their binding to the surface. Factor XIIa cleaves prekallikrein to form kallikrein, and factor XI to form activated factor XI (factor XIa).

Solid-phase activation is followed by fluid-phase activation. Kallikrein molecules produced as a result of solid-phase activation play a major role in this step. Unlike prekallikrein, kallikrein molecules have a low affinity for HMWK, and, therefore, leave the surface to enter the fluid phase. Kallikrein is a potent activator of fluid-phase factor XII, and this reaction is severalfold more efficient than the auto-activation reaction. Kallikrein-induced activation of factor XII results in the formation of factor XIIa, which may be surface-bound, and factor XII fragments (factor XIIf), which are released into the fluid phase. Factor XIIf is a strong activator of prekallikrein. Fluid-phase activation of factor XII thus initiates a positive feedback loop to amplify factor XII activation, in which kallikrein activates factor XII, and activated factor XII fragments induce further prekallikrein activation [3, 4].

In addition to their role in initiation and amplification of contact activation, factor XIIa and factor XIIf can directly activate leukocytes. They induce polymorphonuclear leukocyte degranulation and decrease the expression of FcγRI receptors on monocytes, possibly retarding the clearance of immune complexes. Factor XIIa and factor XIIf are also activators of C1, and can potentially activate the classical complement pathway via direct cleavage of C1 [4].

Activation of the Coagulation Cascade

Surface coagulation is favored on the biomaterial surface because of the absence of the active coagulation inhibitory mechanisms of normal endothelium, such as thrombomodulin, heparin-like molecules and tissue-type plasminogen activator [5]. Coagulation is initiated on such a surface by the adsorption and auto-activation of factor XII. Leukocytes activated by contact with the biomaterial surface [6], and damaged vascular tissue in the vicinity of the implanted biomaterial may elaborate tissue factor, which activates the extrinsic pathway of coagulation. There is some evidence that this may be a major pathway for coagulation during cardiopulmonary bypass [7]. Activation of factor VII by factor XIIa can also induce activation of the extrinsic pathway [3]. In renal failure patients on hemodialysis, a hypercoagulable state induced by recombinant erythropoietin treatment, may contribute further to coagulation [8].

Adsorption and activation of factor XII is followed by sequential activation of the coagulation enzymes factor XI and factor IX, and, eventually, of the common pathway of coagulation (Figure 23-2). Alternatively, factor XI could be activated by thrombin, or autoactivated by factor XIa. Intrinsic or extrinsic pathway activation results in the generation of thrombin and the formation of fibrin.

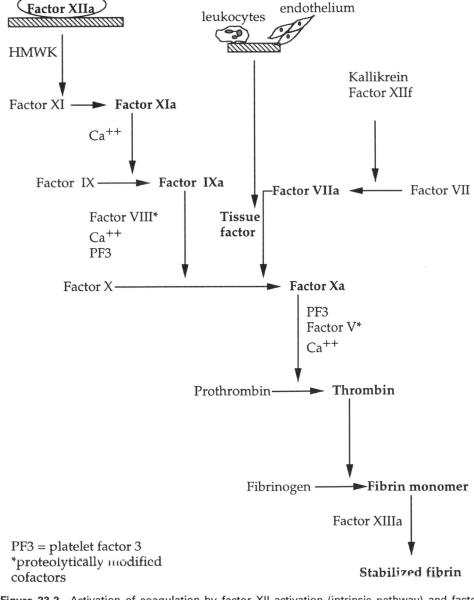

Figure 23-2 Activation of coagulation by factor XII activation (intrinsic pathway) and factor VII/tissue factor activation (extrinsic pathway).

Thrombin is the enzyme responsible for conversion of fibrinogen into fibrin. Thrombin molecules generated as a result of activation of the coagulation cascade on a biomaterial surface may be bound to surface-adsorbed proteins. This protects the thrombin from in-activation by heparin/antithrombin III, prolonging its activity [9]. Thrombin is a potent platelet agonist and can contribute to surface thrombosis by promoting platelet activation. Thrombin is also required for activation of factor XIII, which is responsible for crosslinking and stabilization of the fibrin network [3].

The formation of fibrin can have different implications on different surfaces. On a fabric prosthesis made of a material such as woven polyester, fibrin formation on the surface is a part of the healing process that promotes tissue ingrowth and graft incorporation. In certain applications, however, fibrin formation may compromise device function (e.g., oxygenator membranes) and is generally considered undesirable. Furthermore, on any type of surface, the presence of fibrin provides a surface for platelet adhesion and aggregation. In addition, it provides a surface for adhesion and trapping of bacteria, explaining the frequent association of surface thrombosis with biomaterial-related infection [10].

Activation of Fibrinolysis

The fibrinolytic cascade is activated when kallikrein, directly or via activation of prourokinase, induces the activation of the plasma proenzyme, plasminogen, to the proteolytic enzyme, plasmin. Plasmin degrades fibrin clots into fibrinogen/fibrin degradation products (FDP). FDP have an antithrombin effect, and form incoagulable complexes with fibrinogen/fibrin monomers. They impair further fibrin formation and platelet function, and may cause capillary injury and bleeding. Plasminogen can also be activated by enzymes released from activated leukocytes, notably elastase and cathepsin [3]. In patients undergoing cardiopulmonary bypass, retransfused mediastinal blood may possess considerable fibrinolytic and tissue factor activity, thus worsening the abnormal coagulation/fibrinolysis induced by exposure to biomaterial surfaces [11]. The fibrinolytic activity in such cases is chiefly due to a tissue-type plasminogen activator (t-PA) produced by damaged mediastinal tissue. t-PA binds avidly to fibrin, and requires fibrin in order to trigger fibrinolysis. Therefore, inadequate heparinization of the patient could lead to coagulation-induced fibrinolysis. In children undergoing cardiopulmonary bypass procedures, an additional problem is created by the use of large volumes of priming fluids relative to the total blood volume, which dilutes coagulation factors and contributes to bleeding. The bleeding tendency could be further worsened by biomaterial-induced platelet dysfunction.

Activation of the Kinin Cascade

Activation of prekallikrein to kallikrein occurs both on the surface of the biomaterial and in the fluid phase. Surface activation is induced by factor XIIa, with HMWK as the cofactor, whereas fluid-phase activation is induced by factor XIIf. The major function of kallikrein is to amplify the activation of factor XII. In addition, kallikrein can also activate the fibrinolytic cascade by activating plasminogen and prourokinase to produce plasmin and urokinase, respectively. Kallikrein is a more efficient activator of plasminogen than is factor XIIa, but is less efficient than urokinase. It inhibits the activity of the plasma anti-protease, C1-inhibitor, thus preventing inactivation of the contact proteins, and can also activate prorenin under certain circumstances. Kallikrein promotes chemotaxis and degranulation of polymorphonuclear leukocytes, and primes them for superoxide release. Kallikrein-induced leukocyte activation requires the presence of HMWK bound to the leukocyte surface [4].

Kallikrein cleaves HMWK to produce bradykinin, a potent inflammatory mediator that produces vasodilatation and increases capillary permeability [3, 4]. Bradykinin appears to act synergistically with cytokines from activated mononuclear cells to produce a systemic inflammatory response [12]. Anaphylactoid reactions in patients dialyzed with AN69 hemodialyzers have been attributed to activation of the contact system on the negatively-charged membrane, followed by the generation of bradykinin. The reaction is more severe in patients taking angiotensin-converting enzyme (ACE) inhibitors, because these drugs inactivate plasma kininase and allow bradykinin to accumulate in the circulation [13, 14].

As mentioned earlier, HMWK is an essential cofactor in the initial steps of contact activation. HMWK also has some independent effects at the blood-biomaterial interface that may be important in limiting blood cell activation at the blood-material interface. HMWK is an anti-adhesive protein, and it inhibits cell adhesion on biomaterial surfaces. The anti-adhesive effect of HMWK is believed to be due to its ability to displace adsorbed fibrinogen from the surface [15]. Additionally, HMWK can bind to platelets and prevent thrombin-induced platelet aggregation [16].

Regulation of Contact Activation

Thrombin activity in plasma is inhibited chiefly by fibrin, FDP and antithrombin III. Other enzymes of the contact system, including factor XIIa and kallikrein, are inhibited by the plasma proteins C1 inhibitor, α_2-macroglobulin, α_1-antitrypsin and antithrombin III [4]. Bradykinin is inactivated by plasma kininase II, which is identical to angiotensin-converting enzyme [14].

ACTIVATION OF THE COMPLEMENT SYSTEM

Complement activation is part of the primary host mechanism for the immediate recognition and elimination of foreign particles. Since implanted biomaterials are foreign surfaces, they can activate complement. Activation of complement represents the host inflammatory response, and activated complement fragments mediate leukocyte responses to the biomaterial surface. Therefore, complement activation is an important indicator of the blood compatibility of the surface.

Biomaterial-induced complement activation has been described in the context of a variety of blood-contacting devices, including hemodialysis membranes, cardiopulmonary bypass circuits and vascular grafts. Uncontrolled complement activation may present clinically as transient neutropenia and pulmonary sequestration of leukocytes [17]. Biomaterial-induced complement activation is of particular concern in patients on hemodialysis because multiple episodes of exposure to the hemodialysis membrane can cause a state of chronic complement activation.

Initiation and Amplification
of the Complement Cascade

Activation of complement is triggered by blood contact with a foreign surface. On biomaterial surfaces, complement activation generally occurs via the alternative pathway [17–19]. The key components of this pathway are complement protein C3, the positive regulatory proteins, factor B and factor D and the negative regulatory proteins, factor H and factor I. The alternative pathway is initiated by C3 adsorption on the surface of the material, followed by spontaneous hydrolysis of its intramolecular thioester bond, to form C3b, or a C3b-like molecule, $C3(H_2O)$ (Figure 23-3). The proenzyme, factor B, binds to the C3b (or $C3(H_2O)$) molecule and is cleaved by the plasma enzyme, factor D, to form a C3 convertase. The C3 convertase is capable of cleaving additional molecules of C3 to generate surface-bound C3b and fluid-phase C3a fragments. This is a continuous, slow process that results in the deposition of small amounts of C3b on the surface in the body's attempt to target the foreign surface for phagocytosis.

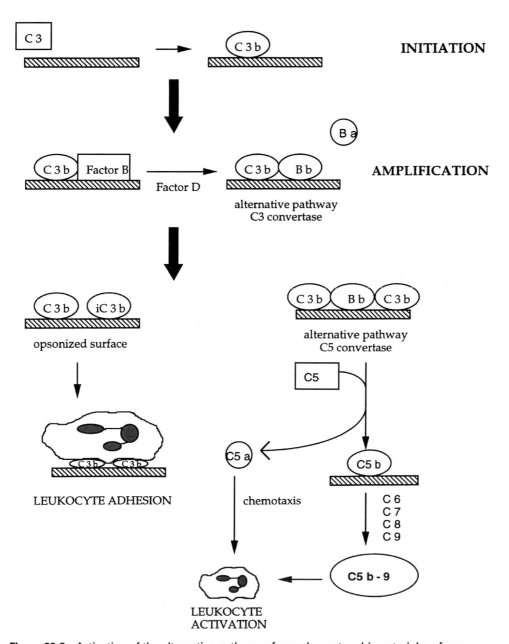

Figure 23-3 Activation of the alternative pathway of complement on biomaterial surfaces.

The ability to initiate and amplify complement is determined by the biochemical characteristics of the biomaterial surface. Surfaces containing amino and hydroxyl groups are considered good activators of complement. These surfaces promote the binding of factor B to surface-bound C3b, and provide a micro-environment in which C3b is protected from inactivation by the negative regulatory proteins, factor I and factor H [19]. Therefore, on such an "activating" surface, C3 cleavage is accelerated, resulting in the formation of large numbers of active C3 fragments. Contributing to the complement-activating effect of the biomaterial are air bubble nuclei trapped in the surface roughness of biomaterial surfaces. Complement activation in this case is believed to be directed against denatured plasma proteins on the surface of the bubble [20]. In patients with chronic renal failure, the accumulation of the intrinsically active enzyme, factor D, in plasma provides an additional mode of complement activation. The increased levels of factor D can enhance spontaneous turnover of C3, further accelerating complement activation on the surface of hemodialysis membranes [21].

The C3a fragment produced by cleavage of C3 is an anaphylatoxin and is often used as a marker of complement activation. The surface-bound C3b fragment (opsonic fragment) promotes adhesion of leukocytes to the biomaterial surface and acts as the non-catalytic subunit of the C3 convertase, C3bBb. In the presence of additional C3b molecules, the C3 convertase can change its specificity to form a C5 convertase, which cleaves complement protein C5 into fluid-phase C5a and surface-bound C5b. C5a, like C3a, is an anaphylatoxin. It is also a potent activator of leukocytes, and blocking antibodies against C5 have been shown to inhibit upregulation of leukocyte and platelet receptors during simulated extracorporeal circulation [22]. C5b binds complement protein C6 and participates in the assembly of the cytolytic multimolecular complex C5b-9. The site of assembly of C5b-9 molecules on the biomaterial surface is not clear. The complex is, however, eventually released into the fluid phase, where it may bind to plasma protein S (vitronectin) to form inactive protein S/C5b-9 complexes.

Complement-Induced Cellular Activation

The most important consequences of complement activation on biomaterial surfaces are leukocyte activation and adhesion resulting from interactions between active complement fragments and specific leukocyte surface receptors. C5a molecules induce chemotaxis of neutrophils and monocytes, upregulate their adhesion receptors, and prime the cells for oxidative metabolism and cytokine release [19]. This effect manifests as increased adhesiveness and aggregation of leukocytes, which are responsible for the syndrome of pulmonary leukostasis. However, chronic complement activation, with consequent prolonged exposure of leukocytes to C5a, is believed to desensitize the cells to further C5a chemotactic stimulation. This observation has led to speculation that prolonged exposure to activated complement may predispose the patient to infection [23].

C5b-9 molecules can provide an additional powerful stimulus for leukocyte activation. Free C5b-9 is normally prevented from inserting into host cell membranes by the membrane-bound regulatory protein, homologous restriction factor. Additionally, nucleated host cells have the capacity to internalize and eliminate C5b-9 molecules, thus protecting themselves from membrane damage. However, fluid-phase C5b-9 may overcome these protective mechanisms and insert into the membranes of bystander blood cells [19]. C5b-9 complexes have been demonstrated on blood cells during cardiopulmonary bypass and hemodialysis [24, 25]. They can cause hemolysis of red cells and sublytic damage to leukocytes, inducing the formation of small hydrophilic transmembrane channels. Passive influx of calcium through the transmembrane channels stimulates arachidonic acid metabolism in neutrophils, cytokine release from monocytes, and platelet degranulation [17, 26, 27].

The opsonic fragments C3b and iC3b are ligands for specific receptors on leukocyte surfaces, and thus mediate the adhesion of leukocytes to biomaterial surfaces. The complement receptors CR3 (CD11b/CD18) and CR4 (CD11c/CD18) are members of the integrin family and bind to iC3b molecules, while the receptor CR1 (CD35) binds preferentially to C3b molecules. CR3 receptors recognize a variety of ligands other than complement fragments, including fibrinogen, ICAM-1 and factor X [17, 19].

Regulation of Complement Activation

Complement activation is amplified by the binding of factor B to surface-bound C3b, and inhibited by the binding of factor H to surface-bound C3b. Factor H competitively inhibits the binding of factor B to C3b, and displaces bound Bb from convertase complexes, thus inactivating the convertases. Factor H also acts as a cofactor in the factor I-mediated degradation of C3b to iC3b, a fragment that retains opsonic activity, but is incapable of forming an active C3 convertase. Hydrophobic surfaces and surfaces containing sialic acid, sulfonate groups and heparin [18, 19, 28] promote the binding of factor H to C3b, and thus prevent amplification of the complement cascade. Surface adsorption of plasma proteins on the surface is another mechanism for decreasing complement activation. Adsorbed proteins are believed to block active sites on the biomaterial surface; therefore, reused hemodialysis membranes are generally less complement-activating than are new membranes [29].

Classical Pathway Activation
on Biomaterial Surfaces

Activation of the classical pathway may contribute to complement activation on biomaterial surfaces [30]. Non-immunological activation of the classical pathway can potentially be induced by factor XIIf-induced cleavage of complement protein C1, or by heparin-protamine complexes formed as a result of protamine sulfate administration at the end of cardiopulmonary bypass [19]. Alternatively, immunoglobulin molecules adsorbed on the biomaterial surface may provide a means of activating C1 [31].

DETECTION OF PLASMA ENZYME ACTIVATION
ON BIOMATERIAL SURFACES

Table 23-1 lists the assays generally used for detecting activation of the contact and complement systems [14, 32, 33]. Short-term activation of the contact system can be detected by measuring the levels of plasma enzymes and degradation products. However, increased turnover of plasma enzymes may compensate for chronic coagulation and fibrinolysis; therefore, they may not be detected by these tests. Assays for activation of the kinin system are not widely available, and their use appears to be limited to the experimental setting.

Complement activation can most conveniently be detected by measuring plasma levels of activation fragments. C3a and C5a tend to adsorb on biomaterial surfaces, particularly on negatively-charged surfaces, or to bind to cell surfaces. Therefore, plasma levels of C3a and C5a may underestimate the extent of complement activation. Plasma C5b-9 or protein S/C5b-9 are considered more accurate indicators of complement activation. In the experimental setting, measurement of fluid-phase indicators can be combined with measurement of surface-bound C3 neoepitopes exposed only upon conversion of C3 to C3b [34]. This

Table 23-1   Assays for Detecting Activation of the Plasma Enzyme Cascades

Coagulation		
Thrombin generation	Fibrinopeptide A	RIA, EIA (Ref. 32)
	TAT complex	EIA (Ref. 32)
	Prothrombin fragment F_{1+2}	EIA (Ref. 35)
	D-dimer	EIA (Ref. 35)
Fibrinolysis		
Plasmin activity	Fibrinogen/fibrin degradation products latex agglutination	EIA, RIA (Ref. 35)
	Plasma plasminogen	COL, EIA, enzyme assay (Ref. 32)
	Plasmin:antiplasmin complex	EIA
Kinin cascade		
Kallikrein generation	Plasma bradykinin	RIA (Ref. 14)
	Plasma kallikrein	RIA (Ref. 14)
	Plasma kallikrein: C1 inhibitor	RIA (Ref. 14)
Complement activation		
C3 conversion	Plasma C3a	RIA, EIA (Ref. 33)
	Plasma C3bi, C3dg	EIA (Ref. 33)
	Surface-bound C3 neoepitopes	EIA (Ref. 34)
C5 conversion	Plasma C5a	RIA, EIA (Ref. 33)
	Plasma S/C5b-9	EIA (Ref. 33)
Alternative pathway	Plasma Bb fragment	EIA (Ref. 33)
Classical pathway	Plasma C4d	EIA (Ref. 33)

COL = colorimetric assay; EIA = enzyme immunoassay; RIA = radioimmunoassay
For sources of test kits, refer to Linscott's Directory of Immunological and Biological Reagents, Santa Rosa, 1996.

approach gives a composite view of complement activation on the surface, and allows correlations with other surface phenomena, such as leukocyte adhesion. However, the selection of tests most appropriate for detecting contact or complement activation in an individual case depends upon the known surface properties of the biomaterial, its intended application, and the information being sought.

APPROACHES TO LIMIT PLASMA ENZYME ACTIVATION ON BIOMATERIAL SURFACES

A knowledge of the mechanisms of plasma enzyme activation can be applied to the design of non-activating biomaterial surfaces. Since the contact system and the complement system are closely linked with each other, inhibition of one cascade may limit activation of the other. The administration of parenteral heparin has long been the standard method for limiting coagulation due to blood contact with the biomaterial surface. Heparin forms a complex with plasma antithrombin III and acts as a cofactor in the antithrombin III-mediated inactivation of thrombin. In recent years, heparin-like compounds such as hirudin and low molecular weight heparins have received more attention because of the possibility that their effects may be more specific than those of heparin. An extension of the anticoagulant approach is the use of heparin-coated biomaterials in applications such as cardiopulmonary bypass [35]. These materials improve anticoagulation to some extent, but it is not yet clear whether they can decrease the requirement for parenteral heparin. Heparinized biomaterials have shown promise in decreasing complement activation at the surface [34, 36]. The mode of heparin attachment to the surface is critical, since the immobilized heparin molecule must retain catalytic activity. Covalent end-point attachment of heparin gives good results in terms of inhibiting both coagulation and complement activation [34]. Aprotinin, an inhibitor of plasmin and kallikrein, is widely used to prevent fibrinolysis during cardiac surgery, and its benefits may extend into the immediate post-operative period [37]. Aprotinin also preserves platelet function by preventing the loss of GPIb receptors from the platelet surface.

Complement activation can be decreased by using biomaterials that inhibit the binding of C3b or promote specific binding of factor H to surface-bound C3b. This has been achieved by chemical modification of the biomaterial surface to reduce the number of active hydroxyl groups [38]. The number of hydroxyl groups on the surface does not correlate with the extent of complement activation, and it may be necessary to modify only a few groups to achieve the desired effect. For hemodialysis applications, surfaces that adsorb and deplete factor D would be particularly useful in decreasing complement activation in renal failure patients with high levels of plasma factor D [39]. The biomaterial surface can also be modified to prevent the biological consequences of complement activation. For example, negatively-charged surfaces capable of adsorbing the cationic anaphylatoxins can be used to prevent complement-mediated leukocyte activation on biomaterial surfaces [38].

Endothelialization of biomaterial surfaces can be promoted experimentally by immobilizing the receptor-binding domain peptides of adhesive molecules, such as fibronectin and laminin, followed by the seeding of endothelial cells on the surface. An alternative approach is to encourage endothelial cell migration through the wall of the biomaterial by incorporating growth factors, such as basic fibroblast growth factor and endothelial cell growth factor [40]. Endothelialization of the biomaterial surface may be the most effective method of inhibiting plasma enzyme activation. It would not only eliminate contact of blood with the artificial surface, but also provide the natural anticoagulant properties of the endothelium.

CONCLUSION

Blood contact with a biomaterial surface activates the enzymes of the contact and complement systems. The extent and consequences of activation depend upon the characteristics of the material, its intended application, and the duration of its use, as well as on patient factors such as drug therapy and the nature of the underlying illness. The clinical context and site of application of the biomaterial will determine the selection of assays for detecting activation of the plasma enzyme systems. Several strategies have been described to inhibit biomaterial-induced activation of the plasma enzyme systems, but the design of a truly non-activating surface remains a challenge.

REFERENCES

1   Vroman L. The life of an artificial device in contact with blood: Initial events and their effect on its final state. *Bull NY Acad Med*, 64 (1988), 352–357.
2   Hanson SR. Device thrombosis and thromboembolism. *Cardiovasc Pathol*, 2 (1993), 157S–165S.
3   Bithell TC. Blood coagulation. In Lee GR, Bithell TC, Foerster J, Athens JW, Lukens JN (Eds.), *Wintrobe's Clinical Hematology*. Philadelphia, PA: Lea and Febiger, 1993, 566–615.
4   Wachtfogel YT, DeLa Cadena RA, Colman RW. Structural biology, cellular interactions and pathophysiology of the contact system. *Thromb Res*, 72 (1993), 1–21.
5   Colman RW. Mechanism of thrombus formation and dissolution. *Cardiovasc Pathol*, 2 (1993), :23S–31S.
6   Kappelmayer J, Bernabei A, Edmunds LH, Edgington TS, Colman RW. Tissue factor is expressed on monocytes during simulated extracorporeal circulation. *Circ Res*, 72 (1993), 1075–1081.

7   Boisclair MD, Lane DA, Philippou H, Esnouf MP, Sheikh S, Hunt B, Smith KJ. Mechanisms of thrombin
      generation during surgery and cardiopulmonary bypass. *Blood*, 82, (1993), 3350–3357.
8   Malyszko J, Malyszko JS, Borawski J, Rydzewski A, Kalinowski M, Azzadin A, Mysliwiec M, Buczko
      W. A study of platelet functions: Some hemostatic and fibrinolytic parameters in relation to serotonin in
      hemodialyzed patients under erythropoitin therapy. *Thromb Res*, 77 (1995), 133–143.
9   Brister SJ, Ofosu FA, Buchanan MR. Thrombin generation during cardiac surgery: Is heparin the ideal anti-
      coagulant? *Thromb Haemost*, 70 (1993), 259–262.
10   Mohammed SF. Association between thrombosis and infection. *ASAIO J*, 40 (1994), 226–230.
11   de Haan J, Boonstra PW, Monnink SHJ, Ebels T, van Oeveren W. Retransfusion of suctioned blood during
      cardiopulmonary bypass impairs hemostasis. *Ann Thorac Surg*, 59 (1995), 901–907.
12   Casey LC. Role of cytokines in the pathogenesis of cardiopulmonary-induced multisystem organ failure. *Ann
      Thorac Surg*, 56 (1993), S92–S96.
13   Schaefer RM, Schaefer L, Horl WH. Anaphylactoid reactions during hemodialysis. *Clin Nephrol*, 42 (1994),
      Suppl. 1, S44–S47.
14   Lemke HD. Hypersensitivity reactions during hemodialysis: The choice of methods and assays. *Nephrol
      Dial Transplant*, 9 (1994), Suppl. 2, 120–125.
15   Asakura S, Hurley RW, Skorstengaard K, Ohkubo I, Mosher DF. Inhibition of cell adhesion by high molecular
      weight kininogen. *J Cell Biol*, 116 (1992), 465–476.
16   Puri RN, Zhou F, Hu CJ, Colman RF, Colman RW. High molecular weight kininogen inhibits thrombin-
      induced platelet aggregation and cleavage of aggregin by inhibiting binding of thrombin to platelets. *Blood*,
      77 (1991), 500–507.
17   Johnson RJ. Complement activation during extracorporeal therapy: Biochemistry, cell biology and clinical
      relevance. *Nephrol Dial Transplant*, 9 (1994), Suppl. 2, 36–45.
18   Hakim RM. Complement activation by biomaterials. *Cardiovasc Pathol*, 2 (1993), Suppl., 187S–197S.
19   Jahns G, Haeffner-Cavaillon N, Nydegger UE, Kazatchkine MD. Complement activation and cytokine pro-
      duction as consequences of immunological bioincompatibility of extracorporeal circuits. *Clinical Materials*,
      14 (1993), 303–336.
20   Kalman PG, McCullough DA, Ward CA. Evacuation of microscopic air bubbles from Dacron reduces com-
      plement activation and platelet aggregation. *J Vasc Surg*, 11 (1990), 591–598.
21   Miyata T, Inagi R, Hong K, Iida Y, Oda O, Kinoshita T, Inoue K, Miyama A, Maeda K. Fluid-phase activation
      of the alternative pathway of complement by excess factor D in regularly dialyzed patients. *Nephron*, 60
      (1992), 144–149.
22   Rinder CS, Rinder HM, Smith BR, Fitch JCK, Smith MJ, Tracey JB, Matis LA, Squinto SP, Rollins SA. Block-
      ade of C5a and C5b-9 generation inhibits leukocyte and platelet activation during extracorporeal circulation.
      J Clin Invest, 96 (1995), 1564–1572.
23   Lewis SL. C5a receptors on neutrophils and monocytes from chronic dialysis patients. *Adv Exp Med Biol*,
      297 (1991), 167–181.
24   Salama A, Hugo F, Heinrich D, Hoge R, Muller R, Kiefel V, Mueller-Eckhardt C, Bhakdi S. Deposition
      of terminal C5b-9 complement complexes on erythrocytes and leukocytes during cardiopulmonary bypass.
      N Engl J Med, 318 (1988), 408–414.
25   Deppisch R, Schmitt V, Bommer J, Hansch GM, Ritz E, Rauterberg EW. Fluid phase generation of terminal
      complement complex as a novel index of bioincompatibility. *Kidney International*, 37 (1990), 696–706.
26   Morgan BP. Complement membrane attack on nucleated cells: Resistance, recovery and non-lethal effects.
      Biochem J, 264 (1989), 1–14.
27   Deppisch R, Ritz E, Hansch GM, Schols M, Rauterberg E-W. Bioincompatibility: Perspectives in 1993.
      Kidney International, 45 (1994), S77–S84.
28   Lin YS, Hlady V, Janatova J. Adsorption of complement proteins on surfaces with a hydrophobicity gradient.
      Biomaterials, 13 (1992), 497–504.
29   Hakim RM. Clinical implications of hemodialysis membrane biocompatibility. *Kidney International*, 44
      (1993), 484–494.
30   Kottke-Marchant K, Anderson JM, Miller KM, Marchant RE, Lazarus H. Vascular graft-associated com-
      plement activation and leukocyte adhesion in an artificial circulation. *J Biomed Mater Res*, 21 (1987), 379–
      397.
31   Uchida T, Hosaka S, Murao. Complement activation by polymer binding IgG. *Biomaterials*, 5 (1984), 281–
      283.
32   Lindhout T. Biocompatibility of extracorporeal blood treatment. Selection of haemostatic parameters. *Nephrol
      Dial Transplant*, 9 (1994), 83–89.
33   Cheung AK. Complement activation as index of haemodialysis membrane biocompatibility: the choice of
      methods and assays. *Nephrol Dial Transplant*, 9 (1994), 96–103.

34 Mollnes TE, Riesenfeld J, Garred P, Nordstrom E, Hogasen K, Fosse E, Gotze O, Harboe M. A new model for evaluation of biocompatibility: Combined determination of neoepitopes in blood and on artificial surfaces demonstrates reduced complement activation by immobilization of heparin. *Artif Organs*, 19 (1995), 909–917.

35 Boonstra PW, Gu YJ, Akkerman C, Haan J, Huyzen R, van Oeveren W. Heparin coating of an extracorporeal circuit partly improves hemostasis after cardiopulmonary bypass. *J Thorac Cardiovasc Surg*, 107 (1994), 289–292.

36 Pekna M, Hagman L, Halden E, Nilsson UR, Nilsson B, Thelin S. Complement activation during cardiopulmonary bypass: Effects of immobilized heparin. *Ann Thorac Surg*, 58 (1994), 421–424.

37 Lu H, Du Buit C, Soria J, Touchot B, Chollet B, Commin PL, Conseiller C, Echter E, Soria C. Postoperative hemostasis and fibrinolysis in patients undergoing cardiopulmonary bypass with or without aprotinin therapy. *Thromb Haemost*, 72 (1994), 438–443.

38 Johnson RJ, Lelah MD, Sutliff TM, Boggs DR. A modification of cellulose that facilitates the control of complement activation. *Blood Purif*, 8 (1990), 318–328.

39 Pascual M, Schifferli JA, Pannatier JG, Wauters JP. Removal of complement factor D by adsorption on polymethylmethacrylate dialysis membranes. *Nephrol Dial Transplant*, 8 (1993), 1305–1311.

40 Hubbell JA. Pharmacologic modification of materials. *Cardiovasc Pathol*, 2 (1993), 121S–127S.

Chapter 24

Genotoxicity

J. Barry Phelps

WHAT IS GENOTOXICITY?

In a living organism, the smallest unit capable of independent existence is the cell. Each cell has specific functions that it must maintain in order to sustain its life. Instructions for these specific functions are encoded within genes, defined as sections of DNA with a specific function. Many genes strung together, along with large amounts of DNA whose function is largely unknown, form a long thread called a chromosome. The chromosome is divided into two halves called chromatids and the chromatids are joined together at a junction called a centromere. Cells within the human body each contain 46 chromosomes. Alterations in the structure of DNA resulting in permanent, heritable changes in function are called mutations. Agents that cause mutations are genotoxic agents. Genetic toxicology is the study of these agents [1].

To understand how genotoxic agents work, a knowledge of DNA is helpful. The DNA molecule is composed of two strands held together by hydrogen bonding. Each strand is composed of a string of nucleotides. A nucleotide has three parts (deoxyribose, a phosphate group and a nitrogenous base, either a purine or a pyrimidine) joined by covalent bonds. A nucleotide from one strand matched with a nucleotide from a second strand is called a base-pair. Three nucleotides from the same strand grouped together are called a codon, which instructs its cell to produce a specific protein from available amino acids. Proteins are responsible for the structure of a living organism and for its hormones and enzymes. The functional sections of the DNA molecule responsible for the production of the proteins are called genes. Genes ultimately determine the characteristics of an organism.

Most cells periodically divide to create new cells. During cell division, DNA is duplicated for the new cell. At division, it is essential that the cell accurately reproduce its DNA so that the new cell can function like the old one. If an exact DNA duplication is not made, there are several mechanisms that may come into play to correct the error. If the error is not corrected and becomes permanent in a section of DNA that controls cellular form or function, then the result is called a mutation. Mutations change the genetic makeup of a cell, which may be beneficial or detrimental to the organism, depending upon the nature of the change.

Mutations may occur spontaneously or they may be induced by environmental factors such as radiation, chemicals or heat. Resulting mutations may affect either somatic or germinal cells and can be classified according to the level of the genetic lesion. Thus, a clastogenic mutation is a change in the structure of the chromosome, which may lead to chromosomal rearrangement. An aneuploid mutation alters chromosomal replication, which may lead to a loss or gain in the number of chromosomes. Alterations in the nucleotide sequences on the DNA molecule are called point mutations. Clastogenic and aneuploid mutations are called macrolesions because they can be observed microscopically. Point mutations are called microlesions because they are microscopically invisible.

Although a variety of environmental genotoxic agents exist, only chemical agents will be discussed here, since the subject of concern is the extractable chemicals present in biomaterials. Some genotoxins act directly, while others must be converted metabolically by mammalian enzyme systems into derivatives that are genotoxic. This metabolic activation can be achieved in the in vitro test system by using an homogenate prepared from the livers of rodents treated with enzyme-inducing agents. The liver homogenate (called S-9) is mixed with the testing article and placed in direct contact with the test system.

WHY TEST BIOMATERIALS FOR GENOTOXICITY?

The toxicology of medical devices deals largely with the toxicology of the extractable chemicals contained within their component materials. The nature of the toxic effects that can be produced by these chemicals ranges from acute to chronic and from local to systemic. Although most adverse effects caused by medical device materials can probably be classified as irritant or sensitizing, there is growing recognition that some of the chemical components of devices may exert genotoxic effects. Any attempt to assess the safety of medical devices, particularly those having intimate and/or prolonged contact with the body, would be incomplete without considering the presence of genotoxins. This has been made clear in the Tripartite Guidance, which served as a regulatory standard in the U.S. until 1995. It has been reiterated in the ISO 10993 standards that are becoming accepted worldwide for biocompatibility testing. Until development of the ISO standards, a single genotoxicity test was usually considered adequate to satisfy regulators. The ISO standards identify the need to assess genotoxicity in more than one model, in order to increase the likelihood of detecting a genotoxic agent. ISO 10993-3 specifies that "when the genetic toxicity of a medical or dental material or device has to be experimentally assessed, a series of in vitro tests shall be used. This series shall contain at least three assays. At least two of these should preferably use mammalian cells as a target. The tests should preferably cover the three levels of genotoxic effects: DNA effects, gene mutations, and chromosomal aberrations" [2].

LEVELS OF GENOTOXIC EFFECTS

Genotoxicity tests are generally grouped according to the genotoxic effects they are designed to detect. The groups are those noted in the ISO standard: DNA effects, gene mutations, and chromosomal aberrations. Another group, which is usually discussed with the others but is not truly a genotoxic effect, is oncogenic transformation. Chromosomal aberration and gene mutation assays are true measures of genotoxicity. They detect actual lesions in the DNA molecule. Assays designed for DNA effects detect events that may lead to genotoxicity. Oncogenic transformation assays measure the ability of a test article to transform normal cells to tumor cells [3, 4].

So-called "point mutations," that is, gene mutations affecting a small portion of the DNA molecule, include "frameshifts" or "base-pair substitutions." A frameshift mutation is an addition or deletion of a base-pair in the codon sequence, which makes nonsense of the encoded message it contains. Similar results can occur with base-pair substitutions, in which one base pair in the code is inappropriately substituted for another [5, 6, 7].

Assays in the chromosome aberration category detect structural or numerical changes in DNA. Structural changes may be grouped into two types depending on the nature of the change; chromosome-type and chromatid-type. Chromosome-type aberrations affect both sister chromatids, whereas chromatid-type aberrations affect only one chromatid of a pair. Generally, chromosome-type aberrations occur when exposure to a genotoxic chemical occurs in one phase of the cell cycle and chromatid-types occur in another. Variation in the chromosome number can result from incomplete dissociation of chromosomes at metaphase. This may result in cell aneuploidy, monosomy, trisomy, etc.

Assays in the DNA effect category are miscellaneous tests that do not logically fit in any other categories. They all detect chemically-induced DNA damage but through different mechanisms. One assay detects newly synthesized DNA which is used to replace the damaged region of the DNA molecule. This is referred to as unscheduled DNA synthesis, which is different from the synthesis occurring during normal cell division. Another assay detects reciprocal exchanges of DNA at homologous loci between two sister chromatids of duplicating chromosomes. The exchanges presumably involve DNA breakage and reunion.

SAMPLE PREPARATION

Preparation of a biomaterial for testing is different from preparation of a soluble chemical substance. As for in vivo studies of materials, suitable fluid extracts of materials must be prepared for dosing the test system. Most genotoxicity testing methods are designed to test soluble chemicals and thus start with a known concentration of test article. Since most biomaterials are insoluble, detection of suspect mutagens is limited to extractable chemicals; therefore, consistency in the preparation of samples is important. The United States Pharmacopoeia has established standard preparation methods for materials testing that can be employed in genotoxicity testing. An international standard, ISO 10993-12 also describes standard methods for sample preparation [2].

Fluid extracts are prepared by placing the appropriate amount of material in an inert container and covering it with a corresponding volume of extraction medium. The amount of extraction vehicle needed to cover the material for extraction depends on the surface area or mass of the material. If the material thickness is less than 0.5 mm, a ratio of 120 cm^2 to 20 ml of vehicle is used to cover the material. If the thickness is greater than or equal to 0.5 mm, a ratio of 60 cm^2 to 20 ml is used. If the surface area of the material cannot be determined, a ratio of 4 g to 20 ml is used. These ratios of material to extraction medium have become established by convention [2].

If the test article is a soluble liquid or solid, the highest possible concentration that achieves complete dissolution of the material and is non-toxic to the test system is used for testing. Concentrations of the solution are reported in volume-to-volume or weight-to-volume ratio. All extracts and preparations of soluble materials should be prepared the day of the test to minimize loss of activity due to extract instability.

Vehicles

The choice of vehicle varies with the testing system. Bacterial test systems are frequently conducted using two different types of vehicles, one for water-soluble and the other for water-insoluble extractables. The most commonly used vehicles are 0.9 percent USP sodium chloride (SC) for injection, ethanol (ETOH), and dimethyl sulfoxide (DMSO). In mammalian test systems, the medium used to support cell growth is used as the vehicle.

Extraction Conditions

By convention, the temperature and time of the extraction process vary with the vehicle being used. The temperature and time for SC is 121°C for 1 hour, 50°C for 72 hours, 37°C for 24 hours or 70°C for 24 hours. Room temperature for 72 hours or 37°C for 24 hours is recommended for DMSO. ETOH extraction is carried out at room temperature (various times can be used). Based on the U.S. Pharmacopoeia, selections of condition should be based on the highest temperature that will not degrade the test material [8]. If a cell growth medium is used, extraction is usually carried out for 24 hours at 37°C since higher temperatures can degrade heat-sensitive components of the medium.

Controls

Negative and positive controls are used in all tests. The negative control is frequently the vehicle in which the sample was extracted or solubilized. In the case of such "blank" controls, the vehicle is subjected to the same temperature conditions as is the test extract. Alternatively, known, non-genotoxic polymer samples can be used as negative controls. Positive controls vary with the test method. Usually the positive controls are known mutagens. Special precautions should be taken when handling these compounds. Disposable latex gloves, safety glasses, and designated laboratory clothing should be worn at all times.

TEST SYSTEMS

Many methods of testing for genotoxic agents exist. The methods make use of different types of test systems including bacterial (Salmonella typhimurium, Escherichia coli) and mammalian (Chinese Hamster Ovary, Mouse Lymphoma L5178Y and V79 Hamster) cells for in vitro testing. In addition, but not covered in this section, mice and rats (bone marrow or hepatocytes) may be used as test systems for in vivo testing. Generally, an in vitro test system should be used first to determine if potential genotoxic agents are present. If genotoxic agents are present, then in vivo test systems can be used to confirm the in vitro results [9].

Test Models

There are many variations of test procedures used to detect potential genotoxins in biomaterials. The following three examples were selected from a list suggested by the Organization for Economic Co-operation and Development (OECD) Guidelines for testing of chemicals [10]. The three examples satisfy the ISO 10993-3 requirement for one bacterial and two mammalian models. Each procedure addresses a different genotoxic mechanism.

Ames Assay—Salmonella typhimurium reverse mutation   The *Salmonella typhimurium* histidine reversion system [11–13] is an assay that detects a mutation in the gene of a histidine-dependent bacterial strain. The bacterial strains used require a source of histidine for their growth. When the bacteria are exposed to a genotoxic agent, point mutations occur. This mutation results in a bacterial strain that no longer requires histidine for growth. Following exposure to the test article, the organisms are plated on a solid, histidine-free growth medium. Mutagenic activity of the test article is indicated by an increase in growth of colonies of the mutated Salmonella strains. In the absence of genotoxicity, only sparse growth occurs, representing spontaneous mutations. All resulting mutant strains can grow in the histidine-free media. In a variation of the test, the test article and tester strains are combined in the presence of S-9, active rat liver microsomes, capable of converting pro mutagens into active mutagens, simulating metabolic activation within the mammalian body. Figure 24-1 shows the appearance of typical plates.

Salmonella typhimurium tester strains TA98, TA100, TA1535, TA1537 and TA1538 are the primary strains used in testing. Each tester strain contains different types of mutations that increase their ability to detect mutagens. In addition to the histidine requiring mutation

A

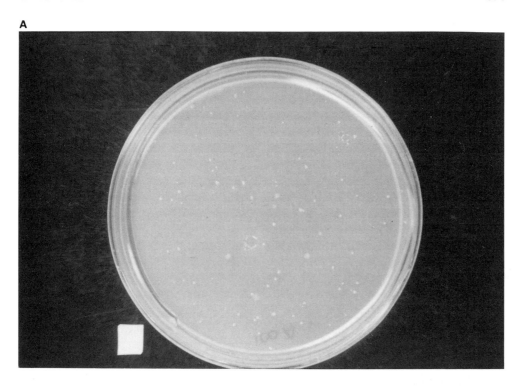

B

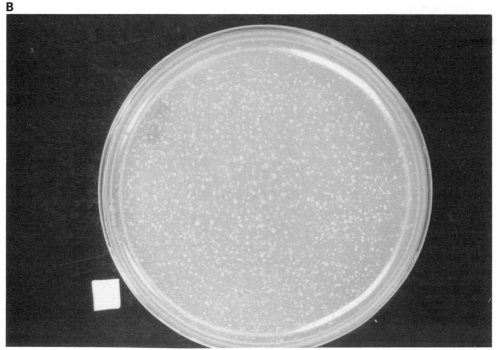

Figure 24-1 Plate A is a negative control. The visible colonies on the plate are spontaneous reversion colonies. Plate B is a positive control. A valid positive control must contain three times as many colonies as the negative control.

(his), one mutation (rfa) causes partial loss of the lipopolysaccharide wall, which increases permeability of the cell to large molecules. Another mutation (_uvrB) is a deletion of a gene coding for the DNA excision repair system which also increases the system's ability to detect mutagens. Tester strains TA 98 and TA100 contain an R-factor plasmid (pKM101), which makes them resistant to ampicillin. This R-factor is used to verify the genotype of the tester strain. TA100 and TA1535 tester strains detect mutagens that cause base-pair substitutions, and tester strains TA98, TA1537 and TA1538 detect mutagens that cause frameshift mutations.

Negative controls (vehicle containing no test material) are used for each tester strain with and without S-9 activation. Besides the commonly used DMSO or SC, other vehicles are compatible with the tester strains: glycerol, formal, dimethyl formamide, formamide, acetonitrile, 95 percent ethanol, acetone ethylene glycol dimethyl ether, 1-methyl-2-pyrrolidinone, p-dioxane, tetrahydrofurfuryl alcohol and tetrahydrofuran.

Since each tester strain responds differently, there is no single positive control chemical that can be used to demonstrate a mutagenic response in all strains. Therefore the assay is conducted with multiple positive controls. Dexon is a positive control for TA98, TA100 and TA1537. Sodium azide is used for TA1535 and 2-nitrofluorene for TA1538. These chemicals are direct-acting compounds. To demonstrate metabolic activation, 2-aminofluorene is used with TA100 and TA1538. Other positive controls that have been used include Mitomycin C, methyl methanesulfonate, 4-nitro-o-phenylenediamine, and 4-nitroquinoline-N-oxide.

To confirm the genotype of each tester strain, a strain characteristic control is conducted at the beginning of each test. To confirm the histidine dependent requirement, each tester strain is streaked onto a plate that contains agar supplemented with biotin. There should be no growth on the plates after incubation at 37° overnight. To confirm the rfa mutation for each tester strain, a filter disc saturated with crystal violet is placed on a seeded nutrient agar plate. A zone of bacterial death should be produced around the filter disc after 12 hours of incubation at 37°C. The ΔuvrB mutation is confirmed by demonstrating UV sensitivity by streaking the tester strains on nutrient agar plates. Strains TA98 and TA100 are exposed for 6 seconds and TA1535, TA1537, and TA1538, for 8 seconds. Before exposure, half of each plate is covered to prevent exposure. The plates are incubated for 12 to 24 hours at 37°C. Strains with the ΔuvrB mutation will grow only on the un-irradiated side of the plate. To confirm the R-factor, the strains are streaked on an ampicillin plate and incubated at 37°C for 12 to 24 hours. There should be growth with TA98 and TA100 and no growth with TA1535, TA1537 and TA1538.

Erlenmeyer flasks containing sterile growth medium are inoculated with each of the five tester strains of *Salmonella typhimurium* from frozen permanent stocks or from master plates. Cultures are incubated overnight in a 37°C rotary shaker for 10–12 hours. Because mutational events are rare, it is essential to use large populations of bacteria. Therefore populations should be at least 1×10^8/ml when testing is started.

The S-9 homogenate is mixed with a buffer containing 0.4 M $MgCl_2$/1.65 M KCl, 1.0 M Glucose-6-phosphate, 0.1 M NADP, 0.2 M sodium phosphate buffer and sterile deionized or distilled water.

The following screen is used to evaluate for toxicity, which defines non-inhibitory concentrations of test solutions. Tubes containing 2 ml of melted top agar supplemented with histidine-biotin solution are inoculated with each of the five tester strains. After mixing, the agar is poured across the surface of separate agar plates. Once the agar solidifies, sterile filter discs are placed in the center of each plate. A 0.1 ml aliquot of the test article is added to the filter discs on each of the plates. Parallel testing is conducted with a negative control, and to demonstrate a positive zone of inhibition, 10x stock Dexon is used. Inoculated plates are incubated at 37°C for 48–72 hours and the zone of growth inhibition recorded. If significant inhibition of the background lawn occurs, the solubilized material or extract concentration is adjusted by preparing one or more dilutions and repeating the inhibition screen to find a nontoxic concentration.

Standard plate incorporation assays are conducted using nontoxic concentrations of test article. Tubes containing 2 ml of melted top agar supplemented with histidine-biotin solution are inoculated with 0.1 ml of culture for each of the five tester strains, and 0.1 ml of the test material. A 0.5 ml aliquot of S-9 homogenate mixture may be added at this stage. The mixture is poured across triplicate agar plates. Parallel testing is conducted on a negative control and four positive controls.

A typical assay should be conducted on histidine-free agar plates in triplicate for each tester strain as follows:

Test article without S-9 activation
Test article with S-9 activation
Negative control without S-9 activation
Negative control with S-9 activation
Dexon without S-9 activation with strains TA98, TA100, and TA1537
2-nitrofluorene without S-9 activation with strain TA1538
2-aminofluorene with activation with strains TA100 and TA1538
Sodium azide without S-9 activation with strain TA1535

Plates are incubated at 37°C for 48–72 hours and colonies on each plate (test, negative and positive) are counted and recorded.

Test materials that cause a two-fold or greater increase over controls in the number of colonies are considered positive in the test. Any apparent "positive response" must be confirmed by evaluating the dose-response relationship using three nontoxic concentrations. There should be a range of concentrations that produce a linear dose-response. A test material is judged mutagenic if it causes a dose-related increase in the number of colonies over a minimum of two dose concentrations.

For an assay to be considered valid, it must meet the following criteria:

Tester strain genetic characteristics All tester strains (TA98, TA100, TA1535, TA1537 and TA1538) must exhibit sensitivity to crystal violet (rfa mutation), and ultraviolet light (_uvrB), and must exhibit no growth on biotin plates, and growth on histidine-biotin plates. Tester strains TA 98 and TA 100 must exhibit resistance to ampicillin (R-factor), tester strains TA1538, TA1535, and TA1537 must exhibit sensitivity to ampicillin.

Positive Control Values Each positive control mean must exhibit at least a three-fold increase over the respective mean of the tester strain employed.

Tester Strain Titer Organism populations should not be less than 1×10^8/ml.

Toxicity Screen Only samples that are non-inhibitory to the tester strains by the spot-plate technique should be tested by the standard plate incorporation method. In the event a test material is inhibitory, dilutions must be performed to identify a nontoxic concentration.

Spontaneous Reversion Rates Each tester strain must exhibit a characteristic number of spontaneous revertants based on historical laboratory data. If spontaneous reversion rates exceed these ranges, the assay should be repeated with a fresh isolate of the tester strain in question.

Sister Chromatid Exchange in Chinese Hamster Ovary Cells   Sister Chromatid Exchange or SCE [14–20], a DNA effect, takes place when a segment of DNA from one chromatid has reciprocated or exchanged with the corresponding segment of DNA of its sister chromatid. By exchanging segments, the cell attempts to repair the chromosome from some form of damage. The mechanism of this event is unfortunately not fully understood. An increased incidence of SCEs can be correlated with greater DNA damage and therefore a greater chance of a mutation.

In order to recognize an exchange, chromatids must be labeled and then differentially stained. DNA can be labeled by incubating cells for two divisions in the presence of bromodeoxyuridine (BrDU). Cells incorporate BrDU, a thymidine analog, into DNA in place of thymidine. When the cells are stained, one chromatid with BrDU appears light while the other is dark in color. A banding effect can be seen in the chromosome where exchanges have taken place (see Figure 24-2). This test is specifically designed to detect primary DNA effects and should be used in conjunction with other tests that characterize potential mutagenic properties. Goto [19] developed the method described below using Chinese Hamster Ovary (CHO) cells.

CHO cells are used in genetic toxicology testing because of their small number of relatively large chromosomes per cell, which facilitates evaluation [21]. CHO-WBL is the clone that will be described in this procedure. Note any reference to CHO will imply CHO-WBL. CHO cells have an average generation time of 12 to 13 hours and 21 chromosomes.

Cell cultures are maintained in 75 cm^2 flasks and are identified by type and passage number. Sterile McCoy's 5a medium for propagation of cells is supplemented with 10 percent Fetal Bovine Serum (FBS), 1 percent L-glutamine, 2 percent N-2-Hydroxyethylpiperazine-N'-2-Ethane buffer (HEPES), and nontoxic concentrations of the antibiotics penicillin, streptomycin and amphotericin B. If an open flask system in conjunction with a CO$_2$ incubator is used, HEPES buffer should not be supplemented.

The negative control is McCoy's 5a medium. The positive control is Mitomycin C (MMC), used for the portion of the assay without metabolic activation and cyclophosphamide (CP), for the portion of the assay with metabolic activation.

The S-9 homogenate is mixed with a buffer containing NADP and isocitric acid. The final concentration of each per ml of media is 20 μl, 3.4 mg and 4.5 mg, respectively.

CHO cells are grown to 40–60 percent confluence in each culture flask used for testing. Tests are conducted in the presence and absence of metabolic activation in triplicate. For the portion of the assay conducted without metabolic activation, the growth medium in the culture flask is replaced with ten ml of the test extract or solution. The positive control flask contains a 100 μl aliquot of MMC and 9.9 ml of growth medium. The growth medium in each negative control flask is replaced with ten ml of McCoy's 5a medium. The test and control flasks are then incubated at 37°C for 2 hours, at which time 100 μl of BrDU at 0.1 Mm is added to cultures and incubated for an additional 24 hours. The cultures are then rinsed twice with five ml of Calcium Magnesium Free-Phosphate Buffered Saline (CMF-PBS). A 10 ml portion of McCoy's 5a medium containing BrDU and a spindle fiber inhibitor such as Colcemid (0.1 μg/ml) are added to each test and control flask and incubated for 2 to 3 hours at 37°C.

For the portion of the assay conducted with metabolic activation, 9.2 ml of the test extract or solutions, positive control, and negative control are added to the S-9 mixture (800 μl) and incubated for 2 hours at 37°C. All culture flasks are rinsed twice with 5 ml

A

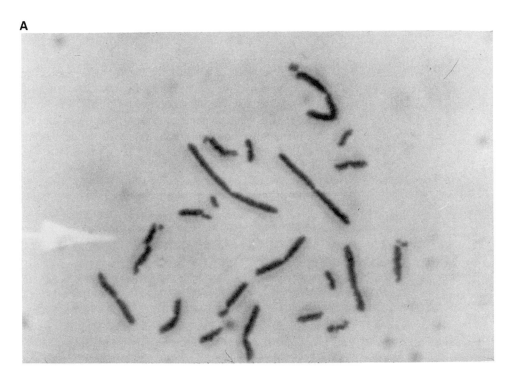

B

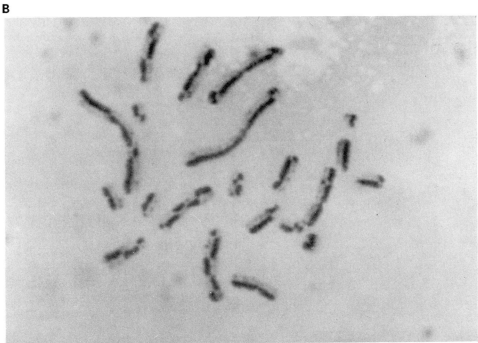

Figure 24-2 (A) is a negative control. The arrow is pointing to a chromosome which has 2 exchanges. (B) is a positive control. Note the checkerboard effect caused by the exchanges.

of CMF-PBS. A 10 ml portion of fresh McCoy's 5a growth medium supplemented with BrDU (10 μM) is added to all cultures and incubated 26 hours with Colcemid (100 μl) for the final 2 to 3 hours.

After the final 2 to 3 hours, cells are collected by shaking the flasks to detach the cells which have been arrested in metaphase by the spindle fiber inhibitor. Collected cells are pelleted by centrifugation and exposed to a hypotonic solution (0.075 KCl) for 3 minutes to cause swelling of the cell membrane. The suspension is then centrifuged and the cell pellet washed with fixative (3:1 methanol:acetic acid) three times. Two slides (A and B) from each culture flask are prepared. The chromosome spreads are stained, cover-slipped, and examined microscopically for sister chromatid exchanges at 100X magnification.

A typical assay is conducted in triplicate as follows:

Test article without S-9 activation
Test article with S-9 activation
Negative control without S-9 activation
Negative control with S-9 activation
Positive control without S-9 activation
Positive control with S-9 activation

Slides are stained with Hoechst 33258 (50 μg/ml) for 15 minutes at room temperature. The staining jars must be covered with foil to reduce exposure to light. Excess stain is removed by washing slides with tap water and blotting them dry with bibulous paper. The slides are then exposed to "black light" and heat for 22 minutes at 55°C. To protect the cells during this period, a few drops of MacIlvanes's buffer are placed on the slides along with a cover slip to aid in spreading the buffer. The final step is to rinse the slide in tap water to remove the cover glass, blot dry, stain with 10% Giemsa for 8 minutes and then cover-slipped.

Only CHO cells that have undergone two cell divisions and are in the metaphase stage of the second division (referred to as M_2) and have a chromosome number of 21 ± 2, are evaluated. Possible observable metaphases are:

A. M_1 No differential staining in chromatids.
B. M_{1+} Chromatids appear "fuzzy" or not clear as in M_2 metaphase.
C. M_2 Chromatids have a clear differential staining. This category is the only one scored for SCE.
D. M_{2+} Small sections of chromatid differentially stained.
E. M_3 Only 1/4 of chromosome differentially stained.

Fifty M_2 cells from each culture flask (test, negative and positive control) are evaluated. If the positive control exhibits a positive response after evaluating twenty-five M_2 cells, the evaluation may stop. The number of observances of M_1, M_{1+}, M_2, M_{2+}, and M_3 metaphases is recorded to determine the average generation time (AGT) for each slide. The average generation time is the hours BrDU was present (usually 26 hours) divided by the sum of the products of $1(M_1)$, $1.5(M_{1+})$, $2(M_2)$, $2.5(M_{2+})$, and $3(M_3)$ times 100, where () is the percentage of observable metaphases. If an increase is noted from the negative control, this is an indication of toxicity and dilutions should be tested. The average of the three replicates for SCE per cell and corresponding standard error are calculated for all test and control cultures and the percent increase over the negative control.

For an assay to be considered valid, it must meet two criteria. First, the positive control SCE average for the three replicates must be 15 or more. Second, the negative control SCE average for the three replicates must be 10 or less. If a control differs from the expected, the test should be repeated.

If the test article produces an average SCE response that is more than 20 percent above the negative control value, the article is considered positive in the test. A positive response should be confirmed by demonstrating a dose-response relationship using three nontoxic dose levels of the test article extract or solution. There should be a range of concentrations that produce a linear dose-response. A test material is judged mutagenic if it causes an increase of 20 percent or more over negative controls in the number of SCEs.

Chromosomal Aberration Assay   The Chromosomal Aberration (CA) assay [21–24] detects damage induced after one cellular division. Most aberrations are structural changes of either chromosome- or chromatid-type. Chromosome-type aberrations are induced when a test article is active during the first resting (GAP1 or G1) phase of the cell cycle. Chromatid-type aberrations are induced when a test article is active during the DNA synthesis (S) phase or the second resting (GAP2 or G2) phase of the cell cycle. The same cell line and culture medium is used in the CA assay as in the SCE assay. The negative control is McCoy's 5a medium; the positive controls are the same as those used for the SCE assay. An example is shown in Figure 24-3.

Each culture flask used for testing should contain a (40–60 percent) confluent cell monolayer. When the assay is conducted without metabolic activation, the growth medium in the culture is simply replaced with 10 ml of the test extract or solution. For positive control cultures, 100 μl of MMC are added to 9.9 ml of growth medium. For negative control cultures, the growth medium in each flask is replaced with 10 ml of McCoy's 5a medium. All cultures are incubated for 10 hours, then rinsed twice with 5 ml of Calcium Magnesium Free-Phosphate Buffered Saline (CMF-PBS). Finally, 10 ml of McCoy's 5a medium containing Colcemid (0.1 μg/ml) are added to each test and control flask, and incubation is continued for an additional 2 to 3 hours at 37°C.

When the assay is conducted with metabolic activation, 9.2 ml of the test extract or solutions, positive control, and negative control are added to the S-9 mixture (800 μl) and incubated for 2 hours at 37°C. All culture flasks are rinsed twice with 5 ml of CMF-PBS. Then 10 ml of McCoy's 5a growth medium are added to all cultures, and the flasks are incubated for 10 hours at 37°C with Colcemid for the final 2 to 3 hours, after which cells are harvested. Slides of cells are prepared, stained with 10% Giemsa, and examined microscopically for chromosomal aberrations at 100X magnification.

A typical assay should be conducted in triplicate as follows:

Test article without S-9 activation
Test article with S-9 activation
Negative control without S-9 activation
Negative control with S-9 activation
Positive control without S-9 activation
Positive control with S-9 activation

Only CHO cells which have undergone one cell division and are in the metaphase stage of the first division (referred to as M_1) and which have 21 ± 2 chromosomes are evaluated. Aberrations are recorded and grouped into three categories: simple, complex, and other. Simple aberrations are chromatid breaks, chromosome breaks, and double minutes. Complex aberrations are interstitial deletions, triradials, quadraradials, complex rearrangements, dicentrics, rings, and chromosome intrachanges. A cell with >10 aberrations or one which

A

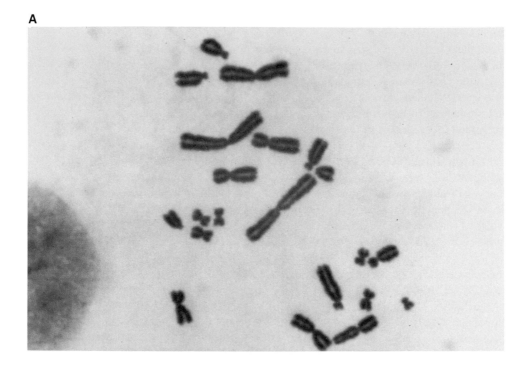

B

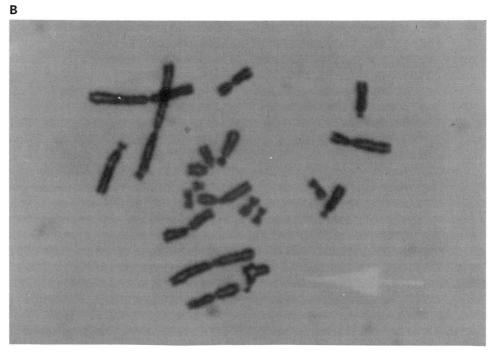

Figure 24-3   (A) is a negative control. No aberrations are noted. (B) is a positive control. The arrow is pointing to a triradial, one of several forms of chromosomal aberrations.

is pulverized is placed in the other category. Gaps are recorded but not included in the statistics.

One hundred M_1 cells from each culture flask (test, negative and positive control) are evaluated. If the positive control exhibits a positive response after evaluating fifty M_1 cells, evaluation may stop. The percentage of cells with aberrations is calculated for the simple, complex and other categories and a combined or total percentage of cells with aberrations is calculated.

For an assay to be considered valid, it must meet two criteria. First, positive control cells must average 15 percent aberrations or more. Second, negative control cells must average 6 percent aberrations or less. If a control differs from the expected, the test should be repeated.

If the percent of cells with aberrations from one or the sum of all three categories is not significantly higher than the negative control using the chi-square test, then the assay results in a negative response. If any one category or the sum of all three categories is significantly higher than the negative control, then the assay results in a positive response.

A positive response should be confirmed by demonstrating a dose-response relationship using three nontoxic dose levels. There should be a range of concentrations that produce a linear dose-response. A test material will be judged mutagenic if it causes the percent of cells with aberrations to be significantly higher than the negative control over a minimum of two increasing dose concentrations.

DEALING WITH GENOTOXIC POSITIVE BIOMATERIALS

If one, two or all three tests are positive, a careful evaluation of the device is needed. Since most devices are a composite of several materials, the first step may be to examine each major part of the device and determine which one (or more) is or contains the genotoxin. Once the source of the problem is known, a literature review may provide the background information needed to conduct an appropriate risk assessment. In most cases, it will be difficult to justify the clinical use of a positive genotoxic biomaterial unless the material possesses essential, unique properties and the patient population that will be exposed is at serious risk without its use.

A second option is to proceed to in vivo testing. There are several assays that can be conducted to confirm in vitro responses: the chromosomal aberration assay using either mouse or rat bone marrow detects structural aberrations; the mouse micronucleus test detects chromosomal or spindle fiber damage. Materials that produce a positive response in vitro but a negative response in vivo must be subjected to careful risk assessment, but, in general, in vivo test results are most persuasive.

REFERENCES

1   Brusick D (Ed.). *Principles of Genetic Toxicology*. New York: Plenum Press, 1987.
2   International Organization of Standardization, International Standard ISO 10993-3.
3   Rundell JO. In Douglass JF (Ed.), *In Vitro Cell Transformation, An Overview In Carcinogenesis and Mutagenesis Testing*. Clifton, NJ: Humana Press, 1984, 39–62.
4   Dipaolo JA, Takano K, Popescu NC. Quantitation of chemically induced neoplastic transformation of BALB/3T3 cloned cell lines. *Cancer Research*, 32 (1972), 2686–2695.
5   Clive D, Spector JFS. Laboratory procedures for assessing specific locus mutations at the TK locus in cultures of L5178Y lymphoma cells. *Mutation Research*, 31 (1975), 17–29.

 6   Clive D, Flamm WG, Patterson JB. Specific locus mutational assay systems for mouse lymphoma cells. In
     Hollaender A (Ed.), *Chemical Mutagens: Principles and Methods for Their Detection*, Vol. 3. New York:
     Plenum Press, 1973, 79–103.

 7   Clive D, Johnson KO, Spector JFS, Batson AG, Brown MMM, Maron, DM, Ames BN. Revised methods for
     the salmonella mutagenicity test. *Mutation Research*, 113 (1983), 73–215.

 8   The United States Pharmacopeia. Mack Publishing.

 9   Butterworth BE, Golberg L (Eds.). *Strategies for Short-Term Testing of Mutagens/Carcinogens*. West Palm
     Beach, FL: CRC Press, 1979.

10   *Guidelines for Testing of Chemicals*. OECD (Organization for Economic Co-operation and Development),
     1981; revised May 1983.

11   Ames BN. The detection of chemical mutagens with enteric bacteria. In Hollaender A (Ed.), *Chemical
     Mutagens, Principles and Methods for Their Detection*, Vol. 1. New York: Plenum Press, 1971, 267–282.

12   Ames BN, McCann J, Yamasaki E. Methods for detecting carcinogens and mutagens with the salmonella/
     mammalian-microsome mutagenicity test. *Mutation Research*, 31 (1975), 347–364.

13   Maron D, Ames BN. Revised methods for the salmonella mutagenicity test. *Mutation Research*, 113 (1983),
     173–215.

14   Galloway SM, Bloom AD, Resnick M, Margolin BH, Nakamura F, Archer P, Zeiger E. Development of a
     standard protocol for *in vitro* cytogenetic testing with Chinese Hamster Ovary cells: Comparison of results
     for 22 compounds in two laboratories. *Environ Mutagen*, 7 (1985), 1–51.

15   Gulati DK, Whitt K, Anderson B, Zeiger E, Shelby MD. Chromosome aberration and sister chromatid
     exchange tests in Chinese Hamster Ovary Cells in vitro. III: Results with 27 chemicals. *Environmental and
     Molecular Mutagenesis*, 13 (1989), 133–193.

16   Stetka DG, Carrano AV. The interaction of Hoechst 33258 and BrdU substituted DNA in the formation of
     sister chromatid exchanges. *Chromosoma*, 63 (1977), 21–31.

17   Okinaka RT, Barnhart BJ, Chen DJ. Comparison between sister chromatid exchange and mutagenicity fol-
     lowing exogenous metabolic activation of promutagens. *Mutation Research*, 91 (1981), 57–61.

18   Kato H. Induction of sister chromatid exchanges by chemical mutagens and its possible relevance to DNA
     repair. *Experimental Cell Research*, 85 (1974), 239–247.

19   Goto K, Maeda S, Kano Y, Sugiyama T. Factors involved in differential Giemsa-staining of sister chromatids.
     Chromosoma, 66 (1978), 351–359.

20   Wolff S, Perry P. Differential Giemsa staining of sister chromatids and the study of sister chromatid exchange
     without autoradiography. *Chromosoma*, 48 (1974), 342–353.

21   Savage JRK. Classification and relationships of induced chromosomal structural changes. *Journal of Medical
     Genetics*, 12 (1975), 103–122.

22   Raj AS, Heddle JA. Simultaneous detection of chromosomal aberrations and sister chromatid exchanges:
     Experience with DNA intercalating agents. *Mutation Research*, 78 (1980), 253–260.

23   Nishi Y, Mori M, Inui N. Chromosomal aberrations induced by maleic hydrazide and related compounds in
     Chinese Hamster Cells in vitro. *Mutation Research*, 67 (1979), 249–257.

24   Heddle J. A rapid in vitro test of chromosomal damage. *Mutation Research*, 18 (1973), 187.

ADDITIONAL READING

 1   Kilbey BJ, Legator M, Nichols W, Ramel C. *Handbook of Mutagenicity Test Procedures*. Amsterdam: Elsevier
     Science Publishers, 1984.

 2   Venitt S, Parry JM. *Mutagenicity Testing: A Practical Approach*. Washington, DC: IRL Press, 1984.

 3   Evaluation of short-term test for carcinogens. In de Serres FJ, Ashby J (Eds.), *Progress in Mutation Research*,
     Vol. 1. Amsterdam: Elsevier Science Publishers, 1981.

 4   Evaluation of short-term test for carcinogens. In Ashby J, de Serres FJ, Draper M, Ishidate M, Jr., Margolin
     BH, Matter BE, Shelby MD. *Progress in Mutation Research*, Vol. 5. Amsterdam: Elsevier Science Publishers,
     1985.

 5   Hollaender A (Ed.). *Chemical Mutagens: Principles and Methods for Their Detection*, Vol. 4. New York:
     Plenum Press, 1976.

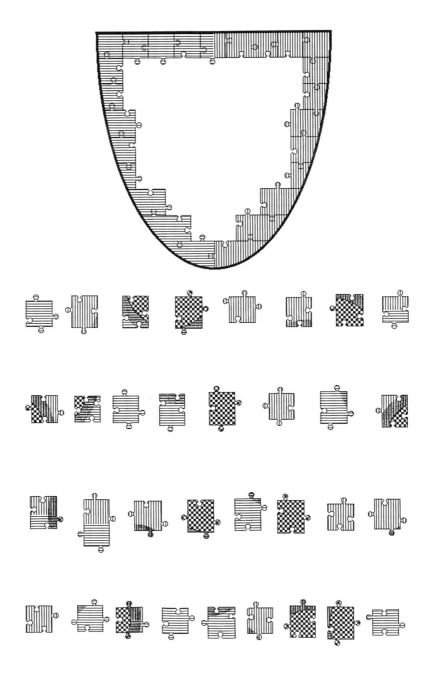

Section Five

Active Implants

Antonios G. Mikos

INTRODUCTION

This section includes four chapters and addresses critical issues related to the design, fabrication, testing, and evaluation of bioactive implants.

The first chapter focuses on the biomaterials component of tissue engineered implants comprised of combinations of materials, cells, and tissue induction factors, with particular emphasis on synthetic biodegradable polymers. The methodologies for the fabrication of bioactive implants and the incorporation of signals to modulate cellular response are thoroughly presented. Moreover, the evaluation studies of tissue engineered implants, most of which are in pre-clinical stage, are systematically classed for a plethora of tissues.

The biomaterials utilized in immunoisolation devices either as membranes or as matrices for the transplantation of allogeneic or xenogeneic cell populations are discussed in the second chapter. The detailed methodologies for assessment of the transport and mechanical properties of devices, as well as the cell function and biomaterial stability are further reviewed. The considerations for evaluation of devices including product release are also analyzed.

The characterization and testing of polymeric and ceramic carriers for bioactive agents is presented in the third chapter. The biological, physical, and chemical requirements of drug delivery implants are examined for the different release mechanisms. In addition, the design characteristics of the clinically available drug delivery devices including bioerodible and swelling controlled release systems are very comprehensively reported.

The last chapter of this section deals with biosensors. It includes a complete and critical review of the literature on in vivo sensor performance and biocompatibility, and uses the indwelling glucose sensor as a paradigm. The methodologies to assure reliable sensor function are considered in view of the factors that can limit its in vivo performance. The testing schemes for bio/sensocompatibility assessment of devices are finally elucidated for new or improved biosensors.

Biomaterials play a key role in most bioactive implants. They are utilized as supportive scaffolds for cells, as conduits for guided tissue growth, as barriers for immunoisolation, as carriers for growth factors, or as biosensors for monitoring. Until recently, most research in the biomaterials field has focused on making the material invisible to the body. However, innovations that use the inverse approach of programmed extensive interaction of the material with biological tissue will give biomaterials research a new focus.

Chapter 25

Tissue Engineering Concepts

Horst A. von Recum
Michael J. Yaszemski
Antonios G. Mikos

INTRODUCTION

At a bioengineering panel meeting for the National Science Foundation in 1987, the term "tissue engineering" was coined. A working definition was established the next year at a Keystone Symposium in Lake Tahoe, California:

> Tissue engineering is the application of the principles and methods of engineering and the life sciences toward the fundamental understanding of structure-function relationships in normal and pathological mammalian tissues and the development of biological substitutes to restore, maintain, or improve functions [1].

Even though the term was new, many researchers discovered that work they had been doing for years fell under the title of tissue engineering. This can perhaps be referenced as far back as 1933 when Bisceglie implanted encapsulated cells to determine if protection against host attack could be achieved [2]. Tissue engineering in its simplest form involves modifying artificial materials (which have been used in medical applications since the dawn of man) to assist cells in reconstruction, regeneration and repair of damaged tissue as well as restoring lost function.

Several important characteristics of tissue must be understood before the directions of research in tissue engineering can be clear. Organs are the centers in our body designated to provide specific functions. Organs are composites of one or more tissues, with some ubiquitous types, such as connective tissue, and others which are much more specific such as hepatic tissue. Tissue, at the most fundamental level, is made up of cells. However, since all somatic cells contain the same genetic material and potential, clearly there are other elements of tissue that allow differentiated function; for example, the cells in a pancreas islet are different from adjacent exocrine cells or connective tissue fibroblasts.

The three parts of tissue that regulate how a cell will behave and perform in vivo are the cells themselves; non-soluble factors within the extracellular matrix (ECM), such as collagens, glycosaminoglycans (GAGs), laminins, fibronectin, and other molecules; and soluble factors either created in the matrix or transported to it, such as cytokines and hormones, as well as nutrients, vitamins, minerals, ions and waste products. The roles of all three components of tissue must be elucidated before tissues can be reconstructed to operate functionally.

MATERIALS

While the cell is always present in modern tissue engineering constructs, it is often difficult to find the presence of the other two required elements of tissue engineering. The matrix used for cell delivery is designated as a scaffold and forms the bare backbone over which reconstruction will occur. Some engineering constructs use the scaffold only as a physical mechanism to hold cells together in the proper orientation, or to provide mechanical properties. While this may be the simplest property of ECM, it is definitely not the only one. Since tissue engineering constructs of the future will require extensive signaling to recreate functional tissue, it is becoming more and more imperative that the scaffold takes on the signaling properties of both the insoluble and soluble components of the ECM. Some attempts to include these factors have been made, especially in use of natural material scaffolds, or incorporation of natural materials into a scaffold [3]. Care must be taken, however, in analyzing what signals must be transmitted to cause cell growth as well as restoration of differentiated function. To some extent, proper matrix signaling can be developed by the cell culture's own matrix deposition, since each cell type will generate its own characteristic ECM. Biochemical and mechanical stimuli may also affect signaling. Normally passive, the ECM of the connective tissue in blood vessel media exhibits massive wound healing response when the endothelium is removed and it is exposed to blood [4].

Most materials which will be discussed in this chapter are polymers, both natural and synthetic. Among the polymers, biodegradable ones are of critical importance because they can be manipulated to temporarily assume properties of tissue, but will gradually disappear. Moreover, they allow incorporation of various factors which can be delivered to growing or existing tissue. In addition, natural and synthetic materials such as inorganic matrices found in bone have been used in tissue engineering applications. While these may not be biodegradable per se, they are usually resorbable and can be replaced by their natural counterparts.

Natural

Natural materials exist in many different forms and are made of many different building blocks. Most natural materials are biodegradable; that is, they can be broken down by many different cellular processes such as hydrolysis or specific enzyme attack. The major disadvantage is that natural materials are difficult to shape and form: they may not have suitable mechanical properties, may not maintain those properties after implantation, or allow them to be tailored. Natural materials have potential, however, not as mechanical materials, but as signaling molecules that are present naturally in the ECM of most tissues. The following three categories are samples of natural materials most abundantly found in ECMs and most commonly used in tissue engineering constructs.

Proteins   Some of the most abundant proteins in ECMs are collagens which, with the exception of Collagen IV, are fibrillar in nature. Collagen IV has its own unique structure and is found mostly in the basement membranes of epithelial tissue [5]. Collagens are polymeric chains which form the skeletons of most ECMs. Because of their frequency, their role may be more structural, as are the elastins found in the more elastic connective tissues. Other smaller proteins may be more active in the signaling of ECM. Investigated proteins of this nature include fibronectin, vitronectin, and the family of laminins. While the signaling element of the ECM may come from any of these molecules, it may also come from growth factors and paracrine hormones secreted by cells attracted or stimulated by the ECM.

Examples of proteins used strictly as engineering materials have been collagen or collagen-graft-glycosaminoglycan matrices. Often these matrices are cross-linked by using such agents as dialdehydes or carbodiimide to improve mechanical properties and degradation. Cross-linked matrices have better mechanical properties than non-cross-linked ones, but there is a danger of leachable agents remaining in the scaffold. In tissues where mechanical properties and formability of scaffold material are less necessary, proteins such as collagen may be ideally suited; however, most often the combination of the adjustable properties of synthetic polymers with the signaling capabilities of such natural proteins work best [6].

Glycosaminoglycans As previously stated, glycosaminoglycans were used in conjunction with collagen matrices to make tissue induction scaffolds. There are many families of these, including the chondroitin sulfates, dermatan sulfates, keratin sulfates, and hyaluronic acids. These are sometimes used as mechanical substrates, but are more often fillers of other scaffolds added to improve the cellular signaling capability of the construct. Although much research has been done, the actual cellular response to their presence in ECMs still needs to be determined [7, 8].

Polysaccharides There are many types of polysaccharides as well, ranging from the dextrans to gelatins, starches, and hydroxyethylstarches. These also range in biodegradability from almost none, to immediate, depending on the implanted site. They have poor mechanical properties, but are praiseworthy for their good biocompatibility and degradation into key nutrients (monosaccharides) which do not have as significant a dose effect as other degradation by-products [9, 10].

Synthetic

Synthetic materials, of which mainly the polymers are important to the tissue engineering field, also have incredible diversity [11]. While synthetic polymers will always show some amount of polydispersity, they can be produced in a purity which is unattainable with natural products. Their main advantage is the range of mechanical properties, and the ease with which these can be manipulated, by adjusting chain length, side chains, and amount of cross-linking.

Degradable Polymers Of greatest importance to the field of tissue engineering are the biocompatible, degradable polymers (see also Chapter 6). With these polymers it is possible to make a synthetic construct in which cells are cultured. The construct upon implantation mimics the mechanical properties of the replaced tissue, allowing the implanted cells to grow and divide. As the cells begin to fill the implant, the polymer breaks down until it is entirely dissolved, and only the newly formed cell conglomerates remain. Timing this sequence of events remains one important challenge in tissue engineering, as degradation may vary from individual to individual, and definitely varies in different tissue systems.

There are two main types of polymers, following either zero- or first-order degradation kinetics. The first type are those which degrade only on the surface, such that the implant gets smaller and smaller until it is finally gone while polymer chain length and density remain constant throughout the undegraded implant. The second type are those which degrade uniformly throughout the polymer. The implant does not change size during degradation, but polymer chain length decreases steadily in all areas throughout the polymer as random chain cleavage events occur.

The degradation process may be also categorized as random (such as hydrolysis), or specific (such as enzyme-catalyzed cleavage). While random degradation may be more consistent from trial to trial (as the amount of water in a certain tissue remains constant, as does its fluid transport into and away from the implant), specific degradation may be preferred for more controllable rates. Again, the choice needs to be determined individually for each system.

Finally, although most degradable polymers are made to cleave down to their inherent monomers which then can be utilized in metabolic processes or excreted as necessary, this need not be the only degradation mechanism. Some degradable non-crosslinked hydrogels "dissolve" slowly as chains slip out of the matrix [12]. If these chains are small enough, they can be cleared by the kidney. Likewise, copolymer chains of non-degradable sequences with degradable ones can be fabricated and will be removed from the body so long as the clearance threshold (approximately 40–50,000 Mw) is observed [13]. When the term "degradable polymer" is used in this chapter, it could mean any degradable types and combinations, including the degradable natural polymers mentioned in the previous section.

Poly(α-Hydroxy Esters)   These polymers share the distinct advantage of being the first polymers holding Food and Drug Administration (FDA) approval for implantation in the human body (namely in the form of degradable sutures) [14]. Early investigations in degradable scaffolds primarily used these materials to simplify FDA approval of such devices, as well as for the range of their mechanical properties and degradation times. While these polymers may be well suited in some applications, they may be less suitable in others.

Constructs are mostly made from the two members of this family: poly(glycolic acid) (PGA), poly(lactic acid) (made from the L isomer, PLLA; or the D,L racemic mixture, PD,LLA), or copolymers of the two, poly(lactic-co-glycolic acid) (PLGA). Within a certain range, mechanical properties can be adjusted by copolymer ratio [15], chain length [16], and degree of crystallinity [15]. Likewise, the degradation rate can be adjusted in response to these factors. PGA is fairly hydrophilic, endowing it with more elastic properties, but low solubility in many solvents [17]. The poly(lactic acids) show better solubility, but their hydrophobicity makes them more brittle [18].

Both degrade by random hydrolysis of the ester linkage, releasing the monomer acids which are part of natural metabolic pathways and can be absorbed by cells and digested. Bulk degradation follows first-order kinetics and is dependent only upon water entering the matrix (easier in non-crystalline regions than crystalline ones). A local accumulation of the monomer acids leads to a drop in pH which, in addition to damaging tissue [19], causes autocatalysis, as the hydrolysis is pH-dependent [20].

Poly(ε-Caprolactone)   From a similar family of polyesters, poly(ε-caprolactone) (PEC) degrades by bulk hydrolysis, although some enzymatic cleavage, possibly by non-specific esterases, occurs [21]. PEC has rubbery properties similar to PGA and undergoes similar pH-dependent autocatalysis. Its main advantage is a degradation rate that is about three times slower than PGA [22].

Poly(Ortho Esters)   This group of amorphous hydrophobic polymers does not undergo hydrolysis under normal conditions, but is sensitive to hydrolysis under low pH conditions. Their degradation can be facilitated by incorporation of differing quantities of acidic groups onto the polymer backbone. Poly(ortho esters) exhibit a large range of mechanical properties and all undergo degradation by zero-order surface erosion [23].

Poly(Anhydrides)   This group of polymers undergoes surface erosion as well. Although they show good biocompatibility, they are highly reactive, especially with nucleophilic groups. These polymers can be made aliphatic or aromatic, resulting in a large range of degradation rates from days to years. Mechanical properties, however, are poor, being very brittle; efforts to improve them are being made [24, 25].

Poly(3-Hydroxybutyrate) Copolymers Chief among these copolymers is the cohydroxyvalerate system. These polymers are naturally occurring energy storage forms of some bacteria, and their breakdown products are natural compounds found in the blood. Mechanical and degradative properties are limited, yet can be adjusted with changes in copolymer ratio. The amorphous hydroxyvalerate adds elasticity with increasing ratios [26].

Poly(Phosphazenes) This group of polymers is formed with alternating backbones of nitrogen and phosphorous, with varying attached functional groups. While several non-degradable versions exist, the degradable ones break into phosphate and ammonium derivatives, with the main disadvantage being the effect this would have on the delicate nitrogen balance of the blood. There are many possible forms of these polymers with an equally large range of degradation rates and mechanical properties [27, 28].

Poly and Pseudopoly(Amino Acids) Varieties of amino acids have been assembled both with the usual amide linkages using the 20 natural amino acids as well as others. Pseudopoly(amino acids) are made of linkages to pendant functional groups either to the carboxyl group or to the amine or to other groups. Their degradation is usually enzyme-dependent and only a few have been characterized [29].

Degradable/Non-Degradable Copolymers As described earlier, constructs made of non-degradable sequences and degradable polymers have the potential of accessing properties available to traditional biomaterials with added desirability for tissue engineering applications. Chief among these are incorporating poly(ethylene oxide) blocks to take advantage of their ability to resist protein deposition and poly(urethane) blocks to take advantage of the microdomain organization of these polymers and their elastic properties [30]. In addition, cyanoacrylates have been used both as cross-linking agents in polymers [31] and as tissue adhesives alone [32]. Although these have degradable properties, care must be taken as to monitor their monomer release rate since the monomers are toxic even in moderately low quantities.

Non-Degradable Polymers

As there are innumerable types of non-degradable polymers, many of which are discussed elsewhere (see Chapter 2), they will only briefly be mentioned here. Often non-degradable polymers are used early in tissue engineering models or in tissue engineering constructs which have no similar replacement in the degradable category of polymers. An example of this is silicone, the elastic impermeable properties of which are difficult to replace in such devices as tube replacements in the esophagus [33] and nerve guides [34], or in skin graft protection [35]. The main problem with keeping non-degradable polymers in a tissue engineering construct is that either the polymer must remain in the host indefinitely, generating perpetual host-material interactions, or a second surgical procedure is required to remove the non-degradable polymer. There are few situations in which resolution of the non-degradable case is advantageous, so biomaterials sought for tissue engineering applications are usually biodegradable. The most obvious exception to this rule is encapsulation materials. These are fabricated from a variety of substrates, and all basically serve to protect the cells contained inside from exposure to immunological elements of the host. This protection must be maintained throughout the life of the implant, so non-degradable materials must be used. This is covered in detail in Chapter 26.

PROCESSING

There are several methods for processing a biomaterial to be suitable for a tissue engineering device [36]. Most methods involve processing the material following polymerization, although theoretically processing can occur simultaneously with polymerization. An example of this is the traditional implant material poly(methyl methacrylate) (PMMA) bone cement which is molded while polymerizing. Polymers used in tissue engineering applications, as in most industrial applications, are often pre-formed and distributed in solid pellet form. This form is often not suitable to fit tissue engineering needs. In fact, the requirements of device processing usually involve shaping to fit anatomical needs, forming pores to allow tissue ingrowth, and incorporating biologically active factors. Processing methods often require a purification step in which biologically non-compatible materials are removed, such as unreacted monomer or material processing agents which exist in the distributed polymer pellet as well as solvents and casting aids used in shaping and pore formation. If this purification is a wash step, this may expose the polymer to water molecules which could begin degradation of hydrolyzable polymers.

Solvent-Casting and Particulate-Leaching

This method works by dissolving the polymer in a solvent (usually organic) and mixing in some non-soluble particulate [37]. The suspension is then put into a mold and the solvent is allowed to evaporate. Once cast, the device is placed in a solvent in which the particulate is soluble, but the polymer is not. The pores form where the original particulate was located, and the size of the pores can be regulated by particulate size. The porosity of the device depends on the relative amount of particulate to polymer. A disadvantage of this method is that the use of solvents may destroy or denature any factors which need to be incorporated into the matrix. Also, since this process is dependent upon solvent evaporation, it is usually limited to a flat sheet.

Phase Inversion Casting

This process involves dissolving the polymer in one solvent, casting the mixture in its respective shape, and immersing the mixture in a non-solvent for the polymer which is miscible with the first solvent [38]. The polymer thus precipitates and forms an asymmetric porous structure of a dense skin with a porous base. This process still has the problem of using solvents which can denature factors or can remain in the construct and leach into the host. Likewise, using this method, polymers can only be cast into flat sheets and tubes. Nevertheless, it is often used for formation of barriers used in encapsulation of cellular or tissue implants to prevent immunological responses by the host [39].

Melt Processing

The need to process scaffolds without using organic solvents brought about the melt process. In this method the polymer is softened at a certain critical temperature and then molded to suitable shapes, or liquified to allow incorporation of particulate and biologically active factors [40]. These processes can expose factors to temperatures above their denaturing point, and therefore may not be ideal for sensitive factors, such as many proteins.

Fiber Bonding

Fiber bonding includes temperature processing in which fiber meshes or felts are heated to partially fuse the fibers [41]. An alternative method involves bonding of the polymer fibers with a solution of another polymer in a non-solvent for the fibers [42]. As before, solvent casting limits the use of incorporated factors which are sensitive to the solvent, and likewise, temperature processing limits the use of temperature sensitive factors.

Membrane Lamination

Not entirely a method of creating initial porous constructs, membrane lamination is usually a method of combining the porous sheets of the previous methods to make a three-dimensional porous construct. This can be achieved by gluing the surfaces of flat sheets using a polymer solvent. This results in formation of laminated structures with interconnecting pores and pore morphologies similar to those of the constituent layers [43–45].

ACTIVE COMPONENTS

Initially, materials used for traditional biomaterials applications were selected to be as inert as possible in an attempt to hide from biological processes (the so-called bio-inert surfaces). Current trends are to use signals from the implant to accomplish functions such as inducing or preventing tissue formation [46], activating cellular processes [47], and maintaining or changing differentiated state [48–50] (the so-called bio-cooperative surfaces). As was stated in the introduction, cells in vivo see signals constantly, whether from the ECM molecules, soluble factors in the fluid environment, or neighboring cells. Much research must be done to elucidate and understand their means of action in order to mimic signals. This has been approached as a trial-and-error process with each system rather than an extensive multisystem evaluation of signals and signal action.

Factors

Various soluble factors are used to direct cellular processes in vivo and replication of their action has been attempted in vitro. The factors can be cytokines, hormones, or even nutrients. Although these can be physically present in the fluid spaces of a tissue engineering construct, diffusion following transplantation would reduce local concentrations of such soluble compounds. In order to make soluble factors available to transplanted cells, several methods from the area of drug delivery have been adopted. For more detailed descriptions of these methods, the reader is referred to Chapter 28.

Embedded Embedding compounds or factors involves entrapping them within a matrix. Once the factors are entrapped, they can either be released slowly through a tortuous matrix, or remain entrapped but exposed to cells or cellular processes. An example of this is thermally reversible hydrogels which allow incorporation of biomolecules in the hydrophobic polymer below the lower critical solution temperature (LCST) and entrapment about the LCST. This has been investigated as a method for releasing heparin to improve hemocompatibility in implanted materials using poly(N-isopropyl acrylamide) [51].

Bound   Another method of modifying a polymer with a soluble factor is by chemically binding the factor to the polymer itself, either directly or with a short chain to allow surface interaction of cells to the bound factor. This is different from protein adsorption onto biomaterials as described by the Vroman effect, in that the bound factors will not be displaced by other molecules, but remain bound and chemically active. A disadvantage of such a system is that the amount of signaling cannot be regulated over time as with a factor delivery system unless the factor is bound to a polymer backbone which is degradable [52].

Surface Modification

Signaling of cells can also be accomplished through actual modification of the implant surface to simulate the ECM component of tissue engineering models. Modifications in this area can be as simple as embedding insoluble ECM components into the base polymer to form interpenetrating networks. Chemical attachment of these ECM components can be similar to that of bound soluble factors. Two other methods described below are artificial means of isolating the signaling element of ECM components.

Chemical   Certain peptide sequences have long been recognized as active signaling elements of ECM components. The most famous of these, the RGD (arginine-glycine-serine) tripeptide, has been found in many adhesion proteins to be specific to integrin receptors. Attachment of the tripeptide to implant surfaces has significantly improved cell attachment. Likewise the YIGSR (tyrosine-isoleucine-glycine-serine-arginine) pentapeptide sequence found in laminin binds to many laminin receptors, and the REDV (arginine-glutamate-aspartate-valine) sequence from fibronectin is specific for the $\alpha4\beta1$ integrin receptor on human endothelial cells [53–55]. Critical parameters for engineers in designing these constructs are peptide concentration, peptide spacer length, and material hydrophilicity.

Physical   Two methods of surface modification are under investigation. The first, micropatterning, involves physico-chemical modification of a surface on a microscopic level. Research in this area has been creating microdomains which are hydrophobic to repel cells, as well as hydrophilic to attract cells. This may be useful in patterning cell processes [56].

The other method, microtexturing, involves physico-mechanical modification of a surface. Research in this area has shown that surfaces of a certain regular texture promote cell attachment while others do not (see also Chapter 13). In fact, similar texturing of many different materials shows similar attachment rates, even on materials with fairly different attachment capabilities. This could be an invaluable discovery in tissue engineering constructs. Rather than finding a material which forms suitable interactions with cells and trying to tailor its mechanical properties, a material with suitable mechanical properties can be modified for improved cell attachment [57, 58].

TISSUE STRUCTURES

One of the evaluations that needs to be made is of the nature of the tissue that is to be replaced. Tissues often involve fairly simple definable organizational schemes. Reconstructing a tissue requires an understanding of its organization and an attempt to physically mimic the tissue to be replaced with synthetic materials, pure cell transplants, or, more commonly, combinations of materials and cells.

In addition to evaluating what type of tissue structure the designated tissue has, the investigator must also determine whether repair or regeneration of the defect can be accomplished by a reconstructed tissue alone, or by a combination of tissues in an artificial organ. Organs are designated here as combinations of several definable tissue schemes. A common example of organ reconstruction is found in tissue engineering constructs to replace small-diameter blood vessels. These are often made with an endothelial cultured cell lining as intima, a smooth muscle cultured cell wrap as media, and a polymer scaffold tube, perhaps with implanted fibroblasts, as adventitia [59]. The following are three distinct tissue schemes, each of which may need to be applied to provide a functional, tissue-engineered blood vessel.

Two-Dimensional Sheets

The first category of tissue organizational schemes is the simple two-dimensional sheet. Although these types rarely exist as flat sheets, they can often be cultured as such and then transplanted to comply to the appropriate surface geometry. Likewise, they do not have solely two-dimensional geometry, but the organization exists mainly in two dimensions, with simple repetition of the planar scheme in the third dimension. The most common examples of this scheme are epithelial sheets, with simple monolayers, but stratified epithelia often fit in this category as well.

Monocellular   The most simple sheets have only one cell type (although continuing research in this field may indicate that several different cell types do, in fact, exist, but may not be as apparent as in other tissues). Among these are the various epithelia of the eye, such as the retinal pigmented epithelium and the corneal endothelium. Transplant of these tissues may involve simple transplant of a monolayer sheet of cells.

Multicellular   Most epithelia exist as co-cultures of several cell types with different functions. Often only one cell type (usually the least differentiated one) is the only one capable of cell division in culture, and, therefore, does not show differentiated function in culture. Transplantation of these epithelia types involves problems both of propagating cells in culture, as well as of causing the differentiation into the various cell types needed in the implant. One example of this transplant type may be the lining of the stomach, to treat chronic ulcers. A transplant for this problem could be cultured as a flat sheet of cells, and then implanted into the damaged site.

Modified Two-Dimensional Cultures

Schemes which are defined as modified two-dimensional sheets involve cells in a non-flat structure which are two-dimensional in their reference frame. Transplants of smaller patches in these areas could involve flat sheets of cells, but often transplantation is required in a non-flat arrangement, necessitating the creation of more complex cell culture vessels than simple flat dishes.

Tubes   The tube is the most common organizational scheme of this type, found in blood vessel endothelium as well as the epithelial lining of the gastrointestinal, urinary, reproductive and respiratory systems. While they appear to be three-dimensional, these schemes can be cultured two-dimensionally, albeit in a non-flat arrangement.

Monocellular   The intima of blood vessels exists as a tube of mainly one cell type. A simple tissue engineering construct for vascular implantation may involve a polymer tube arrangement lined with a layer of cultured endothelium. Urothelium also exists as a monocellular layer of epithelial cells, although its structure is stratified transitional epithelium.

Multicellular   Most other tubular schemes exist as mixtures of several cell types, with the same inherent culture problems as flat, two-dimensional sheets of multiple cell types. Examples of this type are the absorptive, goblet, Paneth, and M cells of the intestinal mucosa, as well as the ciliated columnar, mucous goblet, brush, basal, and small granule cells of the respiratory lining.

Shells   Shells of a two-dimensional cell scheme can either be capsules, with a lumen on the exterior, such as the lens epithelium surrounding the lens matrix, or pouch-like, with a lumen on the interior, such as is found in the gall bladder lining as well as other endocrine and exocrine organs.

Three-Dimensional Constructs

Schemes of a three-dimensional nature do not need the large surface-area-to-volume ratio of simple sheets, but need the organizational geometry of small surface-area-to-volume ratio found in dense three-dimensional organs. One of the inherent problems that exists in a three-dimensional tissue that is not found in the so-called two-dimensional ones is diffusion limitation. Without transport of nutrients and waste, cells in the interior of an implant greater than 1 mm from a nutrient source will die [60]. Attempts to overcome this problem involve some mechanism to allow diffusion into the interior of a large implant, such as implant neovascularization. The implant, however, must be prevascularized before seeding of cells takes place.

Homogeneous Tissue   Not truly homogeneous in nature, tissues of this scheme require little directional geometry. An example is the liver, where each lobule of hepatocytes requires the transport of the portal triad, involving several fluid compartments as well as the bile canaliculi organization, but not directional organization.

Acellular Matrix   These tissues do have a cellular component to maintain and repair, but far more important are the mechanical properties provided by the acellular component, namely the ECM. Clear examples of these tissues are bone, cartilage, tendon, and ligament. Replacement would require both substitutes for the mechanical and structural properties, as well as the small cellular population to regenerate the synthetic matrix with a natural one.

Organized Three-Dimensional Constructs

Tissues of the organized three-dimensional arrangement have a more obviously directional-specific geometry. An example of this is skeletal muscle, which pulls along aligned fibers in a specific directional vector, and kidneys, which have multiple fluid compartments with fluid flow in many directional vectors.

Simple Organizational Matrix   The simplest three-dimensional organizational matrices involve only single cell types, with easily definable directional vectors. Culture of these tissues may begin as a simple two-dimensional culture with some protocol to allow for cellular alignment.

Linear When the directional organization of a tissue is one-dimensional, the tissue can be defined as linear. An example of this is skeletal muscle or peripheral nerve fibers. The pulling force and the electrochemical signal in these cases have a defined direction, while the tissue itself is organized in three dimensions.

Lamellar Smooth muscle cells also have a one-dimensional organization, but are most often composed of lamellar sheets of such tissue, each with its own different directional vector. Reconstruction of these organs might also require reconstruction of other cell layers, such as surrounding circumferential and longitudinal muscle layers in the adventitia of blood vessels.

Complex Organizational Matrix The last organizational scheme involves complex directional organization which is not easily defined. The clear example of this is the kidney, of which the glomeruli, blood vessels and renal tubules each require specific directional geometry. Another example is central nervous system tissue: the brain, ganglia, and neuroretina have a clear, three-dimensional structure with directional specificity.

ENGINEERING METHODS

Tissue engineering methods involve the use of combinations of polymer scaffolds, cells, and induction factors. Currently, several approaches are employed to deliver autogeneic cells to replace functional loss. Autogeneic cells isolated and cultured from the host are free of immunological concerns of graft rejection and pathogen transfer. For those cell types which cannot be cultured or grown in vitro, allogeneic or xenogeneic cells have been used encapsulated in membranes for immunoisolation. As these implants are discussed in Chapter 26, they are only briefly mentioned here. A complication of delivering autogeneic cells is that any inherent cellular defect still exists in the isolated and expanded cells.

Transplantation Scaffolds

A common method of delivering cells to a site is by construction of a cellular scaffold [61]. The scaffold often is designed as a porous degradable sponge in which cells can divide, fill the sponge, and take the place of material as it degrades. Other cell scaffolds have included non-porous rods, tubes, sheets and microspheres, upon which cells are cultured prior to implantation. There have also been many non-degradable implants. While these may serve the same function as degradable ones, the added complication of eventual inflammatory response, including the formation of a tissue capsule, makes these materials a less viable alternative to similar degradable ones. Ideally, a tissue engineering approach would include a temporary scaffold as new tissue forms, but eventually only the new cellular components would remain as the cells restore the lost function.

Cartilage Early efforts with PLLA and PLGA sponges involved reconstruction of cartilage with cultured chondrocytes [62, 63]. Cartilage replacement is necessary both in reconstruction of plastic defects such as in the ears and nose, as well as replacement of articular surfaces found in joints. Current prostheses made of non-degradable polymer and/or metals and ceramics have the complications of wear products. Autograft tissue has been used successfully, but adds an additional wound and ensuing discomfort from the harvest site [64]. Allograft tissue has also been transplanted successfully, with immuno-logical complications being surpassed by irradiation or chemical devitalization [65]. This removes viable chondrocytes from the matrix, so regeneration and remodeling is dependent upon cell induction, making the devitalized allograft similar to a non-cellular, tissue-engineered construct. Any tissue graft transplant is also complicated by the problem of donor scarcity.

In a tissue engineering approach to cartilage reconstruction, the polymer scaffold is required to take the mechanical and physical load of the replaced tissue until the neocartilage is formed. Research to tailor degradable polymers to suit these needs is underway.

Bone   Defects in bone have also been investigated for repair by tissue engineering methods [66, 67]. These defects can be caused by massive trauma (such as motor vehicle accidents), or from resection due to cancerous bone growths. Also, some more traditional fractures can undergo a dysfunctional non-union where surgical intervention may be necessary.

As in cartilage, the synthetic scaffold in bone is required to bear greater physical and mechanical loads than in most tissues. Traditionally materials with high mechanical properties, such as metals and ceramics, have been used. Other than the immediate problems of biocompatibility, interface adhesion, and abrasion, there are also the long-term problems of stress shielding, in which bone undergoes inferior remodeling around the implant. Allograft and autograft bone suffer the same limitations as are found in cartilage transplants [46].

Biodegradable scaffolds of natural origin (sea coral) [68] or inorganic minerals (hydroxyapatite, tricalcium phosphate, and others) [69] were among the first materials studied. These materials are inexpensive, inert, and easily sterilizable. Unfortunately, they are naturally brittle and possess low tensile strength.

Biodegradable porous polymer scaffolds have also been investigated. These materials can easily be shaped to suit the defect, and their mechanical properties can be adjusted within limits. The serious drawback of polymers is their degradation in this fairly avascular environment. The traditional polymers used, namely the poly(α-hydroxy esters), do not undergo resorption by osteoclasts as do the inorganic matrices; rather, they break down by hydrolysis and release the degradation products at a regular rate. Accumulation of these degradation products, due to limited fluid transport away from the area, leads to low local pH which causes additional tissue irritation, even necrosis. While this effect has been observed with dense degradable implants such as screws and plates, no similar effect has been reported with porous degradable sponges. Investigations using copolymers, as well as mixtures of low and high molecular weight chains, may allow a more controlled release of the acidic monomer [16]. Other constructs being investigated involve composites of polymer and inorganic minerals [70]. These allow combinations of the mechanical properties of polymers and the resorbable properties of the inorganic matrix. Porous scaffolds of this nature can be implanted with osteoblasts to begin immediate remodeling upon transplantation.

Liver   Cellular transplantation of liver hepatocytes shows some promise as a treatment for liver deficiencies caused by viral factors, toxicological agents, cancer, or congenital defects. Whole organ transplants have been successful, but are limited by donor scarcity. Since the number of donors has not been increasing at the same rate as the number of individuals requiring treatment, some other viable method for organ replacement must be developed.

Microencapsulation of xenograft [71] and allograft [72] tissue has been tested successfully, but the strength of liver repair and restoration of lost function lies in its ability to regenerate cell mass from autograft tissue. Hepatocytes have been successfully isolated and cultured for transplantation, although susceptibility of surface proteins to enzymatic attack has made routine culture difficult. Originally these cells were grown on naturally occurring ECM proteins to provide an environment similar to that found in vivo, maintaining long-term differentiation [73]. One of the problems with using matrices of this nature is that they could not be tailored physically to provide for ingrowth of the vascular tissue needed to supply cells in the interior of the implant.

Biodegradable polymers were therefore tested for their feasibility as a cellular scaffold. Although they could support implanted cells and be tailored to very specific porous geometries, they lacked initial vascularity [74]. A scheme recently developed involved implanting a porous degradable sponge which would be prevascularized and injection of a cellular suspension once all areas of the implant were supplied [75]. To reach this goal, more and more complex scaffolds have been created, including ones which incorporate angiogenic factors to improve neovascularization as well as ECM proteins to help the hepatocytes maintain a differentiated state [76, 77].

Urothelium   Repair of urothelial injury has been investigated with synthetic [78] as well as natural [79] materials, with limited success. Preliminary trials with biodegradable PGA meshes seeded with rabbit urothelial cells and implanted in athymic mice showed good cell attachment as well as neovascularization and multilayer formation in the implant [80]. This shows the feasibility of a tissue engineering construct for treatment of urothelial injury, but research is only in its early stages.

Respiratory Epithelium   Similarly, respiratory epithelium has been cultured on scaffolds for purposes of defect repair. Preliminary results have had moderate success, with cells showing good attachment maintained in vivo [81, 82]. As is the case in the intestine described below, the mixed cell types of the respiratory system require more extensive investigation into achieving the various differentiated states.

Intestine   Tissue engineering constructs for repair of intestinal defects have also shown some promise. PGA fibers seeded with fetal rat enterocytes showed attachment and neovascularization of the implant, although cell orientation results were not consistent [83]. Clearly reconstruction of whole intestine or urinary or respiratory tract would require more than epithelial transplant. A transplant would need to have composite structure including wall support such as is provided by the smooth muscle cells in vivo. Work in this area has been attempted with vascular grafts.

Vascular Grafts   The search for a suitable vascular graft is perhaps the longest in the history of biomaterials. Some of the earliest materials used in implants were in vascular grafts for treatment of blood vessel occlusion and damage (for more detail see Chapters 5, 35, and 44). Large-diameter grafts for use in high flow vessels have been fairly successful, including both fully synthetic (such as Dacron and expanded poly(tetrafluoroethylene) grafts) and synthetic grafts seeded with endothelial cells [84]. In lower flow conditions dominated by viscous components, as in the small-diameter graft, additional complications arise. Repair in such vessels is fairly successful using autograft tissue (e.g., the great saphenous vein dissected out for coronary bypass surgery). The problems with this use of autograft tissue lie in the inherent inconvenience caused by the second surgical wound, the need for alternative tissue sources for individuals who have such poor vessel health that transplantation is not feasible, and the frequent postoperative pathological changes observed in the autograft called medial hyperplasia.

Recent research has investigated multilayer constructs. Early studies with simple endothelial-lined stents showed poor integration at the anastomosis site. The next generation of transplants was a three-layer construct of bovine vascular tissue, namely an inner layer of endothelial cells, a layer of smooth muscle cells (SMC) and collagen, and a layer of fibroblasts and collagen. These composite vessels showed better biocompatibility but did not have the mechanical properties of native blood vessels and distended too easily [85]. Current efforts on improving SMC contractility have led to a two-layer composite of endothelium and SMC together with appropriate ECM components. These efforts have succeeded in making a suitable model for testing mechanical functionality of developing vascular grafts [86]. Perhaps the future of vascular graft material holds biodegradable polymer composites with suitable mechanical properties to serve as a scaffold for the developing multilayer composite until it is able to assume a mechanical load itself.

Retinal Pigment Epithelium   The retinal pigment epithelium (RPE) is a simple monolayer of single cells which provide a supportive function for the neuroretina in the eye. Loss of this function leads to photoreceptor damage, and possible irreversible blindness. Preliminary research with cell transplantation has shown that an oriented sheet of RPE cells can prevent photoreceptor loss. Experiments with degradable scaffolds of collagen [87] or PLGA [88] are promising in terms of providing a means of cell culture and transplantation. However, since the eye is a very avascular tissue, the accumulation of degradation products may lead to toxic effects as it has in bone. Preparation of a minimal cell implant with little or no scaffold may be necessary [89].

The RPE provides a good model for testing tissue engineering constructs because it is made of a single cell type which is easily isolated and cultured as well as visualized in vivo. The loss of function of RPE is characterized by obvious symptoms, namely vision loss; currently there is no known treatment of many of these dysfunctions. Understanding the many aspects of this simple system may be fundamental in elucidating the various aspects of a more complicated system.

Induction Conduits

In addition to tissue engineering constructs which utilize cultured cells, some constructs encourage cells in the surrounding tissue to grow into a synthetic structure. This concept, long used for vascular grafts, was reported before in the fabrication of the liver construct. In order to obtain suitable nutrient transport into the interior of the implant, it was first allowed to vascularize. That is, the empty scaffold was implanted and vascular tissue was induced to grow into the pores. In some ways this simplifies the cell culture part of tissue engineering in that cell isolation and growth takes place in vivo. It is possible, however, that the scaffold is more supportive to the induction of less desirable cell types, or does not allow the induced cells to remain differentiated. These are problems which would be more difficult to solve in the tissue induction model.

Tissue induction is usually preferred over scaffold/cell composites only in instances when the patient cannot wait for autogenous tissue isolation and culture, or when the tissue cannot be cultured in vitro. Often the more successful tissue induction models involve addition of cells in a secondary procedure.

Skin   There is a significant clinical need for skin replacement for burn patients. Autograft skin is fairly successful, taking a small patch and expanding it several times in size. For a patient with major burns on most of the body it may not be possible to harvest these small patches. Also, the harvest site brings up the same problems of second injury complications. Allograft skin has also been fairly successful, but is limited by the usual problems of donor scarcity and infectious agent transfer.

Early experiments with synthetic skin involved a collagen-glycosaminoglycan (GAG) dermis covered with a silicone layer which prevented dehydration and pathogen entry [35]. Once the dermis was incorporated and tissue was induced into the degradable scaffold, the silicone sheet could be removed. Epithelium could then be induced from the edges of the implant. This model was fairly successful, although newer versions include transplanting a sheet of epithelium at the time of the silicone removal [90] (this could be cultured from a small biopsy at the time of the injury), or a dermal matrix already seeded with fibroblasts [91]. Although these methods work well, the simple induction model is currently the most practical, since burn patients need solutions immediately, and often cannot wait for cell culture expansion as other patients requiring tissue engineering often can.

Synthetic skin is one of the most successful tissue engineering constructs to date. There are at least four companies whose work deals with skin reconstruction and regeneration. Skin has an amazing self-repair capability, but this involves massive scar formation and wound contraction, which is alleviated only after much complicated reconstructive surgery. The synthetic skin equivalents are designed to limit wound contraction and scar formation, giving the burn area time to construct new skin.

Nerve   It was long thought that nervous tissue was unable to undergo self-repair. It is now known that peripheral nerves which are cut at the distal end (away from the cell body) can undergo regeneration. The distal end degenerates (Wallerian degeneration) while the proximal end makes a new axonal process. If it is possible to align and suture the two cut ends, regeneration is simplified as the new process follows the path of the degenerating old one (including the myelin sheaths). In cases where a piece of peripheral nerve has been resected, it may not be possible to appose and suture the two ends. Also, the suturing process produces additional trauma to the nerve, which may be undesirable. Autograft of segments of "less important" nerve fibers has been successful, but this solution is far from ideal, with nerve regrowth and regeneration subsequently required in two systems. Tissue engineering methods for the repair of peripheral nerve (i.e., tissue induction) is mandated.

In early tissue engineering experiments silicone tubes were implanted into 15 mm gaps in rat sciatic nerve (a distance over which no natural regeneration will occur). Extension of new axonal processes through the tube was observed [34]. Filling the tube with various inducing factors such as collagen or GAGs improved ingrowth [92]. Trends in degradable scaffolds led to the use of U-shaped ducts of PGA with a flat cover (to be used in nerves which are not completely transsected) [93]. Ingrowth likewise was observed here, and the scaffold was resorbed. In the era of cellular implants, tubes filled with Schwann cells (which both are required for formation of the myelin sheath, and have been observed to stimulate increased axonal regeneration) were tested as well, with promising results [94]. Although completely transsected peripheral nerves are neither a common problem, nor clinically significant in terms of cost, modeling of their repair may help in understanding repair of other critical nervous tissue, such as the spinal cord.

Esophagus   Similar to intestinal repair, esophageal reconstruction may be required in cases of injury or tumor excision. The use of synthetic biomaterial implants or natural tissue has had limited success. Preliminary work with silicone tubes (for continuous esophageal transport) coated with a porous collagen sponge showed resorption and growth of neoesophageal tissue [33]. The problem of removal of the silicone inner tube still remains, however.

Biodegradable PLGA tubes implanted in dogs were also overgrown with connective tissue and epithelium, and allowed the animals to drink freely and eat semi-solid foods over time [95]. Initial seeding with fetal intestinal cells showed organized epithelial lining with possible mucous secretion [96]. These models, though limited, were successful in showing the feasibility of a tissue induction engineered construct.

Tendon and Ligament   Work on both anterior cruciate ligament and Achilles tendon models has shown good initial results in inducing tissue growth. Collagen fibers were implanted into anterior cruciate ligament models. Although little degradation occurred, the implant quickly lost mechanical properties [97]. Likewise, tendon scaffolds of various degradable materials (polymer [98], carbon fiber [99], and collagen [100] combinations) seeded with bone marrow mesenchymal cells became tendon-like over a period of 12 weeks, but the mechanical properties were not elucidated. As in the other work in this section, rapid repair of defects needs to be accomplished. An inducible scaffold seems to be a feasible method, as long as mechanical properties upon implantation and during degradation are managed.

Bone   Replacement or repair of bone often must be available on demand, in which case an induction model for this system may be required. Currently the only available method for rapid bone repair or cementation is PMMA. This polymer cement has been used clinically for many years, although it has many drawbacks: it is not degradable, polymerization leads to temperatures which can damage neighboring tissue, and unreacted monomer is extremely toxic. The need to develop a bone cement without these drawbacks is apparent.

Biodegradable poly(propylene fumarate)-based composite materials have shown encouraging results for orthopaedic application. They show mechanical properties suitable for replacing bone maintained over 12 weeks [101]. The polymers are degradable to natural metabolites, and have a low polymerization temperature. Additional products have been added, such as a water-soluble salt for initial porosity, and a calcium phosphate matrix for formation of an osteoconductive scaffold for new bone growth [102]. Osteoconduction is defined as allowing bone to grow in areas where it would normally grow (versus osteoprevention), while osteoinduction encourages bone to grow in situations where it is not normally growing. Work on developing osteoinduction is also underway in other systems, by use of bone morphogenic protein (BMP) and transforming growth factor-β (TGF-β) [103, 104].

Primary Culture Models

In some systems cell transplantation models are in the early cell culture stage or cellular implant, but have not reached the point of development into polymer scaffold implants.

Cornea (Endothelium and Epithelium)   Corneal transplants are among the most successful donor allograft transplants to date, and the waiting list for corneas is fairly short. Since the cornea and anterior chamber of the eye are entirely avascular, there is no problem with immunological agents from the blood which makes host-graft rejection extremely uncommon and obviates the need for immunosuppressive therapy. Also, very few pathological agents or conditions have been shown to be passed along into the host following transplantation. It is clear that any tissue engineering construct would have to perform as well as a transplanted allograft cornea if it is to compete in this fairly successful area of transplantation.

Non-degradable hydrogels have been seeded with cultured corneal endothelium and implanted into test animals [105] as have been xenograft stromas seeded with corneal endothelium [106]. These performed well initially, but long-term results were inconclusive. Synthetic constructs have been made with epithelial layers seeded as well, but since the host usually replaces the epithelium (even of allografts) with native epithelium rapidly, this step may not be necessary. Clearly some possibility exists of creating a tissue engineering construct of cornea, but this field is only in its infancy.

Skeletal Muscle   Culture of myoblasts and skeletal muscle satellite cells have both been successful, as well as transplantation of such cells in various models. Healthy myoblasts have been transplanted into patients with Duchenne muscular dystrophy; it was found that dystrophin can be produced for 1 to 6 months after transplant, showing the feasibility of a factor-delivering muscular construct [107]. Satellite cells have been transplanted to dog hearts and resulted in muscle-like tissue, although the results are still too far from organized muscle sheets to be transplanted for lost mechanical function [108]. Work with elastic polymer scaffolds has shown some promise, possibly in aligning muscle fibers.

Kidney   As a first step in creating tissue engineered kidney, renal tubule cells were grown on synthetic porous membranes made of poly(acrylonitrile)-poly(vinyl chloride) copolymer or cellulose nitrate. These constructs showed transport of insulin, glucose, and tetraethylammonium [109], but are far from reaching the organized microstructure of the natural kidney. Other work in formation of kidney-like tubules (tubulogenesis) involved use of induction factors [110].

IMPLEMENTATION

Once the need to engineer a specific tissue or organ has been determined, there are several steps that need to be taken to accomplish this goal: cell isolation, cell culture, scaffold material choice, cell/scaffold co-culture, animal studies, and human trials. In some cases these steps may be less obvious or less rigorous than in others, but all the issues must be addressed to make a viable construct. For example, a construct using non-replicating cells will have minimal cell culture, or simply will involve isolation of cells in situ as the implant is placed in the host. In this case the culture-scaffold interactions are observed in vivo in the animal trials. Such was the case in peripheral nerve tube guides [34]. Other approaches, however, may involve more intensive use of the earlier stages as well, for example in tubes seeded with Schwann cells [94].

Cell Isolation

The active element of all tissue engineering constructs is the living cell. The cell is what constitutes the main difference between tissue engineering and traditional biomaterials. There are many methods of isolating cells for cell culture, although all methods usually involve surgical isolation of tissue, tissue homogenization (whether enzymatic, mechanical or chemical), followed by specific means of purification. Although these methods will be briefly discussed here, the reader may refer to reference [111] for a more detailed text.

Surgical isolation differs from tissue to tissue. Some tissues are easily isolated into their components, such as removing epithelial sheets from their substratum, while others involve complex mixtures of cells with different functions such as the endocrine and exocrine components of pancreas as well as the fibroblasts of pancreatic connective tissue.

Once tissue is dissected out, it needs to be broken into its component cells or cell clusters. The usual method is with enzymatic digestion such as trypsin combined with ethylenediaminetetraacetic acid (EDTA), a $Ca++$ chelating agent which disables calcium-dependent binding proteins. This decreases the association of calcium binding protein, as well as cleaves independent binding proteins. Other enzymes, such as collagenase mixtures or other protein specific proteases, may be more useful in isolating the desired cells while not disturbing undesired cellular contaminants. Some cell types cannot undergo any enzymatic digestion. Most prominent among these is hepatocytes, which lose the ability to make specific receptors at some point in embryogenesis. These cells are isolated by mechanical separation, such as a tissue homogenizer (blender). Although nominally some cell types can survive enzymatic isolation, clearly long exposure to enzymatic attack would be detrimental. Establishing an ideal protocol for such isolation usually involves finding an optimal enzyme, modifying its exposure length and temperature, and then finding an enzymatic inhibitor. The convenience of the trypsin/EDTA system is that the serum component of most media contains a trypsin inhibitor. Experience has found that the most viable isolation schemes involve not necessarily separation into wholly independent cells, but into very small cell clusters.

The final stage of purification isolates the desired cells from various undesirable cells as well as damaged cell fragments or ECM components. There are several methods to accomplish this: filtration, centrifugation, gradient separation, or a combination of the three. More active separation methods such as preferential attachment can also be used. This method can separate attachment-dependent cells from unattachable cells, or even cells which attach and/or migrate at different rates. No isolation method is perfect, however, and the researcher must be on the constant lookout for unanticipated cellular contaminants.

Cell Culture

Mammalian cell culture is an art form which is not fully taught by any educational system, but rather is a trial-and-error process that can only be learned by experience. For example there are many factors which need to be optimized to make the ideal culture medium. Several different media types exist, varying in composition from high sugar, low amino acid/vitamin/mineral mixtures of the Minimal Essential Medium type to the low sugar, high nutrient mixture of the Ham's F-12 type. Moreover, there are many supplements, including growth factors, hormones, minerals and drugs, as well as antibiotics and fungicides which need to be added to the base medium. Some of these supplements come in the serum (usually 5–10%) that is added to most media. Serum has the drawback of containing uncharacterizable elements, but has the advantage of providing such factors in the ratios necessary to support cell growth.

As was stated in the introduction, soluble factors are one of the three elements of tissue engineering; optimizing soluble factors in nutrient media is ongoing work. While it may be an easy process to make a cell grow and divide, the difficulty arises in restoring, maintaining, or establishing differentiated function. There is some considerable debate whether cells that have truly lost differentiated state are able to re-differentiate. Usually cell culture involves a battle to prevent de-differentiation. Investigations of the fluid microenvironment around functioning and non-functioning cells in vivo are essential to make cell cultures resemble in vivo models more closely. It is becoming increasingly obvious that simple flat schemes on solid polymer or glass substrates are far from actual in vivo cellular performance.

Functionality Assay It is common for the tissue engineer to establish a cell transplantation scheme yet have no method for assessing functionality either in vitro or in vivo. While it is key to be able to successfully culture and implant cells to develop a tissue engineering construct, the primary purpose of the construct is to replace lost function. Determining a proper functional assay first requires determining functional parameters of the tissue in vivo, then devising a method of testing it in vitro. The following is a list of commonly used methods of testing functionality. It is far from exhaustive, and in each tissue engineering case the actual function which is lost and needs to be restored has to be determined. While it may be possible to grow non-functional cells, implanting them at the very least will have no effect, but more likely will cause more damage than would exist without the implant.

Mechanical Function In the case of bone, cartilage, tendon and ligament, these functions may be mechanical. While it is essential to transplant cells which will eventually reconstruct and remodel the tissue as before, the cells themselves provide little mechanical function. In this case the purpose of a scaffold which can take up the function is obvious. In other cases the scaffold may be less necessary, as in the cases where a soluble cellular product is missing.

Protein Production One product of functional expression is proteins. In some cells the missing protein may be obvious, such as insulin in pancreatic islet β-cells, or ECM components in connective tissues. Other tissues may have very specific protein expressions, but determining what they are and how they can be detected can be a long process. Proteins can be expressed and detected in the extracellular environment by collection and assay of used media. Expression can be on the surface or interior of a cell and can be detected (although quantitative assays are more difficult) by immunocytochemistry. Protein expression can be assayed on the molecular level by evaluating DNA transcription (by mRNA analysis with Northern blotting) to determine new expression, or translation (by Western blot analysis) to detect the presence of non-new, pre-existing proteins (as with immunocytochemistry).

Cell Viability Some functional assays are determined simply by cell viability. A good test for this is DNA synthesis evaluation (for example by BrdU (5-Bromo-2'-deoxyuridine) labelling), although there are several other methods such as the MTT (3-[4,5-dimethylthiazol-2-yl]-2,5-diphenyltetrazolium bromide; thiazolyl blue) method which tests mitochondrial activity, the fluorescein diacetate which assays activity of the lysosomal components, or trypan blue which detects the integrity of the cell membrane. The mere presence of a viable cell does not guarantee its differentiated function, however (see also Chapter 21).

Cell Morphology Another assay of the condition of a particular culture can be by microscopic evaluation of cell morphology, ascertained histologically by various microscopic methods such as electron microscopy or laser confocal imaging. This rests on the assumption that cells require a certain morphology to maintain differentiated function. While this assumption may be erroneous (there might be non-morphologically sound cells with proper function, or, more importantly, morphologically sound cells without proper function), it is often the first selection criterion made, but should never be the only one.

Some methods of detecting sound morphology look for obvious morphological features such as microvilli, cilia, infolded membranes, or junctional complexes. A more appropriate functional assay may involve gross visualization of a function, such as phagocytosis in RPE cells, which is a key feature lost in some dystrophies. Orientation of cellular components as observed by immunofluorescence microscopy and confocal imaging may give a better indication of proper cell function, especially if this can be determined on a molecular level where protein expression is on one surface but not on another.

Scaffold Material Choice

The choice of polymer to use in any particular system may be the most all-encompassing choice a tissue engineer needs to make, addressing concerns such as biocompatibility, material properties (chemical and physical), ease of manufacture, and cost. Sections I and II provide more details on material selection.

Common concerns the tissue engineer faces are cell adhesion, promotion of cell proliferation and differentiation, and suitable degradation or accommodation characteristics. Cell adhesion is required for many cell types in order for division to occur. Proliferation is necessary to fill the scaffold and replace lost or damaged tissue mass. Differentiation or maintenance of differentiated state allows expression of function whose loss led to disease symptoms. Restoring lost function is the primary goal for any tissue engineer. The ability of a scaffold to degrade or to be "hidden" from the body reduces concerns of long-term, host/material interactions, such as chronic inflammation.

The traditional choice, although increasingly often not the only choice, is a degradable porous sponge whose porosity allows cell ingrowth, organization, and direction [37]. This sponge can be tailored to promote and/or enhance adhesion, proliferation and differentiation, and later to degrade at a controllable rate into natural metabolites.

Cell/Scaffold Interactions

This part of implementing an experimental design is mainly concerned with cell attachment and propagation on a synthetic material as well as biocompatibility of the material. As these are discussed in other chapters, they will only be mentioned briefly here as being an integral component in assessing the viability of a tissue engineering construct on the cellular level (see Chapters 21 and 24).

Animal Studies and Human Trials

Since these are covered in another chapter, they will not be discussed here other than to mention that once the implant has reached this stage, another series of tests to assay functionality and biocompatibility must be established (see Sections VI, VII, VIII, and X). Within limits, one can predict how an implant will be received by the host, but again each system is different; once the implanted cells are exposed to the new environment, they could change protein expression, growth rate, or even state of differentiation. While the early models are informative, they should be viewed only as models, with the final test being how a device performs upon implantation.

CONCLUSIONS

This chapter is not to be taken as a cookbook on making and evaluating a tissue engineering construct, but rather a guide to existing constructs and their cellular systems, as well as a treatise addressing several of the concerns that should be investigated by the tissue engineer. Clearly each cellular system is different, and there can even be functional dystrophies solved in different ways within the same system. The point is that resorting to cookbook ideas will lead only to solutions already available to us. In order to find a place in the newly emerging field of tissue engineering, the researcher must address issues that have not been investigated. This cannot be done alone, and there is no classical education which will provide all the knowledge available to do this; instead, it requires an interdisciplinary effort and an interdisciplinary education. Traditional biomaterials research has involved cooperation of the materials scientist, the pathologist and the surgeon. Tissue engineering has introduced the need for additional disciplines, including but not limited to embryology, developmental biology, molecular biology and biochemistry, genetic engineering, as well as innovative polymer chemistry.

REFERENCES

1   Skalak R, Fox CF (Eds.). *Tissue Engineering.* New York: Alan R. Liss, 1988.
2   Hubbell JA, Langer R. Tissue engineering. *Chem Eng News*, 73 (1995), 42–54.
3   Yannas IV, Burke JF, Orgill DP, Skrabut EM. Wound tissue can utilize a polymeric template to synthesize a functional extension of skin. *Science*, 215 (1982), 174–176.
4   Buchanan MR, Richardson M, Haas TA, Hirsh J, Madri JA. The basement membrane underlying vascular endothelium is not thrombogenic: *In vivo* and *in vitro* studies with rabbit and human tissue. *Thromb Haemost*, 58 (1987), 698–704.
5   Glanville RW. Collagen IV. In Mayne R, Burgeson RE (Eds.), *Structure and Function of Collagen Types.* Orlando, FL: Academic Press, 1987, 43–80.
6   Hubbell JA. Biomaterials in tissue engineering. *Bio/Technology*, 13 (1995), 565–576.
7   Yannas IV. Tissue regeneration templates based on collagen-glycosaminoglycan copolymers. *Adv Polym Sci*, 122 (1995), 219–244.
8   Urman B, Gomel V, Jetha N. Effect of hyaluronic acid on postoperative intraperitoneal adhesion formation in the rat model. *Fertil Steril*, 56 (1991), 563–567.
9   Gray I, Highland GP. Metabolism of plasma expanders studied with carbon-14-labeled Dextran. *Am J Physiol*, 174 (1953), 462–466. .
10 Gruber UF. In *Blutersatz.* Berlin: Springer Verlag, 1968.
11 Suggs LJ, Mikos AG. Synthetic biodegradable polymers for medical applications. In Mark JE (Ed.), *Physical Properties of Polymers Handbook.* Woodbury, MA: American Institute of Physics, 1996, 615–624.
12 Leach RE, Henry RL. Reduction of postoperative adhesion in the rat uterine horn model with poloxamer 407. *Am J Obstet Gynecol*, 162 (1990), 1317–1319.
13 Kopecek J. Soluble polymers in medicine. In Williams DF (Ed.), *Systemic Aspects of Biocompatibility*, Vol. II. Boca Raton, FL: CRC Press, 1981, 159–180.
14 Frazza EJ, Schmitt EE. A new resorbable suture. *J Biomed Mater Res, Biomed Mater Symp*, 1 (1971), 43–58.
15 Miller RA, Brady JM, Cutright DE. Degradation rates of oral resorbable implants (polylactates and poly-glycolates): Rate modification with changes in PLA/PGA copolymer ratios. *J Biomed Mater Res*, 11 (1977), 711–719.
16 von Recum HA, Cleek RL, Eskin SG, Mikos AG. Degradation of polydispersed poly(L-lactic acid) to modulate lactic acid release. *Biomaterials*, 16 (1995), 441–447.
17 Reed AM, Gilding DK. Biodegradable polymers for use in surgery—Poly(glycolic)/poly(lactic acid) homo and copolymers: 2. *In vitro* degradation. *Polymer*, 22 (1981), 342–346.
18 Gilding DK, Reed AM. Biodegradable polymers for use in surgery—Polyglycolic/polylactic acid homo- and co-polymers: 1. *Polymer*, 20 (1979), 1459–1464.
19 Therin M, Christel P, Li S, Garreau H, Vert M. *In vivo* degradation of massive poly(α-hydroxy acids): Validation of *in vivo* findings. *Biomaterials*, 13 (1992), 594–600.

20   Vert M, Mauduit J, Li S. Biodegradation of PLA/GA polymers: Increasing complexity. *Biomaterials*, 15 (1994), 1209–1213.

21   Pitt CG. Poly ε-caprolactone and its copolymers. In Chasin M, Langer R (Eds.), *Biodegradable Polymers as Drug Delivery Systems*. New York: Marcel Dekker, 1990, 71–120.

22   Engelberg I, Kohn J. Physico-mechanical properties of degradable polymers used in medical applications: A comparative study. *Biomaterials*, 12 (1991), 292–304.

23   Merkli A, Heller J, Tabatabay C, Gurny R. Synthesis and characterization of a new biodegradable semi-solid poly(orthoester) for drug delivery systems. *J Biomed Mater Res, Polym Ed*, 4 (1993), 505–516.

24   Domb AJ, Amselem S, Shah J, Maniar M. Polyanhydrides: Synthesis and characterization. *Adv Polym Sci*, 107 (1993), 93–141.

25   Tamada J, Langer R. The development of polyanhydrides for drug delivery applications. *J Biomater Sci, Polym Ed*, 3 (1992), 315–353.

26   Miller ND, Williams DF. On the biodegradation of poly b-hydroxybutyrate (PHB) homopolymer and poly b-hydroxybutyrate-hydroxyvalerate copolymers. *Biomaterials*, 8 (1987), 129–137.

27   Laurencin CT, Norman ME, Elgendy HM, el Amin SF, Allcock HR, Pucher SR, Ambrosio AA. Use of polyphophazenes for skeletal tissue regeneration. *J Biomed Mater Res*, 27 (1993), 963–973.

28   Cohen S, Baño MC, Visscher KB, Chow M, Allcock HR, Langer R. Ionically cross-linkable phosphazene: A novel polymer for microencapsulation. *J Am Chem Soc*, 112 (1990), 7832–7835.

29   Barrera DA, Zylstra E, Lansbury PT, Langer R. Copolymerization and degradation of poly(lactic acid-co-lysine). *Macromolecules*, 28 (1995), 425–432.

30   Gilding DK, Reed AM. Significant variables that must be controlled in the design and synthesis of polyurethanes for use in medicine. *Life Support Syst*, 5 (1987), 19–24.

31   Hill-West JL, Chowdhury SM, Sawhney AS, Patnak CP, Dunn RC, Hubbell JA. Prevention of post-operative adhesions in the rat by *in situ* photopolymerization of bioresorbable hydrogel barriers. *Obstet Gynecol*, 83 (1994), 59–64.

32   Leonard F, Kulkarni RK, Brandes G, Nelson J, Cameron JT. Synthesis and degradation of poly(alkyl a-cyanoacrylates). *J Appl Polym Sci*, 10 (1966), 259–272.

33   Natsume T, Ike O, Okada T, Takimoto N, Shimizu Y, Ikada Y. Porous collagen sponge for esophageal replacement. *J Biomed Mater Res*, 27 (1993), 867–875.

34   Jenq CB, Coggeshall RE. Nerve regeneration through holey silicone tubes. *Brain Res*, 361 (1985), 233–241.

35   Yannas IV. Regeneration of skin and nerve by use of collagen templates. In Nimni ME (Ed.), *Collagen*, Vol. 3. Boca Raton, FL: CRC Press, 1988, 87–115.

36   Thomson RC, Yaszemski MJ, Mikos AG. Polymer scaffold processing. In Lanza RP, Langer R, Chick WL (Eds.), *Principles of Tissue Engineering*. Austin: R.G. Landes, 1997, 263–272.

37   Mikos AG, Thorsen AJ, Czerwonka LA, Bao Y, Langer R, Winslow DN, Vacanti JP. Preparation and characterization of poly (L-lactic acid) foams for cell transplantation. *Polymer*, 35 (1994), 1068–1077.

38   Lo H, Ponticello MS, Leong KW. Fabrication of controlled release biodegradable foams by phase separation. *Tissue Eng*, 1 (1995), 15–28.

39   Galletti PM, Aebischer P, Lysaght MJ. The dawn of biotechnology in artificial organs. *ASAIO J*, 41 (1995), 49–57.

40   Thomson RC, Yaszemski MJ, Powers JM, Mikos AG. Fabrication of biodegradable polymer scaffolds to engineer trabecular bone. *J Biomater Sci, Polym Ed*, 7 (1995), 23–38, 1995.

41   Mikos AG, Bao Y, Cima LG, Ingber DE, Vacanti JP, Langer R. Preparation of poly(glycolic acid) bonded fiber structures for cell attachment and transplantation. *J Biomed Mater Res*, 27 (1993), 183–189.

42   Mooney DJ, Mazzoni CL, Organ GM, Puelacher WC, Vacanti JP, Langer R. Stabilizing fiber-based cell delivery devices by physically bonding adjacent fibers. In Mikos AG, Murphy RM, Bernstein H, Peppas NA (Eds.), *Biomaterials for Drug and Cell Delivery, MRS Symposium Proceedings*, 331. Pittsburgh, PA: Materials Research Society, 1994, 47–52.

43   Mikos AG, Sarakinos G, Leite SM, Vacanti JP, Langer R. Laminated three-dimensional biodegradable foams for use in tissue engineering. *Biomaterials*, 14 (1993), 323–330.

44   Wald HL, Sarakinos G, Lyman MD, Mikos AG, Vacanti JP, Langer R. Cell seeding in porous transplantation devices. *Biomaterials*, 14 (1993), 270–278.

45   Wake MC, Gupta PK, Mikos AG. Fabrication of pliable biodegradable polymer foams to engineer soft tissues. *Cell Transplantation*, 5 (1996), 465–473.

46   Reddi AH. Symbiosis of biotechnology and biomaterials: Applications in tissue engineering of bone and cartilage. *J Cell Biochem*, 56 (1994), 192–195.

47   Adams JC, Watt FM. Regulation of development and differentiation by the extracellular matrix. *Development*, 117 (1993), 1183–1198.

48 Blaschke RJ, Howlett AR, Desprez PY, Petersen OW, Bissell MJ. Cell differentiation by *ECM* components. In Ruoslahti E, Engvall E (Eds.), *Methods in Enzymology: Extracellular Matrix Components*. New York: Academic Press, 1994, 535–556.

49 Watt FM. Cell culture models of differentiation. *FASEB J*, 5 (1991), 287–294.

50 Muramatsu H, Muramatsu T. Purification of recombinant midkine and examination of its biological activities: Functional comparison of new heparin binding factors. *Biochem Biophys Res Commun*, 177 (1991), 652–658.

51 Gutowska A, Bae YH, Feijen J, Kim SW. Heparin release from thermosensitive hydrogels. *J Controlled Release*, 22 (1992), 95–104.

52 Kuhl PR, Cima LG. Fabrication of a tethered growth factor surface. *Ann Biomed Eng*, 23 (1995), S-48.

53 Massia SP, Hubbell JA. An RGD spacing of 440nm is sufficient for integrin aVb3-mediated fibroblast spreading and 140 nm for focal contacts and stress fiber formation. *J Cell Biol*, 114 (1991), 1089–1100.

54 Massia SP, Rao SS, Hubbell JA. Covalently immobilized laminin peptide Tyr-Ile-Gly-Ser-Arg (YIGSR) supports cell spreading and co-localization of the 67-kilodalton laminin receptor with a-actinin and vinculin. *J Biol Chem*, 268 (1993), 8053–8059.

55 Hubbell JA, Massia SP, Drumheller PD. Surface-grafted cell-binding peptides in tissue engineering of the vascular graft. *Ann NY Acad Sci*, 665 (1992), 253–258.

56 Matsuda T, Sugawara T. Development of surface photochemical modification method for micropatterning of cultured cells. *J Biomed Mater Res*, 29 (1995), 749–756.

57 Green AM, Jansen JA, van der Waerden JP, von Recum, AF. Fibroblast response to microtextured silicone surfaces: Texture orientation into or out of the surface. *J Biomed Mater Res*, 28 (1994), 647–653.

58 von Recum AF, van Kooten T. The influence of microtopography on cellular response and the implications for silicone implants. *J Biomater Sci, Polymer Ed*, 7 (1995), 362–374.

59 Weinberg CB, Bell E. A blood vessel model constructed from collagen and vascular cells. *Science*, 231 (1986), 397–400.

60 Folkman J, Hochberg MM. Self-regulation of growth in three dimensions. *J Exp Med*, 138 (1973), 745–753.

61 Thomson RC, Wake MC, Yaszemski MJ, Mikos AG. Biodegradable polymer scaffolds to regenerate organs. *Adv Polym Sci*, 122 (1995), 245–274.

62 Freed LE, Marquis JC, Nohria A, Emmanual J, Mikos AG, Langer R. Neocartilage formation *in vitro* and *in vivo* using cells cultured on synthetic biodegradable polymers. *J Biomed Mater Res*, 27 (1993), 16–23.

63 Vacanti CA, Langer R, Schloo B, Vacanti JP. Synthetic polymers seeded with chondrocytes provide a template for new cartilage formation. *Plast Reconstr Surg*, 88 (1991), 753–759.

64 Amiel D, Coutts RD, Harwood FL, Ishizue KK, Kleiner JB. The chondrogenesis of rib perichondrial grafts for repair of full thickness articular cartilage defects in a rabbit model: A one-year postoperative assessment. *Connect Tissue Res*, 18 (1988), 27–39.

65 Bolano L, Kopta JA. The immunology of bone and cartilage transplantation. *Orthopedics*, 14 (1991), 987–996.

66 Crane GM, Ishaug SL, Mikos AG. Bone tissue engineering. *Nature Medicine*, 1 (1995), 1322–1324.

67 Yaszemski MJ, Payne RG, Hayes WC, Langer R, Mikos AG. The evolution of bone transplantation: Molecular, cellular, and tissue strategies to engineer human bone. *Biomaterials*, 17 (1996), 175–185.

68 Sartoris DJ, Holmes RE, Tencer AF, Mooney V, Resnick D. Coralline hydroxyapatite bone graft substitutes in a canine metaphyseal defect model: Radiographic-biomechanical correlation. *Skeletal Radiol*, 15 (1986), 635–641.

69 Shimazaki K, Mooney V. Comparative study of porous hydroxyapatite and tricalcium phosphate as bone substitute. *J Orthop Res*, 3 (1985), 301–310.

70 Yaszemski MJ, Payne RG, Hayes WC, Langer RS, Aufdemorte TB, Mikos AG. The ingrowth of new bone tissue and initial mechanical properties of a degrading polymeric composite scaffold. *Tissue Eng*, 1 (1995), 41–52.

71 Wong H, Chang TM. The viability and regeneration of artificial cell microencapsulated rat hepatocyte xenograft transplants in mice. *Biomater Artif Cells Artif Organs*, 16 (1988), 731–739.

72 Demetris AJ, Lasky S, Van Thiel, DH, Starzl TE, Dekker A. Pathology of hepatic transplantation: A review of 62 adult allograft recipients immunosuppressed with a cyclosporine/steroid regimen. *Am J Pathol*, 118, 151–161.

73 Moshage HJ, Rijntjes PJ, Hafkensheid JC, Roelofs HM, Yap SH. Primary culture of cryopreserved adult human hepatocytes on homologous extracellular matrix and the influence of monocytic products on albumin synthesis. *J Hepatol*, 7 (1988), 34–44.

74 Vacanti JP, Morse MA, Saltzman WM, Domb AJ, Perez-Atayde A, Langer R. Selective cell transplantation using bioabsorbable artificial polymers as matrices. *J Pediatr Surg*, 23 (1988), 3–9.

75 Mikos AG, Sarakinos G, Lyman MD, Ingber DE, Vacanti JP, Langer R. Prevascularization of porous biodegradable polymers. *Biotechnol Bioeng*, 42 (1993), 716–723.

76 Folkman J, Klagsbrun M. Angiogenic factors. *Science*, 235 (1987), 442–447.

77 Naughton BA, Sibanda B, Weintraub JP, San Roman J, Kamali V. A stereotypic, transplantable liver tissue culture system. *Appl Biochem Biotechnol*, 54 (1995), 65–91.

78 Monsour MJ, Mohammed R, Gorham SD, French DA, Scott R. An assessment of a collagen/Vicryl composite membrane to repair defects of the urinary bladder in rabbits. *Urol Res*, 15 (1987), 235–238.

79 Lebret T, Gobet F, Dallaserra M, Mitrofanoff P. Use of a digestive mucosal graft in urethroplasty. An experimental study—prospective utilization of the appendix mucosa. *Eur Urol*, 27 (1995), 58–61.

80 Atala A, Vacanti JP, Peters CA, Mandell J, Retik AB, Freeman MR. Formation of urothelial structures *in vivo* from dissociated cells attached to biodegradable polymer scaffolds *in vitro*. *J Urol*, 148 (1992), 658–662.

81 Gruenert DC, Finkbeiner WE, Widdicombe JH. Culture and transformation of human airway epithelial cells. *Am J Physiol*, 268 (1995), L347–L360.

82 Yamaya M, Finkbeiner WE, Chun SY, Widdicombe JH. Differentiated structure and function of cultures from human tracheal epithelium. *Am J Physiol*, 262 (1992), L713–L724.

83 Organ GM, Mooney DJ, Hansen LK, Schloo B, Vacanti JP. Transplantation of enterocytes utilizing polymer cell constructs to produce a neointestine. *Transplant Proc*, 24 (1992), 3009–3011.

84 Schmidt SP, Hunter TJ, Hirko M, Belden TA, Evancho MM, Sharp WV, Donovan DL. Small diameter vascular prostheses: Two designs of PTFE and endothelial cell seeded and non-seeded Dacron. *J Vasc Surg*, 2 (1985), 292–297.

85 Hussain S, Glover JL, Augelli N, Bendick PJ, Maupin D, McKain, M. Host response to autologous endothelial seeding. *J Vasc Surg*, 9 (1989), 656–663.

86 Ziegler T, Nerem RM. Tissue engineering a blood vessel: Regulation of vascular biology by mechanical stresses. *J Cell Biochem*, 56 (1994), 204–209.

87 Bhatt NS, Newsome DA, Fenech T, Hessburg TP, Diamond JG, Miceli MV, Kratz KE, Oliver PD. Experimental transplantation of human retinal pigment epithelial cells on collagen substrates. *Am J Ophthalmol*, 117 (1994), 214–221.

88 Thomson RC, Giordano GG, Collier JH, Ishaug SL, Mikos A, Lahiri-Munir D, Garcia CA. Manufacture and characterization of poly(α-hydroxy ester) thin films as temporary substrates for retinal pigment epithelium cells. *Biomaterials*, 17 (1996), 321–327.

89 von Recum HA, Kim SW, Kikuchi A, Okuhara M, Sakurai Y, Okano T. Novel thermally reversible hydrogel as detachable cell culture substrate. *J Biomed Mater Res*, 40 (1998), 631–639.

90 Regnier M, Darmon M. Human epidermis reconstructed *in vitro*: A model to study keratinocyte differentiation and its modulation by retinoic acid. *In Vitro Cell Dev Biol*, 25 (1989), 1000–1008.

91 Yannas IV, Lee E, Orgill DP, Skrabut EM, Murphy GF. Synthesis and characterization of a model extracellular matrix that induces partial regeneration of adult mammalian skin. *Proc Natl Acad Sci USA*, 5 (1989), 933–937.

92 Madison RD, Da Silva CF, Dikkes P. Entubation repair with protein additives increases the maximum nerve gap distance successfully bridged with tubular prosthesis. *Brain Res*, 447 (1988), 325–334.

93 Tountas CP, Bergman RA, Lewis TW, Stone HE, Pyrek JD, Mendenhall HV. A comparison of peripheral nerve repair using an absorbable tubulization device and conventional suture in primates. *J Appl Biomater*, 4 (1993), 261–268.

94 Guénard V, Kleitman N, Morrissey TK, Bunge RP, Aebischer P. Syngeneic Schwann cells derived from adult nerves seeded in semipermeable guidance channels enhance peripheral nerve regeneration. *J Neurosci*, 12 (1992), 3310–3320.

95 Grower MF, Russell EA, Jr., Cutright DE. Segmental neogenesis of the dog esophagus utilizing a biodegradable polymer framework. *Biomater Artif Cells Artif Organs*, 17 (1989), 291–314.

96 Natsume T, Ike O, Okada T, Shimizu Y, Ikada Y, Tamura K. Experimental studies of a hybrid artificial esophagus combined with autologous mucosal cells. *ASAIO Trans*, 36 (1990), M435–M437.

97 Chvapil M, Speer DP, Holubec H, Chvapil TA, King DH. Collagen fibers as a temporary scaffold for replacement of ACL in goats. *J Biomed Mater Res*, 27 (1993), 313–325.

98 Liem MD, Zegel HG, Balduini FC, Turner ML, Becker JM, Caballero-Saez A. Repair of Achilles tendon ruptures with a polylactic acid implant: Assessment with MR imaging. *Am J Roentgenol*, 156 (1991), 769–773.

99 Parsons JR, Weiss AB, Schenk RS, Alexander H, Pavlisko F. Long-term follow-up of Achilles tendon repair with and absorbable polymer carbon fiber composite. *Foot Ankle*, 9 (1989), 179–184.

100 Goldstein JD, Tria AJ, Zawadsky JP, Kato YP, Christiansen D, Silver FH. Development of a reconstituted collagen tendon prosthesis. A preliminary implantation study. *J Bone Joint Surg*, 71 (1989), 1183–1191.

101 Yaszemski MJ, Payne RG, Hayes WC, Langer R, Mikos AG. The *in vitro* degradation of a poly(propylene fumarate)-based composite material. *Biomaterials*, 17 (1996), 2127–2130.

102 Peter SJ, Miller MJ, Yaszemski MJ, Mikos AG. Poly(propylene fumarate). In Domb AJ, Kost J, Wiseman DM (Eds.), *Handbook of Biodegradable Polymers*. Amsterdam: Harwood Academic, 1997, 87–97.

103 Reddi AH, Cunningham NS. Initiation and promotion of bone differentiation by bone morphogenetic proteins. *J Bone Miner Res*, 8 (1993), S499–S502.

104 Elima K. Osteoinductive proteins. *Ann Med*, 25 (1993), 395–402.

105 Mohay J, Lange TM, Soltau JB, Wood TO, McLaughlin BJ. Transplantation of corneal endothelial cells using a cell carrier device. *Cornea*, 13 (1994), 173–182.

106 Lange TM, Wood TO, McLaughlin BJ. Corneal endothelial transplantation using Descemet's membrane as a carrier. *J Cataract Refract Surg*, 19 (1993), 232–235.

107 Karpati G, Pouliot Y, Zubrzycka-Gaarn E, Carpenter S, Ray PN, Worton RG, Holland P. Dystrophin is expressed in MDX skeletal muscle fibers after normal myoblast implementation. *Am J Pathol*, 135 (1989), 27–32.

108 Yoon PD, Kao RL, Magovern GJ. Myocardial regeneration. Transplanting satellite cells into damaged myocardium. *Tex Heart Inst J*, 22 (1995), 119–125.

109 Uludag H, Ip TK, Aebischer P. Transport function in a bioartificial kidney under uremic conditions. *Int J Artif Organ*, 13 (1990), 93–97.

110 Humes HD, Cieslinski DA. Interaction between growth factors and retinoic acid in the induction of kidney tubulogenesis in tissue culture. *Exp Cell Res*, 201 (1992), 8–15.

111 Freshney RI. *Culture of Animal Cells: A Manual of Basic Technique*, 2nd ed. New York: Alan R. Liss, 1987.

Chapter 26

Immunoisolation

Molly S. Shoichet
Michael V. Sefton

INTRODUCTION

Immunoisolation is a means of implementing cell transplantation using selectively permeable membranes to isolate the cells from the host's immune system. The encapsulated cells, from either the same species (allogeneic) or a different species (xenogeneic), produce the desired therapeutic product while the membrane prevents their rejection. Cells of primary (e.g., islets of Langerhans), immortalized (e.g., pheochromocytoma [PC12]) or engineered (e.g., baby hamster kidney [BHK] cells engineered to produce nerve growth factor [NGF]) origins can be used in immunoisolation devices because the membrane protects the cells against immune attack.

The membrane material must ensure diffusion of both nutrients (e.g., oxygen, glucose, etc.) to the encapsulated cells and the therapeutic product to the host system. The membrane may be of natural or synthetic origins; however, all must have the appropriate transport properties and geometry for optimal functioning and survival of cells. Biocompatibility and biostability of the membrane material affect its transport and immunoisolatory properties.

Encapsulated cells are often suspended or immobilized within a hydrogel matrix material within the membrane. The matrix material defines the environment within the membrane with nutrients and cell products that diffuse across it. The matrix material provides a distribution of cells within the membrane, thereby inhibiting the formation of large cell clusters and cell necrosis. The matrix may be tailored to provide the most suitable environment for continued cell viability and cell secretory function. For example, the matrix may provide an attachment site for anchorage-dependent cells.

Immunoisolation may be achieved by two methods. In macroencapsulation, a preformed membrane device such as a tube or hollow fiber is filled with cells and matrix (the macrocapsule); in microencapsulation, the membrane is formed around the cells from a polymer solution [1] or from the monomer [2] in the form of spheres (Figure 26-1). Additional biomaterials may be involved in immunoisolation, depending upon the method of encapsulation. For macroencapsulation, the devices must be sealed with a biocompatible glue to ensure device integrity; a tether can be attached to one end of the device, allowing for device retrievability.

Immunoislation involves the synergistic use of materials with cells and cell products for the treatment of diseases and disorders of the central nervous or endocrine systems. This novel mode of therapy is regulated by the Food and Drug Administration, through both the divisions of Drugs and Devices.

Need and Relevance

Immunoisolation is still in its infancy, despite the tremendous imbalance of organs required and organs available for transplantation. Only in the past decade have companies in

411

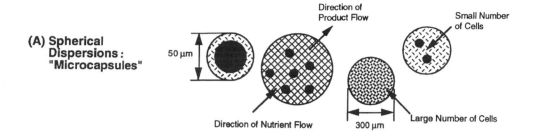

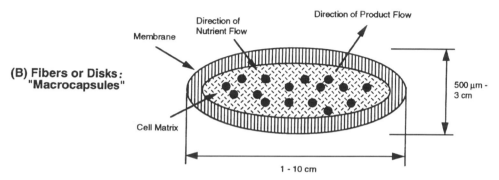

Figure 26-1 (A) Typical microencapsulated device and (B) typical macroencapsulated device. (Reprinted from *Trends in Polymer Science*, 3, M.S. Shoichet, F.T. Gentile, S.R. Winn, "The use of polymers in the treatment of neurological disorders," 374–380, © 1995, with permission from Elsevier Science.)

the United States become involved in immunoisolation for cell transplantation. Given the complexity of cells and the need to control their behavior in an unusual geometry in vivo, novel techniques are needed to understand the behavior of prototype devices, redesign and optimize improvements and provide the necessary data for regulatory authorities.

Factors Affecting Tests and Evaluation Methods

Device evaluation depends critically upon the source and purity of the starting cells and materials. The raw material properties—the method of manufacturing, the amount and type of additives, and material storage—will impact the ultimate functioning and reproducibility of devices prepared. The source and handling of the cells will affect the final device performance. Cells are not static components; features as simple as passage number can dramatically affect device performance. The storage and handling of devices post-fabrication will also affect ultimate functioning. Sterility cannot be over-emphasized. Additionally, the surgeon's handling of the device and the method and site of implantation will have an important impact on device functioning. For example, a device that is deformed or scratched upon implantation will likely evoke a greater host immune response than a pristine one.

Tests and Evaluation Methodologies

The authors have found the following tests and evaluation methodologies of practical value but they do not comprise standard methods due to the infancy of the immunoisolation field. Methods are described for assessing both transport properties and encapsulated cell behavior. In addition, aspects of stability and mechanical strength peculiar to these devices are outlined.

Like other studies in biomaterials, in vitro studies can give some insight to ultimate in vivo functioning, but the in vitro studies cannot substitute for those in vivo. In vivo generated cytokines or the tissue reaction can dramatically alter encapsulated cell behavior, making the in vitro studies useful only as a first step. Even when studies are done in vivo, the implantation site may be dictated by size considerations. In one study [3], poly(acrylonitrile-co-vinyl chloride [P{AN/VC}]) devices were implanted in the rat peritoneal cavity because devices of the appropriate dimensions for material stability analysis were too big to be implanted in the brain (the clinical target site) of the rat. In some cases, such as material stability or permeability, the analytical techniques preclude the presence of cells under the assumption that the cells would not affect the conclusions; this assumption has yet to be proven.

Transport Properties

The transport properties of the device are largely defined by those of the membrane, although the matrix may impart additional barriers to transport. The polymer membrane used for cell encapsulation serves as a selectively permeable (permselective) barrier, providing the appropriate nutrients for cell viability while inhibiting the transport of host immunologic species such as immunoglobulin G (IgG, Mw $\sim$ 150 k), immunoglobulin M (IgM Mw $\sim$ 900 k) and various complement fractions (Mw $\sim$ 150–500 k). The molecular weight cut-off, more loosely described as the "pore size" needed for immunoisolation, is in the process of being redefined [4] as we learn more of the immunology of such devices; the classic attempt to exclude immunoglobulin has focused many individuals on the search for membranes with a 50–100 kD cut-off. Determining the appropriate balance of transport properties required for cell viability (i.e., sufficient nutrient but no immunoglobulin transport) is the key to fabricating the optimal membrane for encapsulation. In addition to being an essential component for successful encapsulation and immunoisolation, the membrane transport properties can be used as a measure of consistency in membrane fabrication.

Convective Transport   The convective resistance of the membrane to water or solutes (i.e., polydisperse proteins or dextrans) is described by hydraulic permeability (HP) and the solute rejection profile (or nominal molecular weight cut-off, MWCO), respectively. For macrocapsules, both measurements can be obtained from the same representative group of hollow fiber membranes. Approximately ten hollow fiber membranes (HFMs) are inserted into an open-ended cartridge and fixed in place with 5-minute epoxy glue. The cartridge is connected to tubing through which water or solute solution flows and thus through the lumens of the HFMs. The water/solute that flows across the membrane is used to measure hydraulic permeability/MWCO, respectively. Careful attention must be paid to the lumenal flow rate used to minimize the concentration polarization caused by boundary layer formation during rejection measurements. For microcapsules MWCO is determined from diffusive transport measurements (see below).

Hydraulic permeability is calculated from the convective water flow at a specific transmembrane pressure and over a given exposed membrane area, resulting in units of flow/area/pressure (e.g., ml/min/m2/mmHg). Molecular weight cut-off is determined from the ratio of filtrate and retentate solute concentrations as a function of solute molecular weight. The membrane rejection coefficient (R) can be described as $R = 1 - C_f/C_r$ where C_f and C_r are the concentrations in the filtrate and retentate, respectively. A membrane with a rejection coefficient of 1 indicates that the species (i.e., protein or dextran) does not pass through the membrane. Proteins used to determine MWCO are detected by UV spectrophotometry or by fluorescence labeling for increased sensitivity. Alternatively, poly-disperse dextran solutions can be used to generate membrane rejection curves. Size exclusion chromatography with refractive index detection is used to analyze reservoir and filtrate concentrations as a function of molecular weight. Fluorescein-tagged dextrans with fluorescence detection enhances this sensitivity. Membrane fouling issues inherent in protein rejection curves are minimized using dextran solutions due to their low binding capacity to many polymeric membranes [10].

Diffusive Transport   While convective characterization is a pressure-driven process that provides information on the hollow fiber's sieving properties, diffusive transport is a concentration-gradient-driven process that governs transport in most immunoisolation devices. Diffusion through hollow fiber membranes can be measured by either filling the lumen of the membrane with a concentrated protein (or dextran) solution and measuring the amount of solute detected in the surrounding bath over time, or immersing the membrane in a concentrated solution and measuring the concentration of solute in the hollow fiber membrane lumen over time. Only the first method is practical with microcapsules which are loaded with solute by immersing them in a concentrated solution, rinsed and then placed in a solute-free "release" medium. The nature of the solute dictates the mode of analysis: radiolabelled solutes [5], UV absorbance [5], enzyme activity [6], and fluorescence have all been used.

For low molecular weight species (Mw $<$ 20,000 g/mole) in hollow fibers, a tracer solution flows around the outside of the fiber, while the sampling solution flows down the fiber lumen. The flow rates are adjusted to minimize boundary layer formation on both the inside and outside of the fiber. Diffusion coefficients are calculated from the concentration difference between lumen and bath at a set lumen flow rate over time. For larger molecular weight species (Mw: 50,000–300,000 g/mole), membrane resistances are far greater than the boundary layer resistances, and thus the experimental design does not involve flow. The measurement can be made by sampling either the bath or the membrane lumen. To enhance the sensitivity of the measurement, fluorescently tagged species such as fluorescein-labeled dextran can be used with fluorescence detection.

Figure 26-2 shows the convective and diffusive transport properties of a poly(acrylonitrile-co-vinyl chloride) hollow fiber membrane that has been used to immunoisolate xenograft tissue. Bovine adrenal chromaffin cells were encapsulated in this membrane and transplanted for several months in human patients suffering from chronic pain. Shown in Figure 26-2 are the rejection coefficient (R), mass transfer coefficient (k_m), and the ratio of diffusion coefficients of a marker in the membrane to that in water ($D_{membrane}/D_{water}$).

Horseradish peroxidase (HRP) was found to be a particularly useful test solute for HEMA-MMA microcapsules, because its enzyme activity (substrate: tetramethyl benzidine) enabled such low concentrations to be detected that the permeability of individual capsules could be measured [6]. HRP (40 kDa) was loaded into the capsules by immersing the capsules in a 5 mg/mL solution for three days to saturate the capsules. Fractional release was then measured by placing capsules, one per well of a 96-well plate, in 60 μL of solute-free PBS. The concentration of HRP was determined as a function of release time (0–24 hours) by taking aliquots and inferring the concentration from its enzyme activity. Calibration curves were linear in the 1 to 100 ng/mL concentration range. This method enabled the capsule-to-capsule distribution in permeability to be measured and controlled through changes in capsule precipitation conditions [7] (Figure 26-3). This method is now

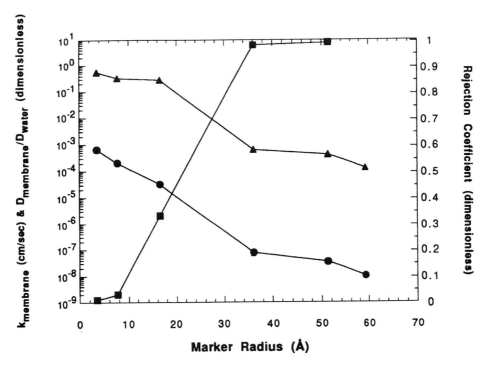

Figure 26-2   Convective rejection coefficient (■), membrane mass transfer coefficient ($K_{membrane}$) (●) and relative membrane diffusivity ($D_{membrane}/D_{water}$) (▲) vs. protein molecular size at 37°C for a poly(acrylonitrile-co-vinyl chloride) membrane [7]. (Reprinted from *Trends in Polymer Science*, 3, M.S. Shoichet, F.T. Gentile, S.R. Winn, "The use of polymers in the treatment of neurological disorders," 374–380, © 1995, with permission from Elsevier Science.)

being adapted to larger molecules using biotin-conjugated test solutes and strepavidin-HRP conjugates.

Mechanical Strength

Tensile strength is important in the event of macrocapsule retrieval, while compressive strength may be important during device implantation. The mechanical fragility of both microcapsules and macrocapsules is a technical limitation of current devices. The limited resilience of the immunoisolatory device in vivo may ultimately limit its success; thus methods to strengthen the device may be necessary after finding a suitable immunoisolatory material that will support cell viability and function.

The hollow fiber membrane provides most of the mechanical strength but the matrix material may impart additional strength to the device. Alternatively, another device component may be used to provide additional strength, as in the case of composite membranes [9]. While membrane strength may be enhanced by manipulating its dimensions and morphology, it should be noted that enhancing membrane strength frequently leads to a reduction in diffusive transport properties [10]. The membrane can be fabricated to have a small ratio of outer to inner diameters and a large wall thickness; however, the diffusion distance of oxygen and glucose (essential to cell viability) is limited and substantially reduced at 500 Å. The membrane morphology within the wall can be one of macrovoids or microvoids ("open-cell foam"). Increasing the isoreticulated structure within the membrane increases

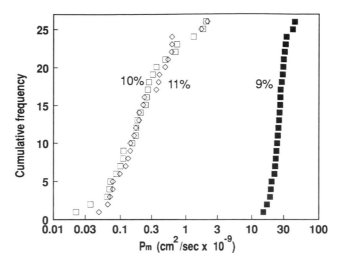

Figure 26-3 Distribution in the permeability coefficient of capsule membranes prepared with different HEMA-MMA concentrations 9% (■), 10% (□), and 11% (◇) polymer in triethylene glycol [8]. (Reprinted from *Journal of Membrane Science*, 108, J.R. Hwang, M.V. Sefton, "Effect of polymer concentration and a pore forming agent (PVP) on HEMA-MMA microcapsule structure and permeability," 257–268, © 1995, with permission from Elsevier Science.)

its tensile strength. Scanning electron microscopy provides both dimensional analysis (i.e., wall thickness, outer and inner diameters) and indicates the nature of the morphology within the membrane walls.

Mechanical strength of the membrane (or device) can be determined in both tensile and compressive modes. A single hollow fiber membrane is tested for tensile strength using an instrument (such as the Vitrodyne) that can measure elongation, yield strength and the force required to break it. Defects in the membrane wall will lead to premature device failure. Compressive hollow fiber membrane strength is determined by a three-point bend method, where the force required to crush the membrane is recorded. For microcapsules, compression methods [11] can be used to compare mechanical properties of similarly sized capsules, but quantitative determination of size-independent mechanical properties is not yet feasible.

Biostability

As for many other biomaterials, the long-term chemical and mechanical stability of an implanted immunoisolation device is essential for its continued functioning *in vivo*. For example, in the event of degradation, the membrane may not continue to isolate the encapsulated cells and thus exposes them to the host's immune system, resulting in device malfunction.

Membrane Biostability   As for other materials [12], the major mechanisms of degradation are typically auto-oxidation, hydrolysis, mechanical loading, and mineralization, all of which can be catalyzed by metal ions or enzymes. All, except possibly oxidation, are unlikely mechanisms of degradation for a poly(acrylonitrile-co-vinyl chloride) membrane implanted in the brain.

Membrane stability should be assessed of a membrane material that shows promise of continued cell viability and functioning in immunoisolation device configurations (micro- or macro-encapsulation devices). The in vivo membrane stability study should be performed on membranes that closely resemble those used for immunoisolation; for example, the membrane configuration, handling, implant location and time of implant should, if possible, be the same as those used for the immunoisolatory devices.

A stability study [13] was performed on poly(acrylonitrile-co-vinyl chloride) [P(AN/VC)] hollow fiber membranes (HFMs). The devices were implanted in the peritoneal cavity instead of the intended central nervous system site because the rat brain could not accommodate an adequate-sized device for material analysis. Cells were not encapsulated in these devices and were not expected to contribute to membrane stability issues except as noted earlier.

Devices were prepared with membranes that had been stored, sterilized and handled like those used in immunoisolation devices. To the hollow fiber membranes was added a hydrogel matrix, sodium alginate, which was crosslinked with calcium chloride. The devices were sealed in a standard fashion and stored for the appropriate time in vitro prior to in vivo implantation. This study assessed membrane stability in rats over a 12-month period. Mechanical and chemical stabilities were assessed by measuring pre-implantation tensile strength and post-explantation molecular weight (by gel permeation chromatography). The stability of the transport properties of the membranes was determined by molecular weight cut-off (MWCO) and hydraulic permeability (HP). In order to measure membrane stability, adsorbed proteins were first removed using a concentrated solution of sodium hydroxide without affecting membrane structure or functioning; adsorbed proteins would have interfered with the analytical tools chosen to monitor membrane stability.

Matrix Biostability   The primary function of the matrix is to provide an optimal environment for continued cell viability and functioning within the membrane. In vivo matrix stability studies are difficult to accomplish due to the minimal volume of matrix material used in cell encapsulation. In vitro studies provide some insight into degradation mechanisms and provide reassurance regarding its safe use in vivo.

A stability study [14] was performed on alginate and agarose hydrogels in vitro; gel strength [15] and protein diffusion [16] were monitored over time and shown to correlate with gel stability. It is most desirable for the materials used in a gel stability study to replicate the configuration and dimensions of gels used in immunoisolation. While the configuration and dimensions used in the in vitro stability study differed from those used in immunoisolation, the matrix concentration and sterilization method were the same. In addition, the effect of cells on stability was assessed.

Gel (compressive) strength was measured over a 90-day period for both agarose and alginate discs in the absence (controls) and presence (samples) of cells. Hydrogel stability was also assessed by following the diffusion of proteins with a range of molecular weights over a 60-day period to track changes in pore size and distribution over time.

The compression test used to monitor gel strength was easy to use and conducive to following the effect of living cells on matrix stability; however, the configuration of the matrix was limited to that of a disc. The geometry and crosslinking conditions encountered in immunoisolation (e.g., the cylindrical geometry) were more easily mimicked by the protein diffusion assay; however, the protein diffusion assay is limited by the exclusion of cells. Both gel stability assays can be used in parallel to better elucidate the mechanism of degradation or de-crosslinking. It is important to correlate indirect measurements of stability with stability using known methods of degradation or de-crosslinking. A correlation between gel strength and gel stability was found for agarose using the degradative enzyme, β-agarase, and for calcium-crosslinked alginate using the calcium chelator, sodium citrate.

The gel strengths of agarose and alginate decreased in the presence of β-agarase and sodium citrate, respectively.

Surface Characterization

Although the cells and matrix likely have a larger influence on the in vivo performance of the capsules, the interface between the capsule and the host tissue is worthy of characterization. X-ray photoelectron spectroscopy (XPS) [17], scanning electron microscopy (SEM), and protein adsorption studies have been used to define immunoisolation device surface properties. Protein adsorption is of interest because of the practice of incubating capsules in serum-supplemented media prior to implantation. The qualitative nature of the protein adsorbate on HEMA-MMA capsules was assessed by eluting the proteins in SDS and using Western blotting to identify which proteins were present [18]. Surface modification post-membrane fabrication with poly(ethylene oxide) was shown to decrease protein adsorption to HFMs and enhance biocompatibility [19].

Cell Number and Viability

The functional effect of immunoisolated cells is directly related to the number and viability of the encapsulated cells. Histological techniques after sectioning (or confocal microscopy) provide qualitative estimates of these parameters; other methods are preferred for quantitative comparisons. In conventional cell cultures, cell number is inferred from DNA or protein content, while viability is assessed either by DNA incorporation rate (using ^{3}H-thymidine) or protein synthesis rate (using ^{35}S-methionine). (See also Chapters 21 and 25.) Unfortunately these methods generally require large cell numbers (more than the few thousand that would be in a single microcapsule), and the capsule membrane can absorb, or interfere with, the reagents in the assays. Regardless of which viability assay is used, some care is needed to interpret the results since each assay measures a particular function of the cells which may or may not correlate with the key function (e.g., protein synthesis) that is being sought. Relating behavior inside the capsule to conventional cell culture can fail to take into account the difference in three-dimensional geometry between the two.

One standard method for cell viability is the MTT assay [20] or more generally any of the formazan product assays (XTT, Alamar Blue). The latter may be preferred since they are non-destructive techniques; however, there are fewer details in the encapsulation literature about these. The MTT assay is based on the ability of metabolically active cells to transform a water-soluble dye (3-(4,5-dimethyl-thiazol-2-yl)-2,5-diphenyl-tetrazolium bromide) into an insoluble formazan. Quantitative determination of the amount of formazan gives an estimate of cell number in capsules. The simplicity and low cost of the assay makes it a valuable tool to screen a large number of encapsulation parameters in a short time. It can be sensitive at a single capsule level, enabling one to look at capsule-to-capsule variations. Care should be taken in using formazan absorbance as a strict measure of cell number in capsules since changes in the metabolic state of the cells (i.e., metabolic deactivation or activation) will affect the results.

MTT solution and fresh medium are added to capsules in a 96-well plate and incubated at 37°C for 5 hours. The supernatant is then removed by aspiration and the capsules dissolved in DMSO; the absorbance in each well is then read on a microplate reader. Blanks consist of microcapsules with only culture medium as the core material. The same general procedure can be followed for macrocapsules where one macrocapsule is assayed per well. However, instead of the membrane being dissolved in DMSO, the capsule is simply cut open and its contents analyzed.

Light and electron microscopy are also used to assess viability [21]. For light microscopy, aqueous toluidine blue staining of nucleic acids and some proteins provides a rapid and easy method to localize cells and generally assess their morphology. HEMA-MMA capsules were fixed, cryoprotected (aqueous glycerol), embedded in OCT compound, frozen and stored on dry ice. Sections were cut using a cryostat. This technique (and that used for SEM [21]) avoided the use of conventional organic solvents such as ethanol or xylene which would dissolve the capsule wall; here the capsule wall remained intact and the cells were well preserved. Similar methods are used for macrocapsules; however, standard histological dehydration steps in ethanol can be followed because the hollow fiber membrane is insoluble in ethanol. Hematoxylin and eosin is a preferred stain in this case since the viable cells are more readily identified.

Confocal microscopy has also been used to examine the three-dimensional arrangement of cells in the capsule without the need for laborious histological sectioning [22]. Intact, unfixed HEMA-MMA microcapsules were washed and stained simultaneously with calcein-AM and ethidium homodimer (Molecular Probes, Live/Dead Viability/Cytotoxicity Kit) at optimal concentrations of 10 g/ml and 50 g/ml, respectively, for 30 minutes, and washed with PBS. Since it was not possible to detect fluorescently stained cells within intact microcapsules (presumably due to light scattering by the capsule), capsules were cut open before examination with a confocal laser scanning microscope at excitation wavelengths of 488 nm and 568 nm, thus exciting calcein and ethidium homodimer, respectively. FITC and Texas red filters for dual-labeled samples were used.

Product Release

Ultimately, product release defines the suitability of the immunoisolated device. The therapeutic products of the encapsulated cells are assayed for constitutive and evoked release by simply incubating capsules in the appropriate release medium in vitro. The number of capsules per mL of medium and the incubation time are determined by the nature of the cell type and the number of cells per capsule. Capsules are typically washed free of the regular culture medium and then placed in fresh medium to mark the beginning of the assay period. Capsules can be assessed at various times after preparation (duration of in vitro or in vivo incubation) or as a function of encapsulated cell number or release medium composition (e.g., presence or absence of cytokines or inhibitors that influence cell behavior). For example, microcapsules containing PC12 cells were incubated in a depolarization K^+/Ca^{2+} release medium to assay dopamine release [23] while encapsulated HepG2 cells [24] (Figure 26-4) were incubated in a well-defined cell culture medium to assay protein production. Dopamine was measured by HPLC while the proteins were assayed by ELISA. When one microcapsule per well is studied it is possible (if the ELISA is sufficiently sensitive and a pre-set dilution is used) to assess the variability in protein release and to identify a sub-group of capsules which had pinholes or defects that were not visible microscopically [6]. The methodology for macrocapsules is similar. Usually only one macrocapsule per well is assayed in a defined medium for a defined time period. Either ELISA (e.g., for baby hamster kidney cells engineered to produce nerve growth factor) or HPLC techniques (e.g., for adrenal chromaffin cells that produce noradrenalins) can be used to quantify the proteins secreted by encapsulated cells.

In Vivo Assessment

In vivo studies are clearly essential to demonstrate the efficacy of the encapsulation device. In addition to functional efficacy data such as dose-response "curves," biochemical (target

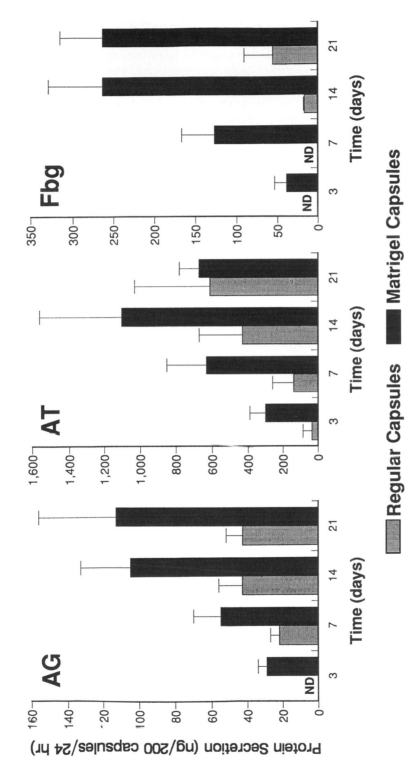

Figure 26-4 Mean +/- SD secretion rate of a1-acid glycoprotein (AG), α1-antitrypsin (AT) and fibrinogen (Fbg) by encapsulated HepG2 cells in regular (□) and Matrigel® capsule (■). ND: not detected. Note the gradual increase in average protein secretion rates with time. On day 21, AG and Fbg secretion rate was higher for Matrigel® capsules, although no difference was observed for AT secretion rate [24]. Used with permission.

molecule levels), biocompatibility, or biostability information can be derived depending on the nature of the study. If the studies are pre-clinical, then the devices are prepared like those which are to be implanted clinically; if the in vivo studies are in an earlier development phase, then the constraints on the device configuration may be deliberately lessened. The biostability study referred to above is a good example of this. In this section, only those features of in vivo studies unique to encapsulation are highlighted; all of the considerations regarding in vivo studies of biomaterials detailed in other chapters are relevant here.

Sterility   An important consequence of cell-containing implants is that they cannot be sterilized before implantation. Thus considerable effort is made to prepare and handle capsules under sterile conditions. All liquids are steam- or filter-sterilized, hollow fiber membranes of macrocapsules are sterilized by exposure to ethylene oxide, and cells are handled without antibiotics under sterile conditions. Because of the viscosity of HEMA-MMA solutions, the polymer is prepared in ethanol as a final step prior to freeze-drying and storage; the polymer is endotoxin-free and bacterial infection has not occurred in animal experiments conducted in the authors' laboratory to date. Standard culture media that are supplemented with serum are usually avoided since the bovine serum is a source of xenoantigens that exacerbate the tissue reaction; a variety of well-defined media are preferred even though the use of human proteins can complicate animal studies.

Implantation Site and Method   Capsules are implanted in the central nervous system, peritoneal cavity (IP) or other locations (e.g., omental pouch [25]) as dictated by the purpose of the study (local or systemic delivery) and the size and number of capsules. The number of capsules needed is often determined by the number of cells per capsule, the extent of secretion per cell or per capsule that is expected in vivo, the secreted molecule bioavailability, and the level needed at the target site for a functional effect. The site dictates the mode of implantation with, for example, stereotactic needles used for intrastriatal implants and surgical incision and direct placement used for some IP sites.

For example [22], the omental pouch in Ethrane-anaesthetized Wistar rats (175–200 g) was prepared by folding the omentum up towards the stomach and suturing (7 "o" silk sutures) along the left and right edges of the omentum and along the top of the pouch but leaving an opening for the placement of 14–17 capsules. After capsule implantation, the opening was sutured closed to completely enclose the implanted capsules within omental tissue.

For intraperitoneal implantation of HEMA-MMA capsules, a small abdominal incision is made and a known number of capsules are placed in defined sites, including the fold of mesenteric membranes, using a micropipette, under direct visual control. Several thousand small capsules can be implanted in this way to achieve the desired therapeutic levels of product.

For intrastriatal implants of macrocapsules [26], animals are anaesthetised with a 1 mL/kg i.m. injection of ketamine, xylazine, and acepromazine mixture (85/5/10 mg/mL, respectively), and positioned in a Kopf stereotaxic apparatus. A sagittal incision is made in the scalp, and two holes drilled from the placement of the polymer capsules into the striatum. Animals received bilateral striatal implants of polymer-encapsulated PC12 cells by placing the capsule in an 18-gauge Teflon® catheter mounted to the stereotaxic frame. A stainless steel obdurator was placed within the cannula, the device lowered into the brain, and the obdurator held in place while the outer cannula was raised to passively place the capsule within the host striatum.

Explantation and Microscopy At the end of the implantation period, rats with HEMA-MMA microcapsules are anaesthetized with an injection of Atravet acepromazine and Rogarsetic ketamine hydrochloride. The ventral area is shaved and wiped with isopropanol solution and, in a sterile laminar flow hood, the peritoneal cavity is exposed. Except for IP implants, the capsules are recovered within the tissue into which they had been placed. Capsules implanted IP are recovered by gently examining the entire peritoneal cavity for free-floating and attached capsules and by removing adhering capsules along with any associated tissue. HEMA-MMA capsules and associated tissue are washed with PBS and then fixed with 3.5% (v/v) glutaraldehyde containing 2% (w/v) tannic acid in 0.1 M Sorenson's phosphate buffer (P-buffer).

The surrounding tissue is fixed, sectioned (5 mm thick) and stained in hematoxylin/eosin or Mason's trichrome for good visualization of the cells in the tissue reaction. Computer-assisted quantification is done using a Zeiss Axiovert microscope and Metamorph software. Fibrous capsule thickness, total cell, neutrophil, macrophage, giant cell, polymorphonuclear cell, mast cell, lymphocyte, plasma cell counts and vascular density (number of vascular structures as a function of distance) are the primary parameters measured, although additional features may be useful as quantitative characteristics of the tissue response. Care is taken to select sections that are free from cutting artifacts and are from the middle of the capsule to minimize the error associated with the sphericity of the capsule. Sections from ~20 capsules per implant per location (1 section quantified/capsule, 5 separate optical fields of the fibrous capsule) provide reasonable statistics.

Device Performance During the implantation period, capsule performance can be monitored by functional or biochemical studies. The extent and duration of normoglycemia with islet capsules in NOD mice or BB rats and the amelioration of amphetamine-induced rotation behavior in hemi-Parkinsonian rats (caused by 6-OHDA) are examples of functional studies. These demonstrate not only that the encapsulated cells are viable but also that the dose is sufficient for the desired therapeutic effect in specific animal model conditions. In the neurologic area, animal behavioral studies are sometimes the best indication of therapeutic performance if the appropriate animal model exists. In cases of sub-therapeutic delivery, evidence of cell viability is obtained by biochemical studies: for example, systemic insulin levels or dopamine concentrations by microdialysis can show that the implant is functioning. Delivering human proteins in animal models can be problematic because neutralizing antibodies may be produced [27] or because some therapeutic molecules (e.g., growth hormone) are species-specific. In both cases, suitable biochemical studies are the only option. Unfortunately, antibody levels are only suggestive of protein delivery since quantitation is difficult; immunocompromised SCID mice are an alternative animal host, provided biocompatibility questions are not being addressed. Alternatively, cell function in vivo can be assessed indirectly by comparing cell function pre- and post-implantation.

Biocompatibility Capsules are implanted for periods ranging from days to weeks or months and explanted along with the surrounding tissue for examination of encapsulated cell viability and host tissue reaction. Histological assessments are carried out with the same techniques as described above, particularly if the presence of the capsule wall is a necessary part of the analysis (see also Section VII). Immunohistological techniques are useful for extracapsular cell identification or for assessment of in vivo-associated changes in encapsulated cell phenotype, such as tyrosine hydroxylase up-regulation. Electron microscopy is also useful here. Otherwise, the standard hematoxylin-eosin or Masson trichrome staining is sufficient. For brain tissue, glial fibrillary acidic protein (GFAP) is a good stain for astrocytes. From a biocompatibility point of view, defining the granulomatous or fibrous character of the tissue reaction (if present) is the typical purpose of examining the tissue surrounding the capsules, although the functional point of view focuses considerable attention on its vascularization [28]. In addition, since the inflammatory response to the capsules may also have a significant immune component, more emphasis is placed on the lymphocyte population (and sub-populations) than for conventional biomaterials (see Chapter 18).

REFERENCES

1   Sefton MV, Broughton RL. Microencapsulation of erythrocytes. *BBA*, 717 (1983), 473–477.
2   Dupuy B, Gin H, Baquey C, Ducassou D. In situ polymerization of a microencapsulating medium around living cells. *J Biomed Mater Res*, 22 (1988), 1061–1070.
3   Shoichet MS, Rein DH. In vivo biostability of a polymeric hollow fibre membrane for cell encapsulation. *Biomaterials*, 17 (1996), 285–290.
4   Colton CK. Implantable biohybrid artificial organs. *Cell Transpl*, 4 (1995), 415–436.
5   Crooks CA, Douglas JA, Broughton RL, Sefton MV. Microencapsulation of mammalian cells in a HEMA-MMA copolymer: Effects on capsule morphology and permeability. *J Biomed Mater Res*, 24 (1990), 1241–1262.
6   Uludag H, Hwang JR, Sefton MV. Microencapsulated human hepatoma (HepG2) cells: Capsule-to-capsule variations in protein secretion and permeability. *J Contrl Rel*, 33 (1995), 273–283.
7   Shoichet MS, Gentile FT, Winn SR. The use of polymers in the treatment of neurological disorders: A discussion emphasizing encapsulated cell therapy. *Trends in Polymer Sci*, 3 (1995), 374–380.
8   Hwang JR, Sefton MV. Effect of polymer concentration and a pore forming agent (PVP) on HEMA-MMA microcapsule permeability. *J Memb Sci*, 108, (1995), 257–268.
9   Brauker J. Polymer science: Engineered biomaterials for the 21st century. *Proc Am Chem Soc*. Palm Springs, CA, 1992.
10 Gentile FT, Doherty EJ, Rein DH, Shoichet MS, Winn SR. Polymer science for macroencapsulation of cells for central nervous system transplantation. *Reactive Polymers*, 25 (1995), 207–227.
11 Klein J, Washausen P. Immobilized whole cells: Pressure stability. In Buchholz K (Ed.), *Characterization of Immobilized Biocatalysts*, DECHEMA Monograph Series No. 1724–1731, Vol. 84. Weinheim, Germany: Verlag-Chemie, 1979, 277–284.
12 Stokes K. Biodegradation. *Cardiovasc Pathol*, 2 (1993), 111S–119S.
13 Shoichet MS. Rein DH. In vivo biostability of a polymeric hollow fibre membrane for cell encapsulation. *Biomaterials*, 17 (1996), 285–290.
14 Shoichet MS, Li RH, White ML, Winn SR. Stability of hydrogels used in cell encapsulation: An in vitro comparison of alginate and agarose. *Biotechnol and Bioeng*, 50 (1996), 374–380.
15 Kirkpatrick FH. Overviews of ararose gel properties. In *Electrophoresis of Large DNA Molecules:* Theory and Applications. Cold Spring Harbor Laboratory Press, 1990.
16 Li RH, Altreuter DH, Gentile FT. Transport characterization of hydrogel matrices for cell encapsulation. *Biotechnol and Bioeng*, 50 (1996), 365–373.
17 Babensee JE, Sodhi RNS, DeBoni U, Sefton MV. XPS surface analysis and in vivo tissue response to HEMA-MMA microcapsules. *Polym Prepr*, 34 (1993), 68–69.
18 Babensee JE, Cornelius RM, Brash JL, Sefton MV. Immunoblot analysis of proteins associated with HEMA-MMA microcapsules: Human serum proteins in vitro and rat proteins following implantation. In preparation.
19 Shoichet MS, Winn SR, Athavale S, Harris JM, Gentile FT. Poly(ethylene oxide)-grafted thermoplastic membranes for use as cellular hybrid bio-artificial organs in the central nervous system. *Biotechnol and Bioeng*, 43 (1994), 563–572.
20 Uludag H, Sefton MV. A colorimetric assay for cellular activity in microcapsules. *Biomaterials*, 11 (1990), 708–712.
21 Babensee JE, DeBoni U, Sefton MV. Morphological assessment of hepatoma cells (HepG2) microencapsulated in a HEMA-MMA copolymer with and without matrigel. *J Biomed Mater Res*, 26 (1992), 1401–1408.
22 Babensee JE. *Morphological Assessment of HEMA-MMA Microcapsules for Liver Cell Transplantation.* Doctoral thesis, University of Toronto, Toronto, Ontario, Canada, 1996.
23 Roberts T, DeBoni U, Sefton MV. Dopamine secretion by PC12 cells microencapsulated in a hydroxyethyl methacrylate-methyl methacrylate copolymer. *Biomaterials*, 17 (1996), 267–275.

24 Uludag H, Horvath V, Black JP, Sefton MV. Viability and protein secretion from human hepatoma (HepG2) cells encapsulated in 400-μm polyacrylate microcapsules by submerged nozzle-liquid jet extrusion. *Biotechnol Bioeng*, 44 (1994), 1199–1206.

25 Ao Z, Matayoski K, Lakey JRT, Rajotte RV, Warnock GL. Survival and function of purified islets in the omental pouch site of outbred dogs. *Transplantation*, 56 (1993), 524–529.

26 Emerich DF, Frydel BR, Flanagan TR, Palmatier M, Winn SR, Christenson L. *Cell Transplantation*, 2 (1993), 241–249.

27 Chang PL, Shen N, Westcott AJ. Delivery of recombinant gene products with microencapsulated cells in vivo. *Human Gene Ther*, 4 (1993), 433–440.

28 Brauker JH, Carr-Brendel VE, Martinson LA, Crudele J, Johnston WD, Johnson RC. Neovascularization of synthetic membranes directed by membrane architecture. *J Biomed Mater Res*, 29 (1995), 1517–1524.

ADDITIONAL READING

1 Christenson L, Dionne KE, Lysaght MJ. Biomedical applications of immobilized cells. In Goosen MFA (Ed.), *Fundamentals of Animal Cell Encapsulation and Immobilization*, Boca Raton, FL: CRC Press, 1993, 7–41.

2 Hubbell JA, Langer R. Tissue engineering. *C&E News*, March 1995, 13.

3 Babensee JE, Sefton MV. Protein delivery by microencapsulated cells. In Park K (Ed.), *Protein Delivery: The Next Generation*. Washington, DC: American Chemical Society (in press).

Chapter 27

Drug Delivery Systems

Surya K. Mallapragada
Balaji Narasimhan

INTRODUCTION

Controlled-release systems are comprised of a bioactive agent incorporated in a carrier which is usually a polymer or a bioceramic. The main objective of a controlled-release device is to maintain the concentration of the drug within therapeutic limits over the required duration. Compared to conventional drug formulations, such systems typically require smaller and less frequent drug dosages and minimize side effects. The release rate is a strong function of the physicochemical properties of the carrier as well as the bioactive agent and may also depend on environmental factors such as pH, ionic strength, or temperature at the site of delivery. Since these devices are implanted, injected or inserted in the body, their toxicity and biocompatibility assume great significance. Once the drug is released, its absorption depends on factors such as its solubility, concentration, local circulation, area of absorbing surface and route of administration (for instance, oral, nasal or vaginal) [1]. On absorption, the drug is distributed into cellular and interstitial fluids, depending on physicochemical and physiological parameters. Viewed in this perspective, such devices need to satisfy a number of biological, chemical, as well as physical objectives before they can be used in the body.

Biological Objectives

Biomaterials [1] used for controlled drug delivery should be non-toxic, non-carcinogenic, non-immunogenic and free of contaminants and leachables. The biological performance of a material depends both on the host response to the biomaterial as well as to the material response to the living system [2]. In vitro testing is usually carried out in physiological or biophysiological conditions only. Biocompatibility testing identifies any reactions that would lead to material failure or would result in disease [3]. These effects include irritation, inflammation, pyrogenicity, mutagenicity, systemic toxicity, sensitization, interaction with blood, carcinogenicity, and reaction to foreign bodies. Shape and size of the implants have an effect on the inflammation produced, and so need to be standardized before comparing the biocompatibility of two specimens. While biocompatibility of implants is thoroughly treated in other chapters, there are issues of special concern in drug delivery implants. Swelling [2] and leaching are modes of drug release from implants, but crazing or intergranular leaching of monomers or drugs themselves can lead to local and systemic biological reactions to the released products.

Physical Objectives

Materials with high strength-to-weight ratio, ease of fabrication, inertness (when suitable polymers are chosen), and wide variation in mechanical properties are excellent carriers for drug delivery [4]. Moreover, some classes of polymers such as hydrogels have physical properties that are very similar to that of body tissue. The mechanical strength depends on the crystallinity as well as on the molecular weight of the polymer.

Chemical Objectives

Depending on the mechanism of release, the carriers might have to be biodegradable [5]. The degradation of polymers can be initiated by heat, oxidation, mechanical energy, electromagnetic radiation, plasma, ultrasound, hydrolysis or enzymatic catalysed hydrolysis. In other cases the carrier might have to swell considerably in the presence of biological fluids to release a drug. These factors need to be taken into account before selecting a biomaterial as a carrier for a particular application.

MATERIALS

The last three decades have witnessed a substantial increase in research developments in the area of controlled release. Polymers and bioceramics that fulfill both biological as well as physicochemical objectives have been utilized as carriers. The polymers that have been used are poly(2-hydroxy ethyl methacrylate) (p-HEMA), poly(N-vinyl pyrrolidone) (p-NVP), poly(vinyl alcohol) (PVA), poly(acrylic acid) (PAA), polydimethyl siloxanes (PDMS), ethylene-vinyl acetate (EVAc) copolymers, poly(lactic acid) (PLA), poly(glycolic acid) (PGA), polyanhydrides, poly(ortho esters), collagen and cellulosic derivatives. Some examples of bioceramics that have been utilized as carriers are hydroxyapatite (HPA), tricalcium phosphate (TCP) and aluminocalcium phosphate (ALCAP).

The mechanism of drug release from polymers can be diffusion-limited, chemically controlled, swelling/dissolution controlled or magnetically controlled [6, 7]. A classification of drug delivery devices based on the mechanism of release is shown in Figure 27-1.

In diffusion-controlled systems, the drug diffuses to the polymer surface and then to the surrounding fluid; this is the controlling transport mechanism. In matrix (monolithic) systems, the drug is uniformly distributed in the polymer, while in reservoir (membrane) devices, the drug or the bioactive agent is enclosed in relatively large quantities within the polymer.

Chemically-controlled systems release drugs either by biodegradation [8–10] of the polymer or by chemical cleavage of the drug from the polymer chain on which it had been bound as a pendant [11].

Drugs can also be released from polymers that swell/dissolve. In these systems, the drug is loaded uniformly in the polymer, which is usually in the glassy state. When brought into contact with body fluids, the polymer swells and releases the drug. This process could be controlled by drug diffusion, polymer dissolution [12–14] or by the morphological structure of the polymer (for instance, crystallinity) [15]. In osmotic systems, the fluid ingresses into the drug-loaded polymer due to osmotic pressure, thereby causing pores to open and facilitating drug release.

Bioceramics can be classified into inert, completely resorbable or controlled surface reactive depending on their stability in the body [16]. Resorbable bioceramics degrade completely with time, and hence should be comprised solely of metabolic constituents. Inert bioceramics do not bond easily with tissues, and therefore, must possess high mechanical strength. Drug release from bioceramics is often controlled by the molecular structure of the drug as well as by the morphology of the bioceramic material. Depending on the

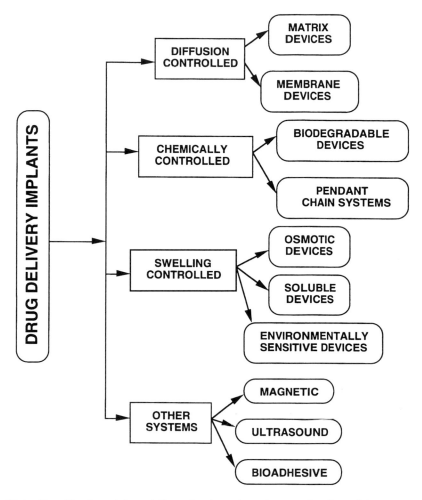

Figure 27-1 Classification of drug delivery implants based on mechanism of drug release.

type of release behavior required, these systems can be manipulated to achieve the desired results.

CHARACTERIZATION AND TESTING

An implant material interacts with the biological environment when material is transferred across the material-tissue interface. This may or may not be accompanied by reaction. The interface produced by the contact of solid biomaterial with body fluids can be characterized in the following ways: bioavailability of the bioactive agent, biocompatibility of the carrier, and structural and mechanical characterization.

Bioavailability

Measurement of Biological Activity Bioassays measure the biological response to a particular compound and indicate the therapeutic potency of a drug. They can be conducted in vitro as well as in vivo. A specific method to measure biological activity in peptides is radioreceptor assays (RRAs) [17].

Purity and Stability   Techniques such as thin film chromatography, gas liquid chromatography, high performance liquid chromatography (HPLC), reversed phase HPLC, ion exchange HPLC and size exclusion HPLC are used to determine the purity of the drug. Electrophoresis techniques [17] may be used to ascertain the stability of high molecular weight compounds, such as proteins and peptides.

Quantitative Detection Methods   These can be classified as radiochemical methods, immunochemical methods (radioimmuno assays, immunoradiometric assays and enzyme immunoassays), optical methods (UV, fluorescence, UV-Vis), and electrochemical methods [17].

Biocompatibility

Biocompatibility is the ability of a material to perform with an appropriate host response in a specific situation [2]. Biomaterials can be classified into four types depending on host response: inert materials which cause little or no host response, interactive biomaterials which elicit specific response such as adhesion or ingrowth, viable biomaterials that incorporate live cells treated by the host as normal tissue matrices, or replants, implantable materials made of native tissue cultured in vitro from cells obtained from the patient. The first two types are generally used for drug delivery. In vitro testing of materials can be carried out either in physiological, biophysiological, biological or pericellular environments. However, it is usually carried out under physiological or biophysiological conditions only. Yet in vitro tests are not conclusive due to the absence of hemodynamic, hematological, and reticuloendothelial compensatory mechanisms. While clotting and thrombosis are the most conspicuous results of incompatibility, they are only the end products of a complex series of events when materials are brought into contact with the body. Plasma proteins, enzymes and clotting factors could all be adversely affected by materials. The absence of adverse toxicological manifestations is only one component of biocompatibility, i.e., non-toxic materials are not necessarily biocompatible. Biocompatibility testing can be one of three types: in vitro (kinetic clotting, Lindholm test, elliptical cell, platelet retention, shear induced hemolysis); ex vivo (stagnation point flow system, arterio-venous shunt system); or in vivo (vena cava ring test, renal embolus test system) [18]. Table 27-1 presents necessary tests to be performed on any biomaterial before it is used as a drug delivery implant.

Structural and Mechanical Characterization of Carrier Materials

Polymers   The viscoelastic nature of polymers complicates the character of the tissue/polymer interface, since many biopolymers exhibit primary and secondary relaxations at and/or below physiological temperatures. Further, polymer processing and sterilization result in conformational as well as morphological changes in the polymer. Also, polymers may contain thermal, oxidizing and UV stabilizing additives, and plasticizers, which may migrate through the interface with time. Hence, meaningful characterization of the polymer becomes a key component of the drug delivery implant design [19]. The length scales involved vary from molecular to "supramolecular" and accordingly, the techniques also

Table 27-1   Necessary Tests for Biomaterials Before Use as Drug Delivery Implants (adapted from ASTM F748-87, 1990)

Implanted Devices Contacting	Cell culture cytotoxicity	Skin irritation	Intramuscular implantation	Blood compatibility	Hemolysis	Carcinogenicity	Long-term implant	Systemic injection acute toxicity	Intracutaneous injection	Sensitization	Mutagenicity	Pyrogen test
Bone	x					x	x	x		x	x	x
Tissue and Tissue Fluid	x	x				x	x	x	x	x	x	x
Blood	x		x	x	x	x	x	x	x	x	x	x

vary. Figure 27-2 provides an explanation of the various length and time scales [20] and the techniques involved (see also Chapter 2).

Techniques such as transmission electron microscopy (TEM), scanning electron microscopy (SEM), and electron probe microscopy (EPM) provide insight into the microstructure of the polymer. Other methods to study polymer morphology include photon beam and ion beam methods.

Dynamic mechanical analysis (DMA) can be used to characterize internal motion in polymers. DMA captures the effect of molecular structure, crystallinity and the presence

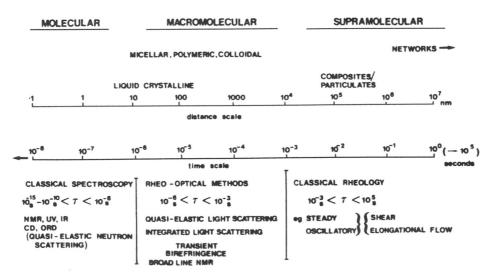

Figure 27-2   Various distance scales, the techniques used to probe them and the approximate time scales involved. (Reproduced with permission from Clark AH, Ross-Murphy SB, Structural and mechanical properties of biopolymer gels, *Adv Polym Sci*, 83 (1987), 57–192, © Springer-Verlag.)

of additives on the dynamics of drug transport within polymers. Important quantities like the storage modulus, G', and the loss modulus, G'', can be obtained from DMA. Other techniques to measure thermomechanical behavior of polymer include differential scanning calorimetry (DSC), thermomechanical analysis (TMA) and thermogravimetric analysis (TGA).

Nuclear magnetic resonance (NMR) spectroscopy is used to characterize polymer structure and dynamics both in solution and in the solid state. While solution NMR is used to characterize monomer content, branching effects and segmental dynamics, solid state NMR provides information about the morphology (crystallinity) and bulk dynamics (for more details see Chapter 2).

In addition, the response of polymers to various kinds of deformation can be studied by testing physical and mechanical properties with an Instron® testing machine. Small deformation rheological measurements provide insight into phenomena like gelation, dissolution and swelling. In addition, large deformation measurements lead to information about failure modes.

Bioceramics Characterization of bioceramics for drug delivery involves studying both the ability of the device to bond to the tissues as well as mechanical stability [21]. The chemical composition of the bioceramic is very critical as it affects the rate of bonding and hence the bioactivity of the implant. X-ray fluorescence analysis is suitable for this measurement. X-ray diffraction studies provide information on the degree of crystallinity of the implant, while either optical or scanning electron microscopy is used to analyze the microstructure of the implant. Characterization involves the determination of the size distribution of the grains, volume fraction of porosity, phase boundary area and phase connectivity in multi-phase microstructures (for details, see Chapter 1).

Characterization of surface features are of great concern for the implant to achieve reliable long-term behavior as the bioceramic surface forms an interface with biological fluids upon implantation. FTIR is used to characterize the surface in a non-destructive manner. In addition, SEM with energy-dispersive x-ray spectroscopy is useful to analyze the composition of the surface microstructure. Electron microprobe analysis (EMP) is an excellent technique to determine the thickness and compositional gradient of reaction layers formed on bioceramic implants. Other techniques for surface characterization include auger electron spectroscopy (AES), secondary ion mass spectroscopy (SIMS) and various surface charge analysis methods. The surface charge of an implant affects the adsorption of proteins and the response of the tissues in contact with it. A useful technique to measure the surface charge is the zeta potential method.

DRUG DELIVERY DEVICES

Based on the mechanisms discussed in the previous section, several drug delivery implants have been designed and approved for commercial use. This section presents details of various implant systems.

Membrane (Reservoir) Systems

Membrane systems depend on the diffusion of the bioactive agent across a polymer membrane. The rate of release in this case is governed by the molecular weight of the polymer or by the degree of crystallinity or the crosslinking ratio, if the polymer is either crystalline or crosslinked.

Membrane systems have been used for ocular therapy, contraception and transdermal applications. For instance, Ocusert® and Progestasert® (both from Alza Corporation, Palo Alto, CA) are EVAc-based reservoir systems which have been used for the release of pilocarpine and progesterone, respectively [22].

Matrix (Monolithic) Systems

Matrix systems are comprised of a polymeric matrix with the bioactive agent uniformly distributed in it. The polymer carrier can be either degradable, such as lactic acid, glycolic acid copolymers, or nondegradable, such as PDMS, EVAc or hydroxylalkyl methacrylate polymers.

It has been shown that bovine serum albumin (BSA) can be released from EVAc systems [23]. Copolymers of HEMA and methyl methacrylate (MMA) were shown to release lutenizing hormone-releasing hormone (LH-RH). It was shown that copolymer composition and crosslinking density control the release of the peptide [24]. Other drugs that have been shown to release from p-HEMA based systems are cyclazocine, erythromycin, tetracycline and progesterone [25].

Collagen is the principal structure protein in vertebrates. Purified bovine type I collagen has been studied as a parenteral delivery system due to its history of safe usage in humans and also due to its biodegradable properties. Collagen-based microspheres have been shown to release IL-2 [26], polylysine [27], and cisplatin [28] for cancer treatment. Chemically modified collagen has been shown to release gentamicin and pilocarpine in vivo [29]. Factors affecting tissue reaction to collagen are sterilization, crosslinking method, physical characteristics such as pore sizes and shape of the device, chemotactic properties of the products of collagenolysis, collagen-cell interaction, resorption mechanism of the collagen implant, antigenicity and the implantation site.

Bioerodible Systems

The advantage of bioerodible systems is that the implants need not be surgically removed and provide direct delivery to systemic circulation for long periods of time. The drug can be attached to the polymeric backbone; the device can be in the form of a reservoir system where the polymer degrades, releasing the drug; or the device can constitute a drug dispersed in a bioerodible matrix.

In hydrophobic systems, such as those based on PLA or PGA or their copolymers, the release is predominantly diffusion-controlled. Implant-based systems called Zoladex® (Zeneca Pharmaceuticals, Wilmington, DE) are based on PLA and are used for the treatment of prostate cancer using LH-RH agonists [30]. Poly(D,L-lactic acid)-based implants have been developed to treat tumors [31]. The local chemotherapy of malignant brain tumors showed that high local concentrations of cytostatics can be attained. Triamterene release from poly(D,L lactide-co-glycolide) microspheres was dependent on the drug loading and the lactic acid/glycolic acid ratio [32]. Release of cisplatin from PLA-PGA microspheres was shown to be feasible and the release kinetics were a strong function of the distribution of drug crystals [33]. An important factor to be taken into consideration while using micropar-ticles is the particle size required for effective drug delivery. Particulates do not cross most epithelial barriers, and particulates greater than 0.4 mm do not leave the vascular system. Biodegradable microspheres prepared from PLA-PGA are well suited for subcutaneous or intramuscular administration. They may not be suited for intravenous administration because they are rapidly cleared from the circulation by the reticuloendothelial system.

In hydrophobic systems such as polyanhydrides and poly(ortho esters), drug release is dictated by polymer hydrolysis. The hydrolysis mechanism in poly(ortho esters) is described in detail by Heller [34]. The release of naltrexone and contraceptive steroids from bioeroding Alzamer® (Alza Corporation, Palo Alto, CA), a poly(ortho ester), was investigated in dogs, rats and baboons and shown to be feasible. The only adverse effects were itching and some redness, which rapidly resolved when the device was removed. The hydrolysis rate of poly(ortho esters) can be accelerated by using more hydrophilic monomers like triethylene glycol (TEG). This effect was studied during 5-fluorouracil release from crosslinked polymers based on a prepolymer formed from 3,9-bis(ethylidene 2,4,8,10-tetraoxaspiro [5, 5] undecane) by varying proportions of the hydrophobic diol, 1,2 propylene glycol and the hydrophilic diol, TEG. The crosslinking agent was 1,2,6-hexanetriol. The release rate was higher when the percentage of TEG was the highest. Other methods of manipulating the hydrolysis rate include the combination of hydrophilicity and the use of diols that contain a pendent carboxylic acid [35]. Other drugs that have been shown to release from various poly(ortho esters) are insulin, hydrocortisone, 4-homosulfanilamide, ganciclovir and polypeptides.

Drug release from a class of erodible polyanhydrides consisting of sebacic acid (SA), 1,3-bis (p-carboxyphenoxy) propane (CPP) and a fatty acid dimer was studied by Langer and co-workers [36, 37]. Polyanhydrides differ from other polymers due to the reactivity of the anhydride bond [38]. Carboxylic acid anhydrides are the most reactive bonds ($t_{0.5}$ = 6 minutes). The faster a polymer erodes, the higher the probability that the drug release will be erosion-controlled. This makes polyanhydrides attractive candidates for the design of erosion-controlled drug delivery systems. Release of tetanus toxoid from non-coated and coated (with poly (D,L-lactic acid)) microspheres of polyanhydrides was studied [39]. It was observed that coating decreased the rate of release of the drug. Gopferich et al. showed that the release of indomethacin from p(CPP-SA) is controlled by dissolution and diffusion effects, even though the polymer biodegrades [40]. In the treatment of osteomyelitis, an infectious bone disease, polyanhydride implants loaded with gentamicin were used for local delivery of antibiotics. In addition, polyanhydride-based implants have been used to treat tumors [41].

Swelling-Controlled Release Systems

Swelling-controlled release systems are usually based on hydrophilic, glassy polymers which undergo swelling in the presence of biological fluids or in the presence of environmental stimuli such as pH or temperature change. Some of the swelling-controlled release hydrogels include those based on PMMA and PAA, PVA, p-NVP, poly(ethylene oxide/urethane) and cellulose derivatives such as Methocel A® (Dow Chemical, Midland, MI), and Cellosize WP (Union Carbide, Danbury, CT). Eudragit® (Rohm Pharma, Darstadt, Germany) is a hydrogel which is mainly a copolymer of methacrylic and acrylic esters with or without quarternary ammonium ions. Release of theophylline from crosslinked PVA was studied by Peppas and co-workers [42]. They investigated the effect of various system parameters like the crosslinking ratio, degree of crystallinity and film thickness on the amount of drug released. Physiologically relevant drug release amounts were shown to be feasible in such systems. Metronidazole release from uncrosslinked PVA devices was studied by Mallapragada et al. [15]. It was shown that the degree of crystallinity of the polymer could be used as a tuning parameter to achieve the desired drug release behavior.

Another commercially available system for drug release called Geomatrix® (Jago, Zug, Switzerland) was developed by Colombo and co-workers [43–45]. This system is based on hydroxy propyl methyl cellulose (HPMC) and is coated on different sides with cellulose acetate propionate, which is impermeable to biological fluids. Diltiazem hydrochloride release from Geomatrix® systems was observed to exhibit zero-order release.

Hydrogels used in pulsatile delivery systems can be either single-pulse systems or multi-pulse systems. The single-pulse systems can be osmotically controlled, dissolution-controlled or melting-controlled [46]. Potassium chloride release from cellulose derivatives (CA latex or ethyl cellulose acetate) was shown to be activated by transport of water through the semipermeable membrane, thus creating an internal osmotic pressure. It was demonstrated that drug release by osmotic pressure control could be achieved by creating porosity in the polymer [47].

Multiple-pulse systems are controlled by environmental changes (temperature [48, 49], pH [50], ionic strength [51], magnetic fields [52], or ultrasound). Environmentally responsive hydrogels can be obtained by using anionic or cationic hydrogels. Hydrogel copolymers of N-Isopropyl acrylamide (NIPAAm) and MAA have been used to release anti-thrombotic agents. It was demonstrated that hydrogels composed of 75 percent NIPAAm or greater were temperature-sensitive, while those with as little as 12 percent MAA showed pH-sensitive behavior. Streptokinase release from such hydrogels revealed that the release was controlled by changes in the swelling behavior, especially when both temperature and pH were altered [48, 49].

Transdermal Delivery Systems

Transdermal delivery is useful for drugs with low dosage requirement and high skin permeability. This type of delivery reduces first pass metabolism, but there is usually a lag time to reach steady state. For effective transdermal delivery, the molecular weight of the bioactive agent should be less than 1,000 and the dosage should not exceed 10 mg/ml. The human stratum corneum is 15–20 mm thick and contains lipid bilayers, which are the major barrier to permeation. Different techniques to enhance permeation include iontophoresis, electroporation and ultrasound. The permeation rate is also a strong function of the site of permeation.

Some transdermal products include Transderm-Scop® (multilaminate system where microporous polypropylene is the rate limiting barrier) and Transderm-Nitro® (ethylene-vinyl acetate copolymer) (both from Alza-Ciba, Palo Alto, CA) and Nitrodisc® (silicone membrane) (Searle, Skokie, IL). Estraderm® (Ciba-Geigy, Ardsley, NY) and Catapres-TTS® (Boehringer, Ingelheim, Germany) are transdermal, membrane-controlled release systems for delivery of estradiol and clonidine, respectively.

Other polymers used as carriers in bioadhesive systems include carboxymethyl cellulose, PAA, poly(vinyl sulfate), PVA and poly-L-aspartic acid [53]. PVA gels prepared by a freeze-thaw technique exhibited bioadhesive properties and were used to release ketansarin, a wound-healing enhancer. It was shown that the number of freeze-thaw cycles and the degree of crystallinity of the polymer controlled the bioadhesiveness and the drug release rate [54].

Other Implant Devices

Sintered EVAc copolymer, inserted subcutaneously in diabetic rats, has been used to release insulin [55] and was found to control glucose levels over a period of 100 days.

Polymeric matrices consisting of EVAc copolymer together with magnetic beads made of chromium steel or samarium-cobalt alloy have been used [56] to deliver BSA. It was shown that the mechanical properties of the polymeric device are influenced by the extent of the magnetic field. In the presence of an oscillating magnetic field, the drug is "squeezed out" of the pores in the polymer containing the magnetic beads. It was also shown that the drug release rate was enhanced in the presence of the beads.

Liposomes have also been used for drug delivery. These are microvesicles made up of a bilayer of amphipathic molecules surrounding an aqueous compartment. Liposome stability is influenced by lipid composition, storage conditions (light, temperature, oxygen etc.) and the presence of stabilizers such as cholesterol (30 mol%) or a-tocopherol. The permeability of the encapsulated compounds in turn depends on the lipid composition, molecular weight of the compound, and amount of cholesterol present in the liposome. Water-soluble compounds with molecular weights greater than 1000 may escape from the liposomes when the liposome bilayer breaks down. Liposomes with sizes greater than 8 μm go to lung, liver or spleen and those with sizes less than 0.15 μm show reduced uptake in liver and spleen, and increased carcass disposition and half-life in blood. Extended circulation time can also be obtained by appropriate surface modifications [57]. Delivery of agents to the lysosomal compartment of the cells of the reticuloendothelial system is the most effective use of liposomes. Antifungal agents have been released from natural phospholipids (Itraconazole®, Cilag Pharmaceuticals Ltd., Sao Paolo, Brazil). Other commercially available systems include Amphocil™ (Liposome Technology, Inc., Menlo Park, CA), ABLC™ (The Liposome Company, Princeton, NJ) and AmBisome™ (NEXstar Pharmaceuticals, San Dimes, CA), all liposome-based devices to deliver Amphotericin B.

Polymeric carbon can be used as a host for several drugs whose ions can be incorporated inside the pores and released in a controlled manner. Resol converts to fully cured phenolic resin on heating at 150–200°C. This resin transforms into a porous but impermeable glass-like polymeric carbon on heating to 1000°C. The final product consists of long, chain-like molecules of carbon atoms aggregated locally [58] to form crystalline domains which are randomly arranged in space. The release of lithium ions, well known for treatment of nervous disorders, from such systems has been reported [59].

Bioceramic Devices

Ceramic reservoirs composed of HA, TCP, inorganic bone meal, or ALCAP can be used as carriers for drug delivery due to their biocompatible nature. Ceramic capsules prepared using the above materials have been shown to be capable of delivering steroids such as testosterone and dihydrotestosterone [60, 61] and drugs such as norepinephrine [62] in a sustained manner. Ceramic tablets made of ALCAP have also been used as effective, long-term delivery devices for proteins, amino acids, enzymes, nucleosides [63] and phenolics [64]. McFall and Bajpai reported that during subcutaneous implantation of ALCAP discs in rat brain, spleen, liver and other major organs, no toxic accumulation of the ceramic components occurred for as long as 3 months [65]. PLA-impregnated ALCAP implants were shown to decrease the rate of release of steroids, thus providing implants that can achieve the steroid levels necessary to inhibit spermatogenesis.

CONCLUSIONS AND FUTURE DIRECTIONS

Controlled drug release implants have already significantly improved the delivery of existing drugs. But these systems have an even greater role to play in the future. The minimization of side effects, prolonging biological lifetimes of the devices, advances in surface coating technology to enable intravenous administration of microspheres, drug targeting to specific cells or organs and increased bioadhesive performance are all formidable challenges that need to be addressed. In addition, the toxicity, biocompatibility and immunogenicity of the drug delivery implants are important due to the direct interfacing of the devices with the biological environment. The development of new materials like polyanhydrides and bioceramics to effectively administer drugs is another major thrust area. Rapid advances in the fields of biomaterials science and engineering, clinical medicine, pharmacology, polymer and materials chemistry, characterization and testing have led to the exciting developments discussed in this chapter. Breakthroughs in successfully meeting the challenges discussed above will only be possible if researchers working in the above areas collaborate to develop systems that will further revolutionize drug therapy.

REFERENCES

1 Bruck SD. Pharmacological basis of controlled drug delivery. In Bruck SD (Ed.), *Controlled Drug Delivery, Vol. 1, Basic Concepts.* Boca Raton, FL: CRC Press, 1983, 1–13.

2 Black J. *Biological Performance of Materials: Fundamentals of Biocompatibility.* New York: Marcel Dekker, 1992.

3 Lord GH. Regulation and reasons for biocompatibility testing. In Williams DF (Ed.), *Techniques of Biocompatibility Testing Vol. I.* Boca Raton, FL: CRC Press, 1986, 5–34.

4 Williams DF. Biomaterials and biocompatibility. In Williams DF (Ed.), *Fundamental Aspects of Biocompatibility Vol. I.* Boca Raton, FL: CRC Press, 1981, 1–10.

5 Gilding DK. Degradation of polymer: Mechanisms and implications for biomedical applications. In Williams DF (Ed.), *Fundamental Aspects of Biocompatibility Vol. I.* Boca Raton, FL: CRC Press, 1981, 43–66.

6 Langer RS, Peppas NA. Chemical and physical structure of polymers as carriers for controlled release of bioactive agents: A review. *J Macromol Sci, Rev Macromol Chem Phys*, C23 (1983), 61–126.

7 Narasimhan B, Peppas NA. The role of modeling in the development of future controlled-release devices. In Park K (Ed.), *Controlled Drug Delivery: The Next Generation.* Washington, DC: American Chemical Society, 1996.

8 Gopferich A. Polymer degradation and erosion: Mechanisms and applications. *Eur J Pharm Biopharm*, 42 (1996), 1–11.

9 Gopferich A, Langer R. Modeling monomer release from bioerodible polymers. *J Contr Rel*, 33 (1995), 55–69.

10 Hopfenberg HB. In Paul DR and Harris FW (Eds.), *Controlled Release Polymeric Formulations*, ACS Symposium Series, Vol. 33. Washington, DC: American Chemical Society, 222, 1976.

11 Tani N, Van Dress M, Anderson JM. In Lewis DH (Ed.), *Controlled Release of Pesticides and Pharmaceuticals.* New York: Plenum Press, 1981.

12 Lee PI, Peppas NA. Prediction of polymer dissolution in swellable controlled-release systems. *J Contr Rel*, 6 (1987), 201–215.

13 Harland RS, Gazzaniga A, Sangani ME, Colombo P, Peppas NA. Drug/Polymer Matrix Swelling and Dissolution. *Pharmaceut Res*, 5 (1988), 488–494.

14 Narasimhan B, Peppas NA. Development of a dissolution-controlled, zero-order release, drug delivery system. *Polym Prepr Am Chem Soc, Div Polym Chem*, 36 (1995), 160–161.

15 Mallapragada SK, Peppas NA, Colombo P. Crystal Dissolution Controlled Release Systems: II. Metronidazole Release from Semicrystalline Poly(vinyl alcohol) Systems. *J Biomed Mater Res*, in press.

16 Hench LL. Stability of Ceramics in the Physiological Environment. In Williams DF (Ed.), *Fundamental Aspects of Biocompatibility Vol. I.* Boca Raton, FL: CRC Press, 1981, 67–86.

17 Randall CS, Malefyt TR, Sternson LA. Approaches to the analysis of peptides. In Lee VHL (Ed.), *Peptide and Protein Drug Delivery.* New York: Marcel Dekker, 1991, 203–246.

18 Bruck SD. Evaluation of blood compatibility of polymeric materials. In Bruck SD (Ed.), *Controlled Drug Delivery, Vol. II. Clinical Applications.* Boca Raton, FL: CRC Press, 1983, 45–64.

19 Barrenberg SA, Brozoski-Varnell B, English AD, Hassel RL, Johnson, Jr., RE, Kelley MJ, Starkweather, Jr., HW. Structural and chemical characterization of polymers. In Williams DF (Ed.), *Techniques of Biocompatibility Testing, Vol. II.* Boca Raton, FL: CRC Press, 1986, 1–48.

20 Clark AH, Ross-Murphy SB. Structural and mechanical properties of biopolymer gels. *Adv Polym Sci*, 83 (1987), 57–192.

21 Hench LL. Characterization of bioceramics. In Hench LL, Wilson J (Eds.), *An Introduction to Bioceramics.* Singapore: World Scientific, 1993, 319–334.

22 Ueno N, Refojo MF. Ocular pharmacology of drug release devices. In Bruck SD (Ed.), *Controlled Drug Delivery, Vol. II, Clinical Applications.* Boca Raton, FL: CRC Press, 89–110.

23 Rhine WD, Sukhatme V, Hseih DST, Langer RS. In Baker R (Ed.), *Controlled Release of Bioactive Materials.* New York: Academic Press, 1980.

24 Davidson GWR, III, Domb A, Sanders LM, McRae G. Hydrogels for controlled release of peptides. *Proc Intern Symp Control Rel Bioact Mater*, 15 (1988), 66–67.

25 Ratner BD. Biomedical applications of hydrogels: Review and critical appraisal. In Williams DF (Ed.), *Biocompatibility of Clinical Implant Materials, Vol. II.* Boca Raton, FL: CRC Press, 1981, 145–176.

26 Matsuoka J, Sakagami K, Shiozaki S, Uchida S, Fugiwara T, Gohchi A, Orita K. Development of an IL-2 slow delivery system. *Trans Am Soc Artif Intern Organs*, 34 (1988), 729–731.

27 Singh MP, Lumpkin JA, Rosenblatt J. Effect of electrostatic interactions on polylysine release rates from collagen matrices and comparison with model predictions. *J Contr Rel*, 35 (1995), 165–179.

28 Daniels J, Daniels A, Quinn M. Phase I trials with cisplatin or mytomycin hepatic chemoembolization with angiostat collagen for embolization in patients with colo-rectal cancer. *Proc ASCO*, 7 (1988), 385–386.

29 Miyata T, Rubin AL, Stenzel KH, Dunn MW. Collagen Drug Delivery Device. U.S. Patent 4,164,559 (1979).

30 Gopferich A. Polymer degradation and erosion: Mechanisms and applications. *Eur J Pharm Biopharm*, 42 (1996), 1–11.

31 Stricker H, Remmele T, Ludwig H, von Buren H, Wowra B, Sturm V, Zeller WJ. Polymerabbau und methotrex-atfreigabe von poly (D, L-laktid) implantaten. *Eur J Pharm Biopharm*, 37 (1991), 171–174.

32 Ouellette AD, Peppas NA. Controlled release of triamterene from poly(DL-lactide-co-glycolide) micro-spheres. In Mikos AG, Murphy RM, Bernstein H, Peppas NA (Eds.), *Biomaterials for Drug and Cell Delivery. Mater Res Soc Symp Proc*, 331 (1994), 91–96.

33 Spenlehauer G, Vert M, Benoit J-P, Chabot F, Veillard M. Biodegradable cisplatin microspheres prepared by the solvent evaporation method: Morphology and release characteristics. *J Contr Rel*, 7 (1988), 217–229.

34 Heller J. Poly(ortho esters). *Adv Polym Sci*, 107 (1993), 41–92.

35 Heller J, Penhale DWH, Fritzinger BK, Ng SY. The effect of copolymerized 9,10-dihydroxystearic acid on erosion rates of poly(ortho esters) and its use in the delivery of Levonorgestrel. *J Contr Rel*, 5 (1987), 173–178.

36 Tamada J, Langer R. The development of polyanhydrides for drug delivery applications. *J Biomater Sci, Polym Ed*, 31 (1992), 315–353.

37 Gopferich A, Langer R. The influence of microstructure and monomer properties on the erosion mechanism of a class of polyanhydrides. *J Polym Sci, Polym Chem*, 31 (1993), 2445–2458.

38 Park K, Shalaby SW, Park H. *Biodegradable Hydrogels for Drug Delivery.* Lancaster, PA: Technomic Pub., 1993.

39 Gopferich A, Alonso MJ, Langer R. Development and characterization of microencapsulated microspheres. *Pharm Res*, 11 (1994), 1568–1574.

40 Gopferich A., Shieh L, Langer R. Aspects of polymer erosion. In Mikos AG, Leong KW, Radomsky ML (Eds.), *Polymers in Medicine and Pharmacy. Mater Res Soc Symp Proc*, 394 (1995), 155–160.

41 Gopferich A, Karydas D, Langer R. Predicting drug release from cylindric polyanhydride matrix discs. *Eur J Pharm Biopharm*, 42 (1995), 81–87.

42 Korsmeyer RW, Peppas NA. Effect of the morphology of hydrophilic polymeric matrices on the diffusion and release of water soluble drugs. *J Membr Sci*, 9 (1981), 211–227.

43 Colombo P, Catellani PL, Peppas NA, Maggi L, Conte U. Swelling characteristics of hydrophilic matrices for controlled release: New dimensionless number to describe the swelling and release behavior. *Int J Pharm*, 88 (1992), 99–109.

44 Colombo P, Gazzaniga A, Sangalli ME, La Manna A. In vitro programmable zero-order release drug delivery systems. *Acta Pharm Technol*, 33 (1987), 15–20.

45 Conte U, Colombo P, Gazzaniga A., Sangalli ME, La Manna A. Swelling-activated drug delivery systems. *Biomaterials*, 9 (1988), 489–493.

46 Doelker E. Cellulose derivatives. *Adv Polym Sci*, 107 (1993), 199–265.

47 Zentner GM, Rork GS, Himmelstein KJ. Osmotic flow through controlled porosity films: An approach to delivery of water soluble compounds. *J Contr Rel*, 2 (1985), 217–229.

48 Brazel CS, Peppas NA. Temperature and pH-sensitive hydrogels for controlled release of antithrombotic agents. In Mikos AG, Murphy RM, Bernstein H, Peppas NA (Eds.), *Biomaterials for Drug and Cell Delivery, Proc Mater Res Soc Symp*, 331 (1994), 211–216.

49 Dong L-C, Hoffman AS. A novel approach for preparation of pH-sensitive hydrogels for enteric drug delivery. *J Contr Rel*, 15 (1991), 141–152.

50 Bell CL, Peppas NA. Poly(methacrylic acid-g-ethylene glycol) hydrogels as pH-responsive biomedical materials. In Mikos AG, Murphy RM, Bernstein H, Peppas NA (Eds.), *Biomaterials for Drug and Cell Delivery. Proc Mater Res Soc Symp*, 331 (1994), 199–204.

51 am Ende MT, Hariharan D, Peppas NA. Factors influencing drug and protein transport and release from ionic hydrogels. *React Polym*, 25 (1995), 127–137.

52 Kost J, Wolfrum J, Langer R. Magnetically enhanced insulin release in diabetic rats. *J Biomed Mater Res*, 21 (1987), 1367–1373.

53 Park K, Ch'ng HS, Robinson JR. Alternative approaches to oral controlled drug delivery: Bioadhesives and in situ systems. In Anderson JM and Kim SW (Eds.), *Recent Advances in Drug Delivery Systems*. New York: Plenum Press, 1983, 163–184.

54 Mongia NK, Anseth KS, Peppas NA. Mucoadhesive poly(vinyl alcohol) hydrogels produced by freezing/thawing processes: Applications in the development of wound healing systems. *J Biomater Sci, Polym Ed*, in press.

55 Brown L, Munoz C, Siemer L, Edelman E, Langer R. Controlled release of insulin from polymer matrices: Control of diabetes in rats. *Diabetes*, 35 (1986), 692–697.

56 Hsieh D, Langer R. Zero-order drug delivery systems with magnetic control. In Mansdorff Z, Roseman TJ (Eds.), *Controlled Release Delivery Systems*. New York: Marcel Dekker, 1983, 121.

57 Senior J. Fate and behavior of liposomes in vivo: A review of controlling factors. *CRC Critical Reviews in Therapeutic Drug Carrier Systems*, 3 (1987), 123–195.

58 Jenkins GM, Kawamura K. *Polymeric Carbon-Carbon Fiber, Glass, and Char.* Cambridge, UK: Cambridge University Press, 1976.

59 Ila D, Jenkins GM, Zimmerman RL, Evelyn AL. High porosity carbon ware for controlled release of drugs. In Mikos AG, Murphy RM, Bernstein H, Peppas NA (Eds.), *Biomaterials for Drug and Cell Delivery. Proc Mater Res Soc Symp*, 331 (1994), 281–285.

60 Benghuzzi HA, Bajpai PK. The use of ceramics as drug delivery systems. *Proc South Biomed Eng Conf*, 1989.

61 Benghuzzi HA, Bajpai PK, England BG. The delivery of testosterone and dihydrotestosterone by ALCAP ceramic implants in rats. *J Invest Surgery*, 3 (1990), 197–215.

62 Benghuzzi HA, Tucci MA, Parsell D, Bajpai PK. Sustained release of norepinephrine by four different resorbable and biodegradable ceramic delivery devices. *Proc World Biomater Conf*, 1996, 153.

63 Bajpai PK, Benghuzzi HA. Ceramic system for long-term delivery of chemicals and biologicals. *J Biomed Mater Res*, 22 (1988), 1245–1266.

64 Strasser J, Bajpai PK. Polymer impregnated ALCAP ceramics: Delivery of gossypol acetic acid. *Proc Northeast Bioeng Conf*, 1987, 566–569.

65 McFall F, Bajpai PK. Fate of resorbable alumino-calcium-phosphorus oxide (ALCAP) ceramic implants in rats. *Biomaterials*, 7 (1984), 354.

ADDITIONAL READING

1 Park K (Ed.). *Controlled Drug Delivery: The Next Generation*. Washington, DC: American Chemical Society, 1996.

2 Chasin M, Langer R. *Biodegradable Polymers as Drug Delivery Systems*. New York: Marcel Dekker, 1990.

3 Cleland J, Langer R (Eds.). *Formulation and Delivery of Proteins and Peptides*. ACS Symposium Series, Vol. 567. Washington, DC: American Chemical Society, 1994.

4 Biomaterials for cell and drug delivery. In Mikos AG, Murphy RM, Bernstein H, Peppas NA (Eds.), *Proc Mater Res Soc Symp*, 1994, 331.

Chapter 28

Biosensors

W. Monty Reichert
Adam A. Sharkawy

INTRODUCTION

This chapter reviews the biocompatibility issues most pertinent to long-term implantable biosensors. Particular emphasis is placed on how the in vivo environment affects sensor performance rather than on the conventional view of biocompatibility, which is how the body responds to an implanted artificial material. The glucose sensor is used as an example of the indwelling sensor paradigm throughout this chapter because of its therapeutic importance and because the in vivo performance issues associated with this device is pervasive.

BIOSENSORS

A good overview of biosensors is provided by Hall [1] who uses the term "biosensor" to describe those devices that use a biological component to *specifically* and *selectively* detect the concentration of analyte molecules in the ambient. Although we will adopt Hall's terminology, a more precise descriptor of these devices is "bioanalytical sensors." Arnold and Meyerhoff [2] classify biosensors into two categories: biocatalytic-based sensors in which the velocity of an enzyme-catalyzed reaction is governed by the ambient concentration of analyte, and receptor-based sensors in which the total amount of analyte bound by a bioreceptor molecule at equilibrium is proportional to the analyte concentration. In both cases, the detection mechanism is a chain of three events: biorecognition, perturbation and transduction, where a perturbation is necessary lest the biorecognition event goes undetected. In general, receptor-based sensors are ill-suited for indwelling applications because they respond slowly, if at all, to dynamic fluctuations in analyte concentration.

The most prevalent biocatalytic-based biosensor is the amperometric glucose electrode, such as the Glucose Analyzer marketed by Yellow Springs Instruments (Yellow Springs, OH). This device consists of a hydrogen peroxide electrode with a glucose oxidase (GO) containing layer placed at the electrode tip (Figure 28-1A). The enzyme layer is separated from the electrode and test solution by inner and outer membranes (dashed lines) that are permeable to glucose and hydrogen peroxide, respectively. Biorecognition occurs when the analyte, β-D-glucose, diffuses into the enzyme layer and binds with the active site of the enzyme [3]. The perturbation event comprises two coupled redox reactions shown below: the oxidation of glucose to glucolactone (which spontaneously combines with water to form gluconic acid) by reduction of the enzyme, and the reoxidation of the enzyme by reduction of oxygen to hydrogen peroxide. Transduction is achieved when the Pt anode, biased at +700 mV relative to a Ag/AgCl reference electrode, oxidizes hydrogen peroxide, in the process abstracting $2e^-$ that are detected as a current.

$$\beta\text{-D-glucose} + \text{GO} \underset{k_{-1}}{\overset{k_1}{\rightleftharpoons}} \beta\text{-D-glucose/GO complex} \xrightarrow[\text{O}_2]{k_2} \text{glucolactone} + \text{GO} + \text{H}_2\text{O}_2$$

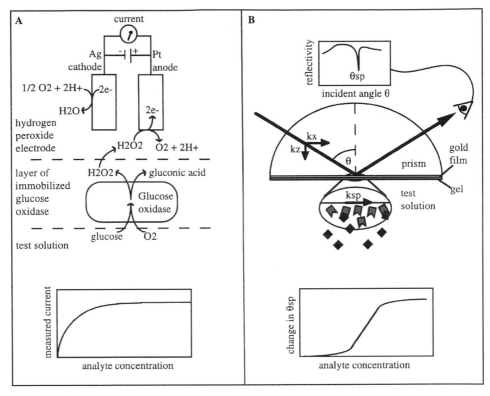

Figure 28-1 Schematic illustrations of common biosensors: (A) amperometric glucose sensor based on glucose oxidase immobilized to the tip of a hydrogen peroxide electrode; (B) surface plasmon resonance immunosensor based on antibody layer immobilized to a metal film deposited at the prism base.

$$H_2O_2 \xrightarrow{\text{hydrogen peroxide electrode}} 2H^+ + O_2 + 2e^-$$

Figure 28-2 is an example of an indwelling "needle-type" glucose electrode that is intended for use in conjunction with an insulin infusion pump to form an artificial pancreas.

The response of the sensor is determined by the rate of production of H_2O_2 which is equal and opposite to the rate of glucose consumption. As H_2O_2 diffuses to the electrode, the measured current is given by [1]:

$$i_{\text{meas}} = K K_e \delta \{d[H_2O_2]/dt\} = K K_e \delta \{-d[\text{glucose}]/dt\}$$

where K is a proportionality constant, δ is the diffusion layer thickness, and K_e is a constant characteristic of the electrode equal to nFA where n is the mols of electrons generated per mol of glucose consumed, F is Faraday's constant, and A is the electrode area. Assuming Michaelis-Menten kinetics, the rate of hydrogen peroxide generation is given by:

$$d[H_2O_2]/dt = -d[\text{glucose}]/dt = \frac{k_2[\text{GO}][\text{glucose}]}{K_m + [\text{glucose}]}$$

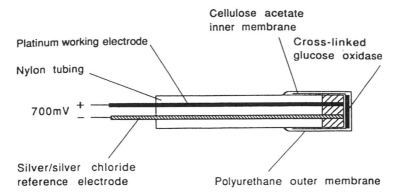

Figure 28-2 Schematic illustration of the glucose sensor showing the needle-type construction commonly used for subcutaneous insertion. Note the presence of the inner and outer membranes, the enzyme layer and the lead insulation. (Reprinted from Pickup JC, In vivo glucose monitoring: Sense and sensorability, *Acta Diabetol*, 1993; 30:143–148. With permission.)

where K_m is the Michaelis-Menten constant $[(k_{-1} + k_2)/k_1]$, and the rate constant k_2 is as defined above. In most instances, however, the enzyme layer is coated with an outer polymer membrane that slows the diffusion rate of glucose into the enzyme layer to much less than the rate of the enzyme-catalyzed reaction. In this diffusion-limited case, the measured current is governed by [1]:

$$i_{\text{meas}} = K'K_e[\text{glucose}]D/\delta$$

where K' is another proportionality constant, K_e is as described above, D is the diffusion coefficient of glucose in the membrane and δ is now the membrane thickness.

The majority of receptor-based biosensors are adaptations of solid phase immunoassays. The dominant optical immunosensor on the market is the surface plasmon resonance (SPR) BIAcore system marketed by Pharmacia Biosensor AB (Uppsula, Sweden). This sensor is an attenuated total reflection device consisting of a glass prism with a very thin gold film (ca. 50 nm) deposited at the prism base (Figure 28-1B). Monochromatic light totally reflected off the prism base has a reflectivity of nearly 100 percent except at a very specific incident angle, θ_{sp}, at which the illuminating radiation comes into resonance with the electrons at the exposed surface of the gold film. This resonance, called a surface plasmon, produces a drastic drop in the reflectivity of the prism.

SPR is observed when the momentum of an incident photon parallel to the prism base (k_x) matches the momentum of the surface plasmon (k_{sp}) (Figure 28-1B). This matching condition can be achieved only with totally reflected parallel polarized incident light, and only with highly reflective metals such as silver and gold with a large density of free electrons. Under these constraints, $k_x = k_{\text{sp}}$ occurs when [1]

$$\sqrt{\varepsilon_p}\sin\theta_{\text{sp}} = \sqrt{\frac{\varepsilon'_m \varepsilon_a}{(\varepsilon'_m + \varepsilon_a)}}$$

where ε_a and ε_p are the dielectric constants of the ambient and prism, respectively, and ε'_m is the real part of the gold film's dielectric constant ($\varepsilon_m = \varepsilon'_m + i\varepsilon''_m$). For example, a clean gold film ($\varepsilon_m = -13.15 + i1.16$) at the base of a glass prism ($\varepsilon_p = 2.30$) and adjacent to an aqueous test solution ($\varepsilon_a = 1.78$) exhibits SPR at $\theta_{sp} = 71.1°$. (Note: the refractive index is the square root of the dielectric constant.)

In the BIAcore immunosensor, the gold film at the prism base is coated with a thin layer of dextran gel impregnated with antibody (Figure 28-1B). As analyte binds with antibody (biorecognition), the gel densifies (perturbation), thus raising the effective dielectric constant of the ambient. This produces a more sluggish surface plasmon that cannot be launched unless the momentum of incident photons in the plane of the gold film increases, which requires θ_{sp} to shift upwards (transduction). Since the change in ε_a with analyte binding is very small, the shifts in the resonance angle are linear with respect to the mass change of the gel layer

$$\Delta\theta_{sp} = \theta_{sp} - \theta_{sp}^{\circ} = K_{sp}\Gamma$$

where θ_{sp} is the shifted plasmon angle upon analyte binding relative to the initial condition θ_{sp}°, Γ is the surface density of bound analyte, and K_{sp} is a proportionality constant. BIAcore reports a K_{sp} equal to a $0.1°$ shift in θ_{sp} for every $1 ng/mm^2$ of mass added to the gold film (see BIAcore commercial literature). Assuming Langmuirian binding, the angle shift at equilibrium is related to the solution analyte concentration $[A]$ and analyte binding site density Γ_0

$$\Delta\theta_{sp} = K_{sp}\Gamma_0 \frac{K_a[A]}{1 + K_a[A]}$$

where K_a is the affinity constant. The rate at which equilibrium or quasi-equilibrium is achieved is nominally transport-limited.

BIOSENSOR BIOCOMPATIBILITY

Sensors immersed long-term in aqueous but non-physiological environments eventually fail from lead detachment, corrosion, component delamination, or loss of hermetic sealing [4]. Thus, before consideration is given to biocompatibility testing, the sensor first must be capable of long-term function in corrosive environments (e.g., Ringer's solution at 37°C for 4 weeks) and be sufficiently rugged to withstand the physical demands of implantation. The device must also remain fully functional after sterilization. Most of the biosensors described in the literature do not meet these criteria.

For a biosensor, or any sensor for that matter, to function in a physiological environment it must meet two requirements. First, it must be biocompatible in the conventional sense, meaning the sensor must minimally perturb, and be accepted by, the in vivo environment in which it is placed [5]. Second, the environment must minimally perturb the performance of the sensor. Sharkawy et al. [6] recently coined the term "sensocompatibility" as a measure of how well a sensor meets the second performance criterion. For example, an implanted biosensor that is encapsulated with a thin fibrous tissue may be biocompatible by definition, but if it ceases to function due to protein deposition on the sensing region, then it is biocompatible but not sensocompatible. In this chapter we will focus on evaluating the performance aspect of sensor biocompatibility rather than examining the biocompatibility of the sensor materials.

The sensocompatibility expectations for a given biosensor fall into three categories of increasing severity: single-shot disposable sensors, sensors for in vitro measurements with prolonged or repeated exposure to sample, and indwelling sensors. Disposable biosensor test strips designed for in vitro measurements, such as pin prick glucose monitoring and urine pregnancy detection kits, have minimal sensocompatibility requirements. Glucose is small and abundant, allowing it to freely diffuse to the enzyme layer, producing a measurement in less time than it takes the blood to foul the sensor. In the case of pregnancy test kits, urine is relatively free of cells and proteins, allowing unencumbered access of hCG analyte to the antibody layer. Sensocompatibility does not really come into play until the in vitro measurements are slow to develop or are repetitive. In the case of immunoassay of blood serum samples, sensocompatibility necessitates the prevention of non-specific protein adsorption long enough to make the measurement, which is usually 5–15 minutes. If the measurement is to be made in whole blood, or if the same sensor is to be used repeatedly or continuously, then the term "sensocompatibility" must encompass resistance to biofouling, the loss of sensor function which occurs when cells or proteins clog or block analyte access to the sensing surface. With the possible exception of periodic ex vivo blood glucose monitoring, which usually protects the electrode tip with a dialysis membrane, a completely satisfactory solution to the biofouling problem has not yet been identified.

Depending on their placement in vivo, indwelling biosensors are subject to a whole host of proteins and cellular agents that can and do hinder sensor function:

- deposition of blood plasma proteins and fibrin formation during hemostasis
- attack by cells and proteins of the immune response
- invasion of inflammatory cells
- growth of a foreign body capsular tissue around the sensor
- calcification and thrombus formation if implanted intravascularly.

It is important that aggressive attack be resisted at all of the tissue/biofluid contacting surfaces, i.e., the sensing surface, the sensor-encapsulating layer and the lead insulation (Figure 28-2). For implantable sensors, one should select materials that will not elicit strong host responses or are biocompatible. The conventional biocompatibility of polymer, metal and ceramic materials is discussed extensively elsewhere in this handbook. Previously, we reviewed the materials considerations in the selection, performance and adhesion of polymeric encapsulants for implantable sensors; therein, we discuss indwelling sensor failure modes as well as the tissue and blood compatibility of implanted sensors [4]. In general, there has been very little change in the menu of suitable sensor encapsulants in the last 20-plus years. Metals and ceramic encapsulants, primarily titanium and glass, offer the best hermeticity and mechanical protection, but are not amenable to the processing of many sensing devices. This leaves polymeric encapsulants, all with limited hermeticity, but several with acceptable biocompatibility, e.g., PTFE, epoxies, SR, PI, PU, PE and parylene. A common lead configuration, for example, is PTFE- or PE-coated wires encased in SR or PU outer layers.

REVIEW OF IN VIVO PERFORMANCE

Although the occasional sensor continues to function in vivo for weeks to months, no biosensors are capable of *reliably* surviving long-term implantation, primarily due to analyte transport and biofouling consequences of the foreign body response [4, 6]. The avascular fibrous capsule that forms around an implanted sensor can impose a transport limitation on the diffusion of analyte to the sensor surface, especially for blood-borne analytes. Access to the analyte is diminished by the adhesion of cells, deposition of proteins and calcification of the sensing region. Hydrolytic enzymes released during inflammation and immune reaction further degrade the sensing tip. Until these long-term implantation hurdles are overcome, biosensors will not transcend in vitro or short-term applications. Because indwelling glucose sensors encompass all aspects of sensor biocompatibility, from sensor tip fouling to transport issues associated with encapsulation tissue, the remainder of the chapter will discuss only these devices.

In order to get a sense for the body of research on this topic, the Medline data base was searched from 1985 to 1995 using the keywords "biosensor" and "biocompatibility" separately, yielding 402 and 1536 papers, respectively. Confining the search to biosensor *and* biocompatibility yielded 3 papers. Broadening the search to sensor *and* biocompatibility yielded 12 English language papers that actually dealt with some aspect of biosensor biocompatibility. Extending the search back to 1966 and using various combinations of multiple key words (sensor, biosensor, in vivo, biofouling, biocompatibility, packaging, hemocompatibility, blood, blood compatibility, electrodes, subcutaneous, glucose, capsule and implant) identified 54 English language papers that at least mentioned the biocompatibility of biosensors. Not surprisingly, 36 of 54 papers were on glucose sensing. We also identified several recent reviews on the potential for closed loop glucose monitoring [7–13]. The two reviews by Fischer [8, 12] are particularly informative. Only one review specifically addressed glucose sensor biocompatibility [12], but just in a cursory fashion. The structure of the GO enzyme itself is described by Hecht et al. [3].

Of the papers retrieved, 24 examined some aspect of in vivo glucose sensor performance [12, 14–36], describing a total of 18 different sensors (Table 28-1). Fourteen sensors were needle-type (Figure 28-2), ten of which were GO coupled hydrogen peroxide electrodes (HPE), two were GO coupled oxygen electrodes (OE), one was a GO redox hydrogel electrode, and one was a metal-catalytic sensor that directly oxidized glucose at the working electrode. Two sensors were cathetcrized, microfabricated, planar GO HPE sensors, and two were GO HPE integrated into a sensor/transmitter packet. One needle-type sensor was connected via catheter to a transmitter. Fourteen sensors were implanted subcutaneously (SQ); four were implanted intravascularly (IV); one was implanted intraperitoneally (IP). Implantation subjects were dogs (seven), rats/mice (five), humans (five), sheep (two), and rabbits (one). Implant durations ranged over minutes (one), hours (five), days (five), weeks (five), months (four), and years (one).

Nineteen of 24 papers had either some description of the host response and/or analyzed the effect of implantation on sensor performance (Table 28-2). Only the studies of Pickup et al. [14], Moatti-Sirat et al. [21], Rebrin et al. [22], Clark et al. [23], Ertefai and Gough [26], Armour et al. [27], Gilligan et al. [31], Updike et al. [32] and Lager et al. [34] were reasonably serious in characterizing the in vivo response. The sensor/transmitter systems of Armour et al. and Updike et al. had perhaps the best in vivo results. Armour et al. had four of six sensors placed IV still functioning after 50, 62, 88 and 108 days. The three sensors implanted SQ by Updike et al. functioned in vivo for 42, 83 and 94 days.

Although some success is evident from these studies, the fact remains that only the rare sensor survives longer than 10–14 days in vivo. Thus a comprehensive summary of findings of the studies in Tables 28-1 and 28-2 is as follows:

- Inflammatory cells bind to and degrade sensor performance.
- Protein adsorption hinders sensor function by lowering permeability to glucose and/or oxygen.
- Fibrous tissue and exogenous pool of FBC presents a transport barrier to glucose.

Table 28-1 In Vivo Studies of Glucose Sensors

Reference	Sensor type	Implantation site and duration	Tissue/biofluid contacting materials
Fischer et al. [12]	Needle-type GO HPE	SQ in necks of non-diabetic dogs for up to 20 h.	PU or regenerated cellulose outermost sensing membrane. Insulation material not specified.
Pickup et al. [14]	Needle-type GO HPE	SQ in abdomen of non-diabetic humans for up to 5 h.	PU outermost sensing membrane. Nylon insulation.
Kerner et al. [15]	Needle-type GO HPE	SQ in abdomen of diabetic humans for 15 h.	PU outermost sensing membrane. Teflon insulation.
Poitout et al. [16]	Needle-type GO HPE	SQ in forearm of non-diabetic humans for 15 h.	PU outermost sensing membrane. Teflon insulation.
Moussy et al. [17–19]	Needle-type GO HPE	SQ in non-diabetic dogs for 10–14 d [20, 22]; IV jugular vein of non-diabetic dogs for 14 d. [31]	Nafion outermost coating of entire sensor.
Shichiri et al. [20]	Needle-type GO HPE	SQ intrascapular of non-diabetic humans for 3 d.	PU/PVA laminate outermost sensing membrane. Insulation material not specified.
Moatti-Sirat et al. [21]	Needle-type GO HPE	SQ intrascapular of non-diabetic rats up to 10 d.	GO/CA outermost sensing membrane. Telfon insulation.
Rebrin et al. [22]	Needle-type GO HPE	SQ into neck of normal and non-diabetic dogs for up to 4 d.	Regenerated cellulose outermost sensing membrane. CA or PU electrode insulation.
Clark et al. [23]	Needle-type GO HPE	IP in non-diabetic mice for up to 600 d.	Cellulose outermost sensing membrane. SR insulation.
Ammon et al. [24]; Eisele et al. [25]	Needle-type GO HPE	IV in jugular vein of non-diabetic rat for up to 3 d.	Bacterial-derived cellulose or wood-derived cellulose outer most sensing membrane. Insulating layer not specified.
Ertefai & Gough [26]	Needle-type GO OE	SQ in dorsal viewing chamber in rat skin fold for 10 d.	GO/albumin gel outermost sensing membrane. SR catheter encases electrodes.
Armour et al. [7]	Needle-type GO/catalase OE with SQ transmitter or percutanous	IV in vena cava of non-diabetic dogs for 1–15 wk.	Crosslinked albumin outermost sensing membrane. SR insulation.
Linke et al. [28]	Needle-type redox hydrogel electrode	SQ in neck of non-diabetic dogs for 3 d.	PC outermost sensing membrane. Teflon insulation.
Johnson et al. [29]	Microfabricated GO HPE	SQ intrascapular tissue of non-diabetic rabbits for 24 h. and SQ in abdomen of non-diabetic humans for 72 h.	PU outermost sensing membrane. PE insulation.
Bobbioni-Harsch et al. [30]	Microfabricated GO HPE	SQ intrascapular of diabetic rats for up to 8 d.	Sensor configuration not described.
Gilligan et al. [31]; Updike et al. [32]	GO HPE sensor/transmitter packet	SQ in paravertebral thoracic tissue of non-diabetic dogs for up to 3 months.	PU "glucose restriction" outer sensing membrane. PE insulation with velour outer coating.
Wilkins et al. [33]	GO HPE sensor/transmitter packet	SQ above shoulder in non-diabetic sheep for 50 min.	Nafion/PC outermost sensing membrane. Unspecified plastic insulation material.
Lagger et al. [34–36]	Needle-type metal-catalytic sensor (not a biosensor).	IV in of non-diabetic sheep for 71 d in carotid artery and 221 d in vena cava.	Pt working electrode covered with "hydrophilized" PTFE membrane. PU or SR insulation.

Table 28-2   In Vivo Sensor Performance and/or Biocompatibility

Reference	Comments pertaining to sensor biocompatibility
Gilligan et al. [31]	FBC of explanted sensors was vascularized on outermost layer and fibrous tissue was well integrated with Dacron or ePTFE velour shell of sensor. 2 of 8 sensors remained fully functional with ~7 min. lag times, indicating that interstitial fluid of FBC is accurate measure of plasma glucose levels. Remaining sensors either failed or exhibited loss of sensor sensitivity attributed to enzymatic degradation and/or biofouling of PU/GO sensing membrane. In some cases, sensitivity of sensors partially restored after explantation. Speculated that decreased vacularity of FBC over time may limit long term sensor performance.
Updike et al. [32]	Enzyme-active PU membranes implanted for 6–12 months SQ in dogs were explanted and tested in sensor, showing 30–80% of preimplantation sensitivity. 3 implanted sensors monitored glucose SQ for 42–94 d. Sensor response drops to near zero in first days following implantation, then rises over several days until it stabilizes. Sensor output monitored telemetrically exhibited lag times of 3–12 min. for accurately monitoring plasma levels. Dacron velour coating of sensor insulation integrated well with vascularized encapsulation tissue. Concludes mature SQ FBC is adequate monitoring site for implanted glucose sensor.
Fischer et al. [12]	Cellular and protein material depositing on sensor increases the diffusion barrier to glucose. Exudative fluid of FBC provides a diffusional barrier and has glucose level significantly lower than plasma level (contradicts introductory remark in same paper). Immunogenicity and sterilizability of sensor outermost membrane influences sensor stability. Reduced sensor size reduces histological reaction to implantation. Permanent skin puncture for SQ sensor provides infection site. Telemetric communication recommended to reduce infection.
Pickup et al. [14]	Only half (7 of 14) sensors responded to increases in plasma glucose level. In those that did respond, in vivo sensitivity dramatically and unpredictably reduced. Sensitivity restored upon explantation. Attributed loss of sensor activity to irreversible coating of proteins and cells at sensor tip. Good images of biofouling.
Kerner et al. [15]	2 of 6 sensors failed with blood clots forming at sensing tip. Response of failed sensors restored in buffer after clot removal. Remaining sensors showed lower sensitivities in plasma and SQ than in buffer. Sensitivity loss attributed to low mwt substances diffusing into PU outermost membrane.
Linke et al. [28]	Redox copolymer gel impregnated with GO deposited on Pt electrode. Gel eliminates sensor dependence on dissolved oxygen. In vivo sensitivity half that in plasma. 10 min. lag time observed between sensor response and change in plasma glucose level. Redox gel and polycarbonate outermost membrane not toxic to cultured cells.
Moussy et al. [17, 18]	Sensor connection percutaneous. Needle-type geometry chosen to minimize biological response. Heat curing of sensors at 120°C stabilized Nafion outermost coat and improved selectivity of sensor. 5–10 min. lag observed between plasma glucose level and sensor response. Lag time decreased after a few days, attributed to resorption of blood clots and formation of stable FBC. Mentioned that explanted sensors exhibited limited inflammatory response after 14 d, and FBC was nonfibrous and vascularized.
Shichiri et al. [20]	5 min. lag time in plasma increased to 13.5 min. in vivo. Increase attributed to protein deposition at sensor tip. Suggested addition of alginate/polyL outermost gel layer would reduce protein adsorption to sensing tip.
Ertefai & Gough [26]	6 min. in vitro lag time increased to 10–15 min. in vivo. FBC tissue surrounding electrodes remained well vascularized with maximum capillary density 75 μm from sensor. Good histological images of encapsulated sensor tip.

Table 28-2 *Continued*

Reference	Comments pertaining to sensor biocompatibility
Moatti-Sirat et al. [21]	Less than 5 min. lag time observed. Minimal sensitivity drift after 10 d in vivo. Miniaturized needle-type sensor invokes minimal wound healing response with little inflammation and considerable neovascularization. Fibrovascular tissue reaction surrounds sensor with few inflammatory cells. No correlation between preimplantation in vitro sensitivity and in vivo sensitivity, suggesting the importance of in situ sensor environment.
Rebrin et al. [22]	Sensor performance continuously degrades 20–40 h after implantation. All implant sites exhibited acute inflammatory reaction. Sensor performance not correlated to section of PU or CA packaging materials. Stability of sensors effected by fluctuations in glucose level caused by inflammatory reaction, i.e. interstitial glucose level at implant site 23% of plasma level. Exudative pool of FBC produces glucose diffusion barrier.
Lagger et al. [34–36]	In vivo sensor measurements differed from enzymatically measured glucose level by 3–6 mM. Some thrombus found at tip of explanted sensor thought to be caused by irregular surface texture. Implanted sensor caused no apparent damage to vessel wall. Sensor implanted in carotid artery for 71 d tested cross-sensitivity of sensor toward cysteine, aspirin and ethanol. No comment of biological response to sensor.
Armour et al. [27]	4 of 6 sensors functional at explantation. 1 telemetry pack lasted life of battery (28 d). Percutaneous sensor functioned 108 d. 3 sensors exhibited nearly same in vitro calibration curves before and after explantation. No adherent clots found on explanted sensors. Sensor tip with longest in vivo lag time (14 min.) had become adherent to vessel wall and encapsulated. Sensors freely floating in center of blood stream not encapsulated. SR sensor leads encapsulated with thin tissue layer that increased distally. Vigorous flow minimized thrombus formation and discouraged encapsulation. Thromboemboli mentioned as a potential problem, but not assessed.
Moussy et al. [19]	Catheterized sensor inserted in jugular vein through skin button in neck. Intravenous lag time of 15 min. was worse than acute SQ lag time of 3 min. Attributed increased lag time to blood pooled around sensing tip. Sensors followed plasma glucose level for 1 wk. Sensor failed after 2 wk. due to degradation of Ag/AgCl ref. electrode. 30–40 min. required for post-implantation in vivo sensor stabilization.
Ammon et al. [24]; Eisele et al. [25]	Measurements made through cannulated access to vein. Between measurements sensor removed, rinsed and placed in saline solution. Bacterial cellulose (BC) membrane adsorbed homogenous layer of albumin adsorption and showed less complement activation than Cuprophan membrane (Cup). Layered membranes with polyamid to increase diffusion resistance to glucose. Glucose sensitivity to in vitro blood samples dropped to 50% in 5 h with Cup membrane and in 25 h with BC membrane. BC coated sensors remained active in ex vivo measurements of venous glucose level over 3 d. Measurement accuracy unknown because independent glucose measurements not shown.
Clark et al. [23]	FBC of explanted sensors was thin, mostly fibrous near sensor membrane and mostly cellular near peritoneal space. Removal of FBC from explanted sensor significantly increased sensitivity and decreased response. Ratio of sensitivities measured before and after implantation and FBC removal decreased steadily with implantation time. Decrease attributed to mechanical microdefects or unknown substances in peritoneal fluid, however some retained activity for 500 days. All sensor responses measured in buffer.

- Vascularization of the foreign body capsule is necessary for good long-term stability of response.
- Sensors inactivated in vivo often regain function when FBC is removed and retested in vitro.
- Sensor baseline and sensitivity gradually degrade with implantation time.
- Sensor performance is erratic for the first hour and then becomes steady upon equilibration.
- SQ glucose levels lag behind plasma levels by 5–20 minutes.
- IV implantation gives immediate glucose readings but suffers from thrombus formation.
- IV implantation is best if the sensor is placed in fast-moving bloodstream.
- IP FBC is thinner than SQ.
- Textured coatings produce vascularized FBC that might ensure long-term SQ sensor accuracy.
- New protective membranes must be developed to improve in vivo sensor performance.
- Chronic percutaneous access sites heal poorly and are prone to infection.

Another interesting point is the apparent time course of in vivo sensor failure, which depends largely on the implant site and the aspect of the implant environment that is inducing failure. Again, we shall ignore component-based failure modes such as lead detachment and membrane delamination. Figure 28-3A shows the drop in the measured current for two different sensors of Kerner et al. [15] immersed in stirred, heparinized blood plasma doped with 5 mM glucose. These sensors exhibit what may be considered as a "classic" biofouling response with an initially rapid drop in sensor activity that tapers off and appears to be approaching steady state, which in this case is approximately 50 percent at 10 hours. It is easy to envision that this behavior results from the loading of the sensor membrane with proteins adsorbing from the plasma solution and progressively retarding analyte transport. For sensors intended for long-term use, it is necessary that they first "stabilize," meaning that the initial biofouling process has run its course without overly compromising sensor activity. Once stabilized, the sensor is then subject to a more-or-less stochastic process where the probability of failure increases steadily with time. Figure 28-3B is a plot from Clark et al. [23] showing the fractional loss in sensor activity as a function of IP implantation time for up to 600 days. In this case, the ratio of sensor currents to a 22 mM (400 Mg%) glucose buffer solution was measured before and after implantation (and FBC removal). Linear regression of the data in Figure 28-3B shows a 50 percent loss of activity would occur on the average at approximately 250 days. Clark et al. attributed the loss of sensor activity to degradative enzymes and inflammatory cells that enter the GO layer through cracks forming in the outer membrane. Interestingly, some of the sensors showed essentially no loss of activity (indicated by the dashed line) after prolonged implantation. It is important to note, however, that Clark et al. did not assess any aspect of in vivo sensor function in their study.

FACTORS THAT LIMIT IN VIVO SENSOR PERFORMANCE

The hope of developing reliable, long-term, indwelling glucose sensors seems to hinge on four key issues which we discuss below: reducing biofouling of tissue/biofluid contacting materials, engineering the wound healing tissue to make it less fibrous and/or more vascular,

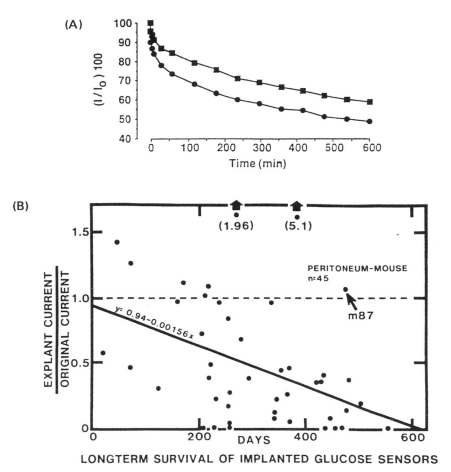

Figure 28-3 Time course of sensor failure: (A) Biofouling in blood. Relative decrease of sensor current (I/I_0) of two sensors immersed in stirred human plasma spiked with glucose. Decay of response attributed to accumulation of blood plasma proteins at the sensor tip. (Reprinted from Kerner W, Kiwit M, Linke B, Keck FS, Zier H, Pfeiffer EF, The function of a hydrogen peroxide-detecting electroenzymatic glucose electrode is markedly impaired in human sub-cutaneous tissue and plasma, *Biosensors and Bioelectronics*, 1993; 8:473–482. With permission.) (B) Decay of sensor function after long-term implantation. Relative response of sensor to in vitro glucose challenge before implantation and after explanation. (Reprinted from Clark LC, Spokane RB, Homan MM, Sudan R, Miller M, Long-term stability of electroenzymatic glucose sensors implanted in mice, ASAIO Trans, 1988; 34:259–265. With permission.)

developing totally implantable sensing systems that eliminate the need for percutaneous access, and performing real-time in vivo sensor recalibration.

Biofouling

Biofouling occurs at any sensor surface exposed to blood or tissue. The extent of biofouling is, in general, less pronounced in the peritoneal cavity or in subcutaneous tissue than in blood. Figure 28-4 provides an example of sensor tip biofouling from Pickup et al. [14] observed after 5 hours SQ implantation. The sensor with minimal biofouling (Figure 28-4B)

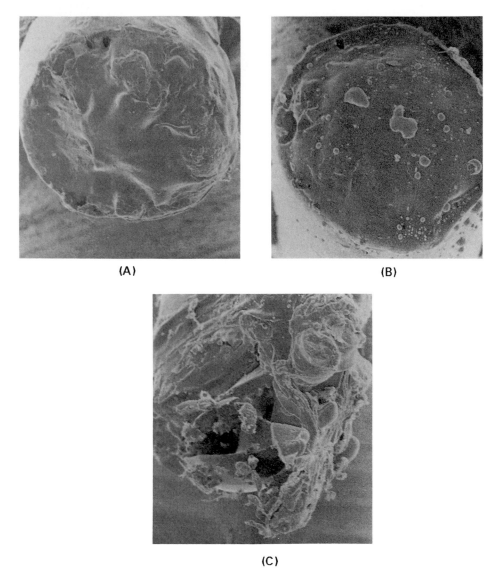

Figure 28-4 Scanning electron micrographs of tips of glucose sensors (ca. 150X): (A) control sensor soaked in buffered glucose and not implanted; (B) functioning sensor examined after 5 hours of implantation showing minimal biofouling; (C) non-functioning sensor examined after 5 hours of implantation showing significant protein and cellular accumulation. (Reprinted from Pickup JC, In vivo glucose monitoring: Sense and sensorability, *Acta Diabetol*, 1993; 30:143–148. With permission.)

was still functioning at explantation. The sensor with significant biofouling (Figure 28-4C) had failed during implantation. The other image (Figure 28-4A) is of a sensor tip prior to implantation.

In our previous treatments of bio/sensocompatibility [4, 6], we reviewed the surface modification schemes designed to enhance sensor biocompatibility as well as the methods used to minimize biofouling of chemically selective transducer surfaces after implantation. In comparison to other areas of biomaterials, very little surface modification work has been done with sensors. A key reason for this is that modifying the transducer surface may adversely affect the sensor's response [4]. For example, co-immobilization of an anti-fouling agent with a receptor protein may reduce the receptor surface loading or sterically hinder receptor-ligand binding. Similarly, the addition of an anti-fouling overlayer may increase the analyte transport barrier, either reducing sensitivity or increasing response time.

Table 28-1 lists the insulating and the outermost sensing layers of the in vivo glucose sensor studies. Not surprisingly, PE, PTFE and SR are the primary insulation materials, and PU and cellulose-based membranes were used most to cover the sensing region. Many such as Updike et al. [32] have added a PU glucose restriction membrane to reduce glucose transport and thus eliminate parasitic dependence on dissolved oxygen levels. Only in a few cases were the outer membranes modified to improve sensor performance. Linke et al. [28] entrapped GO in a redox hydrogel that directly communicates between GO and the Pt electrode, thus eliminating the need to measure hydrogen peroxide production or oxygen consumption. The tissue compatibility of this redox gel layer was assessed in tissue culture. Wilkins et al. [33] and Moussy et al. [17–19] introduced coatings of Nafion, a fluorinated isonomer, to reduce biofouling of the sensing surface and reduce interference from urate and ascorbate. However, Nafion has yet to be shown superior to PU or SR membranes. Shichiri et al. [20] suggested an additional layer of alginate/polylysine gel at the sensor to reduce protein adsorption, but they did not implement this recommendation. Shaw et al. [37] coated their glucose sensors with a layer of PHEMA/PU with the intent of improving biocompatibility, but only tested their devices in buffer solution.

Attempts to improve sensor blood compatibility are even less evident. Armour et al. [27], whose IV sensors functioned in vivo for up to 108 days, coated their sensor tips with crosslinked albumin. This group attempted to minimize thrombus formation on their sensors by placing them in the fast-moving bloodstream of the vena cava. Ammon et al. [24, 25] showed that bacterially derived cellulose membranes, with their more hydrogel-like character, are superior to Cuprophane (a wood-based cellulose) for reducing sensor biofouling in blood. Similar to the findings of Kerner et al. [5], the cellulose-coated sensors decayed to 50% of their original activity in blood after 25 hours. Although not studying biosensors per se, Cosofret et al. [38] attempted to improve the blood compatibility of their K^+ and pH ion-selective membrane sensors by coating them with a protective layer of PHEMA hydrogel. The blood compatibility of gel-coated sensors were assessed by immersing them in refrigerated, heparinized, whole blood plasma and periodically testing the sensor sensitivity and selectivity. Approximately 20 percent and 40 percent of the pH and K^+ gel-coated sensors, respectively, failed after 14 days immersion.

The biomaterials community is beginning to join forces with the sensor community to more seriously address the issue of sensor biocompatibility. Hubbell recently reported the effect of coating one of Heller's redox hydrogel sensors with a PHEMA/PEG copolymer [39]. In this study, the layer of copolymer was photopolymerized on top of the redox hydrogel at the tip of a needle-type sensor. The sensor was implanted SQ in the intrascapular tissue of rats for 3 days to examine whether this coating affected protein adsorption, cellular attachment and tissue encapsulation. Explanted gel-coated sensors had significantly reduced fibrous tissue encapsulation and did not cause noticeable inflammation or tissue necrosis. Uncoated sensors were completely encapsulated by fibrous tissue. A similar team was formed when the inflammation reaction to Buck's K^+ and pH ion selective membrane sensors was assessed using the stainless steel cage implant model of Marchant and Anderson [40]. The effect of sensing membrane plasticizer content and the application of a PHEMA hydrogel coating were examined by placing specimens in cages and implanting them in the dorsal rat subcutis. Using empty cages as controls, this model exposes the implant to exudate and inflammatory cells, but protects the device from direct contact with wound healing tissue. In addition to examining cellular and protein accumulation on the explanted sensor, this system allows one to periodically withdraw aliquots of exudate, and thus quantitatively and temporally assess the inflammatory reaction to the cage with implant.

Unfortunately, neither team examined the in vivo sensor response or the altered response of the explanted sensor, thus ignoring the functional aspect of sensor biocompatibility. The caged implant system could, however, provide an excellent means of examining a functioning sensor in vivo. To our knowledge, this set of experiments has not been conducted.

Fibrous Capsule Formation

Blood-borne analytes are most accurately monitored in the vascular lumen; however, IV placement is surgically risky and requires percutaneous venipuncture. Moreover, the combined impact of thrombosis, emboli formation, immune reaction, septicemia, and wound healing creates a very aggressive sensor environment [9]. Consequently, most indwelling glucose sensors are designed for SQ use where the surgical placement is simpler and the device has only to survive hemostasis and acute inflammation before it is enveloped in a FBC that becomes increasingly fibrous with time.

Figure 28-5 is a histological section from Ertefai and Gough [26] showing FBC formation around a glucose electrode after 10 days of SQ implantation. The fibrous connective

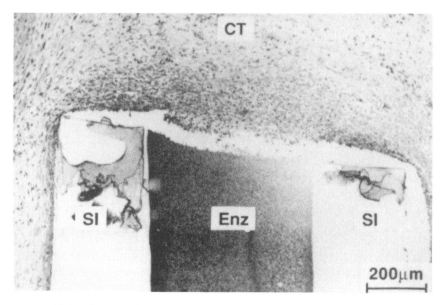

Figure 28-5   Light micrograph image of glucose sensor tip after 10 days of implantation in subcutis. Note dense connective tissue (CT) of FBC surrounds sensor, but is separated from sensor tip by a pool of exudate. Enz denotes enzyme layer. SI denotes remnants of the silicon rubber housing that disintegrated during sample fixation. (Reprinted from Ertefai S, Gough DA, Physiological preparation for studying the response of subcutaneously implanted glucose and oxygen sensors, *J Biomed Eng*, 1989; 11:362–368. With permission.)

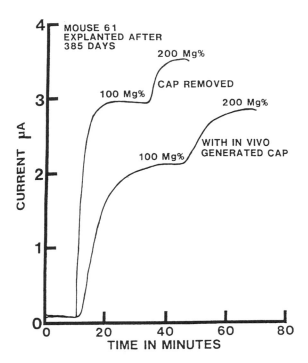

Figure 28-6 Example of how FBC can impede analyte transport and thus compromise sensor function. Sensor was removed after 385 days of implantation and tested against buffered glucose solutions before and after FBC removal. Mg% denotes mg/dL of glucose. Note that FBC removal increases sensor response and reduces sensor response time.

tissue (CT) of the FBC that surrounds the sensor is separated from the sensing tip of the electrode by a few microns of interspacial fluid. For glucose to be detected by this sensor, it must exit a capillary and then serially diffuse through subcutis, the fibrous connective tissue, and the exudate fluid before reaching the surface of the implanted sensor. While providing a relatively stable sensor environment, the absence of capillaries, the fibrous content of the FBC, and the fluid pocket all retard analyte transport to the sensor surface. Figure 28-6 from Clark et al. [23] provides an excellent in vitro illustration of how the FBC can affect sensor response by comparing measurements made by an explanted glucose electrode before and after FBC removal. Specifically, sensor current was measured to a serial sampling of 5.5 mM (100 Mg%) and 11 mM (200 Mg%) glucose buffer solutions. In the case of the 100 Mg% glucose challenge, FBC removal increased the measured current by 50% and decreased response time twofold. This difference clearly results from the additional transport barrier imposed by the capsular tissue.

According to Woo and Henry [41], it is "unanimously agreed" that the glucose level measured SQ lags behind blood glucose levels by 5–15 minutes. The diffusion of glucose from capillaries into the SQ space is responsible for approximately 5–7 minutes of this delay. The FBC that forms around a sensor can increase the lag time by an additional 5–7 minutes [6]. This problem was articulated nearly 15 years ago by Woodward [42] who reasoned that the best tissue environment for an indwelling glucose sensor is a vascularized one. In brief, smooth-surfaced, non-degradable implants are destined to be encapsulated by a densely fibrous and avascular FBC, whereas porous or textured, non-degradable implants are encapsulated with highly vascular granulation tissue for up to several months. Since

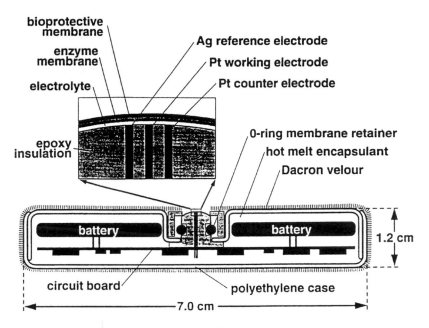

Figure 28-7 Schematic cross section of a totally implantable glucose sensor/transmitter system. Note Dacron™ velour added around sensor housing for tissue integration and smooth polyurethane bioprotective membrane that covers enzyme layer, electrolyte layer and electrodes encased in epoxy. (Reprinted from Gilligan BJ, Rhodes RK, Shults MC, Updike SJ, Evaluation of a subcutaneous glucose sensor out to 3 months in a dog model, *Diabetes Care*, 1994; 17:882–887. With permission.)

sensors normally have smooth surfaces, Woodward recommended that sensors be embedded in non-degradable porous polymer sponges to produce a vascularized, wound-healing tissue.

Porous textiles like Dacron® and Teflon® (E. I DuPont de Nemours & Co., Inc., Wilmington, DE) felts and velours have long been used as tissue integration patches for prosthetics like breast implants and percutaneous skin buttons [5]. Figure 28-7 is a schematic cross-section of the sensor/transmitter device of Gilligan et al. and Updike et al. [31, 32] showing a Dacron® velour with 90-micron pore size that surrounds the sensor housing. The implanted sensors became stable 4–18 days after implantation, which was attributed to a well-vascularized FBC providing "sufficient blood supply to support the needs of their sensor." Examination of the explanted sensors indeed showed a vascularized FBC that was "tightly attached to the Dacron coating . . . and had no attachment to the sensor membrane." Note that smooth-surfaced implants like those used by Armour et al. [27] are more desirable for IV applications because textured surfaces are likely to become matted with thrombus that fouls the sensor and/or breaks away as thromboemboli. This is not to say, however, that a smooth surface will eliminate this problem.

The concept of texture-induced changes in the FBC was further elaborated upon by Campbell and von Recum [43] who showed that implants with 1–3-micron pore sizes produced pronouncably thinner capsular tissue than did either smooth implants or implants of larger pore size. Sharkawy et al. [44] recently characterized the transport properties of the FBC that formed around smooth and porous implants. It was found that after 4 weeks SQ implantation in rats, the smooth-surfaced implants produced densely fibrous and avascular

FBCs, while the porous implants produced less fibrous and vascularized FBCs. It was also observed that a model analyte diffused twice as slowly through smooth-surfaced implant FBCs than it did through porous implant FBCs and through normal subcutis. Brauker et al. [45] showed that FBC capillary density varied in porous implants with greater than 0.8-micron pore size. They also demonstrated that the vascularization is stable and can persist for prolonged periods. A proprietary expanded PTFE bilayer membrane with an outer tissue integration layer of micron-sized porosity and a sub-micron porosity inner immunoisolation layer is currently being developed by Brauker and coworkers to support insulin-producing beta cells in a small subcutaneously implanted pouch [46]. This bilayer pouch becomes encapsulated with a well-vascularized FBC, and has been capable of gluco-regulating diabetic animals for more than a year. Such a pouch-like structure could prove useful for tissue integration layers of implantable sensors.

Percutaneous Access

A significant problem that remains with implantable sensors is that sites of percutaneous access are excellent routes for infection. The best solution to this problem is transcuta-neous telemetric monitoring of sensor response. Again, the device of Gilligan et al. and Updike et al. (Fig. 28-7) provides an example of a sensor/transmitter where both com-ponents are integrated into a single packet. Armour et al. [27] and Wilkins et al. [33] have developed sensor/transmitter devices in which the two components are separated, in one case via a catheterized lead and by radio in the other. One of three devices im-planted by Updike et al., and three of five devices implanted by Armour et al., failed due to problems with the transmitter. The problems cited were battery discharge, encasement leakage, and component failure. The in vivo measurements of Wilkins et al. were too short to tax the transmitter. In spite of the success experienced with smart pacemakers, the analogously reliable sensor/transmitter system is yet to be realized. Unfortunately, a sen-sor/transmitter system can function telemetrically only as a complete package. Thus, even if transmitter component failure is eliminated as a problem (a likely prospect), one still has to contend with the less reliable sensor which is the Achilles heel of the totally implantable concept.

Real-Time Sensor Recalibration

The general method for calibrating for glucose sensors occurs in two stages. Prior to implantation, a pre-calibration is conducted by measuring sensor current against known in vitro glucose standards, usually in buffered solution. After implantation, the in vivo sensor response is checked by performing a glucose tolerance test (administering a load of glucose) that is monitored by the sensor and independently verified by determining the glucose level of withdrawn blood samples. The sensitivity drift of the implanted sensor is periodically determined by taking independent measurements of blood glucose level and adjusting the monitor used to convert sensor current to glucose concentration. If the sen-sor drift occurs slowly or consistently, then performing occasional sensitivity checks is a feasible solution. However, if the sensor drift is erratic, then the frequency of calibration checks obviates the advantage of an implantable glucose sensor. Thus, one cannot rely upon a recalibration scheme to make up for a sensor that does not behave in a predictable and con-sistent manner in vivo. If the sensor communicates via a transmitter, and if the transmitter gives glucose levels directly, then the transmitter must be capable of in situ adjustment.

Poitout et al. [16] and Pickup et al. [14] both describe linear two-point algorithms intended eventually for in situ sensor recalibration without having to repeatedly draw blood samples. In both cases, the current corresponding to a baseline plasma glucose level is recorded along with the maximum current measured after a known amount of glucose has been administered to the patient. Plotting the baseline current and maximum current (I_b, I_{max}) on the ordinate and the baseline and maximum blood glucose levels on the abscissa (C_b, C_{max}) yields a straight line with a slope and y-intercept equal to the sensor sensitivity and background current, respectively. Assuming that C_b and C_{max} are constant and need only be determined at the outset, then periodic determination of I_b and I_{max} can be used to assess shifts in sensor sensitivity (proportional to shifts in slope) and baseline current (proportional to shifts in y-intercept).

Wilkins et al. [33] alternatively proposed addressing what they felt is the primary cause of the sensor drift: degradation of the enzyme layer. Rather than repetitively recalibrating a continuously degrading device, their device has inlet and outlet "recharge tubes" for removing spent enzyme and replacing it with fresh enzyme. The recharging is accomplished without removing the device via extracorporeal septa.

RECOMMENDATIONS

In spite of the fact that the technology exists for an artificial pancreas, the current state of bio/sensocompatibility prevents these devices from becoming functionally suitable for long-term implantation. Even when confined to real-time glucose monitoring, with its potential $100 billion plus market, the approaches toward preventing or assessing biocompatibility are rather ordinary. Suffice it to say that the race between the artificial pancreas, with its glucose sensor, and the bioartificial pancreas, with its transplanted beta cells [47], may be won or lost solving biosensocompatibility problem (or ultimately the biomaterial/biocompatibility problem).

How can the biosensocompatibility of these devices be improved? First of all, a paradigm shift is necessary to prevent us from expecting different results when we do the same things over and over again. For example, be assured that an SQ implanted needle-type GO HPE with a PU outer membrane (Table 28-1) will function reasonably well for 10–14 days, or possibly even up to a month, in vivo, and then fail. Sharkawy et al. [6] describe novel design considerations that may result in improved sensor performance. Second, new and better materials are needed primarily for the membranes that protect the sensing surfaces. At the very least, a more rigorous investigation of surface modification of conventional materials should be investigated. Some very interesting results currently being obtained on hydrogel or protein modification of polymers may prove relevant to biosensocompatibility. Third, more proactive means of "engineering" the wound healing process should be investigated. One possible reason for the "magical" period of 10–14 days may be that this is the typical time during which vascularized granulation tissue is replaced with fibrous connective tissue. Fourth, the overall approach toward assessing biosensor suitability for in vivo use needs to be conducted in a more hierarchical fashion.

A suggested scheme for biosensocompatibility assessment is presented in the flow chart of Figure 28-8. First, the sensor must withstand the rigors of sterilization. Second, the sensor must remain functional for up to a month in corrosive in vitro environments at physiological temperatures. Lindner et al. [48] and Cosofret et al. [38] display the appropriate testing sequence from buffer, to blood, to in vivo; however, the duration of the

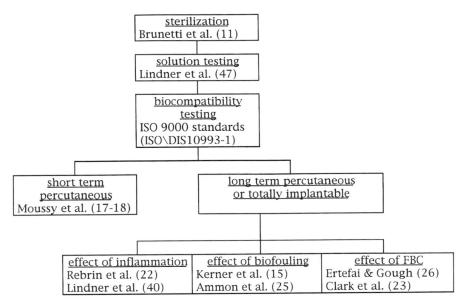

Figure 28-8 Flow chart of recommended approach toward assessing sensor biosensocompatibility. Referenced are illustrative examples of each category as they pertain to glucose sensors.

buffer studies were just minutes to hours. Third, the sensor must pass a standardized battery of preliminary biocompatibility tests (e.g., cytotoxicity, mutagenicity, clotting time, complement activation, biodegradation; see Sections III and IV). Fourth, it must be decided whether the sensor is intended for percutaneous or totally implantable use. For short-term percutaneous use, the current state of biosensor biocompatibility may be adequate, and effort should go into designing a device that is easily replaced when it begins to fail. This is the tack taken by Moussy [49] with his percutaneous/SQ needle-type sensor. For long-term percutaneous or totally implantable devices, however, one needs to take a hard look at in vivo sensocompatibility assessment.

In our view, sensocompatibility assessment really boils down to examining three categories: the effects of inflammation, biofouling, and the FBC on sensor performance. Figure 28-8 cites relevant examples for each category. The most effective approach towards in vivo characterization would employ a "bifunctional" implant system capable of tracking the host response to the sensor while simultaneously monitoring the sensor function. The dorsal viewing chamber of Ertefai and Gough [26] was designed for direct viewing of the tissue reaction to an implanted functioning sensor. Although not yet implemented with a "live" sensor, the caged implant model described by Marchant et al. [50] also has potential for simultaneous assessment SQ- and IP-implanted sensors. It may also be possible to use the cage concept to obtain in situ information on the diffusion of analyte through an FBC by periodically drawing aliquots of exogenous fluid. Developing the analogous bifunctional system for sensor characterization in blood would also be a useful, but a more challenging task.

ACKNOWLEDGMENTS

Financial support from the NSF Engineering Research Center grant CDR-8622201 is gratefully acknowledged. The literature survey of glucose sensors was conducted with thoroughness by Duke engineering undergraduate Ms. Ann Lam. We also gratefully acknowledge insightful discussions with Drs. Michael Neuman, Vasile Cosofret and Erno Lindner.

REFERENCES

1   Hall EAH. Biosensors. Englewood Cliffs, NJ: Prentice Hall, 1991.
2   Arnold MA, Meyerhoff ME. Recent advances in the development and analytical applications of biosensing probes. *CRC Crit Rev Anal Chem*, 20 (1988), 149–196.
3   Hecht HJ, Kalisz HM, Hendle J, Schmid RD, Schomberg D. Crystal structure of glucose oxidase from *Asperigus niger* refined at 2.3 Å resolution. *J Mol Biol*, 229 (1993), 153–172.
4   Reichert WM, Saavedra SS. Materials considerations in the selection, performance, and adhesion of polymeric encapsulants for implantable sensors. In Williams DF (Ed.), *Medical and Dental Materials*. New York: VCH Publishers, Inc., 1992, 303–343.
5   Park JB, Lakes RS. *Biomaterials*, 2nd ed. New York: Plenum Press, 1992.
6   Sharkawy AA, Neuman MR, Reichert WM. Sensocompatibility: Design considerations for biosensor-based drug delivery systems. In Park K (Ed.), *Controlled Drug Delivery: The Next Generation*. Washington, DC: American Chemical Society, in press.
7   Pfeiffer EF. The glucose sensor: The missing link in diabetes therapy. *Horm Metab Res Suppl*, 24 (1990), 154–164.
8   Fischer U. Fundamentals of glucose sensors. *Diabetic Medicine*, 8 (1991), 309–321.
9   Reach G, Wilson GS. Can continuous glucose monitoring be used for the treatment of diabetes? *Anal Chem*, 64 (1992), 381A–368A.
10 Pickup JC. In vivo glucose monitoring: Sense and sensorability. *Diabetes Care*, 16 (1993), 535–539.
11 Brunetti P, Massi-Benedetti M, Calabrese G, Reboldi GP. Closed-loop delivery systems for insulin therapy. *Int J Artif Organs*, 1991, 216–226.
12 Fischer U, Rebrin K, van Woedtke T, Abel P. Clinical usefulness of the glucose concentration in the subcutaneous tissue—Properties and pitfalls of electrochemical biosensors. *Horm Metab Res*, 26 (1994), 515–522.
13 Kyrolainen M, Rigsby P, Eddy S, Vadgama P. Bio-haemocompatibility: Implications and outcomes for sensors? *Acta Anasthe Scand*, 104 (1995), 55–60.
14 Pickup JC, Claremont DJ, Shaw GW. Responses and calibration of amperometric glucose sensors implanted in the subcutaneous tissue of man. *Acta Diabetol*, 30 (1993), 143–148.
15 Kerner W, Kiwit M, Linke B, Keck FS, Zier H, Pfeiffer EF. The function of a hydrogen peroxide-detecting electroenzymatic glucose electrode is markedly impaired in human sub-cutaneous tissue and plasma. *Biosensors and Bioelectronics*, 8 (1993), 473–482.
16 Poitout V, Moatti-Sirat D, Reach G, Zhang Y, Wilson GS, Lemonnier F, Klein JC. A glucose monitoring system for on-line estimation in man of blood glucose concentration using a miniaturized glucose sensor implanted in the subcutaneous tissue and a wearable control unit. *Diabetologia*, 36 (1993), 658–663.
17 Moussy F, Jakeway S, Harrison DJ, Rajotte RV. In vitro and in vivo performance and lifetime of perfluorinated ionomer-coated glucose sensors after high-temperature curing. *Analytical Chemistry*, 66 (1994), 3882–3888.
18 Moussy F, Harrison DJ, Rajotte RV. A miniaturized Nafion-based glucose sensor: In vitro and in vivo evaluation in dogs. *Internatl J Artif Org*, 17 (1994), 88–94.
19 Moussy F, Harrison DF, O'Brien DW, Rajotte RV. Performance of subcutaneously implanted needle-type glucose sensors employing a novel trilayer coating. *Anal Chem*, 65 (1993), 2072–2077.
20 Shichiri M, Yamasaki Y, Nao K, Sekiya M, Ueda N. In vivo characteristics of needle-type glucose sensor-measurements of subcutaneous glucose concentrations in human volunteers. *Horm Metab Res Suppl*, 20 (1988), 17–20.
21 Moatti-Sirat D, Capron F, Poitout V, Reach G, Bindra DS, Zhang Y, Wilson GS, Thévenot DR. Towards continuous glucose monitoring: in vivo evaluation of a miniaturized glucose sensor implanted for several days in rat subcutaneous tissue. *Diabetologia*, 35 (1992), 224–230.
22 Rebrin K, Fisher U, Hahn von Dorsche H, von Woetke T, Abel P, Brunstein E. Subcutaneous glucose monitoring by means of electrochemical sensors: Fiction or reality? *J Biomed Eng*, 14 (1992), 33–40.
23 Clark LC, Spokane RB, Homan MM, Sudan R, Miller M. Long-term stability of electroenzymatic glucose sensors implanted in mice. *ASAIO Trans*, 34 (1988), 259–265.

24 Ammon HPT, Ege W, Oppermann M, Göpel W, Eisele S. Improvement in the long-term stability of an amperometric glucose sensor system by introducing a cellulose membrane of bacterial origin. *Anal Chem*, 67 (1995), 466–471.

25 Eisele S, Ammon HPT, Kindervater R, Gröbe A, Göpel W. Optimized biosensor for whole blood measurements using a new cellulose-based membrane. *Biosensors and Bioelectronics*, 9 (1994), 119–124.

26 Ertefai S, Gough DA. Physiological preparation for studying the response of subcutaneously implanted glucose and oxygen sensors. *J Biomed Eng*, 11 (1989), 362–368.

27 Armour JC, Lucisano JY, McKean BD, Gough DA. Application of chronic intravascular blood glucose sensor in dogs. *Diabetes*, 39 (1990), 1519–1526.

28 Linke B, Kerner W, Kiwit M, Pishko M, Heller A. Amperometric biosensor for in vivo glucose sensing based on glucose oxidase immobilized in a redox hydrogel. *Biosensors and Bioelectronics*, 9 (1994), 151–158.

29 Johnson KW, Mastrototaro JJ, Howey DC, Brunelle RL, Burden-Brady PL, Bryan NA, Andrew CC, Rowe HM, Allen DJ, Noffke BW, McMahan WC, Morff RJ, Lipson D, Nevin RS. In vivo evaluation of an electroenzymatic glucose sensor implanted in subcutaneous tissue. *Biosensors and Bioelectronics*, 7 (1992), 709–714.

30 Bobbioni-Harsch E, Rohner-Jeanrenaud F, Koudelka M, de Rooij N, Jeanrenaud B. Lifespan of subcutaneous glucose sensors and their performances during dynamic glycemia changes in rats. *J Biomed Eng*, 15 (1993), 457–463.

31 Gilligan BJ, Rhodes RK, Shults MC, Updike SJ. Evaluation of a subcutaneous glucose sensor out to 3 months in a dog model. *Diabetes Care*, 17 (1994), 882–887.

32 Updike SJ, Shults MC, Rhodes RK, Gilligan BJ, Luebow JO, von Heimburg D. Enzymatic glucose sensors, improved long-term performance in vitro and in vivo. *ASAIO J*, 40 (1994), 157–163.

33 Wilkins E, Atansov P, Muggenburg BA. Integrated implantable device for long-term glucose monitoring. *Biosensors and Bioelectronics*, 10 (1995), 485–494.

34 Lager W, von Lucadou I, Nischik H, Nowak T, Preidel W, Ruprecht L, Stanzel MJ, Tegeder V. Electrocatalytic glucose sensor for long-term in vivo use. *Int J Artif Org*, 17 (1994), 183–188.

35 Lager W, von Lucadou I, Nischik H, Nowak T, Preidel W, Ruprecht L, Stanzel MJ, Tegeder V. Implantable electrocatalytic glucose sensor. *Horm Metab Res*, 26 (1994), 526–530.

36 Lager W, von Lucadou I, Preidel W, Reprecht L, Saeger S. Electrocatalytic glucose sensor. *Med Biol Eng Comp*, 32 (1994), 247–252.

37 Shaw GW, Claremont DJ, Pickup JC. In vitro testing of a simply constructed, highly stable glucose sensor suitable for implantation in diabetic patients. *Biosensors and Bioelectronics*, 6 (1991), 401–406.

38 Cosofret VV, Erdosy M, Buck RP, Johnson TA, Bellinger DA, Buck RP, Ash RB, Neuman MR. Electroanalytical and surface characterization of encapsulated implantable membrane planar microsensors. *Analytica Chim Acta*, 314 (1995), 1–11.

39 Quinn CP, Pathak CP, Heller A, Hubbell JA. Photo-crosslinked copolymers of 2-hydroxyethyl methacrylate, poly(ethylene glycol) tetra-acrylate and ethylene dimethacrylate for improving biocompatibility of biosensors. *Biomaterials*, 16 (1995), 389–396.

40 Lindner E, Cosofret VV, Ufer S, Buck RP, Kao WJ, Neuman NR, Anderson JM. Ion-selective membranes with low plasticizer content: Electroanalytical characterization and biocompatibility studies. *J Biomed Mater Res*, 28 (1994), 591–601.

41 Woo J, Henry JB. The advance of technology as a prelude to the laboratory of the twenty-first century. *Clin Laboratory Med*, 14 (1994), 459–471.

42 Woodward SC. How fibroblasts and giant cells encapsulate implants: Considerations in design of glucose sensors. *Diabetes Care*, 5 (1982), 278–281.

43 Campbell CE, von Recum, AF. Microtopography and soft tissue response. *J Investigative Surg*, 2 (1989), 51–74.

44 Sharkawy AA, Klitzman B, Truskey GA, Reichert WM. Engineering the diffusion properties of tissue which encapsulates subcutaneous implants. *J Biomed Mater Res*, submitted.

45 Brauker, JH, Carr–Brendel VE, Martinson LA, Crudele J, Johnson WD, Johnson RC. Neovascularization of synthetic membranes directed by membrane microarchitecture. *J Biomed Mater Res*, 29 (1995), 1517–1524.

46 Brauker JH. Personal communication, 1995.

47 Bodziony J. Bioartificial endocrine pancreas: Foreign-body reaction and effectiveness of diffusional transport of insulin and oxygen after long-term implantation of hollow fibers into rats. *Res Exper Med*, 1992, 305–316.

48   Lindner E, Cosofret VV, Ufer S, Johnson, TA, Ash BR, Nagle HT, Neuman MR, Buck RP. In vivo and in vitro testing of microelectronically fabricated planar sensors designed for applications in cardiology. *Fresenuis J Anal Chem*, 346 (1993), 584–588.

49   Bionics for Diabetics. Interview with Dr. Francis Moussy. *AHFMR Newsletter*, June/July 1993, 5.

50   Marchant RE, Hiltner A, Hamlin C, Rabinovitch A, Slobodkin R, Anderson JM. In vivo biocompatibility studies. I. The cage implant system and a biodegradable hydrogel. *J Biomed Mater Res*, 17 (1983), 301–325.

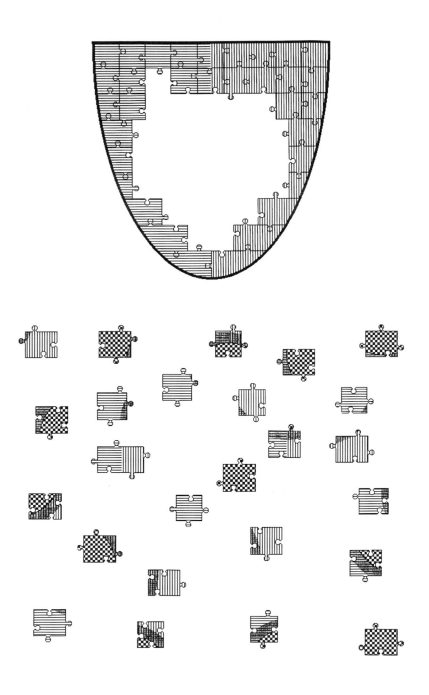

Section Six

Implantology

Andreas F. von Recum

INTRODUCTION: THE EVOLUTION OF IMPLANT DEVELOPMENT AND TESTING IN ANIMAL TRIALS

Evaluating surgical methods or implants in animals is a relatively recent concept in medicine. For centuries new procedures were tried immediately in patients and therefore, willingly or not, intended or not, many of them became a sacrifice to the goal of medical progress. From the 18th century onwards animals served more and more as surrogates for the study of anatomy and physiology but human experimentation proceeded well into the mid-twentieth century. Modern warfare produced increasing numbers of war victims that survived but needed replacement or repair of major body parts and functions. Since advancing technology was not only improving the destructive power of the war machinery but was also advancing technology for medical use, new materials and fabrication methods offered options for replacement or repair of body functions. As a direct consequence of these two developments, surgical research laboratories evolved in academic medical centers worldwide, the so-called "dog labs," which were used for surgical training and experimentation. For a historical review of this evolution I highly recommend Markowitz's *Experimental Surgery* which was published in many editions by Williams & Wilkins Company starting in 1937.

In the 1940s sudden advances were made in a variety of surgical disciplines initiating the development and testing of many prosthetic means including intra-ocular lenses, hip joints, vascular grafts, heart valves, blood transfusion, cardiopulmonary bypass, cardiac assist and replacement devices, dialysis, and fracture fixation and bone replacement devices. Almost all of these devices went through extensive animal testing and have long been accepted as very successful surgical treatment methods prolonging life and improving its quality in many millions of patients. Starting in the 1960s professional efficacy and general safety concerns generated scientific and governmental efforts to formalize bench trials and animal testing as a pre-requisites for the use of implantable materials and devices in patients (as presented in Section IX).

MAN'S CONCERN FOR ANIMALS IN BIOMEDICAL TESTING

During the same time frame the Western societies evolved an increasing concern for the well-being of companion animals. Opponents of the use of animals for medical research organized themselves and became a powerful lobby for their cause. As a direct result of their societal and political pressure, humane treatment of experimental animals was enforced through laws and regulations (see Chapter 29). This has resulted in significant reductions of animal experimentation. Most medical research centers have now abandoned their "dog labs" and no longer teach and practice surgical skills in live animals. But, at the same time, general health and quality of life of used experimental animals has been improved drastically and this has led to better research results with higher predictive power. Today's animal experiments, by decree, are highly focused prospective studies, guided by valid scientific queries, and concerned with the well-being of the test animal itself. Biocompatibility studies are predominately concerned with efficacy and safety testing in the common laboratory animals (see Chapter 30).

FACTORS INFLUENCING BIOCOMPATIBILITY RESULTS IN ANIMAL STUDIES

Sections I and II deal with the effect of material properties on biocompatibility and this effect needs to be established for every material and device in animals before the latter can be used in patients. Therefore Section VI focuses on animal testing. But beyond material properties there are other factors influencing biocompatibility outcome studies: *animal species* as generally treated in Chapter 30; *surgical knowledge and skills* as dealt with in Chapters 31, 32 and 33; *implantation site* and *implant function* as illustrated in Chapters 34, 35, and 36; and *test period* as treated in all the chapters of Section VI.

THE FUTURE OF BIOCOMPATIBILITY STUDIES IN ANIMALS

The last ten years have evidenced significant progress in biocompatibility research and this progress may allow us to venture that, within the next 10 years, the advances in the understanding of fundamentals of biocompatibility will lead to the development of truly (site- and function-specific) biocompatible materials. We may then realize that the modifying role of the experimental animal and the surgical technique may have little importance and that the natural healing power of tissue will be very forgiving and will quickly integrate the "acceptable" implant into its tissue bed as has been postulated by Brånemark's bone-specific term of "osteointegration" (see Chapter 36).

My personal research experience spans most of the above-described surgical research evolution. Based on my surgical career, I speculate that the experimental animal will remain the guarantor to mankind for efficacy and safety of surgical implants. However, many alternative research models are developing and will continue to evolve that can reduce the need for animal experiments and glean additional information on the principles and mechanistic interrelationships of biocompatibility. Such analytical models currently include cell and tissue culture studies (see Sections III and IV), cell genetic studies of explanted tissues (see Chapter 34), and micro-biological and gene-technological models (see Chapter 32). Researchers will undoubtedly rehabilitate animal trials to confirm the efficacy and safety of medical innovations for human use and benefit.

Chapter 29

Protection of Research Animals

Melvin B. Dennis, Jr.

RATIONALE FOR TESTING BIOMATERIALS IN ANIMALS

The process of development and licensing of biomaterials or implantable devices will invariably involve research or testing in animals at some point. Even when research and development begins in vitro, animal studies are eventually required to assess safety, efficacy, and interactions with the intact, living organism. The approval process for devices requires testing in animals prior to testing in humans. These requirements are designed to protect people from exposure to ineffective or dangerous agents. They have evolved as a result of problems encountered with using human subjects for research and development studies. The problems were rooted in lack of informed consent, coercion of subjects, and use of prisoners, handicapped, or indigent people in studies of untested ideas. The most notorious incidents were brought to light in the investigation of Nazi atrocities following World War II and resulted in the Nuremburg Code which stated that any experiments on humans "should be designed and based on results of animal experimentation." The concept was reinforced in the Helsinki Declaration, adopted by the 18th World Medical Assembly in 1964, and revised in 1975. It states that medical research on human subjects "should be based on adequately performed laboratory and animal experimentation."

Dependence upon animal testing is due, in part, to the large disparity between what is testable in non-animal models and the degree of assurance of safety and efficacy that is necessary to begin testing in people. There is interest in replacing animal studies with computer models and other in vitro methods. There is even discussion regarding use of tissue from aborted human fetuses for research purposes. This concept is very controversial, with some arguing that it would diminish the need for using animals and others asserting that unborn fetuses have a right to the same protection as they would have after birth. At the present time, safety and efficacy must ultimately be tested in intact animals.

One of the few examples of alternatives replacing intact animals in testing is the assay for endotoxin in which rabbits have been replaced by the limulus lysate test [1]. However, animal testing continues to be required to determine biocompatibility, safety, and efficacy of implant devices and materials prior to testing in human beings until better alternative tests are devised.

The amount of testing required prior to human trials is expanding. The investigator with a promising new device or material has a daunting task to accumulate the data necessary to obtain permission to begin clinical testing. The proliferation of requirements comes from experiences such as those encountered with the drug thalidomide, which was cleared for human use in Europe without any teratogenicity studies in animals. When pregnant women took the drug, it produced severe birth defects. Opponents of the use of animals for research have used the incident to argue that the animal testing that was done failed to predict the problems that occurred in humans and are, therefore, a waste of money, time, and animal lives. However, subsequent research showed that proper teratogenicity studies in animals would have predicted the problems that were encountered. The thalidomide episode illustrates the danger of allowing a drug to be used without complete testing [2].

ETHICAL CONSIDERATIONS OF ANIMAL USE

The use of animals in research, teaching, and testing is a subject of considerable controversy. Views range from the belief that animals have the same rights as humans to the belief that animals have no rights at all. The former assert that it is a violation of an animal's rights even to keep it as a pet, and the latter maintain that animals can be used and exploited without regard for humane considerations. The majority of people have views somewhere between these extreme views. Toward the center of the spectrum are those who believe that in questions about the use of animals in research, one must consider the cost-benefit ratio of studies. These people weigh the value of the information that will be learned against any pain or distress to the animals being studied. They believe that animals may be used to benefit people and other animals, but that humans have a stewardship obligation to the animals. There is considerable agreement in both the scientific community and the population at large regarding the duty to ensure laboratory animals are treated in a humane fashion. As a result, research animals are protected by regulations and guidelines to ensure their humane treatment.

The Interagency Research Animal Committee in the U.S. has provided guidance for the proper use of animals in research, teaching, and testing supported by government funds. It published the *U.S. Government Principles for the Utilization and Care of Vertebrate Animals Used in Testing, Research, and Training* in the Public Health Services (PHS) Policy and the *Guide for the Care and Use of Laboratory Animals*. They are also presented in Table 29-1. Animal use should be designed so as to conform to these principles.

The 3-R's of Animal Research

Russell and Burch [3] proposed the 3-Rs of animal research (refinement, replacement, and reduction) as guiding principles when using animals in research, teaching, and testing. Refinement refers to methods used to minimize pain and distress, such as anesthesia and analgesia. In the LD50 test in which death is the end-point of the study, animals are required to suffer through the agonal process. Refinements such as the "Limit Test" involve selecting end-points earlier than death, so that animals can be euthanized when they become comatose or when body temperature drops to certain levels [4]. Refinement also refers to the design of studies so as to maximize the data collected from each animal. An example of this is use of crossover study design, so that animals can act as their own controls.

Reduction refers to methods to decrease the numbers of animals required for a study. Examples include selecting test animals within tight limits of age, weight, sex, and genetic variability to cut down the scatter of data and achieve statistical significance with smaller numbers. Reducing numbers can also be accomplished by consultation with a statistician to ensure proper sample size and statistical analysis. It is good to remember that it can be more wasteful to use too few animals as to use too many, if the results fail to achieve statistical significance.

Replacement of animals can be accomplished by substitution of in vitro for in vivo studies. Some researchers resist the use of in vitro replacement tests; they privilege certain animals for a study simply because they consider those animals to be more like humans.

Table 29-1   U.S. Government Principles for the Utilization and Care of Vertebrate Animals Used in Testing, Research, and Training

The development of knowledge necessary for the improvement of the health and well-being of humans as well as other animals requires in vivo experimentation with a wide variety of animal species. Whenever U.S. Government agencies develop requirements for testing, research, or training procedures involving the use of vertebrate animals, the following principles shall be considered; and whenever these agencies actually perform or sponsor such procedures, the responsible Institutional Official shall ensure that these principles are adhered to:

I   The transportation, care, and use of animals should be in accordance with the Animal Welfare Act (7 U.S.C. 2131 et seq.) and other applicable Federal laws, guidelines, and policies.

II   Procedures involving animals should be designed and performed with due consideration of their relevance to human or animal health, the advancement of knowledge, or the good of society.

III   The animals selected for a procedure should be of an appropriate species and quality and the minimum number required to obtain valid results. Methods such as mathematical models, computer simulation, and in vitro biological systems should be considered.

IV   Proper use of animals, including the avoidance or minimization of discomfort, distress, and pain when consistent with sound scientific practices, is imperative. Unless the contrary is established, investigators should consider that procedures that cause pain or distress in human beings may cause pain or distress in other animals.

V   Procedures with animals that may cause more than momentary or slight pain or distress should be performed with appropriate sedation, analgesia, or anesthesia. Surgical or other painful procedures should not be performed on unanesthetized animals paralyzed by chemical agents.

VI   Animals that would otherwise suffer severe or chronic pain or distress that cannot be relieved should be painlessly killed at the end of the procedure or, if appropriate, during the procedure.

VII   The living conditions of animals should be appropriate for their species and contribute to their health and comfort. Normally, the housing, feeding, and care of all animals used for biomedical purposes must be directed by a veterinarian or other scientist trained and experienced in the proper care, handling, and use of the species being maintained or studied. In any case, veterinary care shall be provided as indicated.

VIII   Investigators and other personnel shall be appropriately qualified and experienced for conducting procedures on living animals. Adequate arrangements shall be made for their in-service training, including the proper and humane care and use of laboratory animals.

IX   Where exceptions are required in relation to the provisions of these principles, the decisions should not rest with the investigators directly concerned but should be made, with due regard to Principle II, by an appropriate review group such as an institutional animal care and use committee. Such exceptions should not be made solely for the purposes of teaching or demonstration.

Mammalian models are preferred for toxicity testing, which in this view must comprise an exhaustive search for ways in which a chemical might be toxic, even in ways that cannot yet be imagined. This bias is called the "High Fidelity Fallacy" by Russell and Burch [5]. However, contrary to this opinion, replacement can be effectively accomplished in the testing of biomaterials by limiting animal testing to those materials and devices that have shown promise in preliminary in vitro studies. An alternative in vitro screening test does not need to meet the rigid criteria of a definitive test. It can be designed to answer fewer and less complex questions. The definitive animal tests could be limited to those devices that appear safe to tissue culture cells.

Studies in which animals are euthanized to provide cells for tissue culture or organs for ex vivo a experiments are referred to as "relative replacement," because higher animals are used as the source. Studies in which higher animals are not required at any stage are said to be "absolute replacements." The limulus lysate test, in which amebocytes harvested from horseshoe crabs are used instead of rabbits to test for pyrogenicity, is an absolute replacement.

The desire to replace animals in the testing of cosmetics led the European Economic Community Council of Ministers to approve the 6th amendment to Directive 76/768/EEC, on June 14, 1993. It bans testing of cosmetics on animals as of January 1, 1998, unless alternative methods have not been scientifically validated [6].

REGULATIONS PROTECTING LABORATORY ANIMALS

In the United States, laboratory animals are protected by a series of laws, regulations, and guidelines to ensure humane care and use. Because regulations from different agencies can appear to be in conflict with each other, the investigator is faced with a formidable task to understand and comply with all of them. However, the investigator can generally comply by ensuring that every procedure performed on animals is approved by the local Institutional Animal Care and Use Committee (IACUC), because it is charged with ensuring compliance. In a situation where a deviation from the provisions of regulations and guidelines is required in order to accomplish a study, the IACUC can approve an exception if the investigator provides adequate scientific justification. The investigator should contact the IACUC prior to starting studies to learn the local procedures for acquiring training and approval to use animals. It is also imperative that the investigator remain in communication with the IACUC throughout the study because of requirements that any significant changes to a protocol be approved.

Animal Welfare Act

The Animal Welfare Act of 1966, as amended in 1970, 1976, and 1985, directed the Secretary of the U.S. Department of Agriculture (USDA) to promulgate regulations governing the use of animals in research, teaching, and testing. The regulations [7] apply to all warm-blooded animals, alive or dead, which are used in research, teaching, and testing, except for birds, rats, mice, and horses and farm animals used in studies to improve production of food and fiber.

Research laboratories are required to register with the USDA and to adhere to published standards for the care of animals. The regulations also require research institutions to obtain dogs and cats only from dealers licensed by the USDA. An IACUC of at least 3 members, including an attending veterinarian, is required for each research institution. The law also requires an annual report to the Secretary of the USDA to certify the facility uses acceptable standards in the care and treatment of animals, report the total number of animals used, and list the numbers used in activities involving pain or distress and for which anesthetic, analgesic, or tranquilizing drugs were not administered. The justification for withholding of such agents must also be explained.

The USDA regulations prescribe requirements for employees, facilities, cages, feed, water, sanitation, grouping of animals, veterinary care, and transportation. They require that alternatives to animal use be considered and that studies not be unnecessarily duplicative. They stipulate that institutions provide training for personnel performing animal use procedures. The regulations also require development of a plan for environment enhancement to promote psychological well-being of nonhuman primates and a plan to provide dogs with the opportunity for exercise.

Public Health Service Policy

The Public Health Service Policy on Humane Care and Use of Laboratory Animals [8] applies to institutions receiving PHS awards for studies using vertebrate animals. It requires institutions to provide written assurance to the Office for Protection from Research Risks (OPRR) that they are committed to follow the *Guide for the Care and Use of Laboratory Animals* [9]. The policy requires an IACUC of at least 5 members to oversee animal facilities and procedures.

Guide for the Care and Use of Laboratory Animals. The *Guide for the Care and Use of Laboratory Animals* [9] was prepared by a committee of the National Research Council to provide information on proper methods of oversight, husbandry, and veterinary care of animals used in teaching, testing, and research. Its recommendations regarding methods and practices are advisory in nature and are subject to professional judgment in their application. The latest edition is dated 1985, but a proposed 1996 revision has been published.

The *Guide* recommends that the attending veterinarian provide a program of adequate veterinary care. The American College of Laboratory Animal Medicine has stated that such programs should include daily observation of all animals; programs for the detection, surveillance, prevention, diagnosis, and treatment of disease; monitoring of handling and restraint; proper use of anesthetics and analgesics; and proper euthanasia [10].

Endangered Species Act

The Endangered Species Act of 1973 requires a permit from the Department of Interior Fish and Wildlife Service in order to import or use animals listed as endangered. Unless there is compelling scientific justification, animals on the endangered species list should be avoided when planning biomaterials evaluations.

Marine Mammal Protection Act

The Marine Mammal Protection Act of 1972 requires a permit from the Department of Commerce to import, possess, sell or transport a marine mammal. The use of marine mammals in research should be avoided unless there are strong scientific reasons for choosing them over other species.

Animal Enterprise Protection Act

The Animal Enterprise Protection Act of 1992 is a law to protect facilities using animals in biomedical research from animal rights terrorists. It prohibits breaking and entering or obtaining unauthorized access to an animal facility; stealing or causing intentional loss of animals; or receiving or having knowledge of any stolen materials. However, if an intruder finds incriminating evidence of true animal abuse, the facility or the investigator can be held liable.

Good Laboratory Practices Regulations

Other regulations, such as the Good Laboratory Practices Regulations of the Food and Drug Administration [11], may apply to biomaterials testing. These regulations govern preclinical studies for research or marketing permits from the Food and Drug Administration. They are designed to protect people who might participate in subsequent human trials, rather than animals used in research or testing.

REGULATORY COMPLIANCE

To comply with regulations and ensure the protection of research animals, the investigator should ensure that all animal use procedures are approved by the IACUC. In order to accomplish this, the proposed use must be described completely and consideration given to the following:

1   Housing of research animals should be in accordance with the provisions of the *Guide*. Psychological well-being of nonhuman primates can be addressed by providing for interaction with conspecific animals, toys, and foraging for food. Housing must also ensure dogs are provided with adequate exercise. If animals are to be exempted from these programs, the attending veterinarian must concur.

2   Animals should be observed on at least a daily basis. More frequent observation and perhaps administration of medication may be required for certain animals such as postsurgical animals or those that are models of pathologic conditions.

3   Close monitoring, including assessing pain and distress, is required if procedures will involve more than momentary pain. Appropriate anesthetics or analgesics must be administered. If a study requires that anesthetics or analgesics must be withheld, the investigator must provide scientific justification in writing and obtain approval from the IACUC.

4   Proper monitoring, care, and record keeping are the responsibility of the investigator.

5   Euthanasia of animals should be accomplished by a method approved by the American Veterinary Medical Association Panel on Euthanasia [12] or the investigator must provide scientific justification for the method to be used and it must be approved by the IACUC.

Association for the Assessment and Accreditation of Laboratory Animal Care

The Association for the Assessment and Accreditation of Laboratory Animal Care (AAALAC) is a non-profit, non-governmental, voluntary accrediting body for laboratory animal programs and facilities. Accreditation is based on peer review using the *Guide* for standards. The U.S. Public Health Service accepts accreditation as evidence that facilities are in compliance with the PHS policy. Thirty-two academies, associations, and foundations sponsor AAALAC and each has a representative on its governing body, the Board of Trustees. The Council on Accreditation is composed of 18 members appointed by the Trustees. It reviews site visit reports and determines accreditation status, subject to confirmation by the Board of Trustees.

To apply for accreditation, an institution submits a self-description of its facilities and programs. An initial site visit is conducted by one or more members of the Council, often augmented by one or more ad hoc site visitors who are often selected because of expertise in a particular area. Site visitors write a report describing their findings and giving recommendations to the Council regarding accreditation and to the institution regarding improvement of the program. Additional site visits are conducted, usually every three years, with annual reports submitted by the institution the other years.

PROTECTION OF ANIMALS FROM INFLUENCES AFFECTING THE VALIDITY OF RESEARCH

There is increasing evidence that in addition to ethical and regulatory considerations, there are scientific reasons for protection of research animals from infection and exposure to stressful conditions. Studies reveal that the most accurate data come from animals that are healthy and not under stress. Factors affecting the validity of data have been extensively reviewed [13, 14].

Effects of Disease

When data are being collected to assess the safety of materials or devices, the effects of any intercurrent disease must be considered. Some infections which can alter parameters being assayed can be present in animals without producing overt signs of disease. Even though animals may appear to be healthy, hemogram, clinical chemisty, histology, and other measurements could be altered by the body's attempt to combat microorganisms that are present, but not producing signs of overt disease. There are numerous examples of this in rodents, where it has been found that the immune response can be altered by lactic dehydrogenase virus, mouse hepatitis virus, mouse thymic virus, murine cytomegalovirus, pneumonia virus of mice, rat coronavirus, rat parvoviruses, and Sendai virus. Similarly, altered tumorigenesis in rodents has been attributed to the presence of lactic dehydrogenase virus and *Citrobacter freundii*. Subclinical infections have been studied more in rodents than in other laboratory animals, but their occurrence in the other commonly used laboratory animal species must be assumed. At the minimum, investigators should ensure that animals are free from overt signs of disease.

In addition to protection of the animals used in research and testing, it is vital that research team members be aware of situations in which animals can carry diseases which pose a threat to humans. Among the many zoonotic diseases that have caused mortality in people are hantavirus, Q fever, yellow fever, hepatitis A virus, herpes virus B, lymphocytic choriomeningitis virus, rabies, salmonellosis, and tuberculosis [15]. In addition, a multitude of organisms are capable of causing non-fatal illness in the people who come into contact with them.

Effects of Stress

Investigators evaluating the carcinogenicity of materials should be aware of studies linking increased tumor incidence with increased stress. It has been reported that rats handled frequently as neonates had improved ability to cope with stress, and these animals had a lower incidence and later onset of 7,12-dimethylbenz(a)anthracene (DMBA) induced mammary tumors than did rats raised without neonatal handling [16]. Aarstad and Sejelid [17] found that when mice were subjected to water stress, they had increased tumor size and tumor growth rate of transplanted intradermal Meth A fibrosarcomas compared to non-stressed controls.

Increased stress has also been found to affect other types of animal studies. Holson et al. [18] demonstrated that when rats were handled frequently, group-housed, and reared in plastic cages, they showed fewer abnormalities in behavioral tests than did those raised in isolation in hanging metal cages. Marti et al. [19] found that increasing stress caused reduced food intake in adult rats. This study illustrates that investigators must ensure that all groups in comparative tests are raised under similar conditions, especially in tests which compare weight gain. Brodin et al. [20] found increases in the somatostatin levels of rats euthanized fourth in a group as compared to those decapitated first. They concluded that being present when the first were euthanized was stressful and altered the hormone levels. They also reported that isolation of rats individually in metal cages for as little as 24 hours significantly increased the substance P levels in brain tissue. Landi et al. [21] found that corticosterone levels of mice were elevated and immune function assays were lessened for

48 hours after shipment. Reese and Wahlstrom [22] found that time of blood sample relative to feeding and degree of excitement resulted in significant hemoconcentration in dogs, as measured by packed cell volume. Rasko and Hood [23] studied the effects of stress on retinoic-acid-induced teratogenesis. They reported increased incidence of short tails, fused ribs, supernumerary ribs, fused vertebrae, and exencephalies in litters when the retinoic acid administration was combined with maternal restraint stress, as compared to identical doses of retinoic acid administered without restraint.

These studies indicate that factors which might increase stress should be considered in the design of studies to test biomaterials and implantable devices. It is conceivable that adverse outcomes, such as increased tumor incidence or decreased weight gain, could occur in tests and be attributed to a particular device, when, in fact, the difference is due to inadvertent stress of the test group.

In addition to disease and stress, factors such as cage design, lighting cycles and intensity, temperature, air quality, nutrient content of feed, and quality of water and air have been shown to produce changes in animals that can be confused with effects due to experimental manipulation [14]. The investigative team, animal caretakers, and veterinary personnel should remain cognizant of the possibility of such considerations.

It is in the best interests of all concerned to work to ensure that laboratory animals are afforded the maximum protection. As studies have become increasingly sophisticated, defining factors that can affect the data obtained in animal studies are becoming increasingly important. As discussed in this chapter, there are compelling ethical, humane, and scientific reasons for scientists to ensure that laboratory animals are shielded from exposure to disease, pain, and distress.

REFERENCES

1   Roth RI, Levin J, Behr S. A modified limulus amebocyte lysate test with increased sensitivity for detection of bacterial endotoxin. *J Lab Clin Med*, 114 (1989), 306–311.
2   Hendricks AG, Binkerd PE. Nonhuman primates and teratological research. *J Med Primatol*, 19 (1990), 81–108.
3   Russell WMS, Burch RL. *The Principles of Humane Experimental Technique*. London: Methuen, 1959.
4   Soothill JS, Morton DB, Ahmad A. The HID50 (hypothermia-inducing dose 50): An alternative to the LD50 for measurement of bacterial virulence. *Int J Exp Pathol*, 73 (1992), 95–98.
5   Balls M. Replacement of animal procedures: Alternatives in research, education and testing. *Lab Anim*, 28 (1994), 193–211.
6   Council Directive 93/35/EEC, amending for the sixth time Directive 76/768/EEC on the approximation of the laws of the Member States relating to cosmetic products. *Official Journal of the European Communities*, L151 (1993), 32–36.
7   CFR (Code of Federal Regulations), Title 9; Parts 1, 2, and 3 (Docket No. 89-130). *Federal Register*. Vol. 54, No. 168, August 31, 1989, and 9CFR Part 3 (Docket No. 90-218). *Federal Register*. Vol. 56, No. 32, February 15, 1991.
8   Office of Protection from Research Risk. *Public Health Service Policy on Humane Care and Use of Laboratory Animals*. Revised, 1996.
9   Committee on the Care and Use of Laboratory Animals, Institute of Laboratory Animal Resources. *Guide for the Care and Use of Laboratory Animals*. NIH Publ. No. 86-23. Bethesda, Maryland: Public Health Service, U.S. Department of Health and Human Services, 1985.
10 Report of American College of Laboratory Animal Medicine on adequate veterinary care. *ACLAM Newsletter*, October, 1986.
11 CFR (Code of Federal Regulations), Title 21; Part 58 (Docket No. 8324-0142). *Federal Register*. Vol. 52, No. 172, September 4, 1987.
12 1993 report of the AVMA panel on euthanasia. *JAVMA*, 202 (1993), 230–249.
13 Waggie KS, Kagiyama N, Allen AM, Nomura T. *Manual of Microbiologic Monitoring of Laboratory Animals*, 2nd ed. NIH Publ. No. 94-2498. Bethesda, Maryland: Public Health Service, U.S. Department of Health and Human Services, 1994.

14 Pakes SP, Lu YS, Munier PC. Factors that complicate animal research. In Fox JG, Cohen BJ, Lowe FM (Eds.), *Laboratory Animal Medicine*. Orlando, FL: Academic Press, 1984, 649–660.

15 Fox JG, Newcommer CE, Rozmiarek H. Selected zoonoses and other health hazards. In Fox JG, Cohen BJ, Lowe FM. *Laboratory Animal Medicine*. Orlando, FL: Academic Press, 1984, 614–648.

16 Hilakivi-Clarke L, Clarke R, Lippman ME. Perinatal factors increase breast cancer risk. *Breast Cancer Res and Treat*, 31 (1994), 273–284.

17 Aarstad HJ, Seljelid R. Effects of stress on the growth of a fibrosarcoma in the nu/nu and conventional mice. *Scand J Immunol*, 35 (1992), 209–215.

18 Holson RR, Scallet AC, Ali SF, Turner BB. "Isolation Stress" revisited: Isolation-rearing effects depend on animal care methods. *Physiol & Behav*, 49 (1991), 1107–1118.

19 Marti O, Marti J, Armario A. Effects of chronic stress on food intake in rats: Influence of stressor intensity and duration of daily exposure. *Physiol & Behav*, 55 (1994), 747–753.

20 Brodin E, Rosen A, Schott E, Brodin K. Effects of sequential removal of rats from a group cage, and of individual housing of rats, on substance, cholecystokinin and somatostatin levels in the periaqueductal grey and limbic regions. *Neuropeptides*, 26 (1994), 253–260.

21 Landi MS, Krieder JW, Lang CM, Bullock LP. Effects of shipping on the immune function in mice. *Am J Vet Res*, 43 (1982), 1654–1657.

22 Reece WO, Wahlstrom JD. Effect of feeding and excitement on the packed cell volume of dogs. *Lab Anim Care*, 20 (1970), 1114–1117.

23 Rasco JF, Hood RD. Enhancement of the teratogenicity of all-trans-retinoic acid by maternal restraint stress in mice as a function of treatment timing. *Teratologys*, 51 (1995), 63–70.

Chapter 30
Animal Selection

H. Vince Mendenhall

ANIMAL MODEL SELECTION

The decision regarding which test system (animal model) to use for a specific study must come from an extensive review of the literature. This review must be related not only to the specifics of the system into which the new device is to be implanted, but also to the physiological and chemical nature of the system to be studied. All this must refer to its final relation and applicability to the target species: humans.

The ideal animal model should have consistently reproducible features that simulate an analogous or homologous condition where the biomaterial would be used in man. The scientific criteria for animal model selection depend upon the intended application of the biomaterial. More specifically, anatomical, biochemical, physiological, pathological, and/or psychological characteristics need to be considered.

Over the years it has been found by trial and error—and keen relational observation—that human systems resemble similar systems in various animal species. Delineation of all of the subjective "proof" for these physiological and anatomical similarities and differences would take up many volumes, and is out of the range of this chapter.

The American College of Laboratory Animal Medicine has sponsored several reference texts on spontaneous animal models of human disease [1–2], and the Armed Forces Institute of Pathology has developed a series of publications that summarize nearly 300 animal models [3]. Several other publications frequently list newly developed animal models, some of which may be applicable to biomaterial technology [4–6].

The following is a summary of suggested test systems for study of implants according to the surgical specialty for which the device may be used. It also provides examples of the factors which enter into the selection process. This list is by no means complete, and largely represents my own bias, gleaned from over 25 years' experience in these areas and from periodic literature review.

ABDOMINAL

The anatomy and physiology of the abdominal contents of the dog is more similar than other laboratory animals to that of humans, making this species the ideal animal model for any experimental surgery involving the abdomen [7].

Studies involving the development of an artificial pancreas for treatment of diabetes mellitus have primarily been conducted in the dog [3]. Dogs are easily rendered diabetic either by surgical pancreatectomy or by the administration of streptozocin. Implantation of the prosthetic device into the omentum mimics the venous drainage of the pancreas.

The evaluation of anti-adhesion products is usually conducted in rats or rabbits, with definitive studies again being performed in dogs. The animal model of choice is the rat cecal abrasion model, or secondarily, the rabbit uterine horn model. In the former, the cecum and peritoneum are mechanically abraded in a reproducible fashion. The wounded edges are treated with the candidate material, and opposed. The degree of adhesions between the two structures is determined at necropsy, usually 14 days after the insult. A similar procedure is performed in the latter model.

CARDIOVASCULAR

There are many considerations in cardiovascular research, and nearly all laboratory species have been used. The choice of the model depends upon the objective of the experiment. Briefly, arterial healing and vascular grafts are best studied in goats [8, 9], thrombogenicity in pigs and non-human primates [10], hemodynamics in dogs and secondarily in non-human primates [11], heart valves in sheep [3, 12–13], and artificial hearts and left ventricular assist devices in calves [14].

A new area of vascular research involving "restenosis," the smooth muscle cell proliferation in an artery subsequent to endothelial cell removal and rupture of the internal elastic lamina, as seen following balloon angioplasty or placement of intra-luminal stents, is now being extensively studied. The pig femoral and coronary artery seem to resemble most closely the situation in man. Unfortunately, all treatments so far determined to be efficacious in animals have not proven to be so in humans. Other test systems used in this area of research have included the rat internal carotid artery, the rabbit aorta, and the non-human primate saphenous artery.

NEUROLOGY

The rat sciatic nerve is a good model for preliminary testing of the effects of new treatments designed to improve peripheral nerve regeneration [15]. However, the non-human primate should be used for validation of the efficacy of the treatment because of the similarity in complexity of the peripheral nerves in higher animals [16]. The spinal cord and brain of the cat, rat and non-human primate are the best mapped and understood [17]. Hydrocephalus shunts are best tested in dogs, however, because of the relatively large size of the lateral ventricle in this species.

OPHTHALMOLOGY

The testing of new ophthalmological devices or pharmacological agents can potentially involve three animal models: rabbits, white domestic geese, and cynomolgus monkeys. The rabbit eye is very sensitive to irritation, and should be the primary source of information regarding the toxicology of a new ophthalmic material [18]. The anterior segment is, however, too large and reactive for the evaluation of intra-ocular devices. From my own experience, this type of work is best done in the white domestic goose. The lens capsule of the goose is nearly identical in size to that of the human, and the reaction of the eye to intraocular surgery is quite similar, but accelerated. Evaluation of a new intraocular lens haptic design or for a potential treatment and/or prophylaxis of posterior capsular opacity can thus be completed in a relatively short time (12 weeks). For long-term studies, the cynomolgus monkey is the most appropriate, because of its similarity to the human with regard to the size of the anterior segment in general, the reactivity to intraocular surgery, and healing time and processes. Glaucoma shunts and other treatments for increased intraocular pressure are commonly performed in dogs or monkeys.

ORTHOPEDICS

The healing of bone and its reaction to biomaterials in the goat has been shown to very closely resemble that seen in the human with regard to cell type, collagen structure, organization of both hard and soft tissue structures, and time. Sheep, on the other hand, tend to calcify soft tissue structures. Beagle dogs tend to be chondrodystrophic [8].

These three animal models have been extensively utilized in the evaluation of artifical ligaments and tendons, bone graft substitutes, aids to spinal fusion, artificial joints, and evaluation of various medical treatments for osteoarthritis. Animal models for osteoarthritis include dogs in which the anterior cruciate ligament has been sectioned, sometimes followed by dorsal root rhizotomy. Surface arthroplasty of the femoral head in dogs, sheep and goats has also been reported to be a useful model for evaluation of drug therapy for osteoarthritis.

Tendon healing is best studied in chickens or turkeys. Apart from management considerations, goats and sheep, as well as rats, tend to develop ectopic ossification in these structures [3], making them poor models for the study of candidate artificial tendons or research into the healing characteristics of these structures.

A test system commonly used in orthopedic research is the rabbit. Despite a large body of literature that indicates the inadequacy of this animal model in predicting the outcome of similar biomaterial implants in humans [3], it is still used extensively. The reasons are probably more historical and economical than scientific.

Dental

Dental implants have been extensively studied in dogs, monkeys, baboons and pigs. Although the specific anatomy is quite different between these species and humans, the tissue response to periodontal disease and gingival recession is quite similar [3].

OTOLOGY

The microscopic anatomy of the temporal bone and its contents in cats and chinchillas bears a remarkable resemblance to that of the human. This is especially true of the auditory ossicles and the cochlea. These characteristics have made these species the test systems of choice for the evaluation of cochlear implants, artificial stapes, and other otologic prostheses. The development of surgical techniques for the treatment of otosclerosis and otitis media have been developed and refined in these animals, especially the cat [3].

RESPIRATORY

Again, because of similar anatomical size and healing characteristics, the animal models most frequently used for evaluation of materials to be implanted into the respiratory system include the dog and pig. There is an extensive amount of literature regarding the dog as an animal model for evaluation of candidate artificial tracheas [3]. The pig has also been extensively used for testing of tissue adhesives and sealants following lung resection.

UROGENITAL

The evaluation of various urological prosthetic devices has been limited to stent-like devices to help prevent stenosis following ureteral or urethral anastomosis. Primarily because of the size of these structures, the animal models utilized have again included dogs and pigs.

The microscopic anatomy and healing characteristics of these structures appears to be quite similar to those of humans [3]. Surgical techniques and instrumentation for transurethral prostatectomy were developed and evaluated in dogs. Intrauterine contraceptive devices have been extensively studied in rabbits. This work revealed similar effectiveness and tissue reaction to that subsequently observed in humans.

WOUND HEALING

Wound healing studies designed to study the effectiveness of various treatments on "donor site" wounds are best performed in the young domestic pig. The rate of reepithelialization of partial thickness (<0.5 mm deep) blade (dermatome) wounds or burns is largely dependent upon the concentration per square centimeter of keratinocytes. This concentration in the skin of young pigs is nearly identical to that of humans (11 hair follicles/cm^2) [19]. The use of other test systems for wound healing studies should be limited to studying the effect of materials on the healing of incisional wounds.

Beyond the anatomic, pathologic, and physiologic similarities to man that must be looked for in selection of an animal model, the experimental surgeon may have to limit his or her choice by practical considerations. The size and conformation of the animal may be an important one. Small animals cost less and are easier to handle. Surgical procedures in large animals, however, are more easily performed. Body conformation is especially important where long-term restraint is required. For example, as mentioned above, pigs and non-human primates both have cardiovascular systems similar to that of man; however, for a study requiring long-term catheterization and continuous monitoring, the primate may in fact be the animal model of choice.

The choice of experimental animal to be used in implant research should be based on considerations other than the risk of infection. There are no reliable data indicating that one species is more susceptible to septic complications than another [20, 21].

Realistically, it must be admitted that all the results of an experiment involving the implantation of a material either as the raw material, or as the finished device, will never exactly duplicate those seen when the material or the device is finally implanted in man. However, it is certainly possible to predict the safety of the material in use, and from there, to be able to extrapolate presumed efficacy, if the final use of the implant under study is accurately stated and similar work properly reviewed.

REFERENCES

1   Andrews EJ, Ward BC, Altman NH (Eds.). *Spontaneous Animal Models of Human Diseases*, Vol. I. New York: Academic Press, 1979.
2   Andrews EJ, Ward BC, Altman NH (Eds.). *Spontaneous Animal Models of Human Disease*, Vol. II. New York: Academic Press, 1979.
3   *Animal Models of Human Disease*, Vols. 1–23. Washington, DC: The Registry of Comparative Pathology, Armed Forces Institute of Pathology, 1972–1995.
4   *ILAR News*. Institute of Laboratory Animal Resources, National Research Council (published quarterly).
5   *Veterinary Pathology*. Washington, DC: American College of Veterinary Pathologists Inc. (published bimonthly).
6   *Comparative Pathology Bulletin*. Registry of Comparative Pathology, Armed Forces Institute of Pathology (published quarterly).
7   Markowitz J, Archibald J, Downie HG. *Experimental Surgery*, 5th ed. Baltimore: Williams & Wilkins, 1964, 6.
8   Gibbons DF. Personal communications, 1982–1991.

9 Clowes AW. Pathobiology of arterial healing. Strandness DE, Didisheim P, Clowes AW, Watson JT (Eds). *Vascular Diseases. Current Research and Clinical Applications.* Orlando, FL: Grune and Stratton, Inc., 1987, 351–362.

10 Parks PJ, Ericson DG. Testing and evaluation of thrombogenicity. *Evaluation and Testing of Cardiovascular Devices. Short Course.* Minneapolis: Society for Biomaterials, 1993.

11 Rushmer RF. *Cardiovascular Dynamics,* 2nd ed. Philadelphia, PA: W. B. Saunders Co., 1961.

12 Levy RJ, Schoen FJ, Anderson HC, Harasaki H, Koch TH, Brown W, Lian JB, Cumming R, Gavin JB. Cardiovascular implant calcification: A survey and update. *Biomaterials,* 12 (1991), 707–714.

13 Levy RJ. Calcification models and evaluation of the efficacy of controlled release drug delivery for anticalcification. In *Evaluation and Testing of Cardiovascular Devices. Short Course.* Minneapolis: Society for Biomaterials, 1993.

14 Schoen FJ, Anderson JM, Didisheim P, Dobbins JJ, Gristina AG, Harasaki H, Simmons RL. Ventricular assist device (VAD) pathology analyses: Guidelines for clinical studies. *J Appl Biomat,* 1 919900, 49–56.

15 Seckel BR, Ryan SE, Gagne RG, Chiu TH, Wadkins E. Target specific nerve regeneration through a nerve guide in the rat. *Plast Reconstr Surg,* 78 (1986), 793.

16 Tountas CP, Bergman RA, Lewis TW, Stone HE, Pyrek JD, Mendenhall HV. A comparison of peripheral nerve repair using an absorbable tubulization device and conventional suture in primates. *J Appl Biom,* 4 (1993), 261–268.

17 Nauta WJH, Karten HJ. A general profile of the vertebrate brain, with sidelights on the ancestry of cerebral cortex. In Schmitt RO (Ed.), *The Neurosciences.* New York: Rockefeller University Press, 1970, 7–25.

18 Beckley JH. Comparative eye testing: Man vs. animal. *Toxicol Appl Pharmacol,* 7 (1965), 93–101.

19 Winter GD. Oxygen and epidermal wound healing. *Adv Exp Med Biol,* 94 (1977), 673–8.

20 Brown MJ, Pearson PT, Tomson FN. Guidelines for animal surgery in research and teaching. *Am J Vet Res,* 54 (1993), 1544–1559.

21 Dougherty SH. Implant infections. In von Recum AF (Ed.), *Handbook of Biomaterials Evaluation,* 1st ed. New York: Macmillan, 1986, 276–289.

ADDITIONAL READING

1 References 1–7 are recommended for further in-depth reading on the subject of this chapter.

Chapter 31

Surgical Procedures

H. Vince Mendenhall

INTRODUCTION

The determination of the in vivo safety and efficacy of a potential biomaterial or combination of materials into a new medical device will, by definition, require surgery. As opposed to pharmacology, surgery is that branch of medicine concerned with the treatment of disease (or in this case, the evaluation of a new medical device) by manual and instrumental interventional procedures. These procedures occur first when the tissue reactivity to the material is determined in routine TriPartite and/or ISO 9000 Phase I and II biocompatibility testing, and secondly when the efficacy and safety-while-in-use of the completed device is determined (Phase III) [1]. Efficacy and safety-while-in-use testing involves true experimental surgery, which often requires the development of a new procedure.

Everyone involved in a surgical research project must embrace the idea that the requirements for successful survival experimental surgery on animals are more rigid than those for clinical surgery. Medical device evaluation in particular requires a multi-disciplinary approach to the experiment. Research studies must demonstrate an appreciation of all elements of the perioperative care of the animal, not just the surgical technique itself. A knowledge of the anatomy, physiology, anesthesia, and basic care of the specific animal test species is mandatory. The related differences from the human target species must be clarified. All operative procedures must be scrupulously planned and executed. The surgeon and his/her team must have an intimate knowledge of the procedures and routines required to ensure aseptic results, as well as possess adequate surgical skills.

Animal surgery must be ethical and humane, while meeting the research objectives, and it must be performed using sound professional, scientific knowledge and judgement. Any research proposal must demonstrate a scientific rationale for the use of animals, the appropriateness of their use as a model, and a justification for the number of animals to be used [2] (for details see Chapter 30).

PERSONNEL

It is the responsibility of the research institution to ensure that all personnel concerned with biomaterial implantation and evaluation studies (regardless of academic degrees) are qualified and trained to conduct surgical procedures. A multi-disciplinary approach is most likely to produce the best results, and should include the following categories of personnel [3]:

(1) *Scientist/Study Director*: A person with a degree in any of a number of disciplines who plans and conducts the study. The scientist may or may not participate in the performance of the surgical procedures.

(2) *Laboratory Animal Veterinarian*: The individual who oversees veterinary care at the institution and ensures that adequate veterinary care is provided to all animals.

(3) *Peri-operative Care Technician*: The individual who prepares the animal for surgery, and who monitors the animal throughout the surgery and recovery periods.

(4) *Anesthetist*: The person who administers the anesthetic agents necessary for the procedure, and who monitors the animal during the procedure to ensure adequate analgesia and physiologic homeostasis.

(5) *Surgeon*: The person performing the operation. Although not necessarily required to be so, this person should have a broad range of experience in both animal and human clinical surgery. He/she should also possess a thorough appreciation of the differences between clinical and experimental surgery, as described later.

Each category may involve one or more persons and, in some instances, one person may perform more than one task.

PROTOCOL

The most important step in establishing a research program is to develop the protocol. The research objective in studies involving animals should be prospective: surgical experiments should not be performed in animals just to see what happens. A well-considered hypothesis and a carefully-developed protocol should be written by the research team, and approved by the IACUC, before the first "pilot" animal is anesthetized.

The protocol should include the following:

(1) A descriptive title, plus a statement of the objective of the study. The protocol must state the rationale for the animal use and describe the operative procedures.

(2) Identification of the material by name, chemical abstract number, or code number. For the conduct of any one experiment, all materials should come from the same lot number.

(3) The proposed starting and completion points. Protocols that do not include an end-point are not prospective.

(4) Justification for selection of the particular species and the approximate number of animals to be used. The selection of the animal model should be one that, it is hoped, will give results appropriate to the end use of the data. Extensive literature review and cadaver dissection of proposed species should lead to the final animal model selection.

(5) Animal specifications including number, body weight range, sex, source of supply, species, strain, sub-strain, and age. It should be known whether sex, species or age of the animal may influence the results of the experiment. If so, these variables should be controlled or eliminated.

(6) The procedure of identification of each animal used in the study.

(7) A description of the experimental design, including the methods for the control of bias. The institution must ensure that professionally-acceptable standards governing the care, treatment, and use of animals will be followed, including appropriate aseptic technique and appropriate use of anesthetic, analgesic, and tranquilizing drugs.

(8) The route of administration of all drugs, and the reason for their choice. If anesthetic and/or analgesic drugs cannot be administered during pain-causing procedures, the protocol must include a scientific justification, which must be approved by the IACUC before the study can begin. The Animal Welfare Act prohibits the use of paralytic drugs without general anesthesia for procedures that may cause more than momentary or slight pain or distress.

(9) The type and frequency of tests, analyses, and the measurements to be made.

(10) The records to be maintained.

(11) The method of euthanasia, the tissues to be processed, the methods of processing, and the specific tests and observations to be performed on the implant and its surrounding tissues.

(12) A statement of the proposed statistical methods.

Although cumbersome at first to novice investigators, the exercise of writing the protocol is crucial to the outcome of an experiment, especially when the study involves a team including scientists other than the surgeon. It helps to clarify which procedures can, and should, be done in one animal model and prevents impulsive changes or additions of further procedures.

PRINCIPLE CONSIDERATIONS FOR EXPERIMENTAL SURGICAL PROCEDURES

Consideration of eight major factors will ensure that all surgical operations will be performed to a uniformly high and reproducible standard. Inattention to any one of these points will invalidate the positive effects of the others. These principal areas of concern include the following:

(1) The operating room environment
(2) The equipment necessary to perform the operation
(3) Appropriate anesthesia and the equipment for its delivery
(4) Aseptic technique
(5) Preparation of the animal
(6) The operating room personnel
(7) The operative technique
(8) Postoperative care

Operating Room Environment

The specific type and extent of the experimental surgical facilities needed depend to some extent on the animal species and complexity of the surgery. However, it should be designed similarly to that of facilities used for human clinical operations. The suite should be located at the end of a hallway. It should have only one entrance, and it should have positive pressure in relation to other areas of the facility, attained by at least 10–15 non-recirculating air changes per hour, introduced into the suite through HEPA filters. The ambient temperature in the suite should be approximately 19°C, with 30–50 percent humidity. If inhalation anesthetic agents are to be used, a mechanism for scavenging waste gases must be provided.

All furniture in the suite, and the operating lights, should be wiped down with antiseptics prior to the animal entering the room, between cases, and at the end of the day. The floors should be similarly treated. At least monthly, and preferably weekly with heavy use, the room should be fogged with a disinfectant. The specific type of disinfectant used for this purpose should be changed twice a year to prevent the development of bacterial resistance [4].

Equipment

Simplicity and standardization are essential in every successful operating room, but the instrument cabinet of the experimental surgical suite should never be the repository of antiquated or discarded instruments. It is economical to purchase only instruments of the best quality, and only those that are needed to perform the required operation. Compromises can be made in other areas, but should be minimized in the selection of instruments.

Instrument packs should be double-wrapped prior to autoclaving, using appropriate indicator tape and expiration dates. The effectiveness of the autoclave should also be checked periodically with appropriate indicators. Packs wrapped in linen are sterile for only 3–4 weeks, while those wrapped in paper or plastic may retain sterility for 9–12 months. Instruments sterilized with ethylene oxide will retain their integrity almost indefinitely. Wrapping of the instruments and sterilizing by this method is preferable to keeping them in cabinets and steam autoclaving immediately prior to use [5].

Anesthesia

General anesthesia is a state induced by one agent, or a combination of agents, providing controlled, reversible unconsciousness of the central nervous system. Often, insufficient attention is paid to the selection of the most appropriate anesthetic method. Anesthesia is a form of temporary, controlled poisoning, and should, therefore, be treated with the utmost respect. The anesthetic regime with which the anesthetist is most familiar may be the safest, but may not necessarily be the best. Each anesthetic agent has individual advantages and disadvantages, both with respect to the actions elicited by the agent in different species, and with respect to the various effects that the agent can cause within a single species. The operating team must be aware of all these effects, and be able to choose the anesthetic best suited to the animal model and procedure. Laboratory animal veterinarians are generally knowledgeable in this field and should be consulted when the protocol is being designed.

A comprehensive list of specific agents and methods of anesthesia is beyond the scope of the current discussion; however, there are many excellent texts that deal with this subject [6–7]. It is no longer acceptable to anesthetize every animal, regardless of species, with sodium pentobarbital. In fact, unless the situation absolutely warrants it, pentobarbital should only be used for euthanasia. Endotracheal intubation to deliver inhalant anesthetic agents, in conjunction with controlled or assisted respiration utilizing an automatic ventilator, is the best choice for all larger animals. Gas inhalation anesthesia requires a thorough understanding of its actions and animal responses, sophisticated equipment, and well-trained anesthesia personnel to administer it and maintain the equipment. This anesthetic method is very safe, and is easily controlled and reversed. The initial costs associated with acquisition of gas anesthesia equipment and training personnel for its administration are greatly outweighed by the long-term costs of uncontrolled animal losses due to inadequate or inappropriate anesthetic methods.

A number of drugs are currently available to induce what is thought to be the safest method of anesthesia, commonly termed "balanced anesthesia." In general, this term implies the use of multiple agents. These agents include: (a) pre-anesthetic administration of narcotics or tranquilizers; (b) barbiturates, dissociative agents, or narcotics for induction of anesthesia; and (c) the use of muscle relaxants in addition to the inhalation anesthetic agents for maintenance of anesthesia. Such combinations reduce the required dosage of each agent and in general provide a safer state of anesthesia. Each species reacts slightly differently to these agents, and it is therefore important that the implantation team be thoroughly aware of the actions of each drug intended for use, not only on the animal, but also on the tissue into which the device will be implanted. Table 31-1 provides examples of suitable anesthetic drugs and recommended dosages for most of the commonly used laboratory animals.

Table 31-1   Anesthetics, Tranquilizers, and Analgesics

Drug	Mouse, hamster, guinea pig	Rat
Pentobarbital	40 mg/kg IP or IV (Sedation) 90 mg/kg IP (Surgical Anesthesia)	40 mg/kg IP or IV (Sedation) 100 mg/kg IP (Surgical Anesthesia)
Ketamine	200 mg/kg IP	100 mg/kg IP
Ketamine + Xylazine	150 mg/kg IP + 10 mg/kg IP	80 mg/kg IP + 8 mg/kg IP
Halothane or Isoflurane	1–4%	1–4%
Buprenorphine	1.0 mg/kg SQ	1.0 mg/kg SQ

Drug	Rabbits	Swine
Atropine (pre-op)	1.0 mg/kg SQ	0.04 mg/kg IM
Pentobarbital	60 mg/kg IV	25 mg/kg IV
Ketamine	50 mg/kg IM	20 mg/kg IM
Ketamine + Xylazine + Oxymorphone	35 mg/kg IM + 10 mg/kg IM + NA	20 mg/kg IM + 2 mg/kg IM + 0.75 mg/kg IM
Halothane or Isoflurane	1–4%	1–4%
Buprenorphine	1.0 mg/kg SQ	0.05–0.1 mg/kg IM
Butorphanol	1.0 mg/kg SQ	0.2 mg/kg IM
Tiletamine-Zolazepam (Telazol)	NA	5.0 mg/kg IM

Drug	Dogs	Cats
Atropine (pre-op)	0.02 mg/kg SQ, IM	0.02 mg/kg SQ, IM
Acetylpromazine (pre-op)	0.1 mg/kg IM, SQ	0.025 mg/kg SQ, IM
Pentobarbital	33 mg/kg IV	33 mg/kg IV
Thiopental or Thiamylal	20 mg/kg IV	20 mg/kg IV
Methohexital	7–12 mg/kg IV	7–12 mg/kg IV
Ketamine	15 mg/kg IM	17.5 mg/kg IM (Not recommended for use by itself)
Ketamine + Xylazine	2.5 mg/kg IM + 0.45 mg/kg IM	2.5 mg/kg IM + 0.45 mg/kg IM
Halothane, Isoflurane	1–4%	1–4%
Buprenorphine	0.02 mg/kg IM	0.005 mg/kg SQ
Flunixin meglumine	1.0 mg/kg IM	NA

Drug	Ruminants
Pentobarbital	33 mg/kg IV
Thiopental or Thiamylal	20 mg/kg IV
Methohexital	15 mg/kg IV
Halothane or Isoflurane	1–4%
Flunixin meglumine	1.0 mg/kg IV

Drug	Birds
Ketamine	25 mg/kg IM
Xylazine	10 mg/kg IM
Isoflurane	0.5–1.5%

Drug	Non-human primates
Ketamine	10–15 mg/kg IM
Ketamine + Diazepam	10 mg/kg IM + 0.5 mg/kg IM
Ketamine + Xylazine	7 mg/kg IM + 0.6 mg/kg IM
Butorphanol	0.025 mg/kg IM every 3–6 hours
Buprenorphine	0.01–0.03 mg/kg IM every 8–12 hours
Isoflurane	1.5–2.5%

Monitoring   Some classic descriptions of biological response to certain anesthetics in specific species can be found, and may serve as general guidelines in evaluating the anesthetic status of an animal patient. However, a simple description of an animal's response to a particular anesthetic that is applicable to all conditions and all individuals within that species does not exist. Each animal, therefore, should be evaluated individually, and the anesthetic regimen must be controlled by graded administration of anesthetic drugs on the basis of monitoring of clinical signs and certain vital parameters.

Accepted surgical protocol requires repeated assessment of the physiologic status of the animal throughout the surgery. Circulatory and respiratory function, as well as core body temperature, need to be monitored during the anesthetic and surgical episodes. The degree of monitoring sophistication required depends on the species undergoing surgery, the extent and duration of the surgical procedure, whether it is a survival or terminal procedure, and the anesthetic regimen used. Because most anesthetics depress the function of the cardiovascular and respiratory systems, these systems must be monitored to accurately balance the need to provide sufficient anesthesia to prevent pain perception, while limiting the total dose of the anesthetic. These systems should be monitored throughout the anesthetic period. Monitoring can be qualitative, using the anesthetist's sense of touch, sight, and hearing to evaluate the patient, or quantitative, using instruments for periodic measurement of specific vital organ performance. This monitoring is essential to the successful outcome of the surgery. Physiological monitoring parameters should include oxygen saturation, pulse, heart rate, oxygen saturation, and end-tidal CO_2.

Fluid Therapy   Unless specific conditions dictate alternate fluid regimens, which should not be the case in experimental surgical situations, polyionic isotonic maintenance fluids should be used when the procedure is anticipated to exceed one hour, or is likely to involve considerable tissue manipulation. The purpose of fluid therapy during anesthesia and surgery is to inhibit antidiuretic hormone levels and induce mild diuresis so as to counterbalance anesthetic-drug-related oliguria and to maintain urinary output during the operative and postoperative period. Also, the metabolic response to surgical trauma itself includes increased plasma levels of cortisol, catecholamines, glucagon, aldosterone, and antidiuretic hormone. The net effects of these hormones also include oliguria with sodium retention. This injury phase may persist for as long as 48–72 hours postoperatively. If not corrected, they may predispose the surgical patient to further renal impairment. Attenuation of this antidiuresis can be achieved by replacement fluid therapy during surgery.

Tissue desiccation, evaporative losses from the lungs and surgical site, redistribution of extracellular fluid (third space loss), and fluid deficits from the preoperative fasting period are iso-osmotic losses and therefore can be replaced with the intravenous administration of iso-osmotic solutions. A polyionic fluid, such as lactated Ringer's solution, retards the formation of excess free water that occurs with dextrose base fluids or hypotonic preparations. It is, therefore, the fluid of choice. As mentioned earlier, an infusion rate of 5–15 ml/kg/hr will fulfill all maintenance requirements [8].

Asepsis

Surprisingly little experimental work has been done on the problem of implant infection. It still appears to be a generally held belief that animal surgery does not require as stringent an adherence to aseptic technique as does human surgery. This erroneous belief may be perpetuated by the lesser importance placed on casualties in animal surgery. Even the belief that rodents are not affected by surgical infections, or that they are more resistant to infection than are other laboratory animals, has not been supported [9–10]. No species is really any different in its susceptibility to the infective process [2]. In fact, rodents often serve as effective animal models for studying bacterial infections [9].

Animal surgery in general, but particularly that involving implanted materials, demands the most rigid aseptic technique. Biomaterials or devices are implanted into animals to evaluate the tissue/body response to the foreign object and to assess its safety for therapeutic use. Colonization by bacteria, or the presence of very few particulate contaminants on the implant, can alter the cellular response to the device. Contamination of the implant at the time of implantation will create severe histological reactions that will camouflage or abolish characteristic reactions to it. Consequently, infected implants do not accomplish the objective of the experiment [9]. State-of-the-art biomaterial histopathologic techniques allow the research team to observe the interface between the tissue and the implant with the implant still in place. Experimental surgeons need to remember that the cellular response observed by the pathologist will allow him/her to judge not only the quality of the surgical technique, but also the adequacy of the aseptic procedures employed in the operating room.

Aseptic routine can, indeed, be both time-consuming and inconvenient, but these considerations are inconsequential when weighed against the cost of compromise to the study. A subclinically-infected implant results in a total waste: waste of the animal's life, of the investigative team's time, of the money spent to place the implant, and of the statistical information that would have been provided by the animal and its implant. It must be the surgical team's very specific goal to perform the implantation procedure under the most strictly aseptic conditions possible.

Antibiotics The clinical literature is replete with animal studies demonstrating the efficacy of systemic antibiotic prophylaxis. Systemic antibiotic prophylaxis in experimental animals undergoing implant surgery is therefore probably advisable; however, parenteral prophylaxis should be started within 2 hours of the operation and should be continued for no more than 48 hours. More prolonged administration may be justified in procedures involving prostheses of large surface area. Currently, cephalosporins should be used because they have relatively long serum half-lives (50–120 minutes) and an extended spectrum of effectiveness against both gram-positive and gram-negative organisms and, most importantly, they act directly in the surgical wound [9]. If topical antimicrobial products are used, they should be free of serious local or systemic side effects. The topical use of penicillin or other antibiotics alone has long been known to be of little value in preventing secondary subcutaneous infections [17]. Their use should be discontinued in favor of topical antiseptics, especially *undiluted* povidone-iodine. This product is remarkable in its ability to prevent (and treat) secondary subcutaneous infections without any harm to the subcutaneous tissues. However, if the product is diluted with water prior to its subcutaneous application, it reverts to a free inorganic iodine solution, and as such can then be quite toxic to the tissues with which it comes in contact.

Animal Preparation

Although the skin of animals is invariably dirty, with proper preparation, nosocomial infections can be reduced to a minimum and wounds (i.e., surgically-induced incisions) will heal by first intention.

All hair clipping and initial preparation of the animal must be done outside the operating area with an electric clipper and fine blades. Hair removal should be done as near the time of operation as possible, preferably immediately before. Nicks inflicted in the skin several hours before operation have been shown to promote wound infection [11]. The hair should be generously removed before draping so that none will become exposed during the operative procedure. Following hair removal, the general area of the operation should be washed thoroughly with antiseptic soap and water before moving the animal to the operating room for the definitive preparation of the skin.

Methods of skin preparation vary and change with the introduction of new products. In general, however, skin preparation is accomplished with an antiseptic detergent applied in a circular motion starting from the proposed line of incision and working out, never going over the same area more than once, to avoid recontamination. The detergent is then wiped off and 70 percent alcohol sprayed on the site. This procedure is repeated three times. The final application of alcohol should be allowed to dry. Finally, a solution of povidone-iodine is sprayed on the entire area and also allowed to dry [12].

Skin preparation must be appropriate to the species. Rabbits, rats, and guinea pigs are very sensitive to strong antiseptics. In these animals it is sufficient to clip the hair, wash the skin with soap and water, and swab once with 70 percent alcohol. When the alcohol has dried, povidone-iodine solution is sprayed on the site and allowed to dry [13].

Draping of the animal is of utmost importance. No area of the animal except the incision site should be visible, and all furniture with which operative personnel might come into contact should also be draped. Plastic impermeable drapes are preferred to linen because once linen gets wet, it no longer functions as a bacterial barrier [14]. Initially, four small drapes are placed around the incision site, with larger ones then used to cover the animal and furniture. Plastic "incise" drapes are useful for draping of the incision site, not only for isolating the skin from the tissues beneath, but also for holding the drapes around the operative area in place. If applied after the antiseptic solutions have been allowed to dry, or if "tackifier" is applied to the skin before their application, they adhere well to animal skin.

Operating Room Personnel

Traffic in the operating room should be kept to a minimum [14]. Prior to entering the surgical suite, all personnel must don a scrub suit, cap, mask, and shoe covers. No hair should be visible on any person entering the operating room. This requires the additional provision of hoods designed to cover long hair and beards. The anesthetist and circulating nurse should wear a "warmup" jacket over the scrub suit to ensure arm hair coverage. Observing personnel should wear surgical gowns (that need not necessarily be sterile) over the scrub suit. All laboratory personnel should wear only shoes that are dedicated for use in the surgical area and that are routinely sterilized in ethylene oxide.

Members of the team who are to touch the sterile field should scrub their hands and arms to the elbows with an antiseptic (chlorhexidine, iodophors, hexachlorophene) before each operation. Scrubbing should be done before every procedure and for at least five minutes before the first procedure of the day (two minutes for subsequent procedures). Hand scrubbing by the surgeon and his assistants should be done in essentially the same manner as preparation of the animal's skin for surgery. A sterile gown is donned, and gloves put on using the closed technique or with the assistance of a previously gloved person. The gloves must be washed of all powder before handling any of the instruments or drapes, particularly in an experiment involving histology. Powder contamination of the implant will not give a true histological picture of the tissue's response [15]. Gloves punctured during the operation should be promptly changed. For orthopedic or cardiovascular implant operations of long duration two pairs of gloves should be worn [16].

The Operative Technique

Biomaterial evaluation is dependent upon the classic sequence of events that characterizes normal wound healing. Local environmental conditions must be optimal for cellular metabolism, because almost all biological phenomena associated with healing require the active participation of cells. The majority of technical advances in wound care over the past century have been based on a "minimal interference" concept: the less "surgery" the surgeon does, while removing all impediments to normal wound healing processes, the better the result. Indeed, all technical considerations in surgery may be viewed as methods of minimizing the surgeon's interference with normal healing. Clearly, the duration and intensity of the inflammatory response to surgery alone depends upon the amount of local tissue damage. Rapid and complete invasion of the wound space by fibroblasts is a critical step in normal healing. Extensive tissue injury and/or the presence of foreign materials and/or bacteria can prolong the inflammatory phase for months. Large amounts of fibrin, dead tissue fragments, hematomas, and fluid collections due to dead space formation act as physical barriers, preventing normal fibroblast penetration and delaying collagen fiber production. The evaluation of the material under study can therefore be significantly affected by the surgery used to implant that material. The minimization of the 3 T's (Time, Trash and Trauma) will help lead to a successful outcome.

To the clinical surgeon, surgery is a craft involving skilled, prescient dissection in the presence of pathologic anatomy, with the intent of correcting that pathology. To the research surgeon, and more particularly the biomaterials scientist, surgery is an evaluation tool. It also requires skilled, prescient dissection, but with the added intent of creating specific pathologic anatomy and the substitution of a foreign material for normal tissue. This alteration of the normal requires the strictest attention to all principles that relate to minimization of trauma. These principles must be followed so that, despite the nearly infinite number of variables in the in vivo milieu, this implantation will allow the study not only of differences in biological response to basic materials, but also of subtle, induced changes in surface chemistry or morphology of a material when in use as an artificial internal organ or device.

The maxim of implantation surgery is to leave the animal as a system, and the tissue into which the biomaterial is implanted, as normal as possible after the implantation. Maintaining tissue viability is the essence of proper surgical technique. Good surgical technique includes gentle tissue handling, effective hemostasis, maintenance of sufficient blood supply to tissues, asepsis, accurate tissue apposition, proper use of surgical instruments, and expeditious performance of the surgical procedure. Optimum care of the wound starts prior to wounding and ends months later. It includes gentle surgical technique, post-operative protection, cleanliness, and superior nutrition.

The purpose of excellence in surgical technique is to diminish the depth and duration of the injury components, thus diminishing endocrine and metabolic changes and reducing the likelihood of local or systemic complications. If the operative technique is ideal and the appropriate operation well conceived and executed, there will be minimal catabolic change induced in the animal's composition. There is no question that a smoothly-done operation reduces the magnitude and duration of pathological disorders. The maintenance of a very low level of tissue trauma results in a minimal amount of bleeding or hematoma formation in the tissue planes. Also, postoperative edema is reduced by avoiding extensive dissection and by the precise use of noninjurious methods of handling tissue. In summary, a successful result depends upon clarity of concept, expeditious and meticulous handling of tissues, aggressive pursuit of the objective, careful wound management, avoidance of contamination, and careful wound closure.

Postoperative Care

Three overlapping phases characterize the post-operative period: recovery from anesthesia and short- and long-term post-operative care. The animal's welfare and the validity of the experiment are vitally dependent upon good communication, which will minimize complications through the teamwork it inspires. Effective, constructive communication creates an environment in which the postoperative care program—tailored to the animal's needs, the study's objectives, and the institution's capabilities—can be managed productively. The appropriately-trained personnel involved in postoperative management need to be identified *in advance* of surgery in order to ensure effective animal care, and prevent potential problems.

Since it is the period of greatest physiologic disturbance, recovery from the anesthesia is the most critical time in post-operative care. This period is, of course, handled and monitored by the primary operative team, particularly the anesthetist. The animal should be positioned properly to prevent any impediments to normal respiratory and cardiovascular functioning, the physiologic condition should be monitored regularly, and the body temperature maintained.

With respect to the need for postoperative analgesics, an important principle prepared by the Interagency Research Animal Committee and used by the United States Public Health Service (USPHS) is that, "unless the contrary is established, investigators should consider that procedures that cause pain and distress in human beings may cause pain or distress in other animals" [18].

Long-term recovery of the animal from the trauma of the implantation is, of course, vital to the success of the study. This period will be greatly facilitated by a management program that is as well organized as the implantation procedure itself. The key to postoperative management is, again, good communication among the members of the team, and careful observation by trained and caring personnel. The nature of the surgical procedure and the stage of recovery will determine the frequency and type of monitoring performed. At the very least, body temperature, food intake, locomotion, behavior, and signs indicative of pain should be monitored. The wound should be observed for signs of infection, dehiscence, or self-inflicted trauma. Percutaneous cannulae and catheters should be cleaned and disinfected daily. They should also be examined daily for proper operation and lack of interference with the animal's physiologic functions. Complications such as acute renal failure, intestinal hypermotility or paralytic ileus, can be identified early by careful monitoring of food and water intake and the quantity and character of urine and feces.

The institution and the implantation team must always be flexible enough to re-evaluate all aspects of the study, including the pre-operative, operative and postoperative plans and their implementation, at any time during the study. In a new study, some changes often need to be made for subsequent procedures, as the specifics of the study may never have been done before. This evaluation requires the input of the surgical team, attending veterinarian, research technicians and animal care staff. The feeling of teamwork is never more important than in these evaluation sessions. The study environment must reflect an attitude in which all constructive suggestions, from all members of the team (regardless of their position), are taken seriously, and are given due consideration. Changes to the procedures must arise from group discussion, not authoritarian mandate. Modifications that do result from these meetings need to be reviewed with all other personnel involved and, when significant changes are to be made, with the IACUC.

The postoperative care program must be tailored to the individual study and procedure, and be individualized for the well being of each animal.

Of paramount importance in this activity is thorough and accurate documentation of all aspects of the study, using appropriate medical records and logs, with regular evaluation of the entire program, carried out by trained personnel during all phases of the work.

RESULTS

If the device was well designed, based on extensive literature review, early toxicity testing, and sufficient cadaver dissection; if the protocol was well thought out and the experiment performed accordingly; and if the operation was well performed, then the results of the experiment will be useful. Significant data will be obtained, and the animal will have served the purpose of improving health care for both mankind and animals.

REFERENCES

1   Park JJ. Biocompatibility of medical devices: Tripartite biocompatibility for medical devices. Toxicology Subgroup, Tripartite Subcommittee on Medical Devices of Canada, the United Kingdom, and the United States; International Standard ISO/DIS 10993: Biological Testing of Medical and Dental Materials and Devices. *Regulatory Requirements of Medical Devices*, FDA Publication 92-4165. Washington, DC: Department of Health and Human Services, 1992, A1–A24.

2   Brown MJ, Pearson PT, Tomson FN. Guidelines for animal surgery in research and teaching. *Am J Vet Res*, 54 (1993), 1544–1559.

3   Academy of Surgical Research. Guidelines for training in surgical research in animals. *J Invest Surg*, 2 (1989), 263–268.

4   Atkinson LJ. Physical facilities. In *Berry & Kohn's Operating Room Technique*, 7th ed. St. Louis: Mosby, 1992, 36–45.

5   Atkinson LJ. Sterilization and disinfection. In *Berry and Kohn's Operating Room Technique*, 7th ed. St. Louis: Mosby, 1992, 126–153.

6   Flecknell PA. *Laboratory Animal Anesthesia: An Introduction for Research Workers and Technicians.* London: Academic Press, Inc., 1987.

7   Lumb WV, Jones EW. *Veterinary Anesthesia*, 2nd ed. Philadelphia, PA: Lea & Febiger, 1984.

8   Raffe MR. Fluid Therapy in the surgical patient. In Slatter DH (Ed.), *Textbook of Small Animal Surgery.* Philadelphia, PA: W. B. Saunders, 1985, 90–102.

9   Dougherty SH. Implant infections. In von Recum AF (Ed.), *Handbook of Biomaterials Evaluation*, 1st ed. New York: Macmillan, 1986, 276–289.

10 Committee on Pain and Distress in Laboratory Animals, Institute of Laboratory Animal Resources, Commission on Life Sciences, National Research Council. *Recognition and Alleviation of Pain and Distress in Laboratory Animals.* Washington, DC: National Academy Press, 1992.

11 Alexander JW, Fischer JE, Boyajian M. The influence of hair-removal methods on wound infections. *Arch Surg*, 118 (1983), 347.

12 Atkinson LJ. Preoperative preparation of surgical patients. In *Berry & Kohn's Operating Room Technique.* St. Louis: Mosby, 1992, 265–272.

13 Mendenhall HV. Principle considerations for experimental surgical procedures. In von Recum AF (Ed.), *Handbook of Biomaterial Evaluation*, 1st ed. New York: Macmillan, 1986, 265–274.

14 Polk HC, Simpson CJ, Simmons BP. Guidelines for prevention of surgical wound infection. *Arch Surg*, 118 (1983), 1213.

15 Gibbons DF. Personal communications, 1982–1991.

16 Atkinson LJ. Attire, surgical scrub, gowning and gloving. In *Berry and Kohn's Operating Room Technique.* St. Louis: Mosby, 1992, 192–205.

17 Halasz NA. Wound infection and topical antibiotics. *Arch Surg*, 112 (1977), 1240.

18 *U.S. Government Principles for Utilization and Care of Vertebrate Animals Used in Testing, Research, and Training.* Office of Science and Technology Policy. Federal Register, 50 (1985), 20864–20865.

Chapter 32

Implant Infections

Julie M. Higashi
Roger E. Marchant

INTRODUCTION

Over 35 million surgical procedures involving the extensive use of artificial implants and devices are completed each year in the United States [1]. Unfortunately, infection is a potentially serious complication with implants and devices and a major impediment to the long-term clinical success of complex devices [2]. Even though the incidence of infection is relatively low, the morbidity and mortality associated with these infections is high (Table 32-1). Additionally, implanted devices have become so numerous that implant-centered infection is now a very costly problem. Clinical treatment of implant infections can be 5 to 7 times the cost of the initial implantation [3].

Most microorganisms infecting implants are either present in the host flora or nosocomial in origin (Table 32-2). The most frequent etiologic agents are *Staphylococcus aureus* and the coagulase negative staphylococci of which *S. epidermidis* is the most predominant. Methicillin resistant *S. aureus* and *S. epidermidis* are also becoming more prevalent [4]. Gram negative organisms, particularly enteric bacteria, as well as nosocomially acquired *Pseudomonas aeriginosa* are frequent pathogens that are particularly virulent [5–9]. Fungi Candida spp and Aspergillus spp are the etiologic agents in only 8 percent of implant infections, but are emerging as formidable pathogens with a survival rate of only 50 percent [10].

Implant-centered infections have several characteristic traits which set them apart from infections not involving biomaterials. A consequence of device implantation is the resulting tissue damage, which disrupts natural physical barriers and provides an opportunity for invading pathogens. Indeed, the inoculum of microbes needed to establish an infection in the presence of a biomaterial is several orders of magnitude less than that needed to establish an infection otherwise [11]. The implanted biomaterial may impair host immunity, making it extremely difficult for the host to mount an effective response. Nonpathogenic commensals like *S. epidermidis* or opportunistic pathogens like *Candida albicans* can become virulent organisms in the presence of an implant. While neutrophil chemotaxis to an infection nidus is unaffected, phagocytosis and oxidative burst of the cell is attenuated, resulting in inefficient microbial killing. Lastly, the majority of implant infections are resistant to antibiotic treatment, and unless the infected implant or device is removed or replaced, the infection rarely resolves [12, 13].

On a cellular level, the critical initial step in the pathogenesis of implant infection is the adhesion of the microbe to the implant, which is determined by interactions between the implant, host, and pathogen [5]. Once attached, the microbe can divide and colonize the surface, developing microcolonies which may elaborate and extrude an exopolysaccharide substance called slime, produced by some strains of bacteria like *S. epidermidis*, forming a protective "biofilm" [12]. Extruded slime may serve as an ion exchange resin that acts to trap important nutrients for continued microbial growth. It is a potent virulence factor, since slime-encased bacteria are significantly more resistant to antibiotics [14]. The biofilm

Table 32-1   Clinical Incidence of Implant-Associated Infections

Implant or device	Number used or implanted	Incidence of infection	Morbidity/ mortality	References
Intravascular catheters (peripheral, central venous)	150–200 million/year	<.1% 3–7%	15–20% mortality	[7, 60]
Urethral catheters	4–5 million/year	5–10% daily risk	1–2% gram negative sepsis	[60]
CNS shunts	>80,000/year	10–15%		[60]
Hemodialysis grafts		10%	28% mortality	[6]
Pacemaker leads	115,000– 130,000/year	2–11%	2% mortality	[9]
Vascular graft	>60,000/year	0–3%	40% mortality; 20–30% amputation	[5, 60]
Prosthetic heart valve	>100,000/year	1–5%	34% mortality; 25–30% CNS complications	[61]
Total artificial heart	230 (1969– 1991)	36%	34% mortality	[2, 62]
Genitourinary prosthesis	150,000 total	5%	72% permanent device removal	[63]
Total artificial hip	222,000/year	<1%	7–63% mortality	[8]
Total knee arthroplasty	110,000/year	1–2%	2.5% mortality; 80% non-functioning	[3]

Table 32-2   Etiology of Implant Infections [64]

Microorganism	Potential source of inoculum	Pathogenic features or complications	References
Gram positive cocci		predominant implant infecting organisms	[7]
Staphylococcus aureus	nasal pharanx (40–50%)	associated with metallic implants	[3, 8, 13]
Staphylococcus epidermidis	skin, respiratory, gastrointestinal tract	associated with polymer implants; exudes slime	[5, 13, 61]
Gram negative rods			
Enterobacteriaceae (E. coli, klebsiella, enterobacter, morganella, serratia)	gastrointestinal tract	anastomotic hemorrhage in vascular grafts; graft-enteric fistulas	[5]
Pseudomonas aeriginosa	nosocomial, gastrointestinal tract	extremely virulent, associated with polymer implants	[2, 5, 13]
Fungi			
Candida spp	respiratory, gastrointestinal, and female genital tracts	rare, but extremely virulent	[7]

is thought to decrease the efficacy of antibiotics both by presenting a physical barrier and containing extracellular beta-lactamases. Exuded slime may be one source of this immune response deregulation, since slime is thought to inhibit B and T cell blastogenesis, immunoglobulin production, bacterial opsonization, and phagocytosis, thus enabling the microorganisms to survive [15]. The scope of implant infections is quite broad. In this chapter, we review current in vivo and in vitro methods of studying implant infections. We emphasize that the interactions between the biomaterial surface, host molecules and cells, and microbe which result in microbial adhesion may differ from one implant to another. Although the chapter is largely discussed from the point of view of blood contact implant infections, the same general principles can be applied analogously to infections involving any kind of biomedical implant or device.

IN VIVO MODELS OF IMPLANT CENTERED INFECTION

In vivo models are utilized for studying the long-term course (days to months) of implant-centered infections, particularly in the assessment of the host response and potential antibiotic treatment regimens [16–18]. In vitro and ex vivo tests are appropriate for studying the acute development of infection or short-term response to a microbial challenge on the order of minutes to hours. Ex vivo tests, that involve the shunting of blood directly from a test animal to a test chamber offer the advantage of studying events under physiological flow conditions with native blood, but they are far more expensive than in vitro tests which are good for screening a large number of parameters [19, 20].

The most appropriate and useful animal model is determined by its ability to mimic the analogous clinical course in humans, but other factors such as species size and cost can greatly contribute to the design of the model. Larger animals are often necessary because they can support human-sized implant devices. In the study of cardiovascular device-centered infection, nonhuman primates like baboons have similar blood values and reactivity to humans, but device testing in nonhuman primates may be prohibited [21]. A canine, swine, or calf model is often utilized instead. The calf is used extensively in the United States for total artificial heart studies (TAH), because of its size and rapid post-implantation recovery. Moreover, the incidence, etiologic organisms, and onset of bacterial infection in calves are similar to those in humans, indicating that this is also a good animal model for studying TAH-related infection [22].

There is extensive literature devoted to characterizing the blood compatibility of vascular grafts in canine models, which are also invaluable in the study of implant infection [19, 23, 24]. However, healing characteristics and bloodstream clearance of bacteria in swine more closely resemble those of humans than do the same measured values in dogs. For example, platelet adhesion, thrombosis, and hemolysis occurs much more readily in dogs than in humans [21]. A comparative study of vascular graft infection showed that the same graft was much more susceptible to infection in dogs than in swine [24]. In this study, the infrarenal aorta was replaced with a 6 mm woven double velour Dacron® (E. I. DuPont de Nemours & Co., Inc., Wilmington, DE) graft, with *Staphylcoccus aureus* infused intravenously. Grafts were retrieved 1 week after implantation; both native tissue and graft were cultured and examined histologically and by scanning electron microscopy (SEM). Porcine explanted grafts showed a smooth, compacted fibrinous surface with occasional bacteria trapped on the surface, while grafts from dogs had a more irregular surface with loose fibrin, bare fibers, and numerous trapped bacteria particularly in areas with bare fibers or thrombi. Such studies suggest that swine may provide a better animal model than dogs for in vivo graft infection studies.

Small animals are often appropriate for in vivo studies on candidate biomaterials rather that the larger complete devices, and are particularly useful for studying long-term host responses over a period of months. The tissue cage implant model (see Chapter 42) allows the assessment of the host response to an implant material as well as the evaluation of antibiotic treatment regimes [18, 25]. This is particularly useful since standard in vitro antibiotic susceptibility tests like the minimum inhibitory concentration (MIC) do not accurately reflect the susceptibility of microorganisms involved in implant-related infections. The tissue cage is implanted subcutaneously into the flanks of rats or guinea pigs, and 10^4 cfu inoculated directly into the cage or via hematogenous seeding [26]. The interstitial wound fluid, cells, and bacteria in the tissue cage are analyzed periodically during the implantation time period [18]. Antibiotics may be administered intraperitoneally or intramuscularly to evaluate their effectiveness in clearing the infection in the tissue cage. The results from these in vivo experiments have been used as a standard to develop an in vitro method to test antibiotic efficacy in implant infections [26].

A common site for implantation in small animal models is the peritoneum, which offers an accessible site for monitoring as well as a confined space that discourages adventitious contamination from other sources. These studies are particularly relevant to peritoneal catheter infections which occur in patients who undergo continuous ambulatory peritoneal dialysis (CAPD). A mouse model has been developed in which a segment of a peritoneal catheter with adherent *S. epidermidis* biofilm is inserted intraperitoneally and secured to the lateral abdominal wall with a single suture [16]. Animals are examined at 2 weeks and 3 months, and by 6 months 80% of the mice retain a stable, localized, implant infection postoperatively as determined by animal survival, recovery of the inoculated bacterial strain from catheter scrapings, cellular response in the peritoneal cavity and circulating blood, and direct examination of catheter surface by SEM [16, 27]. A clinically relevant porcine model for peritoneal catheter-associated infection includes partial nephrectomization to reproduce the uremic state observed in humans undergoing CAPD as well as implantation of the peritoneal catheter through the abdominal wall. An exit site infection is produced by inoculating 10^9 cfu/mL *S. epidermidis* between the exit site and catheter. The systemic host immune response to the catheter associated bacteria is assessed by determining white blood cell counts, antistaphylococcal IgG concentration by ELISA, and immunoblots of antisera against extracted *S. epidermidis* cell wall proteins. The catheters and surrounding tissue are harvested for the recovery and verification of the inoculated strain as well as characterization of the bacterial cell wall protein profile [28]. Results indicated that uremia had no effect on the serological response of the pigs to the infection, but significant increases in antistaphylococcal antibody and peripheral neutrophil count were observed. Such studies are invaluable for developing criteria to aid diagnosis and treatment of these infections in humans.

Several models for cardiovascular implant infection have been developed, including a rabbit model of bacteremia and endocarditis [17, 29]. A silicone elastomer catheter is dipped in a 10^8 cfu/mL *S. epidermidis* suspension, immediately inserted into the right jugular vein of the animal, and then attached to a subcutaneous osmotic pump filled with heparin to ensure blood flow through the catheter. Bacteremia is evaluated by culturing blood from an ear vein daily for seven days. Supernates of positive cultures are checked by Ouchterlony immunodiffusion to evaluate the immunity of immunized and nonimmunized rabbits toward specific surface antigens on *S. epidermidis*. In the endocarditis model which examines post-implantation infection, a Teflon® (E. I. DuPont de Nemours & Co., Inc., Wilmington, DE) catheter is inserted via the carotid artery into the left ventricle in order to simulate aortic valve leaflet vegetations. After a one-week healing period, bacteria are inoculated into the catheter. The rabbits are maintained for 20–22 days, after which they are sacrificed and the cardiac vegetations examined and cultured.

IN VITRO METHODS OF STUDYING MICROBIAL ADHESION

The physicochemical surface properties of an implant influence the host response by affecting the composition and conformation of adsorbed proteins and activation state of adhering cells. If the inoculation occurs at or near the time of implantation, the pathogen has an opportunity to bind directly to the biomaterial surface; otherwise the pathogen may only interact with the host-modified surface [12, 13]. Figure 32-1 illustrates the basic interactions that result in microbial adhesion to a blood-contacting device or implant. A blood-contacting device is usually a synthetic polymer on which plasma proteins will immediately adsorb, followed by the deposition of cellular elements [30]. Microbial adhesion to orthopaedic implants such as a total artificial hip often involves a metallic alloy, extracellular matrix proteins, and connective tissue cells in a relatively quiescent flow environment. Both cardiovascular and orthopaedic implants are colonized by microbes, but the cell and molecular interactions leading to microbial adhesion are distinct because of differences in the biomaterials and the host environments.

Adhesion between a microbe and biomaterial surface result from nonspecific and/or specific interactions between the microbe and either the biomaterial or adsorbed host proteins and cells. Intermolecular forces at surfaces are determined by surface chemical composition and surface free energy of the microbe and biomaterial, influenced by properties of the local fluid environment such as pH and ionic strength [13]. Surface topography and local interfacial shear forces are also important, nonspecific factors affecting microbial adhesion. This is illustrated in Figure 32-2, which shows the result of a study that examined the roles of surface physicochemistry, topography, and shear forces in determining *S. epidermidis* adhesion to biomaterials. Bacterial adhesion to a woven Dacron® vascular graft was

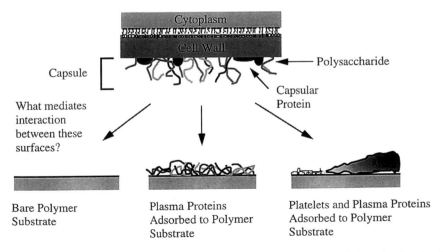

Figure 32-1 Microbial adhesion to blood contact devices. The surfaces of the microbe, implant, and the surrounding media continuously interact with each other. Adsorption of elements from the blood like plasma proteins and platelets on the surface greatly influences the interactions which result in microbial adhesion.

A

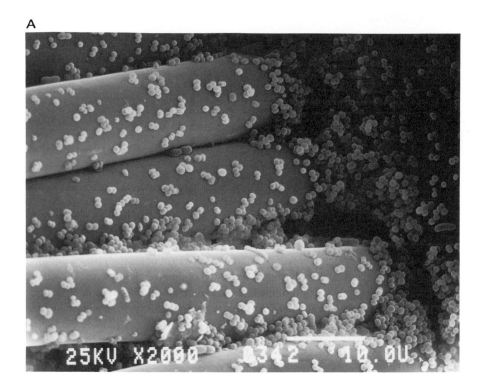

B

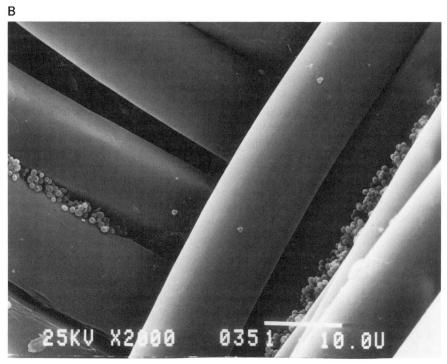

Figure 32-2 Role of surface topography in determining bacterial adhesion to Dacron®. Scanning electron micrograph (2000X) showing turbulent-flow-induced physical entrapment of *S. epidermidis* in Dacron® fiber interstices (A). The inclusion of plasma proteins in solution which adsorb to the Dacron® fiber significantly decreases overall microbial adhesion (B). (Reproduced from the *Journal of Biomedical Materials Research*, 1995, 29:485-403).

dominated by topography-induced turbulent flow, causing physical entrapment of the bacteria in fiber interstices [30].

Specific interactions result in a ligand receptor recognition and subsequent adhesion between the microbe and implant surface. This may involve protein-protein interaction, lectin (protein-carbohydrate) interaction, or carbohydrate-carbohydrate interaction. The conformations of the ligand and receptor are important, as the microbe may not interact specifically with the molecule in both its soluble and surface adherent forms [31]. Specific interactions with microbes usually involve blood plasma proteins, extracellular matrix molecules, or host cell surface molecules [32]. Bacterial cell surface molecules which bind to extracellular matrix molecules have been classified as a family of adhesins called MSCRAMMs (microbial surface components recognizing adhesive matrix molecules) [33].

Transport of Pathogen to Device Surface

Most bacterial adhesion studies have been conducted under conditions of fluid stasis, and are appropriate for preliminary screening and testing of implants materials. However, microbial adhesion to cardiovascular devices occurs in the bloodstream, and adhesion mechanisms should be studied under dynamic flow conditions. For example, it has been demonstrated in static assays that neutrophil adhesion to endothelial cells is mediated by the neutrophil adhesins, P-Selectin and ICAM-1, while only P-Selectin is an effective adhesin under fluid flow [34]. Analogously, the absence of shear forces may affect the conformations of surface molecules and proteins on the bacteria and biomaterials, thus influencing subsequent adhesion.

In vitro adhesion experiments involving blood-contacting materials should include an appropriate flow chamber to provide a controlled dynamic flow conditions. If the fluid flow is well controlled and characterized, i.e., laminar, then shear stresses at the interface between substrate and fluid are known, and this can provide information on the strength of the microbial adhesion. Several flow chambers in current use are depicted in Figure 32-3. The flow chamber most used in cell adhesion studies is the parallel plate flow chamber. It can be mounted on an optical microscope, allowing for in situ, real time observations and assessment of adhesion kinetics with either an opaque or transparent biomaterial substrate [35, 36]. Its major limitation is that only one shear stress can be evaluated per experiment. The radial flow chamber provides a laminar axisymmetric flow which results in a continuous range of shear stresses within one experiment. It may be mounted on an optical microscope for direct in situ observation of cellular adhesion with transparent substrates [37]. The rotating disk produces a laminar flow environment over a range of shear stresses while maintaining constant transport of microbes to the disk surface. The efficiency of microbial adhesion may be assessed by counting microbes attached to the disk surface compared with the total number of microbes transported to the disk. In situ, real time observation of microbial adhesion is not feasible with the rotating disk, but both opaque and transparent biomaterials may be evaluated [30, 38].

The Biomaterial Surface

Bacterial adhesion studies may include a reference material, a model surface, or a candidate material, to be compared against an existing, clinically used biomaterial. Knowledge of the physicochemical surface properties of the biomaterial is essential in designing appropriate experiments that examine microbial adhesion. Techniques frequently used to characterize surface chemical composition of biomaterials include electron spectroscopy

Flow Chamber	Features	Shear Stress (τ) Equation
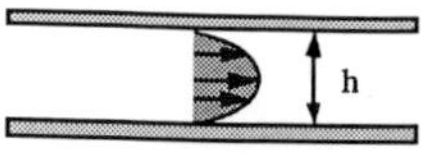 Parallel Plate Flow Chamber	• in situ real time observation • one shear stress • opaque and transparent substrates	$\tau = \mu \dfrac{6Q}{wh^2}$
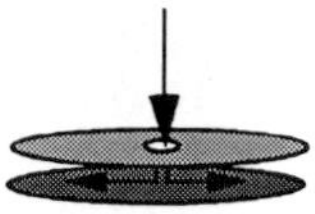 Radial Flow Chamber	• in situ real time observation • range of shear stresses • transparent substrate only	$\tau = \dfrac{3Q\mu}{\pi r h^2}$
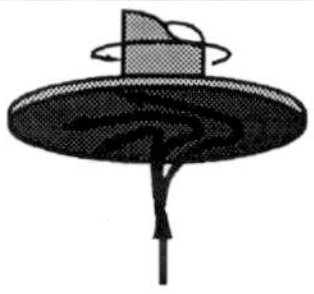 Rotating Disk	• adhesion efficiency • range of shear stresses • opaque and transparent substrates	$\tau = .800\mu r \sqrt{\dfrac{\omega^3}{\nu}}$

μ-absolute viscosity, Q-volumetric flow, ω-angular velocity, r-radius, w-width, h-height, and ν-kinematic viscocity

Figure 32-3   Flow chambers for studying microbial adhesion under dynamic fluid flow.

for chemical analysis (ESCA) and Fourier transform infrared spectroscopy (FTIR). Measurement of contact angles enables calculation of the interfacial free energy and assessment of hydrophobicity, or wettability [39]. Surface charge may be assessed by measuring the streaming potential on flat surfaces and calculating the zeta potential [40, 41]. SEM and atomic force microscopy (AFM) enable evaluation of biomaterial topography, the latter on a three-dimensional nanometer scale [39].

A good reference material is one that is identical or closely related to commonly used biomaterials, stable, well characterized, smooth, available in many forms (sheet, tube, microsphere), and sterile or sterilizable. NHLBI low density polyethylene (LDPE) is a good reference because of its simple surface chemistry relative to other biomedical polymers like the polyurethanes and its simple topography compared with woven Dacron® fiber or expanded PTFE [39]. Unfortunately, the surface chemistry of clinical biomedical polymers is often variable, and correlating particular interactions with microbial adhesion is often extremely difficult. To address this issue, model surfaces containing well-defined terminal head group functionality can be prepared from self-assembled monolayers (SAMs) on glass or gold substrates. By varying the terminal head group, SAMs with uniform and well defined surface properties can be prepared [42]. Wiencek et al. employed mixed and single SAMs with hydroxyl and methyl terminal groups in different proportions to explore the effects on bacterial adhesion and found that decreasing the percentage of hydroxyl head groups increased surface hydrophobicity and bacterial adhesion [43]. In developing candidate biomaterials resistant to microbial adhesion, investigators have capitalized on the finding that attaching hydrophilic, non-ionized polymers such as poly(ethylene oxide) (PEO) or dextran to existing clinical materials significantly reduces protein and cellular adhesion [44, 45]. However, much work remains to optimize the molecular weight, crosslinking, stability, manufacture and processing of these modified surfaces before they become a clinical reality.

The Microbe

Characterization of a microbe's surface is a daunting task, as factors like growth phase, environmental conditions, growth media, and strain type may alter the surface properties and components substantially [46]. Nevertheless, numerous techniques are used effectively to characterize both the surface properties of pathogens associated with implant infections. Surface hydrophobicity has an important influence on microbial adhesion and can be assessed in several ways. Microbial adherence to hydrocarbons (MATH) measures the migration of cells from an aqueous phase to an organic interface in a two-phase water/hydrocarbon system. The percentage of cells depleted from the water phase, which corresponds to increasing surface hydrophobicity, is assessed by changes in optical density. MATH is simple and quick, although it is not quantitative and is difficult to standardize. MATH is best used for qualitatively grouping strains as either hydrophobic or hydrophilic [47]. A more quantitative assessment is obtained using hydrophobic interaction chromatography (HIC), which measures microbe retention on a hydrophobic packing matrix, reflecting the interaction between nonpolar hydrocarbon ligands attached to the column matrix and nonpolar regions of the microbial surface. The percentage of bacteria retained on the column is correlated with the bacteria's surface hydrophobicity. Varying either the length or structure of the hydrocarbon ligand on the gel, or the ionic strength of the solvent, affects the strength of the interaction enabling the detection of differences in microbe hydrophobicity [41]. Contact angle measurements on microbial lawns also are used extensively to assess the surface hydrophobicity and interfacial free energy of both bacteria and fungi in order to correlate results with microbial adhesion on material surfaces [41, 48]. However, these measurements should be approached with care, as it is difficult to obtain reliable contact angles, and data interpretation depends on several underlying assumptions that may be invalidated. For example, it is assumed there is no interaction between the probe liquid and the surface so that the surface tension of the liquid remains constant, but components from microbial lawns may desorb into the probe liquid, changing its surface tension, and hence the contact angles obtained.

Surface charge might be expected to play an important role in determining microbial adhesion to biomaterials, although this issue is not well understood on a molecular scale because of the complexity of cell surface molecules and the presence of other intermolecular forces. Microbial surface charge can be determined from electrophoretic mobility, and electrostatic interaction chromatography (EIC) [41]. Electrophoretic mobility is determined from the velocity of microbes through a buffer of known ionic strength under the application of an external electric field [35]. The zeta potential can be calculated from electrophoretic mobility using the Helmholtz-Smoluchowski equation, and the isoelectric point may be determined from electrophoretic mobility measured as a function of pH [41, 48]. Surface charge also may be analyzed quantitatively using EIC which is analogous to HIC, except that the gel matrix is an ion exchange resin. Usually, both cationic and anionic columns are run simultaneously to assess the relative contributions to the total surface charge.

A challenging task is identification of microbial surface molecules that interact specifically and recognize either implant or host-modified implant surfaces. This information is important in the development of new strategies for preventing implant infection. Sjollema et al. demonstrated the importance of proteinaceous bacterial surface molecules from differences in deposition rates between *Streptococcus salivarius* and a spontaneous mutant bald strain [49]. Studies involving the treatment of coagulase negative staphylococci with proteolytic enzymes or antibodies reduced bacterial adhesion to polymer surfaces [50]. However, this effect might arise from either a difference in physicochemical surface properties and/or the loss of the specific ligand. To account for this possibility, molecular genetics techniques involving transposon mutagenesis have successfully produced mutant strains of bacteria deficient in the expression of specific surface molecules and used to study specific microbial surface molecules as putative mediators of adhesion. The technique involves incorporating a transposon, a self-integrating piece of DNA, into the wildtype genome, creating a mutant strain genetically identical to the parent except for the transposon interruption. Use of isogenic strains of bacteria in adhesion studies enables the assessment of the putative adhesion mediator in the absence of phenotypic differences which arise between genetically different strains of bacteria. However, the transposon interruption may result in the absence of more than one surface molecule, obscuring the contributions of the respective molecules to microbial adhesion [51].

Detection of Bacteria on Test Surfaces

In situ, real time enumeration of adherent bacteria and fungi requires an optical microscope connected to a video or digital camera that can quickly grab images for processing and analysis [35, 37]. Detection is most straightforward on transparent materials so that the microbes do not have to be labelled. Real time epifluorescent microscopy on opaque surfaces is possible, provided the fluorescent probe does not easily photobleach. For samples which are not imaged in real time, care should be taken to minimize introduction of artifacts as the processing and fixation may cause detachment or spatial rearrangement of adhering cells [52]. Once fixed, cells can be labelled with histochemical stains, fluorochrome dyes, or antibodies conjugated to fluorescent probes or gold beads [53]. The results may be compared with complimentary techniques such as AFM (see Figure 32-4) and SEM. Total internal reflection fluorescence microscopy (TIRF) allows close scrutiny of the interface between cells and surfaces through analysis of focal contacts between the adherent cell and the substrate [54]. SEM is used extensively to evaluate microbial adhesion, particularly on

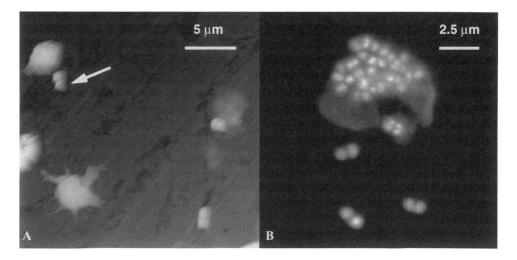

Figure 32-4 Detection of *S. epidermidis* and platelets on NHLBI low density polyethylene (PE) by atomic force microscopy (A) and fluorescence microscopy (B). A representative bacterium has been designated with the arrow in (A). Bacteria and platelets were stained with acridine orange in (B) and can be differentiated from each other by staining intensity. Note the large number of bacteria associated with the platelet relative to the PE surface.

implants with complex topography [30]. TEM is used for ultrastructural studies of adherent bacteria, and enables visualization of the interface between cell and material. However, both SEM and TEM require elaborate sample preparation which may alter the polymer and/or microbial surfaces and introduce artifacts [53].

For evaluation of microbes on large or complex surfaces, indirect techniques coupled with appropriate calibration can be used to quantify cell numbers [53]. The simplest approach is to culture the sample. This entails dislodging cells by scraping or sonication, resuspending the cells in buffer, and determining cfu/mL by viable counts. Sample surfaces can then be examined by SEM to assess the remaining microorganisms. A more quantitative approach involves radiolabelling microbes with ^{3}H-thymidine or ^{3}H-leucine added to growth media, and then measuring by scintillation counts. Finally, a bioluminescence assay can quantify the amount of ATP extracted from adherent bacteria by measuring the emitted light after the addition of luciferin-luciferinase.

Host Contribution to Microbial Adhesion

Protein adsorption on a biomaterial in blood is so rapid that complete surface coverage occurs within seconds. Therefore, the host contribution to microbial adhesion is considerable, since the microorganism will likely interact with adherent proteins or cells and not with the bare biomaterial. Adsorbed proteins will generally decrease bacterial adhesion relative to adhesion on the bare biomaterial (Figure 32-2B) [30, 38]. This effect is largely attributed to adsorbed albumin, which accounts for 50 percent of all plasma proteins [50]. To study the effects of adsorbed proteins, one can either preadsorb, or "condition" the surface with proteins. Alternatively, proteins can be included in the test media with cells, as the kinetics of microbial adhesion are orders of magnitude slower than protein adsorption. It is only necessary to include enough proteins in the test media to achieve surface coverage; microbial adhesion in platelet poor plasma (PPP) or 1 percent PPP to LDPE under hemodynamic shear are not significantly different [30, 38].

The binding of *S. aureus* to fibrinogen and fibronectin are examples of specific, ligand-receptor interactions between a microorganism and host protein [20, 55]. To demonstrate saturation, one must show that by increasing the concentration of the microbe in test media, there is a concomitant increase in microorganisms adhering to the protein adsorbed surface which eventually levels off, indicating maximum binding and saturation. Specificity is demonstrated by showing that the interaction between the microorganism and the adsorbed protein can be inhibited or blocked with a receptor antagonist [56]. *S. aureus* adhesion to adsorbed fibrinogen can be inhibited with an antibody to fibrinogen in a dose dependent manner in a competitive binding assay [57]. Antibodies are large molecules, so they may not only inhibit the interaction by occupying the active site, but may also change the physicochemical properties of the test surface. It is preferable to use smaller blocking agents like peptide analogs to minimize competing effects [55].

A similar approach can be used to study specific binding of microbes to surface adherent cells such as platelets or leukocytes. For example, *S. aureus* adhesion to platelets on surfaces may involve fibrinogen as a bridging molecule. In addition, *S. aureus* adhesion was inhibited by three different antibodies to the platelet receptor GPIIb/IIIa, but not by antibodies to four other platelet receptors. Another important consideration is the activation state of the cell, as this may change the conformation and distribution of cell surface receptors and alter bacterial binding [20]. Platelets are also potential mediators of *S. epidermidis* adhesion to biomaterials [38, 58]. These studies help solidify the link between thrombosis and infection, which has been implicated clinically.

FUTURE DIRECTIONS

The treatment and prevention of implant-centered infections remain a serious and problematic clinical complication. The original approach of designing implants with chemically "inert" surfaces is being reexamined, as these implants tend to elicit a chronic inflammatory response which results in incomplete tissue integration and provides opportunities to the invading pathogen. Researchers in the field of tissue engineering are developing biomimetic materials designed to promote improved tissue integration via programmed biological and cellular interactions. This approach shows great promise for the future development of infection resistant implants. Other avenues of study involve developing new techniques to study the fundamental mechanisms of microbial adhesion. AFM is currently being technically refined to measure adhesion forces between individual specific ligand-receptor pairs [59]. The combination of efforts in clinical medicine, basic science, and engineering make the study of implant infections a truly interdisciplinary endeavor.

ACKNOWLEDGEMENTS

The authors acknowledge the financial support of NIH Grants HL-47300 and T32GM07250-19. SEM images of bacteria on Dacron® were provided by I.-W. Wang, and the AFM image of bacteria on low density polyethylene was provided by N. B. Holland, Center for Cardiovascular Biomaterials, Case Western Reserve University, Cleveland, OH.

REFERENCES

1   Malchesky P, Chamberlain V, Scott-Conner C, Salis B, Wallace C. Reprocessing of reusable medical devices. *ASAIO Journal*, 41 (1995), 146–151.

2   Nosé Y. Is a totally implantable artificial heart realistic? *Artif Organs*, 16 (1992), 19–42.

3   Bengston S. Prosthetic osteomyelitis with special reference to the knee: Risks, treatment, and costs. *Ann Med*, 25 (1993), 523–529.

4   Witte W, Braulke C, Heuck D, Cuny C. Analysis of nosocomial outbreaks with multiple and methicillin-resistant *Staphylococcus aureus* (MRSA) in Germany: Implications for hospital hygiene. *Infection*, 22 (1994, Suppl. 2), S128–S134.

5   Bandyk D, Esses GE. Prosthetic graft infection. *Surgical Clinics of North America*, 73 (1994), 571–590.

6   Ballard J, Bunt T, Malone JM. Major complications of angioaccess surgery. *Am J Surg*, 164 (1992), 229–232.

7   Collignon PJ. Intravascular catheter associated sepsis: A common problem. *Med J Aust*, 161 (1994), 374–378.

8   Fitzgerald RH. Total hip arthroplasty sepsis. *Orthop Clin N Am*, 23 (1992), 259–264.

9   Pfeiffer D, Jung W, Fehske W, et al. Complications of pacemaker defibrillator devices: Diagnosis and management. *Am Heart J*, 127 (1994), 1073–1080.

10 Johnston B, Schlech III WF, Marrie TJ. An outbreak of *Candida parapsilosis* prosthetic valve endocarditis following cardiac surgery. *J Hospital Infection*, 28 (1994), 103–112.

11 Elek S, Connen PE. The virulence of *Staphylococcus pyogenes* for man: A study for the problems of wound infection. *Br J Exp Path*, 38 (1957), 573–586.

12 Gristina A, Giridhar G, Gabriel B, Naylor P, Myrvik QN. Cell biology and molecular mechanisms in artificial device infections. *Int J Artif Org*, 16 (1993), 755–764.

13 Gristina A, Giridhar G, Myrvik QN. Bacteria and biomaterials. In Greco RS (Ed.), *Implantation Biology*. New Brunswick, NJ: CRC Press, 1994, 131–148.

14 Arizono T, Oga M, Sugioka Y. Increased resistance of bacteria after adherence to polymethyl methacrylate. *Acta Orthop Scan*, 63 (1992), 661–664.

15 Gristina A, Naylor P, Myrvik Q, Wagner WD. Microbial adhesion to biomaterials. In Szycher M (Ed.), *High Performance Biomaterials*. Lancaster, PA: Technomic Publishing, 1991, 143–154.

16 Gagnon R, Richards GK. A mouse model of implant-associated infection. *Int J Artif Organs*, 16 (1993), 789–798.

17   Takeda S, Pier G, Kojima Y, et al. Protection against endocarditis due to *Staphylococcus epidermidis* by immunization with capsular polysaccharide/adhesin. *Circ*, 84 (1991), 2539–2546.

18   Zimmerli W. Experimental models in the investigation of device-related infections. *J Antimicrob Chemother*, 31 (1993, Suppl. D), 97–102.

19   National Heart, Lung, and Blood Institute Working Group. Guidelines for Blood-Material Interactions. Bethesda, MD: U.S. Department of Health and Human Services, 1985.

20   Herrmann M, Albrecht R, Mosher D, Proctor RA. Adhesion of *Staphylococcus aureus* to surface-bound platelets: Role of fibrinogen/fibrin and platelet integrins. *J Infect Dis*, 167 (1993), 313–322.

21   Biological evaluation of medical devices. *AAMI Standards and Recommended Practices*, Volume 4. Arlington, VA: Association for the Advancement of Medical Instrumentation; 1993:

22   Burns GL, Olsen DB. Patterns of bacterial infection in calves implanted with artificial hearts. *ASAIO Trans*, 36 (1990), M138–M140.

23   Mehran RJ, Ricci M, Graham A, Carter K, Symes JF. Porcine model for vascular graft studies. *J Invest Surg*, 4 (1991), 37–44.

24   Ricci MA, Mehran R, Petsikas D, et al. Species differences in the infectability of vascular grafts. *J Invest Surg*, 4 (1991), 45–52.

25   Marchant R, Hiltner A, Hamlin C, et al. In vivo biocompatibility studies. I. The cage implant system and a biodegradable polymer. *J Biomed Mater Res*, 17 (1983), 301–325.

26   Blaser J, Vergeres P, Widmer A, Zimmerli W. In vivo verification of in vitro model of antibiotic treatment of device-related infection. *Antimicrob Agents Chemother*, 39 (1995), 1134–1139.

27   Gallimore B, Gagnon R, Subang R, Richards GK. Natural history of chronic *Staphylococcus epidermidis* foreign body infection in a mouse model. *J Infect Dis*, 164 (1991), 1220–1223.

28   McDermid KP, Morck D, Olson M, et al. A porcine model of *Staphylococcus epidermidis* catheter-associated infection. *J Infect Dis*, 168 (1993), 897–903.

29   Kojima Y, Tojo M, Goldmann D, Tosteton T, Pier GB. Antibody to the capsular polysaccharide/adhesin protects rabbits against catheter-related bacteremia due to coagulase-negative staphylococci. *J Infect Dis*, 162 (1990), 435–441.

30   Wang I-W, Anderson J, Jacobs M, Marchant RE. Adhesion of *Staphylococcus epidermidis* to biomedical polymers: Contributions of surface thermodynamics and hemodynamic shear conditions. *J Biomed Mater Res*, 29 (1995), 485–493.

31   Westerlund B, Korhonen TK. Bacterial proteins binding to the mammalian extracellular matrix. Mol Microbiol, 9 (1993), 687–694.

32   McDevitt D, Francois P, Vaudaux P, Foster TJ. Molecular characterization of the clumping factor (fibrinogen receptor) of *Staphylococcus aureus*. *Mol Microbiol*, 11 (1994), 237–248.

33   Patti J, Höök M. Microbial adhesins recognizing extracellular matrix macromolecules. *Curr Op Cell Biol*, 6 (1994), 752–758.

34   Lawrence M, Springer TA. Leukocytes roll on a selectin at physiological flow rates: Distinction from and prerequisite for adhesion through integrins. *Cell*, 65 (1991), 859–873.

35   Meinders J, Van der Mei H, Busscher HJ. Physicochemical aspects of deposition of *Streptococcus thermophilus B* to hydrophobic and hydrophilic substrata in a parallel plate flow chamber. *J Colloid Interfac Sci*, 164 (1994), 355–363.

36   Alevriadou BR, Moake JL, Turner NA, et al. Real time analysis of shear dependent thrombus formation and its blockade by inhibitors of von Willebrand factor binding to platelets. *Blood*, 81 (1993), 1263–1276.

37   Dickinson R, Nagel J, McDevitt D, et al. Quantitative comparison of clumping factor and coagulase-mediated *Staphylococcus aureus* adhesion to surface-bound fibrinogen under flow. *Infect Immun*, 63 (1995), 3143–3150.

38   Wang I-W, Anderson J, Marchant RE. *Staphylococcus epidermidis* adhesion to hydrophobic biomedical polymer is mediated by platelets. *J Infect Dis*, 167 (1993), 329–336.

39   Marchant R, Wang I-W. Physical and chemical aspects of biomaterials used in humans. In Greco R (Ed.), *Implantation Biology: The Host Response and Biomedical Devices*. Ann Arbor, MI: CRC Press, 1994, 13–38.

40   Van Wagenen RA, Andrade JD. Flat plate streaming potential investigations: Hydrodynamics and electrokinetic equivalency. *J Colloid Interfac Sci*, 76 (1980), 305–315.

41   Krekeler C, Ziehr H, Klein J. Physical methods for characterization of microbial surfaces. *Experentia*, 45 (1989), 1047–1055.

42   Ullman A. Self-assembled monolayers. In *An Introduction to Ultrathin Organic Films: From Langmuir Blodgett to Self Assembly*. New York: Academic Press, Inc., 1991, 237–304.

43   Wiencek KM, Fletcher M. Bacterial adhesion to hydroxyl and methyl terminated alkanethiol self-assembled monolayers. *J Bacteriol*, 177 (1995), 1959–1966.

44 Desai N, Hubbell JA. Biological responses to polyethylene-oxide-modified polyethylene terephthalate surfaces. *J Biomed Mater Res*, 25 (1991), 829–843.

45 Marchant R, Yuan S, Szakalas-Gratzl G. Interactions of plasma proteins with a novel polysaccharide surfactant physisorbed to polyethylene. *J Biomater Sci Polymer Edn*, 6 (1994), 549–564.

46 McDermid K, Morck D, Olson M, Dasgupta M, Costerton JW. Effect of growth conditions on expression and antigenicity of *Staphylococcus epidermidis* RP62A cell envelope proteins. *Infect Immun*, 61 (1993), 1743–1749.

47 Rosenberg M. Basic and applied aspects of microbial adhesion at the hydrocarbon/water interface. *Crit Rev Microbiol*, 18 (1991), 159–173.

48 Van der Mei HC, Brokke P, Dankert J, et al. Physicochemical surface properties of nonencapsulated and encapsulated coagulase negative staphylococci. *App Environ Microbiol*, 55 (1989), 2806–2814.

49 Sjollema J, Van der Mei C, Uyen H, Busscher HJ. The influence of collector and bacterial cell surface properties on the deposition of oral streptococci in a parallel plate flow cell. *J Adhesion Sci Technol*, 4 (1990), 765–777.

50 Paulsson M, Kober M, Freij-Larsson C, et al. Adhesion of staphylococci to chemically modified and native polymers, and the influence of pre-adsorbed fibronectin, vitronectin, and fibrinogen. *Biomaterials*, 14 (1993), 845–853.

51 Muller E, Hubner J, Gutierrez N, et al. Isolation and characterization of transposon mutants of *Staphylococcus epidermidis* deficient in capsular polysaccharide/adhesin and slime. *Infect Immun*, 61 (1993), 551–558.

52 Busscher HJ, Sjollema J, vanderMei HC. Relative importance of surface free energy as a measure of hydrophobicity in bacterial adhesion to solid surfaces. In Doyle R and Rosenberg M (Ed.), *Microbial Cell Surface Hydrophobicity*. Washington, DC: American Society for Microbiology, 1990, 335–359.

53 Fletcher M. Methods for studying bacterial adhesion and attachment to surfaces. *Methods in Microbiol*, 22 (1990), 251–283.

54 Burmeister J, Truskey G, Yarbrough J, Reichert WM. Imaging of cell/substrate contacts on polymers by total internal reflection fluorescence microscopy. *Biotechnol Prog*, 10 (1994), 26–31.

55 Raja R, Raucci G, Hook M. Peptide analogs to a fibronectin receptor inhibit attachment of *Staphylococcus aureus* to fibronectin-containing substrates. *Infect Immun*, 58 (1990), 2593–2598.

56 Limbird L. *Cell Surface Receptors: A Short Course on Theory and Methods*. Boston, MA: Martinus Nijhoff Publishing, 1986.

57 Herrmann M, Vaudaux P, Pittet D, et al. Fibronectin, fibrinogen, and laminin act as mediators of adherence of clinical staphylococcal isolates to foreign materials. *J Infect Dis*, 158 (1988), 693–701.

58 Wang I-W, Anderson J, Marchant RE. Platelet-mediated adhesion of *Staphylococcus epidermidis* to hydrophobic NHLBI reference polyethylene. *J Biomed Mater Res*, 27 (1993), 1119–1128.

59 Florin E, Moy V, Gaub HE. Adhesion forces between individual ligand-receptor pairs. *Science*, 264 (1994), 415–417.

60 Sugarman B, Young EJ. Infections associated with prosthetic devices: Magnitude of the problem. *Infec Dis Clin N Am*, 3 (1989), 187–197.

61 Fang G, Keys T, Gentry L, et al. Prosthetic valve endocarditis resulting from nosocomial bacteremia: A prospective multicenter study. *Ann Int Med*, 119 (1993), 560–567.

62 Johnson K, Liska M, Joyce L, Emery RW. Registry report use of total artificial hearts: Summary of world experience, 1969–1991. *ASAIO J*, 38 (1992), M486–M492.

63 Randrup ER. Clinical experience with 180 inflatable penile prostheses. *South Med J*, 88 (1995), 47–51.

64 Brooks G, Butel J, Ornston LN. *Jawetz, Melnick, and Adelberg's Medical Microbiology*. Norwalk, CT: Appleton & Lange, 1991, 1–632.

ADDITIONAL READING

1 Doyle R, Ofek I. Adhesion of microbial pathogens. In Abelson JN, Simon MI (Eds.), *Methods in Enzymology*. Boston, MA: Academic Press, 1995, 253.

2 Gristina A, Giridhar G, Myrvik QN. Bacteria and biomaterials. In Greco RS (Ed.), *Implantation Biology*. New Brunswick, NJ: CRC Press, 1994, 131–148.

3 Doyle R, Rosenberg M. *Microbial Cell Surface Hydrophobicity*. Washington, DC: American Society for Microbiology, 1990.

4 Bisno AL, Waldvogel FA. *Infections Associated with Indwelling Medical Devices*. Washington, DC: American Society for Microbiology, 1989.

5 Sugarman B, Young EJ. *Infections Associated with Prosthetic Devices*. Boca Raton, FL: CRC Press, 1984.

Chapter 33

General Compatibility

Neal R. Cholvin
Norman R. Bayne

TESTING OBJECTIVES

Biological Objectives

Implantation techniques are used for three categories of studies leading to new biomaterials or devices: (1) for safety (biocompatibility) assessments of biomaterials or devices; (2) for developmental studies; and (3) for efficacy studies. This chapter will concentrate on safety testing and will frequently use sutures as examples of implants.

Examples of safety evaluations are tissue reaction, absorption, irritation, and mechanical strength studies. In these evaluations, standard sample shapes are implanted in contact with soft tissues because one then is able to take advantage of knowledge derived from past investigations on similarly shaped materials. There are some cases in which safety test samples may take the form of a marketed product, e.g., some specimens may be implanted as sutures. Developmental studies are scheduled between safety and efficacy studies. These are for optimizing device designs leading to final products. Efficacy (functionality) studies, the last of the preclinical series, utilize material samples that are shaped and used exactly like the intended clinical products.

Physical Objectives

In vivo exposure of biomaterials tests for changes in physical properties induced by a living system. Parameters for evaluation include: (1) weight measurements to detect material loss due to biodegradation; (2) mechanical testing for retention of breaking or tensile strength, Young's modulus, and elongation to break (e.g., of a suture); and (3) examination of surface appearance (e.g., as determined from scanning electron micrographs). For physical studies, explantation of implants must be performed carefully so that the retrieval process does not damage the specimens (for details see Section I).

Chemical Objectives

Chemical determinations are conducted after in vivo exposure to characterize the effects (or lack thereof) of the biological environment on a biomaterial's chemical makeup. Determinations may be made for loss of components by elution, uptake of natural substances (e.g., lipid imbibition by silicone rubber in a heart valve), changes in molecular weight, and other assays to trace the fate of manufacturing additives or substances formed as a result of biological degradation (see Section II). Generally, it is necessary to remove tissue residues from explanted specimens to prevent interference with chemical analytical procedures.

STUDY PARAMETERS

Two types of reaction are incited when a test material is deposited into tissue. Both processes run simultaneously from the time of implantation. One is the inflammatory and healing response to the vascular disruption and mechanical trauma of the surgery. Unless implantation is performed crudely and roughly, with or without bacterial contamination leading to infection, the most dramatic elements of an uncomplicated healing response usually subside within 10–20 days.

The second reaction is, of course, the one of primary interest in the study, i.e., the tissue response to the test material itself. The nature of this response depends upon the chemical and physical properties of the biomaterial. Nonabsorbable biocompatible materials may remain inert in the implant site after wound healing has been completed. Slowly absorbable materials manifest their properties after that time. On the other hand, tissue response to rapidly absorbing specimens may be completed within three weeks, thus masking desired experimental information.

When rapid absorption causes one to suspect that it will be difficult to differentiate responses due to healing from those induced by the implant, then sham surgical procedures (without implants) can be performed, either on a separate group of animals, or using bilateral sites in each animal where one side is sham-operated and the other receives an implant. The sham site reactions will provide baseline information about the uncomplicated healing response. Comparisons then can be made between this and the implanted group.

Study Duration

The end-point of a study should either be when responses reach steady state or endpoint approximates clinical residence time. For truly nonabsorbable, nonreactive materials, 90-day studies are sufficiently long. For absorbable, or more reactive nonabsorbable materials, in which a prolonged reaction consisting of a succession of different cellular responses may occur, longer end-points may be required.

Biocompatibility studies can be classified according to duration into two types: acute and chronic. Acute studies generally are less than 30 days in length. Choice of study length depends upon factors which may include: (1) the degree of biodegradability of the test material; (2) the temporal information desired about the tissue response at an implant site; and (3) the type of test sought. For example, the duration of a study to characterize tensile strength of a rapidly absorbing material may be relatively short, whereas that to determine carcinogenicity of a nonabsorbable material intended for contact with a patient's tissue for a lifetime might span several years in an experimental animal. Chronic tissue reaction studies of nonabsorbable biomaterials generally are thought to be complete in 3 months, although for some materials, e.g., silicones which might migrate, up to 2 years may be specified. Studies of absorbable biomaterials must span time sufficient for complete absorption of the test material. Duration for carcinogenicity studies ideally would span the remainder of the lifetime of the test species. For simulating applications in man, the objective would be to expose the biomaterial to animal tissue for a maximum length of time.

In the design of both short- and long-term studies, intermediate time periods frequently are included in order to document changes in absorption or degradation, or to ascertain qualitatively or quantitatively the dynamics of cell populations and intercellular matrix surrounding implants during the postoperative period.

Implant Parameters

Before any material is considered for implantation, its bulk and surface properties should be thoroughly characterized. Furthermore, the source of the material, and its treatment and handling should be carefully documented to increase chances for achieving reproducible results in follow-up studies.

IMPLANTS

Sources of Tissue Reactivity in Biomaterials

Tissue reactions are incited either by an implant's base material or by substances added to facilitate the manufacturing process. If an implant consists only of a pure, nonabsorbable, and impenetrable polymer, then it only contacts tissue at its surface. Surface area of an implant varies with geometry and surface texture (rough surfaces offer greater contact area than do smooth ones). If an implant is chemically pure and does not resorb, its size remains constant, and it contributes little to the tissue's chemical environment. If the material is absorbable, however, it releases breakdown products and the contact area becomes quite variable as it is affected by degradation of its surface (increasing area) and reduction in implant size (decreasing area).

Implants containing leachable materials (e.g., plasticizers, antioxidants, stabilizers, unreacted monomer, etc.) present additional stimuli for tissue reaction. These components can, and usually do, diffuse from the implant's interior to its surface, and the tissues are exposed at rates depending upon material diffusivity, remaining mass, and surface area (which decreases with time as the material resorbs). If irritants from the implant emerge at rates easily handled through tissue fluid dilution and transport, tissue reaction can be minimal. However, if irritants accumulate more rapidly and these mechanisms are overwhelmed, severe tissue reaction can occur.

Specimen Geometry Implant shape has been reported to affect tissue responses to implants. For example, it was found that tissue reaction intensity was homogeneous around disk-shaped implants, while it was more pronounced at the ends than in the middle of rod-shaped implants [1]. Others reported that tissue reaction was more intense around extruded rods having triangular, rather than circular, cross-sections [2].

Size of the test object normally implanted necessarily is limited by the dimensions of the tissue bed. For routine studies, it is recommended that standard-sized and -shaped specimens be implanted in order to cancel out differences in mass and geometry. Typical standard specimens are rods 0.02–2.00 mm in diameter and 1–2 cm in length. In order to minimize implantation trauma, test samples can be inserted through trocars or hypodermic needles. For biomaterials destined to become sutures, actual product configurations can be tested.

Implants for biocompatibility testing best utilize configurations that induce minimal mechanical stimulation to their tissue beds. It has been observed that pulverized samples tend not to be carcinogenic, whereas films of the same material can be carcinogenic [3]. Others have noted the tendency for disproportionately large masses to contribute to solid state carcinogenesis [4].

Irregular shapes also may be implanted. If no dimension is more that 3 mm, intramuscular implantation may be easily achieved in rat or rabbit gluteal muscle. Larger specimens might better be implanted subcutaneously.

More than one size of implant may intentionally be included in studies, if sizes of the marketed product will range widely.

Control Materials   Control materials, for which much previous information about tissue reactions exist, generally are included in experiments in order to make comparisons. A control material that incites either a minimal or maximal reaction, or one of each type, may be employed depending upon the objectives of a study.

Representative nonabsorbable control materials which have been recommended for biocompatibility comparisons include both metals and polymers [5]. Iron, soft steel, copper rods and plasticized PVC with 0.3% organotin are recommended for positive (strongly reactive) controls, while tantalum rods and marketed nonabsorbable polymers are recommended for negative (minimally reactive) controls.

Representative absorbable test specimens which have been recommended for biocompatibility comparisons include surgical catgut for positive controls and selected marketed synthetic absorbable polymers for negative controls.

Implants of both test and control materials should be as similar in size and shape as possible in order to eliminate dimensional factors as causes for differences in responses.

IMPLANT SITES

Subcutaneous and muscle tissues of rodents and lagomorphs provide acceptable implant sites for most routine safety studies. These sites in both the rat and the rabbit have been used extensively for tissue reaction and absorption studies. Abundant historical data are available for comparing tissue responses.

Other tissues may be selected in order to expose implants to special cell populations, e.g., the mesenchymal cells of the peritoneal cavity, where a tendency to incite carcinogenesis or adhesion formation may be investigated.

Some important clinical sites, e.g., cornea, coronary artery, dura mater, and urethra, which are known to react differently to biomaterials than do subcutis or muscle, may be included in special studies. In most instances, test samples can be secured in these sites only if implanted in the form of the clinical product.

EXPERIMENTAL DESIGN

Ideally, adequate numbers of subjects should be included in each test group of an experiment to establish significance in delineating responses. The ultimate experimental objective is to obtain scientifically relevant data from which unequivocal conclusions can be drawn to test a hypothesis.

Number of subjects per group can be estimated if observations are to be quantitative in nature, and if the expected ranges of responses between the control and experimental treatments are known. These values may be estimated by judicious pilot experimentation.

However, for studies that are descriptive, subjective, and/or qualitative in nature, statistical significance may not be achieved. Even so, the experimental objective should be to accurately describe the nature of the tissue response to the implant. Experience has shown that in the more qualitative tissue reaction or absorption studies at least four rabbits or dogs, or six to eight rats, usually will define the response.

The prediction of the tissue reaction's nature can be improved if the experimental design includes same-animal paired sites for each test and control specimen. Paired comparisons thus can minimize between-animal variations as sources of experimental error. Pairing also may reduce the number of animals required for statistical analyses.

To recapitulate, experimental designs and implantation schemes should be carefully constructed to fulfill study objectives. Resources (materials, animals, personnel) must be carefully allocated to achieve study objectives while recognizing moral and ethical responsibilities in animal research. Protocols and designs for all studies must be carefully composed to maximize retrieval of interpretable data with the smallest animal group sizes as possible, and with minimal harm and distress [6]. When options exist, the cost of animals, housing space required, and personnel time required may affect the choice of animal numbers per experimental group for a study.

PREPARATION OF TEST MATERIALS FOR IMPLANTATION

The surfaces and interiors of implants must be free of foreign matter and viable microbial agents to ensure that resultant tissue responses are due solely to the test biomaterial. Two types of decontamination processes must be undertaken to make samples acceptable for implantation: cleansing and sterilization. Biomaterial properties must be taken into account when designing these procedures; otherwise, implants may be irreversibly altered.

Cleansing

The first process consists of physically dislodging particulates left as a result of the manufacturing process, and chemically dissolving manufacturing process contaminants and handlers' skin oils. An acceptable procedure is initial washing with a nonfilming detergent solution to remove particulates and water-soluble materials, followed by numerous rinsing steps with distilled or deionized water. Next is treatment with an appropriate nonpolar organic solvent (e.g., reagent grade isopropyl alcohol) to dissolve organic material including oils. The final cleaning step is drying.

In order to preserve cleanliness and ensure subsequent sterility after cleaning, the samples then should be wrapped in at least two layers of a suitable barrier.

Sterilization

The second process is sterilization. Depending upon the properties of the implant material, one of several sterilization methods may be chosen. The proper choice depends upon the biomaterial's properties, i.e.: (1) stability in the presence of water vapor (moist heat in an autoclave); (2) stability when exposed to moist or dry heat; (3) absorption and desorption of volatile sterilizing gases (ethylene oxide or formaldehyde vapors); and (4) radiation sensitivity to ^{60}Co or electron beam sources (for more details see Chapter 15). For most biomaterials one of the above methods can be employed. In case none of these procedures are acceptable, then the last resort is treatment for an adequate period of time in an aqueous chemical disinfectant solution suitable for antiseptic treatment of the skin, followed by thorough rinsing with sterile distilled water or physiological saline, and then enclosure in a sterile wrap.

GENERAL COMMENTS ON IMPLANTATION TECHNIQUES

Well-conceived implantation protocols take into account objectives, compliance with guidelines for humane use of animals in research, the extent of surgical trauma anticipated, and the nature of the biomaterial.

Extensive surgical dissection may be required in order to implant relatively large, irregular test samples. Because surgery itself incites considerable tissue reaction, separation of healing responses from those induced by an implant may be difficult.

In experiments where responses to induced trauma must be kept to a minimum, and/or where precision of placement may not be critical, implantation may be facilitated with minimum tissue disruption through the use of "introducers." Introducers are injector-type devices. An example in which minimum tissue disruption is desirable is a chronic study to detect biodegradation of a suture that must function as a permanent tissue fastener (e.g., one employed to maintain an intraocular lens in position). An example where placement is not critical would be routine subcutaneous implantation for screening absorbability of new polymers.

Types of introducers include needles (both suture and hypodermic), trocars and cannulas, and assorted injectors. Injectors specifically for implantation may be obtained commercially or may be made by removing the tip end of resterilizable polypropylene hypodermic syringes. The latter are useful for implanting large masses of test material as in chronic toxicity testing, where the amount of material implanted approaches 100X (on a body weight basis) that utilized in human clinical procedures.

EUTHANASIA

The ideal agent and/or method for euthanasia of experimental animals should fulfill the following criteria: (1) able to rapidly induce unconsciousness rapidly, and death without causing pain, distress, anxiety, or apprehension; (2) reliable; (3) safe for attending personnel; (4) minimum emotional effect on observers and operators; (5) irreversible; (6) compatible with subsequent evaluations of tissues and materials; (7) appropriate for species and age of subjects; and (8) equipment for administration easily maintained in proper working order [7].

An acceptable agent for euthanatizing small numbers of laboratory animals of most species is sodium pentobarbital. The euthanatizing dose recommended usually is three times that employed to produce a surgical plane of anesthesia. The desired route of administration is intravenous when practical, as in the case of rabbits, dogs, and larger species. For small rodents, intraperitoneal administration is acceptable. Commercial pentobarbital euthanasia solutions are available at concentrations about three times greater than that of anesthesia grade solutions.

Where it is necessary to euthanatize large numbers of rats and mice and even larger species, carbon dioxide narcotization humanely induces insensibility prior to asphyxiation. Carbon dioxide chambers can be constructed to handle animal groups conveniently. Facilities in which CO_2 is used must be well ventilated in order not to expose laboratory personnel to accumulated gas. In situations where space permits, this type of operation may be performed in an exhaust hood.

Other agents which have been found acceptable are carbon monoxide (CO), nitrogen and argon [7].

GENERAL IMPLANTATION METHODOLOGIES

Subcutaneous Implantation—Rat Dorsal Subcutis

The subcutis commonly serves as an in vivo environment for test samples which subsequently are tested for mechanical strength retention.

Preparation   The anesthetized animal is placed in ventral recumbancy and the dorsal trunk region is clipped, shaved, and swabbed with an antiseptic agent.

Incision   A transverse dorsal skin incision 1.5 cm in length is made directly caudal to the scapulae.

Dissection   A tissue pocket can be made either prior to, or simultaneously with, the act of implantation. In the former case, the areolar subcutaneous space between the skin and muscle fascia is separated by inserting and spreading the tips of a blunt-tipped, nontraumatic instrument, e.g., Carmalt forceps or Metzenbaum scissors. In the latter case (see below) the pocket is made as the forceps are inserted, while grasping the ends of the test biomaterial.

Insertion   Prior to insertion, the specimens are removed from the package using sterile technique, taking care that they do not touch the naked or gloved hand. Using forceps, they are hydrated in a bowl of sterile saline until they are inserted. Upon insertion the sample is advanced caudally into the subcutaneous space lateral to the midline and deposited sufficiently distant from the incision itself so as not to contact the healing wound. Care must be exercised in grasping the sample for subsequent mechanical testing so that it is not weakened. The forceps then are opened to release the sample in the implant bed. Two implants can be sited bilaterally through this one incision.

Closure   The skin is closed with stainless steel wound clips (or staples) only if the incision site is inaccessible to the animal's teeth. If self-mutilation of the wound site may occur, a subcuticular closure may be made with a nonabsorbable suture instead. Multiple housing of rodents may not be desirable if one animal is apt to disturb another's incision.

Explantation   After the desired in vivo residence time, the animal is euthanatized, and the skin lateral to both implant sites and the healed incision is incised and carefully retracted to expose the specimen(s). Each specimen is removed in a manner consistent with the objectives of the study. If only mechanical testing is to be performed, the tissues are carefully stripped away without damaging the implant. But if tissue reaction is to be evaluated, the implant, along with a generous zone of tissue surrounding the implant and healing tissue, is removed en bloc.

Subcutaneous Implantation—Screening Method for Estimating Absorption Rate

The macroscopic subcutaneous absorption (MSA) method provides a semiquantitative, macroscopic screening method for assessing the time rate of absorption of polymer candidates in tissues. It is especially useful for screening sets of prototypes to identify those worthy of further testing in more quantitative, microscopic biocompatibility tests. Convenient-sized (2 cm) segments of sutures, thin fibers, or rods are implanted.

Preparation   An anesthetized rat or rabbit is positioned in dorsal recumbancy and the ventral abdominal skin is prepared for surgery.

Emplacement   A saline-wetted test sample is extruded percutaneously through a hypodermic needle into the subcutaneous space, parallel to and 1.5 cm from the midline. An alternative method would be manual insertion through a small skin incision.

Recovery   At designated time intervals, groups of animals are euthanized. The skin is treated with a chemical depilatory agent, and then a large rectangular piece is isolated and carefully removed so that the specimen is centered in the explanted portion. The test sample invariable adheres to the underside of the skin. The skin is then trimmed, to display the implant site, mounted on a cork board, and dried in a 37°C oven.

Evaluation   Dried specimens representing initial implant time (baseline) and various implant periods are examined by both direct lighting and transillumination under a dissecting microscope. Visual examinations are made of each sample, to compare (with respect to unimplanted samples) sample shape, amount of dye retention, estimated percentage of sample remaining, etc. Photographs may be taken and stored for future examinations with the specimens themselves.

Caged Implant—Subcutaneous Tissue of the Rat

The caged implant technique [8] utilizes a capped cylindrical cage of medical grade 0.8×0.8 mm stainless steel wire mesh, 3.5 cm long by 1 cm in diameter. The cage, containing the test material, is implanted dorsolaterally in lumbar subcutaneous tissue. During the course of the in vivo period, chamber fluid can be aspirated for cellular and enzymatic serial determinations, employing strictly sterile procedures. Terminally the cage can be removed and the test material examined for mechanical and chemical properties (for details, see Chapter 43).

Incision   A 2 cm longitudinal incision is made on the dorsal midline extending craniad from a point 3 cm from the base of the tail.

Dissection   Two bilateral implant sites may be prepared by bluntly dissecting the subcutaneous tissue craniolaterally from the skin incision.

Insertion   One cylinder may be implanted in each tissue pocket. The implants should be carefully placed at least 2.5 cm from the incision in order to avoid irritating the healing skin wound. This precaution minimizes the possibility for erosion of the implants through the skin.

Closure   The skin may be sutured or closed with stainless steel wound clips.

Intramuscular Implantation—Rodent Gluteal Muscle or Rabbit Paravertebral Muscle

Muscle, a highly vascularized tissue, possesses highly capable vascular transport mechanisms and is capable of responding more vigorously to the presence of reactive foreign materials, with less toxic result, than is less vascular subcutaneous tissue.

In the rat and rabbit, both intramuscular sites can be conveniently accessed through the skin and relatively fat-free tissues of the body wall. The rat may be preferred for many biocompatibility studies ranging up to 2 years in duration. For experiments requiring more than 2 years (to more closely simulate human clinical usage the rat's life span may be insufficient), or if implant size may preclude placing implants in rats, the rabbit may be the preferable choice.

Preparation   The anesthetized animal is placed in ventral recumbancy and the skin over the lumbar and pelvic regions is clipped, shaved, and swabbed with an antiseptic.

Incision   A 4-cm longitudinal incision, long enough to provide bilateral exposure of the gluteal muscles, is made over the sacral spine.

Dissection   The skin is separated from underlying fascia and connective tissue and is spread with a retractor to expose the superficial gluteal muscle on each side of the midline. If the sample to be implanted is a suture, there is no need to incise the fascia overlying the muscle. A needle, with the sample either attached or passed through its eye, can be used to pull the sample through the fascia down into the muscle. The protruding suture ends then can be clipped at the fascial surface. Fascia need not be incised if the sample is implantable through a hypodermic needle or small trocar. If the sample cannot be implanted by either of these techniques, the fascia and muscle are incised and the sample then is emplaced. The sample can be anchored in place with a fascial suture.

Closure   The retractors are removed and the skin is closed with stainless steel wound clips or sutures.

Intraperitoneal Implantation—Rodents

Intraperitoneal implantation of a bare test sample generously exposes it both to the fluid and a variety of mesenchymal cell types of the abdominal cavity. The connective tissue capsule which eventually invests the implant can be examined microscopically at explantation. During the implantation period paracentesis can be employed to obtain peritoneal fluid and free-floating cells from the peritoneal cavity, cells whose state of differentiation may be affected by the implant [9].

Preparation   The anesthetized animal is secured in dorsal recumbancy and the ventral abdominal skin is clipped, shaved, and swabbed with an antiseptic.

Incision   A ventral midline incision is made through the skin and linea alba at the level of the umbilicus.

Dissection   The incision is extended to provide access into the desired location in the peritoneal cavity.

Insertion   The specimen is advanced into the abdominal cavity to a location which will least interfere with organ function during normal visceral movements. In some instances, the implant may be anchored to the body wall or to a viscus with a suture.

Closure   The linea alba is closed with nonabsorbable size 3-0 or 4-0 suture material. Closure of the skin may be with stainless steel wound clips or a subcuticular suture pattern.

Diffusion Chamber Method for Determining
Absorption Rate of Polymers

A diffusion chamber, described below, bathes the enclosed biomaterial in tissue fluid while protecting it from cell contact and encapsulation. Encapsulation would coat a retrieved implant with proteinaceous material that might interfere with subsequent chemical analyses and/or physical testing. The sample may be implanted either intraperitoneally or subcutaneously. Prior to implantation, and employing aseptic technique, the specimen is placed in an implantable observation chamber shaped like a thick washer. The chamber sides are sealed with adhesive-edged Nucleopore® (Nucleopore Corp., Pleasanton, CA) filter disks of 0.5–5 mm porosity. These disks must be handled carefully because they are delicate and their integrity is easily breached.

Preparation   The animal is prepared in the same manner as for previously described intraperitoneal or subcutaneous implantations.

Emplacement   The surgical techniques for implanting the chamber in either site are similar to those described earlier for caged implants.

Recover and Evaluation   The animal is euthanatized and the chamber is carefully extracted. If chemical analyses are to be conducted upon the solid and liquid contents of the chamber, the external surfaces must be handled carefully to remove proteinaceous material.

The fraction of a biodegradable sample remaining can be determined quantitatively by removing, washing, drying and then comparing it with its preimplant weight.

Mucous Membrane Irritation—Hamster Cheek Pouch Model

Mucous membrane irritation studies are conducted to evaluate materials intended for clinical and/or personal application to oral, vaginal, or ophthalmic epithelium.

The hamster cheek pouch model provides a convenient, relatively large, demarcated area of oral mucous membrane onto which samples of various forms may be intermittently applied. The hamster cheek pouch epithelium, unlike human buccal epithelium, is keratinized in order to withstand the abrasive action of stored food materials [10]. Consequently, interpretation of responses must account for this difference in epithelial type.

Because there are no practical methods to appose a test sample to an animal's buccal surface for long periods of time, multiple contact exposures usually are made on successive days, during anesthesia or sedation, until it is deemed that an adequate contact interval has been attained.

Cheek pouch irritation responses to mechanical or chemical irritant properties of a test material may vary from mild, with kyperkeratinization and increased vascularity of submucous tissue, to severe, with depression of cell replication and thinning of the membrane. In the most severe reactions, ulceration of the surface is manifest, due to actual cell necrosis.

Cutaneous Irritation Model

This procedure seeks to evaluate the potential irritant properties of products being developed for topical use. Prolonged contact of specimens, or extracts thereof, directly with skin is achieved by apposing the sample to a test site with tape or film overlaid with gauze. If the sample is a solid, then a 0.5 ml volume may be applied. If it is a film, a 2.5 × 2.5 cm square is placed in contact with skin. If leachable agents are to be evaluated, an extract is prepared [11] and 0.5 ml is flowed onto gauze, which is applied to the site. If the bandage that apposes the specimen to the skin itself causes reaction, then sham treated sites, i.e., those exposed to the bandage alone, should be included in the experimental design for comparison purposes.

Species utilized for this test commonly include the rabbit and guinea pig, but the mouse, pig, dog, baboon and even human volunteers also have been employed. Differences in dermal responses between species have been reported [12]. Criteria for selection of test species may include availability of an adequate expanse and quality of skin desired, previous test results with similar agents, and typical clinical applications anticipated. The test is commonly performed on the dorsolateral trunk region, both sides of the midline, of the rabbit.

Skin Preparation   The aforementioned site, preferably unpigmented, is clipped or shaved in a nontraumatic fashion 24 hours prior to initiating the experiment. A chemical depilatory agent may be employed instead.

Prior to application of test material the next day, the skin region is cleansed with a swab dipped in ethanol. If the eventual clinical product is apt to be applied to inflamed skin, it may be appropriate to abrade the subject's skin in one half of the sites to increase absorption. Abrasion may be accomplished by gently scraping the skin surface with a perpendicularly-held scalpel blade.

Specimen Application   Various specimens are emplaced on the skin in the designated areas, and a bandage is applied.

Time of Exposure   This can depend upon the projected clinical use of the product candidate. If momentary contact is intended, exposure times of several hours may be sufficient, whereas 24 hours or more may be recommended for materials intended for prolonged use.

Specimen Removal   This step should not induce irritation by itself. If removal is difficult because an adhesive has been used to attach the specimen to the skin, one should verify that any solvents used during the removal, such as acetone or alcohol, will not affect the results.

Evaluation   A grading system [13], modified from Draize [14], may be used to score the severity of reaction. Reactions range from erythema (reddening), edema (swelling), and superficial necrosis leading to excoriation and eschar (scar) formation and swelling. Others [15] also have described gradations of edema or erythema/eschar formation.

Guinea Pig Maximization Test

Human skin normally is much more sensitive to topically applied substances than are skins of most experimental animal species. This makes extrapolation of animal test results difficult. The Guinea Pig Maximization Test [16] was developed to raise the sensitivity of guinea pig skin to a level approaching that of human skin. Increased sensitivity is attained by preliminary series of sensitizing intradermal injections. Topical applications of test substances follow. Good correlation between "G. P." results and those from human preclinical trials has improved the validity of animal testing for evaluating topically applied product candidates.

Intracutaneous Irritation Model

This model is utilized to evaluate the irritant potential of substances that may leach from a biomaterial in the presence of biological fluids. A liquid extract from a test biomaterial is injected intracutaneously, and the resultant reaction is evaluated at appropriate time intervals.

Components of biomaterials that may cause undesirable biological reactions include plasticizers, catalysts, unreacted monomer, etc. Since solubilities of leachates are highly variable, it is prudent to include in the protocol solutions or suspensions [11, 15] in several aqueous and lipid solvents or carriers. Each carrier should simulate a corresponding tissue or tissue fluid "solvent." Polyethylene glycol or physiological saline (0.9% sodium chloride in distilled water) mimics the aqueous properties of interstitial fluid. Five percent ethanol in physiological saline emulates aliphatic biological compounds. Pure vegetable oil (e.g., sesame or cottonseed) simulates lipid components of living tissue. Because these solvents may themselves invoke reactions when applied either topically or intracutaneously, it is imperative to include additional test sites for both positive and negative controls of solvent alone. Negative control agents are the solvents themselves, 0.9% saline, vegetable oil, polyethylene glycol and 5% ethanol in 0.9% saline [15]. Positive control agents are 20% ethanol in 0.9% saline and pure vegetable oil.

Because reactions may be augmented by infection, it is recommended that all solutions and suspensions be sterilized prior to injection and that injections be performed using antiseptic technique.

The rabbit is the most common species utilized for this test. Again, the reasons for utilizing rabbits are the same as those mentioned for the cutaneous irritation model. The site locations are also the same. Because the test materials are introduced into the dermis, no bandaging is required. As with the cutaneous irritation test procedure, the hair is removed from the site 24 hours in advance of the injections to allow any irritation to subside.

Standard Test Procedure A line of intradermal injections are made bilaterally on centers approximately 3/4 inch (2 cm) apart. Two-tenths ml of the experimental samples, as well as positive and negative controls, are introduced for readouts 24, 48, and 72 hours after administration. Evaluation of the reactions is facilitated by using the Draize scale previously cited [14].

Trypan Blue Modified Test Procedure A variation on the standard methodology, one which reduces testing time, has been employed [17]. Irritant materials cause increased vascular permeability, so that if a vital stain such as Trypan Blue is injected intravenously, it may extravasate and dye the skin, thus facilitating visualization of irritation. Trypan Blue solution (1%) is given approximately 15 minutes following the last test site injection. The dye escapes from permeable capillaries and stains the surrounding tissue. Twenty percent ethanol in 0.9% saline induces vascular damage and can act as a positive control. The size and intensity of stained areas should be graded at frequent intervals, in no case exceeding 90 minutes post-injection.

SPECIAL IMPLANTATION PROCEDURES

Tissue evaluations of test materials implanted in muscle and subcutaneous tissue suffice for predicting suitability of wound closure biomaterials in most surgical sites. However, in tissues with unique mechanical or physiological properties, protocols analogous to those used in clinical procedures may be required to obtain bona fide tissue responses. As mentioned earlier, the special cases that require implantation in target tissue are cornea, coronary artery, dura and urethra. In these sites, secure placement of the implant is facilitated if it is in the form of the anticipated marketed product, e.g., a suture. The implantation technique then can be closely designed to simulate a clinical procedure.

Tissue Reaction Studies in Cornea

The reaction to a new suture intended for use in corneal surgery is obtained by implanting the test sample, a short segment of properly needled fine suture, approximately size 7-0, in the cornea without positioning a knot in the cornea or at the limbus, either of which would cause excessive corneal vascular reaction. The rabbit eye is the preferred model for this type of study. It is not possible to use surgical disinfectants in ophthalmic procedures because of the extreme sensitivity of ophthalmic tissues. Supplies and instruments used in the surgery should be sterile, however, so as not to introduce pathogenic microorganisms into the surgical field.

Preparation   The anesthetized rabbit is placed in lateral recumbancy with the head propped upon a pad for convenient access to the eye. An eye drape is placed to provide a sterile surface. Over this is placed a sterile rubber dam with 0.5 cm slit in the center. By proptosing the eye through this slit, surgical exposure and immobility of the eyeball is achieved.

Emplacement   A mattress-like suture is emplaced as follows. A 3–5 mm wide pass is made centripetally in the sclera to emerge 1 mm from the limbus. The suture is carried over the limbus and a similar width pass is made in the cornea, parallel to the limbus, and partially through the thickness of the cornea. The pattern is completed by reversing direction and making the final pass through scleral tissue, completing the interrupted mattress suture. A knot is made with the free end of the suture over the sclera. The result is a knot located well away from the limbus.

Tissue Reaction Studies in Dura Mater

The intimate juxtaposition of bone, blood vessel, dura, cerebrospinal fluid, and brain tissue presents a very complex and sensitive environment in which to study new suture biomaterials. Interpretation of tissue responses is complicated. In this preparation, it is advisable to implant both negative and positive suture controls in order to compare reactions. Negative and positive control materials may be selected from among those products that are recommended or contraindicated, respectively, for clinical dural closures. The dog is the most commonly used test subject.

Preparation   A dog anesthetized with isoflurane [18] is placed in sternal recumbancy. The dorsal scalp area is clipped, scrubbed and disinfected in standard fashion, and carefully draped to bar contamination from nonscrubbed areas.

Incision.   A midline incision is made in the dorsal cranial skin and underlying fascia, both of which are reflected. The temporalis muscle on one side then is incised parallel to, and 1 cm lateral to, the frontal crest. Then it is reflected to expose the cranium. A craniotomy approximately 1.5 cm in diameter is made with a trephine, and the bone is removed. The dura mater is exposed and a linear incision, approximately 1.5 cm long, is made in it.

Implantation   The dural incision then is sutured with the test material (suture size approximately 5-0), employing either simple interrupted sutures or a continuous suture pattern. During the entire intracranial procedure, extreme care is exercised in order to avoid traumatizing brain tissue. Needle handling must be precise, and tensioning of the strands must be performed so that emplacement of stiff suture coils do not embed ("cheesewire"), then or postoperatively, in brain tissue. Implantation of a selected control material can be done through a craniotomy on the opposite side of the cranium.

Closure   A discoid tantalum plate may be positioned over each craniotomy site if it is desired to mechanically protect the underlying site, and to isolate the healing response of the overlying muscle from that of the dura. If a disc is not used, the temporalis muscle merely is sutured over the bony defect.

Recovery   At the designated time, the animal is euthanized and the dural tissue is carefully exposed. Adhesion of the temporal muscle to healing dural tissue requires extremely delicate dissection. In order to evaluate tissue reaction both above and below the dural closure, recovery technique must include precise sectioning of the cranial vault.

Infection Potentiation Studies

Refractive bacterial infections frequently develop in surgical sites where biomaterials have been employed clinically. Persistent infections occur even when antibiotic agents, specifically active against the invading pathogenic organisms, are employed locally and/or systemically.

The chemical nature of some biomaterials appears to contribute to inflammatory exudates which support bacterial growth. Also, porous or braided biomaterials harbor bacterial growth within an implant's interstices. In some cases there is increased adhesion between tissue and biomaterial. All these mechanisms seem to contribute to infection refractivity.

An objective of infection potentiation studies (beyond tissue reaction, etc.) is to investigate the impact of a biomaterial upon the ability of body defense mechanisms to overcome bacterial infection. Carefully metered numbers of selected pathogenic microorganisms, with or without chemotherapeutic agents, are administered concurrently with implantation. The body is challenged to prevent the inoculum from inciting a bona fide infection.

Implantation protocol for an infection potentiation study generally mimics that for simple subcutaneous implants in the rat, with the added step of instilling a measured dose of an appropriate bacterium into both test and sham-operated sites.

Potentiation is noted either when a frank infection develops or, should clinical signs of infection be absent, when a bacterial culture taken later from the site confirms the continued presence of the same microorganisms. The test would be especially convincing if the bacterial doses had been titrated so that responses were negative in sham-operated animals, and positive in animals with implants. Positive results support the hypothesis that a given biomaterial interferes with resistance to infection.

At least two problems are encountered in conducting definitive infected wound studies. First, the defense mechanisms of healthy experimental animals may be too effective to permit pathogenic microorganisms to thrive, the same microorganisms that produce infections in traumatized or diseased human subjects. Second, animal-to-animal variations in resistance make it extremely difficult to establish an unique dose at which the organisms invariably will thrive.

REFERENCES

1 Wood NK, Kaminski EJ, Oglesby RJ. The significance of implant shape in experimental testing of biological materials: Disc vs. rod. *J Biomed Mater Res*, 4 (1970), 1–12.

2 Matlaga BF, Yashenchak LP, Salthouse TN. Tissue response to implanted polymers: The significance of sample shape. *J Biomed Mater Res*, 10 (1976), 391–397.

3 Oppenheimer ET, Wilhite M, Danishefsky I, et al. Observations on the effects of powdered polymer in the carcinogenic process. *Cancer Res*, 21 (1961), 132–154.

4 Bischoff F, Bryson G. Carcinogenesis through solid state surfaces. *Prog Exp Tumor Res*, 51 (1964), 85–133.

5 Gourly SJ, Rice RM, Hegyeli AF, et al. Biocompatibility testing of polymers: In vivo implantation studies. *J Biomed Mater Res*, 12 (1978), 219–232.

6 Russell WMS, Burch RL. *The Principles of Humane Experimental Technique*. Springfield, IL: Charles C. Thomas, Publisher, 1959, 239.

7 Andrews EJ, et al. Report of the AVMA Panel on Euthanasia. *JAVMA*, 202 (1993), 229–249.

8 Marchant R, Hiltner A, Hamlin C, et al. In vivo biocompatibility studies. I. The cage implant system and a biodegradable hydrogel. *J Biomed Mater Res*, 17 (1983), 301–325.

9 Keller JC, Marshall GW. An in vivo method for biological evaluation of metal implants. *J Biomed Mater Res*, 18 (1984), 829–844.

10 Bernstein ML, Carlish R. The induction of hyperkeratotic white lesions in hamster cheek pouches with mouthwash. *Oral Surg, Oral Med, Oral Path*, 48 (1979), 517–522.

11 Extraction of medical plastics. *1995 Book of ASTM Standards*, Vol. 13.01. Philadelphia, PA: American Society for Testing and Materials, 1994, No. 619-79.

12 Davies RE, Harper KH, Kynoch SR. Interspecies variation in dermal reactivity. *J Soc Cosmetic Chem*, 23 (1972), 371–381.

13 Testing biomaterials in rabbits for primary skin irritation. *1995 Book of ASTM Standards*, Vol 13.01. Philadelphia, PA: American Society for Testing and Materials, 1994, No. F719-81.

14 Draize JH, Woodard G, Calvery H. Methods for the study of irritation and toxicity of substances applied topically to the skin and mucous membranes. *J Pharmac Exp Ther*, 82 (1944), 377–390.

15 *The United States Pharmacopeia USP XXII—National Formulary NF XVII*. Rockville, MD: United States Pharmacopeial Convention, Inc., 1990.

16 Magnusson B, Kligman AM. Development of a standard procedure for identifying contact allergens (the guinea pig maximization test). In Magnusson B, Kligman AM, *Allergic Contact Dermatitis in the Guinea Pig*. Springfield, IL: Charles C. Thomas, Publisher, 1970, 102–123.

17 Hoppe JO, Alexander EB, Miller LC. Use of the trypan blue and rabbit eye tests for irritation. *J Amer Pharmaceut Assoc*, 39 (1950), 147–151.

18 Werner RE. Isoflurane anesthesia: A guide for practitioners. *Compendium Small Animal*, 9 (1987), 603–606.

Chapter 34

Hemocompatibility

Yoshito Ikada

INTRODUCTION

A variety of biomaterials have been used in contact with fresh blood although thrombi are formed on their blood-contacting surfaces, often followed by embolization. A series of events occurring in blood as a result of interactions with biomaterials are shown in Table 34-1 as a function of the time of exposure ranging from a few hours to many years [1]. Medical devices of short-term blood contact include catheters, hemodialyzers, and cardiopulmonary bypasses, while those of long-term blood contact are intravenous access lines for parenteral nutrition, artificial heart valves, arterial grafts, and artificial hearts. Regarding biocompatibility of biomaterials, hemocompatibility seems to be the most difficult in assessment, because it greatly depends on the time of blood exposure and involves a large number of interrelated parameters. An example is cardiopulmonary bypass which triggers a massive defense reaction that is mediated by production and circulation of more than 25 vasoactive hormones, electrolytes, eicosanoids, autocoids, cytokines, and enzymes which influence coagulation and that alter contraction of endothelial cells, vascular smooth muscle cells, or cardiac mycocytes [2]. In addition, the body is bombarded with a variety of microemboli, as shown in Table 34-2 [2].

An ideal method for the hemocompatibility assessment is to evaluate the biomaterial under the same conditions as it will be used in clinical applications. In such a situation, the blood around the biomaterial to be tested must simulate clinical blood flow patterns since blood flow has a great influence on the clinical performance of the blood-contacting biomaterial. It follows that in vitro methods cannot provide good assessment results although they often help in screening of hemocompatible candidate materials. Thus, medical devices used in combination with an extracorporeal circuit should be assessed with ex vivo methods, while in vivo assessments will be essential for medical devices used as long-term implants. In addition, it should be pointed out that even ex vivo and in vivo methods are not perfect in a strict sense for the hemocompatibility assessment if animals are used for the assessment, because hematologic properties of animal blood are different from those of human blood. Even blood of human donors varies depending on their age, physical condition, disease conditions, and administered drugs.

Because medium- and large-sized animals are generally required for the hemocompatibility assessment of blood-contacting implants, recent developments in animal welfare regulations have made it quite difficult to carry out animal experiments in sufficient numbers. This chapter describes ex vivo and in vivo methods for hemocompatibility assessments, referring to information mostly published after the first edition of this book [3].

EX VIVO ASSESSMENT

As shown in Table 34-1, the initial major events occurring on a foreign surface in contact with blood include protein adsorption and cell adhesion, which may ultimately determine

Table 34-1   Time Course of Blood-Material Interaction Events

Hours	Water and ion interactions
	Proteins are absorbed
	Cell adhesion/content release
	Fibrin production
	Platelet aggregation
	Fibrinolysis
	Activation of white cells and complement
	Embolization off the surface
Days	Coagulation activation
	Cell adhesion
	Recurrence of platelet/fibrin emboli
	Depletion of some coagulation factors
	Inflammatory response stimulation
Months	Changes in local tissues (fibrosis)
	Calcification
	Continued embolization
	Physical and chemical properties of the implant are altered
	Growth of endothelial cells to form a neointima

1) Courteny JM, Forbes CD. Thrombosis on foreign surfaces. British Med Bull, 1994; 50:966–981.

the hemocompatibility of the biomaterial. These blood components adherent to a foreign surface can be studied with in vitro methods using protein solutions and cell suspensions. The results of these in vitro studies provide valuable information for understanding mechanisms of the initial blood interactions with biomaterials, but may be far from predicting the in vivo performance of biomaterials which is associated with numerous parameters. The simplest method for the hemocompatibility assessment using fresh, flowing blood is an ex vivo shunting method. Arteriovenous (A-V), arterioarterious (A-A), and venovenous (V-V) shunts have been utilized in the rabbit, dog, sheep, and baboon to study deposition of plasma proteins, platelets, white blood cells, and fibrin on the luminal surface of shunt tubings made from biomaterials. Also, single pass, ex vivo procedures using human blood have been established for the evaluation of hemodialysis membranes.

Figure 34-1 represents an example of A-V shunts [4]. Sample tubes are connected with a silicone tube using a small silicone sheath. The loop part of this shunt circuit is also made of the silicone tube. To facilitate cannulation and avoid turbulence of blood flow, both ends

Table 34-2   Emboli Formed by Cardiopulmonary Bypass

Gas (nitrogen, oxygen)
Fibrin
Fat (free fat, denatured lipoproteins, chylomicrons)
Denatured protein
Platelet aggregates
Leukocyte aggregates
Red cell debris
Foreign material (calcium, tissue debris, fibrin, clot, fat, etc.)
Spallated material (primarily roller pumps)

2) Edmunds LH Jr. Breaking the blood-biomaterial barrier. ASAIO J. 1995; 824–830.

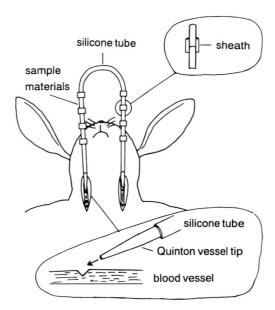

Figure 34-1 Rabbit with the A-V shunt connected using vessel tips. Reprinted from Fujimoto K, Minato M, Tadokoro H, Ikada Y. Platelet deposition onto polymeric surfaces during shunting, *J Biomed Master Res*, 1993; 27:335–343. With permission.

of this shunt circuit are connected tightly to an arterial vessel tip. An animal is anesthetized and the carotid artery and jugular vein are dissected free. Both the vessel tips, connected to each end of the shunt tube, are inserted through a small incision in the blood vessel wall and externally secured with sutures. In the case of the V-V shunt model, both the vessel tips are inserted into the proximal and distal limb of the jugular vein. The clamp of the shunt tube is removed to start blood flow in the shunt. After removal of the sample tubes from the shunt at the prescribed time interval, the material surfaces contacted with blood are processed for radio-chemical and morphologic analyses.

An important procedure in this shunting experiment is to insert the tube ends into the artery or vein without creation of turbulent blood flow. The sample material to be tested should be flexible enough to build an extracorporeal loop and large enough to be compatible with the diameter of the animal's cannulated blood vessel.

Caix et al. used a canine ex vivo shunt for the hemocompatibility assessment of artificial surfaces using radiolabeled blood cells and proteins [5]. Figure 34-2 shows white blood cell radioactivity profiles on different materials including two poly(vinyl chloride)(PVC) samples: PVC provided by IUPAC Working Party (PVC. IUPAC) and a medical grade PVC (PVC control), and an NHLBI primary reference silica-free poly(dimethyl siloxane) (PRM. PDMS). The sudden initial increase observed for PVC control seems to be due to a variation of the extracorporeal circuit length under the isotope detector or of the extracorporeal circuit position. Indeed, when the respective evolution of the radioactivity ratios (red blood cells/white blood cells) was plotted for each type of material, the behavior of white blood cells in blood exposed to PVC control did not feature any sudden variation during the same period of time. Red blood cells are known not to be involved in the initial steps of thrombogenic phenomenona and hence provide a permanent reference index for blood volume and blood flow. This canine ex vivo shunt with the use of labeled proteins and cells gives results as summarized in Table 34-3. As judged from the platelet affinity and fibrinogen

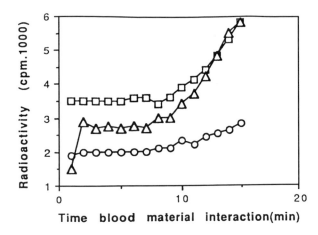

Figure 34-2 White blood cell radioactivity profiles on PVC.IUPAC (circles), PRM.PDMS (squares) and PVC control (triangles). Reprinted from Caix J, Janvier G, Legault B, Bordenave L, Rouais F, Basse-Cathalinat B, Baquey C. A canine ex vivo shunt for isotopic hemocompatibility evaluation of a NHLB1 DTB primary reference material and of a IUPAC reference material, *J Biomater Sci Polymer Ed,* 194; 5:279–291. With permission.

adsorption data, the most hemocompatible material appears to be the PVC control followed by PRM. PDMS and PVC. IUPAC. As judged from white blood cell affinity, PRM. PDMS behaves worse than PVC. IUPAC but better than PVC control. The authors questioned whether these hierarchies were relevant in terms of thrombogenicity, and concluded that long-term testing would probably be more appropriate than the acute ex vivo experiment described here.

Another ex vivo shunt model that allows much longer exposure to blood than that shown in Figure 34-1 was reported by Fong Ip et al. [6]. The schematic representation is given in Figure 34-3. As can be seen, the total shunt length is approximately 100 cm. Each limb of the shunt is inserted 10 cm into the blood vessel, anchored with grommets to the vessel wall at the cannulation site, and tunnelled under the skin at each side of the body to exit separately on the back of the animal.

IN VIVO ASSESSMENT

For long-term assessment of hemocompatibility, implantation of biomaterials in animals is required. Such in vivo testing for designated periods will provide the most useful information for the clinical application of biomaterials. Widely known assessments by implantation include the vena cava ring test and the renal embolus test. However, they have largely been

Table 34-3   Result of Hemocompatibility Evaluation by Canine *Ex Vivo* Shunting

Platelet affinity	PVC.IUPAC > PRM.PDMS > PVC control
Leukocyte affinity	PVC control > PRM.PDMS ≥ PVC.IUPAC
Fibrinogen adsorption	PVC.IUPAC ≥ PRM.PDMS > PVC control

5) Caix J., Janvier G, Legault B, Bordenave L, Rouais F, Basse-Cathalinat B, Baquey C. A canine *ex vivo* shunt for isotopic hemocompatibility evaluation of a NHLB1 DTB primary reference material and of a IUPAC reference material. *J Biomater Sci Polymer Ed.* 1994; 5:279–291.

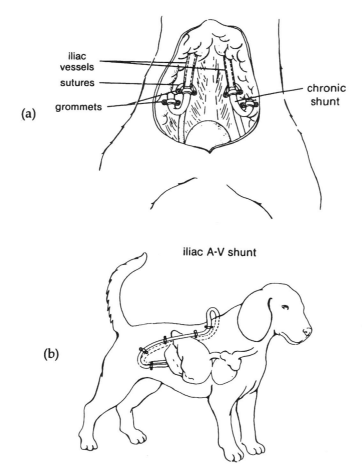

Figure 34-3   (a) Position of shunt in iliac artery and vein, showing the use of gromments to anchor the shunt to the adjacent tissue. (b) Position of shunt anchored to tissue along the subcutaneous tunnels and externalized from the back of the animal (without the test section). Reprinted from Fong Ip W, Zingg W, Sefton MV. Parallel flow arteriovenous shunt for the ex vivo evaluation of heparinized material, *J Biomed Mater Res*, 1985; 19:161–178. With permission.

abandoned now because the test period was not sufficiently long to effectively evaluate the material surface per se, and because blood flow patterns, created by the configuration of the cava ring, affected the test results. Consequently it is now recommended that biomaterials be tested in their end-use configurations.

Indwelling Catheters

Catheters are often indwelled in the central vein for purposes which include administration of intravenous fluid, parenteral nutrition, and chemotherapy. Thrombus formation takes place most commonly on the outside surface of indwelling catheters (sleeve thrombus). The sleeve thrombi composed of platelets and fibrin may be dislodged when the catheter is removed, and may result in embolization downstream from the vascular entry site. Therefore, for the assessment of hemocompatibility of a catheter indwelling in veins or arteries, it should not be removed from the animal for surface analysis. Otherwise, the thrombi formed on

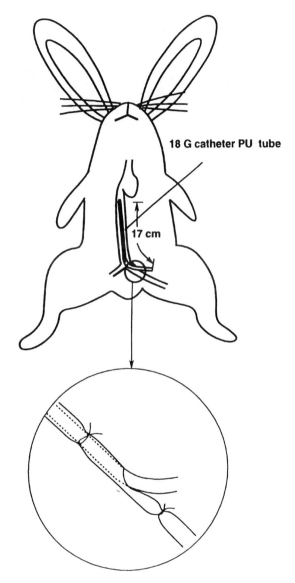

Figure 34-4 Schematic representation of catheter implantation in the rabbit inferior vena cava. Reprinted from Inoue H, Fujimoto K, Uyama Y, Ikada Y. Ex vivo and in vivo evaluation for the blood compatibility of surface-modified polyurethane catheter, *J Biomed Mater Res*, submitted. With permission.

the outside of the catheter would be stripped off and retained in the catheterized vessel, resulting in clear appearance of the external catheter surface.

Figure 34-4 shows a schematic representation of an assessment method for an indwelling catheter [7]. Its implantation in the femoral vein is performed as follows. A catheter tubing of about 20 cm in length, 0.7 mm in inner diameter, and 1.2 mm in outer diameter is prepared for implantation in the inferior vena cava of an anesthetized rabbit. The femoral groin of a rabbit is shaved, disinfected, draped, and incised to expose the femoral vein. After distal ligation and proximal incision of the vein, the catheter is inserted proximally into the vein and passed forward until its tip is located in the inferior vena cava. Then the proximal portion of the vein is ligated over the inserted catheter. The external part of the catheter tube

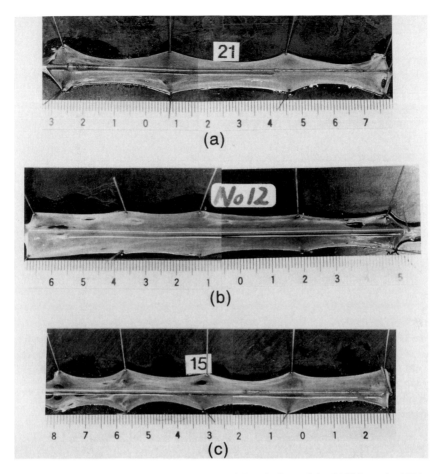

Figure 34-5 Clot formation on the outer surface of the virgin and the DMAA-grafted PU catheter with a graft density 30 μg/cm^2 after implantation in the rabbit inferior vena cava for different periods of time. (a) Virgin, 2 weeks, and grade; (b) DMAA-grafted, 2 weeks, and grade 5; (c) DMAA-grafted, 1 month, and grade 4. Reprinted from Inoue H, Fujimoto K, Uyama Y, Ikada Y. Ex vivo and in vivo evaluation for the blood compatibility of surface-modified polyurethane catheter, *J Biomed Mater Res*, submitted. With permission.

is cut to an appropriate length and the incised skin is closed. After predetermined implant duration, the catheter is removed together with the femoral vein and vena cava from the sacrificed rabbit and the catheter lumen is flushed with physiological saline to remove the blood remaining inside. The outer surface of the catheter is inspected with the naked eye and scanning electron microscopy (SEM) to evaluate the clot formation on the surface.

Figure 34-5 shows representative optical photographs of the outer appearance of the virgin and surface-modified polyurethane catheters which had been in contact with blood for 2 weeks and 1 month, respectively. The surface modification was conducted by surface graft polymerization of dimethylacrylamide (DMAA), a nonionic hydrophilic monomer. It is seen that clots of various sizes are formed discontinuously on the surface of the implanted catheters. Large clots noticed at the distal end of the catheters must be due to stagnant flow of the blood resulting from ligation of the femoral vein. For quantitative hemocompatibility assessment numerical grading on the clot formation is desirable. Although the number of clots and the clot diameter vary in some complex manner, one may roughly grade the extent of clot formation for comparison, as presented in Table 34-4. The assessment result of

Table 34-4   Grading for Blood Compatibility Evaluation

Grade	Clots formed	
	Diameter (mm)	Number on one catheter surface
1	>1.0	5<
2	1.0–1.5	3–4
3	1.0–1.5	1–2
4	0.5–1.0	2–5
5	<0.5	0

7) Inoue H, Fujimoto K, Uyama Y, Ikada Y. Ex vivo and in vivo evaluation for the blood compatibility of surface-modified polyurethane catheter. J Biomed Mater Res. submitted.

hemocompatibility for different surfaces based on this 5-graded level is given in Table 34-5 as a function of implantation time. As can be seen, the evaluation results are widely scattered even on the surface brought into contact with blood for the same period, but apparently the poorest hemocompatibility is noticed on the unmodified surface. Clot formation on the grafted surfaces is likely to become more remarkable as blood exposure to the catheters is prolonged.

Vascular Grafts

In vivo hemocompatibility has been assessed most commonly by directly anastomosing the tubing to be tested to arteries or veins, because the major purpose of current development of long-term blood-contacting biomaterials is for substitution of defective blood vessels, especially vessels of small diameter (less than 6 mm) such as coronary and popliteal arteries. The biocompatibility of vascular grafts is evaluated on the basis of a variety of standards including thrombus formation, patancy rate, neointima coverage, endothelial coverage, intima hyperplasia, aneurysm-like expansion, and tube kinking. Most of these features are closely related to the hemocompatibility of vascular grafts. In this hemocompatibility assessment with the anastomotic method, care should be taken in connecting the test tubing to the host blood vessel. Otherwise, acute thrombus formation at the anastomotic site, resulting in occlusion, would readily take place because of the blood flow turbulence due to graft luminal mismatch and exposure of vascular tissues to the blood stream, especially collagenous tissues.

The work of Marois et al. is a good example to demonstrate the hemocompatibility assessment of vascular grafts [8]. They selected four chemically processed biological grafts, anastomosed them to the infrarenal aorta of dogs, and retrieved them at 4, 24, and 48 hours (short-term), 1, 2, and 4 weeks (medium-term), as well as 3 and 6 months

Table 34-5   *In Vivo* Evaluation for the Blood Compatibility of the Grafted Surfaces Implanted for Different Periods of Time

Surface	Implantation time	Evaluation grade
DMAA-grafted PU	1 week	4, 4(average = 4.0)
DMAA-grafted PU	2 weeks	5, 4, 4, 5, 4, 4, 3, 4 (average = 4.1)
DMAA-grafted PU	1 month	4, 3 (average = 3.5)
Virgin PU	2 weeks	3, 2, 4, 4, 3, 3, 3, 3 (average = 3.1)

7) Inoue H, Fujimoto K, Uyama Y, Ikada Y. Ex vivo and in vivo evaluation for the blood compatibility of surface-modified polyurethane catheter. *J Biomed Mater Res.* submitted.

(long-term) after anastomosis. The four biological grafts included Omniflow® (Bionova, Melbourne, Australia), adapted from the Sparks-mandril grown in the subcutaneous tissue of sheep; Biopolymeric® (St. Jude Medical Inc., St. Paul, MN), originated from bovine carotid; Dardik-Biograft® of the second generation (Meadox Medicals Inc., Oakland, NJ), originated from human umbilical cord vein; and BIMA® (Biocor Industries Ltd., Nova Lima, Brazil), originated from bovine internal mammary artery. All of them were tanned in glutaraldehyde.

Before implantation, dogs were anesthetized and given 1mg/kg of heparin. One 5 to 6 cm long segment, 6 mm in diameter, of each graft was interposed as a substitute for the infrarenal abdominal aorta. Under sterile conditions, end-to-end anastomoses were done with 5/0 or 6/0 running stitches. The dogs were also administered 15,000 units of prolonged-effect antibiotic and fed on a normal diet without further treatment. At the predetermined time of death, the dogs were anesthetized, and the grafts were excised and opened longitudinally. Patency was assessed by macroscopic observation. The grafts were photographed and the thrombus-free surface of the graft was evaluated by a computerized digitized image analysis. The grafts were fixed in a buffered glutaraldehyde solution for histological examination and SEM study.

The explanted grafts were evaluated in terms of patency and macroscopic healing characteristics as schematically shown in Figure 34-6. It is still extremely difficult to evaluate the healing process in a quantitative manner. One Omniflow® graft was occluded at 6 months and two Dardik-Biografts® were thrombosed, one at 24 hours and one at 1 month. All explanted grafts in the Biopolymeric® series and in the BIMA® were patent at the animals' time of sacrifice. The BIMA® graft performed the most satisfactorily and retained its blood compatibility best; that is, the luminal surface was smooth, with only minor thrombotic deposits and a thin pannus along the anastomotic lines. The BIMA® graft originated from bovine internal mammary artery, whose endothelium had almost disappeared, but the basement membrane was well preserved, apparently providing the host with the least thrombogenic surface.

The protocols adopted for hemocompatibility assessment of vascular grafts should be those which satisfy the needs of those surgeons who make the decisions on selection of vascular grafts for clinical use.

Artificial Heart Valves

Prosthetic valves, currently in use as substitute cardiac valves, include two types, mechanic and biologic. The greatest concern of mechanical valves is thrombus formation, while that of biological valves is biostability and calcification. These same problems are associated also with valves in artificial hearts.

Calcific deposits are the principal single cause of the clinical failure of bioprosthetic heart valves. Several hypotheses are proposed for the calcification; one hypothesis involves an impaired balance between positively and negatively charged amino acids, exposing affinity sites to Ca^{2+} ion [9] and another a release of glutaraldehyde from bioprosthetic cardiac valves [10]. Surfactants such as polysorbate and sodium dodecyl sulfate [11, 12], diphosphonates [13, 14], polyacrylamide [11], and toluidine blue [12] have been reported to decrease the calcification. Jones et al. evaluated the effectiveness of these agents in mitigating the calcification that develops in bioprosthetic valves implanted in young sheep [15]. They used 247 bioprostheses including 229 valves implanted in the mitral position and 18 implanted in the tricuspid position. Whenever possible, the valves were allowed to

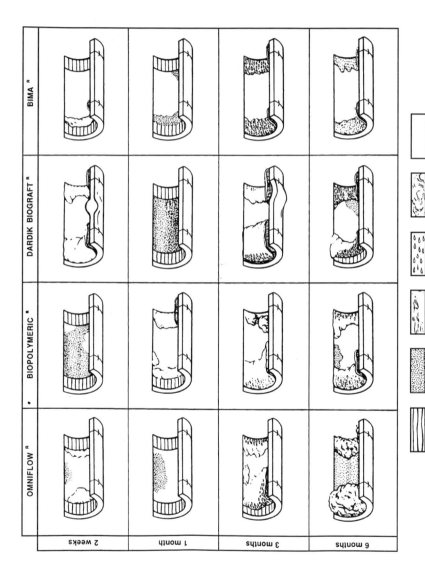

Figure 34-6 Schematic representation of the healing sequences observed in the four chemically processed biological grafts implanted for 2 wk, 1, 3 and 6 months. Reprinted from Marois Y, Boyer D, Guidoin R, Donville Y, Marois M, Francisco-Javier T, Paul-Emile R. In vivo evaluation of four chemically processed biological grafts implanted as infrarenal arterial substitutes in dogs, *Biomaterials*, 1989; 10:368–379. With permission.

Table 34-6   Calcium Content of Valves Treated with Anticalcification Agents

Valve Type	N	mg Ca/gm tissue dry weight, mean ± S.E.M.
Baxter Edwards CVS Divsion		
Standard PAVs (controls for PV2 and PV2′)	22	99.8 ± 11.1
Polysorbate-80 treated (PV2) PAVs	15	7.6 ± 2.6 (P < 0.001)
Triton X-100 and N-lauryl sarcosine (PV2′) treated PAVs	14	12.7 ± 3.8 (P < 0.001)
Standard BPVs (PV2 controls)	18	73.1 ± 10.3
Polysorbate-80 treated (PV2) BPVs	11	55.2 ± 12.7
Standard BPVs (PV3 controls)*	10	66.1 ± 15.5
Polyacrylamide treated (PV3) BPVs*	8	112.9 ± 15.3 (P < 0.005)
Hancock Laboratories		
Standard PAVs	28	64.7 ± 9.6
Sodium dodecyl sulfate treated PAVs (Hancock-II-T6)	17	17.7 ± 4.2 (P < 0.001)
Standard BPVs	12	136.2 ± 3.6
Sodium dodecyl sulfate treated (T6) BPVs	24	117.7 ± 5.3
Mitroflow/Mitral Medical		
Standard BPVs	17	104.3 ± 9.1
Diphosphonate (ADP) treated BPVs	12	126.6 ± 7.3 (P < 0.07)
Xenotech Laboratories		
Standard PAVs	17	139.3 ± 14.7
Toluidine blue treated PAVs	21	81.6 ± 12.0 (P < 0.05)

*Implanted in the tricuspid position; all other valves implanted in the mitral position. PAVs, porcine aortic valves; BPVs, bovine pericardial valves.

15) Jones M, Eidbo EE, Hilbert SL, Ferrans VJ, Clark RE. The effects of anticalcification treatments on bioprosthetic heart valves implanted in sheep. *Trans. Am. Soc. Artif. Intern. Organs.* 1988; XXXIV: 1027–1030.

remain in place for 20 weeks. However, in the case of certain types of bioprostheses, this period of time had to be reduced because of morbidity and mortality associated with calcification and degeneration. At the time of death, echocardiography, Doppler ultrasound evaluation, cardiac catheterization, ventriculography, and a complete necropsy were performed on each animal. Techniques used for analysis of the explanted bioprostheses included radiography, macroscopic and histologic evaluation, transmission and scanning electron microscopic studies, and quantitative analyses for calcium and phosphate. One half of each leaflet, selected in a systematic manner, was used for the quantitative measurements of calcium and phosphate. The results obtained with each type of treatment were compared with those from matched control valves from the same manufacturer. All infected valves were excluded from the study because these often contained calcified vegetations. The results of quantitative analyses for calcium in the different groups of explanted valves are given in Table 34-6. All calcium analysis data are presented in milligrams of calcium per gram of tissue dry weight ± SEM. The calcium analyses were considered, together with the radiographic studies, to be the most sensitive indicators of the degrees of calcification present in explanted bioprostheses.

Artificial Hearts

The number of donors available for heart transplantation is much smaller than necessary. In addition, there is a high incidence of left ventricular failure in patients who have suffered myocardial ischemia. These problems have encouraged the use of cardiac assist devices to supplement the action of the left ventricle and use of the artificial heart while patients are waiting for heart transplantation. Nevertheless, the ideal artificial heart has not yet become available primarily because of thrombus formation, platelet consumption, and the pumping action which results in hemolysis of red blood cells with liberation of ADP which accentuates the thrombotic tendency.

The cardiac assist device and the total heart replacement are generally composed of a pumping chamber, blood conduits, and blood flow regulating valves. Over the past 20 years a number of artificial heart research centers have developed and optimized pumping characteristics, blood flow patterns, material choices, pump cycles and synchronization, connections to the host circulation, and implantation sites in large series of animal trials. Predominately calves, sheep, and goats were used for short- and long-term trials to assess long-term hemocompatibility but also reliability and effectiveness. Hemocompatibility should be assessed for all of these device components. The assessment of blood conduits and heart valves was already described above.

Most hemocompatibility assessments on the pumping chamber have been performed by observing the morphological changes on the blood-contacting surface with optical, isotope techniques and electron scanning microscopes, similar to assessment techniques used for vascular grafts. However, in the case of the pumping chamber, occlusion does not take place.

Menconi et al. have recently reported gene expression for matrix composition of cellular linings formed on blood-contacting surfaces of clinically implanted cardiac assist devices in addition to morphological observations [16]. They characterized the biological linings associated with blood-contacting surfaces of 11 of left ventricular assist devices (Heartmate-1000 LVAD®, from Thermo Cardiosystems Inc., Woburn, MA) implanted as schematically shown in Figure 34-7. The LVAD is an implantable, pneumatically driven pusher-plate type blood pump composed of an outer rigid titanium housing and a flexible polyurethane diaphragm. The pump was positioned intraperitoneally in the left upper quadrant of the patient's abdomen and, when implanted for temporary use, was powered by an external console. Programmed pulses of pressurized air were delivered to the implanted pump chamber via a percutaneous drive line. The inflow and outflow conduits of the device contain 25 mm porcine xenograft valves.

The blood-contacting surfaces of both the titanium housing component and the flexible polyurethane diaphragm were textured to encourage the formation and adherence of a biologic lining. The flexible diaphragm consists of a fibrillar surface integral with the base material to eliminate detaching of the fibrils. The nonflexing housing surface was fabricated from titanium microspheres sintered together to form a textured nonpermeable topography. These textured structures were quite different from those of other heart assist devices which are designed to have smooth blood-contacting surfaces, primarily consisting of elastomeric biomaterials, as a means of preventing thrombogenesis.

When this device with textured, blood-contacting surfaces was clinically implanted for durations ranging from 21 to 324 days, it was found that no clinical thromboembolic events or pump-related thromboembolism occurred. Biologic linings developed on the textured surfaces were composed of patches of cellular tissue intermingled with areas of compact fibrinous material. In addition, islands of collagenous tissue containing fibroblast-like cells appeared after 30 days of implantation. Many of these cells contained microfilaments with dense bodies indicative of myofibroblasts.

Protein deposition on the diaphragm was highly variable, depending on the diaphragm flexure patterns and blood flow conditions within the pump chamber. The flexure patterns and blood flow conditions within the pump chamber were roughly classified as schematically

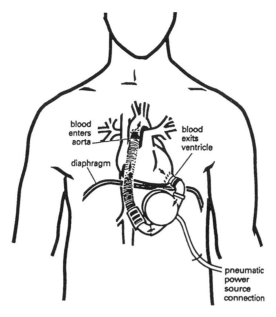

Figure 34-7 Schematic illustration of the LVAD implanted in patient. The pump is positioned intraperitoneally in the upper left quadrant of the abdomen. Dacron conduits are used to connect the pump between the apex of the left ventricle and the ascending thoracic aorta. The LVAD is pneumatically driven via a percutaneous drive line powered by an external console. Porcine valves placed in the inflow and outflow conduits ensure the unidirectional flow of blood (arrows). Reprinted from Menconi MJ, Pockwinse S, Owen TA, Dasse KA, Stein GS, Lian JB. Properties of blood-contacting surfaces of clinically implanted cardiac assist devices: gene expression, matrix composition, and ultrastructural characterization of cellular linings, *J Cell Biochem*, 1995; 57:557–573. With permission.

shown in Figure 34-8. The greatest shear rates of blood along the walls of the device were found in the region between the inflow and outflow ports (regions A and B). Flexure of the diaphragm was uniformly high around the circumference of the diaphragm (regions A and D), but very low within the central area bonded to a pusher plate. This central region (region C) was exposed to the lowest combination of shear rates and diaphragm flexure. Figure 34-9 shows the quantities of total protein deposited on the diaphragm surfaces.

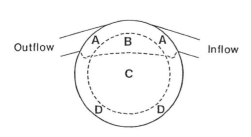

Figure 34-8 Hemodynamic conditions and mechanical flexure patterns within the LVAD pumping chamber. A: High-shear/high-flex region. B: High-shear/low-flex region. C: Low-shear/low-flex region. D: Low-shear/high-flex region. Reprinted from Menconi MJ, Pockwinse S, Owen TA, Dasse KA, Stein GS, Lian JB. Properties of blood-contacting surfaces of clinically implanted cardiac assist devices: gene expression, matrix composition, and ultrastructural characterization of cellular linings, *J Cell Biochem*, 1995; 57:557–573. With permission.

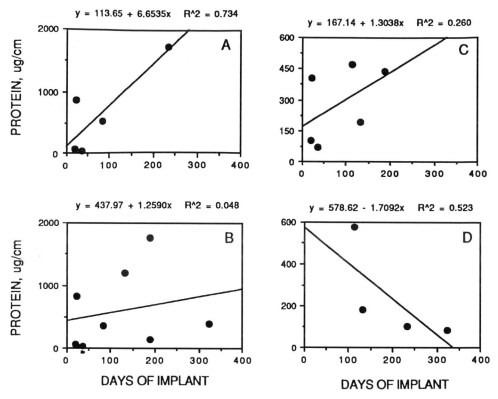

Figure 34-9 Relationship of protein deposition of flex/shear conditions and implant duration. Tissue deposits on diaphragm samples exposed to various combinations of hemodynamic and mechanical flexure conditions were hydrolyzed and subjected to amino acid analysis as described. A: High shear/high flex. B: High shear/low flex. C: Low shear/low flex. D: Low shear/high flex (Fig. 34.7). Reprinted from Menconi MJ, Pockwinse S, Owen TA, Dasse KA, Stein GS, Lian JB. Properties of blood-contacting surfaces of clinically implanted cardiac assist devices: gene expression, matrix composition, and ultrastructural characterization of cellular linings, *J Cell Biochem*, 1995; 57:557–573. With permission.

Generally, protein content per cm^2 was greater in the high shear regions (Figures 34-9A, B). In low-flex regions, no significant correlations as a function of implant duration were found with either high-shear (Figure 34-9B) or low-shear (Figure 34-9C) conditions. In high-flex regions, there were trends toward increased protein accumulation in the high-shear areas (Figure 34-9A) and a decrease in the low-shear regions (Figure 34-9D) as a function of increasing implant duration.

To characterize cellular growth properties and synthesized products of cells associated with the titanium and polyurethane surfaces, RNA was extracted from the tissue linings harvested from both the housing and diaphragm surfaces. The isolated RNA samples were subjected to hybridization analyses to determine if the cells colonizing the pump surfaces expressed genes encoding proteins for cell proliferation (histones), cell adhesion (fibronectin), cell shape (actin, vimentin), and extracellular matrix (collagen types I and III). Relative levels of mRNA transcripts of cell growth-, cytoskeletal-, and extracellular matrix-related genes in cells colonizing the LVAD diaphragm as a function of implant duration are shown in Figure 34-10. It is seen that the colonizing cells actively express genes encoding proteins for cell proliferation, adhesion, cytoskeleton, and extracellular matrix. Type I collagen mRNA levels synthesized by cells populating the housing surfaces of the

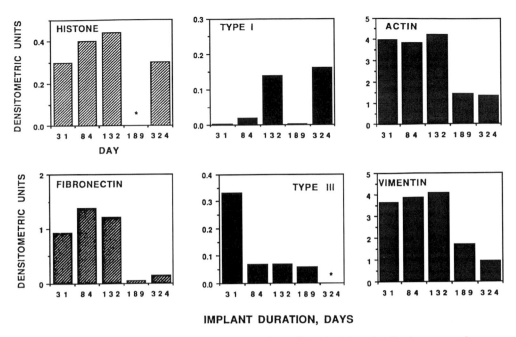

Figure 34-10 Relative levels of gene expression by cells colonizing the diaphragm surface as a function of implant duration. Equal quantities of total cellular RNA from each sample were applied to Zeta-Probe membranes using a slot-blot apparatus (2 or 4 μg RNA/slot). The blots were then hybridized to gene-specific ³²P-labeled cDNA probes. Resultant autoradiograms were quantitated by scanning laser densitometry. Asterisks (∗) indicate not analyzed. Reprinted from Menconi MJ, Pockwinse S, Owen TA, Dasse KA, Stein GS, Lian JB. Properties of blood-contacting surfaces of clinically implanted cardiac assist devices: gene expression, matrix composition, and ultrastructural characterization of cellular linings, *J Cell Biochem*, 1995; 57:557–573. With permission.

84- and 132-day implants are 28- and 3.6-fold greater, respectively, than mRNA levels synthesized by cells populating the corresponding diaphragm surfaces within the same implant. A similar result was obtained for the type III collagen mRNA levels. This finding is not surprising since cytoskeletal architecture [17, 18] and extracellular matrix production [19, 20] are known to be modulated by exposure to shear forces and mechanical flexure stresses.

Based on the above results, together with morphological and ultrastructural features of the blood-contacting surfaces, Menconi et al. concluded that textured surfaces induced the formation of a thin, tightly adherent, viable lining which exhibited excellent long-term hemocompatibility.

SUMMARY

Although numerous assessment procedures have been proposed for investigating the response of blood to artificial foreign surfaces, there is no ideal procedure for linking the hemocompatibility assessment of a biomaterial to its potential clinical performance [1]. Nevertheless, for the development of improved biomaterials, in vitro, ex vivo, and in vivo hemocompatibility assessment procedures are required. They range from those relevant to an initial screening of biomaterials to those designed for a detailed investigation and clinical trials of end-use devices. Basic features to be considered in any hemocompatibility assessment are the nature of blood, the method of achieving blood-material contact, and parameter selection. The parameter selection may require a compromise between the advantages of multiparameter assessment and the benefit of determining a single parameter by a consistent methodology. Data acquired from animal experiments must be interpreted on the basis of species-related differences for blood components. *In vitro* procedures allow the use of human blood but ignore the inter-relationships between the donor and the clinical use of the material. In vivo hemocompatibility assessment requires almost inevitably a certain number of animals in order to produce statistically significant results. We should try to present the results obtained by animal experiments in a quantitative manner as much as possible. In this connection, gene expression of cells populating blood-contacting surfaces and composition determination of biologic lining, as demonstrated above, may be very useful in future methods for the quantitative assessment of hemocompatibility.

REFERENCES

1   Courtney JM, Forbes CD. Thrombosis on foreign surfaces. *British Med Bull*, 50 (1994), 966–981.
2   Edmunds LH, Jr. Breaking the blood-biomaterial barrier. *ASAIO J*, 1995, 824–830.
3   Sawyer PN, Sophie Z, O'Shaughnessy AM. Systems implantology: Hemocompatibility assessment. In von Recum AF (Ed.), *Handbook of Biomaterials Evaluation*, 1st ed. New York: Macmillan, 1986, 306–320.
4   Fujimoto K, Minato M, Tadokoro H, Ikada Y. Platelet deposition onto polymeric surfaces during shunting. *J Biomed Mater Res*, 27 (1993), 335–343.
5   Caix J, Janvier G, Legault B, Bordenave L, Rouais F, Basse-Cathalinat B, Baquey C. A canine *ex vivo* shunt for isotopic hemocompatibility evaluation of a NHLBI DTB primary reference material and of a IUPAC reference material. *J Biomater Sci, Polymer Ed*, 5 (1994), 279–291.
6   Fong Ip W, Zingg W, Sefton MV. Parallel flow arteriovenous shunt for the ex vivo evaluation of heparinized materials. *J Biomed Mater Res*, 19 (1985), 161–178.
7   Inoue H, Fujimoto K, Uyama Y, Ikada Y. Ex vivo and in vivo evaluation for the blood compatibility of surface-modified polyurethane catheter. *J Biomed Mater Res*.
8   Marois Y, Boyer D, Guidoin R, Donville Y, Marois M, Teijeira FJ, Roy PE. In vivo evaluation of four chemically processed biological grafts implanted as infrarenal arterial substitutes in dogs. *Biomaterials*, 10 (1989), 369–379.
9   Golomb G, Ezra V. Covalent binding of protamine by glutaraldehyde to bioprosthetic tissue: Characterization and anticalcification effect. *Biomater Artif Cells Immobilization Biotechnol*, 20 (1992), 31–41.
10 Grimm M, Eybl E, Grabenwoger M, Spreitzer H, Jager W, Grimm G, Bock P, Muller MM, Wolner E. Glutaraldehyde affects biocompatibility of bioprosthetic heart valves. *Surgery*, 111 (1992), 74–78.
11 Carpentier A, Nashef A, Carpentier S, Ahmed A, Goussef N. Techniques for prevention of calcification of valvular bioprostheses. *Circulation*, 70 (1984, Suppl. 1), 1–165.
12 Lentz DJ, Pollock EM, Olsen DB, et al. Inhibition of mineralization of glutaraldehyde-fixed Hancock bioprosthetic heart valves. In Cohn LH, Gallucci V (Eds.), *Cardiac Bioprostheses*. New York: Yorke, 1982, 306–319.
13 Levy RJ, Schoen FJ, Lund SA, Smith MS. Prevention of leaflet calcification of bioprosthetic heart valves with diphosphonate injection therapy. Experimental studies of optimal dosages and therapeutic durations. *J Thorac Cardiovasc Surg*, 94 (1987), 551.
14 Levy RJ, Wolfrum J, Schoen FJ, et al. Inhibition of calcification of bioprosthetic heart valves by local controlled release diphosphonate. *Science*, 228 (1985), 190.
15 Joens M, Eidbo EE, Hilbert SL, Ferrans VJ, Clark RE. The effects of anticalcification treatments on bioprosthetic heart valves implanted in sheep. *Trans ASAIO*, 34 (1988), 1027–1030.
16 Menconi MJ, Pockwinse S, Owen TA, Dasse KA, Stein GS, Lian JB. Properties of blood-contacting surfaces of clinically implanted cardiac assist devices: Gene expression, matrix composition, and ultrastructural characterization of cellular linings. *J Cell Biochem*, 57 (1995), 557–573.
17 Ives CL, Eskin SG, McIntire LV. Mechanical effects on endothelial cell morphology: In vitro assessment. *In Vitro Cell Dev Biol*, 22 (1986), 500–507.
18 Sumpio BE, Banes AJ, Buckley M, Johnson G, Jr. Alterations in aortic endothelial cell morphology and cytoskeletal protein synthesis during cyclic tensional deformation. *J Vasc Surg*, 7 (1988), 130–138.
19 Sumpio BE, Banes AJ, Link GW, Iba T. Modulation of endothelial cell phenotype by cyclic stretch: Inhibition of collagen production. *J Surg Res*, 48 (1990), 415–420.
20 Sumpio BE, Banes AJ, Link WG, Johnson G, Jr. Enhanced collagen production by smooth muscle cells during repetitive mechanical stretching. *Arch Surg*, 123 (1988), 1233–1236.

Chapter 35

Osteocompatibility

Allan F. Tencer

Orthopedic devices are generally implanted to perform some load-bearing function within the musculoskeletal system. Implants may be classified as temporary or permanent in terms of their load-bearing function. An example of a temporary implant is a fracture fixation device which bears load until the bone fragments it supports heal. Prosthetic hip or knee joints are examples of permanent orthopedic implants, designed for a long functional life as joint replacements. Implants may be grouped in terms of their functions, as devices to maintain alignment of bone fracture or osteotomy components, to resurface or replace synovial joints, and to act as graft materials for soft or hard tissue regeneration.

Evaluations of orthopedic materials usually are related to determining the mechanical strength of the implants themselves as a result of exposure to the in vivo environment, or their ability to develop a high strength attachment to bone. Nonfunctional evaluations of their characteristics are normally performed to optimize a material or geometric variable, such as the effect of surface pore size or texture on the bone ingrowth and ultimate fixation of porous-surfaced prosthetic devices. Nonfunctional testing can provide a quantitative measure of the effect of an isolated parameter, uncomplicated by the physiological and mechanical variables inherent in load bearing, typical of functional evaluations. Parameters which are commonly tested in nonfunctional osteocompatibility assessments are outlined in the first part of this chapter. Functional evaluations are concerned with the determination of the performance of a device, usually as an in vivo simulation of its actual use. The load-bearing performance of an artificial hip is an example of functional testing. Evaluation methods and the types of models used for these studies are described in the second part of this chapter.

GENERAL OSTEOCOMPATIBILITY NONFUNCTIONAL PROPERTY TESTING

Evaluation Parameters

The evaluation parameters to be described in this chapter were chosen based on two criteria. First they must be quantifiable, and second they must be responsive to the in vivo environment when implanted. For example, basic material properties such as the grain size of a metallic implant which would not be affected by the in vivo environment are not considered in this discussion, since they are treated in Chapters 2, 4, and 7 (although there could be an effect of grain boundaries on corrosion). However, basic material properties such as the elastic modulus are included because in biodegradable or porous materials this property might be modified by the biological environment. Also, the evaluation parameters listed here can be subdivided into mechanical or biological.

Interface Ultimate Shear Stress This parameter is calculated by measuring the ultimate strength at failure, usually determined from a mechanical pushout test [1–4], divided by the average surface area of the interface, which is approximately calculated by

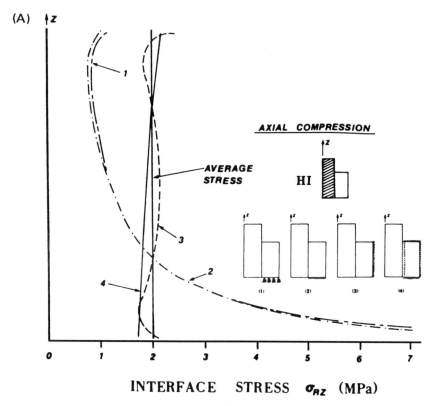

Figure 35-1 (A) Actual shear stress distribution along the interface of a cylindrical specimen undergoing pushout testing, with different specimen support conditions (from Shirazi-Adl A, *J Biomech Eng*, 114:111–118, 1992). (B) Typical load/deformation result of mechanical testing showing various parameters which can be used to define behavior (from Tencer AF, Johnson KD, *Biomechanics in Orthopedic Trauma, Bone Fracture and Fixation*, Lippincott-Raven, 1994).

multiplying the perimeter of the implant times its length of engagement in bone (typically the material in which it is evaluated). It should be noted that stresses at this interface, assumed to be uniform for this calculation, are actually very dependent on specimen interface and test fixture geometry (Figure 35-1A). Therefore, this test is best used only for comparing specimens of very similar geometries, loaded in specific types of fixtures [5, 6]. The implants used, and therefore the interface, are usually cylindrical. A typical application in which ultimate shear stress would be evaluated is in determination of fixation strength of an implant in bone, which is critical for evaluating its load-bearing capacity.

Ultimate Compressive or Tensile Stress   This parameter is determined from the maximum tensile or compressive load that a specimen can support, Figure 35-1B, divided by the average cross-sectional area over which the force is applied. Dividing the measured force by the applied load normalizes the measured value for differences in specimen geometries. This provides a direct measure of load capacity and might be used, for example, to measure the strength of a bone graft material (compression) or a healing ligament (tension) [7, 8] at some time after in vivo implantation.

Yield Compressive or Tensile Strength   This is the stress magnitude (measured load divided by loaded surface area) at which the behavior of the material changes from linearly

(B)

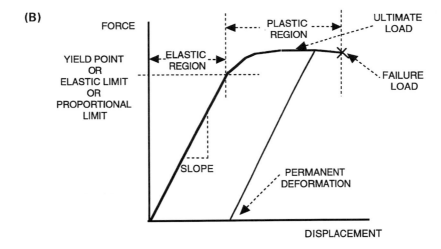

STIFFNESS = SLOPE = FORCE / DISPLACEMENT

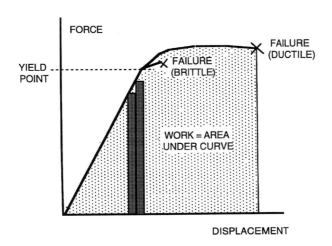

Figure 35-1   Continued.

elastic to plastic or elastoplastic (Figure 35-1B). This parameter defines the functional stress limit of a material because beyond this stress, permanent (as opposed to elastic and recoverable) deformation occurs in the implant, which is usually undesirable. In some cases there is no sharp transition from elastic to plastic behavior; therefore some arbitrary deformation may be defined at which the yield stress is measured.

Stiffness and Elastic Modulus   These parameters define the ratio of applied load to measured displacement (stiffness) (Figure 35-1B), or stress to strain (elastic modulus), where stress is load-divided by surface area and strain is the measured change in specimen length divided by its original unloaded length. These measures allow matching of mechanical properties of biomaterials with those of biological tissues, such as the cancellous bone beneath the articular surface of a joint. Elastic modulus is a more standardized parameter, allowing comparison between different materials without requiring knowledge of the specific geometry of the materials tested. In soft tissues, stress may be hard to define because of significant changes in specimen cross-sectional area under load. Stiffness, or more commonly elastic modulus are basic properties usually defined for all load-bearing orthopedic materials.

Strain Energy or Energy Absorbed to Failure   These parameters define the mechanical work done in deforming a material to failure (Figure 35-1B). Tough or ductile materials are able to absorb considerable energy before failure, as opposed to brittle materials which typically allow little deformation. Energy absorption is particularly important to characterize in materials which might be loaded beyond their elastic limit, such as ligament substitutes, or materials subjected to repeated high stress loading, where fatigue due to crack growth could occur.

Radiographic Appearance   This evaluation consists of defining both gross and microradiographic images of the implant in its biological environment. While not strictly quantifiable, grading systems have been devised to measure the relative degree and location of ossification (since a radiograph defines the presence of calcified tissues). Microradiography provides a detailed image of a region of interest in a calcified tissue sample (Figure 35-2), and if an image analysis system is employed, can provide quantitative data regarding the rate of bone formation within an implant (see also Chapter 49).

Scanning Electron Micrograph Appearance   This technique provides a three-dimensional image of implant surface geometry and permits precise measurement of cellular and biomaterial features at high magnifications (Figure 35-3). In addition a technique known as backscattered electron imaging provides an alternative method to microradiography for

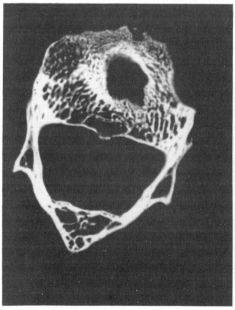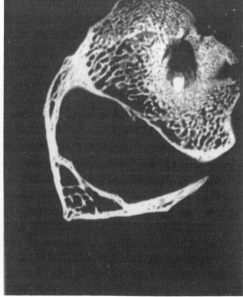

Figure 35-2   Microradiographs of bone formation within two vertebral bodies of the rabbit, one containing a biodegradable polymer implant (left) and the other, the same implant with sodium fluoride (right) (from Guise JM, McCormack A, Anderson PA, Tencer AF, *J Orthop Res*, 10.588–595, 1992.

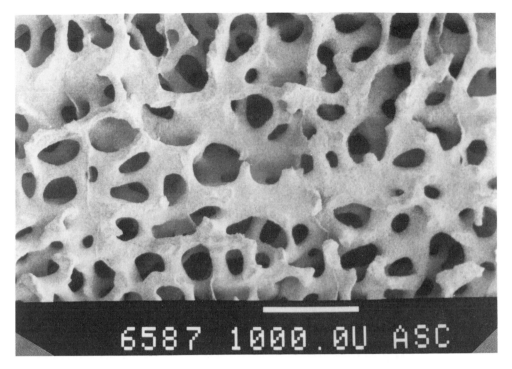

Figure 35-3 Geometric features of a porous hydroxyapatite implant demonstrated by electron microscopy.

imaging calcified tissues [9], which allows calcified tissues of different densities to be easily distinguished. This is particularly useful for distinguishing the amount of bone ingrowth into a porous hydroxyapatite implant, for example, which would otherwise be hard to determine.

Histological Appearance   Using histological stains which are specific to certain tissues or components of those tissues (collagen, hydroxyapatite) provides a qualitative image of cross-sections through the implant and surrounding tissues, including cellular structures. Histological sections are valuable for demonstrating the biological response to an implant, such as direct calcified tissue apposition, formation of a fibrous capsule, or an inflammatory reaction. Quantitative measurements can be made using histomorphometric techniques [9–14]. For more details, see Section VIII.

Bone Formation or Resorption Rate   The rate of bone turnover in response to a biomaterial can be determined quantitatively by tetracycline or other fluorescent markers which are absorbed only into sites of active bone formation (Figure 35-4). By knowing the time at which markers were administered and measuring the distance between labels microscopically, the rate of bone formation can be determined [15]. For more details, see Chapter 47.

Bone Blood Flow   The blood flow to a biomaterial is important since it provides information on the potential for bone formation, among other things. Typically bone blood flow changes with mechanical operations such as drilling holes and placing screws. A radioisotope such as SrC1 can be injected into the carotid artery and used to label blood

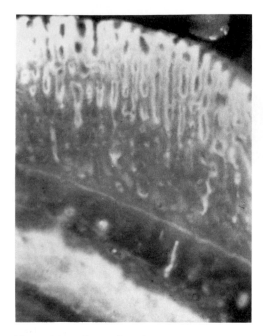 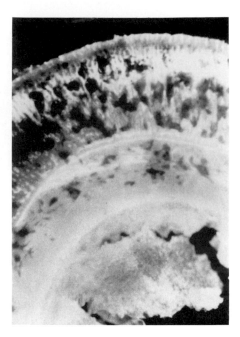

Figure 35-4 Examples of florescent dye (tetracycline) labeled sections of the femoral corticies of two rabbits, demonstrating new bone formation on the periosteal surfaces (less dense, light-colored regions) in response to controlled release of sodium fluoride (from Tencer AF, Allen BL, Woodard PL, Self J, L'heureux, Calhoun JH, *J Biomed Mat Res*, 23:571–589, 1989).

volumes in the region of interest [16]. An alternative method uses a microprobe which sends and receives a pulse of helium-neon laser light. The shift in frequency of the reflected (received) light can be used to measure the rate of blood flow past the probe tip [17]. This method determines real-time blood flow but is restricted to measurement over a very small area and may require a sampling scheme in which the probe is located in a variety of locations within the area of interest.

Surface Area and Volume Ratio   These geometric parameters can also be used to define tissue ingrowth or biodegradation rates of an implant. Quantitative values are obtained by scanning histological slides [9–14] or microradiographs [18–20], from which the presence of soft tissue, bone, and implant material can be defined in three dimensions. The use of geometric probability permits the determination of volume and surface area ratios of the various materials from randomized measurements from histological cross sections. For more details, see Chapter 48.

Calcium Distribution   The concentration of calcium ions along a boundary between growing bone and implant can be used to determine the penetration of bone into a porous material or porous interface. Measurements can be made from prepared cross sections using an electron probe microanalyzer [4].

Ion Distribution   Concentrations of ions released from a biomaterial into various body organs such as the liver, spleen, kidney, lung, or skeletal muscles can be measured. Implants may be radioactively tagged to aid in the detection of released ions.

Implantation Methods

Methods used to implant biomaterials into animals should be designed to minimize the number of animals required, the trauma of the implantation procedure, and the risk of post-operative complications (see Chapters 29, 30, and 31). Consideration should be given to optimizing variables using benchtop testing, before implantation is performed. Use of multiple implantation sites minimizes the number of animals but may increase operative times and post-operative complications. Because the typical response of an orthopedic biomaterial is dependent upon healing time, this additional variable tends to increase the number of specimens required to characterize the complete behavior of the implant. The quantity of animals used should reflect a number sufficient to provide valid statistical comparisons, and encompass at least the early and late stages of bone healing response. Small sample non-parametric comparisons using matched pairs [21] provides the most powerful method of statistical comparisons with the fewest number of specimens. Since most orthopedic implants are placed into forelimbs or hindlimbs, matched pair comparisons are easy to perform for orthopedic evaluations. In some cases it is beneficial to design an experiment which allows a sham surgery to be performed so that the effect of the surgical trauma can be evaluated (see also Chapter 31).

Surgically induced infection, dislodgment of the implant, or mechanical failure, either of the implant or the bone into which it is placed, are the most common orthopedic complications which are not related to the biomaterial itself. In cases where the bone is to be subjected to load bearing, even if the biomaterial will not be, it is prudent to simulate the situation biomechanically on the benchtop to ensure mechanical stability before expending a large amount of effort in surgery and possibly wasting valuable in vivo experiments. Benchtop evaluation may consist of developing the surgical approach and implantation technique, as well as loading an implant placed into a trial bone to expected in vivo loads and measuring strength and deformation of the construct (the implant/bone/and bone fixation if it is used). It should also be noted that placing a hole into a bone may significantly weaken it (Figure 35-5), and can result in disastrous complications such as fracture after implantation

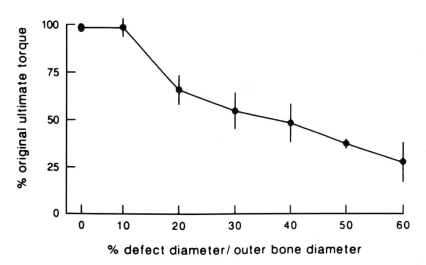

Figure 35-5 Effect on the torsional strength of the radius of a dog with different radii holes drilled through a single cortex (from Edgarton BC, An K-N, Morrey BF, *J Orthop Res*, 8:851–855, 1990).

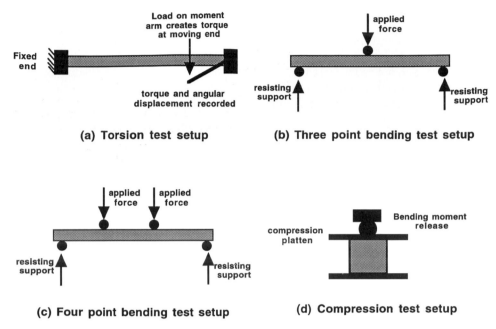

Figure 35-6   Alternatives for mechanical testing of biomaterials, (A) torsion, (B) three-point bending, (C) four-point bending, (D) compression.

[22]. In some cases, where a fixation device is used to stabilize a bone, for example if a central segment is removed (this model will be discussed in detail) the fixation (plate or rod) used to stabilize the bone may be too flexible and may overshadow any expected effect of the implanted biomaterial.

When post-implantation testing of mechanical strength properties is desired, consideration should be given to the type of test method to be employed, since this will affect the shape and location of implantation of the biomaterial. Samples with a uniform circular cross section can be tested in torsion (Figure 35-6), which allows uniform loading of the entire specimen (between the grips of the mechanical tester), and simulates a common loading condition in vivo. Tension testing of specimens also allows uniform loading to be applied (so that all regions of the implant are equally likely to fracture). Both types of specimens are usually dumbbell-shaped so that higher stresses, and failure, occur in the central region and are not affected by the grips. Long bones may also be tested in three- or four-point bending. Bending is a functional loading mode, and problems with gripping the specimens are eliminated. In four-point bending (Figure 35-6), the load is uniform only between the two central loading points, while three-point bending produces a completely non-uniform load which is greatest under the central loading point. Compression testing (Figure 35-6), is used for specimens which are either subjected to primarily compressive loading in vivo (e.g., being located under the articular cartilage of a joint or within a vertebra) or are wide relative to their length, making them impractical to test by other methods.

Species

A variety of animal species have been employed in testing orthopedic biomaterials. A number of factors govern the selection of the appropriate species (see also Chapter 30). The life span of the animal must be sufficient to encompass the time span of the experiment. (Some experiments involving the long-term function of orthopedic implants been conducted for several years). The animal used should be healthy and tolerant of anesthesia, blood loss, and surgical trauma. The tissue histology should be similar to that of the human, and the gross anatomy and biomechanical loading situation should be similar to that in which the biomaterial is expected to be used. Intraspecies variability increases the number of animals required, especially if a contralateral control cannot be used. Finally, practical considerations such as cost, availability, housing requirements, and bone size may be important factors in determining the final choice of species to be used. A comparison of species in terms of these parameters is given in Table 35-1.

Implantation Sites

The following provides a discussion and illustrations of various specific methods of non-functional biomaterials implantation techniques. These descriptions are limited to the actual procedure. General principles of surgery such as anesthesia, sterile procedure, closure, and post-operative care are discussed in Chapters 31 and 33. Table 35-2 provides information on the advantages and disadvantages of each implantation site for nonfunctional orthopedic implants for biomaterials evaluation. The procedure should be chosen to be as little traumatic as possible, by locating implants away from major nerves and blood vessels, and highly stressed regions of bone. Copious irrigation should be used to decrease temperatures at bone surfaces during cutting and drilling, reducing the zone of thermally created bone necrosis. Soft tissues should be protected, and any devitalized tissue should be removed to reduce post-operative necrosis and the additional potential for infections.

Implants that are nonfunctional should be designed to fit well, using either a frictional interference fit, or other fixation devices. Loose-fitting implants will tend to migrate, and motion of the implant may result in formation of a fibrous capsule, isolating it. On the other hand, it should be recognized that bone is quite brittle and that excessively tight-fitting implants may result in fracture of bone. The following discusses the techniques and specific risks and benefits of common implantation sites for nonfunctional orthopedic biomaterials evaluations.

Transcortical (Femur, Tibia, Radius)   An example of this implantation site [1, 22–33] is shown in Figure 35-7. The location of muscles, major blood vessels, and nerves in the region should be identified from anatomical textbooks. After anesthesia, sterile draping, and preparation, an incision is made, exposing an area just large enough to permit implantation of the biomaterial. Retraction of the muscles is followed by incision and reflection of the periosteum in some cases. This is an important step to consider because this membrane is the site of osteogenic cells. Excessive trauma to the periosteum may cause bone responses, regardless of the presence of the implant. As mentioned previously, the effect of the surgical trauma may have to be evaluated by performing sham procedures in the contralateral limb. Drilling with bone drills made for humans has a tendency to shatter bones in some small animals (rabbits, for example), especially if the diameter of the drill is larger than 1/2 of the diameter of the bone [34]. A machine shop center drill (a small, flat, fluted drill bit which expands gradually to a larger diameter) has been found to be effective in both locating drill hole sites since this bit does not tend to wander on the surface, and in gradually enlarging the hole to its final diameter. Copious irrigation should be used during these processes. The implant should fit snugly into the drilled hole, which requires that the implant diameter be 0.025–0.076 mm (0.001–0.003 inches) oversize compared with the hole diameter, depending on the flexibility of the implant and the thickness of the bone cortex into which it is placed.

Table 35-1 A Comparison of Common Animal Species Used in Orthopedic Biomaterials Research

Type of animal	Average life span* (years)	Susceptibility to disease	Average weight* (kg)	Typical cost# per animal	Housing requirements*	Ease of handling	Comments
Rat (Sprague-Dawley)	2	Highly resistant to most bacteriological and viral diseases	0.2–0.3	$13 $7 shipping	Single cages, 1 × 1 1/2 ft Temp. 22° C+/− 3°C	Docile	Inexpensive, permits use of large numbers
Rabbit (New Zealand White)	7	Susceptible to pasteurellosis, which is highly contagious and may be fatal	3–5	$5/lb $10 shipping	Single cages 2×3 ft, Temp 22°C relative humidity 40–60%	Variable, frighten easily and may kick	Relatively inexpensive, bones are larger permitting larger implants compared with the rat
Dog (Numerous Breeds)	11	Susceptible to distemper, canine hepatitis, toxoplasmosis, histoplasmosis, heartworm, parvovirus	10–20 depends on breed	$$675–$1000 (class A) $200–500 shipping	Single kennels, 6 × 3 ft w/exercise area	Respond well to firm but kind handling	Bone Mechanics are similar to that in man but bone turnover rate is 2–3 times as fast. Most commonly used orthopedic model for this reason
Sheep (Merino)	12.5	Susceptible to scrapie, sheep pox which may be fatal as well as a variety of other diseases	70	$100–200 $100 shipping	Well-ventilated, constant temp., floor space up to 18 ft², single pens not needed	Variable, heavy animals may require 2 handlers	Permits study of materials at physiological loads approaching those of humans
Pig (Domestic White Skinned)	17	Generally not as susceptible as above breeds, however swine fever can be fatal	20–40	$85 $75 shipping	Pens for up to 6 animals, 3.5–7.0 ft² per pig	Usually restrained in specially designed crates	Not commonly used, except for work in soft tissue reconstruction

*Mitruka et al. listed in Additional Reading, provides detailed information on care, handling, and feeding of various species.
#Typical Costs, Animal Medicine, University of Wahsington, 1996.

Table 35-2   Advantages and Disadvantages of Various Nonfunctional Implantation Sites

Implantation site	Advantages	Disadvantages	Parameters evaluated
Transcortical	Permits implantation of multiple specimens in the same animal. Easy surgical approach with limited exposure and disruption of the periosteum and endosteal vasculature. Applicable in both large and small animals.	Not applicable to implants where a response to trabecular bone of importance. Multiple bones may weaken the bone shaft leading to fracture. Applicable only to hard tissue implants.	(a), (f)–(m)
Subchondral	Permits study of trabecular bone response or combined trabecular and cortical bone response to the biomaterial.	Number of specimens implantable in one animal is limited.	(b)–(m)
Metaphyseal transarticular	Permits determination of effect of implants of differing stiffness on articular cartilage.	Potential for articular surface disruption exists. Possibility of protective response if joint is disrupted.	
Cranium	Non-load-bearing eliminating problems of fracture found with long bone models. Permits the evaluation of onlay response.	Not applicable to specimens designed for mechanical testing. Only for tissue response and compatibility. Lower inherent healing ability.	(f)–(m)
Mandible	Permits study of mucosal response. Response is easy to observe compared with other sites.	Region of high bending moments due to chewing action requiring additional fixation for protection of implant.	(b)–(m)
Intramuscular Subcutaneous Abdominal wall	Ease of access. Permits study of biological response and degradability.	Not applicable to study of mechanical properties or osseous response.	(f)–(m)
Intramedullary	Permits study of trabecular and cortical response. Does not weaken bone shaft or disturb joint.	Limited number of specimens implantable in one animal. Greater vascular alteration than in some other methods (intramedullary vascular disruption).	(b)–(m)

As shown in Figure 35-5, consideration should be given to the effect of the hole drilled into bone on its structural integrity [22]. Burstein et al. [34], using whole rabbit tibiae tested in torsion, showed that the ratio of the energy absorbed to failure in a bone with a 2.3 mm diameter hole, compared with a contralateral intact bone, was less than 50 percent immediately after surgery. They considered this ratio to be a measure of torsional strength, thus demonstrating the effect of even a small stress concentrator. Energy to failure ratios returned to 100 percent only after about 8 weeks, by which time the hole was filled with new bone. In rabbits, given to strong kicking actions, bone fracture is a definite possibility. Decreasing the hole size or locating the holes in the metaphyseal ends instead of the mid-diaphyseal cortex can reduce this problem.

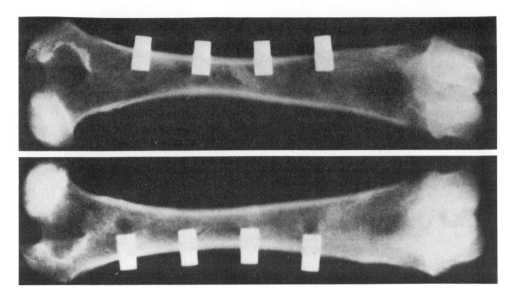

Figure 35-7 A transcortical implantation method for evaluating porous surface interface strengths (from Bobyn JD, Pilliar RM, Cameron HU, Weatherly GC, *Clin Orthop*, 150:265, 1980).

The implant should be aligned so that its longitudinal axis is perpendicular to the bone surface. Leaving a distance equal to three hole diameters between holes provides sufficient material for holding specimens during cutting and embedding procedures for histological evaluation, and supporting specimens for a mechanical pushout test, the usual method of evaluation of these implants. Placing a specimen through both cortices results in double the number of specimens after sacrifice, if the bone is cut down its centerline, allowing one to be used for mechanical testing and one for histology. Implants should not be left prominent to the bone surface since this may cause abrasion and irritation to the overlying soft tissues, including skin, resulting in additional wound-healing reactions. When specimens are used in a push out test, alignment of the specimen in the test apparatus is important. Leaving a tail of the implant protruding into the medullary canal can aid in centering the implant in the test fixture.

Intramedullary For this nonfunctional evaluation, cylindrical specimens are fabricated and sized to fit the isthmus or narrowest part of the medullary canal, usually as determined by a pre-operative radiograph [35]. Normally, implantations of this type are limited to the femurs and are performed in larger animals, because of size restrictions of the medullary canal. The benefit of this type of implantation is that it allows access to cells along the complete length of the bone. The medullary canal is reamed (passing a flexible drill down the center region of the bone) starting at the greater trochanter, and reamers of progressively increasing size are used to enlarge the canal diameter to the appropriate size. Reamer size is usually increased in very small steps. Irrigation is used to decrease bone necrosis due to the cutting action of the reamer. Also, since some reamers have very thin flutes, there is a significant rise in pressure ahead of the reamer. To reduce the pressure ahead of the reamer, either the force applied to the reamer should be reduced or it should be backed out occasionally and suction used to remove bone chips and marrow which are trapped ahead of the reamer.

In some systems, a guide pin is placed down the medullary canal. The reamers are cannulated so they can be slipped over the guide pin, reducing the potential for eccentric reaming of the intramedullary canal, which can thin the cortex of the bone shaft on one side excessively. In other cases, a transverse osteotomy is made at the midshaft of the bone and the medullary canal is reamed both proximally and distally from the osteotomy site. This reduces the potential of the reamer passing near or through an articular joint.

Subchondral (Femur, Tibia)   For this evaluation [24, 36–38], typically of materials to be used around joints, the medial surface of the proximal tibial metaphysis or the distal femoral metaphysis is exposed, taking care to preserve the ligamentous capsule surrounding the joint. A drill of appropriate size can be used to create a defect. The defect size in this case is less critical than when using the transcortical model, because it will usually be significantly smaller than the diameter of bone in that region. Also there is less chance of shattering bone when drilling because the metaphyseal bone around the joint is less brittle than diaphyseal cortex. Because of fragmentation of trabeculi, the fit of the implant will not usually be as tight as when placed into cortex.

An example of a subchondral procedure, involving also the articular cartilage, was described by Chiroff et al. [38]. After anesthesia and surgical preparation, the knee joint of the rabbit was exposed by a longitudinal incision, anterolaterally, about 2.5 cm long. Dissection of the subcutaneous tissue, extensor retinaculum, joint capsule, and synovium was performed to expose the lateral femoral condyle. The tendon of the digital extensor muscle was released from its origin on the anterior aspect of the condyle, exposing the articular surface. Using a scalpel, a 2 mm ellipse of cartilage was removed in order to provide a starting location for a 1 mm diameter drill bit. The hole was drilled through the articular cartilage, perpendicular to the joint surface and into subchondral bone. Implants were then press fit so that they lay just below the articular surface. The soft tissues were then progressively sutured, including tendon, synovium, subcutaneous tissue, and skin. In this model, the response of articular cartilage as well as subchondral bone could be studied.

Cranium   Frame [39] described an animal model for testing biomaterials in flat bones. In the rabbit a semilunar incision is created though the scalp, and muscle and periosteum are raised to expose the midline of the cranial vault. Circular holes are then made using a hole cutter along the midline, taking care not to damage the underlying dura. The implants are then positioned and overlying soft tissues repaired, including replacement of the periosteum.

Mandible   In this model, the mandibular premolar and carnassial teeth are extracted 8 weeks before implantation surgery. During implantation surgery a subperiosteal approach is used. A segmental osteotomy of the mandible is performed using a pneumatic cross cut burr, and the basal part of the mandible is left intact. The neurovascular segment is ligated and excised, and a mesh tray is screwed into place to maintain alignment and bear loads across the segmental gap (see Figure 35-8). The implant is then cut to fit snugly to fit within the defect and is supported by the mesh tray [40–43].

Intramuscular and Subcutaneous   The biochemical properties, degradation rates, ion release rates, and histological responses can be studied by locating implants in various soft tissue areas such as the sacrospinalis muscle pocket [44], the presacral adipose pocket [45], or within the abdominal wall [46]. Standardized methods for these soft tissue implantation models have been proposed [47] and are presented elsewhere.

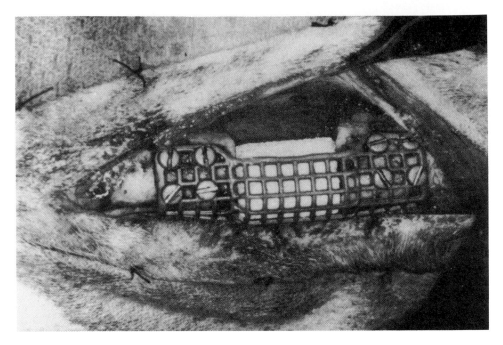

Figure 35-8 A mandibular implantation method (from Holmes RE, *Plast Reconstr. Surg*, 63:628, 1979).

FUNCTIONAL MATERIALS TESTING OF ORTHOPEDIC DEVICES

Evaluation Parameters

The parameters considered in functional testing encompass those specific to the proposed function of the implant, and are evaluated in a load-bearing setting. Some parameters discussed under the heading of nonfunctional evaluation, such as mechanical strength or radiographic appearance, can also be used to evaluate the characteristics of the biomaterial in a functional device form. Defined here are additional parameters related to functional in vivo performance.

Fatigue Life The fatigue or functional life of a device is defined as the number of loading cycles experienced at a particular stress level at the time of failure. Functional fatigue life of an implant depends on the type and properties of the material, the type of loads it is exposed to, the surface finish and geometry, and nicks and scratches which may result from implantation surgery. Stress corrosion, the action of two parts of an implant (such as a screw and plate) rubbing together, creates both mechanical wear and accelerated corrosion since the rubbing action eliminates the protective oxide layer. This property is of importance in many load-bearing orthopedic implants, and frank failure of the implant during service, while not common, does occur. Fatigue testing may be performed in bench studies but is best evaluated using animal experiments.

Cold Flow or Creep Continuous plastic deformation, cold flow, or creep of an implant occurs with repeated loading (see Chapters 1 and 2), particularly with certain polymers such as polyethylene. This parameter, measured in terms of a linear or area deformation compared with the original shape of the material, is usually of concern in polymer components of joint replacement devices.

Wear Volume Rate   This is the volume rate of loss of material between articulating surfaces of a total joint prosthesis. The wear rate should be minimized so that migration of wear particles into neighboring tissues is minimized. This parameter may be measured in benchtop testing but is a functional property based on the geometry and the load conditions to which the implant is subjected.

Flexural Rigidity or Bending Stiffness   Flexural rigidity is the product of the elastic modulus and section moment of inertia of a structure in the plane of the applied bending load. Actual constructs, consisting of an implant and the bone to which it is attached, have geometries which are too complex to analyze to allow accurate calculation of this property. Instead, the bending stiffness of the construct (which is related to flexural rigidity but is not normalized for the length of the construct between its supports in bending) is measured by determining experimentally the deformations under defined loads that the implant/bone construct is likely to experience in vivo. Bending stiffness can then be calculated as the ratio of applied load to deformation measured. This parameter applies mainly to implants used to stabilize fractured bones since the magnitude of deformation at the fracture site determines the type and quality of tissues that healing produces.

Bending Strength   This parameter is the ultimate strength under bending loads, which are the most common loading conditions found in vivo in long bones, and is similar in concept to ultimate tensile or compressive loading discussed previously. The difference is that the complete construct (implant and bone to which it is attached) is usually tested in this case and the loads simulate those expected in vivo as opposed to more fundamental loads such as tension and compression.

Stress Corrosion Fatigue Failure   This type of failure is the result of the combination of fatigue due to cyclic mechanical loading and galvanic corrosion of an implant due to immersion in a bodily fluid (electrolyte). Abrasion of two components of the implant (for example a screw head on a fracture plate) causes elimination of the passivating oxide layer on the implant locally, which creates a galvanic corrosion cell between the more passivated and less passivated regions of the implant. Stress corrosion can accentuate the fatigue process and can lead to early mechanical failure of the implant.

Prosthetic Joint or Fracture Component Alignment   The alignment of the components of a joint or bone fragments in the case of a fracture after implantation and functional use are a measure of its functional load-bearing performance. Implant loosening and migration indicate loss of a mechanically strong interface, while misaligned bone fragments demonstrate impending failure of a fracture implant. Parameters such as angulation (with respect to the centerline of a long bone for example), shortening, rotation, migration, radiolucency (loss of bone around the implant) or settling can be determined by direct measurements from a radiograph.

Tissue Quality   Bone tissue may be removed and tested mechanically, histologically, and radiographically as described in the section on nonfunctional assessment techniques. In addition whole bones may be tested in bending or torsion, the two most common modes.

IMPLANTATION METHODS

Experimental Considerations

The experimental considerations for functional testing of biomaterials are similar to those discussed for nonfunctional assessments, with the major exception being that functional assessments are usually performed on optimized implants, bearing functional loads, and using fewer animals which are maintained over longer time intervals. Typically, fracture healing devices may be left in dogs for at least 6 months, while prosthetic joints may be monitored for several years in order to simulate their actual use as closely as possible. Less common animal models may be employed to more closely simulate human load-bearing functions [48–50].

Implantation Methods

Bone healing after a simulated fracture or osteotomy is used to test the performance of novel devices, which may degrade or stimulate fracture healing mechanically by micromovement or ultrasound for example. Other uses of this model include measuring the rate of bone ingrowth into defect filler materials, or determining the effects of various growth factors or other biochemical agents on healing. The objective of many of the studies cited in this chapter was the determination of the quality of the resulting bone both mechanically and histologically. Table 35-3 provides information on the typical types of constructs used for immobilization after bone osteotomy or fracture in order to determine the properties of the healing tissues.

Plate Fixation of Bone Osteotomies   Fracture plates, Figure 35-9 [51–71] find application in the fixation of long bone defects, or in spinal fusion studies. Typical sites of application include the radius, femur, tibia, and spinal vertebrae. For the case of the femur, the lateral aspect of the thigh is exposed by separation of the gluteus maximus and the

Table 35-3   Advantages and Disadvantages of Functional Implantation Methods with Immobilization

Method of immobilization	Advantages	Disadvantages
Plate Fixation	Easy operative access and placement	Fatigue failure of plate may occur if apposition of bone ends is lost (implant at mechanical disadvantage). Screw holes form large stress concentrations in bone. Disturbs periosteal vasculature.
Pin, rod fixation	Loading on implant is centralized, reduced compared with plates	Provides alignment but is least stable in torsional and bending loading. Disturbs endosteal vasculature. Poor for cortical defects in weight bearing.
External fixation	Permits fixation of various types of structural defects. Structural stability of device can be easily modified for animal size.	Pin tract infection and pin loosening are common occurrences.

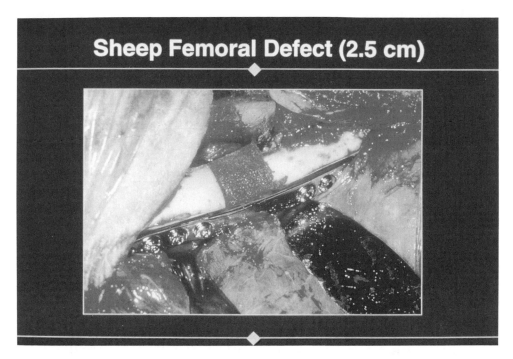

Figure 35-9 A segmental defect in a sheep tibia filled with bone morphogenic protein and fixed with a plate.

anterior fascia lata, and by splitting or elevating the lateral musculature. The periosteum may be stripped or simply nicked in the areas where screw holes are to be placed. Removal of the periosteum reduces the potential for new bone formation since it is the local source for osteogenic cells.

Depending on the objective of the experiment, fixation of the bone by a plate may be accompanied by an osteotomy to create a segmental defect in the bone, usually at its mid-diaphysis. A transverse osteotomy, creating a defect which would not heal by itself (at least 1 cm wide) reduces the confounding effect of the natural potential for bones to heal in most young adult animals. One side typically receives no treatment except for the sham surgery while the contralateral limb will receive the treatment being studied, which could be a bone graft substitute, or a material releasing a growth factor, for example. It is important to test the fracture fixation construct to be used biomechanically, especially on the side where nothing will be placed in the defect. It is well known that bone-to-bone contact across a fracture site significantly increases the stiffness and strength of the construct, so loss of cortical contact may produce unacceptably low construct strength (Figure 35-10). A plate placed on the lateral side of the bone surface without cortical contact across the osteotomy results in high bending loads on the plate. Intramedullary rods without some form of crosslocking are typically quite unstable when subjected to torsional loads. Excessive movement of the fixation can far overshadow the potential effect of the treatment under study.

A commonly accepted fixation technique involves the use of the self-compressing or dynamic compression plate [72]. This plate has been designed with oval screw holes and spherical head screws. If the screw is located at one end of the slot and is tightened, it displaces the plate away from the screw body, resulting in a compressive effect at the

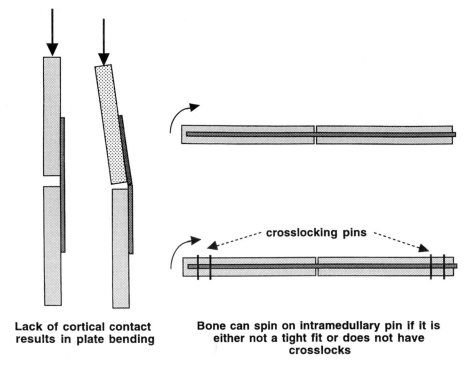

Lack of cortical contact   **Bone can spin on intramedullary pin if it is**
results in plate bending   **either not a tight fit or does not have**
                                     crosslocks

Figure 35-10 Problems with fixation using plates or IM rods in long bones: (A) lack of cortical contact creates high bending stresses in the plate; (B) an unlocked intramedullary rod is non-resistant to torsional loading.

osteotomy site which significantly increases the stability of the construct to physiological loading.

The principles of this technique have been well outlined in the fracture surgery literature [72]. Briefly, the plate is always located on the tensile side of the bone (typically the lateral side of the tibia or femur). A special drill guide, supplied with the plate, is used to locate the screw holes offset from the center of the slot in the plate, if compression is desired. The screw holes are drilled and tapped using instruments supplied and screws are used which are long enough to span both corticies. Following fixation of the plate, which maintains alignment, the gap osteotomy can be made in the bone. Care should be taken to avoid scratching the plate during this step since scratches or notches can lead to a significant decrease in fatigue life of the implant. If set up for compression, further tightening of the screws lead to closing of the osteotomy gap or compression of the material placed within the gap. Since this system has a large mechanical advantage, care should be taken not to overtighten the screws as the material plated within the gap has been known to crack from the compressive force applied, especially if it is brittle. As mentioned previously, contact relieves some of the load on the implant and increases the stiffness and strength of the construct. Longer plates with multiple holes (at least six) should be considered for heavier or more active animals, or cases in which cortical contact is not possible.

Intramedullary Fixation of Bone Osteotomies Intramedullary pin fixation [16, 58, 59, 73–79] (see Figure 35-11), is an alternative to plate fixation and is commonly used in

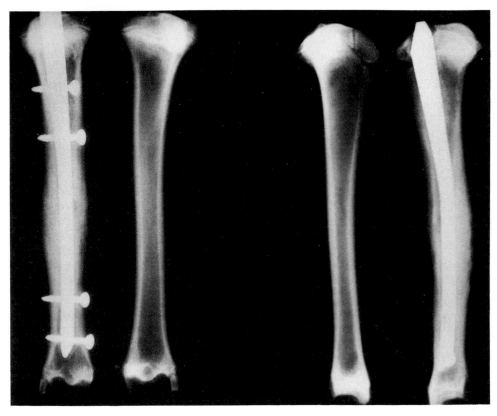

Figure 35-11   Fixation using an intramedullary rod and crosslocking pins (from Schemitsch EH, Kowalski MJ, Swionkowski MF, Harrington RM, *J Orthopedic Res*, 13:382–389, 1995.

smaller animals where plate and screw fixation would not be feasible. The pin must be a tight fit to maintain alignment of the fracture components, especially due to rotation around the long axis of the pin. The pin must be flexible enough to accommodate the curve from the entrance point into the medullary canal, since the entrance point must be placed away from the bone centerline to avoid its being located within the joint space. Determining the pin to use and the entrance location is a significant aspect which should be addressed by benchtop biomechanical study before in vivo application.

In this fixation procedure, in the femur of the rat as a typical example, a lateral approach is used so that the osteotomy can be created and the material being evaluated can be inserted. A longitudinal incision is made lateral to the fascia and the muscles around the lateral aspect of the femur retracted. An oscillating saw can be used to create a transverse osteotomy. In order to obtain a tight fit, retrograde reaming may be performed to open the isthmus or narrowest part of the femoral canal. Retrograde reaming involves reaming from the osteotomy site both proximally and distally within the canal, taking care not to violate the joints on either end. Suction should be maintained to prevent pressurization of the medullary canal ahead of the reamer and copius irrigation should be employed to prevent thermal necrosis. Alternatively, the pin may be inserted from the greater trochanter proximally in the femur or from the anterolateral aspect distally, near the knee joint. These approaches reduce the trauma around the insertion site and more closely simulate the method

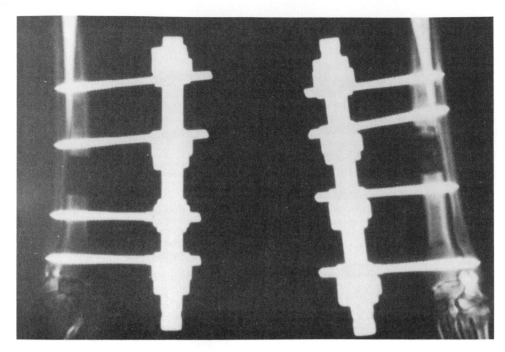

Figure 35-12   A half-pin external fixation used in a dog tibial segmental defect model.

of insertion of the fixation device in humans. Once placed, the pin may be secured with crosslocking pins (Figure 35-10).

External Fixation of Osteotomies   External fixation [80, 81] (see Figure 35-12) is a third form of immobilization which can be used for functional biomaterials evaluations. It has the advantage of the hardware being located far away from the site at which the evaluated material is located, and because it is external, it can be adjusted. However, it is restricted to use in larger bones, such as the radius, tibia, and femur of larger species. The tibia, as an example, may have external fixation pins percutaneously applied by limited stab incisions to bone on the anteromedial aspect, minimizing the trauma to the osteotomy or fracture site. The most distal pin is applied by pre-drilling a pilot hole and using a self-tapping pin. Pins are driven into and through the far cortex until they protrude a short distance through it, taking care that the pin end does not abrade muscle tissue. Partly threaded pins with just enough thread to engage the cortices provide the best combination of purchase in bone and stiffness of the construct [82]. Depending on the actual device used, the clamps and bar can be used as a drill guide to locate the rest of the holes. Pin position and number affect the rigidity of the system [82, 83]. Half-pin systems (the pin does not pass out the other side) are favored because there is less possibility of piercing the muscle belly than with full pins. However, half-pin systems are eccentrically loaded by forces acting through the bone and can have quite low rigidities, especially in torsion and in bending in a direction perpendicular to the plane of the fixator. In addition, since there is a significant possibility of necrosis or infection around a pin site if only four pins are used, half-pin systems can lead to complete loosening of the fixation.

To maximize the rigidity of the system, at least six pins should be used. The inner pins should be placed as close to the osteotomy site as possible to reduce the bending span of the external fixator bar, and the outer pins as far from each other as possible. The connecting bar should be placed as close to the bone as possible, to reduce the span of the pins. Serious consideration should be given to attaching a second half-pin frame, with one placed nearly anterior and the other anterolateral, and connected together, since this will significantly improve the torsional stiffness of the construct, especially if there is a segmental defect in the bone. Benchtop biomechanical testing comparing an intact bone in bending and torsion and after osteotomy and use of the proposed fixation can significantly reduce the potential for failure of these constructs. Also, meticulous attention should be paid to postoperative care for the pin sites because pin tract infection and subsequent loosening are common occurrences.

Soft Tissue Evaluations   Functional assessment of soft tissue biomaterials typically involves study of their performance as ligament or tendon replacements [84–90]. In a typical procedure, the biomaterial tendon replacement is inserted into a hole in the muscle, 0.5 cm proximal to the level of the origin of the actual tendon, and through a hole in the os calcis (the insertion of the tendon). Another model involves the anterior cruciate ligament [89] (see Figure 35-13), where an oblique drill hole is made through the femoral cortex at the origin of the ligament and a second oblique hole is made through the tibial cortex at the ligament insertion site, after removal of the actual ligament. The biomaterial is then located proximally with a large knot, a button, or washer and screws placed into bone. In order to maintain the correct initial tension in the ligament with the knee in a

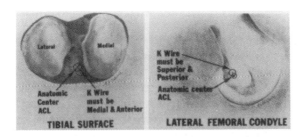

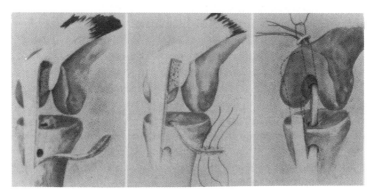

Figure 35-13   Anterior cruciate ligament assessment model (from Clancy WG, Narechania RG, Rosenberg TD, et al., *J Bone Jt Surg*, 63A: 1271, 1981).

specific position, it is fixed to the tibia only after testing for a negative anterior drawer sign (no forward displacement of the tibia with respect to the femur) but retaining full knee flexion and extension motion range. Knee mechanics are significantly affected by both the locations of attachment and tension of the anterior cruciate ligament, and these aspects should be appreciated in simulated surgery before actual implantations are performed.

The flexor profundus and flexor digitorum sublimis tendons of the chicken are reported to have anatomical features similar to those of the human finger [87], and therefore have been used as models for tendon procedures. The extensor radialis tendon of the dog has been described as a site for testing tendon biomaterials as well [88]. In one experiment, the chicken is restrained and digital nerve blocks made in the second and fourth toes. Blood is then expressed from the limb using a tourniquet and the flexor tendons are exposed through mid-lateral incisions. Both tendons may then be removed, or sectioned, depending on the objective of the experiment, and the implant fixed to the tendon ends by suturing. It should be appreciated that the weak link in the tendon apparatus after reconstruction is the suture connection between biomaterial and natural tendon, which may be too bulky to slide effectively within its sheath or may stretch, unloading the tendon. Again, adequate pretest biomechanical testing can avoid these problems.

Joint Prostheses   Evaluation of the functional biomaterials aspects of total joint replacements include studies of cement properties, bone prosthesis interface strength and ingrowth, formation of wear particles, and creep deformation in polyethylene components [91–93]. Canine hip prostheses are commercially available, or custom-designed devices may be supplied [48, 49] for these studies. Implantation of a femoral prosthesis involves a lateral approach to the hip joint [91]. The abductor muscles and their bony attachment to the greater trochanter are severed by osteotomy. The joint capsule is incised, the femoral head dislocated from the acetabulum, and the femoral neck is severed by osteotomy. Gauze sponges are packed into the acetabulum to protect it from debris and mechanical injury. The intramedullary cavity of the femur is drilled and reamed to appropriate diameter and depth, and finished with a broach having the shape of the prosthetic stem. If acrylic cement is to be used for fixation, the material is mixed and may be centrifuged to eliminate air bubbles. It is then placed into a needless syringe and the intramedullary cavity rinsed with saline and suctioned. A plug may be placed down the canal to aid in maintaining pressure during cement insertion if this technique is being used. A vent tube can be used to aid the escape of trapped blood and air as the cement is injected into the medullary cavity. With the cement in place, the vent tube is removed and the femoral stem inserted while the cement is still a viscous liquid.

Once the cement has hardened, extraneous cement and the acetabular sponges are removed and the joint reduced, unless the study involves acetabular replacement as well. In this case a hemispherical reamer is used to ream the articular cartilage and pelvic bone, gaining sufficient depth for the implant but not sacrificing excessive bone stock or penetrating the pelvis. Five mm holes may be drilled into the ilium, ischium, and pubis (to aid cement attachment to the pelvis if used) and the particular acetabular component and screwed, cemented, or press fit in place, with 45^{α} lateral and 5^{α}–10^{α} anterior orientation. The joint is then reduced. The greater trochanter and attached muscles are relocated and fixed with a lag screw and surgical wire as a figure-eight tension band, anchored also to the cortex of the femoral shaft. Following this, muscle, subcutaneous, and skin layers are closed in standard procedure. Alternatives to the dog, the most common model used, include the goose since it is a biped [48, 49].

EXPERIMENTAL CONSIDERATIONS

Defect Size

If the biomaterial is to be tested for its effect upon bone regeneration, a defect of sufficient size must be created which will not heal spontaneously. In the rat, complete regeneration of bone is reported to take place in cavities less than 5 mm in diameter [94, 95]. Key [96] observed that a defect 1 1/2 times the diameter of the shaft of a long bone with the periosteum removed will consistently produce a nonunion. Although choosing the size of a defect for implantation involves arresting spontaneous healing, consideration should also be given to the effect of the defect in creating a stress concentrator (if a cavity type defect is being used), reducing the strength of the remaining structure. As discussed previously, Burstein et al. [34] demonstrated significant losses in torsional strength of whole rabbit bones due to a hole drilled through the cortex.

Time Duration

The time duration required to observe a response depends on the particular behavior of the biomaterial to be tested. The time for complete remodeling of bone varies between species. Porous-coated implants are normally evaluated for interface ingrowth at 2–3 weeks, 4–6 weeks, and 12 weeks in dogs because the interface is relatively thin so ingrowth happens rapidly [1–4]. Implants used as defect fillers in dog long bones may be left for as long as 12 months [36] to observe long-term remodeling and degradation.

Sham Procedures

Depending on the type of implant and evaluation, either a sham procedure should be performed or a control implant implanted on the contralateral side in the same animal, if the long bones are chosen as implantation sites. The sham operation disrupts the blood supply and the periosteum, which in itself creates a healing response apart from the effect of the biomaterial. The actual effect of the biomaterial can be more easily distinguished through comparison.

Biological Variation

No matter how closely bred, different animals will produce different responses to the same biomaterial due to biological variation, differences in surgical technique, effects on blood flow, as well as other, often unidentifiable factors. It is desirable if at all possible to use a matched pair design, where implants are placed in the same manner in opposite limbs when comparing biomaterials. As discussed above, depending on the experiment, performing the same procedure on the contralateral limb but without the biomaterial or other treatment produces an effective control. In some cases, for example if the treatment has a systemic effect, this scheme cannot be used.

Using a matched pair design reduces the number of animals required because biological variability will be diminished. Large standard deviations are usually anticipated (at least 30 percent of the mean value) because of inherent biological variations, reducing the ability to detect a statistically significant difference. Practical considerations, especially in pilot studies, usually limit the number of animals to less than 20, typically 6 animals each at three time intervals, or 10 each at early and late stages post-implantation. Post-implantation fracture, infection or other complications may further reduce the numbers, to a point where it is very difficult to demonstrate a significant difference unless the effect is very large. These factors make the use of biomechanical and biological simulations of the surgery beforehand necessary to reduce unanticipated problems.

SUMMARY

Osteocompatibility assessment of biomaterials is usually performed with the objectives of stimulating bone tissue formation across a gap or defect, or creating ingrowth into a porous interface to produce a permanent mechanism of prosthetic attachment. Therefore, assessments are focused on biomechanical as well as biological properties. Nonfunctional assessments focus more on optimizing a certain feature of an implant while functional assessments are used to define the performance of an implant in its proposed setting. Biomechanical properties usually measured relate to the strength of attachment at an interface, or the strength of either a whole bone with a repaired defect or a sample of the healing tissue. Many biological assessments are concerned with the degree of calcification, which defines the load-bearing properties of the biomaterial or the tissue which it has affected in some way, since load bearing is the primary purpose of implants meant for orthopedic use.

REFERENCES

1   Bobyn JD, Pilliar RM, Cameron HU, et al. The optimum pore size for the fixation of porous-surfaced metal implants by the ingrowth of bone. *Clinic Orthop Rel Res*, 150 (1980), 263–270.
2   Cameron HU, Pilliar RM, MacNab I. The rate of bone ingrowth into porous metal. *J Biomed Mater Res*, 10 (1976), 295–302.
3   Welsh RP, Pilliar RM, MacNab I. Surgical implants: The role of surface porosity in fixation to bone and acrylic. *J Bone Joint Surg*, 53A (1971), 963–977.
4   Nilles JL, Coletti JM, Wilson C. Biomechanical evaluation of bone: Porous material interfaces. *J Biomed Mater Res*, 7 (1973), 231–251.
5   Shirazi-Adl. A finite element stress analysis of a pushout test, Part 1: Fixed interface using stress compatabile elements. *J Biomech Eng*, 114 (1992), 111–118.
6   Harrigan TP, Kareh J, Harris WH. The influence of support conditions in the loading fixture on failure mechanisms in the pushout test: A finite element study. *J Orthop Res*, 8 (1990), 678–684.
7   Butler DL, Noyes FR, Grood ES. Measurement of the mechanical properties of ligaments. In Bahnink G, Burstein AH (Eds.), *CRC Handbook of Engineering in Medicine and Biology*, Vol. 1, Section B. Boca Raton, FL: CRC Press, 1978, 297–314.
8   Aragona J, Parson JR, Alexander H, et al. Soft tissue attachment with a filamentous carbon-absorbable polymer tendon and ligament replacement. *Clin Orthop Rel Res*, 160 (1981), 268–278.
9   Holmes RE, Hagler HK, Coletta CA. Thick-section histometry of porous hydroxyapatite implants using backscattered electron imaging. *J Biomed Mat Res*, 21 (1987), 731–739.
10 Freree RH, Weibel ER. Stereologic techniques in microscopy. *J Microsc Soc*, 87 (1967), 25.
11 Underwood EE. *Stereology*. Reading, MA: Addison Wesley, 1970.
12 Chalkley HW. Method for the quantitative morphologic analysis of tissues. *J Natl Cancer Inst*, 4 (1943), 47–53.
13 Recker RR. *Bone Histomorphometry: Techniques and Interpretation*. Boca Raton, FL: CRC Press, 1983.
14 Aherne W. Quantitative methods in histology. *J Ed Lab Technol*, 27 (1970), 160–170.
15 Frost HM, Villanueva AR, Roth H, et al. Tetracycline bone labeling. *J New Drugs*, 1 (1961), 206–216.
16 Rand JA, An KN, Chao EYS, et al. A comparison of the effect of open intramedullary nailing and compression plate fixation on fracture-site blood flow and fracture union. *J Bone Joint Surg*, 63A (1978), 427–442.
17 Swionkowski MF, Tepic S, Perren SM, Moor R, Ganz R, Rahn BA. Laser Doppler flowmetry for bone blood flow measurement: Correlation with microsphere estimates and evaluation of the effect of intracapsular pressure on femoral head blood flow. *J Orthop Res*, 4 (1986), 362–371.
18 Lloyd F, Hodges D. Characterization of bone: A computer analysis of microradiographs. *Clinic Orthop Rel Res*, 78 (1971), 230–250.

19 Lloyd E, Rowland RE, Hodges D, et al. Surface-to-volume ratios of bone determined by computer analysis of microradiographs. *Nature (London)*, 218 (1968), 365–366.

20 Whitehouse WJ. The quantitative morphology of anisotropic trabecular bone. *J Microsc*, 101 (1974), 153–168.

21 Siegel S, Castellan NJ, Jr. *Nonparametric Statistics for the Behavioral Sciences*, 2nd ed. New York: McGraw Hill, 1988.

22 Edgarton BC, An K-N, Morrey BF. Torsional strength reduction due to cortical defects in bone. *J Orthop Res*, 8 (1990), 851–855.

23 Carvalho BA, Bajpai PK, Graves GA. Effect of resorbable calcium aluminate ceramics on regulation of calcium and phosphorus in rats. *Biomedicine*, 25 (1976), 130–133.

24 Vert M, Christel P, Chabot R, et al. Bioresorbable plastic materials for bone surgery. *Macromolecular Biomaterials*. Boca Raton, FL: CRC Press, 1983.

25 Brooks M, Gallennaugh SC. Circulatory changes in bone after implantation of metal. In Uhthoff UK (Ed.), *Current Concepts of Internal Fixation of Fractures*. Berlin: Springer-Verlag, 1980, 277–285.

26 Griss P, Krempien B, von Andrian-Werburg HF, et al. Experimental analysis of ceramic-tissue interactions: A morphologic, fluorescenseapptic and radiographic study on dense alumina oxide ceramic in various animals. *J Biomed Mater Res Symp*, 5 (1974), 39–48.

27 Hulber SF, Matthews JR, Klawitter JJ, et al. Effect of stress on tissue ingrowth into porous aluminum oxide. *J Biomed Mater Res Symp*, 5 (1974), 85–97.

28 McGee TD, Wood JL. Calcium-phosphate magnesium-aluminate osteoceramics. *J Biomed Mater Res Symp*, 5 (1974), 137–144.

29 Clemow ATT, Weinstein AM, Klawitter JJ, et al. Interface mechanisms of porous titanium implants. *J Biomed Mater Res*, 15 (1981), 73–82.

30 Sauer BW, Weinstein AA, Klawitter JJ, et al. The role of porous polymeric materials in prosthesis attachment. *J Biomed Mater Res Symp*, 5 (1974), 145–153.

31 Park JB, von Recum AF, Kenner GH, et al. Piezoelectric ceramic implants, a feasibility study. *J Biomed Mater Res*, 14 (1980), 269–277.

32 Gross UM, Strunz U. The anchoring of glass ceramics of different solubility in the femur of the rat. *J Biomed Mater Res*, 14 (1980), 607–618.

33 Denissen HW, deGroot K, Makkes PCN, et al. Tissue response to dense apatite implants in rats. *J Biomed Mater Res*, 14 (1980), 713–721.

34 Burstein HH, Currey J, Frankel VH, et al. Bone strength. The effect of screw holes. *J Bone Joint Surg*, 54A (1972), 1143–1156.

35 Nilles JL, Karagianes MT, Wheeler KR. Porous titanium alloy for fixation of knee prostheses. *J Biomed Mater Res Symp*, 5 (1974), 319–328.

36 Holmes RE, Mooney V, Bucholz RW, et al. A corraline hydroxyapatite bone graft substitute. *Clin Ortho Rel Res*, 188 (1984), 282–292.

37 Chiroff RT, White RA, White EW, et al. The restoration of articular surfaces overlying replamineform porous biomaterials. *J Biomed Mater Res*, 11 (1977), 165–178.

38 Chiroff RT, White EW, Weber JN, et al. Tissue ingrowth of replamineform implants. *J Biomed Mater Res Symp*, 6 (1975), 29–45.

39 Frame JW. A convenient animal model for testing bone substitute materials. *J Oral Surg*, 38 (1980), 176–180.

40 Holmes RE. Bone regeneration within a corraline hydroxyapatite implant. *Plast Reconst Surg*, 63 (1979), 626–633.

41 Freeman MJ, McCullum DE, Wolf D, et al. Reconstruction of mandibular bone with alumino-calcium-phosphorous oxide (ALCAP) ceramics. *Trans 7th Ann Meet Soc Biomater*, 4 (1981), 109.

42 Getter L, Cutright DE, Bhaskar SN, et al. A biodegradable intraosseous appliance in the treatment of mandibular fractures. *J Oral Surg*, 30 (1972), 344–348.

43 Boyne PJ. Methods of osseous reconstruction of the mandible following surgical resection. *J Biomed Mater Res Symp*, 4 (1973), 195–204.

44 Jacobs ML, Black J. Composite implants for orthopaedic applications: In vivo evaluation of candidate resins. *J Biomed Mater Res Symp*, 6 (1975), 221–225.

45 Geret V, Rahn BA, Mathys R, et al. In vivo testing of tissue tolerance of implant materials: Improved quantitative evaluation through reduction of relative motion at the implant tissue interface. In Uhthoff HK (Ed.), *Current Concepts of Internal Fixation of Fractures*. Berlin: Springer-Verlag, 1980, 160–164.

46 Brady JM, Cutright ED, Miller RA, et al. Resorption rate, route of elimination and ultra-structure of the implant site of polylactic acid in the abdominal wall of the rat. *J Biomed Mater Res*, 7 (1973), 155–166.

47 Kallus T, Eklund G. Instrumentation for preparation and placement of subcutaneous implants. *J Biomed Mater Res*, 17 (1983), 735–740.

48 von Recum AF, Wroblewski TJ, Bryant CC. Experimental coxofemoral replacement hemi-arthroplasty in the goose (Anser sp.) *Vet Surg*, 10 (1981), 101–105.

49 Wroblewski TJ, Park JB, Kenner GH, et al. Prosthetic coxofemoral joint replacement in the goose (Anser sp) II. Histologic and mechanical interface evaluations. *Vet Surg*, 10 (1981), 106–112.

50 Daum WJ, Chang SL, Simmons DJ, et al. Healing of canine femoral osteotomies. Effects of compression plates versus Eggers' plates. *Clin Orthop Rel Res*, 180 (1983), 291–300.

51 Woo SLY, Akeson WH, Coutts RD, et al. A comparison of cortical bone atrophy secondary to fixation with plates with large differences in bending stiffness. *J Bone Joint Surg*, 58A (1976), 190–195.

52 Uhthoff HK, Bardos DI, Liskova-Kiar M. The advantages of titanium alloy over stainless steel plates for the internal fixation of fractures. *J Bone Joint Surg*, 63B (1981), 427–434.

53 Stromberg NEL. Diaphyseal bone in rigid internal plate fixation. *Acta Chir Scand Suppl*,. 456 (1975), 1–34.

54 Uhthoff HK, Dubuc FL. Bone structure changes in the dog under rigid internal fixation. *Clin Orthop Rel Res*, 81 (1971), 165–170.

55 Slatis P, Karaharju E, Holmstran T, et al. Structural changes in intact tubular bone after application of rigid plates with and without compression. *J Bone Joint Surg*, 60A (1978), 516–522.

56 Olerud S, Danckwardt-Lilliestrom G. Fracture healing in compression osteosynthesis in the dog. *J Bone Joint Surg*, 50B (1968), 844–851.

57 Graves GA, Hentrich RL, Stein HG, et al. Resorbable ceramic implants. *J Biomed Mater Res Symp*, 2 (1971), 91–115.

58 Anderson LD. Compression plate fixation and the effect of different types of internal fixation on fracture healing. *J Bone Joint Surg*, 47A (1965), 191–208.

59 Rand JA, An KN, Chao EYS, et al. A comparison of the effect of open intramedullary nailing and compression-plate fixation on fracture-site blood flow and fracture union. *J Bone Joint Surg*, 63A (1981), 427–442.

60 Hutzchenreuter P, Mathys R, Walk H, et al. Polyacetal plates with a metal core. In Uhthoff HK, (Ed.), *Current Concepts of Internal Fixation of Fractures*. Berlin: Springer-Verlag, 1980, 149–155.

61 Hutzchenreuter P, Walk H, Brummer H, et al. Strength of cortical bone following experimental osteotomy with plaster cast or internal plate fixation. In Uhthoff HK (Ed.), *Current Concepts of Internal Fixation of Fractures*. Berlin: Springer-Verlag, 1980, 292–297.

62 Burns H, Artmann M, Grobpeter K. Load-stable osteosynthesis in animal tests under limited preloading. In Uhthoff HK (Ed.), *Current Concepts of Internal Fixation of Fractures*. Berlin: Springer-Verlag, 1980, 298–305.

63 Schatzker J, Manlev PA, Sumner-Smith G. In vivo strain gauge study of bone response to loading with and without internal fixation. In Uhthoff HK (Ed.), *Current Concepts of Internal Fixation of Fractures*. Berlin: Springer-Verlag, 1980, 306–314.

64 Brown SA, Merritt K, Mayor MB. Internal fixation with metal plates and thermoplastic plates. In Uhthoff HK (Ed.), *Current Concepts of Internal Fixation of Fractures*. Berlin: Springer-Verlag, 1980, 306–314.

65 Tonino AJ, Klopper PJ. The use of plastic plates in the treatment of fractures. In Uhthoff HK (Ed.), *Current Concepts of Internal Fixation of Fractures*. Berlin: Springer-Verlag, 1980, 342–347.

66 Zenker H, Bruns H, Hepp W, et al. Long-term results of animal investigations with elastic fixation plates for osteosynthesis. In Uhthoff HK (Ed.), *Current Concepts of Internal Fixation of Fractures*. Berlin: Springer-Verlag, 1980, 363–374.

67 Phillips T. The non-rigid fixation plate. In Uhthoff HK (Ed.), *Current Concepts of Internal Fixation of Fractures*. Berlin: Springer-Verlag, 1980, 375–378.

68 Comtet JJ, Moyen BJL, Meyrueis JP, et al. Plate of variable flexibility: Mechanical and biologic study on intact femora of dogs. In Uhthoff HK (Ed.), *Current Concepts of Internal Fixation of Fractures*. Berlin: Springer-Verlag, 1980, 379–387.

69 Nunamaker DM, Perren S. Pure titanium plates in sheep: The effect of rigidity and compression. In Uhthoff HK (Ed.), *Current Concepts of Internal Fixation of Fractures*. Berlin: Springer-Verlag, 1980, 389–397.

70 Liskova-Kiar M, Uhthoff HK. Radiologic and histologic determination of the optimal time for the removal of titanium alloy plates in beagle dogs—Results of early removal. In Uhthoff HK (Ed.), *Current Concepts of Internal Fixation of Fractures*. Berlin: Springer-Verlag, 1980, 404–410.

71 Muller ME, Allgower M, Willenegger H. *Technique of Internal Fixation of Fractures*. Berlin: Springer-Verlag, 1965.

72 Muller ME, Allgower M, Willenegger H. *Manual of Internal Fixation*. Berlin: Springer-Verlag, 1970.

73 Danckwardt-Lilliestrom G. Reaming of the medullary cavity and its effect on diaphyseal bone: A fluorchromic, microangiographic, and histologic study on the rabbit tibia and dog femur. *Acta Orthop Scand Suppl*, 1969, 128.

74 Danckwardt-Lilliestrom G, Lorenzi L, Loerud S. Intramedullary nailing after reaming: An investigation on the healing process in osteotomized rabbits. *Acta Orthop Scand Suppl*, 1970, 134.

75 Gothman L. The arterial pattern of the rabbit's tibia after application of an intramedullary nail. *ACTA Chir Scand*, 120 (1960), 211–219.

76 Trueta J, Cavadias AX. Vascular changes caused by the Kuntscher type of nailing. An experimental study in the rabbit. *J Bone Joint Surg*, 37B (1955), 492-505.

77 Waelchi-Suter C. Vascular changes in cortical bone following intramedullary fixation. In Uhthoff HK (Ed.), *Current Concepts of Internal Fixation of Fractures*. Berlin: Springer-Verlag, 1980, 411–415.

78 Klopper PJ, Tonino AJ. Internal fixation of femur fractures with plastic rods—An experimental study. In Uhthoff HK (Ed.), *Current Concepts of Internal Fixation of Fractures*. Berlin: Springer-Verlag, 1980, 416–422.

79 Brown SA, Mayor MB. Intramedullary nailing with metals and plastics. In Uhthoff HK (Ed.), *Current Concepts of Internal Fixation of Fractures*. Berlin: Springer-Verlag, 1980, 423–428.

80 Wu JJ, Shyr HS, Chao EYS, et al. Comparison of osteotomy healing under external fixation devices with different stiffness characteristics. *J Bone Joint Surg*, 661 (1984), 1258–1264.

81 Panjabi MM, White AA, Wolf JA, Jr. A biomechanical comparison of flexible and rigid fracture fixation. In Uhthoff HK (Ed.), *Current Concepts of Internal Fixation of Fractures*. Berlin: Springer-Verlag, 1980, 324–333.

82 Tencer AF, Claudi B, Pearce S, et al. Development of a variable stiffness external fixation system for stabilization of segmental defects of the tibia. *J Orthop Res*, 1, 395–404.

83 Briggs BT, Chao EYS. The mechanical performance of the standard Hoffman-Vidal external fixation apparatus. *J Bone Joint Surg*, 64A (1982), 566–573.

84 Forster IW, Ralis ZA, McKibbin B, et al. Biological reaction to carbon fiber implants: The formation and structure of a carbon-induced neotendon. *Clin Orthop Rel Res*, 131 (1977), 299–307.

85 Jenkins DHR, Forester IW, McKibbin B, et al. Induction of tendon and ligament formation by carbon implantation. *J Bone Joint Surg*, 59B (1978), 53–57.

86 Jenkins DHR. The repair of cruciate ligaments with flexible carbon fiber. *J Bone Joint Surg*, 60B (1978), 520–522.

87 Salisbury RE, Mason AD, Levine NS, et al. Artificial tendons: Design, application, and results. *J Trauma*, 14 (1974), 580–586.

88 Bader KF, Curtin JW. A successful silicone tendon prosthesis. *Arch Surg*, 97 (1968), 406–411.

89 Claney WG, Jr., Narechania RG, Rosenberg TD, et al. Anterior and posterior cruciate ligament reconstruction in Rhesus monkeys. *J Bone Joint Surg*, 63A (1981), 1270–1284.

90 Salisbury RE, McKell D, Pruitt BAJ, et al. Morphologic observations of neosheath development of undifferentiated connective tissue development around artificial tendons. *J Biomed Mater Res Symp*, 5 (1974), 175–184.

91 Barb W, Park JB, Kenner GH, et al. Intramedullary fixation of artificial hip joints with bone-cement-precoated implants: Interfacial strengths. *J Biomed Mater Res*, 16 (1982), 447–458.

92 Walker PS, Mendes DG, Figarola F, et al. Total surface replacement of the hip joint. *J Biomed Mater Res Symp*, 5 (1974), 245–260.

93 Esslenger JO, Rutkowski EJ. Studies on the skeletal attachment of experimental hip prostheses in the pygmy goat and dog. *J Biomed Mater Res Symp*, 4 (1973), 187–193.

94 Melcher AH, Irving JT. The healing mechanism of artificially created circumscribed defects in the femoral of albino rats. *J Bone Joint Surg*, 44B (1962), 928–936.

95 Pallasch TJ. The healing pattern of an experimentally induced defect in the rat femur studied with tetracycline labeling. *Calcif Tiss Res*, 2 (1968), 334–342.

96 Key JA. The effect of a local calcium depot on osteogenesis and healing of fractures. *J Bone Joint Surg*, 16 (1934), 176–184.

ADDITIONAL READING

1 American Dental Association. Recommended standard practices for biological evaluation of dental materials. *J Am Dent Assoc*, 99 (1979), 697–698.

2 Bahnink G, Burstein AH (Eds.). *Handbook of Engineering in Medicine and Biology*. Boca Raton, FL: CRC Press, 1978.

3 *Methods of Biological Assessment of Dental Materials*, BS 5828. London: British Standards Institution, 1980.

4 Federation Dentaire Internationale. Recommended standard practices for biological evaluation of dental materials. *Int Dent J*, 30 (1980), 140–188.

5 Geret V, Rahn BA, Mathys R, et al. A method for testing tissue tolerance for improved quantitative evaluation

through reduction of relative motion at the implant-tissue interface. In Winter GD, Leray JL, deGroot K (Eds.), *Evaluation of Biomaterials*. London: Wiley, 1980.

6   Hobkirk JA. Standardization of intraosseous implantation testing in small laboratory animals. In Winter GP, Leray JL, deGroot K, (Eds.), *Evaluation of Biomaterials*. London: Wiley, 1980.

7   Kerker AE, Murphy HT. *Comparative and Veterinary Medicine, A Guide to the Resource Literature*. Madison, WI: University of Wisconsin Press, 1973.

8   Marion L, Haugen E, Major IAJ. Methodological assessment of subcutaneous implantation techniques. *J Biomed Mater Res*, 14 (1980), 343–357.

9   Mitruka BM, Rawnsley HM, Vadehra DV. *Animals for Medical Research, Models for the Study of Human Disease*. New York: Wiley, 1976.

10 Müller ME, Allgower M, Willenger H. *Manual of Internal Fixation*. Berlin: Springer-Verlag, 1970.

11 Piermattei DL, Greeley RG. *An Atlas of Surgical Approaches to the Bones of the Dog and Cat*, 2nd ed. Philadelphia, PA: W. B. Saunders, 1966, 198.

12 *The UFAW Handbook on the Care and Management of Laboratory Animals*, 5th ed. London: Churchill Livingstone, 1976.

13 Williams, D (Ed.). *Biocompatibility of Implant Materials*. London: Sector Publishing, 1976.

Chapter 36

Odontocompatibility

Joseph R. Natiella

INTRODUCTION

Since 1970 there has been a proliferation in the use of dental implants and implantable materials designed to augment diseased atrophic or deficient jaw bone. Presently, there are over 30 companies that manufacture and distribute dental implants [1]. There is a considerable variation in implant designs and materials and a wide range of indications for use of implants and jaw-augmenting materials. Consequently, biomaterials evaluation has become an integral part of the daily practice of dentistry. The practitioner must choose a device or material that meets complex biocompatibility requirements and which is associated with a reasonable benefit/risk ratio. The responsibility for determining safety and efficacy does not end in the pre-market phase of development but continues through assessment of short- and long-term clinical success or failure. The criteria for this determination are continuing to be defined. The dentist may function as both surgeon and prosthodontist in implant cases. To do so requires an understanding of many aspects of host response and important properties of the different biomaterials used in this field.

This chapter is written to provide some pertinent discussion on the regulations affecting dental implants, an update on usage testing in biocompatibility studies, and practical applied clinical assessments of implant function. The references given reflect several elements of the present state of the art of dental implantology.

REGULATORY & ADVISORY AGENCIES

The dentist is guided in many aspects of dental implantology by two primary agencies, the American Dental Association (ADA) and the Food and Drug Administration (FDA). Since 1972, the American Dental Association provides updated status reports assessing the application of implants to general dental treatment [2]. An important joint symposium co-sponsored by the ADA Council on Dental Materials and Devices and the National Institute of Dental Research (NIDR) was held in 1973. The status of several implant systems was examined from several perspectives which included important initial discussions on criteria for success of implant devices. A provisional acceptance program for dental implants was established by the ADA in 1980 and 1981 [3, 4]. However, as late as 1986 only one implant type was provisionally accepted by the Council and the updated Council report continued to emphasize the need for longitudinal clinical studies and basic science and applied research investigation [5]. In 1987 two ADA categories were created for dental implants fully and provisionally acceptable. Five years of clinical study were required for full acceptance, three years for provisional. Specifics are vague relative to the documentation required and study criteria necessary. In June 1988 the NIDR sponsored a second Consensus Conference on Dental Implants. The effect of current regulation and pending regulatory changes on approval of dental implants was reflected in the panel recommendations.

Dental implants were included into regulatory classification by the FDA when the Medical Devices Amendments to the Food, Drug and Cosmetic Act were implemented in 1976. Final classification of dental implants appeared in the Federal Register in 1987 [6]. Currently, the Code of Federal Regulations defines an endosseous implant as a device made of a material such as titanium intended to be surgically placed in the bone of the upper or lower jaw arches to provide support for prosthetic devices such as artificial teeth and to restore the patient's chewing function. Endosseous implants are classified as Class III devices. Devices placed in this class are subjected to rigorous standards and there is a requirement for pre-market approval. This approval includes verification of the safety and effectiveness of the product before distribution. The focal points of the pre-market approval process are summarized by Eckert [1]. These concern safety and effectiveness and technical studies. A partial listing of the pertinent information required includes intended use of the device, types of indications (edentulous, partially edentulous), prosthodontic applications, medical and dental contraindications, description of osseous and soft tissue repair, design features that make the device unique, chemical constituents of implant and coatings, long-term evaluation of toxic effects, potential for carcinogenicity, alternative clinical procedures, foreign market development, mechanical laboratory studies, animal studies, human clinical investigations and design characteristics. Animal studies require "an appropriate animal model." The FDA does not specify a specific animal test system. Specific requirements are inclusive of a 1 year study period with observations at 1, 2, 3, 6 and 12 months, undecalcified and decalcified section bone histomorphometry. Also required are the histologic assessment of bone response, vascularity, gingival attachment, inflammation, foreign body reactions and bone-implant interface; implant mobility; gingival health; standard biocompatibility studies; and radiographic assessment. Controlled, human clinical trials involve two independent centers with 50 patients each. The study period is for three years of implant function under load. Assessment of patients within the studies must include gingival health, radiographic evaluation and implant mobility.

In 1988 the "Guidance for Arrangement and Content of a Pre-market approval (PMA) Application for Endosseous Implants" was developed and published and in 1989 the FDA proposed a rule that required a modified PMA based on the 1988 guidance [7]. Presently, although endosseous implants are classified as Class III medical devices, they may be approved for use and marketed under a 510(k) pre-market notification. Section 510(k) of the Federal Food, Drug and Cosmetic Act allows determination of equivalence to marked predicate devices [8]. The summary submitted must contain comprehensive information relative to safety and effectiveness of the preamendment device. It is interesting to note that the Code of Federal Regulation classifies subperiosteal implants as Class II.

The dentist who uses a particular dental implant must understand that the comprehensive testing requirements in a pre-market approval of a Class III device are designed to insure safety and efficacy. Since current implants have achieved market status on the basis of "equivalent materials properties and host response," it is important to request documentation of the acceptable biocompatibility status of the device. It may be advisable to determine to what extent testing as specified in pre-market approval application guidelines has been done.

Dental implants are evaluated in the Dental Devices Branch within the FDA. There are six centers in the FDA. The Center for Devices and Radiological Health (CDRH) has eight offices. The Office of Device Evaluation (ODE) is responsible for evaluation of the safety and effectiveness of dental devices. The ODE has five divisions. The Dental Devices branch is a part of the Division of General and Restorative Devices [9]. Presently, there is no

Table 36-1   Recommended Biocompatibility Tests for Dental Materials

Initial tests	Secondary tests	Samples of usage tests—preclinical
1. Cytotoxicity*	9. Mucous membrane irritation test (hamster's pouch)*	14. Irritation of pulp
2. Hemolysis*		15. Pulp capping (includes pulpotomy)
3. Ames'*	10. Dermal toxicity from repeated exposures	16. Endodontic usage test
4. Styles' cell transformation	11. Subcutaneous implantation in guinea pigs)	17. Dental implant*
5. Dominant lethal	12. Implantation in bone of guinea pigs*	
6. Oral LD_{50} (acute systemic toxicity test by the oral route)* *	13. Sensitization (guinea pigs)	
7. IP-LD_{50} (acute systemic test by the IP route)*		
8. Acute inhalation test		

*Suggested for implant materials.
Source: Seventeen tests recommended by the ADA Document No. 41.
Addendum to American National Standards Institute American Dental Association Document No. 41 for Recommended Standard Practices for Biological Evaluation of Dental Materials.

requirement that the ADA must approve a product prior to marketing. However, the ADA has significant representation on the FDA American National Standards Committee MD 156 for Dental Materials. This committee organizes subcommittees that write and approve ANSI standards. In 1979 the ADA published ANSI/ADA document No. 41 for Recommended Standard Practices for Biological Evaluation of Dental Materials [10]. Specific tests for dental implants were included in this document. Eleven of the recommended 17 tests are shown in Table 36-1. To some degree, these mirror biomaterials testing formats requested in PMA documentation.

DENTAL IMPLANTS: MATERIALS AND DESIGN

There are three types of dental implants: endosseous, subperiosteal and transosseous. The endosseous implant is placed into bone in a vertical plane and consists of a variety of root forms and plates or blades. Root form implants may be smooth, threaded, textured, hollow, solid or include perforations [11]. Subperiosteal implants consist of custom cast-metal frames which rest on cortical bone beneath the fibrous periosteum. Transosteal implants combine a subperiosteal plate and an endosteal component. All dental implants have a transmucosal segment termed the abutment which may be fixed to the implant (or fixture) by screws or cement.

Materials commonly used in dental implants include commercially pure titanium, titanium alloy (Ti6Al4V) chrome cobalt molybdenum (subperiosteal implants) and ceramics. Ceramics are used as coatings for both endosseous and subperiosteal implants in the form of hydroxylapatite (HA). There are also root forms of Al_2O_3 (single crystal α alumina and sapphire). Some implant surfaces are plasma flame-sprayed with titanium powder.

The variation in implant design reflects a lack of agreement in the optimum implant shape and material. The range of design was shown by Wennerberg and associates who studied 13 commercially available dental implants by measuring surface topography and found considerable variation [12]. Some implant manufacturers claim enhanced host response and long-term function on the basis of the implant design, the base material or coating, and the accessories for prosthodontic restoration. Certain materials such as titanium and titanium alloy are favored because they form a surface coating of titanium dioxide in the form of a stable ceramic-like surface which minimizes biodegradation [13]. Again, it is recommended that the user of a particular implant understand the data that exists to support the specific claims of a manufacturer.

BIOCOMPATIBILITY/ODONTOCOMPATIBILITY EVALUATION OF THE HOST/IMPLANT RELATIONSHIP

The biocompatibility of dental implants can be considered a condition of successful function as a tooth replacement without adverse long-term effects on the host. The vast majority of testing dental implants involves usage tests in multiple species of animals and clinical evaluation of longitudinal human studies which are analyzed for "success" or implant survival over time. Detailed basic biocompatibility studies are not routinely continued since the necessary tests to determine safety and efficacy have been done during development of the biomaterial used.

Dental implant materials tested and used in designs and uses comparable to present prototypes appear to be safe when assessed on the basis of toxicity and carcinogenicity. An International Workshop on the Biocompatibility, Toxicity and Hypersensitivity to Alloy Systems Used in Dentistry was convened in 1985 [14]. A review of dental implant systems, especially concerning the safety of dental implants, was a part of this workshop. There have been reports that document soft tissue hypersensitivity to dental alloys and prosthetic appliances. The reactions have included stomatitis and lichenoid eruption possibly associated with wear phenomena, corrosion, and host/ion complexes formed at the interface [15, 16]. Only exceedingly rare reports of malignancy developing at sites of a dental implant may be found. To date, little evidence exists to suggest that the long-term exposure of dental implants to the oral environment will cause the formation of carcinogenic substances or locally or distant toxic effects. There appears to be no consensus protocol for long-term evaluation of ion release from currently used implant systems. There are examples of techniques that study this potentially critical phenomenon. Schliephake and associates used scanning electron microscopy, energy dispersive X-ray analysis, and backscattered electron imaging to determine ionic release from titanium dental implants in pigs [17]. While titanium particles initially found in the bone interface disappeared after five months, the lungs, liver and kidneys contained values with significant differences over the control group. The use of human and animal primary cultures exposed to particulate matter from implants may be used to screen for toxicity and neoplastic potential [18, 19]. Ionic release in muscle sites may be monitored by electrothermal atomic adsorption spectrometry and neutron activation analysis [20]. Tests developed for orthopedic implants that monitor long-term ion release can be applied to dental implant investigations [21–24]. Continued evolvement of tests to monitor the significance of these findings are warranted and leading investigators in the field have indicated the importance for continued long-term basic compatibility tests to monitor such long-term effects. Black has advocated large-scale epidemiologic studies of dental implant recipients [25]. Others have suggested that additional, continuous, long-term tests be done. These are designed to elucidate any neoplastic potential of implants, comprehensively define host/implant environments and determine the rate of ion release and the mode of host chemical binding of implant substances [26–29].

USAGE TESTING

Table 36-1 provides a listing of recent usage tests which primarily study tissue response to endosseous implants [30–51]. Studies of titanium, titanium alloy and titanium-coated implants predominate. Various recommended test methodologies can be found in these studies. Host response characterization includes clinical assessment of survival tissue, analysis of critical areas of the implant crypt and peri-implant tissues, and mechanical testing.

The Peri-Implant Soft Tissue Zone

Study of the permucosal soft tissue zone around dental implants has included varied microscopic techniques. These include detailed ultrastructural characterization [52, 53]. The pioneer work of McKinney and associates characterized regenerating peri-implant epithelial components which produced a sulcular area reminiscent of the zone around natural teeth [54, 55, 56]. The identification of certain epithelial cell organelles which included basal lamina hemi-desmosomes and desmosomes fostered the concept that an attachment apparatus similar in structure to that associated with natural teeth is possible around biocompatible dental implants (see also Chapter 45). However, definition of an epithelial attachment has not yet been realized. Recent studies suggest that potential epithelial attachment and maintenance of an underlying connective tissue that would support a non-migrating and sufficiently keratinized "sulcular" epithelium may in part depend on the surface condition of the implant neck. For example, Lin and associates examined gingival attachment properties of endosseous implants with varied levels of hydroxyapatite coatings [41]. There is continued discovery of new structures within this important part of the implant. Extensive transmission and scanning electron microscopic analysis of the peri-implant mucosa done by Schupback and co-workers showed a supracrestal connective tissue component that possessed an interlacing network of collagen [46]. This was supported by fibrous tissue and delicate endothelial-lined structures with an associated junctional epithelium. An "unidentified material" was seen in a narrow zone between the termination of functionally oriented collagen fibrils and the implant surface. Despite long years of study of the permucosal segment of the implant, there is still no general agreement on the optimum "collar area" of the implant body. A surface that does not colonize plaque, allows an abating tissue relationship that resembles attachment, and is easily maintained with preventative dental methods would be optimum.

Additional correlations between peri-implant soft tissue and the periodontium can be made through animal studies that examine the peri-implant microflora and the biophysiology of this tissue. These investigations have indicated that the counts of microflora around endosseous implants mirror those around teeth in both health and disease [40]. A superb example of a comprehensive animal study that studied ligature-induced peri-implantitis was done by Lang and associates [38]. These techniques mirrored those used in human clinical studies and assessment of peri-implant tissue included determination of plaque index (PI), gingival index (GI), probing depth (PD) and standardized radiographs.

Peri-Implant Bone

Bone repair and remodeling against the endosseous implant surface has been described for most every type of implant used. Emphasis is on the "osseointegration" of the implant interface which was postulated by the work of Branemark as "a direct structural and functional connection between ordered, living bone and the surface of a load-carrying implant" [57].

Table 36-2   Animal Studies

Author	Year	Implant	Model	Tests
Becker et al. [30]	1991	Endos-guided tissue regen	Dogs	Histology
Carr et al. [31]	1995	Endos	Baboons	Torque failure
Caudill & Meffert [32]	1991	Endos-guided tissue regen	Dogs	Histology
Cook et al. [33]	1993	Endos, HA-coated	Dogs	Mechanic histology
Ericsson et al. [34]	1994	Endos, titanium	Dogs	Histo-morphometry
Hurzeler et al. [35]	1995	Guided tissue regen & bone graft material	Dogs	Histology
Hurzeler et al. [36]	1995	Endos	Dogs	Clinic radiol, histology
Kardo et al. [37]	1995	Endos, HA-coated	Monkey	Histology
Lang et al. [38]	1993	Endos	Monkey	Clinical & radiographic
Lekholm et al. [39]	1993	Endos, guided tissue regeneration	Dogs	Histology
Leonhardt et al. [40]	1992	Endos	Dogs	Clinic & microbiol
Lin et al. [41]	1992	Endos, HA-coated	Dogs	Histology
Parr et al. [42]	1992	Endos, root forms, blades	Dogs	Clinical & radiographic
Parr et al. [43]	1992	Endos, ceramic	Dogs	Clinical
Parr et al. [44]	1993	Endos, titanium	Dogs	Histo-morphometry
Ptolzke et al. [45]	1993	Polymeric composite particles	Dogs	Histo-morphometry
Schliephake et al. [17]	1993	Endos, titanium	Pigs	SEM, back scattered electron imaging, atomic absorption spectroscopy
Schupback et al. [46]	1994	Endos & guided tissue regen	Dogs	SEM, TEM, histology
Sennerby et al. [47]	1993	Endos, titanium	Pigs	Histology
Steflik et al. [48]	1992	Endos, titanium	Dogs	TEM
Warren et al. [49]	1993	Endos, titanium	Monkeys	Histology
Weinlander et al. [50]	1992	Endos, titanium	Dogs	Histo-morphometry
Yan et al. [51]	1994	Endos, titanium	Dogs	Histology

The hunt continues to the present day for the implant of optimum shape, material, porosity, length, width and load-bearing characteristics that will accomplish "osseointegration." Incredibly, it is only recently that animal studies have been used to qualitate and quantitate this fibrous tissue and bone component described around many implants. Advancements in the knowledge of the properties of the implant bone crypt have resulted from recent animal studies. Table 36-2 shows several studies that include morphometric analysis of bone responses often expressed in hard tissue/soft tissue ratios (bone/marrow ratios). These baseline data allow extension to other test protocols which involve determining the relationship of force on maintenance of tissue ratios and to the surface topography of the implant [44]. The integrity of osseous components around implants have also been measured by torque-failure tests. Carr et al. used the baboon to evaluate the anchorage properties of endosseous screws composed of titanium, titanium alloy and HA-coated surfaces [31]. Four months after placement the implants were torqued to failure with an electronic torque driver. Push-out tests done on dental implants correlate with other general biocompatibility tests. The canine-femur model has been used to evaluate effect of surface roughness on shear strength [33]. Transcortical push-out tests on HA-coated implants have indicated the critical points of failure. The sites of failure were also learned which often occur in the coating substrate, not the bone/coating interface [58]. Marani used histomorphic backscattered electron microscopy to compare HA-coated and uncoated implants [59]. This technique gave an accurate assessment of depth of bone penetration. Most usage tests of bone response focus on light microscopic tissue morphology, but the transmission electron microscope is important in refining the understanding of the bone/implant interface. Steflik and co-investigators described a dynamic interface of mineralized bone at the interface of titanium cylinders in dogs [48]. Of particular interest was the 100 nm zone of mineralized collagen at the implant surface associated with a 20–50 nm electron dense zone. Histologic analysis is important in usage tests that compare and contrast modifications in implant design. Morphometry (see Chapter 47) can provide a technique for identifying differences in the volume of osseous tissue when implant superstructures are designed with stress-absorbing material [37]. For example, in the work of Ericsson et al., histomorphometry was used to compare titanium implants with standard machined surfaces with a TiO_2-blasted surface [34]. Ground, undecalcified sections illustrated the highest bone-to-metal ratio in the machine-prepared specimens. Similar studies have been done to demonstrate the significantly enhanced rates of osteogenesis and osseointegration at implant surfaces exposed to bovine bone morphogenic protein and bovine serum albumin [48, 51].

CLINICAL ASSESSMENTS OF DENTAL IMPLANTS

Clinical Studies

The biocompatibility assessment of dental implants ultimately depends on the performance of the device in function. It is important that clinical evaluation includes many of the tests that are found in animal usage studies. There is an apparent trend to construct clinical tests that replace the requirement for animal experiments.

The reader is referred to Table 36-3 that lists recent longitudinal clinical studies, many of which extend through a 5-year period and contain acceptable methods for implant/case evaluation [60–79]. Generally, these reflect a high "success rate" for many of the currently used endosseous implants. Fewer reports can be found regarding subperiosteal implants. There are still lively discussions in the field regarding the definition of "success." One list of criteria proposed in 1986 has been adopted by some large dental specialty groups [71, 80]. The parameters include (1) implant tested separately is clinically immobile; (2) no radiolucent peri-implant zone appears on a retroalveolar radiograph; (3) the average vertical bone loss is 1.0 mm during the first year and less than 0.2 mm actually after the first functioning year of the implant; (4) no persistent or irreversible sign or symptom of pain, infection, necrosis, paresthesia or piercing of the mandibular dental canal is caused by the implant; (5) the relative location of the implant does not rule out the fitting of a crown or

Table 36-3   Clinical Studies

Author	Year	Implant	Number	Duration	Success Rate
Arvidson et al. [60]	1992	Endos, titanium (Astra)	310	3	98%
Babbush & Kirch [61]	1991	Endos, titanium IM2	561 802	3 4	97% 98%
Babbush & Shimura [62]	1993	Endos, titanium IM2	1059	5	95%
Fugazzotto et al. [63]	1993	Endos, titanium	513	5	96%
Hahn [64]	1991	Endos, titanium (Steri Oss)	470	3.5	96%
Jemi & Patterson [65]	1993	Endos, titanium Branemark	430	1	84%
Jemi, et al. [66]	1992	Endos, titanium Branemark	430	1	84%
Lill et al. [67]	1993	Endos, titanium Branemark & IM2	683	—	—
Naert et al. [68]	1992	Endos, titanium Branemark	589	7	95%
Quirynen et al. [69]	1992	Endos, titanium Branemark	589	6	92%
Rominger & Triplett [70]	1994	Endos, guided tissue regen	61	—	97%
Saadown & LeGall [71]	1992	Endos, Steri Oss	673	5	92%
Salonen et al. [72]		Endos, TPS, ITI	204	1–60 mo.	—
Small I [73]		Mandibular staple, bone plate	102	6	100%
Stvrtecky et al. [74]	1993	Subperiosteal	115	5–10	58%
Spickerman et al. [75]	1995	Endos, IMZ & TPS	300	5.7 yrs.	90%
Takarada & Kinebruchi [76]	1993	Endos, titanium with HA spray	227	4	99%
van Steenberghe et al. [77]		Endos,	160	3	94%
Wedgewood et al. [78]	1992	Endos, ITI, titanium	451	3	94%
Yanese et al. [79]	1994	Subperiosteal		10	53%

prosthesis; (6) there is a minimum success rate of 85 percent at the end of the fifth year of observation and 80 percent at the end of the tenth year.

Somewhat similar criteria for success are utilized by five dental implant centers in the United Kingdom [81]: (1) satisfactory healing of the implant site and stabilization of the implant with no mobility; (2) absent or minimal gingival inflammation with a gingival crevice not more than 4 mm deep; (3) radiographic and clinical ankylosis with no signs of vertical bone loss after 6 months other than saucerization of the crest of the alveolus around the implant neck; (4) satisfactory function, appearance, and comfort of the prosthesis.

Percentages of successful implants are calculated by different methods. Many studies may use basic input-output methods. It is now recommended that survival analysis be derived from time-life methods with random accrual methods and random censoring. Weyant and Burt designed exemplary statistical methods for a large multicenter study in the Veterans Administration Hospital System [82]. Lill and associates, also reporting on a large study, discuss the discrepancy between input-output statistics and life table analysis [83]. Mow supports the recommendations for time-life approaches to statistical analysis of implant cases. It is proposed that time-life methods would adjust failure percentages for mean time of follow-up and would alter the high percentages of success reported in some studies [84].

Clinical Assessment of Peri-Implant Zone

Since the peri-implant sulcus health is critical for long-term survival, it is recommended that the evaluation of this site include several tests which are standard in the evaluation of periodontal health in the natural dentition [85]:

1   Suppuration Index: expressed as the presence or absence of an exudate produced by gentle finger pressure.
2   Plaque Index: modification of the method of Sibness and Loe may be used:

Score	Criteria
0	No plaque
1	A film of plaque adhering to the post and free peri-implant tissue; this may be identified only after application of disclosing solution or use of a probe
2	Moderate accumulation of soft deposits within the peri-implant soft tissue or on the post visible with the naked eye
3	Abundant deposits within the peri-implant soft tissue or on the post of the implant

Each of the 4 surfaces of the post (buccal, lingual, mesial, distal) are scored from 0 to 3. The scores from the 4 areas are divided by 4, giving the plaque index.

3   Probe Depth Measurement: measured to nearest mm using a PGF-GFS periodontal probe inserted with moderate pressure into the peri-implant sulcus.
4   Bleeding Index (sulcus bleeding index or SBI): following probing, 0 = none, 1 = moderate, 2 = severe.
5   Calculus Index: gentle stream of air and probing with fine-pointed probe or ball-end probe, 0 = none, 1 = minimal, 2 = moderate, 3 = abundant.

6 Gingival Margin Index (GMI): probe passed around upper portion of implant sulcus. 0 = no redness, no bleeding; 1 = marginal inflammation, no bleeding; 2 = bleeding after probing; 3 = spontaneous bleeding from the crevice, visible inflammation.

7 Mobility: assessment of movement when tapped between two instrument handles.

Additional evolving methods of determining gingival health around implants include crevicular fluid flow rates and identification of Interleukin-1-beta levels [87, 88]. An example of comprehensive studies of the peri-implant tissue are illustrated in the report of Niini and Veda [86].

Microbiology

It is now known that there is a similarity between the microbial flora around failing implants and microorganisms that are classically associated with periodontal disease. Mombelli has shown that implants are colonized predominately by gram-positive facultative organisms, and when evaluated over a 5-year period there is little alteration in these populations [89]. However, bone loss and increased peri-implant pocket depths are accompanied by increases in gram negative anaerobes, fusobacteria, spirochetes and black pigmenting organisms such as *Prevotella intermedia*. The severity of periodontal disease affecting the dentition is correlated with similar increases in spirochetes to mobile rods and spirochetes and therefore, it is reasonable to include diagnostic testing as an important adjunct to biocompatibility assessment of dental implants. Adherence and propagation of significant microorganism populations are related to implant surface properties, design and ease of maintenance.

Newer methods of diagnosis of periodontal pathogens are adapted to provide practical plaque analysis. Comprehensive analysis of samples sent to diagnostic centers may require specific transport protocols. Other more simple test modes use identification of DNA sequences which allow characterization of specific pathogens such as *Actinobacillus actinomycetemcomitans*, *Porphyromonas gingivalis*, and *Prevotella intermedia*, selectively [90].

Radiographic Evaluation

Radiographic techniques are designed to show bone levels in relation to easily located landmarks of the implant. The intra-oral film is positioned parallel to the threads of the fixture or measured reference points. Parallel long cone techniques are used with the film packet positioned orthoradially in a parallel plane to the long axis of the implant. The bone crest position may be measured to the nearest 0.3 mm (1/2 the width between 2 threads). Significant radiographic features recorded are saucerization, a reference to a particular cupped radiolucency around the neck of the implant. Representative studies using these techniques are available for review. Quirynen et al. demonstrated techniques that facilitate serial radiographic and clinical assessment of bone loss around endosseous implants. These were useful in determining "marginal bone loss" [91]. Computer-assisted methods are being developed to more accurately determine crestal-bone levels [92]. Animal research of digital subtraction methods also has excellent potential for adaptation to clinical studies [93].

Mechanical Assessment

There has been an increase in the adaptation and use of instrumentation to measure forces on implants in the clinical setting. Methodologies can be found in several current reports [94]. These studies explain measurement of bite forces and bending movements on a fixed prosthesis on a single endosseous implant. It is possible to identify load-sharing conditions between the flexible screw joint of the implant [95]. Masticatory force can be measured with transducers incorporated into endosseous implants supporting fixed prostheses or single crowns. Some investigations have exhibited occlusal forces which ranged from 200–300 N depending on the site studied [94]. Other studies which positioned transducers within the implant showed a differential in maximum vertical forces between self-standing molar position implants (120–150N) and molar position endosseous implants fixed to adjacent premolars (60–120N) [97].

Other methods are used to elucidate the significant force distribution around implants and to consider these points in design of the devices. Stress and finite analysis around implant/bone areas have shown that the neck area and crestal cortex of the implant site is subject to high stress under lateral and axial loads and compression stresses directed at the cortex adjacent to the implant [98]. Adequate bone density must form at this region of the implant to withstand peak stresses and local fatigue failure which is associated with bone resorption. A greater understanding of force relationships is important since long-term observation of implant cases have shown significant altered occlusion and/or intrusion of roots of natural teeth associated with rigid connectors [99, 100]. The design of full arch restorations on implants and the positioning of proper numbers of implants are based on the desire to have the masticatory forces directed in a predominantly axial direction and directed toward large bone mass zones such as the cortex [101].

The mechanical behavior of dental implants is incompletely described and difficult to understand because of the lack of fundamental understanding of the forces and distribution of forces that are present during the function of the teeth. Attempts to model the jaws and to design and test implants have included finite-stress analysis and photoelastic stress analysis [102, 103]. These methods have been useful in the design of implants in relation to optimum conical shapes and size of the cervical/cortical segment [104]. These methods can also identify strain shielding at the implant neck and distribution of critical stress points to minimize bone resorption around the implant [104]. Techniques of photoelastic stress analysis that utilize computed tomographic scanning help demonstrate desirable bone morphology necessary to reduce apical strain and achieve higher cortical stresses [103].

Additional Factors That Influence Implant Success

There are critical factors of implant site preparation, implant handling and maintenance that influence the successful long-term use of dental implants. Many implant systems include instruments tipped with metal similar to the implant. Site preparation is done with complex systems of guide drills, twist drills to achieve final depth, taps to finish thread areas and slow speed drills (15–12 rpm) to place the implant in the final position. Bone cutting is done with copious irrigation. Some drills provide internal irrigation. Healing periods for the submerged implant range from 3 to 6 months [107]. Previous publications have emphasized the importance of careful sterilization techniques and handling before and during insertion. Faulty steam sterilizer, glass bead or salt sterilizers, substances from trays, trimming instruments, packages, gloves, residues from detergents, and lubricant aerosol residues all affect the optimum surface passivation of the implant [108–111].

Implant Retrieval

The benefits of examining failed implants and associated tissue are obvious. While there are several centers that receive explanted specimens, a defined protocol for retrieval analysis is not in general use [113, 114]. Re-examination of the implant surface with SEM and EDAX may provide information about the efficiency of coatings or produce evidence of corrosion [113]. Rare cadaver studies are an opportunity to assess tissue after long-term successful use and to compare the tissue finding with previous radiographic assessment. Not all implants are removed because of inflammatory disease. Mechanical failures with subsequent implant removal have allowed analysis of bone/implant interfaces [114].

RECOMMENDATIONS AND CONCLUSIONS

There are basic questions the dentist should ask about any dental implant device selected for use. It is essential to know what previous testing has been accomplished on the material and design that examines the potential toxicity or hypersensitivity to the material used. Data should exist that indicate rationale for the design used, the surface finish, and the components that allow optimum distribution of masticatory forces. The surface chemical properties of the implant should be known, especially in relation to maintenance of gingival health, sterilization, and the potential for corrosion, biodegradation or alteration of surface coatings. Equally important is the effect of oxidation products on the adjacent tissue or the mode of transfer from the site to distant vital organs. Lastly, the result of clinical studies should be evaluated on the basis of compliance with standardized, accepted methods determining success.

REFERENCES

1   Eckert SE. Food and Drug Administration requirements for dental implants. *J Prosthetic Dent*, 74 (1995), 162–168.
2   Natiella JR, Armitage J, Meenaghan M, et al. Current evaluation of dental implants. *J Am Dent Assoc*, 84 (1972), 1358–1372.
3   American Dental Association Council on Dental Materials, Instruments and Equipment. Current evaluation of dental endosseous implants. *J Am Dent Assoc*, 100 (1980), 274.
4   American Dental Association Council on Dental Materials, Instruments and Equipment Association Reports. Expansion of the acceptance program for dental materials, instruments and equipment: endosseous implants. *J Am Dent Assoc*, 102 (1981), 350.
5   American Dental Association Council on Dental Materials, Instruments and Equipment. Dental endosseous implants. *J Am Dent Assoc*, 113 (1986), 949–950.
6   U.S. Code of Federal Regulations 21: CFR 872.3640; 872.3645.
7   Schumann D. FDA and ADA evaluation of dental implants. *J Public Health Dent*, 52 (1992), 373–374.
8   U.S. Food and Drug Administration. *The Safe Medical Devices Act of 1990 and the Medical Device Amendments of 1992*, HHS Publication 93–4243. Washington, DC: Department of Health and Human Services, 1992, 9.
9   Tylenda CA. FDA regulation of dental devices. Past, present & future. *J Public Health Dent*, 52 (1992), 364–368.
10 American National Standards Institute/American Dental Association. *Recommended Standard Practices for Biological Evaluation of Dental Instruments*, ANSI/ADA Document No. 41. New York: American National Standards Institute, 1979.
11 Misch CE. Implant terminology. In *Contemporary Implant Dentistry*. St. Louis, MO: Mosby; 1993, Chapter 2.
12 Wennerberg A, Albrelktsson T, Andersson B. Design and surface characteristics of 13 commercially available oral implant systems. *Int J Oral & Maxillofac Impl*, 8 (1993), 622–633.
13 Lemons J, Bidez M. Endosteal implant biomaterials and biomechanics. In McKinney RV (Ed.), *Endosteal Dental Implants*. St. Louis, MO: Mosby Year Book, 1991, Chapter 4.
14 Lang BR, Morris HF, Razzoog ME (Eds.). *International Workshop on the Biocompatibility, Toxicity and Hypersensitivity to Alloy Systems Used in Dentistry*. Ann Arbor, MI: University of Michigan, 1985, 191–223.

15 Merritt K. Biochemistry, hypersensitivity, clinical reaction. In Lang BR, Morris HF, Razzoog ME (Eds.), *International Workshop on the Biocompatibility, Toxicity & Hypersensitivity to Alloy Systems Used in Dentistry*. Ann Arbor, MI: University of Michigan, 1985, 191–223.

16 Natiella JR. Local tissue reaction: Carcinogenesis–Review of the literature. In Lang B, Morris H, Razzoog M (Eds.), *International Workshop: Biocompatibility, Toxicity and Hypersensitivity to Alloy Systems in Dentistry*. Ann Arbor, MI: University of Michigan, 1986, 247.

17 Schliephake H, Reiss G, Urban R, et al. Metal release from titanium fixtures during placement in the mandible: An experimental study. *Int J Oral & Maxillofac Impl*, 8 (1993), 502.

18 Rae T. The biological response to titanium and titanium-aluminum-vanadium alloy particles 1: Tissue culture studies. *Biomaterials*, 7 (1986), 30.

19 Rae T. The biological response to titanium and titanium-aluminum-vanadium alloy particles 2: Long-term animal studies. *Biomaterials*, 7 (1986), 37.

20 Reuling N, Wisser W, et al. Release and detection of dental corrosion products in vivo: Development of an experimental model in rabbits. *J Biomed Mater Res*, 24 (1990), 979.

21 Memoli V, Woodman J, et al. Long-term biocompatibility of porous titanium fiber composites. *Trans Orthop Res Soc*, 8 (1983), 237.

22 Memoli V, Woodman J, et al. Malignant neoplasms associated with orthopedic implant materials. *Orthop Trans*, 6 (1987), 264.

23 Woodman J, Jacobs J, et al. Titanium release from fiber metal composites in baboons: A long-term biocompatibility study of porous titanium fiber metal composites. *Trans Orthop Res Soc*, 7 (1982), 166.

24 Woodman J, Jacobs J, et al. Metal ion release from titanium-based prosthetic segmental replacements in long bones in baboons. *J Orthop Res*, 1 (1984), 421.

25 Black J. Systemic effects of biomaterials. *Biomater*, 5 (1984), 11–18.

26 Williams DF. Titanium and titanium alloys. In Williams DF (Ed.), *Biocompatibility of Clinical Implant Materials*, Vol. 1. Boca Raton, FL: CRC Press, 1981, 9–44.

27 Autian J. Carcinogenic potential of metals. In *Workshop on Biocompatibility of Metals in Dentistry*. National Institute of Dental Research, National Institutes of Health. Chicago, IL: American Dental Association, 107 (1984), 113.

28 McNamara A, Williams, DF. Enzyme histochemistry of the tissue response to pure metal implants. *J Biomed Mater Res*, 18 (1984), 395–402.

29 Salthouse T. Observations of implanted biomaterials. *J Biomed Mater Res*, 18 (1984), 395–402.

30 Becker W, Becker B, Handelsman M, et al. Guided tissue regeneration for implants placed into extraction sockets. A study in dogs. *J Periodontol*, 62 (1991), 703.

31 Carr A, Papazoglou, Larsen P. The relationship of periotest values, biomaterials and torque to failure in adult baboons. *Int J Prosthod*, 8 (1995), 15–20.

32 Caudill R, Meffert R. Histologic analysis of the osseointegration of endosseous implants in simulated extraction sockets with and without e-PTFE barriers. *J Periodont Rest Dent*, 11 (1991), 201.

33 Cook SD, Salkeld SL, Gaisser DM, et al. An in vivo analysis of an elliptical dental implant design. *J Oral Implantol*, 19 (1993), 307.

34 Ericsson I, Johansson, CB, Bystedt H, et al. A histomorphometric evaluation of bone-to-implant contact on machine prepared and roughened titanium dental implants. *Clin Oral Impl Res*, 5 (1994), 202.

35 Hurzeler M, Quinones C, Morrison, et al. Treatment of peri-implantitis using guided bone regeneration and bone grafts. *Int J Oral & Maxillofac Impl*, 10 (1995), 474–494.

36 Hurzeler M, Quinones C, Schupback P. Influence on the superstructure on the peri-implant tissues in beagle dogs. *Clin Oral Impl Res*, 6 (1995), 139–148.

37 Kaida H, Akagawa Y, Hashimoto M, et al. The effects of a stress-absorbing system involved in the superstructure supported by hydroxyapatite-coated implants in monkeys. *Int J Oral & Maxillofac Impl*, 10 (1995), 213.

38 Lang N, Bragger U, Walther D, et al. Ligature-induced peri-implant infection in Cynomologus monkeys. *Clin Oral Impl Res*, 4 (1993), 2–11.

39 Lekholm U, Becker W, Dahlin C, et al. The role of early vs late removal of GTAM-membranes on bone formation around oral implants placed in immediate extraction sockets. *Clin Oral Impl Res*, 4 (1993), 121–129.

40 Lionhardt A, Berglundh T, Ericsson I, et al. Putative periodontal pathogens on titanium implants and teeth in experimental gingivitis and periodontitis in beagle dogs. *Clin Oral Impl Res*, 3 (1992), 112–119.

41 Lin H, Vant V, Klein CP. Permucosal implantation pilot study with HA-coated dental implants in dogs. *Biomater*, 13 (1992), 825–831.

42 Parr GR, Gardner LK, Steflik DE, et al. Comparative implant research in dogs: Prosthodontic protocol using two-stage endosseous dental implants. *Int J Oral & Maxillofac Impl*, 7 (1992), 508–512.

43 Parr GR, Gardner LK, Steflik DE, et al. Comparative implant research in dogs: A prosthodontic model. *J Prosthodontic Dent*, 68 (1992), 509–514.

44 Parr GR, Steflik DE, Sisk AL. Histomorphometric and histologic observations of bone healing around immediate implants in dogs. *Internat J Oral & Maxillofac Impl*, 8 (1993), 534.

45 Plotzke AE, Barbosa S, Nasjleti C, et al. Histologic and histomorphic responses to polymeric composite grafts. *J Periodontal*, 54 (1993), 343–348.

46 Schupback P, Hurzeler M, Grunder O. Implant tissue interfaces following treatment of peri-implantitis using guided tissue regeneration. *Clin Oral Impl Res*, 5 (1994), 55–65.

47 Sennebry L, Odman J, Lekholm V, et al. Tissue reaction toward titanium implants inserted in growing jaws: A histological study in the pig. *Clin Oral Impl Res*, 4 (1993), 65.

48 Steflik D, Parr G, Sisk A, Hanes P, et al. Electron microscopy of bone response to titanium cylindrical screw type indosseous dental implants. *Int J Oral & Maxillofac Impl*, 7 (1992), 497–507.

49 Warren K, Karring T, Gotfredsen K. Periodontal ligament formation around different types of dental titanium implants. *J Periodontol*, 64 (1993), 29–34.

50 Weinlander M, Kenney E, Lekovic V, et al. Histomorphometry of bone apposition around three types of endosseous dental implants. *Int J Oral & Maxillofac Impl*, 7 (1992), 491–496.

51 Yan J, Xiang W, Baolin L, et al. Early histologic response to titanium implants complexed with bovine bone morphogenic protein. *J Prosthet Dent*, 71 (1994), 389.

52 Hashimoto M, et al. Single-crystal sapphire endosseous dental implant loaded with functional stress-clinical and histological evaluation of peri-implant tissues. *J Oral Rehab*, 15 (1988), 65.

53 Hashimoto M, et al. Ultrastructure of the peri-implant junctional epithelium on single crystal sapphire endosseous dental implant loaded with functional stress. *J Oral Rehab*, 16 (1989), 261.

54 McKinney R, Steflik D, Koth D. Ultrastructural surface topography of the single crystal sapphire endosseous dental implant. *J Oral Impl*, 11 (1984), 327.

55 McKinney R, Steflik D, Koth D. Evidence of a biological seal at the implant-tissue interface. In McKinney R, Lemons J (Eds.), *The Dental Implant*. Littleton, MA: PSG Publishing, 1985, 25.

56 McKinney R, Steflik D, Koth D. Evidence for a junctional epithelial attachment to ceramic implants. *J Periodontol*, 56 (1985), 579.

57 Albrektsson T, Lekholm V. Osseointegration: Current state of the art. In Berman C (Ed.), *Osseointegration*. Philadelphia, PA: W. B. Saunders, 1989, 538.

58 Inadomo T, Hayashi K, Nakashima Y, et al. Comparison of bone implant interface shear strength of hydroxyapatite-coated alumina-coated metal implants. *J Biomed Mater Res*, 20 (1995), 10–24.

59 Marani A, Caja V, Egger C, et al. Histomorphometry of hydroxyapatite coated and uncoated porous titanium bone implants. *Biomater*, 15 (1994), 11.

60 Arvidson K, Bystedt H, Frykholm A. A three-year clinical study of Astra dental implants in the treatment of edentulous mandibles. *Int J Oral & Maxillofac Impl*, 7 (1992), 321–329.

61 Babbush CA, Kirsch A. The IMZ-Interpore osseointegrated implant system. In McKinney RV (Ed.), *Endosteal Dental Implants*. St. Louis, MO: Mosby Year Book, 1991, 331–347.

62 Babbush CA, Shimura M. Five-year statistical and clinical observations with the IMZ two-stage osseointegration implant system. *Int J Oral & Maxillofac Impl*, 8 (1993), 245.

63 Fugazzoto PA, Wheeler S, Lindsay J. Success and failure rates of cylinder implants in type IV bone. *J Periodontol*, 61 (1993), 1085–1087.

64 Hahn JA. The Steri-Oss implant system. In McKinney RV (Ed.), *Endosteal Dental Implants*. St. Louis, MO: Mosby Year Book, 1991, 349–361.

65 Jemi T. Implant treatment in older patients. *Int J Prosthodont*, 6 (1993), 455–461.

66 Jemi T, Book K, Linden B, et al. Failures and complications in 92 consecutively inserted overdentures supported by Branemark implants in severely resorbed edentulous maxillae. *Int J Oral & Maxillofac Impl*, 7 (1992), 162–167.

67 Lill W, Thornton B, Reichsthaler J, et al. Statistical analysis on the success potential of osseointegrated implants: A retrospective single-dimension statistical analysis. *J Prosthetic Dent*, 69 (1993), 176–185.

68 Naert I, Quirynan M, van Steenblerghe D, et al. A study of 589 consecutive implants supporting fixed prostheses. *J Prosthetic Dent*, 68 (1992), 949–958.

69 Quirynan M, Naert I, van Steenblerghe D, et al. A study of 589 consecutive implants supporting fixed prostheses. Part I: Periodontal aspects. *J Prosthetic Dent*, 68 (1992), 655–663.

70 Rominger J, Triplett RG. The use of guided tissue regeneration to improve implant osseointegration. *J Oral Maxillofac Surg*, 52 (1994), 106–112.

71 *Proc World Workshop in Clinical Periodontics, American Academy of Periodontology*, Chicago, 1989.

72 Salonen MA, Oikarien K, Vertanen K, et al. Failures in the osseointegration of endosseous implants. *Int J Oral & Maxillofac Impl*, 8 (1993), 92–97.

73 Silness J, Loe H. Periodontal disease in pregnancy. II Correlation between oral hygiene and periodontal condition. *Acta Odontol Scand*, 1964, 533–538.

74 Stvrtecky RO, Bergette ZA, Manzano M. Subperiosteal implants. *J Oral Implantol*, 19 (1993), 48.

75 Spickerman H, Jansen V, Richter E. A ten-year followup study of IMZ and TPS implants in the edentulous mandible using bar-retained overdentures. *Int J Oral & Maxillofac Impl*, 10 (1995), 231–243.

76 Takarada H, Kinebuchi T. Clinical evaluation of hydroxylapatite-coated titanium artificial tooth root. *J Stomatol Soc Japan*, 60 (1993), 532.

77 van Steenberghe D, Klinge B, Linden V, et al. Periodontal indices around natural and titanium abutments: A longitudinal multicenter study. *J Periodontol*, 64 (1993), 538–541.

78 Wedgewood D, Jennings KJ, Critchlow HA, et al. Experience with ITI osseointegrated implants at five centers in the UK. *Brit J Oral & Maxillofac Surg*, 30 (1992), 377–381.

79 Yanase RT, Bodine RL, Tom JF, et al. The mandibular subperiosteal implant denture: A prospective survival study. *J Prosthet Dent*, 71 (1994), 369.

80 Albrektsson T, Zarb G, Worthington P, et al. Long-term efficacy of currently used dental implants. A review and proposed criteria for success. *J Oral Maxillofac Impl*, 1 (1986), 11–25.

81 Wedgewood D, Jennings KJ, Critchlow HA, et al. Experience with ITI osseointegrated implants at five centres in the UK. *Brit J Oral & Maxillofac Surg*, 30 (1992), 377–381.

82 Weyant R, Burt B. An assessment of survival rates and within-patient clustering of failures for endosseous oral implants. *J Dent Res*, 72 (1993), 2–8.

83 Lill W, Thornton B, Reichsthaler J, Schneider B. Statistical analyses on the success potential of osseointegrated implants: A retrospective single-dimension statistical analysis. *J Prosthet Dent*, 69 (1993), 176–185.

84 Mau J. On statistics of success and loss for dental implants. *Internat Dent J*, 43 (1993), 254–261.

85 Morris H, Ochi S. The influence of implant design, application and site on clinical performance and crestal bone. *Implant Dent*, 1 (1992), 49–55.

86 Niimi A, Veda M. Crevicular fluid in the osseointegrated implant sulcus–A pilot study. *Int J Oral & Maxillofac Impl*, 10 (1995), 434.

87 George K, Zafiropoulos G, Murat Y, et al. Clinical and microbiological status of osseointegrated implants. *J Periodontol*, 65 (1991), 766–770.

88 Kao R, Curtis D, Richard D. Increased interleuken-1 beta in the crevicular fluid of diseased implants. *Int J of Oral & Maxillofacial Impl*, 10 (1995), 696–701.

89 Mombelli A. Microbiology of the dental implant. *Adv Dent Res*, 7 (1993), 202–206.

90 Schwartz M, Lamster I, Fine J. *Clinical Guide to Periodontics*. Philadelphia, PA: W. B. Saunders Co., 1995, Chapter 10.

92 Pham AN, Fiorellini J, Paquette D, et al. Longitudinal radiographic study of crestal bone levels adjacent to non-submerged dental implants. *J Oral Implantol*, 20 (1994), 26–34.

93 Jeffcoat M, Reddy M. Digital subtraction radiography for longitudinal assessment of peri-implant bone change: Method and validation. *Adv Dent Res*, 7 (1993), 196–201.

94 Glantz PO, Rangert B, Svensson P, et al. On clinical loading of osseointegrated implants. A methodological and clinical study. *Clin Oral Impl Res*, 4 (1993), 99.

95 Rangert B, Gunne J, Glantz PO, et al. Vertical load distribution on a three-unit prosthesis supported by a natural tooth and single Branemark implant. An in-vivo study. *Clin Oral Impl Res*, 6 (1995), 40.

96 Mericske-Stern R, Assal P, Mericske E, et al. Occlusal force and oral tactile sensibility measured in partially endentulous patients with ITI implants. *Int J Oral & Maxillofac Impl*, 10 (1995), 343.

97 Richter EJ. In vivo vertical forces on implants. *Int J Oral & Maxillofac Impl*, 10 (1995), 98.

98 Lozada JL, Abbate MF, Pizzarello FA, et al. Comparative three-dimensional analysis of two finite-element endosseous implant designs. *J Oral Implantol*, 20 (1994), 315.

99 English C. Root intrusion in tooth-implant combination cases. *Implant Dent*, 2 (1993), 79–85.

100 Dario LJ. How occlusal forces change in implant patients: A clinical research report. *J Am Dent Assoc*, 128 (1995), 1130.

101 Rangert B. Mechanical and biomechanical guidelines for the use of the Branemark system–Clinical studies. *Aust Prosthodont J*, 7 (1993 Suppl.), 45.

102 Clelland NL, Gilat A, McGlumphy EA, Brantley WA. A photoelastic and strain gauge analysis of angled abutments for an implant system. *Intern J Oral & Maxillofac Impl*, 8 (1993), 541.

103 Clelland NL, Lee JK, Bimbenet OC. The use of an axisymmetric finite element method to compare maxillary bone variables for a loaded implant. *J Prosthodon*, 1993, 183–189.

104 Deines DN, Eick JD, Cobb CM. Photoelastic stress analysis of natural teeth and three osseointegrated implants. *Int J Perio Restor Dent*, 13 (1993), 540.

105 Brunski J, Hipp J. In vivo forces on dental implants. *J Biomech*, 17 (1984), 855–860.

106 Cleft SE, Fisher J, Watson C. Finite element stress and strain analysis of the bone surrounding a dental implant: effect of variations in bone modules. Proceedings of the Institution of Mechanical Engineers. Part H. *J Engin Med*, 206 (1992), 233–241.

107 Goldman BM, Sisk AL. In McKinney RV (Ed.), *Endosteal Dental Implants*. St. Louis, MO: Mosby Year Book, 1991, 293–314.

108 Baier R, Meyer A. Implant surface preparation. *Int J Oral Maxillofac Impl*, 1 (1988), 9.

109 Baier R, Meyer A, Natiella J, et al. Degradative effects of conventional steam sterilization on biomaterials. *Biomat*, 3 (1982), 241.

110 Baier R, Meyer A, Natiella J, et al. Surface properties determine biohesive outcomes. *J Biomed Mater Res*, 18 (1984), 337.

111 Baier R, Natiella J, Meyer A, et al. Importance of implant surface preparations for biomaterials with different intrinsic properties. In van Steenberghe D (Ed.), *Tissue Integration in Oral and Maxillofacial Reconstruction*. Amsterdam: Excerpta Medica, 1985, 13.

112 Carter J, Natiella J, Baier R, et al. Fibroblastic activities postimplantation of cobalt chromium alloy and pure germanium in rabbits. *Artif Organs*, 8 (1984), 102.

113 Lemons J. Dental implant retrieval analyses. *J Dent Ed*, 52 (1988), 748–755.

114 Steflik D, Parr G, Singh B. Light microscopic and scanning electron microscopic analysis of dental implants retrieval from humans. *J Oral Implantol*, 20 (1994), 9–24.

115 Takeshita F, Kuroki H, Yamasaki A, et al. Histopathic observation of seven removed endosseous dental implants. *Int J Oral & Maxillofac Impl*, 10 (1995), 367.

116 Rohrer M, Bulard RA, Patterson M. Maxillary and mandibular titanium implants one year after surgery: Histologic exam in a cadaver. *Inter J Oral & Maxillofac Impl*, 10 (1995), 466–473.

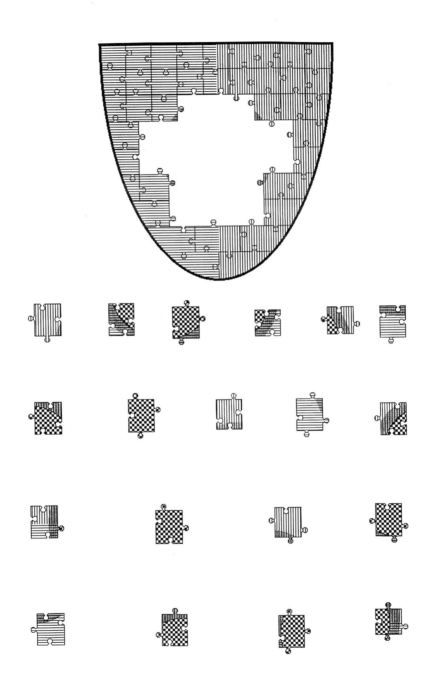

Section Seven

Soft Tissue Histology

James M. Anderson

Dedicated to Thomas N. Salthouse,
pioneer in the histological evaluation of biomaterials

INTRODUCTION

Since publication of the first edition of this handbook, significant advances have been made in microscopic techniques and molecular and cellular biology approaches to soft tissue reactions with biomaterials. Thus, this section is a blend of the old, tried-and-true techniques together with new technologies and approaches which not only identify the blood and tissue components interacting with biomaterials but also address issues related to function and physiology.

The visual, morphological and pathological analysis of tissue and implant site sections by light microscopy remains the foundation of the histological evaluation. Approaches to the utilization of standard histological evaluation are presented in the first three chapters, which have been revised from the first edition.

For information about evaluation by transmission electron microscopy, readers are referred to the section on hard tissue histology, a field in which transmission electron microscopy has been used extensively to evaluate the tissue/implant interface.

Scanning electron microscopy evaluation of biomaterials is a useful technique for appreciating cellular interactions with materials as well as material surface changes. The development of new technologies has enhanced the usefulness of scanning electron microscopy in the evaluation of biomaterials.

Over the past decade or so, advances in molecular and cellular biology have provided techniques which begin to address the physiology and function of cellular components of tissue interacting with biomaterials. Perspectives on the utilization of molecular and cellular biology techniques are provided in a new chapter in the edition. A new chapter describing the utilization of the in vivo cage implant system has been included to provide information on a technique which provides in vivo perspectives of the temporal responses in tissue in a sensitive and quantitative fashion. A chapter on the pathological evaluation of explanted cardiovascular prostheses has been included as an example of how these various techniques may be combined in a structured program to address tissue and blood responses to a specific type of device.

These approaches and the utilization of these techniques not only provide a basis for the safety and efficacy testing necessary in the determination of the biocompatibility of a biomaterial, but they also may be utilized to develop an understanding of tissue/

material interactions which then may be used in understanding the individual roles or contributions by the biomaterial and the tissue components. Moreover, information derived from the utilization of these techniques and approaches may provide insight into previously undiscovered relationships which may form the basis for the development of new materials.

Chapter 37

Tissue Preparation

Barbara F. Matlaga

This chapter deals with the methodology of preparing devices or material specimens that had been implanted in patients or animals for light microscopic evaluation. It includes techniques of retrieval, fixation, trimming, tissue processing, embedding, sectioning, and staining.

IMPLANT RETRIEVAL

Specimens should be removed from the animal as soon after euthanasia as possible. The prosector should be aware that as soon as the animal is sacrificed, vital cellular processes cease and autolysis begins due to enzyme activity within cells. In order to preserve cells in as lifelike a state as possible, it is imperative that tissue containing implants be removed and placed into a fixative solution immediately. At the time of recovery, all gross descriptions of the specimens (appearance, color, size) should be made because fixation will alter the original appearance and cause some minor shrinkage. Care must be taken not to dislodge the implant within the tissue specimen prior to fixation. During specimen recovery, the prosector should follow the study protocol and ensure proper animal and specimen identification. The Good Laboratory Practice (GLP) regulations require traceability of specimens from fixed tissue to the finished slide.

SPECIMEN FIXATION

The process of fixation involves the coagulation and stabilization of cellular proteins within cells and tissue. This is the most critical aspect of histological processing because subsequent techniques cannot improve a poorly fixed tissue specimen. The aims of fixation are to preserve organs or parts of organs so that microanatomical arrangements are not destroyed or altered; preserve the intracellular anatomy of cells so that cytologic conditions can be studied; stop autolysis; bring out differences in the refractive index of tissue types; and render tissue components insoluble so they will not be removed during subsequent processing procedures. Fixation also hardens tissue so it can be trimmed and can act as a chemical mordant to aid in the staining process. Ten percent neutral buffered formalin is the most common fixative used in routine histology for light microscopy. The fixative stabilizes tissue proteins by forming cross-links with the basic amino acid residues. Other fixatives can be used for selected tissue types or special staining procedures [1]. Buffered glutaraldehyde solutions are sometimes used, but usually only when tissue may be evaluated by scanning or transmission electron microscopy. These fixatives are toxic substances and should be handled in a fume hood while wearing gloves and eye protection. Formalin sodium acetate solution is recommended for routine use [2].

Immersion Fixation

The tissue specimen should be immersed in a volume of fixative at least 15 to 20 times the volume of tissue. Since fixatives only penetrate 2–3 mm into solid tissue, the specimens should be approximately 3–4 mm thick, if possible. If specimens are larger than this, then deep cuts should be made into the tissue specimen to provide more surface area for penetration and adequate fixation. Several days of fixation at room temperature will usually be adequate but larger specimens may take weeks. When fixation is complete, tissues can be trimmed to expose the implant.

Vascular Perfusion Fixation

In perfusion fixation, the fixative is perfused through the vascular system. This is accomplished by catheterizing a major blood vessel, usually the aorta [3], or through the heart. Fixative is then pumped through the blood vessels under physiological pressure, and fixation of the tissues occurs in situ. This process is most often used to preserve tissues for electron microscopy where immediate fixation is imperative (see Chapters 42 and 43). However, these techniques may be necessary for adequate fixation of some biomaterial implants, namely, small-diameter vascular grafts or other sites where penetration could be a problem. One advantage of perfusion fixation is that soft tissues around an implant are hardened by the process, which would minimize movement of the implant during recovery and more adequately preserve the implant tissue interface if this is critical. If tissues are being prepared for light microscopic evaluation, perfusion with 10 percent neutral buffered formalin is adequate. Buffered glutaraldehyde is required for electron microscopy fixation.

Tissue Trimming

Once the specimen is adequately fixed, it often needs to be trimmed for further processing. The thickness should not exceed 4 mm in order to allow for adequate penetration of subsequent processing chemicals. Tissue dimensions will also be dependent on the size of the embedding molds used. If possible, the implant should be surrounded by tissue on all sides. This location may facilitate the sectioning of some implant materials and allow the implant to be retained within the tissue section. During trimming, care must be taken to preserve adequately the important anatomic locations of the implant.

TISSUE PROCESSING

Once tissues are fixed, further processing is necessary for the specimen to be in a form that will faciliate sectioning on a microtome. These processes require impregnation with some supporting media to furnish stability and allow cell structures to remain in proper relationships to each other within the tissue block. Biomaterial implants also require support in media that will hold them during the sectioning process. The most commonly used embedding medium is paraffin wax. More recently, plastic embedding medium, namely, glycol methacrylate, has been introduced. The size, texture, and hardness of the implant may influence which medium is chosen.

Treatment of Absorbable Polymers

The synthetic absorbable polymers are generally difficult to section at early periods, when little or no polymer degradation or absorption has occurred. From our experience with lactide/glycolide copolymers we have found a technique to hydrolyze these implants in vitro prior to tissue processing. These methods involve incubation of a piece of formalin-fixed tissue containing the implant in a solution of 10 percent buffered formalin for several days at 37°–56°C. During this process, the implant undergoes further hydrolysis, which "softens" the implant, making it easier to section. The structure of the tissue surrounding the implant is preserved. Cellular morphology and staining are not adversely affected by this treatment. Depending on the polymer type and its absorption profile, the incubation time and temperature will have to be arrived at by trial and error on a test specimen. Similarly, other polymers can be softened or even dissolved prior to embedding and sectioning [15].

Paraffin Processing and Embedding

In order to allow paraffin to impregnate, tissues need to be dehydrated and cleared. The dehydration process removes water from tissues and is usually carried out through a graded series of ethanol. Ethanol is used in routine histology because it is reliable, nontoxic, fast-acting, and causes relatively little tissue shrinkage if a graded series is used. However, it is expensive, may be prohibitively taxed, and hard to obtain. Prolonged exposure to absolute ethanol may cause excessive tissue shrinkage and hardening. Despite these disadvantages the use of ethanol is recommended for routine paraffin processing.

Once tissue is completely dehydrated, a clearing agent which is miscible with both alcohol and paraffins is used. Clearing agents remove the alcohol, make tissue transparent, and allow impregnation with melted paraffin. Xylene is the solvent of choice for clearing in routine paraffin embedding procedures because it clears quickly and makes tissues transparent so the end-point of clearing can be easily determined.

Xylene is less expensive and less toxic than alternatives such as toluene and benzene. Xylene should be handled with caution since it is flammable. Exposure to vapors and skin contact should be minimized. Recently several "xylene substitutes" have been marketed that are advertised to be less toxic and claim to have a similar chemical action to xylene. They are, however, more expensive than xylene, and modifications in processing schedules may be required to obtain optimum preparations.

Although these embedding processes can be carried out manually, they are more conveniently accomplished overnight on a commercial automatic tissue processing unit. Fixed and trimmed tissue specimens are placed in small plastic cassettes that can be labeled with proper specimen identification and then placed onto a tissue processor. The processor can be programmed to the desired schedule so that specimens in paraffin will be ready for embedding the next morning.

Tissues infiltrated with molten paraffin have to be manually embedded into a mold that can be placed onto the microtome for sectioning. Commercial embedding centers are available that hold liquid paraffin and have warming and cold plates. Embedding molds and embedding rings are available commercially. Care should be taken to ensure proper temperature of the liquid paraffin. Too high a temperature can destroy the cutting properties of the paraffin (see manufacturer's directions). Care must be taken to allow the liquid paraffin to solidify properly. Too slow or too rapid hardening of paraffin causes crystallization. The formation of large crystals will make the block difficult to section properly. Cooling of blocks prepared in a metal mold and placed on the cooling plate of a commercial processor allows hardening to proceed from the surface of the mold to the top of the embedding ring. Cold water between 10° and 15°C can be used, but water colder than 10°C will cause blocks to contract too quickly and crack. A perfect block is one in which the paraffin crystals are contiguous and the paraffin appears clear and homogeneous. If the paraffin does crystallize, the block is difficult to section; the only alternative then is to melt down the block and repeat the embedding process.

Glycol Methacrylate Processing and Embedding

In recent years, the popularity of plastic embedding of tissues has grown [4–7]. Methacrylate offers many advantages over paraffin processing. There is less shrinkage and distortion of tissues in methacrylate because no clearing agent or heat is required. Cellular morphology and tissue relationships are better preserved in glycol methacrylate sections and are generally superior to paraffin sections. Sections can also be cut much thinner than paraffin blocks, 2 to 3 μm. Polymerized methacrylate is harder than paraffin wax, which will allow sectioning of some hard polymer implants. Some soft polymeric materials, such as polyurethanes, are chemically affected by glycol methacrylate monomer. During the processing sequence, these materials may swell. The physical properties of some polymers are changed in such a way as to make them more easily sectioned than when paraffin-embedded. The disadvantage of glycol methacrylate techniques are that reagents are more expensive than routine paraffin, and not all special stains can be readily accomplished on methacrylate sections.

Once tissues are infiltrated with glycol methacrylate monomer, they are embedded in a mixture of monomer and catalyst that initiates the polymerization reaction. The polymerization is exothermic, takes several hours, and produces a block that is easily sectioned with glass knives. Kits are available that supply glycol methacrylate reagents (JB-4 Plastic Embedding Kit, Polysciences, Inc., Warrington, Pennsylvania). However, the solutions can also be prepared as described below. Glycol methacrylate monomer and mixtures with catalyst are referred to as "Hema" in histological methods.

Glycol Methacrylate Solutions   All solutions should be handled in the fume hood. Skin allergies have been reported to develop on repeated exposure to methacrylate solutions. Gloves should be worn at all times. All solutions should be stored in the refrigerator and allowed to come to room temperature before opening, since polymerization may be affected if solution absorbs too much atmospheric moisture.

Uncatalyzed Solution A.   This solution is used for making catalyzed Solution A.

1   160 ml low acid Hema glycol methacrylate
2   32 ml 2-butoxyethanol
3   Mix and store in refrigerator, keeps several months.

Catalyzed Solution A.   This solution is used for infiltrating and embedding.

1   100 ml uncatalyzed solution A
2   0.9 gm benzoyl peroxide
3   Mix and store in brown bottle in refrigerator, keeps several weeks.

Solution B.

1   15 ml polyethylene glycol 400
2   1 ml *N,N*-dimethylaniline

3   Mix and store in brown bottle in refrigerator. Solution may freeze at this temperature; thaw before using.

Final Embedding Media.

1   Mix 40 parts catalyzed solution A with 1 part solution B *or* Mix 25 parts catalyzed solution A with 1 part solution B for faster polymerization.

2   Increase the ratio of catalyzed solution A to solution B to decrease rate of polymerization in final embedding media. Slower polymerization may be preferred because this minimizes the formation of bubbles on voids in tissue.

The following glycol methacrylate processing procedures are recommended:

1   Trim formalin-fixed tissue no larger than $10 \times 5 \times 2$ mm thick. (Larger pieces or dense tissue types may require longer infiltration times.)

2   Wash 90 minutes in running tap water to remove excess fixative which may affect polymerization.

3   Dehydrate through graded ethyl alcohols:

   70 percent 1 hour or hold overnight
   95 percent 10 minutes
   95 percent 10 minutes

4   Infiltrate in three changes of catalyzed solution A. These solutions must be brought to room temperature before opening.

   Catalyzed solution A (Hema I)—1 hour in vacuum at 13–16 psi
   Catalyzed solution A (Hema II)—1 hour in vacuum at 13–16 psi
   Catalyzed solution A (Hema III)—1 hour in vacuum at 13–16 psi

5   Embed. Embedding trays, molds, and block holders are available from Polysciences, Inc., Warrington, Pennsylvania.

6   Place approximately 1.5 ml of embedding medium into molds ($6 \times 12 \times 5$ mm).

   Orient tissue in mold
   Place aluminum holder over mold
   Place embedding trays in nitrogen atmosphere for polymerization

If specimens float in the final embedding media, prepare a block of glycol methacrylate and polymerize. Cut to fit over the specimen in the mold and fill with the embedding medium. This polymerized block will hold the tissue down and prevent it from floating. The polymerization process is exothermic. The aluminum block holders are designed to dissipate heat away from the specimen. Polymerization is more efficient when oxygen is excluded. This can be done by using nitrogen atmosphere or by sealing out oxygen from the block by ringing around the aluminum block holder with liquid paraffin. The formation of air bubbles in the final block usually indicates too rapid polymerization. The rate of polymerization can be changed by lowering the concentration of solution B in the final embedding mixture. If bubbles occur on the face of the block, remove the block from the metal holder and soak in catalyzed solution A overnight or several days as needed to remove polymerized methacrylate and reembed.

SECTIONING

Microtomy (sectioning with a microtome) is an art that can only be learned by experience. Microtomy of soft tissue blocks containing implant materials is especially difficult because the implant can vary in dimensions and hardness. To minimize problems, the histologist should begin with a properly prepared specimen, a sharp microtome knife, a properly functioning microtome, and a determined attitude. For the uninitiated, a tissue block without an implant should be attempted first to gain experience in these techniques.

Paraffin Sectioning

The goal in paraffin sectioning is to obtain a thin section (6–7 μm) of embedded tissue that is free from cutting artifacts. Routine paraffin sectioning requires the following equipment: a microtome, a microtome knife, heated water bath, and a hotplate. The rotary microtome is the most commonly used in the histology laboratory. The mechanism allows the block to move up and down vertically in front of the knife by the turning action of the fly wheel at the side of the microtome. All microtomes have thickness scales that can vary the forward traveling distance of the block, allowing different section thicknesses. A description of other microtome types is available [8]. The wedge-type steel microtome knife, which can be resharpened, is most commonly used for paraffin work. A sharp cutting edge is critical to success in producing sections free of cutting artifacts. Steel knives can be resharpened when they become dull, and commercial knife sharpening equipment is available. A good description of microtome knives and knife sharpening is available elsewhere [9]. Recently, disposable knifes of the safety razor type have been introduced. These blades do not keep their sharpness as well as steel knives, but offer the advantage of being disposable. In the biomaterial histology laboratory, this blade type may offer time savings by eliminating the need for resharpening of standard steel blades that dull easily in the process of cutting hard polymeric materials. A thermostatically controlled water bath is required that can be set at approximately 45°C $\pm$ 5°C. A hotplate for drying sections is recommended and should be capable of being set to a temperature between 37° and 56°C.

The following technique is recommended for block trimming and sectioning:

1   Mount trim knife and tissue block in microtome.
2   Trim into block to expose tissue and implant.
3   Place paraffin block on ice to cool for 10–15 minutes. This hardens the paraffin to facilitate sectioning.
4   Mount sharpened knife into microtome. Mount paraffin block from ice tray into microtome chuck. Set thickness setting at 6–7 μm.
5   Using a smooth even rhythm, cut a ribbon of 10 or more sections while holding it away from knife edge with a fine forceps.
6   Carefully remove edge of ribbon from the microtome knife edge and place on preheated water bath 44°–46°C containing gelatin (2 teaspoons of 5 percent gelatin solution in approximately 2 liters of distilled water). Place one edge of ribbon first and then gently lower rest of ribbon onto water surface.
7   Isolate desired section and mount on a clean glass slide. This is best accomplished by allowing the top of the paraffin section to make contact with the glass slide and then pulling the slide from the waterbath vertically.
8   Properly identify the slide with the specimen identification number and allow to drain.
9   Transfer slides to a hot plate set at approximately 45° until dry. Place slides in rack and into a 56°C oven overnight.
10   Remove slides from oven and allow to come to room temperature before staining.

When sectioning problems occur, the experienced microtomist recognizes the difficulty, the causes, and the remedies. An excellent review of these problems is available [1] and is recommended reading for the novice. Some additional hints are listed below that may be especially helpful in sectioning biomaterial implants.

1   Use low knife angle setting at approximately $2°-2\frac{1}{2}°$.

2   Always clean disposable knives with xylene before using to remove any adherent grease. Mount blade in holder and section a blank paraffin block to establish knife angle and ribboning characteristics with each blade.

3   If difficulty is encountered in sectioning an implant, remove block from chuck and turn block 180°. Remount in chuck, reface block to knife edge, soak, ice, and recut. This procedure may help in sectioning "problem" implants.

4   If problems are encountered in retaining biomaterial implants within the cut section, try coating the slide with a thin layer of albumin. Another technique uses slides coated with a solution of 5 drops of Elmer's Glue in 50 ml of water. Dip slides in solution and allow to dry before using.

Glycol Methacrylate Sectioning

Similar microtomy skills are required for methacrylate block sectioning, although the novice may find it easier than paraffin sectioning. Plastic blocks are harder than paraffin and can be sectioned at room temperature. The equipment needs for glycol methacrylate (GMA) sectioning are somewhat different than those of routine paraffin work. Blocks of GMA can be sectioned on routine paraffin rotary microtome using steel knives or disposable blades. However, several manufacturers now produce rotary microtomes especially designed for plastic sectioning using glass knives. Manufacturers also supply glass knife makers that produce quality knives easily and quickly. Glass knives can be produced by hand from sheet glass using a scoring wheel and knife-breaking pliers [10, 11]. Methacrylate sections do not form ribbons so each cut section needs to be lifted off the knife edge with fine forceps. A heated water bath is not necessary for GMA sectioning because the sections flatten easily at room temperature. A thermostatically controlled hot plate is recommended because the drying temperature for GMA sections may vary greatly depending on the tissue and implant type.

The following techniques are recommended for GMA sectioning:

1   Mount used glass knife onto microtome and trim into tissue block to expose tissue and implant.

2   Mount new glass knife in microtome and set thickness setting to desired level, between 3 and 5 μm.

3   Approach block face and cut a section. Glycol methacrylate sections *do not form ribbons*. Remove section carefully from knife edge with fine forceps and place onto room temperature distilled water bath.

4   Mount on glass slide and properly identify. Place onto hot plate and observe during drying. Check dry section under microscope. If cracks are formed in the section, the hot plate temperature is too high. If folds remain in sections, temperature of hot plate is too cool.

5   Place dried slides in 50°C oven overnight before staining.

The following list of hints may be useful for methacrylate sectioning work.

1   If block appears to crack during sectioning, the block is probably too dry. Breathe gently onto the block face and cut another section. Moisture will penetrate a few microns into the surface and allow for easier sectioning.

2 If block face is too sticky, section will be compressed at knife edge. Dry blocks by storing them overnight in a closed container containing silica gel desiccant.

3 If the block face is rough or scratched from previous knife defects, remove a few, very thin (1 micron) sections. Then return to proper thickness setting and cut a section.

4 Do not place methacrylate slides in oven with paraffin sections. A thin coating of paraffin will be deposited onto the GMA slides and prevent stains from penetrating.

STAINING

The purpose of staining is to color various components of tissue sections so they can be optically differentiated during microscopic evaluation. The most commonly used dye types are acid and basic dyes. Acid dyes are anionic and stain cationic tissue components. Basic dyes are cationic and stain anionic components of tissue sections. The most commonly used general diagnostic stain in histology is hematoxylin (a basic dye) and eosin (an acid dye). The hematoxylin stains nuclear material blue, while the cytoplasm stains pink with eosin. This coloration of tissues allows a general microscopic overview of tissue components. Other special stains that are selective for a variety of tissue types are available. Van Gieson stain for collagen and Gomori's aldehyde fuchsin stain for elastic tissues are useful in the microscopic study of sections of biomaterial implants.

Paraffin Sections

Prior to staining, the sections must be freed from paraffin using xylene and hydrated using a graded series of diluted alcohols. Stains can then be applied. Thereafter the slides are dehydrated again in ethanol, cleared in xylene, and covered with glass slips using a permanent resinous mounting media.

Hematoxylin-eosin (H&E) is the general oversite stain for tissue morphology [2]. It is the most widely used stain in histology because it is simple and clearly demonstrates numerous different tissue structures. Hematoxylin is a natural dye extracted from the logwood tree and has little affinity for tissues unless oxidized to hematein by the action of chemical oxidants. Metal salts, such as aluminum or potassium alum, are added to the solutions to form dye mordants that act to link the dye to tissue components. The Mayer's hematoxylin listed below acts as a progressive stain that will not overstain nuclear material and requires no differentiation. All hematoxylin-stained sections require "bluing" in either tap water or solutions at a slight alkaline pH. This treatment changes the red mordant-dye complex to blue. Following hematoxylin staining, the acid dye combination of eosin/phloxine is used to stain cytoplasmic components. Specific stains for collagen or elastin may be useful for evaluation of biomaterial implant sites. Van Gieson stain for collagen and Gomori's aldehyde fuchsin stain for elastic tissues are recommended [2].

The Staining of Methacrylate Sections

There are several differences in techniques for staining GMA sections compared to routine paraffin methods. The embedding medium, GMA, does not require removal from the sections prior to staining. Modifications in staining times and dye concentrations are often needed in order to accomplish staining of GMA sections. The number of special stains for GMA sections is limited. Many stains do not work on these sections because of undesired chemical reactions between the GMA polymer and the staining chemicals used. Variations in dye permeability into the polymer may also affect stains that work well for paraffin but not for methacrylate sections. Some dye or alcohol solutions will tend to lift sections off glass slides. Fortunately, special techniques for H&E and picro-fuchsin stain have been developed that give excellent results and are described below.

H&E Stain for Glycol Methacrylate The hematoxylin used for methacrylate sections in our laboratory is a strong half-oxidized hematoxylin based on Gill's formula [12]. Similar formulations are marketed as GILL Hematoxylin and are available from Lerner Laboratories, Stamford, Connecticut. Aqueous eosin is employed in order to dilute alcohols that may lift sections from the glass slides.

Hematoxylin Half-oxidized by Gill. Add ingredients in order:

1 365 ml distilled H_2O
2 125 ml ethylene glycol
3 2 gm anyhydrous powdered hematoxylin
4 0.2 gm sodium iodate (Na_2IO_3), weigh out accurately
5 40.25 gm ($Al(SO_4)_3 \cdot 16H_2O$) aluminum sulfate
6 0.5 gm anhydrous citric acid

Stain can be used after 1 hour of mixing. Filter through Whatman No. 1 filter paper before using.

Scott's Tap Water Substitute (pH 8.02).

1 liter H_2O distilled
10 gm magnesium sulfate, $MgSO_4$
2 gm sodium bicarbonate

Eosin-Phloxine (0.5 percent eosin Y, 0.1 percent phloxine in 0.2 percent acetic acid).

1 Add 0.6 ml glacial acetic acid to 500 ml distilled water.
2 Add 2.5 gm eosin Y and 0.5 gm phloxine.
3 Mix until dissolved, and filter before use.

Staining Procedure

1 Place slides directly into hematoxylin and stain 20–30 minutes.
2 Rinse in distilled water, three changes.
3 Blue in Scott's tap water substitute, 3 minutes.
4 Rinse in distilled water, two changes.
5 Stain in eosin-phloxine for 6–8 minutes.
6 Rinse in two changes of 95 percent ethanol, and one rinse in 100 percent.
7 Place in 100 percent ethanol 1 minute.
8 Clear in xylene, two changes, 2 minutes each.
9 Mount in synthetic mounting medium (Permount).

Staining times of the H&E will vary with the thickness of the sections. Thinner sections will require longer staining times. Bluing in tap water is not recommended because chlorine in the water may bleach out the stain.

Van Gieson (Picro-Fuchsin Stain) for Glycol Methacrylate [13]   This stain gives similar results to that used on paraffin sections. The combined nuclear stains of Celestine blue and Mayer's hematoxylin provide a more acid-fast stain that will not be removed by exposure to subsequent acidic solutions. Acid fuchsin stain that stains all tissue components red in GMA sections is applied. The sections are then allowed to dry. The red dye is then selectively removed from noncollagenous proteins in the picric acid differentiation. This step must be carefully controlled to avoid overdifferentiation. The picric acid also acts as a counterstain for muscle tissue and cytoplasm.

Solutions.

1   Celestine Blue
     Ferric ammonium sulfate   2.5 gm
     Distilled water   50.0 ml
     Add Celestine blue (CI No. 51050)   0.25 gm

Boil for 3 minutes, cool, filter and add 7 ml glycerol. This solution should be made up weekly. Old solutions will tend to cause precipitate to be deposited on slides.

2   Mayer's Hematoxylin
3   Acid Fuchsin/Ponceau S
     Acid Fuchsin (CI No. 42685)   0.5 gm
     Ponceau S (CI No. 27195)   0.5 gm
     1 percent Acetic Acid   100.0 ml
4   Picric Acid Differentiator
     SATURATED Aqueous Picric   65.0 ml
     Absolute ethanol   35.0 ml
5   Aqueous acetic acid   2 percent

Staining Method.

1   Place slides in Celestine blue, 10 minutes.
2   Rinse in distilled water.
3   Stain in Mayer's hematoxylin, 5 minutes.
4   Blue in running tap water, 5 minutes.
5   Stain in acid fuchsin-Ponceau S solution 4–5 minutes.
6   Rinse in distilled water; slides can air dry at this point if necessary.
7   Differentiate in alcoholic picric acid, 1 minute or less.
8   Rinse very quickly in 2 percent acetic acid.
9   Immediately blow dry with air. This is easily done with a blast of air from a can of Dust Off.
10   Coverslip dry section with Permount.

Results.

Collagen—red
Muscle—yellow orange
Nuclei—brown

THE HISTOLOGY ARCHIVES

With the advent of the Good Laboratory Practice (GLP) legislation that went into effect in 1979, safety studies for submission to the Food and Drug Administration (FDA) require special recording and filing procedures for specimens. These guidelines require traceability of any histology specimen from necropsy to the finished microscope slide. Appropriate written documentation is necessary including necropsy sheets; fixed tissue trim sheets; and embedding, section and staining records. These forms should be maintained on each animal in the study. All histological material, such as fixed tissue, paraffin or methacrylate blocks, and glass slides, is required to be properly labeled and retained in the designated archives. The blocks and slides can usually be stored indefinitely because no deterioration of these materials will occur under proper temperature conditions. Long-term storage of tissue in formalin is accompanied by a gradual decrease in pH that renders the tissue inadequate for evaluation. The GLP regulations state that wet tissue specimens should be retained for a period of at least 5 years after the date of an FDA submission or "as long as the quality affords evaluation" [14].

REFERENCES

1 Sheenan DC, Hrapchak BB. *Theory and Practice of Histotechnology*, 2nd ed. St. Louis: Mosby, 1980.
2 Luna LG. *Manual of Histologic Staining Methods of the Armed Forces Institute of Pathology*, 3rd ed. New York: McGraw Hill, 1968.
3 Matlaga BF, Salthouse TN. Ultrastructural observations of cells at the interface of a biodegradable polymer: Polygalactin 910. *J Biomed Mater Res*, 17 (1983), 185–197.
4 Bennett HS, Wyrick DA, Lee SW, et al. Science and art in preparing tissues embedded in plastic for light microscopy with special reference to glycol methacrylate, glass knives, and simple stains. *Stain Technol*, 51 (1976), 71–97.
5 Philpotts CJ. Plastic embedding for light microscopy. *Lab Equip Dig*, 5 (April, 1980), 81–87.
6 Janes RB. A review of three resin processing techniques applicable to light microscopy. *Med Lab Sci*, 36 (1979), 249–267.
7 Matlaga BF. Glycol methacrylate: Embedding, sectioning and staining for light microscopy. *Bull Soc Pharmacol Environ Pathol*, 4 (1976), 9–11.
8 Brown GG. *Primer of Histologic Technique*. New York: Appleton-Century-Crofts, 1969, 78–98.
9 Bancroft JD, Stevens A. *Theory and Practice of Histological Techniques*. New York: Churchill Livingstone, 1977, 46–55.
10 Griffin RL. *Ultramicrotomy*. Baltimore, MD: Williams and Wilkins, 1972, 22–34.
11 Glauert AM (Ed.). *Practical Methods in Electron Microscopy*, Vol. 3. New York: American Elsevier, 1974, 246–260.
12 Gill GW, Frost JK, Miller KA. A new formula for a half-oxidized hematoxylin solution that neither overstains nor requires differentiation. *Acta Cytol*, 18 (1974), 300–311.
13 Matlaga BF. A modified van Gieson type stain for glycol methacrylate sections. Unpublished paper.
14 *Federal Register*, December 22, 1978, 60019.

ADDITIONAL READING

1 Bancroft JD, Stevens A. *Theory and Practice of Histological Techniques*. New York: Churchill Livingstone, 1977.
2 Brown GG. *Primer of Histologic Technique*. New York: Appleton-Century-Crofts, 1969.
3 Glauert AM (Ed.). *Practical Methods in Electron Microscopy*, Vol. 3. New York: American Elsevier, 1974.
4 Luna LG. *Histopathologic Methods and Color Atlas of Special Stains and Tissue Artifacts*. Gaithersburg, MD: American Histolabs, Inc., 1992.
5 Sheenan DC, Hrapchak BB. *Theory and Practice of Histotechnology*, 2nd ed. St. Louis: Mosby, 1980.

Chapter 38

Evaluation by Light Microscopy

Stephen C. Woodward

CELLULAR RESPONSES TO IMPLANTED MATERIALS

The response to a biological implant is a specialized version of inflammation and repair, the mammalian reaction to local injury [1]. This response to local injury is nonspecific. The implant may contribute to the inflammatory response or simply may be located within a site of inflammation caused by the implantation procedure itself.

It is impossible to understand and evaluate the local response to an implant without understanding the inflammatory response evoked by the implant or caused by its implantation. An acute inflammatory response attends any implant for a few days. All chronically persistent, non-degraded implants elicit a foreign body response. These responses cannot be placed in context if they are not understood as inevitable local responses.

The testing of a new biomaterial in man, regardless of its proposed specialized use, generally includes the gross and microscopic examination of the response to the material implanted in test animals. The extent and duration of the acute and chronic inflammation response evoked by subcutaneous or intramuscular implants anticipates the response to them in parenchymal organs or other specialized sites [2]. Furthermore, the extent and duration of the inflammatory response in the rodent, dog, or rabbit are comparable to those found in man, allowing prediction of the response in man.

Introducing an implant itself incites an inflammatory response; hence, during the first 24 to 48 hours following implantation, the implant will be seen within a field of acute inflammation, the result of the procedure itself. During this period, the cardinal signs of acute inflammation develop: *redness* (generalized local vascular dilatation), *heat* (increased local blood flow), *swelling* (increased local vascular permeability), and *pain* (local accumulation of chemical mediators). After 2–3 days, any persistent local inflammatory response to the implant usually can be distinguished from the resolving, declining response to the procedure itself. Because an inflammatory process always develops, the events characterizing inflammation will be examined.

When a "nonabsorbable" material is implanted, transient acute inflammation persisting less than a week and slowly developing encapsulation by fibrous connective tissue follows, requiring one month or longer to develop. The capsule surrounding an implant generally is static. In rodents, however, the implant capsule may become transformed into a sarcoma after 6 months, an outcome to be considered in long-term testing. The induction of fibrosarcomas in rats, mice and hamsters by films or discs implanted subcutaneously must never be forgotten in planning tests lasting six months or longer. This problem is peculiar to rats, mice and hamsters but not other species and is reviewed elsewhere [3, 4] and detailed in Chapter 19.

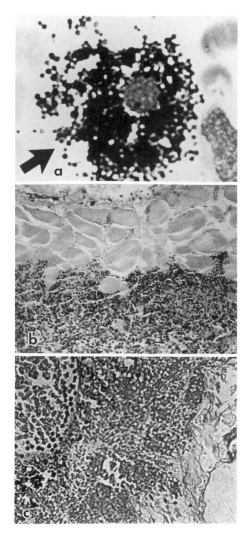

Figure 38-1 Necrosis and acute inflammation. (A) Degranulating mast cell. Mast cells are fragile, containing vascular mediators serotinin and histamine, as well as anticoagulant heparin. Their degranulation initiates the inflammatory response. Giemsa, X500. (B) Necrosis of tissue cells is the principal trigger of the inflammatory response. Pink, necrotic muscle cells at top were chemically killed by cyanoacrylate. Inflammatory response (bottom) is adjacent to necrotic muscle. Injury is 2 weeks old. Hematoxylin and eosin, X50, (C) Inflammatory cells are delivered to site of injury through dilated, permeable blood vessels, mostly postcapillary venules. Injury is 5 days old. Leukocytes marginate and escape through intercellular pores, migrating toward site of injury. Dilated venule with adherent leukocytes, top left, site of necrosis on right. Hematoxylin and eosin, X127.

Necrosis of Cells and Tissues—The Trigger of Inflammation

Necrosis, the death of cells, starts a series of events leading to healing and restitution of function. Morphological changes identifying necrotic cells are well described [5]. Necrosis sets the inflammatory response in motion, permitting the removal by digestion of dead cells. Persistent or intensifying acute inflammation with accumulation of necrotic cells or stromal cells, as contrasted with resolution of these events, suggests that the implant is releasing chemical products that are locally toxic (Figure 38-1A).

Mast Cells and Vascular Responses

Degranulation of mast cells triggers inflammation. Mast cells are permanent residents of perivascular connective tissue. These 15 μm granule-rich cells contain heparin (an anticoagulant), histamine (a potent agent increasing vascular permeability and transvascular passage of leukocytes), and serotonin (which is also vasoactive). The degranulation of mast cells (Figure 38-1B) causes increased vascular permeability followed by the local accumulation of protein-rich edema fluid.

Increased vascular permeability causing increased viscosity of the blood as protein is lost to the extracellular space. Progressive stasis of blood flow and the development of edema follow. Local cellular necrosis developing at the same time damages nearby capillary microvasculature. Prolonged leakage of red blood cells, fibrin, and other proteins accompanied by thrombosis of the microvasculature is characteristic of necrotizing inflammatory responses. As the acute inflammatory response subsides, dilatation of the preexisting vascular bed diminishes, and a new capillary bed develops. The newly forming capillaries are part of the granulation tissue that will repair the site of injury.

Granulocytes and Acute Inflammation

Polymorphonuclear leukocytes (neutrophils) predominate in early inflammation. These bone-marrow-derived cells are attracted by chemoattractants released locally by damaged cells or by the implant and migrate through the walls of venules (Figure 38-1C). Neutrophils are the first defense against bacteria, releasing peroxidases, lysozyme, and other proteolytic and hydrolytic enzymes contained within their granules. These enzymes contribute to the degradation of such materials as catgut and silk sutures [6].

Remove the cause for a persistent acute inflammation, and granulocytes disappear from the site in a few days. Under a variety of circumstances including infection and degradation of biomaterials, persistent acute inflammation is found [7]. The usual causes of persistent, local leukocytes include infection and biodegradation of the implant. Infection can be established as the cause by identifying microorganisms utilizing tissue Gram stain, or other histological stains for microorganisms, or with greater sensitivity by culturing the site. Biodegradation (or the release of materials being leached from the implant) can be inferred when the site is found to be sterile. Biodegradation can be established as the cause of persistent acute inflammation by measuring the excretion products of isotopically tagged polymeric implants. The inflammatory properties of the degradation products can be determined if these degradation products can be chemically isolated, characterized, and directly tested by implantation. In tissue sections, extravascular neutrophils before their degranulation exhibit a characteristic trilobular nucleus resembling a three-leafed clover, a feature distinguishing them from the slightly larger monocyte.

The persistence of neutrophils in tissues implies their continued accumulation there, because of their 48-hour or shorter viability extravascularly. The persistent and progressive accumulation of leukocytes, whether caused by infection or a toxically-degrading implant, leads to abscess formation, with leukocyte-mediated proteolytic digestion of local tissue structures.

Monocytes and Macrophages—Cells of Subacute Inflammation

Macrophages arrive at inflammatory response somewhat more slowly than do neutrophils, but their persistence and phagocytosis promote the transformation of an exudate into vascularized connective tissue and lead to repair. More robust than neutrophils in resisting the acidic conditions resulting from degranulation of neutrophils, the macrophage is the ultimate scavenger cell of the host [1, 2]. The mononuclear phagocytes develop in the bone marrow, circulate in the blood as monocytes, and finally reside in the tissues as the tissue macrophage.

Macrophages generally exhibit an ovoid or irregular shape, with plentiful cytoplasm and with an oval or kidney-shaped nucleus. In electron microscopic preparations, projections from the cell surface are often prominent. Fingerlike projections (pseudopodia) or platelike projections (lammellipodia) are characteristic. Utilizing enzyme histochemical preparations, macrophages demonstrate much higher hydrolase activity than either the granulocytes or fibroblasts.

The enzyme activity of macrophages is contained within intracellular lysosomes. These enzymes effect enzymatic intracellular digestion. In this process, phagocytosis, the macrophage localizes the material within an enzyme-containing digestion vesicle, the primary lysosome, to form the secondary lysosome. The hydrolases within lysosomes will then if possible degrade the ingested material (see Chapter 42, Figure 42-3).

Activated macrophages, those prepared for or engaging in phagocytosis, will be observed at the surface of all implanted biomaterials. Their numbers will be proportional to the toxicity of the implant material. With smooth-walled, nontoxic materials, the macrophage population is never conspicuous, and by two weeks macrophages will be largely replaced by fibroblasts and later by a fibrous capsule. With implants having rough or irregular surfaces, macrophages will remain active at the interface indefinitely. Under these circumstances, macrophages will undergo cell division, and a self replicating population of macrophages will remain adjacent to the implant.

Lymphocytes and Plasma Cells—Cells of Chronic Inflammation

Lymphocytes are round, 5–10 μm cells derived both from the bone marrow and from lymph nodes. They are characteristically present at sites of chronic inflammation. Small numbers of lymphocytes are always present at sites of resolving injury, and large collections of lymphocytes are characteristic of immunological injury.

Plasma cells are produced from bone marrow-derived lymphocytes, and are about 20 μm in diameter. Their characteristic cartwheel nuclei and intensely staining cytoplasm identify them. Plasma cells are the source of immunoglobulins secreted into sites of chronic injury. At sites of chronic inflammation, the numbers of plasma cells and lymphocytes is related to the underlying cause of the inflammation. In conditions of chronic immunological injury, these cells predominate over other inflammatory cells. Implants having antigenic properties, such as amino acid polymers, may incite a response in which plasma cells and lymphocytes are prominent. These cells are also present at sites of persistent chronic inflammation in which granulomas develop.

Giant Cells, Granulomas, and Chronic Inflammation

In addition to macrophages, plasma cells, and lymphocytes, the chronic inflammatory response surrounding nonabsorbable materials contains foreign-body giant cells (Figure 38-2A–C). Giant cells are formed at sites of chronic inflammation from the fusion of monocytes. Giant cells are conspicuous at sites of granulomatous inflammation in chronic infections. A wide variety of agents evoke granulomatous inflammation, including microorganisms causing cell-mediated hypersensitivity. Other materials inciting the formation of granulomas include cotton fibers (Figure 38-2D), silica, talc, beryllium, and zirconium [9].

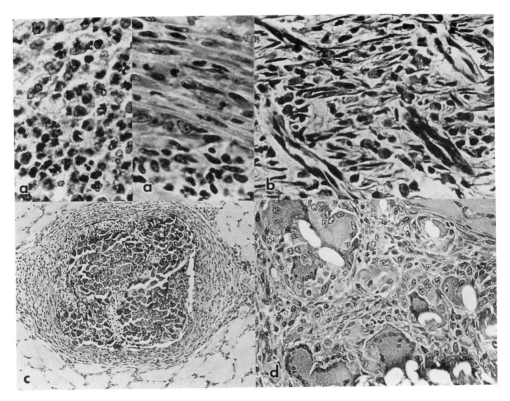

Figure 38-2 Chronic inflammation and repair. (A) Left: acute response at 4 days containing neutrophils and occasional macrophages and plasma cell. Implant below. Hematoxylin and eosin, X160. Right: transition from acute to chronic response. Implant at bottom left. A few neutrophils remain, together with macrophages and an outer population of fibroblasts in the primary stage of capsule formation. Seven days postimplant. Hematoxylin and eosin, X160. (B) Granulation tissue at 14 days. Capillaries and fibroblasts are oriented tangentially, but in an ordered array. Mononuclear cells, plasma cells and pink collagen fibers are visible. Hematoxylin and eosin, X250. (C) Multifilament sutures produce an encapsulated foreign-body response. 7-0 silk suture within rabbit muscle at 7 days. Zone of reaction contains neutrophils, macrophages, and fibroblasts. Suture filaments are being separated by reacting cells. Hematoxylin and eosin, X35. (D) Typical chronic granulomatous response evoked by presence of cotton fibers in rat subcutaneous tissue at 3 weeks. Many multinucleated giant cells surround fibers. Activated macrophages are present, represented as the smaller cells between the giant cells. Hematoxylin and eosin, X160.

No unique contribution of giant cells to chronic inflammation is known. Their phagocytic function is less developed than that of macrophages and their ability to secrete enzymes is similar to those of macrophages. Giant cells represent the boundary between the host and many forms of implants, as will be described.

Granulomatous inflammation heals by fibrous scarring once the inciting cause is localized or eliminated. A special modified form of granulomatous inflammation represents the final host response to nonabsorbable or slowly absorbable implants with irregular surfaces or multiple filaments. This contrasts with the response to implants recognized by the host as smooth surfaced. When multifilament sutures or other sutures with rough surfaces are implanted, irrespective of the site, large, often highly irregular foreign-body giant cells, on occasion containing 100 or more nuclei and measuring up to 200 μm invest every surface irregularity and act as the boundary between the host and the implant. Both macrophages and giant cells phagocytize polymer fragments and cellular debris. When the biomaterial cannot be degraded, this localizing response is permanent, progressing no further, and turnover of cells is indolent.

Encapsulation and Organization—A Specialized Form of Wound Repair

Development of Granulation Tissue and Secretion of Collagen   As acute inflammation subsides, granulation tissue forms at sites of injury. Granulation tissue, a transient, specialized organ of repair, consists of capillaries, collagen-secreting fibroblasts, contractile fibroblasts, and chronic inflammatory cells. Granulation tissue is the site of elaboration of reparative collagen. Rapid blood flow through granulation tissue provides a metabolic environment permitting fibroblasts to proliferate and elaborate collagen. The extent of granulation tissue development adjacent to prosthetic implants relates to their size and surface characteristics, as well as their degree of chemical inertness [10]. Large, rough-surfaced implants evoke extensive granulation tissue development and subsequent broad scars.

In skin wounds, collagen secretion by fibroblasts takes place in three phases, a lag phase (lasting a few days, during which inflammation predominates) a log phase (lasting several weeks, during which the rapid secretion of collagen and the accretion of tensile strength parallel each other), followed by a lengthy phase of remodeling and maturation (during which collagen becomes internally and externally cross-linked and insoluble). This sequence is inhibited when acute inflammation occurs, infection supervenes, or the chemical breakdown products of a biodegradable material cause continuing local necrosis [7].

In wound repair, two principal types of collagen predominate: type I, normally found in skin and tendon, and secreted by fibroblasts, and type III, a normal constituent of the aorta, lung, and embryonal skin. Collagen is a rigid triple helix containing glycine-rich, repeated amino acid triplets as -Gly-AA_1-AA_2, with the signal imino acids hydroxy-proline and hydroxylysine in position AA_2 [11]. The oxidation of the amino acid sequence -Gly-Pro-Pro- to -Gly-Pro-Hypro- by prolyl hydroxylase provides a quantifying, unique amino acid, hydroxyproline. Measures of hydroxyproline permit quantitation of collagen formation at repair sites. Intra- and intercellular cross-linking of collagen provides tensile strength and insolubility [11].

Light and electron microscopy are imprecise in quantitative measurement of the amount of collagen at a repair site, or in estimating the amount of collagen being elaborated, even when special staining procedures are used [12]. By contrast, the collagen content of granulation tissue can be precisely determined by measuring its hydroxyproline content [12]. A sensitive measure of the chemical toxicity of a polymeric implant is its ability to inhibit local collagen formation [12].

Long-Term Encapsulating Responses

Inert Smooth-Surfaced Implants   Chemically nonreactive materials such as monofilament nylon sutures, coupons of stainless steel, silicon disks, or Teflon® rods, are surrounded by circumferentially oriented fibroblasts within 2 weeks of implantation. These fibroblasts secrete collagen oriented parallel to the implant's surface. The final response contains only a few vessels, rare lymphocytes and monocytes and is devoid of giant cells. The zone of repair is more compact in muscle than in subcutaneous tissues and consequently appears more compressed and cellular in muscle. The interface between the host and the foreign body is permanent, and the cells and collagen participating in it turn over extremely slowly after the interfacing response is established (Figure 38-3).

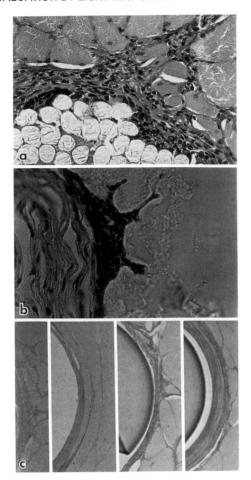

Figure 38-3 Encapsulating responses. (A) Tissue reaction to biodegradable copolymer suture at 2 weeks. Macrophages and giant cell adjacent to implant, with fibroblasts secreting collagen fibers at periphery, X400. (B) Foreign-body giant cells may contain several hundred nuclei, as well as attenuated cytoplasmic processes. This giant cell occupies a portion of the edge of a 4-month deposit of hexyl a-cyanoacrylate, a bland, nondegraded material of irregular contour. Hematoxylin and eosin, X145. (C) Left to right: response to monofilament nylon suture at 1 week, 3 weeks, 3 months, and 6 months in rabbit muscle. The encapsulating collagen follows the contour of the sutures. Methacrylate-embedded preparations pink-stained with iron hemtoxylin-picrofuchsin, X230.

Inert Implants with Irregular Surfaces

Surface irregularities as small as 10–15 μm result in the development of giant cells as the principal cellular interface between the host and nonreactive implant. The cytoplasmic processes of the giant cells adapt to surface irregularities with fidelity, anchoring to the implant. The giant cells are surrounded by irregular, generally circumferentially oriented collagen and small blood vessels. The turnover rate of cells and collagen after this response is established is very slow [2].

Biodegradable Implants

The response to biodegraded materials is controlled by the rate of degradation, but more significantly by the toxicity of the breakdown products [2]. The corrosion products of metallic implants usually are incorporated into macrophages or giant cells and incite little other response from the host. The breakdown products of chromic catgut sutures evoke a moderately persistent inflammatory response that diminishes as the suture degrades. Polyglycolic acid evokes much less of a response than catgut because it slowly disappears [13]. Surprisingly, some materials, such as polyester and silk, generally thought of as nondegradable, appear to degrade slowly, but evoke little or no persistent inflammation [6]. Multifilament silk sutures evoke an unusual response: the suture is "exploded," its filaments being separated by infiltrating monocytes and a few neutrophils. A wide zone of fibroblasts surrounds the suture. Catgut sutures degrade similarly, except that neutrophils persist at the site. Polyglycolic acid and polylactic—polyglycolic copolymer sutures evoke a milder response than catgut, yet sites of their resorption appear active, with persistence of a mixed inflammatory response, as well as occasional giant cells and blood vessels [6].

A still more reactive biodegradable material is poly (methyl 2-cyanoacrylate). The degradation of this tissue adhesive is associated with a necrotizing acute inflammatory response persisting for months in which neutrophils predominate. The degradation of poly-(methyl 2-cyanoacrylate) inhibits the development of collagen and thus retards repair [7].

These examples illustrate how the local response is modified by the surface structure of the implant and its degradation products. The responses described are similar irrespective of the site of implantation [6].

Implant Properties Affecting Tissue Response

The variables that significantly influence the local histological response to an implant include surface characteristics, size (see Section II), chemical composition (see Section I), and location of implantation (see Section VI). Each of these must be taken into account when attempting to compare the reactivity of an uninvestigated material under development with those already in use.

Surface Characteristics   Surface characteristics range from geometrical implant shape configuration to surface topographic irregularities. By comparing the responses to extruded 1-mm diameter cylinders with those to pentagonal and triangular rods of the same surface area composed of various nonabsorbable polymers, including polyvinyl chloride. Salthouse and Matlaga showed that the circular configuration evoked a narrower zone of fibrosis than that seen surrounding the triangular or pentagonal implants, particularly at the apices of their angulations [10]. In addition, lysosomal enzyme activity, as measured by acid phosphatase content of the capsule surrounding a circular implant, at 14 days was only half that found adjacent to a triangular implant. Thus, to control for geometrical effects, materials under development and being evaluated for histocompatibility should be implanted as cylinders or rods.

Surface characteristics also affect the response. Surface topographic irregularities promote the development of a foreign-body giant cell response as contrasted with the circumferentially oriented collagen comprising the wall of a fluid-filled pocket, which is the response to nonreactive, smooth-surfaced materials (Figure 38-3A, B, C). The effects produced by surface irregularities were examined by abrading Teflon® rods and comparing the effects produced by abrasion on the histochemistry of the surrounding capsule. Salthouse and Matlaga [10] observed that the capsules surrounding abraded rods, as compared with smooth-surfaced ones, showed persistently increased levels of acid phosphatase, glucose-6-phosphate dehydrogenase, and succinic dehydrogenase for 90 days. These enzyme activities were localized to the increased populations of macrophages surrounding the abraded rods. Encapsulation was retarded by abrasion. These results strongly suggest, as a standard condition, that in initial tests, the material have as smooth a surface as possible. Obviously materials are also fabricated as meshes, weaves, or other complex geometries, with varying degrees of surface irregularities. The modifying effects of such fabrication can be identified, by comparing the response to that of standard, smooth-surfaced cylinder. The effects of the physical structure of the implant on the response are summarized in Table 38-1.

Table 38-1   Characteristic Responses to the Geometry and Surface of the Implant

Configuration	Ultimate response
Circular, smooth*	Circumferential fibroblasts and collagen, minimal response
Angular, smooth	Collagen and oriented parallel to surface, chronic inflammation at angularities
Rough, irregular	Foreign-body giant cell response, chronic inflammation, and persistent vascularization
Powders* (less than 250 mm)	Foreign-body response with phagocytosis of powder by macrophages and giant cells; granulomatous inflammation
Porous	Infiltration of granulation tissue ultimately producing dense fibrous entrapment

*Both responses can be elicited by the same material, such as PTFE (Teflon®), depending on the physical structure.

Size of Implant   Generally, small implants give more uniform responses than larger ones, in part because they tend to migrate less and their movement is less traumatic to surrounding tissues than movement by a larger implant. If possible, nonabsorbable materials should be fabricated as cylinders 1–4 mm in diameter and 10 mm or less in length. Many such implants can be placed in the same animal and removed sequentially, if necessary. Flat coupons of metal measuring about 10 mm in diameter and 1–2 mm thick are often employed to examine the reactivity and corrosion of the material.

Chemical Composition   In addition to the toxic effects of impurities present on the surface of the implant or plasticizers that may be leached from it, other chemical features related to biodegradation strongly affect the histological response to a degradable material. In general, active enzymatic breakdown of a biodegradable is associated with persistent inflammation, such as the mononuclear response to degrading catgut or the persistent, intense infiltrate of neutrophils attending the degradation of methyl 2-cyanoacrylate [7]. In addition, biodegradable polymers tend to undergo loss of molecular weight with resultant change in physical characteristics, such as increasing brittleness resulting in fracturing and particulate formation. This may result in a previously quiescent capsule being replaced by one of foreign-body response with phagocytosis of the particulate, as was observed in the ultimate degradation of poly (ε-caprolactone) [14]. The degree of reactivity of various materials is given in Table 38-2 which also suggests suitable positive highly reactive controls and nonreactive, negative controls.

Location of Implant   The initial testing of polymeric material is usually carried out in the subcutaneous space or in the deep musculature. The response at these sites is similar and is generally predictive of responses elsewhere. The subcutaneous site measures inflammation, and the intramuscular site predicts necrosis in the cardiovascular system and in parenchymal organs.

Suggestions for Experimental Design

In examining a new chemical formulation, the following questions should be addressed:

    1 Is the material biodegradable? This questions can usually be resolved by observation for persistent acute inflammation at two weeks or the persistence of numerous

Table 38-2   Reactions Produced by Implants, Varying from Inconspicuous (Top) to Intense (Bottom)

Implant	Implantation site	Response
Nonreactive, nonabsorbable		
Monofilament nylon, PTFE (Teflon®) or polypropylene sutures	Muscle or subcutaneous	Narrow, fibrous capsule
Silicone elastomers	Subcutaneous	Fibrous capsule
Nonreactive, biodegradable polyglycolic acid and polyglycolic–polylactic copolymer monofilament sutures	Muscle or subcutaneous	Minimal chronic inflammation, no capsule
Intermediate		
Catgut sutures	Muscle	Persistent mononuclear and giant cell response
Stainless steel monofilament	Muscle	Mononuclear response, first 2-4 weeks
Strongly reactive, biodegradable Methyl 2-cyanoacrylate	Subcutaneous, muscle	Persistent acute inflammation and necrosis
Resins containing organometallics, cadmium, or chromium	Subcutaneous	Persistent acute inflammation

macrophages beyond three-four weeks at subcutaneous or intramuscular implantation sites because persistent inflammation often accompanies biodegradation. Thus, observation at one, two, four and eight weeks generally will suffice to detect early biodegradation or continued reactivity although observations for as long as two years may be required to detect slow breakdown, and physical measures of the integrity and weights of recovered implants, accompanied by studies of excretion of isotopically tagged polymers, ultimately may be required for resolution of the issue of biodegradation.

2   If the implant degrades, does the degradation process evoke an acute inflammatory response? Is the encapsulating response slow to develop, suggesting continuing reactivity or biodegradation? Measuring the zone of acute or chronic inflammation around an implant quantifies reactivity. Similarly, measuring the width of acid phosphatase reactivity can also serve this purpose [10]. Prolonged inflammation, and slow development of a capsule suggests a toxic local response.

3   Does the material inhibit collagen elaboration? The elaboration of collagen is fundamental to wound repair, since during the early phases of this process, increasing tensile strength parallels increasing collagen content of the wound [15].

The inhibition of collagen elaboration can be quantitated by incorporating a powder prepared from biomaterial into polyvinyl alcohol-formal sponges. These are then placed subcutaneously, removed at 7 and 14 days, and compared with controls with respect to wet weight (inflammation), dry weight (connective tissue content), and hydroxyproline content, an identifying imimo acid of collagen [16]. Histological sections of sponges can be examined for their degree of persistent inflammation and organization. Utilizing this procedure, the author has quantified the histotoxicity of several microscopically inflammatory cyanacrylates [7] by measuring their local inhibition of the accumulation of hydroxyproline and shown that polyglycolic acid and poly (ε-caprolactone) [14] powders do not inhibit collagen elaboration by this test and are noninflammatory. Other biochemical measures of collagen elaboration, such as the accumulation of prolylhydroxylase, or of the presence of macrophage enzymes, such as acid phosphatase, can be obtained also from sponge implants. These quantitative measures of inflammation and repair often provide more sensitive indicators of reactivity and local accumulation of collagen than does light microscopy. Microscopic examination contributes unique additional insight into the local response to the biomaterial.

    4   If the material does not degrade, is a smooth-surfaced cylinder encapsulated by a narrow zone of fibrous repair similar to that observed with an appropriate negative control (see Table 38-2 for examples).

Limitations of Light Microscopy

Although light microscopy is the most commonly employed method to evaluate host–biomaterial interactions, it has several significant limitations that should be recognized:

    1   The estimation of collagen production at an implant site is at best semiquantitative; additional chemical determinations are required for quantification.

    2   Intracellular sites of degradation cannot be visualized when particles undergoing degradation are less than 2–4 μm in diameter; electron microscopy is required for this determination [14].

    3   Routine hematoxylin—eosin stains do not allow for quantitative analysis of the chronic inflammatory response adjacent to an implant; they should usually be accompanied by acid phosphatase and other enzyme histochemical techniques.

    4   A false impression that bioabsorption is occurring can result from dissolution of a polymeric material in the solvents used in preparing histological sections. An organizational response surrounding an empty space calls attention to this misleading artifact. Observing this, the solubility of the biomaterial in tissue-processing solutions should be assessed.

RECOMMENDATIONS AND CONCLUSIONS

The evaluation of a biomaterial implant by light microscopy requires an understanding of the local inflammatory response and the various subsequent responses of organization and repair utilized by the host. Light microscopy is technically rapid, and is capable of answering many important questions concerning reactivity, such as the duration and intensity of inflammation, and reveals the type of localizing response to the implant. The sensitivity of light microscopy is enhanced by utilization of appropriate histochemical measures of chronic inflammation. The use of positive and negative controls allows at least a semiquantitative estimate of the reactivity of the material.

    The effects of variations in implant structure, surface characteristics and geometry should be recognized, because of the differences in the host response which can result solely from variations in these physical features.

    Finally, the effects of the implantation procedure, and the understanding of the response of the host by light microscopy is essential to proper toxicological assessment of any biological implant.

REFERENCES

1   Rubin E, Farber JL. *Pathology*, 2nd ed. Philadelphia, PA: Lippencott, 1994, 44–55.

2   Rubin E, Farber JL. *Pathology*, 2nd ed. Philadelphia, PA: Lippencott, 1994, 70–94.

3   Brand GK. Human foreign-body carcinogenesis in the light of animal experiments and assessment of cancer risk at implant sites. In Rubin LR (Ed.), *Biomaterials in Reconstructive Surgery*. St. Louis: Mosby; 1983, 36–39.

4   Woodward SC. How to relate observations of foreign-body oncogenesis in experimental animals to human health risk. In Rubin LR (Ed.), *Biomaterials in Reconstructive Surgery*. St. Louis: Mosby, 1983, 17–26.

5   Majno G et al. Cellular death and necrosis. *Virchows Arch* 333 (1960), 421–441.
6   Salthouse TN. Tissue response to sutures. In Rubin LR (Ed.), *Biomaterials in Reconstructive Surgery*. St. Louis: Mosby; 1983, 131–142.
7   Woodward SC. The effect of cyanoacrylate tissue adhesives upon granulation tissue formation in Ivalon sponge implants in the rat. *Surgery*, 59 (1966), 559–565.
8   Chambers TJ. Multinucleate giant cells. *J Path*, 126 (1978), 125–148.
9   Adams DO. The granulomatous inflammatory response: A review. *Am J Pathol*, 86 (1978), 164–191.
10 Salthouse T, Matlaga BF. Some cellular effects related to implant shape and surface. In Rubin LR (Ed.), *Biomaterials in Reconstructive Surgery*. St. Louis: Mosby, 1983, 40–45.
11 Prockup DJ, et al. The biosynthesis of collagen and its disorders. *N Engl J Med*, 301 (1979), 13–23, 77–85.
12 Woodward SC. Physiological and biochemical evaluation of implanted polymers. *Ann NY Acad Sci*, 146 (1966), 225–250.
13 Miller RA, et al. Degradation rates of oral resorbable implants (polylactides and polyglycolates): Rate modification with changes in PLA/PGA copolymer ratios. *J Biomed Mater Res*, 11 (1977), 711–719.
14 Woodward SC, et al. The intracellular degradation of poly (ε-caprolactone). *J Biomed Mater Res*, 19 (1985), 437–444.
15 Davidson JM. Growth factors in wound healing. *Wounds*, 5 (1995), Suppl. A .
16 Woodward SC, Herrmann JB. Stimulation of fibroplasia in rats by bovine cartilage powder. *Arch Surg*, 96 (1968), 189–199.
17 Sewell WR, et al. New method of comparing sutures. *Surg Gyn Obstet*, 100 (1955), 483–499.
18 Gourlay SJ, et al. Biocompatibility testing of polymers: *In vivo* implantation studies. *J Biomed Mater Res*, 12 (1978), 219–228.
19 Black J. *Biological Performance of Polymers*. New York: Marcel Dekker, 1981, 46–86.

ADDITIONAL READING

Inflammatory Responses, Wound Repair and Biomaterials

1   Liping T, Eaton JW. Inflammatory responses to biomaterials. *Amer J Clin Path*, 103 (1995), 466–471.
2   Davidson JM. Wound repair. In Gallin JI, Goldstein IM, Snyderman R, (Eds.), *Inflammation: Basic Principles and Clinical Correlates*. New York: Raven Press, 1992, 809–819.
3   Davidson JM, Buckley-Sturrock A, Woodward SC. Growth factors and wound repair. In Abatangelo G, Davidson JM (Eds.), *Cutaneous Development, Aging and Repair*. Padova: Liviana Press, 1989, 115–129.
4   Cohen IK, Diegelmann, RD, Lindblad, WJ. *Wound Healing*. New York: W. B. Saunders, 1992, 544–548.
5   Janssen H, Rooman R, Robertson JIS. *Wound Healing*. Petersfield, UK: Wrightson Biomedical Publishers, 1991, 150–160.

In Vivo Evaluation of Biomaterials

6   Black J. *Biological Performance of Materials*. New York: Marcel Dekker, 1981.
7   Williams DF. *Techniques for Examination of Tissues in Implant Retrieval Analysis*. Washington, DC: National Bureau of Standards, 1982, 323–338.

APPENDIX

A Uniform Test Scheme to Evaluate Implants

Various approaches have been suggested to increase objectivity and to evolve a scoring or rating system for the tissue response or reaction to implants. An earlier suggestion by Sewell et al. [17] and later ones by Gourlay [18] Salthouse [10] and Black [19] are useful in ranking the biocompatibility of samples. It is essential that samples to be compared are of identical shape and surface [10]. A selection of methods is given below.

Sample Implantation   Implantation in rat gluteal muscle or rabbit paravertebral muscle is suggested. Samples must be identical in shape and surface. For polymers 10 to 115 mm in length, 0.5 mm diameter can be implanted using a wide-bore needle and trochar. A low reactive control, such as polypropylene, should be included.

Implantation periods of 7, 21, 42, 90, and 180 days will encompass both acute and chronic inflammatory responses. The number of samples and animals should be sufficient for statistical requirements. Adequate controls should be included. Implantation under aseptic conditions is essential. Histological cross sections by either the paraffin or methacrylate procedures should be prepared and stained by hematoxylin and eosin (see Chapter 37).

Rating System

The rating system described below uses samples of 0.5 mm diameters as an example. Such a system can be modified in several ways to suit other sizes and types of implants or requirements.

Grades for Reaction Thickness   The diameter and area of tissue reaction zones can be measured by either point counting eyepiece or by image analysis systems.

Grade 1	0–50 mm zone diameter
2	50–100 mm zone diameter
3	100–500 mm zone diameter
4	500–1000 mm zone diameter
5	1000–2000 mm zone diameter

Cellular Response Grade   Grade 0 to 5 depending on concentration of cells in reaction zone area (cell density).

Weighting Factors   These can be assigned based on the reaction zone characteristics. See tabulation example below.

Reaction zone size	5
Cell density	3
Cell type:	
Neutrophils	5
Giant cells	2
Macrophages	1
Fibroblasts	1
Lymphocytes	1

To continue the example, the final rating might be as follows:

Reaction zone grade 3 × factor 5	15
Cellular response grade 2 × factor 3	6
Cell types Neutrophils 5 × factor 5	25
Macrophages 1 × factor 5	5
Rating:	51

Such a numerical rating can be arbitrarily expressed as follows:

No reaction	0
Minimal	1–10
Slight	11–25
Moderate	26–40
Marked	41–60
Extreme	60+

Chapter 39

Evaluation by Scanning Electron Microscopy

Steven L. Goodman

INTRODUCTION

Microscopy is the only family of scientific instrumentation which provides direct information on the spatial relationships of the biological, chemical, and physical events which occur at biomaterial interfaces. Within the last two decades entirely new microscopies have been developed including atomic force, near field optical, and confocal light, while both light and electron microscopy have undergone a renaissance through improvements in optics, labeling probes, and the application of digital techniques. With these developments it is possible to image dynamic cellular events in real time with light microscopy, and subsequently to examine three-dimensional structure at nanometer-level resolution with electron microscopy [1, 2]. Even though scanning electron microscopy (SEM) is generally incapable of imaging living systems, it is extremely well suited for biomaterials investigations. Since SEM permits the imaging of uncut or bulk samples, this greatly simplifies the study of difficult-to-section ceramic, metal, and polymeric biomaterials. Combined with its wide magnification range, this permits one to relate ultrastructure to the gross morphology of complex, three-dimensional biomaterials (Figure 39-1). Finally, SEM places few limitations on the sample's physical nature, such as the optical or electron transparency required for transmission microscopy, or the need for relatively flat materials for atomic force and scanning tunneling microscopy. Thus, SEM imaging may be applied to virtually any biomaterials investigation.

Since the basic techniques of SEM sample preparation and imaging are generally known, this chapter concentrates on two other areas. The first is to introduce the broad diversity of SEM techniques available to examine biological and biomaterial structure. The second, and potentially more important area, is to assist the biomaterials scientist in developing an eye for the critical interpretation of SEM images. SEM images are often misunderstood, probably because they appear to have such shadow and depth that we are compelled to interpret them as if we are seeing sunlit objects as in the macroscopic world of everyday experience. However, such interpretation can be misleading since the physics of image formation in an SEM is significantly different than the reflection of light.

THE BASICS OF SEM IMAGE FORMATION

A brief outline of SEM image formation is a necessary precondition for understanding sample preparation and image interpretation. Since an in-depth discussion of SEM imaging is well beyond the scope of this chapter, the interested reader is referred to the texts and monographs listed under Additional Reading.

Very briefly, SEM samples are placed in a high vacuum where they are scanned in a raster pattern by a finely focused (1–10 nm diameter) beam of high energy (1–30 keV)

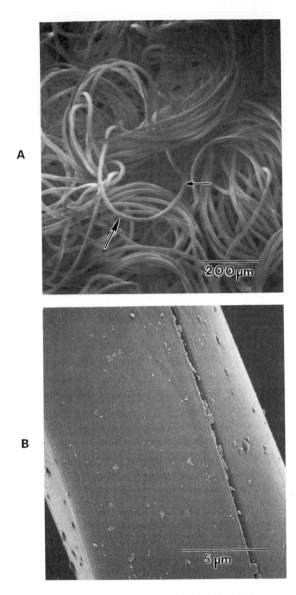

Figure 39-1   Medical grade polyethylene teraphthalate velour fabric. (A) Low magnification image shows the overall structure and demonstrates the large depth of field of SEM. Note that a
single fibril traverses a vertical distance of 400μm between the two arrows, as measured using
stereo photogrammetry. (The larger arrow identifies the upper point.) Thus, the front-to-back
depth of this image is comparable to its full width. (B) At higher resolution the surface structure
of the central fiber above the smaller arrow in Figure 1A is shown at a scale comparable to cellular
size. Ion beam Pt coated and SE imaged at 1.5 keV.

electrons. The energetic electrons of the primary beam induce the emission of electrons,
X-rays, and other signals from the sample. One or more of these emissions are then detected
and used to create an image by modulating the brightness of points on a video screen scanned
in synchrony with the electron beam. Secondary electron (SE) images are what typically
come to mind when one thinks of SEM as these are the most widely used for image formation.

SEs provide information on sample topography because their low energy (50 eV) prevents them from traveling far through solid samples, thus ensuring that the signal is generated near the sample surface. Also of interest in biomaterial investigations are the back-scattered electrons (BSE), primary beam electrons which were scattered following their interaction with the nuclei in the sample. Since BSEs can have an energy up to that of the primary beam, even when interactions occur well below the surface these, can escape from the sample and be detected. Consequently, BSEs are less influenced by sample topography than SEs, and provide images which are strongly dependent upon atomic number and density. Hence SE and BSE images provide complementary information on sample structure. In addition to electron emission, specimens scanned with electron beams also emit X-rays characteristic of elemental content, which may be used to produce maps of elemental distribution. Since the focus on this chapter is morphology, X-ray microanalysis will not be discussed further (see Additional Reading).

Types of SEM Instrumentation

For the purposes of this chapter, three types of SEM instruments can be defined. The first is the conventional SEM (C-SEM), characterized as having a thermionic electron source of tungsten or lanthanum hexaboride (LaB_6), and typically used at accelerating voltages in the 10–30 keV range. The second and newer type of SEM has a field-emission electron source. Because of their increased brightness and lower energy spread, field-emission SEMs (FE-SEM) permit operation at accelerating voltages as low as 1 keV, or less in some instruments. Such low voltage performance is very useful in imaging biological and many biomaterial samples, as will be discussed. The third major type of instrument is the environmental (or variable pressure) SEM. This permits pressures of up to about 1 kPa in the specimen chamber and hence can somewhat minimize specimen preparation since the complete removal of volatile components is not always required in the (reduced) atmosphere, which itself can provide adequate electrical conductivity. However, variable pressure SEM does not obviate specimen preparation, and it complicates the physics of image formation due to the multiple interactions of the imaging electrons with the atmosphere. In addition, its requirement for high electron beam currents can damage samples directly and indirectly by producing reactive intermediates through interactions with water vapor and oxygen. Also, as high accelerating voltages are generally required this leads to reduced surface contrast on uncoated biological and other low atomic number samples. Due to the limited availability and understanding of this relatively new type of instrument, variable pressure SEM will not be further discussed here [3–5]. The remainder of this chapter will be concerned with C-SEM and FE-SEM.

PREPARING AND IMAGING BIOMATERIALS WITH SEM

Because information is inevitably lost or at best becomes more difficult to obtain once a sample is processed, it is important to carefully consider the entire investigation prior to deciding upon a sample preparation and fixation protocol. For example, following chemical fixation of biological samples, it is generally no longer possible to label structures with antibody probes. Similarly, once a sample is conductively coated, it becomes increasingly difficult or impossible to examine atomic density or elemental distributions. A third example is that it becomes more difficult to relate ultrastructure to overall morphology once a sample

Table 39-1   Considerations in Planning an SEM Study

1. What aspects of the sample's biological or biomaterial structure are of interest?
2. What imaging modes and/or instrumentation will be used to provide this information? What constraints on sample preparation or imaging are there in obtaining this information?
3. What type of SEM instrumentation is available for this study? What constraints does this place on experimental design due to limits of instrumental resolution, the size of the sample chamber, and the availability and sensitivity of imaging modes, such as low voltage SE, BSE, and others?
4. Are there any physical characteristics of the sample which require special handling, such as mechanical fragility or interactions with water or solvents?
5. Is the size of the sample consistent with the information sought, and with adequate labeling and fixation?

has been cut to expose an area of interest, and/or to ensure adequate fixation, staining or labeling. Hence, for many studies, sample preparation is necessarily a one-way process which should be carefully planned in order to obtain the maximum amount of information. In planning an SEM study there are many concerns (Table 39-1).

Preparation of Biological Materials

Virtually all biological materials require that volatile water be removed and that the dried sample then be made electrically conductive. Many biomaterials require similar preparation, including synthetic hydrogels and biopolymer matrixes. This is generally accomplished by dehydration, but may also be attained by examining the sample in a frozen-hydrated state. Conductivity is most commonly increased by coating the sample with evaporated or sputtered metals, although chemical modification is sometimes used. Typical SEM preparation procedures for biological samples and biomaterials are outlined in Table 39-2, and discussed below as appropriate for both C-SEM and FE-SEM.

Prior to fixation many samples require a buffer rinse to prevent fixing non-adherent cells and/or proteins onto the biomaterial surface. For most samples, the fixative of choice is 1–2% glutaraldehyde in an iso-osmotic protein-free HEPES, phosphate, or other buffer. For thin layers of cells, 30 minutes of fixation at room temperature is adequate. For thicker tissue samples, overnight or longer fixation is required. In animal studies it is desirable to initiate fixation by whole body or selective organ/tissue perfusion, which is then followed by immersion fixation. For some tissues and for protocols such as for immunolabeling, other

Table 39-2   General Protocol for Preparation of Biological-Biomaterial Samples

1. Rinse in buffer to remove extraneous debris, cells, and/or proteins (optional).
2. Primary fixation (in glutaraldehyde, paraformaldehyde, mixtures, or others).
3. Rinse in buffer to remove unreacted primary fixative.
4. Secondary fixation/staining with OsO_4, and/or other agents (optional).
5. Rinse in distilled water to remove secondary fixative (as required).
6. Dehydrate in ethanol.
7. Dry by critical point procedure, or other methods.
8. Mount sample and make electrically conductive (sputter coat, ion beam coat).
9. Examine sample by SEM

fixatives such as paraformaldehyde and mixtures of glutaraldehyde and paraformaldehyde may be appropriate. All fixatives should be of the highest purity (EM grade) and prepared just prior to use since impure or old glutaraldehyde is often partially polymerized, thereby decreasing its effectiveness and sometimes imparting a contaminating layer which obscures surface details. This is especially noticeable with low voltage FE-SEM at high resolutions. Following fixation, unreacted aldehydes are removed by buffer rinses.

For many samples, a postfixation in freshly-prepared osmium tetroxide (OsO_4) is required, especially for higher resolution imaging of non-aldehyde fixed components. OsO_4 reacts with membranes, cytoskeletal elements, and many cellular organelles, and imparts both electron contrast and a degree of electrical conductivity. It may not be desirable for some studies as it reacts with some biomaterials, although this may also be used to advantage to stain some polymer structures [6, 7]. For thin cell layers, 0.05% OsO_4 in buffer for 15 minutes is adequate. For samples up to a few mm thick, 1% OsO_4 is generally used overnight. The "rule of thumb" is that 1% OsO_4 will perfuse into the sample at the rate of 1 mm per hour. Following this fixation, samples will require additional rinsing to remove residual OsO_4. Distilled water is fine since cellular membranes are no longer osmotically active.

The sample must now be dehydrated. The most common protocol is to dehydrate by immersion in ethanol/water mixtures of increasing ethanol concentrations, followed by multiple changes in absolutely dry 100% ethanol obtained either from a freshly opened bottle or by storing the ethanol over 3Å molecular sieve or desiccant. (Acetone is also used, however it is more toxic, extracts more cellular components than ethanol, can degrade some biomedical polymers such as methacrylates, and is damaging to some critical point dryers.) An alternative method for dehydrating samples is by chemical reaction with acidified 2,2-dimethoxy propane (DMP)[8]. DMP endothermically reacts with water to produce methanol and acetone. To ensure a complete reaction, 2 changes of DMP are used (15–30 minutes each), which may then be followed by 2–3 changes in absolute 100% ethanol. Throughout dehydration in ethanol or DMP, it is imperative that the sample not be allowed to dry out.

To prevent sample collapse due to surface tension drying forces, the ethanol is removed by drying via the critical point drying (CPD) method, by air drying, or (rarely) by freeze drying. For most samples, CPD is used: the sample in water-free 100% ethanol [9] is sealed in a critical point drying apparatus, and the ethanol is exchanged (rinsed out) using water-free liquid CO_2 under pressure at a temperature between 0 and 15°C. Following complete exchange, the temperature and pressure are increased beyond the critical point of CO_2 (31.3°C and 1072 psi $=$ 7.39 MPa), after which the pressure is slowly decreased to atmospheric. Alternative drying procedures are appropriate when a CPD apparatus is not available or when high pressure CO_2 interacts adversely with the material (for example, some silicones swell and bubble). In many cases, air drying from tetramethylsilane or hexamethyldisilazane (available from microscopy suppliers) will provide adequate results. Air drying from solvents such as ethanol will cause fragile biological structures to collapse but may nonetheless be adequate for some studies and with fairly robust samples [10, 11]. Freeze drying of aqueous frozen specimens is another method; however, it is complex and requires special instrumentation to preserve morphology [5, 12, 13]. Once the sample is dried, it is essential that it be kept dry by storing in sealed containers with desiccant or under vacuum.

Using conductive tape or paint, the sample is then mounted onto a conductive support of metal or carbon appropriate for the SEM instrument. Most samples will also require an electrically conductive coating. For C-SEM, typically a 10–20 nm thick layer of Au or AuPd is applied with a sputter coater. A plasma-magnetron or triode-type sputter coater is recommended since older diode types and evaporative coaters can damage some samples by excessive heating. Many sputter coaters incorporate a quartz crystal thickness monitor to measure the coating thickness; otherwise, experience is used to determine the coating time which provides the minimum thickness required to prevent sample charging. Since thick coatings obscure sample features, it is advisable to begin with a thin coating of 5–10 nm. If charging is then a problem, an additional layer may be applied. Since FE-SEM has much higher resolution and surface sensitivity, and as the lower accelerating voltages greatly minimize sample charging, much thinner coatings, or no coating, may be used. While sputtering is appropriate for C-SEM, ion beam coating with platinum (Pt) provides finer grain size and thinner coatings [14]. In many cases even a discontinuous coating is sufficient for thin samples imaged with FE-SEM at low accelerating potentials (1–5 keV).

Preparation of Many Non-Biological Materials

Conductive biomaterials may be imaged with minimal preparation; however, most biomaterials will require the application of a metal coating prior to C-SEM imaging. Since the degree of conductivity necessary for low voltage FE-SEM is considerably less, semiconductors such as silicon and medical carbons often do not require coating [15]. However, metal coatings can be beneficial to minimize electron beam damage of delicate materials, especially when imaged with higher keV C-SEM at high magnification. Coatings can also improve the detection of low atomic density topographic features, such as adherent cells and adsorbed proteins, as described below.

Cryogenic Preparative Procedures

There are a wealth of specialized preparative methods which are appropriate or necessary for some biomaterial studies. Such studies may involve biomaterials which reorganize their structure upon hydration and dehydration (such as hydrogels), materials which are particularly fragile when dehydrated, or alternative procedures to evaluate the possibility of artifacts which may be produced by sample preparation. The "cryo-preparative" methods offer many advantages since chemical fixation and dehydration may be avoided. The major concern with these methods is that large ice crystals can destroy sample structure. In one class of cryo-preparative methods, hydrated samples are rapidly frozen, or frozen in the presence of cryo-protective agents, to reduce ice crystal formation. The samples are then either freeze-dried or alternatively imaged in the frozen hydrated state. However, such studies are difficult and time-consuming, and are not possible for many biomaterials investigations since sample thicknesses are limited to 100 mm to 1 mm at best. Such thin samples are required to ensure sufficiently rapid freezing to prevent or minimize ice crystal formation. A second class of cryo-preparative technique combines cryo-fixation with chemical methods and permits SEM imaging to be done at ambient temperatures. These are generally referred to as freeze-substitution protocols. With these procedures, chemical fixation is performed at cryogenic temperatures to maintain antigenicity, to reduce lipid extraction, and to minimize sample structural reorganization. Such protocols are routinely used for immuno-labeling of sectioned samples for transmission light and electron microscopy, and are also applicable in preserving the hydrated structure of hydrogels and polyurethanes [16]. The cryo-preparative methods also offer the potential for the highest possible resolution, and hence have been extensively reported on in the primary microscopy literature [17–19] and are discussed in the additional reading [5, 13].

SEM IMAGING MODALITIES AND METHODS

Three-Dimensional SEM and Stereo Photogrammetry

SEM images appear so much like the world of everyday experience that one often feels compelled to interpret the third dimension (depth) directly, based upon apparent shadows and other features. However, this is misleading since the real depth cues required for understanding three-dimensional (3-D) structure are absent in routine SEM micrographs. For example, the very large depth-of-field in SEM eliminates focus as a depth cue, thus making it impossible to judge the large front-to-back depth of the textile sample in Figure 39-1. However, true 3-D imaging is easily acquired in the SEM by obtaining two views of the same region at different tilt angles [5, 20, 21]. These stereo pairs are then imaged with a stereo viewer available from vendors of microscopy or cartography supplies. Quantitative measurement of depth may then be calculated from the parallax shift between any two points in the stereo-pair. When this is done with the sample in Figure 39-1, this illustrates that the image depth is comparable to its width. Clearly, measurements made on this micrograph would be erroneous without knowledge of this significant sample depth.

For quantitative 3-D images of biomaterials, stereo-pairs obtained at angles of about $\pm 3.5\%$ from the horizontal (7° total angle) are generally appropriate since this produces an image in which the apparent depth appears visually correct. Measurements of sample height are then calculated from the parallax shift (P) between any two points in the stereo-pair. For applications where the specimen is tilted through zero, hence plus and minus some angle, the specimen height (Z) is calculated using the formula $Z = P/2 \sin(q/2)$, where q is the half angle for the stereo pair [20]. This formula is only appropriate for magnifications above about 1000X, where it can be assumed that the incident electron beam is perpendicular to the sample. There are some benefits in using a larger tilt angle for height measurements, such as $\pm 5°$, since a greater tilt will provide a larger parallax shift to measure, and also enhance the apparent depth. Figure 39-1 demonstrates the considerable depth of the textile material, while Figure 39-2 illustrates that even small platelet aggregates can reach a considerable distance away from biomaterials surfaces and, potentially, well into the flow stream [22].

Surface Sensitivity in SEM Imaging

In biomaterials, the physical nature of the material surface is studied with zeal by contact angles and other methods since biological interactions occur at surfaces. SEM is routinely thought to be a surface analysis method in that it provides images of surface structure. However, this is not strictly true since the primary electron beam has a finite interaction volume with the sample; hence, the secondary or back-scattered electrons which produce images are generated at and below the surface. (SEM surface sensitivity has much in common with ESCA or XPS since both utilize low voltage secondary electron emission, as discussed in Chapter 8). Several factors influence this interaction depth, including sample density, atomic number, topography, and the presence of any coatings. In Figure 39-3 Monte Carlo calculations illustrate the primary beam electron trajectories in carbon at the density of the pyrolytic carbon used in prosthetic heart valves. Immediately apparent is the vast difference in the interaction volume and depth at low and at high accelerating voltages. At 1.5 keV the maximum electron path is about 60 nm, while at 15 keV path lengths are measured in microns. In principle, BSEs and the SEs that they can produce within the sample may arise as a result of interactions occurring anywhere within this excited volume. Hence surface sensitivity is considerably poorer at 15 keV. Since the collected signal is the result

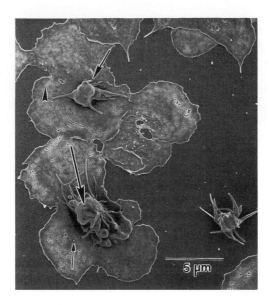

Figure 39-2 One half of a stereo-pair of a cluster of spread and pseudopodial platelets. Stereo photogrammetry was used to measure heights from the flat polymer substrate: a point near the edge of a fully spread platelet is 260 nm high (arrowhead), a point more centrally located on another fully spread platelet is 1.4μm high (small arrow), the tip of a pseudopod is 3.2μm high (medium arrow), and the top of the aggregate is 5.3μm above the substrate (large arrow). Ion beam Pt coated and SE imaged at 1.5 keV. Modified from reference [15].

of a complex average of signals emitting from different sample depths, this is often referred to as "depth averaging." Also note that the resulting signal is "averaged" laterally as well.

Biomaterials vary considerably in their topography, density, and atomic composition; it is useful to examine these influences on surface sensitivity. Most carbon-based polymers have a density of about 1 g/cm^3, while metals and ceramics are of higher density and are composed of higher atomic number elements. The cells and tissues on the biomaterial

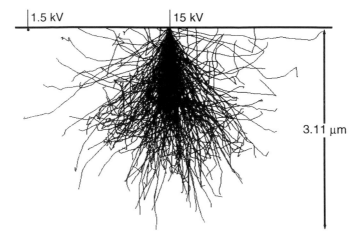

Figure 39-3 Monte Carlo calculation showing electron trajectories in carbon (at a density of 2 g/cm^3, which is equal to that of the pyrolytic carbon used in cardiac valve prosthetics). At 1.5 keV the maximum path length is 60 nm, while it is 3.11μm at 15 keV. From reference [15].

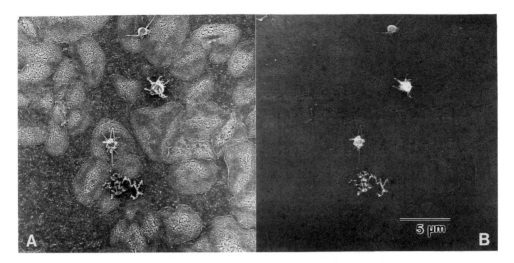

Figure 39-4 Platelets adherent to pyrolytic carbon valve leaflet material imaged with FE-SEM with a 1-2 nm Pt coating. (A) LV-SEM image obtained at 1.5 keV accelerating potential reveals thin, well-spread platelets which form a near-monolayer on the material surface. (B) Same region imaged at 15 keV, as is commonly used in C-SEM. Note that the well-spread platelets imaged at 1.5 keV become nearly invisible, while the scattered round and pseudopodial platelets become much brighter. From reference [28].

surface which have been prepared for SEM (i.e., dehydrated) are of very low density (0.02–0.3 g/cm^3) [17]. Because of their low density, at C-SEM accelerating voltages the range of the primary beam is greater than the thickness of many cells. Thus, in some cases adherent cells may even be undetectable at C-SEM accelerating voltages (Figure 39-4). This is especially a problem on rough materials since low energy secondary electrons produced well below the average surface height are able to escape from the sides of rough features, whereas on smooth surfaces those SEs produced deep within the sample do not have sufficient energy to escape through the solid material. This topographic effect on SE emission can also be used to enhance the imaging of rough surfaces. Tilting the specimen toward the SE detector can increase the visibility of thinly spread platelets and other topographic features, especially with C-SEM (Figure 39-5), since this places more of the excitation volume close enough to the surface to permit SEs to escape.

In practice, low density and low atomic number samples (polymers, cells, tissues) are metal-coated not only to reduce charging, but also to increase the number of SEs emitted near the sample surface. This has the effect of greatly decreasing depth averaging. However, the typical 10–20 nm thick metal coatings can bury fine surface detail, thus significantly altering the appearance of rough surfaces. This can be appreciated by examining two conventional biomaterials, expanded PTFE and pyrolytic carbon, with and without a 15 nm AuPd coating. While the ePTFE material does not appear to be affected by the coating at low magnification (Figure 39-6), it is clear that the coating adds to the apparent thickness of the filaments and obscures the material fine structure at the nodes (Figure 39-6B and D). With respect to pyrolytic carbon, the coating noticeably obscures the rough carbon surface even at a fairly low magnification and even more so at high resolution (Figure 39-7). Although Figure 39-5 shows with C-SEM that the coating structure is not apparent at low magnification, the structure of the sputter-coated AuPd itself is imaged rather than the biomaterial texture when FE-SEM is used (Figures 39-6 and 39-7). In addition, 10–20 nm thick metal

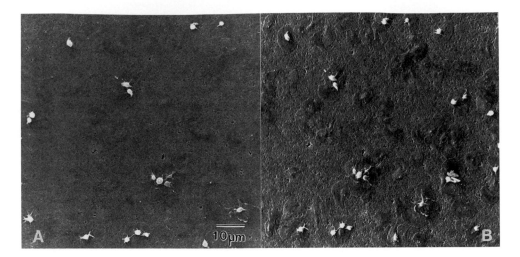

Figure 39-5 Platelets adherent to pyrolytic carbon observed with C-SEM instrumentation at 15 keV and sputter-coated with 10 nm AuPd. (A) At a tilt angle of zero (90° to the primary electron beam) the thin, fully spread, platelets are nearly invisible. (B) In the same general field of view, the visibility of fully spread platelets and the material's surface texture is significantly improved by tilting the specimen 35° towards the secondary electron detector. From reference [15].

coatings prevent imaging small differences in the atomic density of samples and the detection of colloidal gold labels, as discussed below.

There are alternatives to metal coating which can be used to reduce sample charging on some samples. One technique that is always helpful is to ground the sample as close to the region of interest as possible. The method of charge compensation can also be effective with some specimens. As the average SE + BSE yield increases with lower keV, a voltage can be reached where the number of electrons leaving the sample balances those entering. To take advantage of this, one finds by trial and error (usually between 1 and 5 keV) the accelerating voltage where this occurs [5, 23]. Very thin samples (a few hundred nanometers) will also charge less if the primary electron beam can travel entirely through the sample to an underlying conductor. The beam makes the specimen locally and transiently conductive so that excess charge can be conducted away. Finally, with many biological and some polymer samples, bulk conductivity may be produced by (often repeated) reaction with OsO_4 or other metal stains and various mordant agents [5, 24].

Atomic Density Imaging

In addition to imaging surface topography, SEM is also very useful for revealing internal morphology. Sub-surface imaging is accomplished by utilizing atomic density contrast to detect structures labeled with heavy metals or intrinsic high atomic number features. Such contrast is most easily imaged on samples which have not been metal-coated. Consequently, if both internal and surface structures are of interest, either the coating thickness or its atomic number must be reduced. When feasible, the same sample may be examined both before and after a coating is applied. Such sequential examination was used to image a platelet adherent to a thin polymer film supported on a TEM grid (Figure 39-8). Even at a fairly low accelerating voltage of 4 keV, a great deal of the cytoskeletal and organelle structures are visible with SE imaging due to osmium, uranium, and iron staining. Since the entire preparation (cell plus polymer support) is only a few hundred

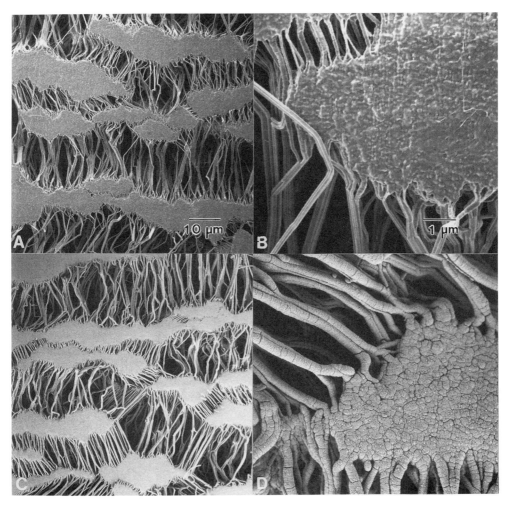

Figure 39-6 Effect of coating on revealing and obscuring the surface structure of expanded PTFE vascular graft material, imaged with FE-SEM at 1.5 keV. Sample was ion-beam coated with 4 nm Pt and imaged at low magnification (A) and the central region at higher resolution (B). Same material sputter coated with 15 nm AuPd coating and also imaged at the same low (C) and higher magnification (D). At low magnification (A and C) there is little apparent difference in the observed structure as a function of the coating. At higher resolution (B and D), the thicker AuPd coating obscures the fine surface structure at the nodes (broad regions) and greatly increases the apparent diameter of the thin filaments.

nanometers thick, and is well grounded by the metal TEM grid support, there is no sample charging on this uncoated sample. Following the application of a 4 nm thick Pt coating, the platelet was then SE-imaged at 2.5 keV with excellent surface resolution. It should also be noted that Figures 39-8A and 39-8B show the specimen viewed at two different tilt angles 20° apart which may be noted due to the smaller apparent width of the platelet in Figure 39-8B. The fact that this is not at all obvious by observation of either micrograph by itself demonstrates the difficulty in estimating specimen surface height from a single image.

High atomic number sub-surface structures may be imaged using BSEs. BSE imaging at higher accelerating potentials (>10–15 keV) is particularly useful for thick samples

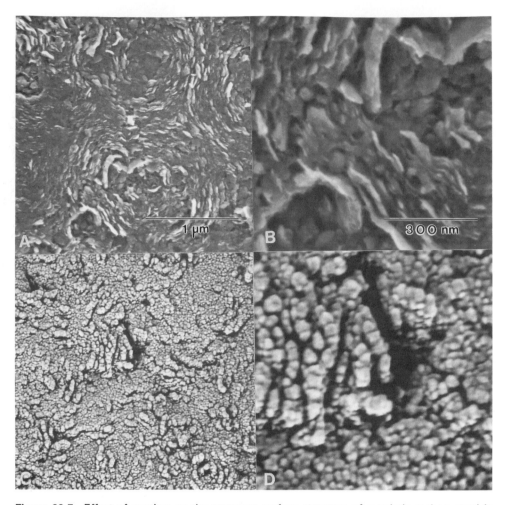

Figure 39-7 Effect of coating on the apparent surface structure of pyrolytic carbon used in prosthetic heart valves imaged with FE-SEM at 1.5 keV. Uncoated pyrolytic carbon valve leaflet imaged at moderate (A) and high (B) resolution (region just below center in A). Same pyrolytic carbon sample imaged after sputter coating with 15 nm AuPd at moderate (C) and high (D) resolution. The effect of the coating on the apparent structure is dramatic even at moderate resolution.

labeled with colloidal gold since higher energy BSEs have sufficient energy to escape from a thinly coated sample where they can be detected. By combining SE and BSE imaging modes, the distribution of colloidal gold-labeled protein can be examined on exposed surfaces, and even in regions hidden under adherent cells (Figure 39-9) [1]. In this case a 4–6 nm thick layer of Pt was required to ensure sufficient conductivity on the glass substrate.

Atomic density contrast can also be used to image the structure of some polymeric biomaterials by staining with appropriate agents. This approach has been used to examine polyurethane block copolymers stained with OsO_4 and RuO_4 [6, 7, 25]. The difference between surface and bulk imaging using SE and BSE imaging is readily observed in a single image of a polyurethane in which the unsaturated double bonds of polybutadiene soft segments were stained with OsO_4 (Figure 39-10A). The SE portion

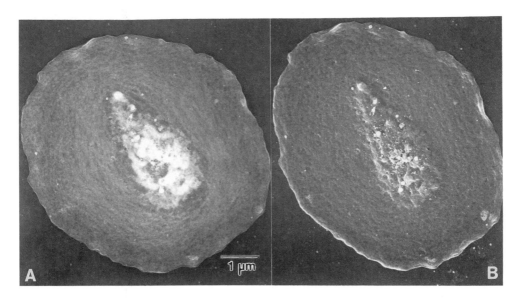

Figure 39-8 Bulk and surface imaging of the same platelet obtained by imaging before and after coating and by using different accelerating voltages. Secondary electron image at 4 keV shows platelet intracellular structure including organelles and the actin cytoskeleton (A). Platelet was fixed in 1% glutaraldehyde containing 1% tannic acid to stain actin filaments (30 min.), and then post-fixed and stained with 0.05% OsO_4 containing 0.8% $K_3Fe(CN)$ (15 min.), and further stained with 5% uranyl acetate (20 min.). The sample was imaged at 0° tilt for Figure 39-8A. To show surface structure, the sample was then ion-beam-coated with 4 nm Pt, and imaged at 2.5 keV (Figure 39-8B) at a tilt angle of 20°.

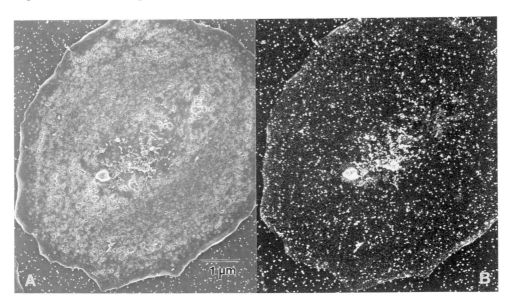

Figure 39-9 Surface and bulk imaging of a platelet adherent to a glass surface covered with 30 nm diameter colloidal gold particles coated with albumin, and ion beam coated with 4 nm Pt. Secondary electron image at 15 keV shows platelet surface structure (A). The colloidal gold is visible as the small white dots surrounding the platelet. Back-scattered electron image at 15 keV shows the location of the colloidal gold unobscured by the overlying platelet.

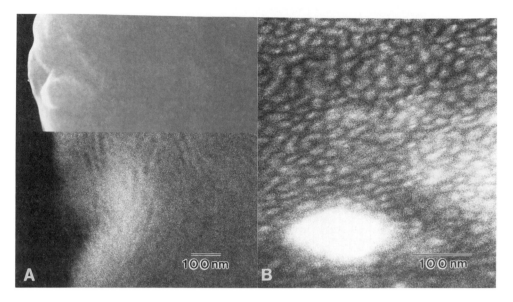

Figure 39-10   Polyurethane microdomain structure detected with SE and BSE imaging. A polybutadiene polyurethane block copolymer stained with dry OsO₄ (A). The SE image in the upper half
reveals little detail of the stained chemical structure compared to the back scattered scan in the
lower half of the image. A similar polybutadiene polyurethane stained with aqueous OsO₄, and
BSE imaged at 5 keV in the hydrated state at −90°C.

of the scan (top half of image) reveals the surface topography of this thin film, while
the lamellar-like chemical morphology is largely undetected until BSE imaging (scanning) was initiated in the bottom half of the image. It is also possible to label the hydrated structure of these and similar materials by staining with aqueous OsO_4 and then
observing the specimen in the hydrated state at a temperature well below the polymer's
glass-transition temperature (Figure 39-10B). BSE imaging was used to examine this
polybutadiene-polyurethane (different than Figure 39–10A) because the presence of an
overlying layer of water (ice) meant that only BSEs carried information on the polymer
structure. Low-voltage SE imaging of the chemical morphology of hydrated polyurethanes
may also be done by examining samples in which aqueous OsO_4 fixes or cross-links the
hydrated structure in place. Then imaging may be done with the dry material at room
temperature [16].

Replicas

It is not possible or desirable to image some biomaterial specimens directly, such as a
functioning implant, or a sample which is too large to fit in the microscope. Techniques using
dental replication polymers and other materials to produce surface replicas by impression
casting have been described and reviewed [5, 26]. Images of replicas can also provide
information in a form which is easier to interpret than images of the original sample. For
example, the internal luminal structure of vascular networks are revealed much more readily
as a replica than by examining the actual tissue (Figure 39-11). Such replicas are prepared by
perfusing the vasculature with monomers or prepolymers which then polymerize in place.
Subsequently, the tissue is removed to reveal the replica, and the sample is dried, mounted

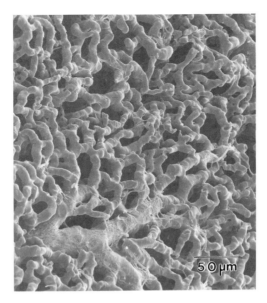

Figure 39-11 The capillary vasculature of a portion of a (rat) lung as seen in a methacrylate micro-corrosion cast.

and coated for SEM imaging in a procedure commonly referred to as vascular casting [27]. It is also possible to create replicas of subendothelial matrix surfaces by removing the endothelium prior to replication. Such replicas are useful to examine matrix morphology and can be used as templates to produce matrix-textured biomaterials [11].

SUMMARY

While SEM is routinely employed to examine biomaterial surface morphology, it is necessary to understand image formation mechanisms in order to ensure proper interpretation. SEM can then be used as a very powerful tool for the evaluation of biomaterials. For example, SEM can enable quantitative three-dimensional imaging of surfaces and even permit the examination of some subsurface structures. Furthermore, the uniquely wide magnification range of the SEM permits understanding macromolecular-scale biological-material interactions in the context of the whole-tissue macroscopic response. By applying SEM methodology with knowledge, foresight, and careful experimental design, it is not only possible to provide a "pretty picture," but also to obtain qualitative and quantitative 3-D information on the chemical, physical, and biological events at the interface between biological systems and biomaterials.

ACKNOWLEDGEMENTS

The author wishes to acknowledge Drs. James B. Pawley and Ralph M. Albrecht (University of Wisconsin, Madison) for helpful commentary; Mr. Paul A. Sims for providing Figure 39-4; Dr. David C. Joy (University of Tennessee, Knoxville) for providing computer programs to simulate SEM electron-solid interactions; the Integrated Microscopy Resource in Madision (NIH RR-570); and the support of the National Institutes of Health (HL-37351) and the Whitaker Foundation.

REFERENCES

1   Goodman SL, Park K, Albrecht RM. A correlative approach to colloidal gold labeling with video-enhanced light microscopy, low voltage scanning electron microscopy and high voltage electron microscopy. In *Colloidal Gold: Methods and Applications*. San Diego: Academic Press, 1990, 369–409.

2   Waples LM, Olorundare OE, Lai QJ, Goodman SL, Albrecht RM. Platelet-polymer interactions: Morphologic and intracellular calcium studies in individual human platelets. *J Biomed Mater Res*, 32 (1996), 65–76.

3   Danilatos GD. Bibliography of environmental scanning electron microscopy. *Microsc Res Tech*, 25 (1993), 529–534.

4   Farley AN, Shah JS. High-pressure scanning electron microscopy of insulating materials: A new approach. *J Microsc*, 164 (1991), 107–126.

5   Goldstein JI, Newbury DE, Echlin P, Joy DC, Romig ADJ, Lyman CE, Fiori C, Lifshin E. *Scanning Electron Microscopy and X-Ray Microanalysis: A Text for Biologists, Material Scientists, and Geologists*, 2nd ed. New York: Plenum Press.

6   Goodman SL, Li C, Pawley JB, Cooper SL, Albrecht RM. Surface and bulk analysis of phase-segregation in polyurethanes by electron microscopies. In *The Surface Characterization of Biomaterials*. Amsterdam: Elsevier, 1988, 281–295.

7   Li C, Goodman SL, Albrecht RM, Cooper SL. Morphology of segmented polybutadiene-polyurethanes. *Macromolecules*, 21 (1988), 2367–2375.

8   Maser MD, Trimble JJI. Rapid chemical dehydration of biologic samples for scanning electron microscopy using 2,2-dimethoxypropane. *J Histochem Cytochem*, 25 (1977), 247–251.

9   Ris H. The cytoplasmic filament system in critical point-dried whole mounts and plastic-embedded sections. 100 (1985), 1474–1487.

10   Albrecht RM, Rasmussen DH, Keller CS, Hinsdill RD. Preparation of cultured cells for SEM: Air drying from organic solvents. *J Microsc*, 108 (1976), 21–29.

11   Goodman SL, Sims PA, Albrecht RM. Three-dimensional bio-mimetic extracellular-matrix textured materials. *Biomaterials*, 17 (1996), 2087–2095.

12   Albrecht RM, MacKenzie AP. Cultured and free living cells. In *Principles and Techniques of Scanning Electron Microscopy*. 1975, 109–153.

13   Lee RE. *Scanning Electron Microscopy and X-Ray Microanalysis*. Englewood Cliffs, NJ: Prentice-Hall.

14   Pawley JB, Erlandsen SL. The case for low voltage high resolution scanning electron microscopy of biological samples. *Scanning Microsc Suppl*, 3 (1989), 163–78.

15   Goodman SL, Tweden KS, Albrecht RM. Three-dimensional morphology and platelet adhesion on pyrolytic carbon heart valve materials. *Cells and Materials*, 5 (1995) 15–30.

16   Goodman SL, Simmons SR, Cooper SL, Albrecht RM. Preferential adsorption of plasma proteins onto a polar polyurethane microdomains, *J Colloid Interface Sci*, 139 (1990), 561–570.

17   Pawley JB. LVSEM for high resolution topographic and density contrast imaging. In *Advances in Electronics and Electron Physics*. Academic Press, 1992, 203–273.

18   Walther P, Chen Y, Pech LL, Pawley JB. High-resolution scanning electron microscopy of frozen-hydrated cells. *J Microsc*, 168 (1992), 169–180.

19   Inoue T, Osatake H. Three-dimensional demonstration of the intracellular structures of mouse mesothelial cells by scanning electron microscopy. *J Submicrosc Cytol Pathol*, 21 (1989), 215–227.

20   Boyde A. Three-dimensional aspects of SEM Images. In Well OC (Ed.), *Scanning Electron Microscopy*. New York: McGraw-Hill, 1974, 277–307.

21   Bozzola JJ, Russel LD. *Electron Microscopy*. Boston: Jones and Barttell, 1992.

22   Goodman SL, Grasel TG, Cooper SL, Albrecht RM. Platelet shape change and cytoskeletal reorganization on polyurethaneureas. *J Biomed Mater Res*, 23 (1989), 105–123.

23   Joy DC, Pawley JB. High-resolution scanning electron microscopy. *Ultramicroscopy*, 47 (1992), 80–100.

24   Allen TD, Jack EM, Harrison CJ, Claugher D. Scanning electron microscopy of human metaphase chromosomes. *Scan-Electron-Microsc*, 1 (1986), 301–308.

25   Goodman SL, Cooper SL, Albrecht RM. Polyurethane support films: Structure and cellular adhesion. *Scanning Microsc Suppl*, 3 (1989), 285–294.

26   Willison JHM, Rowe AJ. General considerations in the replication of specimens. In *Replicas, Shadowing and Freeze-Etching Techniques*. Amsterdam: North-Holland, 1980, 95–105.

27   Hodde KC, Steeber DA, Albrecht RM. Advances in corrosion casting methods. *Scanning Microsc*, 4 (1990), 693–704.

28   Goodman SL, Tweden KS, Albrecht RM. Platelet interaction with pyrolytic carbon heart valve leaflets. *J Biomed Mater Res*, 32 (1996), 249–258.

ADDITIONAL READING

1   Bozzola JJ and Russel LD. *Electron Microscopy*. Boston: Jones and Barttell, 1992.
2   Goldstein JI, Newbury DE, Echlin P, Joy DC, Romig AD, Jr., Lyman CE, Fiori C, Lifshin E. *Scanning Electron Microscopy and X-Ray Microanalysis: A Text for Biologists, Material Scientists, and Geologists*. New York: Plenum Press, 1992.
3   Lee RE. *Scanning Electron Microscopy and X-Ray Microanalysis*. Englewood Cliffs, NJ: Prentice Hall, 1993.
4   Pawley JB. LVSEM for high resolution topographic and density contrast imaging. In Hawkes P (Ed.), *Advances in Electronics and Electron Physics*. New York: Academic Press, 1992, 203–273.

Chapter 40

Evaluation by Histochemical and Quantitative Microscopy

Thomas N. Salthouse

The presence of an implant in the tissues initiates, to some degree, a response in the adjacent cell population. The evaluation of this cellular reaction by light and electron microscopy has been discussed in preceding chapters of this section. There may also be other effects related to implants that are not readily apparent by normal histological means. These effects include changes in cell physiology and function, such as the modification of cellular enzyme activity; materials resulting from the influence of the implant on adjacent tissues; or materials caused by the effects of the in vivo environment on the biomaterial. Histochemical techniques may be required to detect or uncover these types of effects by identifying chemical components of cells and tissues and relating the results to tissue morphology [1].

Some histochemical procedures can be quantitated numerically either by application of some form of densitometry or area measurement, and have been suggested as objective approaches in the evaluation of the acute tissue response to biomaterials. Thus, in a broad sense, histochemistry can be described as functional histology. Some histochemical and related procedures that have proved informative in the author's laboratory for the evaluation of biomaterials are described in this chapter. These include enzyme histochemistry, immunofluorescent procedures, detection of inclusions and deposits, autoradiography, selected microscopical techniques, and approaches to quantitative histochemistry. Because many of the methods are readily available in the literature, only those procedures of most importance in the evaluation of biocompatibility are described in detail. Types of necessary equipment and their use are briefly described. The effect of implant geometry on evaluations is also discussed.

Histology, dependent on descriptive morphology, tends to be a subjective science. Judicious use of histochemical approaches can bolster the objectivity of many studies and supply added dimensions to the histological evaluation of biomaterials.

ENZYME HISTOCHEMISTRY

Application of enzyme histochemistry to sections of tissue from implant sites can supply valuable information on the cellular activity adjacent to the implant-tissue interface. The results will vary with the biocompatibility of the implant. Irritating or toxic implants in soft tissues invariably induce an intense acid phosphatase and aminopeptidase activity in cells (usually macrophages) adjacent to the interface [1, 2]. These enzymes are hydrolases of lysosomal origin [3].

Acid Phosphatase

Acid phosphatase activity is a reliable indicator of the effect of an implant on surrounding tissues and cells. Smooth-surfaced, nonirritating implants elicit only a mild response,

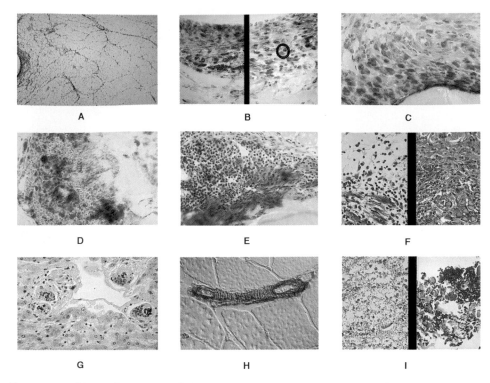

Figure 40-1 Photomicrographs of histochemical procedures at some experimental polymer implant sites: (A) Cryostat-frozen section of PVC implant (on left) in rat muscle treated to demonstrate acid phosphatase (red). Migration of activated macrophages to implant is demonstrated, X25. (B) Two implant sites (rat) at 14 days. On left, PVC rod containing amyl phthalate and right decyl phthalate. Acid phosphatase activity shown as red. Although cell response in both sites is similar, lysosomal enzyme response is much greater than with the amyl-phthalate-containing sample, X150. (C) Collagen implant at 7 days. Acid phosphatase activity shown as red inclusions in activated macrophages adjacent to implant. Neutrophils also present. Counterstained with methylene blue, X350. (D) Hydrolytic enzyme response (red-brown) at site of absorbed collagen implant at 28 days. Activity is prominent. Counterstained methylene blue for cellular response, X50. (E) Similar implant site at 35 days, again with strong proteolytic and mixed cell response, X100. (F) By comparison, 2 silk suture sites at 7 days (left) and 35 days stained hematoxylin and eosin show only morphological detail. Previous examples of hydrolytic enzyme activity provide additional information on the cellular mechanisms involved but not shown by traditional methods, X100. (G) Section of liver from patient with fragmenting silicone implant (courtesy Dr. James M. Anderson) stained with oil red O in polypropylene glycol (see text). Inclusions stained red, cells counterstained hematoxylin (blue), X100. (H) Cryostat section near implant site treated to demonstrate adenosine triphosphase activity (brown), blood vessel smooth muscle shows high activity. Also, photograph by Nomarski optics providing optical relief, X50. (I) Two sections illustrating bacterial infection at implant sites. On the left, a gram stain with presence of staphylococci; on the right, periodic acid Schiff procedure (PAS) demonstrating fungal infection (red hyphae) [Ref. 9], X100.

while rough-surfaced or toxic implants activate a much higher response (Figure 40-1, A, B and C). The red product is easily evaluated on a semiquantitated system or by microphotometry as described later.

The demonstration of acid phosphatase and other enzyme activity requires cryostat-frozen sections. One of the most complete descriptions of cryostat techniques is given by Bancroft [4]. There are several excellent cryostat microtome models available today. A recent model that is adaptable for sectioning implant sites is the Leica CM 1900 cryostat (Leica Inc., Deerfield, IL). Most university and hospital pathology departments have at least one. Basically they are microtomes in refrigerated cabinets kept between $-5°$ and $-30°C$, and are essential for enzyme techniques because tissue processing and embedding in room temperature reduces or destroys enzyme activity. Demonstration requires the incubation of cryostat sections (usually 8–10 μm thick) carried on cover glasses or slides in substrate media at $37°C$ for 20–30 min. Some substrate media and coupling color reagents such as Fast Red TR/naphthol AS-MX and other coupling compounds are available in convenient tablet form (Sigma Chemical Co., St. Louis, MO).

Prior to incubation, cryostat sections on glass slides or cover glasses are placed in cold acetone ($-30°C$) for 15 minutes, transferred to acetone at room temperature for 1 minute, rinsed in saline, and placed in the substrate media. This technique is suitable for acid phosphatase, adenosine triphosphatase, and aminopeptidase preparations. The substrate medium for acid phosphatase is:

Naphthol AS-BI phosphate	10 mg
Dimethylformamide	0.5 ml
Mix	
Acetate buffer [4], pH 5.2, 0.2 M	10 ml
Saline	20 ml
Fast red violet LB salt	15 mg

After incubation, the sections are transferred to formalin fixative overnight, rinsed in distilled water, and counterstained in diluted hematoxylin (1:10) until cell nuclei are lightly stained. Sections can be mounted in an aqueous medium, such as glycerin jelly [4]. Acid phosphatase activity will be colored red and the nuclei blue. Generally, activity will be seen to be associated with the macrophage population from 5 to 30 days postimplantation (Figure 40-1A and B). Activity can be scored on a plus-minus system. Unknown samples should be compared with previously tested samples. The level of phosphatase activity can also be quantitated by use of microphotometry as described later.

Aminopeptidase

The presence of aminopeptidase activity associated with implant sites indicates the presence of proteolytic activity and is usually prominent in areas of tissue damage and necrosis. Activity is high during phagocytosis of tissue affected by irritating or toxic implant materials. It does, therefore, have diagnostic significance. Cryostat sections are prepared in the same manner as for acid phosphatase, including cold acetone fixation, and then incubated in a substrate medium at $37°C$ for 30–60 minutes. The procedure is as follows:

1. Prefix sections in cold acetone ($-30°C$) for 10–15 min.
2. Prepare substrate medium by adding and the dissolving the following in order:
Leucylmethoxy β-naphtholamide (4 mg/ml)	2 ml
Acetate buffer, pH 6.8, 0.2 M	10 ml
Saline	20 ml
Magnesium chloride, sol. 5 percent	2 drops
Fast blue B salt	10 mg
3. Incubate the sections.
4. Fix in formalin overnight.
5. Rinse.
6. Counterstain in hematoxylin.
7. Mount in glycerin jelly [4].

Aminopeptidase activity will be shown as reddish-brown deposits in sections (Figure 40-1, D and E).

Adenosine Triphosphatase

Adenosine triphosphatase plays a pivotal role in the energy transfer and metabolism of the cell and is associated with cell membranes and mitochondria [5]. During increased cellular metabolism, enzyme activity is accelerated. High activity is observed in the developing vascular network adjacent to implants and in vascular endothelium (Figure 40-1H). Thus, it can serve as an excellent marker enzyme for endothelial growth and angioblastic activity. Activity is also observed during the development of the fibrous capsule around implants.

In this approach, cryostat sections are fixed to cover glasses or slides and placed in cold acetone (30°C) for 20–30 minutes. The sections are then rinsed in water and incubated for 30–40 minutes at 37°C in the following medium:

Adenosine triphosphate	10 mg
Tris buffer pH 7.2, 0.2 M (see below)	10 ml
Distilled water	20 ml
Magnesium nitrate 5 percent	2 drops
Lead nitrate 2 percent	0.6 ml

The lead nitrate should be added last, drop by drop, with constant mixing.

The Tris buffer required to make this medium is mixed according to the following steps:

Tris	2.45 gm
Maleic acid	2.32 gm
Sodium hydrozide	0.8 gm
Water	100 gm

Take

1	See above	25.0 ml
2	See above	25.5 ml
3	Water	49.5 ml

Mix, check pH at 7.2.

After incubation the sections are removed, rinsed in three changes of fresh water, and placed for 10 seconds in the following solution:

Ammonium sulfide	2 drops
Water	25 ml

Next the sections are rinsed for about 5 seconds in 0.1 percent acetic acid, rinsed twice in water, and fixed overnight in formalin. They are counterstained with either nuclear fast red, neutral red, or safranin. Sites of adenosine triphosphatase activity are stained dark brown and nuclei red (Figure 40-1H).

Succinic Dehydrogenase

As a major enzyme of the citric acid (Kreb's) cycle, succinic or succinate dehydrogenase serves as a useful indicator of the level of cellular metabolic activity. It is an oxidoreductase mitochondrial enzyme catalyzing the conversion of succinate to fumarate. Increases in succinate dehydrogenase (SDH) activity have been observed at the surface of rough or abraded implants [6] and absorbable suture material. Inhibition of SDH activity has been reported adjacent to toxic implants [7]. Demonstration of this enzyme activity can, therefore, have diagnostic value in evaluating biocompatibility.

To test for SDA activity, unfixed, fresh, cryostat-frozen sections are incubated for approximately 30 minutes at 37°C in the substrate medium described below:

Sodium succinate 0.06 M	3 ml
Nitro blue tetrazolium 0.5 percent (5 mg/ml)	4 ml
Tris buffer 0.2 M, pH 7.4	5 ml
Saline	5 ml
Magnesium chloride 5 percent	1 drop

After incubation, sections are fixed in formalin. A red counterstain, such as nuclear fast red, may be used, but should be light; otherwise, the purple formazan stain marking SDH activity is easily overshadowed.

Lactate dehydrogenase (LDH) is responsible for the interconversion of lactate and pyruvate and an important factor in anaerobic metabolism. Increases in LDH activity have been reported in wound healing and tissue regeneration, and have been associated with implants of absorbable biomaterials (Figure 40-1D) [7]. The procedure to demonstrate LDH activity is relatively simple and similar to that for SDH activity above, but requires the presence of a coenzyme. There are many sources for formulae of the buffer solutions, including Bancroft and Troyer [4, 5].

SPECIAL HISTOCHEMICAL TECHNIQUES

There are a number of miscellaneous histochemical and related procedures that can on occasion be very helpful in the microscopic evaluation of implanted biomaterials, including immunofluorescence, autoradiography, and the rabbit ear chamber.

Immunofluorescent Procedures

Immunofluorescent marking of intracellular details and the use of laser confocal microscopy (LCM) have become very valuable research tools in histological and cell culture evaluations of cellular responses to biomaterials. Fluorescent antibody techniques provide the unique ability to identify specific proteins [10]. An excellent example is the identification of endothelial ingrowth by the immunofluorescent staining of factor VIII-related antigen in frozen sections of implanted vascular grafts [11]. The identification of blood protein fractions adsorbed on the surface of polymers could also be identified by appropriate fluorescent antibody techniques. A number of commercial laboratories will custom-prepare fluorescent antibodies to antigens supplied to them.

Autoradiography

Although autoradiography is not generally considered a routine procedure, it can be a useful research tool. It is the most reliable way to follow cell turnover at the tissue-implant interface. By the use of tritiated thymidine, it was shown that there was significant macrophage cell replication through mitosis at rough or abraded implant surfaces that was absent at smooth surfaces [12] (Figure 40-1E). Implants of absorbable polymers can be synthesized to contain radioisotopic tracers. Carbon-14 and tritium isotopes are commonly employed. The degradation products of the polymer in cells and tissues can be identified and localized by the effect of the low-level radioactivity on a thin layer of photographic emulsion coating the sections. Liquid emulsion autoradiography is the most adaptable and convenient technique for the histologist to apply [13]. (See Reagents section.)

The Rabbit Ear Chamber Model

The transparent plastic ear chamber is a unique system for the continuous observation of biomaterials in an in vivo environment. After surgical implantation into the ear of a laboratory lop-eared rabbit, a thin tissue bed develops in the chamber into which a sample can be inserted and subsequently viewed through the microscope. It is particularly adaptable to the evaluation of absorbable biomaterials. The application of the rabbit ear chamber in biomaterial evaluations and design for a plastic chamber have been described in detail by Matlaga et al. [14].

INCLUSIONS AND DEPOSITS

Occasionally during the microscopic evaluation of tissue sections adjacent to implant sites, unidentified fragments of material may be seen. It is good practice to have polarizing equipment available on the microscope to enable the observer to test for birefringence as will be described later.

The introduction of the energy dispersive X-ray microanalysis (EDX) system to scanning electron microscopy (SEM) has greatly facilitated the recognition of metallic deposits or salts in tissue [8].

Carbon

Deposits of carbon can be identified in a negative manner insomuch as they are not removable by solvents, acid, or alkali treatment of sections.

Iron

Deposits of inorganic iron can be extrinsic or intrinsic due to the breakdown of blood pigments, such as hemosiderin, from areas of earlier hemorrhage. Perl's Prussian blue reaction is the most reliable procedure for chemical identification [5].

Calcium

Calcium deposits are commonly seen as areas of calcification subsequent to necrosis and are not unusual at implant sites. Deposits may be found in association with vascular grafts. The alizarin red S procedure is recommended and is more specific than von Kossa's method [5].

Lipids and Some Polymer Inclusions

The oil red O-isopropanol technique is a reliable method for demonstrating lipids in frozen sections [9]. In other sections from embedded tissues, lipids would be removed by the solvents used in processing. However, this stain can be modified to demonstrate many polymers that might be present as fragments or inclusions in tissue. Nylon, polyethylene, silicone rubber, some cyanoacrylate tissue adhesives, and other polymers have been stained (Figure 40-1G) by this procedure, described below.

One gm of oil red O dye powder is suspended in 100 ml of propylene glycol (or polyethylene glycol), and the solution is left overnight at 60°C with occasional mixing. The mixture is allowed to cool to room temperature and excess dye is allowed to settle. The resulting clear dye solution is carefully decanted and retained.

The following procedure is used for staining the sections:

1   Bring paraffin sections to water.
2   Immerse sections 5 minutes in each of two changes of the pure glycol (no dye).
3   Drain.
4   Place in oil red O glycol solution at 60°C for 1 to 7 days. Check for staining each day.
5   Rinse *quickly* in 50 percent ethanol until tissues are unstained.
6   Place in water.
7   Counterstain *lightly* with hematoxylin (diluted Hx).
8   Mount in glycerin jelly.

Polymeric inclusions will stain pink to red.

OPTICAL AND QUANTITATIVE PROCEDURES

It must be stressed that many studies involving the microscope as a tool tend to be somewhat subjective, relying on visual observations and judgment. However, systems have been developed that, when added to the microscope, can greatly assist in increasing the objectivity of histological and histochemical evaluations. The use of even simple polarizing filters can often provide essential information when examining sections of implant sites. More recently developed optical systems, such as phase contrast and interference contrast, offer new dimensions to microscopy. Finally, when numerical quantitation is required, the investigator can turn to microphotometry and the more recent quantitative digital image analysis. Even the older stage-and-eyepiece micrometer should not be forgotten, together with the point-counting eyepiece reticules. The appropriate application of these systems can add greatly to the confidence of the investigator in light microscopic evaluations.

Polarizing Microscopy

Microscopes used in the investigation of implanted biomaterials should be equipped with a system for polarizing light. A lower linear polarizer under the substage condensor and an upper linear polarizer above the eyepiece or incorporated in it are sufficient for most applications. Polaroid material is a simple and excellent inexpensive polarizing filter. Some provision for rotating the polarizing filter should be made. Manufacturers supply polarizing sets for their own microscopes at various levels of sophistication.

Application of polarized light is particularly valuable in the detection and sometimes the identification of certain crystalline substances and polymeric materials. Birefringence can be observed with most crystalline inclusions and strained noncrystalline materials. Occasionally other foreign materials, such as talc or synthetic textile fibers, are detected by their birefringence. Wear particles or fragments of polymers can migrate considerable distances, and their presence can be recognized by their birefringence patterns. Silica dust is usually recognized by the presence of tiny colorless spicules present in fibrous tissue and showing birefringence by polarized light. Asbestos deposits are not normally birefringent, but can be demonstrated by phase contrast or interference contrast microscopy (see next section).

Glove powder, a possible contaminant from surgery, provokes a chronic inflammatory reaction. Polarized light demonstrates talc as brilliant angular fragments and starch as bright circular bodies with a dark central area. Cholesterol deposits possibly present in atherosclerotic plaques in blood vessels show typical needle-shaped birefringence in frozen sections, also staining with lipid stains. To conclude, the property of birefringence under polarized light of some biomaterials and tissue contaminants should be considered during microscope evaluation of histological sections.

Interference Contrast and Phase Contrast Microscopy

Differential interference contrast (Nomarski) microscopy has great potential in the examination of implanted biomaterials and devices (Figure 40-1H). The older phase contrast system is not of such value and not as easy to apply, and the older system is not recommended for routine use. The great advantage of the Nomarski interference contrast system is that images of phase objects are seen as if they are "shadow cast" as in a medallion. This is a purely optical effect, but it does greatly assist in recognizing the presence of biomaterial inclusions. The author has found it to be an excellent system to distinguish the structure of vascular grafts in association with tissue ingrowth. It is readily adaptable to photomicrography, and excellent demonstration and teaching transparencies can be made by interference contrast optics. The optical principles have been clearly outlined by Allan et al. [15] and the application to histological stained sections in wound-healing studies has been documented [16]. It is a highly recommended system for the delineation of shape and structure of various materials in tissue sections and was applied in Figure 40-1H and I.

Length, Size, Area Measurements, and Image Analysis

It is relatively simple to measure linear length of microscopic objects with the use of a measuring eyepiece, eyepiece micrometer reticule, and slide micrometer. The area of such objects can be measured by the Zeiss integrating eyepiece I or II (Carl Zeiss Inc., Hanover, MD) or by computerized image analysis equipment.

The development of equipment for quantitative digital image analysis has simplified, and increased the accuracy of, measuring geometric magnitudes in tissue sections. Either a direct microscopic image projected with a drawing attachment onto a tablet or a photographic print can be quantitated. It is ideal for evaluating geometric data in both transmission and scanning electron microscope photographic prints. The degradation and/or absorption of biomaterials in stained histological sections can be accurately quantitated. Area and volume of the tissue response to implanted materials are readily obtained.

All histology and histochemistry laboratories involved in the comparative evaluation of implanted biomaterials should consider quantitative image analysis equipment as a basic necessity.

Microphotometry

Photometry and spectrophotometry can also be applied to quantitate the concentration of certain materials in tissue sections. It is an ideal system for measuring the level and rate of enzyme activity in suitable tissue sections. Acid phosphatase and peptidase activity are readily quantitated by microphotometry and have been applied to measure the level of activity associated with a variety of both irritating and biocompatible implants [2, 18]. The methods for demonstrating acid phosphatase, leucine aminopeptidase, and succinic dehydrogenase have been described earlier in this chapter. The procedure of Salthouse and Matlaga [18] employing microphotometry readily gives an objective grading of acute tissue response to implanted polymer samples in soft tissues. Suitable microscope photometers [19] have been designed by the major microscope manufacturers.

The Importance of Implant Shape and Surface

The standardization of both implant shape, surface, and size is a very important factor in conducting truly objective and accurate quantitative in vivo evaluations of biomaterials. When microphotometry was employed to quantitate lysosomal enzyme activity associated with implants, the highest activities were elicited by those with a triangular cross section, and the lowest by circular samples of the same surface area [20]. Likewise, rough and abraded samples were associated with a higher cellular and enzyme response than with smooth-surfaced samples [6]. Therefore, standardization of both sample shape and surface is essential for valid in vivo evaluation of biomaterials. It is certainly crucial if any system of quantitation is employed. Greater differences in tissue responses were found between shapes and surfaces than between different materials [6, 12, 20].

REFERENCES

1   Salthouse TN, Willigan DA. An enzyme histochemical approach to the evaluation of polymers for tissue compatibility. *J Biomed Mater Res*, 6 (1972), 105–113.
2   Salthouse TN, Matlaga, BF, O'Leary RK. Microphotometry of macrophage lysosomal enzyme activity: A measure of polymer implant tissue toxicity. *Toxicol Appl Pharmacol*, 25 (1973), 201–211.
3   Novikoff AB, Holtzman E. *Cells and Organelles*. New York: Holt, Rinehart and Winston, 1976.
4   Bancroft JD. *An Introduction to Histochemical Technique*. London: Butterworth, 1968, 250, 253.
5   Troyer H. *Principles and Techniques of Histochemistry*. Boston: Little, Brown, 1980, 174, 177, 216.
6   Salthouse TN, Matlaga BF. Effects of implant surface on cellular activity and evaluation of histocompatibility. In Winter GD, Leray JL, de Groot K (Eds.), *Evaluation of Biomaterials*. London: Wiley, 1980.
7   Salthouse TN, Matlaga BF. Tissue regeneration associated with lactide-containing implants. *Trans Sec World Cong Biomater*, 1984, 272.
8   Pickett JP. Identification of inorganic particulates in a single histologic section using both light microscopy and x-ray microprobe analysis. *J Histotechnol.*, 3 (1980), 155–158.
9   Lillie RD. *Histopathologic Technic and Practical Histochemistry*. New York: McGraw-Hill, 1965, 431–453.
10   Bentner EH, Nisengard RJ, Albini B. (Eds.). Defined immunofluorescence and related cytochemical methods. *Ann NY Acad Sci*, 420 (1983), 1–432.
11   Dilley R, Herring M, Boxer L, et al. Immunofluorescent staining for factor VIII-related antigen: A tool for study of healing in vascular prostheses. *J Surg Res*, 27 (1979), 149–155.
12   Salthouse TN, Matlaga BF. Some cellular effects related to implant shape and surface. In Rubin LR (Ed.), *Biomaterials in Reconstructive Surgery*. St. Louis, MO: Mosby, 1983.
13   Bogoroch R. Liquid emulsion autoradiography. In Gahan PB, (Ed.), *Autoradiography for Biologists*. New York: Academic Press, 1972.
14   Matlaga BF, Salthouse TN, McTernan MB. The rabbit ear chamber: A unique in vivo model for the continuous observation of implanted biomaterials. *Biomater Med Dev Art Org*, 4 (1976), 359–366.
15   Allan RD, David GB, Nomarski G. The Zeiss-Nomarski differential interference equipment for transmitted-light microscopy. *Zeit Wissen Mikrosk Mik Tech*, 69 (1969), 193–221.
16   Salthouse TN. Nomarski differential-interference contrast microscopy: Application in dermal wound healing studies. *Surgery*, 75 (1973), 59–63.
17   Aherne W. Quantitative methods in histology. *J Med Lab Technol*, 27 (1970), 160–170.

18 Salthouse TN, Matlaga BF. An approach to the numerical quantitation of acute tissue response to biomaterials. *Biomater Med Art Org*, 3 (1975), 47–56.
19 Pillar G. *Microscope Photometry*. Berlin: Springer Verlag, 1977.
20 Matlaga BF, Yasenchak LB, Salthouse TN. Tissue response to implant polymers: The significance of sample shape. *J Biomed Mater Res*, 10 (1976), 391–397.

ADDITIONAL READING

1 Bancroft JD. *An Introduction to Histochemical Technique*. New York: Appleton-Century-Crofts, 1967.
2 Bourne GH. *In Vivo Techniques in Histology*. Baltimore, MD: Williams & Wilkins, 1967.
3 Carr I. *The Macrophage*. New York: Academic Press, 1973.
4 Chayen J. *Practical Histochemistry*. New York: Wiley, 1973.
5 Gahan PB. *Autoradiography for Biologists*. New York: Academic Press, 1972.
6 Goldman M. *Fluorescent Antibody Methods*. New York: Academic Press, 1968.
7 Lojda R, Gossran R, and Schiebler TH. *Enzyme Histochemistry*. New York: Springer Verlag, 1979.
8 Luna LG. *Manual of Histologic Staining Methods of the AFIP*. New York: McGraw-Hill, 1968.
9 Raekallio J. *Enzyme Histochemistry of Wound Healing*. Stuttgart, Germany: Gustav Fischer Verlag, 1970.
10 Sternberg LA. *Immunocytochemistry*. Englewood Cliffs, NJ: Prentice-Hall, 1974.
11 Troyer H. *Principles and Techniques of Histochemistry*. Boston: Little, Brown, 1980.
12 Weissman G. *The Cell Biology of Inflammation*. New York: Elsevier, 1980.

REAGENTS AND EQUIPMENT

Sigma BioSciences, P.O. Box 14508, St. Louis, MO 63178, USA. Substrate for enzyme histochemistry.

AMRESCO, 30175 Solon Industrial Pkwy., Solon, OH 44139, USA. Tissue fixatives and reagents.

Technical Products International, Inc., 5918 Evergreen, St. Louis, MO 63134, USA. Special microtomes.

Eastman Chemical Company, 25 Science Park, New Haven, CT 06511, USA. Autoradiographic detection principles, film selection, exposure principles, processing techniques and bibliography.

Chapter 41

Evaluation Through Molecular and Cellular Biology Approaches

Nicholas P. Ziats

Immunohistochemical and molecular biological techniques for identification of molecules such as growth factors, cytokines, coagulation proteins, extracellular matrix molecules, integrins, oncogenes or other nuclear and cytoplasmic proteins are becoming increasingly important in biomaterials research. The identification of these molecules specific for a particular implanted device or anatomic location may lead to the identification of material-related problems and their elimination through modification of a material and/or pharmacological therapy.

Identification of proteins in tissues by antibodies (immunohistochemistry) is important for detection of protein but does not necessarily indicate which cell is specifically responsible for its production. Concomitant sections stained for cluster of differentiation (CD) markers or specific protein unique to a cell type is beneficial. Molecular biological techniques using hybridization of nucleic acid with recombinant or oligonucleotide probes can be used to indicate the presence of specific deoxyribonucleic acid (DNA) or ribonucleic acid (RNA) sequences within tissues, cells or chromosomes. The technique of Northern (RNA) blot analyses is commonly used to identify expression or upregulated expression of genes in tissues but is not cell-type-specific. However, in some instances the amount of starting material or abundance of messenger RNA (mRNA) is small, and the mRNA needs to be amplified so that identification can be made. The development of the polymerase chain reaction (PCR) for detection of DNA or reverse transcription PCR (RT-PCR) for RNA enables one to detect minute quantities of DNA or RNA in a biologic sample for diagnostic or experimental purposes. Another method, in situ hybridization, is particularly useful to detect specific RNA within cells and therefore indicates the site of production of a certain molecule. In combination with immunohisto- or cytochemistry, identification of a specific cell type responsible for the mRNA and/or protein can be further determined. In addition, the final genetic product of a cell is often a protein that is secreted by cells with biological activity and function. These proteins can be found in the circulation, may adsorb to biomaterials, can be found in the tissue environment surrounding cells and biomaterials, or may bind to specific receptors on cells. Identification of proteins by Western blotting, enzyme-linked immunosorbent assay (ELISA), immunolabeling or immunohistochemistry can be used to qualitatively or quantitatively evaluate the species of protein that may be involved in the initial or final outcome of biocompatibility.

This chapter discusses the different techniques for identification of DNA, RNA (mRNA) and proteins that are currently being used in diagnostic pathology and research laboratories for soft tissue analyses and experimental evaluation of biomaterials. A simplified approach to understanding molecular biology, the necessary tools, and the advantages and limitations of each technique are described. In order to describe the techniques used in this chapter, a brief review of the basic concepts of nucleic and ribonucleic acid structure and function is warranted. For nonmolecular biologists, concise reviews of molecular biology are included [1–4]. A more thorough understanding of molecular and cell biology and the techniques described herein can be obtained from the additional reading list provided at the end of this chapter.

DNA, RNA AND PROTEIN

The genetic material of eukaryotic organisms is deoxyribonucleic acid (DNA), found in the chromosomes in the nucleus of the cell. The genome of an organism is the collection of all of the genes which are the functional units of DNA. In human cells, DNA is a double-stranded helix consisting of two chains that are complementary such that adjacent strands of nucleotide bases (adenine, guanine, cytosine and thymine) always pair in a specific way: adenine with thymine and guanine with cytosine. A sense strand always refers to the sequence of DNA from which mRNA is generated. Therefore, the antisense strand refers to the complementary sequence of the sense strand of DNA. In RNA, the bases are the same except that uracil replaces thymine. In addition, the DNA helix is directional, having a 5′ and 3′ end with nucleotide addition occurring from the 5′ to 3′ end. Since the nucleotides of a typical DNA sequence are added in only one direction, the synthesis of the two strands proceeds in opposite directions and thus, the strands are antiparallel. If the strands are separated (denatured) by boiling, the two separate strands can be reunited to form double-stranded segments by a process called hybridization. During this process of rejoining (annealing), if an excess of labeled (radioactive probe) DNA is added, the radioactive probe will compete with the nonradioactive DNA for binding to the complementary strand. In this manner, specific hybrids of nucleic acid probe and DNA segments can be achieved if nonhybridized material is washed away.

In human and animal cells, DNA is copied into a single strand of ribonucleic acid (RNA) and is referred to as "transcription," which in turn specifies an amino acid sequence to make a protein by a process known as "translation" (Figure 41-1). Thus, encoding a protein from a gene is a complex process involving (1) a transcription step involving copying one DNA strand into a complementary RNA strand (mRNA) by action of an RNA polymerase; (2) processing (including splicing) of this nascent mRNA into mature mRNA and transporting it from the nucleus to the cytoplasm; (3) translation steps to form the final gene product, a protein. A major biological question about this process is how these series of events are regulated. Generally, gene expression as it relates to a pathological or physiological

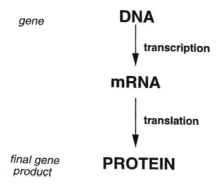

Figure 41-1 The expression of a gene encoding for a protein. This flow of genetic information is known as the central dogma and involves transcription of DNA into RNA and translation of RNA (messenger RNA, mRNA) into protein. The arrow between DNA and mRNA indicates that cellular RNA molecules are made or "transcribed" on DNA templates. All proteins are determined by or "translated" on mRNA templates.

function is of extreme interest and entails the measurement of mRNA levels as they become changed or altered with a change in the physiological state. In this chapter, the evaluation of tissues or cells with respect to qualitative and quantitative measurements of mRNA will be discussed.

IN SITU HYBRIDIZATION

One of the most powerful techniques of molecular biology has been the ability to detect specific DNA or RNA sequences at the tissue, cell or chromosome level. The technique of in situ hybridization is particularly useful to identify a specific RNA (mRNA) within cells and therefore indicates the site of production of a certain molecule [5–7]. The basis of mRNA detection and quantification is the hybridization of a single mRNA species to a specific radioactive or nonradioactive probe. Overall, the most important requirements for in situ hybridization are the retention of nucleic acid and preservation of the morphological structure of the tissue and cells. However, other important considerations for in situ hybridization are choice of fixative and processing of tissue, choice of probe, choice and specific activity of probe label, hybridization procedure, signal detection, and use of appropriate controls (Table 41-1). In combination with immunohistochemistry for specific cell markers, in situ hybridization becomes a more powerful technique because the identity of the cell will be ascertained. This is particularly important since tissues are made up of heterogenous populations of cells and routine histochemistry does not differentiate between cell types.

Table 41-1   In Situ Hybridization Methodology

Choice of Fixatives
  4% Paraformaldehyde, 2% glutaraldehyde, ethanol/acetic acid (95:5), formalin

Tissue Preparation
  Fresh or liquid nitrogen stored after cutting sections
  Paraffin or frozen sections
  Use of poly-L-lysine slides
  Proteinase K or Triton X-100 pretreatment
  Microwave

Choice of Probe
  cDNA: double or single strand (M13 vector)
  Oligonucleotide probes: single strand
  RNA: single strand antisense

Choice of Probe Label
  Radioactive: ^{3}H, ^{35}S, ^{32}P, ^{125}I, ^{131}I
  Nonradioactive: biotin, photobiotin, fluorochrome labeled, digoxigenin, mercury, acetylaminofluorene, colloidal gold

Hybridization
  Salt concentration, formamide, temperature, time, dextrans, polyethylene glycol

Detection
  Radioactive: Autoradiography
  Nonradioactive: streptavidin-biotin, alkaline phosphatase

Controls
  Tissue controls: positive and negative tissues, cell cultures
  Probe controls: Northern blot, sen, sense probes, nonradioactve probe
  Hybridization controls: RNase pretreatment, temperature
  Autoradiogram control: blank slides
  Nonradioactive controls

Retrieval of tissue for in situ hybridization should occur in a fast and efficient manner. Since RNA is rapidly degraded, fresh tissue that is rapidly fixed or immediately frozen in liquid nitrogen provides the best results. In addition, a major problem with RNA is contamination with RNases, which are heat-stable enzymes, present in most tissues, blood, bacteria, molds and on laboratory glassware and human hands. Thus, it is imperative that investigators wear gloves, use sterilized or heat-baked lab ware, and work in an isolated area of a laboratory.

A variety of fixatives have been employed but 4% paraformaldehyde fixation for a short period of 2–4 hours is adequate; other fixatives may distort the tissue and cell morphology. Cytocentrifuge preparations provide the best means for dispersed cells, while cultured cells should be rinsed to remove serum and immediately fixed. The fixed tissue can be stored in buffer solution at 40°C for up to two months while frozen blocks can be stored for a longer time in liquid nitrogen. Sections of tissue are placed on poly-L-lysine-coated glass slides to provide a stickier surface for the sections, which will eventually be exposed to a variety of harsh chemical and temperature treatments. The poly-L-lysine also covers the charge of the glass slides. Finally, prior to hybridization, the slides are pretreated with proteases such as pronase or proteinase K to remove basic proteins, followed by neutralization of the proteases with glycine. In addition, pretreatment with detergents such as Triton X-100 to further permeabilize cells is commonly used by many investigators.

A variety of probes have been utilized for in situ hybridization. Many probes are either commercially available or can be prepared from kits. The most common types of probes are cDNA (double- or single-stranded), RNA (single-stranded antisense) and oligonucleotide (single strand) probes. Nick-translated probes are prepared by cutting (nicking) the cDNA probe first with deoxyribonuclease, which removes nucleotides one at a time; the missing nucleotides are then replaced with radioactive deoxynucleotide triphosphates using a DNA polymerase [8]. The result is a radioactive, double-stranded cDNA probe that is useful for mRNAs that are rather abundant but have the disadvantage of being quite large; single-strand probes have been made from the M13 expression vector. Synthetic oligonucleotide probes are prepared by DNA synthesizers such that large amounts of probe can be made rather easily, are of high specific activity, and are not as susceptible to contaminating RNases. The third type of probe, the RNA probes, are receiving more favor since these asymmetric, single-stranded probe sequences are complementary or antisense to the cellular mRNA. Hybrids of RNA:RNA are more stable than RNA:DNA or DNA:DNA, and therefore higher hybridization and wash temperatures can be used. These probes have the additional advantage of being a constant size and having high specific activity. Furthermore, nonhybridized RNA can be readily removed from tissue sections by ribonuclease digestion. The final consideration for probes is the choice of label to be used, either radioactive or nonradioactive. The ideal label is one of high specific activity, high sensitivity and low energy emission. Radioactive probes such as ^{32}P have high energy and permit rapid and sensitive detection, but have a shorter half-life and poor resolution. Probes such as tritium have lower energy emission and good resolution, but are not as sticky as ^{32}P or ^{35}S and are not of high specific activity. Sulfur 35 has high sensitivity and specific activity, but may produce higher background activity. Iodine-labeled probes are efficient and of high activity, but require special precautions due to their high energy penetration. Nonradioactive probes are becoming more attractive due to the disposal problems of radioactive materials. Biotinylated probes have been used most successfully due to their chemical stability, but are not as sensitive as radioisotopes.

For in situ hybridization to be successful, morphology needs to be preserved with the concomitant prevention of the loss of target nucleic acid. Since the basis for hybridization is the formation of hydrogen bonds between nucleotides (RNA:RNA, RNA:DNA, DNA:DNA), it is important that conditions are favorable for nucleic acid duplex formation. The conditions of hybridization and washing require the use of salts, formamide, temperature, dextrans, and other components to block or reduce non-specific binding of probes and thus reduction in base-pair mismatching. This is referred to as stringency, and the reactions are generally done under low stringent conditions. Generally, increasing the salt concentration will lower the stringency. The use of formamide in the buffers helps to lower the temperature needed for hybridization and reduce the amount of degradation of RNA that can occur at higher temperatures.

Following hybridization, post-treatment of the tissue or cell culture samples is necessary to remove nonspecific binding of the probe and enhance the signal-to-noise ratio. Posthybridization washes are often done at higher stringency to dissociate weakly bound hybrid complexes. Following the posthybridization washes, the slide preparations are dried by processing through increasing alcohol solution and dipped in photographic emulsions until ready for development by autoradiography. After an appropriate period of time (one week for ^{32}P, 2–4 weeks for ^{35}S, one month for 3H), the slides are developed, followed by use of a fixer and then rinsing of the slides. The resultant silver grains over cells are counted and can be quantitatively expressed as number of grains per cell. It is important that the photographic emulsion is not too thick; generally, the thinner the emulsion, the better the resolution.

As appropriate for any diagnostic or experimental protocol, the use of controls will determine the specificity of the procedure. For in situ hybridization, positive and negative tissue controls should be included in the protocol. Additional sections of tissue or cells should be set aside and stained prior to the entire procedure. These should be compared to stained sections after citical steps such as the hybridization steps and after the entire procedure to ensure morphologic integrity. A probe recognizing a constitutive (always expressed) RNA or "housekeeping" gene such as actin is useful in determining the reproducibility of the technique. To determine whether the probe is hybridizing to an intended sequence, Northern blot analysis of the same tissue will give a general idea of the specificity of the target probe. When using RNA (antisense) probes, it is useful to employ sense-oriented probes as a negative control. Hybridization controls are necessary to rule out nonspecific binding of the negatively charged probes to positively charged tissue. Blank slides and nonradioactive probes should be used as additional negative controls as well as nonhybridized tissue for an autoradiographic control.

In situ hybridization technology has been used extensively in embryological development, the detection of oncogene expression in tumors, diagnosis of viral infectious diseases, wound healing, skin disorders, and cardiovascular disease, particularly atherosclerosis [9–13]. Our laboratory has been interested in mechanisms of synthetic vascular graft failure, and we and others have hypothesized that growth factors, cytokines, and extracellular matrix proteins are involved in the pathogenesis of graft failure due to increased anastomotic or intimal hyperplasia. We have evaluated by in situ hybridization, formalin-fixed, paraffin-embedded sections of retrieved human vascular graft prostheses. As shown in Figure 41-2, retrieved human vascular grafts were probed for cytokines Interleukin 1β (IL-1β) and Tumor Necrosis Factor α (TNFα) with ^{35}S-labeled cDNA probes. Other adjacent sections were probed for β-actin as a positive control and no probe or sense strand probes as negative control for these studies. Although there was some nonspecific binding of probe to the materials, the majority of black particles observed on the graft material were small titanium or antimony particles used as catalysts during polymer polymerization for the preparation of this material. This was assessed by comparative observations of non-hybridized

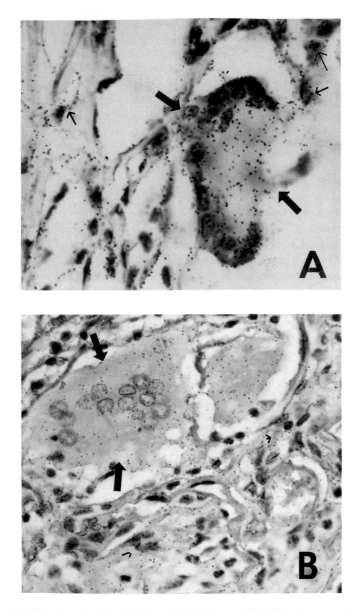

Figure 41-2 In situ (black grains) localization of (A) IL-1β and (B) TNFα in macrophages (thin arrows) and foreign body giant cells (thicker arrows) at sites of a pseudointima/graft boundary of a retrieved human vascular Dacrongraft. Other black grains represent nonspecific binding of probe or titanium and antimony used in fabrication of Dacron® fibers. Original magnification, X240.

adjacent survey sections and negative control hybridization sections. Significant amounts of specifically hybridized probe for IL-1β (Figure 41-2A) and TNFα (Figure 41-2B) were observed to be localized to macrophages and multinucleated foreign body giant cells (FBGC) at the pseudointima/graft boundary. In addition, adjacent sections were stained with the use of monoclonal antibodies to cell markers such as factor VIII antigen (endothelium), HHF-35, smooth muscle specific actin (smooth muscle) and HAM-56 antigen (macrophages) (not shown). These were beneficial in determining the specific cell types expressing these

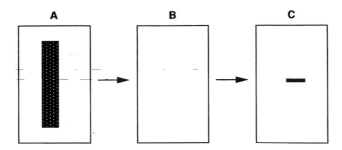

Figure 41-3 Northern blotting analysis for detection of a specific RNA sequence. (A) Total tissue or cellular RNA or poly A$^+$ RNA is isolated by homogenization in extraction buffer containing strong denaturing agents or specific inhibitors of RNase and separated by size using gel electrophoresis. (B) RNA is then transferred and crosslinked to a solid phase such as nitrocellulose or nylon membrane. (C) The membrane is then probed with a radioactive (^{32}P) nucleic acid probe (or oligonucleotide probe) complementary to the RNA sequence of interest. Nonradioactive labeling procedures can also be used. The signal that is generated is visualized by an autoradiogram after X-ray exposure.

molecules and all showed strongly positive reaction with their individual cell types. Interestingly, FBGCs did not stain for the macrophage antigen, HAM-56, but nonetheless were easily identified by their large shape and multinucleation. Therefore, the concomitant use of in situ hybridization with immunohistochemistry addresses issues of gene expression in specific cells of a heterogeneous tissue.

NORTHERN BLOT AND PCR ANALYSIS

Another common method of analyzing RNA is by Northern blotting [14, 15]. Similar to in situ hybridization, the basis of mRNA detection and quantification by Northern blotting is the hybridization of a single mRNA species to a specific probe, usually radioactive ^{32}P. As shown in Figure 41-3, RNA is isolated and separated according to size. The RNA is then transferred to a sheet or membrane-based filter, hybridized with a specific radioactive probe, and finally visualized after X-ray exposure to produce an autoradiogram. The autoradiogram can then be scanned by densitometry to obtain a (semi-) quantitative amount of mRNA. Historically, DNA sequences of genes or gene fragments were identified first by digesting DNA to produce fragments that could be electrophoretically separated according to size and blotted onto nitrocellulose. The fragments were then identified by hybridization with a labeled (^{32}P) probe by E.M. Southern; thus this blotting procedure of DNA was known as a Southern blot [16]. Southern blot analysis is commonly used to determine alterations in gene sequences and are most beneficial for genetic analysis of mutations in the genome. It is useful in prenatal diagnosis of such diseases as cystic fibrosis, α-1 antitrypsin deficiency or sickle cell anemia. Northern blot analyses have been used in numerous applications of soft tissue analysis and often in conjunction with in situ hybridization [9–13, 17–19].

Northern blot analysis can provide information regarding the relative number, size and abundance of RNAs. However, this is not necessarily an easy task since in each cell there may be 10^5 different mRNAs and 10^6 RNA molecules. Since RNA is rapidly degraded, the use of fresh tissue or rapidly frozen tissue in liquid nitrogen provides the best results. Homogenization of tissues or cells with chaotropic agents such as guanidinium thiocyanate and diethylpyrocarbonate in buffer solutions will help reduce contamination by RNase. For abundant RNA species, total RNA may be used but often this is less desirable if smaller samples are obtained. The mRNA (about 2–5 percent of the total RNA) may need to be amplified by a polymerase chain reaction (PCR) or the starting material can be a more purified preparation of the total RNA referred to as poly A^+ RNA [20]. Two other factors in improving Northern blot analysis include optimization of the transfer and coupling of RNA to membranes, and utilization of sensitive probes. Membranes such as nylon are more flexible and tear-resistant. The choice of probe for Northern blotting is similar to in situ hybridization and most commonly is ^{32}P.

One alternative method to Northern blot analysis is the dot or slot blot, in which isolated RNA is directly applied to a membrane without separation by electrophoresis [1,7]. This can be used to determine tissue specificity of the mRNAs with various tissues when the same probe is used. This technique is also useful when analyzing the same tissue but under different experimental conditions (e.g., effect of drug, cytokine or growth factor). However, disadvantages of this technique compared to Northern analysis are that size of the mRNA is not determined and physical attachment to the membrane hinders the ability of the probe hybridization.

A particularly powerful method to amplify small quantities of DNA (or RNA) was described in 1983 by Mullis from Cetus Corporation and referred to as polymerase chain reaction amplification or PCR [21–24]. In this technique (Figure 41-4), genomic DNA is extracted from cells and boiled to separate the two strands. The resulting single strands of DNA are then incubated with two single-stranded oligonucleotide primers complementary to sequences flanking the region of DNA to be studied. It is necessary that the original sequence information with which to design the oligonucleotide primers be known. The primers anneal (join) to the heat-denatured DNA, and then DNA synthesis proceeds in a $5'$ to $3'$ direction with the addition of deoxyribonucleotide triphosphates to cause DNA replication. This is followed by further heat denaturation, and the newly synthesized strand as well as the original DNA combine with additional primers and act as templates for the next round of DNA synthesis. In other words, two double-stranded molecules are yielded from the original parental DNA duplex. The process is repeated using a programmable thermal cycle that automatically carries the samples through numerous cycles (n). Thus, the DNA multiplies exponentially (2^n) as the reaction is repeated, yielding, in theory, 1000 copies of a short set of DNA fragment from one single molecule if the process is repeated 10 times (2^{10}). A disadvantage of PCR is that the sensitivity of the technique, the ability to identify one single molecule of DNA, may also be a limitation. Contamination of the original DNA strands may lead to these species being amplified with the DNA molecule of interest. In addition, there is a risk of introducing experimental mutations during the replication process, resulting in erroneous conclusions concerning the nature of the DNA. In detecting RNA by PCR (referred to as RT-PCR), the first cycle uses a reverse transcriptase to produce a cDNA copy of the mRNA, which is then amplified. An important breakthrough in this technology was the discovery of a heat-stable DNA polymerase obtained from a bacterium (*Thermus aquaticus* or Taq) found in hot springs. In a period of three to four hours, a billionfold amplification can yield microgram quantities of the DNA. This method is particularly applicable to molecular cloning, quantification of mRNA, and genetic linkage analysis.

PROTEIN ANALYSIS

The final product of a gene is a protein. It is advantageous to detect proteins in circulating fluids, adsorbed to biomaterial surfaces, in tissue sites or associated with cell membranes or cell cytoskeleton since it is ultimately proteins that have biologic and pathologic effects.

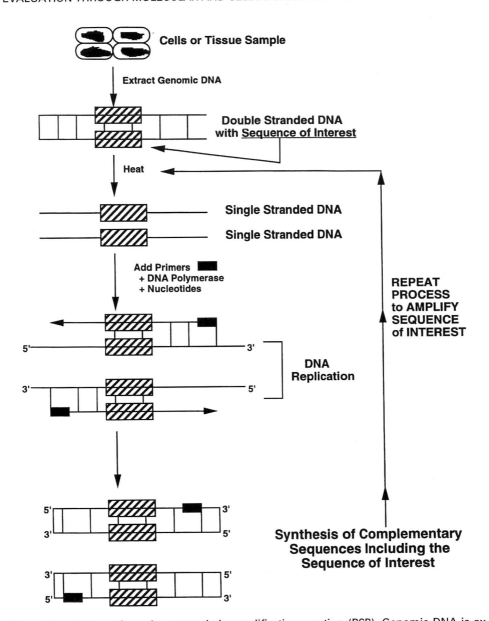

Figure 41-4 Scheme for polymerase chain amplification reaction (PCR). Genomic DNA is extracted from a tissue or cells and heated to denature the double-stranded DNA into two single-stranded DNAs. Oligonucleotide primers (black box) complementary to sequences flanking the the region of interest (striped box) combined with a heat resisitant DNA polymerase (Taq) and nucleotides allow DNA replication to occur. The process is repeated to amplify the sequence of interest. A DNA or RNA strand can be amplified 106- to 107-fold in a few hours.

The numerous functions of proteins require identification by appropriate methods. The basis for these methods is the detection of an antigen (protein) by a specific molecule known as an antibody or immunoglobulin. Antibodies are highly specific in that they bind to short regions, the epitope, of the antigen. Antigens such as proteins may have more than one epitope. Two types of antibodies are used in these protein or immunoassays, either polyclonal or monoclonal. Polyclonal antibodies are isolated from the blood of animals injected

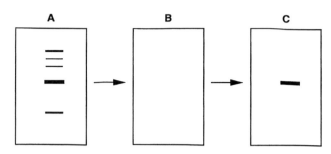

Figure 41-5 Western blotting analysis for identification of specific proteins. (A) Proteins are separated by size using SDS-PAGE gel electrophoresis. (B) Proteins are then passively blotted or electrotransferred to nitrocellulose, nylon or polyvinylidene difluoride membranes. (C) The immunodetection of a specific protein is done by an indirect method using a primary polyclonal or monoclonal antibody against the protein of interest followed by a labeled secondary detecting antibody against the primary antibody. Labeled protein A or G may be alternatively used.

with antigen and are predominately of the IgG class, but also contain smaller amounts of IgM and IgA species; hence, they are polyclonal. Monoclonal antibodies are derived in vitro by hybridoma cells (antibody-producing cells fused with an immortal tumor cell line) producing antibody directed against one specific epitope of an antigen. Both types of antibody must have high binding affinity to the antigen. Polyclonal antibodies are usually of high affinity but may provide more background or variability than monoclonal antibodies. Monoclonal antibodies are more specific, since, by design, they recognize one epitope on the target molecule. Thus, as long as the antigen has not changed its overall structure, an antibody will bind to its specific epitope, whether it be on or within cells, in solution or bound to an inert membrane. Some of the methods for protein identification of biological fluids, tissues, or cells include protein blotting (referred to as Western blotting), immunogold labeling, enzyme-linked immunosorbent assay (ELISA), immunohistochemistry and immunocytochemistry.

Western Blotting

Proteins can be separated from complex mixtures by a qualitative technique referred to as protein blotting or Western blotting [25–27]. The major limitation of Western blotting is the inability of the technique to determine the distribution of protein within cells or tissues. The general aspects of this technique, as depicted in Figure 41-5, include separation of protein by size or isoelectric point by electrophoresis, protein transfer by electroblotting and immunodetection of the isolated protein. The detection of the protein is based upon the recognition of the membrane-bound protein by an appropriate polyclonal or monoclonal antibody. Complex mixtures of proteins can be separated before blotting by at least three different means: (1) sodium dodecyl sulfate (SDS)-polyacrylamide gel electrophoresis (PAGE), in which proteins are denatured with SDS in the presence of β-mercaptoethanol and the negatively charged proteins separated by size by the sieving effect of the gel; (2) urea-PAGE, in which the acidic modification is used to separate very basic proteins; (3) native or nondenaturing gels, in which proteins are dissolved and separated by charge and size using acrylamide gradients (3–20 percent) or by isoelectric focusing, which separates proteins by a pH gradient and accumulates at their isoelectric point. Hydrophobic or amphiphilic proteins are best separated using mild, nonionic detergents, while hydrophilic proteins can be separated by native electrophoresis.

The transfer of proteins to a membrane, or blotting, can be performed by passive diffusion aided by capillary action or vacuum or by an electric field (electrotransfer). Passive transfer is slow and rather incomplete; electrotransfer is faster, but control of the electric force is necessary to retain the protein on the membrane. Membranes must have high protein binding and retention capacity, be mechanically resistant and not interfere with the binding of the antibody. The most commonly used membranes are nitrocellulose, nylon or polyvinylidene difluoride. Nitrocellulose has been the most widely used membrane due to its high binding capacity, retention and ability to be stained with dyes. Nylon membranes are mechanically more stable than nitrocellulose and have found their use in Northern and Southern blot analysis. However, these membranes do not stain with general protein stains. Polyvinylidene difluoride membranes are being more widely used since they have properties characteristic of both nitrocellulose and nylon. Their only drawback is that they must be wetted in methanol prior to use and not be allowed to dry during the blotting or detection procedure.

The detection of protein on the membranes is achieved by an indirect method, use of a primary polyclonal or monoclonal antibody followed by a secondary or detecting antibody. In addition, the membranes can be stained for total protein using a number of different dyes including Amido black, Coomassie blue, Ponceau red, India ink or colloidal gold. A critical step before immunodetection of specific proteins is carried out is the blocking of membranes to eliminate nonspecific adsorption of protein to the membranes. A variety of blocking agents, such as Tween-20, ovalbumin/gelatin, bovine serum albumin or nonfat dry milk solution, have been used. In our experience, a 5–10% solution of nonfat dry milk in phosphate buffered saline with 1 mM disodium EDTA is inexpensive and a superior blocking agent. After blocking, primary antibody against the protein of question is added, followed by blocking again and then detection with a labeled secondary antispecies antibody or with labeled protein A or G. As previously discussed, primary antibodies for immunoassays like Western blotting can be either polyclonal or monoclonal. An important feature is that the antibody must have high binding affinity to the attached protein on the membrane. Polyclonal antibodies are usually of high affinity but may provide more background staining than monoclonal antibodies. Monoclonal antibodies, by design, are more specific but must be able to recognize the epitope on the protein that may be conformationally changed during the binding of protein to the membrane and especially if protein denaturing agents such as SDS are used. Finally, detection of the interaction of the primary antibody with the protein is achieved with a labeled secondary antibody, either antispecies (an anti IgG) or the more global proteins A or G. Protein A has a higher affinity for IgG than protein G but both may not recognize all species of IgG or IgG subtypes. It is often a matter of experience as to which detecting antibody is used. Some of the detecting labels used for the secondary antibody include colloidal gold (with or without silver enhancement), enzymes such as horseradish peroxidase or alkaline phosphatase, and chemi-luminescence. Enzymes exhibit a sensitivity similar to that of colloidal gold and form a colored precipitate with chromogens such as 4-chloro- napthol or 3,3′ diaminobenzidine for peroxidase, 5-bromo-4 chloro-3-indolylphosphate with nitroblue tetrazolium or napthol phosphate with fast red for phosphatase. These enzyme detection systems can be enhanced by use of a bridging antibody which recognizes the primary antibody as well as the antienzyme antibody that is raised in the same species as the primary antibody. The antienzyme antibody will then bind to the enzyme. An example of this is the standard peroxidase-antiperoxidase method commonly used in immunohistochemistry [29]. Colloidal gold beads can be coupled to secondary antibody or to protein A or G. Silver enhancement (gold nucleates silver particles and enlarges them) can increase the sensitivity of the detection of the antibody-antibody (protein A) reaction.

We have used a modification of Western blotting referred to as immunogold labeling with silver enhancement and scanning electron microscopy to identify proteins on the surfaces of retrieved human vascular graft prostheses or from an experimental system of circulating human blood through biomaterials [30–32]. These studies determined if certain blood derived proteins would be present at the endstage of vascular graft failure and showed that proteins such as fibronectin, Hageman factor (factor XII), high molecular weight kininogen, fibrinogen and factor VIII/vWF could be detected on these surfaces. Fibronectin was the most abundant protein detected on either retrieved ePTFE grafts or umbilical vein grafts. Protein deposition was disperse on all surfaces and cellular deposition could be seen in association with proteins identified, in particular, with fibronectin (Figure 41-6A). These studies have contributed to our hypothesis of the importance of protein adsorption to vascular graft

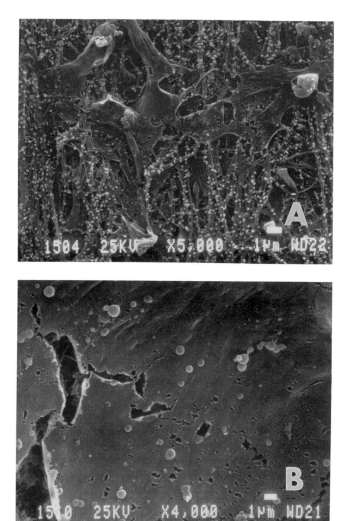

Figure 41-6   Immunogold labeling and scanning electron microscopy of the surface of a retrieved human vascular graft. (A) The surface of a vascular graft stained with an antibody to human fibronectin. There are abundant white beads, approximately 100–200 nm in size. (B) The surface of a retrieved vascular graft not stained with any primary antibody. The large white spherical structures are bacteria, the reason this graft was removed.

materials and indicate the need to study the complex interactions of blood with surfaces as well as understand the molecules present after long-term implantation in failed as well as successful grafts. This technique is especially beneficial for investigating the interactions of proteins with material surfaces.

Immunoassays and Enzyme-Linked Immunosorbent Assay

A useful technique for identification and quantitation of proteins (antigens or antibodies) in solution, particularly from plasma, serum, exudates or cell culture supernatants are the immunoassays [33, 34]. These immunochemical techniques are based upon simple and accurate methods for measuring the quantity of an indicator molecule. If the indicator molecule is labeled with a radioisotope (^{3}H, ^{125}I) and quantified in a scintillation or gamma counter, the assay is referred to as a radioimmunoassay. The indicator molecule may also be covalently coupled to an enzyme and quantified in a spectrophotometer or plate reader by measuring the conversion of a clear substrate to a colored reaction product. This is referred to as an enzyme-linked immunoabsorbent assay, or ELISA [33–36]. The ELISA technique has been particularly useful in biomaterials research for identifying qualitatively and/or quantitatively growth factors or cytokines that may be involved in soft tissue pathology such as myofibroblast, smooth muscle, or epithelial cell growth; angiogenesis; fibrosis; or differentiation of inflammatory cells at implant sites [36, 37].

In general, there are three type of immunoassays: antibody capture, antigen capture, and two-antibody sandwich assays [34]. In an antibody capture assay, the antigen is bound to a solid support (polystyrene plates) and labeled antibody is allowed to bind. After washing, the amount of antibody remaining bound to the antigen is quantified. In an antigen capture assay, the antibody is attached to the solid support, and labeled antigen is allowed to bind. The unbound proteins are removed by washing and the assay quantitated by determining the amount of antigen bound. In a two-antibody sandwich assay such as the ELISA, one antibody is bound to a solid support and antigen is allowed to bind to the first antibody. A second labeled antibody is added and the assay quantified by measuring the amount of labeled second antibody that binds to the antigen. In addition, all of these assays can be performed in antigen or antibody excess, or as an antibody or antigen competition. Antibody excess or antigen competition assays are used to detect and quantitate antigens while antigen excess or antibody competition assays are used to detect and quantify antibodies. All of the immunoassays are relatively easy, rapid, and sensitive. The sensitivity is dependent on the specific activity of the antigen, avidity/affinity of the antibody or antibodies (in the case of the two-antibody sandwich assay), and the type of support. The detection limit for these assays is in the range of 0.1–1.0 fmole or 0.01–0.1 ng. The antibody capture assays are the most versatile of the three since they can determine both antigen and antibody levels as well as compare antibody binding sites. Antigen capture assays are commonly used for antigen detection and quantification using enzyme-linked detection; many commercially available kits for cytokines and growth factors are of this type. The support system for immobilization of antigen or antibody is either polyvinylchloride or polystyrene for microtiter plates, nitrocellulose or diazotized paper for sheets, or activated or protein A-coated beads.

As has been mentioned, the two-antibody sandwich or two-site immunoassay, ELISA, is the basis for many commercially available kits. These kits are of high specificity and sensitivity even among closely related antigenic species. However, high specificity is often obtained at the expense of sensitivity of these types of assays due to many factors including surface effects, polyclonal versus monoclonal antibodies, cross-reactivity of antibodies or antigens, aggregation of antibodies, enzyme interference and validation of statistical significance. This has been a particular problem with cytokine analysis and standardization [38, 39]. However, these assays have been extremely popular since their advent some 25 years ago; because they provide improved sensitivity, specificity, and reduction of time and effort, these assays will still be utilized.

Immunohistochemistry

Immunohistochemical assays are useful for the visualization of cellular antigens by using specific antibodies against the antigen of interest [29, 39, 40]. Once an antibody has bound to its particular protein, a number of methods are available for making the bound antibody visible. This technique is therefore useful in determining whether a particular protein is present within a tissue or cell and with electron microscopy, to localize a protein to a specific organelle. The identification of a protein unique to a organelle, cell or tissue and the change of expression or pattern of expression of the marker protein can be a valuable tool in pathologic diagnoses. By using in situ hybridization on serial sections or combining immuno-histo/cytochemistry and in situ hybridization on the same cell preparation or tissue section, both genetic and phenotypic parameters in the same biological material can be ascertained.

For immunohisto- or cytochemistry, the tissue or cells need to be fixed (formalin, paraformaldehyde or glutaraldehyde) and if they are tissues, need to be imbedded in a support such as paraffin so that thin sections ($5\,\mu$m) for light microscopy or ($<0.1\,\mu$m) electron microscopy can be made. Tissue morphology will be best preserved by crosslinking fixation (formalin, glutaraldehyde) but antibodies may no longer recognize epitopes on the fixed tissue. Therefore, if an antibody cannot be found that reacts with the fixed, embedded tissue sections, tissue can be frozen and sections made for antibody staining. The disadvantage of frozen sections is the loss of cell and tissue architecture; the advantage is antigen preservation.

Detection of antigen in cells or tissues is similar for immunohisto/cytochemistry as described earlier for Western blotting or ELISA. The sections require appropriate primary and secondary antibody applications, washing and blocking techniques. For immuno-histo/cytochemistry the two main detecting systems are either enzymes which give a colored reaction product or fluorescent dyes. Two of the most common enzymes, as mentioned in Western blotting, are horseradish peroxidase and alkaline phosphatase, which when given an appropriate substrate, produce an insoluble, colored reaction product. At our institution we have used a very sensitive immunohistochemical technique known as the labeled streptavidin-biotin system (LSAB). The basis of this technique is the high affinity of avidin (an egg white glycoprotein) for the vitamin biotin. The LSAB method uses an unlabelled primary antibody made specifically against the antigen in question, and a secondary or "link" antibody made against the immunoglobulin of the species in which the primary antibody was developed. The secondary antibody is biotinylated to accept the streptavidin-biotin complex which serves as the tertiary or "labeling" step. Streptavidin (from the bacterium *Streptomyces avidinii*) is capable of binding four molecules of biotin with high and irreversible affinity and can be covalently coupled to horseradish peroxidase or alkaline phosphatase [29, 40]. The last step in the process is the addition of the substrate or chromogen reagent. In this reaction, the enzyme label bound to the streptavidin complexes with the substrate, causing the H_2O_2 to decompose to water and atomic oxygen. The atomic oxygen then oxidizes the chromogen (acting as an electron donor), resulting in a colored electron product at the sites of antigen localization (Figure 41-7). This technique has been successfully used to identify antigens from frozen tissue sections as well as formalin-fixed, paraffin-embedded

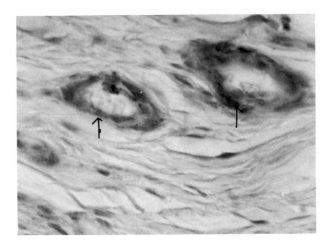

Figure 41-7 Immunohistochemical staining for smooth muscle cell specific actin using a monoclonal antibody, HHF-35, and the labeled streptavidin-biotin system. The reaction product is a brown insoluble precipitate using the chromgen, 3,3' diaminobenzidine and counterstained with hematoxylin. Original magnification, X160.

tissue sections from soft tissues [41]. This has been most useful for serial sections that have also been processed for in situ hybridization to identify specific cell antigens, protein and mRNA species [42].

In addition to enzyme-based methods, immunofluorescent techniques for antigen detection have been commonly used and are based upon fluorophors (fluorescein or tetramethylrhodamine isothiocyanate) that absorb light at one wavelength and emit it at another, longer, wavelength. Although extremely useful in pathologic diagnosis, fluorescent labeling has disadvantages that include appreciable autofluorescence, fading of the fluorochrome upon exposure to light, out-of-focus information degrading the image, and need for additional microscopic equipment. These problems can be overcome with a confocal light microscope with digital imaging to obtain multiple exposures and complex image manipulation and enhancement. Finally, both positive and negative controls are essential to determine the sensitivity and specificity of the technique. Positive controls should include tissue or cell cultures known to express the antigen of interest. Negative controls should include replacement of the primary antibody with a nonimmune antisera or IgG and a buffer solution replacing the primary antibody to determine the extent of nonspecific secondary antibody binding to the tissue or cells.

The use of molecular and cell biology techniques for evaluation of soft tissue (and soft tissue-biomaterial) pathology will be necessary to completely understand the pathologic mechanisms related to device success or failure. As in any scientific discipline, understanding the jargon is often as important as the understanding of the concepts and the techniques. Once the terminology is understood, the techniques for molecular and cellular biological analyses are not implicitly difficult and can provide significant qualitative and quantitative information relevant to soft tissue pathology.

REFERENCES

1   Chirgwin JM. Molecular biology for nonmolecular biologists. *Diabetes Care*, 13 (1990), 188–197.
2   Berk PD, Worman HJ. An introduction to molecular biology and recombinant DNA technology for the hepatologist. *Sem Liver Dis*, 12 (1992), 227–245.

3 Swynghedauw B, Barrieux A. An introduction to the jargon of molecular biology. Part I. *Cardiovasc Res*, 27 (1993), 1414–1420.

4 Swynghedauw B, Moalic J-M, Bourgeois F, Barrieux A. An introduction to the jargon of molecular biology. Part II. *Cardiovasc Res*, 27 (1993), 1566–1575.

5 Terenghi G, Fallon RA. Techniques and applications of in situ hybridization. In Underwood JCE (Ed.), *Current Topics in Pathology*. Berlin: Springer-Verlag, 1990, 289–337.

6 DeLellis RA, Wolfe HJ. New techniques in gene product analysis. *Arch Pathol Lab Med*, 111 (1987), 620–627.

7 Wiesner RJ, Zak R. Quantitative approaches for studying gene expression. *Am J Physiol*, (1991), L179-L188.

8 Rigby P, Dieckmann M, Rhodes C, Berg P. Labeling deoxyribonucleic acid to high specificity in vitro by nick translation with DNA polymerase I. *J Molec Biol*, 113 (1977), 237–251.

9 Boehm KD, Kelley MF, Ilan J, Ilan J. The interleukin 2 gene is expressed in the syncytiotrophoblast of the human placenta. *Proc Natl Acad Sci (USA)*, 86 (1989), 656–660.

10 Engelmann GL, Boehm KD, Haskell J, Khairallah PA, Ilan J. Insulin-like growth factors and neonatal cardiomyocyte development: ventricular gene expression and membrane receptor variations in normotensive and hypertensive rats. *Molec Cell Endocrinol*, 63 (1989), 1–14.

11 Wilcox JN, Smith KM, Williams LT, Schwartz SM, Gordon D. Platelet-derived growth factor mRNA detection in human atherosclerotic plaques by in situ hybridization. *J Clin Invest*, 82 (1988), 1134–1143.

12 Wilcox JN. Analysis of local gene expression in human atherosclerotic plaques by in situ hybridization. *Trends Cardiovasc Med*, (1991), 17–24.

13 Brody JI, Pickering NJ, Capuzzi DM. Interleukin-1a as a factor in occlusive vascular disease. *Am J Clin Pathol*, 97 (1992), 8–13.

14 Krumlauf R. Analysis of gene expression by Northern blot. *Mol Biotechnol*, 2 (1994), 227–245.

15 Naber SP. Molecular pathology-detection of neoplasia. *N Engl J Med*, 331 (1994), 1508–1510.

16 Southern EM. Detection of specific sequences among DNA fragments separated by gel electrophoresis. *J Mol Biol*, 98 (1975), 503–717.

17 Golden MA, Au YPT, Kenagy RD, Clowes AW. Growth factor gene expression by intimal cells in healing polytetrafluoroethylene grafts. *J Vasc Surg*, 11 (1990), 580–585.

18 Golden MA, Au YPT, Kirkman TR, et al. Platelet-derived growth factor activity and mRNA expression in healing vascular grafts in baboons. Association in vivo of platelet-derived growth factor mRNA and protein and cellular proliferation. *J Clin Invest*, 87 (1991), 406–414.

19 Hamdan AD, Aiello LP, Quist WC et al. Isolation of genes differentially expressed at the downstream anastomosis of prosthetic arterial grafts with use of mRNA differential display. *J Vasc Surg*, 21 (1995), 228–234.

20 Boseley PG, Moss T, Birnstiel ML. 5′ labeling and poly(dA) tailing. *Meth Enzymol*, 65 (1980), 478–494.

21 Mullis KB. The unusual origin of the polymerase chain reaction. *Sci Amer*, 264 (1990), 56–65.

22 Bakkenist CJ, O'Leary JJ, Chetty R. The use of recent molecular biology techniques in pathology. *Adv Anat Pathol*, 2 (1995), 306–313.

23 Teo IA, Shaunk S. Polymerase chain reaction in situ: An appraisal of an emerging technique. *Histochem J*, 27 (1995), 647–659.

24 Ma TS. Applications and limitations of polymerase chain reaction amplification. *Chest*, 108 (1995), 1393–1404.

25 Egger D, Bienz K. Protein (Western) blotting. *Mol Biotechnol*, 1 (1994), 289–305.

26 Uhl J, Newton RC. Quantitation of related proteins by Western blot analysis. *J Immunol Meth*, 10 (1988), 79–84.

27 Stott DI. Immunoblotting and dot blotting. *J Immunol Meth*, 119 (1989), 153–187.

28 Hoefakker S, Boersma WJA, Claassen E. Detection of human cytokines in situ using antibody and probe based methods. *J Immunol Meth*, 185 (1995), 149–175.

29 Sternberger LA, Hardy PH, Cuculis JJ, Meyer HG. The unlabeled antibody enzyme method of immuno-histochemistry. Preparation and properties of soluble antigen-antibody complex (horseradish peroxidase-antihorseradish peroxidase) and its use in identification of spirochetes. *J Histochem Cytochem*, 18 (1970), 315–333.

30 Ziats NP, Pankowsky DA, Tierney BP, Ratnoff OD, Anderson JM. Adsorption of Hageman factor (factor XII) and other human plasma proteins to biomedical polymers. *J Lab Clin Med*, 116 (1990), 687–696.

31 Pankowsky DP, Ziats NP, Topham NS, Ratnoff OD, Anderson JM. Morphological characteristics of adsorbed human plasma proteins on vascular grafts and biomaterials. *J Vasc Surg*, 11 (1990), 599–606.

32 Ziats NP, Topham NS, Pankowsky DA, Anderson JM. Analysis of human blood protein adsorption on retrieved human vascular grafts using immunogold labeling with silver enhancement. *Cells & Mater*, 1 (1991), 73–82.

33   Porstman T, Keissig ST. Enzyme immunoassay techniques. An overview. *J Immunol Meth*, 150 (1992), 5–21.
34   Harlow E, Lane D. Immunoassays. In *Antibodies. Laboratory Manual*. Cold Spring Harbor, NY: Cold Spring Harbor Laboratory Press, 1988, 553–612.
35   Crowther JR. ELISA. Theory and practice. *Methods Mol Biol*, 42 (1995), 1–218.
36   Bonfield TB, Colton E, Marchant RE, Anderson JM. Cytokine and growth factor production by monocytes/macrophages on protein preadsorbed polymers. *J Biomed Mater Res*, 26 (1992), 837–850.
37   Anderson JM, Ziats NP, Azeez A, Brunstedt MR, Stack S, Bonfield TB. Protein adsorption and macrophage activation on polydimethlysiloxane and silicon rubber. *J Biomater Sci Polymer Edn*, 7 (1995), 159–169.
38   Pesce AJ, Michael JG. Artifacts and limitations of enzyme immunoassay. *J Immunol Meth*, 150 (1992), 111–119.
39   Falini B, Taylor C. New developments in immunoperoxidase techniques and their applications. *Arch Pathol Lab Med*, 107 (1983), 105–117.
40   Diamandis EP, Christopoulus TK. The biotin-(strept)avidin system: Principles and applications in biotechnology. *Clin Chem*, 37 (1991), 625–636.
41   Anderson JM, Abbuhl MF, Hering T, Johnston KH. Immunohistochemical identification of components of the healing response of human vascular grafts. *ASAIO J*, 8 (1985), 79–85.
42   Speel EJM, Ramaekers FCS, Hopman AHN. Cytochemical detection systems for in situ hybridization, and the combination with immunocytochemistry. "Who is still afraid of red, green and blue?" *Histochem J*, 27 (1995), 833–858.

ADDITIONAL READING

General Molecular and Cellular Biology

1   Lodish H, Baltimore D, Berk A, Zipursky SL, Matsudaira P, Darnell J. *Molecular Cell Biology*. New York: Scientific American Books, Inc., 1995.
2   Watson JD, Hopkins NH, Roberts JW, Steitz JA, Weiner AM. *Molecular Biology of the Gene*, 4th ed. Menlo Park, CA: The Benjamin/Cumming Publishing Company, Inc., 1987.
3   Greco RS. Implantation Biology. *The Host Response and Biomedical Devices*. Boca Raton, FL: CRC Press, Inc., 1994.

General Molecular Biology Techniques

4   Maniatis T, Fritsch EF, Sambrook J. *Molecular Cloning: A Laboratory Manual*, 2nd ed. Cold Spring Harbor, NY: Cold Spring Harbor Laboratory Press, 1989.
5   Berger SL, Kimmel AR. *Guide to Molecular Cloning Techniques*. (Methods in Enzymology, Vol. 152). New York: Academic Press, 1987.

In Situ Hybridization and PCR

6   Hames BD, Higgins SJ. *In Situ Hybridisation, Nucleic Acid Hybridisation. A Practical Approach*. Oxford: IRL Press, 1985.
7   Chesselet M-F. *In Situ Hybridization Histochemistry*. Boca Raton, FL: CRC Press, Inc., 1990.
8   Latchman DS. *PCR Applications in Pathology. Principles and Practice*. Oxford: Oxford University Press, 1995.
9   Nuovo GJ. *PCR In Situ Hybridization. Protocols and Applications*. New York: Raven Press, 1992.
10   Innis MA, Gelfand DH, Sninsky JJ, White THJ. *PCR Protocols: A Guide to Methods and Applications*. San Diego: Academic Press, 1990.

Western Blotting

11   Bjerrum OJ, Heegard NHH. *Handbook of Immunoblotting of Proteins*, Vols. 1 & 2. Boca Raton, FL: CRC Press, Inc., 1988.

ELISA

12 Harlow E, Lane D. *Antibodies. A Laboratory Manual.* Cold Spring Harbor, NY: Cold Spring Harbor Laboratory Press, 1988.

Immunohistochemistry

13 Larsson L-I. *Immunocytochemistry: Theory and Practice.* Boca Raton, FL: CRC Press, Inc., 1988.
14 Furthmayer H. *Immunochemistry of the Extracellular Matrix*, Vols 1 & 2. Boca Raton, FL: CRC Press, Inc., 1982.

Chapter 42

The Cage Implant Testing System

Weiyuan John Kao
James M. Anderson

INTRODUCTION

The objective of in vivo testing of a candidate biomedical material is to determine the safety or biocompatibility of the material in a biological environment. Material biocompatibility can be defined as the ability of a material to perform with an appropriate host response in a specific application. Biocompatibility assessment is considered to be a measure of the magnitude and duration of adverse alterations in homeostatic mechanisms that determine the host response. The International Standards Organization and the American National Standards Institute have developed a multitude of testing protocols for the evaluation of biomedical materials [1, 2]. The test criteria include cytotoxicity, sensitization, irritation, intracutaneous reactivity, implantation, systemic toxicity (sub-acute, acute, sub-chronic, chronic), and biodegradation.

The normal inflammatory events leading to the normal foreign body reaction are categorized into three stages: acute, chronic, and granulation tissue (Figure 42-1). However, the components of the normal foreign body reaction within the implant site may vary. The onset of the inflammatory response to a biomaterial is initiated primarily by the tissue injury due to the invasive surgery procedure (see also Chapter 31). The first phase of the acute inflammatory response is initiated by permeability changes in the adjacent vasculature resulting in the movement of plasma components into the injury area. This leads to exudation which causes the adsorption of blood proteins onto the biomaterials; this is generally considered to be the initial event in tissue-material or blood-material interactions [3]. The preferential migration of neutrophils mediated through chemotactic stimuli is a well known characteristic of the acute inflammatory response. Eventually, monocytes and macrophages become the predominant cell type in the exudate and are the principle cell type responsible for the normal wound healing and the foreign body reaction characteristic of the chronic inflammatory response. Persistent inflammatory stimuli may lead to the development of multinucleated foreign body giant cells (FBGCs) formed from the fusion of adherent macrophages [4]. As the extent of chronic inflammation attenuates, neovascularization, fibroblast proliferation with collagen deposition, and fibrosis constitute the final resolution stage, resulting in the isolation of the material from the physiological environment of the implant site.

The subcutaneous cage implant system has been introduced for in vivo investigations to elucidate the changes in the inflammatory response to biomaterials. The system permits the delineation of the influence between cells and material in a specific, accurate, sensitive, and quantitative manner. Specifically, the cage system provides a standard inflammatory environment in which the biocompatibility of a material can be studied temporally in terms of humoral and cellular responses, enzyme release, cell-material interactions,

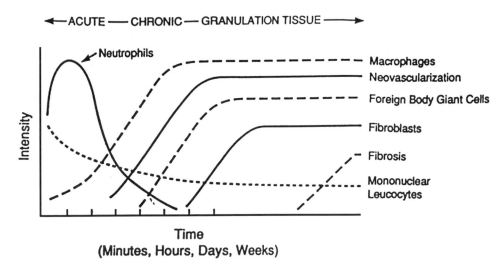

Figure 42-1 Temporal variation in acute, chronic inflammatory response, granulation tissue development, and foreign body reaction to implanted biomaterials. The intensity and time variables depend on the extent of injury created in the implantation and the size, shape, topography, and chemical and physical properties of the biomaterial.

FBGC formation kinetics, and biostability of materials without the mechanical interference of surrounding tissues. Furthermore, this inflammatory environment can be altered by co-implanting additional materials formulated with various pro- or anti-inflammatory substances.

The cage implant procedure is herein briefly described [5–7]. Cylindrical cages (4.0 cm in length and 1 cm in diameter) are constructed from surgical-grade stainless steel mesh (0.25 mm wire diameter, 0.8 mm opening width with 58% open area) (Figure 42-2). A test material is placed inside the cage and the entire specimen is sterilized prior to implantation. The animal is anesthetized and a 1.5–cm incision is made at the posterior region of the animal's back. The specimen is implanted subcutaneously at the level of the panniculus carnosus and the incision is closed with surgical wound clips or sutures. Sterile techniques are used throughout and the implantation of empty cages is used as controls. (The general details of implantations are provided in Chapter 31.) The inflammatory exudate which collected within the cage can be withdrawn for analysis using a 1 cc $17^{1/2}$G tuberculin syringe after 4 days post-implantation as the initial surgical injury subsides. Total and differential exudate leukocyte concentrations can be quantified using standard procedures [5–7]. The exudates can be further analyzed using various immunochemical and biochemical characterization techniques. The results permit quantitative and comparative evaluations of the temporal variation in cellular and humoral components of the inflammatory and immune responses between different types of biomaterials.

Several studies involving the uses of the cage implant system are summarized to demonstrate the extensive applications of the system in evaluating material biocompatibility in vivo. These studies include: inflammatory cell/biomaterial interactions [5–10], intracellular and extracellular enzyme release from leukocytes [9–11], controlled release of bioactive agents from polymer systems [12–14], ion-selective membrane and biosensor evaluation [15, 16], polyurethane biostability and biodegradation [17–22], macrophage adhesion and foreign body giant cell formation [23–25], cytokine-modulated cell-material

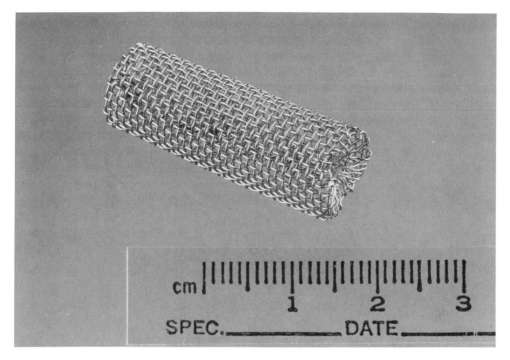

Figure 42-2 Cage for the subcutaneous cage implant system.

interactions [11, 26, 27], and macrophage Ia antigen (major histocompatibility complex II) expression of biomedical polymers [28].

CONTROLLED RELEASE OF BIOACTIVE AGENTS FROM POLYMER SYSTEMS

In the research and development of implantable drug delivery systems, in vivo biocompatibility studies play an important role in determining the safety and efficacy of these devices. As the desired goal of delivery systems is to deliver or release a drug or therapeutic agent either locally or systemically in vivo, studies which concomitantly monitor the delivery of therapeutic agents in conjunction with the biocompatibility of the system are important. From this perspective, the cage implant system offers an ideal testing environment which permits the simultaneous in vivo analysis of the release of therapeutic agents and components of the inflammatory and healing responses. In vivo biocompatibility of several delivery systems has been determined using the cage implant system. Here, two systems will be discussed in detail.

A gentamicin-silicone rubber monolithic delivery system has been developed for insertion in prosthetic heart valves for the treatment of prosthetic valve endocarditis. The exudate leukocyte concentrations showed that the gentamicin-silicone rubber system displayed an increased inflammatory response up to 7 days post-implantation when compared to the silicone rubber specimens alone and empty-cage controls (Table 42-1) [12]. This increased leukocyte concentration was accompanied by an increased neutrophil and exudate extracellular alkaline phosphatase activity. By days 14 and 21 post-implantation, the inflammatory response of the gentamicin-silicone rubber system was comparable to that of the silicone

Table 42-1   Total Exudate Leukocyte Concentrations (Cells/μl) of Gentamicin-Silicone Rubber Monolithic Delivery System

Time (days)	Empty-cage controls	Silicone	Gentamicin-silicone
4	4160 ± 520	3640 ± 510	$6940 \pm 510^{\dagger}$
7	820 ± 180	920 ± 140	$2550 \pm 260^{\dagger}$
14	260 ± 50	$700 \pm 180^{\dagger}$	$750 \pm 10^{\dagger}$
32	120 ± 50	300 ± 80	350 ± 290

Note: All values expressed in mean $\pm$ standard deviation ($n \geq 4$).
† indicates values which are statistically different at 95% confidence level ($p < 0.05$) when compared with the respective values of empty-cage controls as determined by un-paired Student's t-test.

rubber and empty-cage controls. The release of gentamicin into the exudate was monitored and was described by a pseudo first-order characteristic with an initial burst effect at 4 days post-implantation and subsided release at 7 days post-implantation. Thus, it was concluded that the released gentamicin, which had been shown to have clinical nephrotoxic effects, caused the increased inflammatory response.

The cage implant system was also used to identify the effect of hydrocortisone acetate (HA) loaded poly(D,L-lactide) (PLA) film on the inflammatory response [13]. The results showed that the HA/PLA system dramatically inhibited all aspects of inflammation over the 21-day time period when compared with the PLA and empty-cage controls (Table 42-2). This was evident by the decrease in total and differential leukocyte concentrations. The results also indicated that the presence of HA markedly inhibited fibrous capsule formation surrounding the cage implants, indicating a suppressed fibrosis which is the final stage of the healing response.

The utilization of the cage implant system and statistical evaluation of the quantitative results permitted these conclusions to be drawn regarding the broad activity of genta-micin and HA in the in vivo environment. Furthermore, these two examples demonstrate the usefulness of the cage implant system in providing quantitative information regarding the in vivo inflammatory and wound healing responses of drug delivery systems. The tech-nique permits the statistical comparison between drug-carrying materials and the materials themselves, as well as the drug-release profile.

Table 42-2   Exudate Leukocyte Concentrations ($\times$ 10^2 Cells/μl) of Hydrocortisone Acetate (HA) Loaded Poly(D,L-Lactide) (PLA)

Time (days)	Total leukocyte concentration			Neutrophil Concentration			Concentration	Macrophage	
	Control†	PLA	HA/PLA	Control†	PLA	HA/PLA	Control†	PLA	HA/PLA
3	47 ± 7	38 ± 6	25 ± 3	34 ± 1	27 ± 7	8 ± 0	10 ± 5	7 ± 4	6 ± 1
4	22 ± 2	25 ± 4	6 ± 2	15 ± 2	16 ± 3	3 ± 2	5 ± 1	5 ± 1	1 ± 0
7	13 ± 2	13 ± 2	4 ± 2	5 ± 2	5 ± 1	< 1	4 ± 1	4 ± 1	1 ± 0
14	7 ± 2	8 ± 2	1 ± 1	< 1	< 1	< 1	3 ± 1	1 ± 0	1 ± 0
21	7 ± 2	11 ± 6	1 ± 1	< 1	< 1	< 1	1 ± 1	2 ± 0	1 ± 0

Note: All values expressed in mean $\pm$ standard deviation ($n \geq 4$).
† empty-cage controls.

ION-SELECTIVE MEMBRANE AND
BIOSENSOR EVALUATION

Ion-selective sensors have become routine tools in various clinical chemistry laboratories to monitor continuously the ultrafiltrate of blood or blood constituents. However, long-term in vivo applications of ion-selective sensors have been limited due to poor stability (see also Chapter 28 for implantable biosensors). High molecular weight poly(vinyl chloride) (PVC)-based and aliphatic polyurethane-based (Tecoflex®, Thermedics, Inc., Woburn, MA) ion-selective membranes with various plasticizer concentrations were tested to intercorrelate membrane compositions, analytical properties, and biostability [15, 16]. Membranes with decreasing plasticizer content showed improved adhesive properties, fewer anion interferences, extended lifetime, and better biocompatibility. Specifically, the exudate leukocyte concentrations indicated that an increase of plasticizer weight percent in Tecoflex® correlated positively with an increase in leukocyte concentrations, indicating an increased host inflammatory response up to 14 days of implantation. The results also demonstrated that both PVC- and Tecoflex®-based ion-selective membranes with the most common membrane composition (1:2 polymer-to-plasticizer ratio) exhibited a similar acute inflammatory response, but the PVC-based membrane elicited a reduced chronic inflammatory response when compared with the Tecoflex®-based membrane.

The electrochemical properties of the sensor were monitored in situ for various implantation times (data not published). Biosensor electrodes constructed from the membrane were embedded in a cylindrical plug made of a thermoset plastic. Using surgical adhesive, the plug was used to cap the end of a stainless-steel cage using surgical adhesive and prepared for implantation. Lead wires were passed subcutaneously along the dorsal side of the animal to the top of the cranium where an instrumentation interface was mounted with surgical adhesive. At various predetermined post-implantation times, the impedance and other electrochemical properties of the sensor were measured and the exudate was collected to assess the extent of inflammatory response. At the last implantation time, the sensor was retrieved and analyzed with a scanning electron microscope to evaluate sensor integrity and adherent macrophages and FBGCs. There was a significantly higher adherent FBGC density at the sensing element when compared with the substrate. These results offer a optimal design paradigm for ion-selective membranes in the continuous monitoring of electrolytes in vivo.

POLYURETHANE BIOSTABILITY
AND BIODEGRADATION

With the extensive use of polyurethanes in biomedical applications, such as artificial heart diaphragms, ventricular assist bladders, vascular grafts, mammary prostheses, and pacemaker leads, biodegradation of polyurethanes has become an important issue to biomaterials scientists. Proposed mechanisms of polyurethane biodegradation are environmental stress cracking, metal ion oxidation, enzymatic degradation, and electrostatic ion/polymer interactions [22]. Studies in our laboratory have provided the basis for a hypothesis concerning cell/polymer feedback control of in vivo biodegradation [8, 18]. This hypothesis illustrates a sequence of in vivo events leading to polymer surface degradation and to the production of polymer degradation products. Initial biological interactions, i.e., protein adsorption and cellular adhesion, may be influenced by surface properties and characteristics of the biomedical polymer.

The cage implant system allows investigation into the nature of in vivo leukocyte activation, adhesion and FBGC formation on polyurethanes. Cellular characterizations can

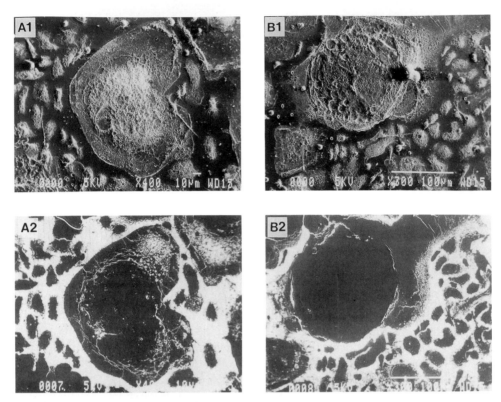

Figure 42-3 Polyether urethane urea/FBGC interphase in vivo after 5 weeks of implantation showing the adherent FBGCs (A1, B1) and cracking/pitting underneath the FBGCs after the removal of FBGCs (A2, B2).

be quantified with enzyme histochemistry and microscopy. The location of FBGCs on the polyurethane surface was correlated to the areas of surface biodegradation in vivo using optical and scanning electron microscopy techniques [19]. Surface cracking and/or pitting were found mostly at the interfacial areas of FBGCs and the polymer surfaces (Figure 42-3). The morphology of surface degradation at the cell/polymer interfacial areas was similar to that observed in an in vitro H_2O_2/Co^{++} oxidative environment [18, 20–22]. Furthermore, the presence of an anti-inflammatory steroid in the implanted cages effectively decreased the adherent leukocyte activation, density, and inhibited polyurethane biodegradation when compared with polymer-only controls [8]. These results further ascertain the important role of adherent macrophages and FBGCs in modulating material biodegradation in vivo.

The chemical changes of the polyurethane as a result of biodegradation were investigated using a micro-attenuated total reflectance-Fourier transform infrared spectroscopy [21, 22]. When compared with untreated controls, degraded surface of implanted polyurethanes showed chemical degradation as evident by large intensity changes: mainly decreases in the methylene bands at 1364 cm^{-1} from the polytetramethyleneglycol soft segment, at 1730 cm^{-1} and 1709 cm^{-1} from urethane carbonyl, and new absorptions at 1670 cm^{-1}, 1255 cm^{-1}, and 1174 cm^{-1} attributed to the formation of carboxylic acid and hydroxyl groups in degradation products. A depth profile analysis was utilized to quantitatively assess the surface degradation with implantation duration. There was a positive relationship between the depth of degradation with increasing implantation time. Furthermore, the higher the penetration depth in the degraded areas, the fewer the changes in spectra relative to the untreated control was observed. This indicated that degradation was a surface phenomenon. The change in molecular weight was determined using gel-permeation chromatography with refractive index and ultraviolet detectors to elucidate the presence and nature of degradation products. The presence of low molecular weight products was observed with increasing implantation time, thus confirming the presence of degradation products. Clearly, these analyses permit the intercorrelations between the cellular/humoral inflammatory responses and the chemical compositions of the biomaterials in vivo and between in vivo and in vitro correlations of degradation mechanisms.

MACROPHAGE ADHESION AND FOREIGN BODY GIANT CELL FORMATION

Since adherent macrophages and FBGCs had been shown to modulate biodegradation by releasing reactive oxygen intermediates which can oxidatively degrade polyurethanes, a quantitative description of FBGC formation on implanted polymer surfaces as a function of time can conceivably correlate cell adhesion with polymer properties and possibly predict the behavior of the polymer in vivo. The formation of FBGCs was studied through theoretical and statistical analysis in terms of cell size distribution, density changes, and kinetics of FBGC formation [23–25]. Two parameters were developed to quantify the dynamic process of FBGC formation: the density of adherent macrophages present initially that participate in FBGC formation (d_0) and the rate constant for cell fusion; both kinetic parameters were used to calculate the time-dependent FBGC density. It was concluded that increase in polyurethane hard segment weight percent, surface hardness, and hydrophobicity increased total protein adsorption and effectively increased d_0 and FBGC density [25]. The presence of mechanical strain in the polyurethane increased the rate of FBGC formation but had no effect on d_0 and FBGC density [25]. The results also indicate that the presence of antioxidant additive in polyurethane, in addition to scavenging oxygen intermediates, increased in vivo biostability by significantly decreasing d_0, FBGC density, and lowering the rate of cell fusion.

CYTOKINE-MODULATED CELL-MATERIAL INTERACTIONS

The host response to implanted biomedical polymers is dynamic and complex. In vitro cell culture systems allow the examination of specific cellular interactions with biomaterials. The cage implant system permits the extension and confirmation of in vitro phenomena in an in vivo environment. In vitro results had suggested that a variety of polymers could differentially activate human monocytes to produce protein(s) of considerable biological significance. Exudate interleukin-1 concentrations were monitored temporally in vivo and were found to be time- and material-dependent (Figure 42-4) [11]. Interleukin-1 mediates various inflammatory processes, regulates fibroblast growth, proliferation, and collagen production. The results indicate the ability of leukocytes in mediating a wide range of host responses to biomaterials in a material-dependent manner in vivo.

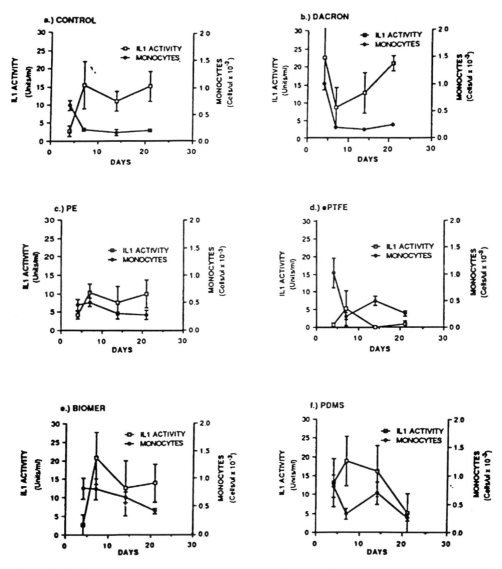

Figure 42-4   Monocyte concentration versus interleukin-1 level in vivo for various biomaterials.

Interleukin-4 was previously shown to induce extensive macrophage fusion to form FBGCs in vitro [27]. The subcutaneous cage-implant system was used to elucidate interleukin-4 participation in mediating FBGC formation in vivo [26]. Exudate leukocyte concentrations from cages containing poly(etherurethane urea) and empty cage controls indicated a similar inflammatory response that turned toward resolution by 14 days post-implantation. Purified goat anti-mouse interleukin-4 neutralizing antibody (IL4Ab) or normal goat nonspecific control IgG (gtIgG) at various concentrations, or recombinant murine interleukin-4 (muIL4) were injected into the implanted cages containing poly(etherurethane urea) every 2 days for 7 days. The injection of IL4Ab significantly decreased the FBGC density on poly(etherurethane urea) cage-implanted in mice, when compared with the non-specific gtIgG or saline injection controls (Table 42-3). Conversely, the FBGC density was

Table 42-3   Adherent Macrophage and FBGC Density on Poly(Ether urethane Urea) in the Presence of Interleukin-4 Neutralizing Antibody (IL4Ab) or Normal Goat Nonspecific Control IgG (gtIgG), or Recombinant Murine Interleukin-4 (muIL4) Injections

Treatment (n-value)	Adherent macrophage density (cells/cm^2)	Adherent FBGC density (cells/cm^2)	Average adherent FBGC size ($\times 10^{-3}$ mm^2)
100 ng muIL4 (3)	80200 ± 12960	$6100 \pm 460^\dagger$	2.90 ± 0.90
250 μg IL4Ab (4)	53040 ± 20170	$1410 \pm 260^\dagger$	2.09 ± 1.80
250 μg gtIgG (4)	63620 ± 13130	4430 ± 1010	2.80 ± 0.49
PBS control (12)	73120 ± 21130	4280 ± 1050	3.58 ± 1.09

Note: All values expressed in mean $\pm$ standard error of means. All injections, in volume of 0.25 ml of sterile PBS, were made every two days for 7 days directly into the cages.
† indicates values which are significantly different at 99% confidence level ($p < 0.01$) when compared with PBS and nonspecific gtIgG controls as determined by independent Student's t-test.

significantly increased by the injection of muIL4 when compared with nonspecific gtIgG and PBS injection controls. Adherent macrophage density, FBGC morphology, FBGC average size and size distribution were not significantly different among IL4Ab, nonspecific control gtIgG, muIL4, and PBS control groups. These data suggest that IL-4 participates in FBGC formation on biomaterials in vivo.

MACROPHAGE Ia ANTIGEN (MAJOR HISTOCOMPATIBILITY COMPLEX II) EXPRESSION

Major histocompatibility complex class II antigens, Ia, are involved in the initiation and control of immune responses regulated by T cells. Activated macrophages display an increased expression of Ia-antigen on the surface membrane. The cage implant system has been used in conjunction with cytofluorimetric analysis of exudate leukocytes to evaluate the monocyte/macrophage cell activation and phenotypic expressions in response to different biomedical materials [28]. Polyurethanes with or without additives, polydimethylsiloxane, polyetherimide, and polyetheretherketone showed maximum numbers of Ia-positive macrophages at 7 days post-implantation. By day 14, the percentage of Ia-positive macrophages decreased, showing 19–32% Ia-positive cells. With the exception of polydimethylsiloxane, the percentages of Ia-positive macrophages for all materials at 14 days post-implantation were higher than the empty-cage controls. These results indicate the multifunctional role of inflammatory leukocytes in the recruitment, activation, and maintenance of immune cells at tissue-material interfaces.

CONCLUSIONS

The subcutaneous cage implant system is a realistic system to evaluate inflammatory cell and material interactions related to biostability and biodegradation phenomena in vivo. Specifically, the system permits quantitative analysis of the temporal variation in cellular and humoral components of the inflammatory and immune response. The quantitative results can be analyzed statistically, allowing comparative evaluations between various types of biomaterials. The cage implant system permits the temporal analysis of biosensor function with concomitant resolution of the inflammatory response. Thus the system is an in vivo model for monocyte and macrophage activation, adhesion, and foreign body giant cell development on biomaterial surfaces.

REFERENCES

1 ISO Standard 10993-1: Biological evaluation of medical devices, Part 1: guidance on selection of tests. In Morrey BF (Ed.), *Biological, Material, and Mechanical Considerations of Joint Replacement*. New York: Raven Press, 1993, 337–392.

2 Anderson JM. Cardiovascular device retrieval and evaluation. In Harker LH, Ratner BD, Didishiem P (Eds.), *Cardiovascular Biomaterials and Biocompatibility: A Guide to the Study of Blood-Material Interactions*. New York: Elsevier, 1993, 199S–208S.

3 Anderson JM, Ziats NP, Bonfield TL, McNally AK, Topham NS. Human blood protein and cell interactions with cardiovascular materials. In Akutsu T, Koyanagi H (Eds.), *Artificial Heart*, 3. Tokyo: Springer-Verlag, 1991, 45–55.

4 Smetana K, Jr. Multinucleated foreign-body giant cell formation. *Exp Mol Pathol*, 46 (1987), 258–265.

5 Marchant R, Hiltner A, Hamlin C, Radinovitch A, Slobodkin R, Anderson JM. *In vivo* biocompatibility studies: I. The cage implant system and a biodegradable hydrogel. *J Biomed Mater Res*, 17 (1983), 301–325.

6 Marchant RE, Phua K, Hiltner A, Anderson JM. *In vivo* biocompatibility studies: II. Biomer®: Preliminary cell adhesion and surface characterization studies. *J Biomed Mater Res*, 18 (1984), 309–315.

7 Marchant RE, Miller KM, Anderson JM. *In vivo* biocompatibility studies: V. *In vivo* leukocyte interactions with Biomer®. *J Biomed Mater Res*, 18 (1984), 1169–1190.

8 Zhao Q, Agger MP, Fitzpatrick M, Anderson JM, Hiltner A, Stokes K, Urbanski P. Cellular interactions with biomaterials: *In vivo* cracking of pre-stressed Pellethane® 2363-80A. *J Biomed Mater Res*, 24 (1990), 621–637.

9 Marchant RE, Anderson JM, Castillo E, Hiltner A. *In vivo* biocompatibility studies: VIII. The effects of an enhanced inflammatory reaction on cast Biomer. *J Biomed Mater Res*, 20 (1986), 153–168.

10 Marchant RE, Sugie T, Hiltner A, Anderson JM. Biocompatibility and an enhanced acute inflammatory phase model. In Fraker AC, Griffin CD (Eds.), *Corrosion and Degradation of Surgical Implant Materials, Second Symposium*. American Society for Testing and Materials, 1985, 251–266.

11 Miller KM, Rose-Caprara V, Anderson JM. Generation of IL-1-like activity in response to biomedical polymer implants: A comparison of *in vitro* and *in vivo* models. *J Biomed Mater Res*, 23 (1989), 1007–1026.

12 Anderson JM, Marchant R, McClurken M. Tissue response to drug delivery systems: The cage implant system. In Zatuchni GI, Goldsmith A, Shelton JD, Sciarra JJ (Eds.), *Long-Acting Contraceptive Delivery Systems*. New York: Harper and Row, 1984, 248–225.

13 Spilizewski KL, Marchant RE, Hamlin CR, Anderson JM, Tice TR, Dappert TO, Meyers WE. The effect of hydrocortisone acetate loaded poly(DL-lactide) films on the inflammatory response. *J Contr Rel*, 2 (1985), 197–203.

14 Anderson JM. *In vivo* biocompatibility of implantable delivery systems and biomaterials. *Eur J Pharm Biopharm*, 40 (1994), 1–8.

15 Lindner E, Cosofret VV, Ufer S, Buck RP, Kao WJ, Neuman MR, Anderson JM. Ion-selective membranes with low plasticizer content: Electroanalytical characterization and biocompatibility studies. *J Biomed Mater Res*, 28 (1994), 591–601.

16 Cosofret VV, Kao WJ, Linder E, Erdosy M, Anderson JM, Neuman MR, Buck RP. Electroanalytical and biocompatibility studies on carboxylated PVC membranes for microfabricated array sensors. *Analyst*, 119 (1994), 2283–2292.

17 Brunstedt MR, Anderson JM, Spilizewski KL, Marchant RE, Hiltner A. *In vivo* leukocyte interactions on Pellethane® surfaces. *Biomaterials*, 11 (1990), 370–378.

18 Anderson JM, Hiltner A, Zhao QH, Wu Y, Renier M, Schubert M, Brunstedt M, Lodoen GA, Payet CR. Cell/polymer interactions in the biodegradation of polyurethanes. In Vert M, Feijen J, Albertsson A, Scott G, Chiellini E (Eds.). *Biodegradable Polymers and Plastics*. Cambridge, England: Royal Society of Chemistry, 1992, 122–136.

19 Zhao Q, Topham N, Anderson JM, Hiltner A, Lodoen G, Payet CR. Foreign-body giant cells and polyurethane biostability: *In vivo* correlation of cell adhesion and surface cracking. *J Biomed Mater Res*, 25 (1991), 177–183.

20 Wu Y, Zhao Q, Anderson JM, Hiltner A, Lodoen G, Payet CR. Effect of some additives on the biostability of a poly(etherurethane) elastomer. *J Biomed Mater Res*, 25 (1991), 725–739.

21 Wu Y, Sellitti C, Anderson JM, Hiltner A, Lodoen G, Payet CR. An FTIR-ATR investigation of *in vivo* poly(ether urethane) degradation. *J Appl Polym Sci*, 46 (1992), 201–211.

22 Frautscki JR, Chinn JA, Phillips Jr RE, Zhao QH, Anderson JM, Joshi R, Levy RJ. Biodegradation of polyurethanes *in vivo*: Comparison of different models. *Colloids Surfaces B: Biointerfaces*, 1 (1993), 305–313.

23 Zhao QH, Anderson JM, Hiltner A, Lodoen GA, Payet CR. Theoretical analysis on cell size distribution and kinetics of foreign body giant cell formation *in vivo* on polyurethane elastomers. *J Biomed Mater Res*, 26 (1992), 1019–1038.

24 Kao WJ, Zhao QH, Hiltner A, Anderson JM. Theoretical analysis of *in vivo* macrophage adhesion and foreign body giant cell formation on polydimethylsiloxane, low density polyethylene, and polyether urethane. *J Biomed Mater Res*, 28 (1994), 73–79.

25 Kao WJ, Hiltner A, Anderson JM, Lodoen GA. Theoretical analysis of *in vivo* macrophage adhesion and foreign body giant cell formation on strained poly(etherurethane urea) elastomers. *J Biomed Mater Res*, 28 (1994), 819– 829.

26 Kao WJ, McNally AK, Hiltner A, Anderson JM. Role for interleukin-4 in foreign-body giant cell formation on a poly(etherurethane urea) *in vivo*. *J Biomed Mater Res*, 29 (1995), 1267–1275.

27 McNally AK, Anderson JM. Interleukin-4 induces foreign body giant cells from human monocytes/macrophages: Differential lymphokine regulation of macrophage fusion leads to morphological variants of multinucleated giant cells. *Am J Pathol*, 147 (1995), 1487–1499.

28 Petillo O, Peluso G, Ambrosio L, Nicolais L, Kao WJ, Anderson JM. *In vivo* induction of macrophage Ia antigen (MHC Class II) expression by biomedical polymers in the cage implant system. *J Biomed Mater Res*, 28 (1994), 635–646.

Chapter 43

Evaluation of Explanted Cardiovascular Prostheses

Frederick J. Schoen

As an updated summary of a previously published [1] set of approaches to analysis of cardiovascular devices explanted after function in either animals or humans, this chapter is intended to be used as a guide to selection rather than performance of procedures. Space limitations necessitate that representative examples be heavily supported by literature citations to sources that comprise detailed discussions and illustrations of specific protocols and methodology.

GENERAL CONSIDERATIONS

Informed analysis of explanted cardiovascular devices (including cardiac valve prostheses, cardiac assist devices, blood vessel grafts, stents, pacemakers and catheters) enhances patient management and recognition of device complications, guides the development and assesses the efficacy and safety of potential improvements, and elucidates the mechanisms of patient-prosthesis and tissue-bio-materials interactions [2–5]. Moreover, pathologic evaluation of FDA-approved medical devices is an important responsibility mandated by the Safe Medical Devices Act of 1990 [6, 7].

The techniques used to study explanted cardiovascular are summarized in Table 43-1. However, not all laboratories have the technical and financial resources to perform all analyses, and not all evaluations are required in each case. Therefore, the components of pathological analysis have been prioritized as Level I (those modalities minimally necessary to characterize the essential safety and efficacy, including device complications, cause of death, and critical patient-prosthesis and tissue-biomaterial interactions) or Level II (those tests that are difficult or expensive to perform or yield more esoteric information). Whenever possible, during the conduct of Level I studies, material should be appropriately preserved, stored and documented for Level II studies, in the event they should subsequently be indicated.

Procedures used to evaluate cardiovascular devices and prostheses after function in animals and humans are largely the same. However, animal studies often permit more detailed in vivo monitoring (subject to humane treatment considerations) and allow in situ observation and procurement of implants following elective sacrifice at desired intervals. In addition, specimens from experimental animals are often obtained immediately after death, thereby minimizing autolytic changes. Furthermore, advantageous technical adjuncts that are impossible in the clinical environment may be feasible in animal studies (e.g., in vivo imaging of radiolabelled platelets to reveal sites and kinetics of their interaction with a device [8], preharvest injection of Evan's blue dye to allow gross assessment of endothelial coverage [9], and physiological pressure perfusion fixation to obtain optimal conditions for electron microscopy [10, 11].

Table 43-1   Techniques Used to Evaluate Explanted Cardiovascular Biomaterials and Prosthetic Devices

Technique	Purpose/information derived
Level I	
Gross examination	Observe local and systemic interactions with a device
Radiographic examination	Detect and localize mineral deposits
Microbiological cultures	Detect and localize infection
Light microscopic histology	Microscopic morphology; special stains may be used as adjuncts to demonstrate specific tissue components
Level II	
Transmission electron microscopy (TEM)	Ultrastructural features of cells and extracellular matrix
Scanning electron microscopy (SEM)	Surface topographic features
Energy dispersive x-ray analysis (EDAX)	Site-specific chemical elemental analysis (e.g., Ca. P. etc.)
Immunohistochemical studies	Identify and localize specific proteins, including cell identification and functional antigens
Chemical and spectroscopic analysis	To assess bulk mineral or other elemental concentrations
X-ray or electron diffraction	Crystal structure
Biochemical assay	Bulk concentration of a specific protein moiety
Molecular studies	Assay cell functions; localize or quantitate DNA or RNA
Functional studies	Device performance in-vitro following in-vivo function

Modified from Schoen FJ, *Interventional and Surgical Cardiovascular Pathology: Clinical Correlations and Basic Principles,* Philadelphia: W.B. Saunders, 1989, with permission.

Studies of pertinent pathology distant from an implant may be informative. In all but the most acute experiments, relevant injury due to emboli is primarily demonstrated by grossly visible active or healing infarcts or scars in the distal circulatory bed; however, because not all emboli produce infarcts, careful gross dissection of major visceral arterial beds (e.g., spleen, kidneys) is advisable. Moreover, the presence of renal iron deposits (hemosiderosis) may be indicative of device-induced blood cell damage (hemolysis) [12], and biomaterials emboli are indicative of device dysfunction [13].

The planning stage of implant experiments should include the preparation of detailed protocols that will maximize information gain. Formulation of such protocols ideally has contributions from all study collaborators, including a pathologist familiar with both the objectives of the study and pertinent methods of evaluation, and includes the development of appropriately detailed diagrams for recording key study data.

Specimen Harvest and Gross Analysis

Pertinent modes of device dysfunction, including thrombus formation, must be anticipated. Location of thrombus should be specifically related, if possible, to areas of flow separation or stasis, or component junctions. Gross examination of implant and associated host tissues (both local and distant) should be done, wherever possible in situ, because removal of the implant from its functional context may impair detection of critical pathological findings (e.g., thrombotic deposits dislodged during removal of a catheter, an endocardial jet lesion in the heart chamber proximal to a substitute heart valve that indicates regurgitation through or around the prosthesis, or a long suture end that precipitates thrombosis of a heart valve prosthesis by extrinsic interference). Generous use of gross photography is encouraged [14]. Microbiological cultures of the device, attached thrombus, and the subject's blood establish whether infectious organisms are present. Additional analyses represent research approaches to the mechanisms of blood-surface interaction and biomaterials degradation processes in unique clinical and experimental situation.

Histological and Special Studies

Histological methods provide near-mandatory documentation in all but the most cursory investigations. Specimen manipulation necessarily varies depending on the information desired from the analysis; limitations and requirements for various types of studies have been described [1, 3, 5]. Because fixation may reduce or eliminate antigen reactivity, sections of rapidly frozen tissue/biomaterial cut on a cryomicrotome may be required for immunohistochemical staining for some (but not all) markers of cell identification and phenotype [15–17], adherent proteins, (such as immunoglobulins or coagulation factors) [18, 19] or histochemical staining for enzymes [20, 21]. In contrast, specimens for routine light microscopy (LM) or scanning or transmission electron microscopy (SEM or TEM, respectively) are generally fixed in solutions that denature proteins by cross-linking (usually 10 percent neutral buffered formalin [a 4 percent formaldehyde solution]) for preservation of gross morphology and for LM, and buffered glutaraldehyde solutions (usually 2–3 percent glutaraldehyde) for SEM and TEM. Division of specimens into frozen and variously fixed portions may allow studies that may otherwise be mutually exclusive.

Formalin penetrates tissue thoroughly and rapidly, despite relatively large specimen size (up to 1 cm thick), but precludes study of tissue by TEM, because preservation of subcellular structures by formalin is poor. In contrast, glutaraldehyde penetrates tissue less well; good fixation necessitates tissue less than approximately 0.1 cm in maximum thickness. Fixatives combining the best features of both glutaraldehyde and formaldehyde fixation, such as Karnovsky's solution, containing 2.5 percent glutaraldehyde and 2 percent paraformaldehyde, yield tissue suitable for both light and electron microscopy [22]. Appropriate fixation in general requires a solution volume approximately ten times that of the specimen.

Specimens for LM are conventionally embedded in paraffin and sectioned to 5–6 μm thick. However, glycolmethacrylate (GMA) embedding medium (JB-4 medium, Polysciences, Warrington, PA) is useful for specimens in which a tissue-biomaterial interface is to be maintained intact, or where calcification is prominent. Tissue morphology revealed by GMA sections cut at 2–3 μm is superior to that in paraffin. However, most special stains demonstrating connective tissue (e.g., collagen or elastin) are not suitable for GMA, and reagent costs and technician effort are greater with GMA than with paraffin.

SPECIFIC DEVICE CONFIGURATIONS

Heart Valve Prostheses

Cardiac valvular replacement enhances functional capacity and prolongs survival of many patients with severe, symptomatic valvular heart disease. Caged-ball, caged-disk and

Table 43-2 Complications of Cardiac Valve Substitutes

Generic	Specific
Thrombotic limitations	Thrombosis
	Thromboembolism
	Anticoagulation-related hemorrhage
Infection	Prosthetic valve endocarditis
Structural dysfunction	Wear
	Fracture
	Poppet escape
	Leaflet immobility
	Cuspal tear
	Calcification
	Commissural region dehiscence
Non-structural dysfunction	Pannus (tissue overgrowth)
	Entrapment by suture or tissue
	Paravalvular leak
	Disproportion
	Hemolytic anemia
	Noise

Modified from Schoen FJ, Levy RJ, Piehler HR. Pathological considerations in replacement cardiac valves. *Cardiovasc Pathol* 1992; 1:29, with permission.

tilting-disk mechanical prostheses fabricated entirely from nonphysiological materials and tissue valves composed of animal or human tissues have been used as cardiac valve substitutes. Of the approximately 172,000 valves implanted each year worldwide (approximately 63,000 in the United States), the great majority are carbon bileaflet tilting disk valves (especially the St. Jude Medical model), and flexible-stent-mounted porcine aortic valve bioprostheses (especially Carpentier-Edwards and Hancock models), each fabricated from a glutaraldehyde-preserved pig aortic valve [23–25].

Despite considerable evolution of surgical techniques and prosthetic valve design over three decades, device failures are common. Valve-related complications not only cause almost half of late deaths but also necessitate reoperation or cause death within 10 years postoperatively in at least 50 percent of patients with either mechanical prostheses or bioprostheses [2, 26–31]. The diverse mechanisms of substitute valve failure and patient-prosthesis interactions (largely summarized in Table 43-2) have been elucidated by many investigators using careful explant analysis [32–42]. Pathologic studies of valve substitutes may also reveal the absence of potential detrimental features and, indeed, may recognize correlates of successful function [43–46].

The high risk of thromboembolic complications in patients with mechanical valve prostheses, including thrombotic valvular malfunction and thromboembolism, necessitates lifetime anticoagulation, usually with warfarin derivatives [23, 24]. Consequently, such patients are at risk for anticoagulation-related hemorrhage. In contrast, the rate of thromboembolic complications in tissue valves remains relatively low, without anticoagulation [23].

As a limitation to the long-term success of clinical and experimental cardiac valve replacement, durability concerns vary widely for mechanical valves and bioprostheses, for specific models of mechanical prostheses and for the same model prosthesis placed in different anatomic sites [2, 28]. Historical intrinsic structural failure modes for mechanical prostheses include ball variance of a silicone elastomer caged-ball valve occluder (due to lipid infiltration and subsequent swelling, distortion, and cracking), cloth abrasion and fragmentation with cloth-covered caged-ball valves, and disk wear in caged-disk valves [2]. Most mechanical heart valve prostheses currently in use have pyrolytic carbon occluders, and some have both carbon occluders and carbon cage components. Except for highly valve-design-specific housing or disk fractures in pyrolytic carbon-containing valves, few mechanical failures have been reported [28, 47].

Infections associated with mechanical prosthetic or bioprosthetic heart valves are often localized to the sewing ring at the site of tissue attachment, causing a ring abscess. Moreover, infection on bioprosthetic heart valves commonly invades and is destructive to the cuspal tissue. Other important valve-related problems (frequently called non-structural dysfunction) include (1) partial separation of the suture line anchoring the valve, leading to a paravalvular leak (regurgitation of blood around the prosthesis), (2) destruction of blood components on their passage through the prosthesis (hemolysis), especially a degraded valve, or around a device with a paravalvular leak, and (3) interference with valve opening or closing by extrinsic structures, such as sutures, valve remnants, or overgrowth of fibrous tissue.

Approaches to the dissection of heart valve explants have been described [2, 5, 28]. A general schema is summarized in Figure 43-1. Valve type identification is facilitated by use of keys and atlases. Inspection of valves for evidence of thrombosis, infection, paravalvular leak or dysfunction, and microbiological cultures of areas suspected of infection should be followed by photography of the prosthesis from both inflow and outflow aspects. Adherent material should be submitted for histological examination to assess tissue reaction and infection. For a tissue-derived prosthesis, the leaflets should be examined for flexibility, uniformity, tears and calcification. Examination of bioprostheses includes radiography (for location and extent of calcific deposits [48]) and usually LM of representative sections. For specific valve types, special analyses and approaches may be appropriate, such as sectioning through whole heart valves [49], SEM of critical wear areas, histology of tissue ingrowth into cloth-covered struts and/or poppet volume analysis [50], and determination of tissue calcium concentrations and spatial distributions in bioprostheses [51, 52]. Unique considerations emerge for studies of prosthetic valve sewing cuffs [53], valvular allografts, trileaflet polymeric prostheses [30, 54, 55] and non-stented aortic (or mitral) valves [56].

Cardiac Assist Devices and Artificial Hearts

Studies of explanted cardiac assist devices or artificial hearts with smooth and textured (fibrillar) pump bladders have been reported, and analytical considerations have been described [57–65]. The most important problems are thrombosis (often with embolism), infection and bladder calcification (in experimental but not clinical devices).

A general schema for analysis of a cardiac assist device or artificial heart is summarized in Figure 43-2. Following disassembly, gross examination of the specimen, cultures and photographic documentation, the pump bladder and valves are radiographed to assess calcification. Sections for LM and SEM should be selected and processed from the inflow, intermediate, and outflow portions of the pump bladder and valves, as well as any other areas suggesting pathology, preferably using GMA embedding to facilitate maintenance of intact tissue-biomaterials interfaces during sectioning. LM of selected embedded and stained cross sections may be used to map pseudointimal thickness variations along the pumping bladder surface and to provide tentative identification of cellular and non-cellular components, such as leukocytes, fibroblasts, endothelial cells, fibrin, collagen, and calcium

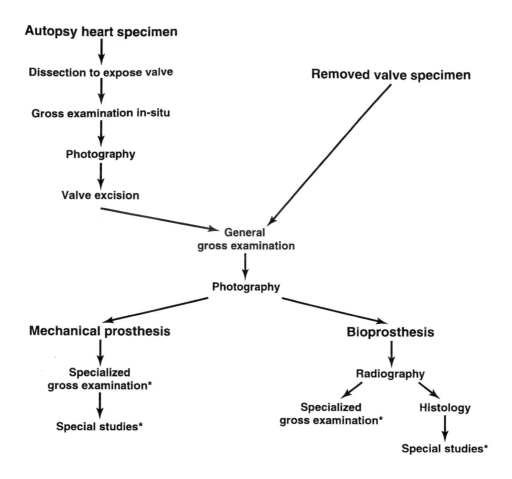

EXPLANT ANALYSIS OF A CARDIAC VALVE PROSTHESIS

* recommended for specific indication only

Figure 43-1   Schema for analysis of retrieved mechanical and bioprosthetic cardiac valves. Evaluations designated by * are Level II tests, recommended for special indication only. (Reproduced by permission from F. J. Schoen, *Interventional and Surgical Cardiovascular Pathology: Clinical Correlations and Basic Principles*, Philadelphia, PA: W. B. Saunders, 1989.)

deposits. Consideration should be given to freezing a portion of the pump bladder for later immunohistochemical or biochemical studies of cell identification and function, in the event they are indicated subsequently. SEM can document surface smoothness, uniformity and the presence of cells and thrombotic elements.

Vascular Grafts

Human autopsy studies over the past three decades have demonstrated that further than 1–2 cm from a vascular graft-blood anastomosis, the blood-surface interface consists of layers of platelet-fibrin aggregate, rather than endothelium [2, 29]. Most experimental animals, in contrast, have a greater ability to endothelialize prostheses than man, both

ANALYSIS OF A CARDIAC ASSIST DEVICE/ARTIFICIAL HEART

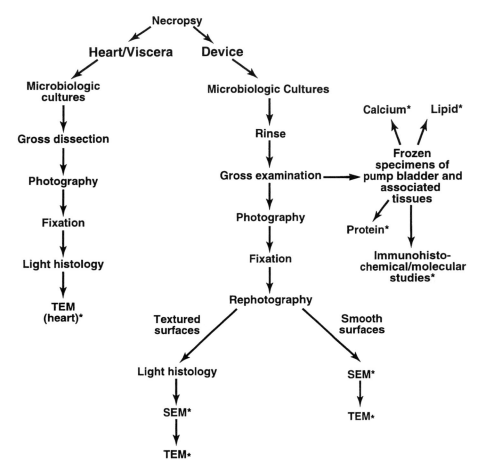

* recommended for specific indication only

Figure 43-2   Schema for pathological analysis of a cardiac assist device/artificial heart. Evaluations designated by * are Level II tests, recommended for special indication only. (Reproduced by permission from F. J. Schoen, *Interventional and Surgical Cardiovascular Pathology: Clinical Correlations and Basic Principles*, Philadelphia, PA: W. B. Saunders, 1989.)

in degree and rapidity. Endothelium in graft healing potentially derives from: (1) growth across anastomotic sites from the host vessel (most important), (2) growth through the interstices of the graft wall, they are if sufficiently large (not a common circumstance), and (3) differentiation of pluripotent mononuclear cells deposited from the flowing blood (however, it is unlikely that this mechanism actually occurs [2, 29]).

Early failure of small (<6–8 mm) diameter vascular grafts is almost entirely due either to technical factors, or poor runoff flow, leading to thrombotic occlusion; late failures are due most often to anastomotic intimal thickening, mechanical failure, infection, or separation at the anastomotic site with hemorrhage (false aneurysm) [66–68].

Gross examination should document the location, type, length, and diameter of the graft, as well as coverage by thrombus fibrous tissue, with particular reference to the anastomoses, and perigraft tissue reaction. The surgeon or pathologist who explanted the specimen should not only have distinguished proximal and distal aspects of the specimen by placement of sutures or notching, but also have provided a key to the designation. For dissection, the graft may be opened longitudinally and pinned out on a cork sheet prior to fixation, or transected at 3–5 mm intervals, the latter superior for occluded biologic or ePTFE grafts. LM histology is used to assess the anastomotic tissue structure, including extent of coverage, cell morphology and type, and the thickness and specific nature of ingrown or deposited layers (see below). Biochemical measurements of endothelial cell synthetic products may serve as an assessment of neointimal function. However, although physiological pressure perfusion in vivo with glutaraldehyde solutions best preserves fine structural detail for SEM or TEM, this technique precludes the subsequent selection of unfixed specimens for immunohistochemical or biochemical analysis.

The most widely used graft type for aortocoronary bypass or peripheral arterial graft surgery is autologous saphenous vein. The internal mammary artery (IMA) is also a popular coronary substitute and expanded polytetrafluoroethylene (ePTFE) is also widely used in peripheral vascular surgery. Aortic grafts are usually fabricated from polyethylene terephthalate fibers. For coronary grafts, postmortem angiographic study by injection of radioopaque material often facilitates assessment of pertinent pathology.

Clinicopathologic correlations, failure modes, histological reactions, and device interaction mechanisms associated with and the methodology appropriate for Dacron, ePTFE, and biological graft materials have been described in detail [2, 70–77]. Following extended function (months to years), saphenous vein grafts suffer intimal fibromuscular thickening (with or without thrombosis); grafts implanted for 3 or more years may show changes analogous to atherosclerosis [2]. High-quality sections of textile grafts are extremely difficult to obtain using paraffin embedding, and GMA techniques are usually required for preservation of the tissue-graft interface. In contrast, ePTFE and tissue grafts are readily processed in either paraffin or GMA.

Stents

Intravascular stents are now widely used as an adjunct to percutaneous transluminal coronary angioplasty (PTCA) and may prevent some of the untoward effects of this procedure, especially the restenosis that occurs over the first 6 months in 25–40 percent of patients [78, 79]. Stents act as a scaffold, intended to minimize thrombus formation and reduce the impact of postangioplasty intimal thickening. The morphologic effects of several types of intravascular stents have been described [80–84]. Since most stent types use metallic wires, methodology for sampling and histologic sectioning to assess adjacent tissue must either initially remove the metallic inclusions or use specialized techniques to section them [83, 84].

GENERIC APPROACHES TO CHARACTERIZATION OF BLOOD-TISSUE-BIOMATERIALS INTERACTIONS
Thrombotic Deposits

Unique to cardiovascular devices, blood-surface interactions, particularly thrombotic phenomena, are important and often dramatic. More than a century ago, the "father of cell pathology," Rudolph Virchow, called attention to the fundamental role of three factors contributing to thrombosis, now bearing the eponym Virchow's triad: (1) an abnormal blood-contacting surface (i.e., not normally-functioning endothelium), (2) local or systemic hypercoagulability and platelet adhesion, and (3) abnormal flow. A consequence of this complex interplay of host and implant biological and physical factors in thrombus formation is the regrettably often-limited predictability of device performance by in vitro or ex vivo tests; indeed, critical pathology is often realized only during function in animal experiments or clinical trials using actual devices.

The need to distinguish between pre- or post-mortem thrombus is a common problem. Pre-mortem thrombi are generally grossly firm, dry, granular, tan, angular or smooth, but clearly layered, uniformly adherent structures. In contrast, post-mortem (artifactual) thrombi are wet, soft, stringy, smooth and poorly adherent. Gross device thrombus can be quantitatively characterized by polar coordinate mapping [61, 85] and regional deposition of platelets can be measured by radioisotopic labeling [86].

In general, histologic organization of thrombotic deposits on valve prostheses and other devices is exceedingly slow, thus making estimates of time of onset extremely difficult and often misleading. Moreover, although patients with cardiovascular devices frequently are therapeutically anticoagulated, the adequacy of this therapy may not be known to the pathologist. In addition, extrinsic interference with function or other influences that might have potentiated thrombus, such as arrhythmias (e.g., atrial fibrillation) or a low flow state, cannot be determined solely from examination of the specimen.

Proteins and Cells at the Blood-Contacting Surface

The blood-contacting surface of a cardiovascular device consists variably of a bare biomaterial, plasma proteins such as fibrinogen/fibrin, inflammatory cells, endothelial cells, and other components of the normal vessel wall, such as smooth muscle cells and extracellular matrix in various combinations. Although the blood-contacting surface of vascular grafts is generally primarily composed of shaggy pseudointima, a smooth, yellow-white, glistening surface of unorganized, compacted fibrin may grossly resemble endothelialized neointima. Thus, investigators should not consider any glistening yellow or white blood-surface interface "endothelialized" without further evidence. In preclinical studies, gross evaluation of the extent of endothelial coverage of blood-contacting surface may be aided by preterminal injection of Evan's blue dye, which stains de-endothelialized surfaces [9]; intact endothelialized surfaces exclude the dye and therefore remain unstained. This facilitates macroscopic assessment of the extent of neointima (surface covered by endothelium) by quantitative morphometric analysis.

Since the morphology of endothelial cells is essentially non-specific, and such cells cannot be absolutely identified by LM, SEM or TEM, verification that a flattened cell layer with the non-specific morphological characteristics of endothelial cells noted on routine histologic examination is required. Most commonly used are immunohistochemical markers for endothelium, including *ulex europaeus* antigen, Factor VIII-related antigen (vWF), CD31 and CD34 [87, 88], their relative merits have been debated [89]. With the recent recognition that endothelial cells may exist in various phenotypes, including dysfunctional states with potentially deleterious properties such as enhanced leukocyte adhesion or reduced thromboresistance [90, 91], future evaluation of blood-contacting surfaces may require assessment of endothelial surface markers indicative of activation.

Other cell types are distinguishable by specific markers smooth muscle cells (e.g., a-actin), macrophages (e.g., HAM-56), T-lymphocytes (e.g., UCHL-1) and B-lymphocytes (e.g., L26). Further immunohistochemical identification of smooth muscle cells, inflammatory cells and accumulated extracellular material can be used to assess the composition and/or sequential development of blood-contacting tissue layers. Ultrastructural immuno-histochemical localization of proteins is also possible.

Fibrous Connective Tissue

Deposition of collagen precursors followed by intermolecular cross-linking and progression in synthesis from Type III to predominantly Type I are fundamental features of sequential tissue repair and healing [92]. Such processes enhance mechanical strength and resistance to degradation.

Collagen is visualized in routine preparations of fixed tissues embedded in paraffin using the Masson's trichrome stain, in which collagen appears blue or green. However, since the routine histological appearance of a collagenous tissue is largely homogeneous and invariant, special techniques must be used to assess maturity or source. The anionic dye picrosirius red markedly increases the birefringence and resolution of collagen under po-larized light, thereby permitting observation of thin collagen fibrils, undetectable in normal microscopy, and distinguishing collagen subtypes I and III [93]. During scar maturation, the subtype synthesis shifts, are accompanied by enhanced birefringence due to increased fi-brillar and molecular organization and loss of tissue water. Therefore, digital image analysis can be used to quantify collagen organization and tissue maturity [94, 95]. Immunohisto-chemical characterization of collagen by species and type-specific antibodies [96] may be particularly useful in studies of highly porous vascular grafts sealed with various forms of collagen, intended to be resorbed [97].

Calcification

Pathological calcification comprises deposition of apatitic calcium phosphate material oc-curring in an ectopic site (i.e., other than normally mineralized tissue, such as bone). It may be further subclassified as metastatic (when the involved tissues are normal, but there is a sys-temic metabolic disorder such as hyper-calcemia) or dystrophic (when overall metabolism is normal, but the involved tissues are necrotic or scarred) [98].

Calcification of cardiovascular implants may be studied in small laboratory animals in extra-circulatory locations. Accelerated calcification of glutaraldehyde-preserved porcine aortic valve cusps occurs after subcutaneous implantation in rabbits, rats, and mice [99] with morphology and biochemistry similar to those which occur in the cardiovascular sys-tem in clinical implants and in large animal models. Subcutaneous models reproduce the basic metabolic processes of mineralization and hence have been used to investigate various host and implant factors in the pathophysiology of degenerative calcification of biopros-thetic tissues. It is logical to use rat subcutaneous implants to investigate the metabolic pathophysiology of bioprosthetic valve calcification and to screen specific hypotheses for its inhibition [100]. The most promising approaches may be investigated in the circulatory environment, such as mitral replacements in sheep [50].

In the analysis of failed biological tissue valves, degree and location of calcification are assessed and documented by gross examination, photography and radiography. Fol-lowing fixation and dehydration according to standard procedures, multiple portions of the specimen are embedded, ideally in both paraffin and GMA, and routinely sectioned and stained. Selected sections are stained by von Kossa's method for calcium salts (which stain brown-black) or by alizarin red for calcium (which stains red). Conventional TEM and SEM may be extremely useful in investigating the morphology of calcific deposits and the relationship of mineral to substrate tissue ultrastructural features. Analysis of frozen tissue by microscopic histochemical staining for alkaline phosphatase has been useful in some studies [20, 21].

Calcium content is most readily measured using atomic absorption spectroscopy (phosphorus can also be determined) [22, 46, 50, 51, 98]. However, while extremely important and useful for comparative studies, bulk chemical studies average mineral content over an entire specimen and do not usually provide details of site specificity. In contrast, SEM with energy dispersive X-ray analysis (EDAX) allows the quantitative mapping of calcium ions and the major anions of their salts [22, 98]. Electron probe microanalysis and high resolution electron energy loss spectroscopy (EELS) provide enhanced spatial resolution and sensitivity for pathophysiological studies of elemental distributions [101].

Physicochemical analysis can be used to characterize other aspects of mineral chemistry and structural properties [102]. With the considerable recent interest in the role of non-collagenous proteins (such as osteopontin) in pathologic mineralization, immunohistochemistry, biochemical analysis or in situ hybridization (see below) may be useful to detect expression of such proteins [103–105].

Determination of Cell Phenotype/Function

Contemporary studies frequently seek detailed data on cellular function. Methods for detection of gene expression fall into two general categories: detection/quantification and mapping. Potential techniques for detection/quantification include: (1) determination of total tissue mRNA levels by Northern blotting and polymerase chain reaction analysis, and (2) determination of total peptide levels by radioimmunoassay and immunoprecipitation assays. Mapping studies include (1) in situ hybridization for localizing RNA and DNA in tissues, and (2) immunohistochemical analyses for cell-specific peptides (described above).

In situ hybridization (ISH) allows the histologic localization of specific messenger RNA (mRNA) transcripts or DNA within tissue sections, while the normal architecture and cytologic features of the tissues being studied are preserved [106, 107]. Cell adhesion will likely be most useful in explant analysis (e.g., probing for mRNA for a particular collagen subtype or molecules that are markers for endothelial cell activation). Frozen or paraffin tissue sections can be used, but the signal from ISH on frozen tissue sections is usually stronger than that with formalin-fixed, paraffin-embedded tissue sections. Nonetheless, because of the greater preservation of morphologic findings, access to retrospective material, and the ease of characterizing new probes, ISH of paraffin sections may be preferred.

Additional approaches that can evaluate cell viability, phenotype, and gene expression will be needed to assess devices that either modify healing, utilize tissue engineering approaches with xenograft or allograft cells, permit tissue regeneration, or utilize gene-therapy techniques [106–112].

ACKNOWLEDGEMENTS

The author is indebted to L. D. Helstowski, S. Murray, R. G. Osol, E. Rabkin and H. Shing, whose expert technical assistance over approximately 15 years has allowed refinement of the methods described. The manuscript was typed by C. Davis.

REFERENCES

1   Schoen FJ. *Interventional and Surgical Cardiovascular Pathology: Clinical Correlations and Basic Principles.* Philadelphia, PA: W. B. Saunders, 1989, 1–415.

2   Schoen FJ, Anderson JM, Didisheim P, Dobbins JJ, Gristina AG, Harasaki H, Simmons RL. Ventricular assist device (VAD) pathology analyses: Guidelines for clinical studies. *J Appl Biomat,* 1 (1990), 49–56.

3   Anderson JM. Cardiovascular device retrieval and evaluation. *Cardiovasc Pathol,* 2 (Suppl), 1993, 199S–208S.

4   Schoen FJ. Approach to the analysis of cardiac valve prostheses as surgical pathology or autopsy specimens. *Cardiovasc Pathol,* 4 (1995), 241–255.

5   Savage RA. New law to require medical device injury report. *CAP Today,* July, 1991, 40.

6   Kahan JS. The Safe Medical Devices Act of 1990. *Med Dev Diagn Ind,* Jan., 1991, 67.

7   Palatianos GM, Dewanjee MK, Panoutsopoulos G, Kapadvanjwala M, Novak S, Sfakianakis GN. Comparative thrombogenicity of pacemaker leads. *PACE Pacing Clin Electrophysiol,* 17 (1994), 141–145.

8   Clowes AW, Gown AM, Hanson SR, Reidy MA. Mechanisms of arterial graft failure. 1. Role of cellular proliferation in early healing of PTFE prostheses. *Am J Pathol,* 118 (1985), 43–54.

9   Davies PF, Bowyer DE. Scanning electron microscopy: Arterial endothelial integrity after fixation at physiological pressure. *Atherosclerosis,* 21 (1975), 463–469.

10 Reidy MA, Chao SS, Kirkman TR, Clowes AW. Endothelial regeneration. VI. Chronic nondenuding injury in baboon vascular grafts. *Am J Pathol,* 123 (1986) 432–439.

11 Roberts WC, Morrow AG. Renal hemosiderosis in patients with prosthetic aortic valves. *Circulation,* 33 (1966), 390–398.

12 Ridolfi RL, Hutchins GM. Detection of ball variance in prosthetic heart valves by liver biopsy. *Johns Hopkins Med J,* 134 (1974), 131–140.

13 Edwards WD. Photography of medical specimens: Experiences from teaching cardiovascular pathology. *Mayo Clin Proc,* 63 (1988), 42–57.

14 Libby P, Schoen FJ. Vascular lesion formation. *Cardiovasc Pathol,* 3 (Suppl.), 1993, 43S–52S.

15 Salomon RN, Hughes CCW, Schoen FJ, Payne DD, Pober JS, Libby P. Human coronary transplantation-associated arteriosclerosis. *Am J Pathol,* 138 (1991), 791–798.

16 Tanaka H, Sukhova GK, Swanson SJ, Cybulsky MI, Schoen FJ, Libby P. Endothelial and smooth muscle cells express leukocyte adhesion molecules heterogeneously during acute rejection of rabbit cardiac allografts. *Am J Pathol,* 144 (1994), 938–951.

17 Anderson JM, Ziats NP. Human blood protein and cellular interactions in the healing responses of vascular prostheses. *J Vasc Surg,* 13 (1991), 750–751.

18 Valenzuela R, Shainoff JR, DiBello PM, Urbanic DA, Anderson JM, Matsueda GR, Kudryk BJ. Immunoelectrophoretic and immunohistochemical characterizations of fibrinogen derivatives in atherosclerotic aortic intimas and vascular prosthesis pseudo-intimas. *Am J Pathol,* 141 (1992), 861–880.

19 Maranto AR, Schoen FJ. Alkaline phosphatase activity of glutaraldehyde-treated bovine pericardium used in bioprosthetic cardiac valves. *Circ Res,* 63 (1988), 844–848.

20 Levy RJ, Schoen FJ, Flowers WB, Staelin ST. Initiation of mineralization in bioprosthetic heart valves: Studies of alkaline phosphatase activity and its inhibition by $AlCl_3$ or $FeCl_3$ preincubations. *J Biomed Mater Res,* 25 (1991), 905–935.

21 Levy RJ, Schoen FJ, Levy JT, Nelson AC, Howard SL, Oshry LJ. Biologic determinants of dystrophic calcification and osteocalcin deposition in glutaraldehyde-preserved porcine aortic valve leaflets implanted subcutaneously in rats. *Am J Pathol,* 113 (1993), 143–155.

22 Grunkemeier GL, Rahimtoola SH. Artificial heart valves. *Ann Rev Med,* 41 (1990), 251–263.

23 Akins CW. Results with mechanical cardiac valvular prostheses. *Ann Thorac Surg,* 60 (1995), 1836–1844.

24 Turina J, Hess OM, Turina M, Krayenbuehl HP. Cardiac bioprostheses in the 1990s. *Circulation,* 88 (1993), 775–781.

25 Schoen FJ, Titus JL, Lawrie GM. Autopsy-determined causes of death after cardiac valve replacement. *JAMA,* 249 (1983), 899–902.

26 Schoen FJ. Surgical pathology of removed natural and prosthetic heart valves. *Human Pathol,* 18 (1987), 558–567.

27 Bloomfield P, Wheatley DJ, Prescott RJ, Miller HC. Twelve-year comparison of a Bjork-Shiley mechanical heart valve with porcine bioprostheses. *N Engl J Med,* 324 (1991), 573–579.

28 Hammermeister KE, Sethi GK, Henderson WG, Oprian C, Kim T, Rahimtoola S. A comparison of outcomes in men 11 years after heart-valve replacement with mechanical valve or bioprosthesis. *N Engl J Med,* 328 (1993), 1289–1296.

29 Schoen FJ, Levy RJ, Piehler HR. Pathological considerations in replacement cardiac valves. *Cardiovasc Pathol*, 1 (1992), 29–52.

30 Schoen FJ. Pathologic considerations in replacement heart valves and other cardiovascular prosthetic devices. In Schoen FJ & Gimbrone MA (Eds.), *Cardiovascular Pathology: Clinicopathologic Correlations and Pathogenetic Mechanisms*. Baltimore: Williams & Wilkins, 1995, 194–222.

31 Roberts WC. Complications of cardiac valve replacement: Characteristic abnormalities of prostheses pertaining to any or specific site. *Am Heart J*, 103 (1982), 113–122.

32 Dollar AL, Pierre-Louise ML, McIntosh CL, Roberts WC. Extensive multifocal myocardial infarcts from cloth emboli after replacement of mitral and aortic valves with cloth-covered, caged-ball prostheses. *Am J Cardiol*, 64 (1989), 410–412.

33 Fernicola DJ, Roberts WC. Frequency of ring abscess and cuspal infection in active infective endocarditis involving bioprosthetic valves. *Am J Cardiol*, 72 (1993), 314–323.

34 Valente M, Bortolotti U, Thiene G. Ultrastructural substrates of dystrophic calcification in porcine bioprosthetic valve failure. *Am J Pathol*, 119 (1985), 12–21.

35 Walley VM, Keon CA, Khalili M, Moher D. Campagna M, Keon WJ. Ionescu-Shiley valve failure. I: Experience with 125 standard-profile explants. *Ann Thorac Surg*, 54 (1992), 111–116.

36 Thiene G, Bortolotti U, Talenti E, Guerra F, Valente M, Milano A, Mazzucco A, Gallucci V. Dissecting cuspal hematomas. A rare form of porcine bioprosthetic valve dysfunction. *Arch Pathol Lab Med*, 111 (1987), 964–967.

37 Walley VM, Rubens FD, Campagna M, Pipe AL, Keon WJ. Patterns of failure in Hancock pericardial bioprostheses. *J Thorac Cardiovasc Surg*, 102 (1991), 187–194.

38 Allard MF, Thompson CR, Baldelli RJ, McNab JS, Babul SA, Betts JM, McManus BM, Jamieson WRE, Ling H, Miyagishima RT. Commissural region dehiscence from the stent post of Carpentier-Edwards bioprosthetic cardiac valves. *Cardiovasc Pathol*, 4 (1995), 155–162.

39 Edwards WD, Agarwal KC, Feldt RH, Danielson GK, Puga FJ. Surgical pathology of obstructed, right-sided, porcine-valved extracardiac conduits. *Arch Pathol Lab Med*, 107 (1983), 400–405.

40 Schwartz L, Scully HE, Silver MD, Azuma J, Wigle ED. Clinicopathological correlations in patients who received an isolated model 104 Beall mitral valve. *Can J Surg*, 23 (1980), 117–120.

41 Silver MD, Butany J. Mechanical heart valves: Methods of examination, complications, and modes of failure. *Hum Pathol*, 18 (1987), 577–585.

42 Silver MD. Wear in Bjork-Shiley heart valve prostheses recovered at necropsy or operation. *J Thorac Cardiovasc Surg*, 79 (1980), 693–699.

43 Silver MD, Koppenhoefer H, Heggtveit HA, Reif TH. Metal wear in Lillehei-Kaster heart valve prostheses. *Artif Organs*, 9 (1985), 270–275.

44 Schoen FJ, Titus JL, Lawrie GL. Durability of pyrolytic carbon-containing heart valve prostheses. *J Biomed Mater Res*, 16 (1982), 559–650.

45 Mitchell RN, Jonas RA, Schoen FJ. Structure-function correlations in cryopreserved allograft cardiac valves. *Ann Thorac Surg*, 60 (1995), S108–S113.

46 Haubold AD. On the durability of pyrolytic carbon in-vivo. *Med Prog Technol*, 20 (1994), 201–208.

47 Schoen FJ, Kujovich JL, Webb CL, Levy RJ. Chemically determined mineral content of explanted porcine aortic valve bioprostheses: Correlation with radiographic assessment of calcification and clinical data. *Circulation*, 76 (1987), 1061–1066.

48 Butany J, d'Amati G, Fornasier V, Silver MD, Sanders GE. Detailed examination of complete bioprosthetic heart valves. *ASAIO Trans*, 36 (1990), M414–M417.

49 Schoen FJ, Goodenough SH, Ionescu MI, Braunwald NS. Implications of late morphology of Braunwald-Cutter mitral heart valve prostheses. *J Thorac Cardiovasc Surg*, 88 (1984), 208–216.

50 Schoen FJ, Hirsch D, Bianco RW, Levy RJ. Onset and progression of calcification in porcine aortic bioprosthetic valves implanted as orthotopic mitral valve replacements in juvenile sheep. *J Thorac Cardiovasc Surg*, 108 (1994), 880–887.

51 Biedrzycki LM, Lerner E, Levy RJ, Schoen FJ. Differential calcification of cusps and associated aortic wall of porcine bioprosthetic valves. *Lab Invest*, 72 (1995), 30A.

52 Tweden KS, Harasaki H, Jones M, Blevitt JM, Craig WS, Pierschbacher M, Helmus MN. Accelerated healing of cardiovascular textiles promoted by an RGD peptide. *J Heart Valve Dis*, (1995), in press.

53 Joshi RR, Underwood T, Frautschi JR, Phillips RE, Schoen FJ, Levy RJ. Calcification of polyurethanes implanted subdermally in rats is enhanced by calciphylaxis. *J Biomed Mater Res*, 13 (1996), 201–207.

54 Hilbert SL, Ferrans VJ, Tomita Y, Eidbo EE, Jones M. Evaluation of explanted polyurethane trileaflet cardiac valve prostheses. *J Thorac Cardiovasc Surg*, 94 (1987), 419–429.

55   David TE, Pollick C, Bos J. Aortic valve replacement with stentless porcine aortic bioprosthesis. *J Thorac Cardiovasc Surg*, 99 (1990), 113–118.

56   Kunin CK, Dobbins JJ, Melo JC. Infectious complications in four long-term recipients of the Jarvik-7 artificial heart. *JAMA*, 259 (1988), 860–864.

57   DeVries WC. The permanent artificial heart. *JAMA*, 259 (1988), 849–859.

58   Pennock JL, Pierce WS, Wisman CB, Bull AP, Waldhausen JA. Survival and complications following ventricular assist pumping for cardiogenic shock. *Ann Surg*, 198 (1983), 469–476.

59   Pennington DG, Samuels LD, Williams G, Palmer D, Swartz MT, Codd JE, Merjavy JP, Lagunoff D, Joist JH. Experience with the Pierce-Donachy ventricular assist device in postcardiotomy patients with cardiogenic shock. *World J Surg*, 9 (1985), 37–46.

60   Schoen FJ, Palmer DC, Bernhard WF, Pennington DG, Haudenschild CC, Ratliff NB, Berger RL, Golding LR, Watson JT. Clinical temporary ventricular assist. Pathologic findings and their implications in a multi-institutional study of 41 patients. *J Thorac Cardiovasc Surg*, 92 (1986), 1071–1081.

61   Fyfe B, Schoen FJ. Pathologic analysis of 34 explanted Symbion ventricular assist devices and 10 explanted Jarvik-7 total artificial hearts. *Cardiovasc Pathol*, 2 (1993), 187–197.

62   Edelman BH, Obrist WD, Wagner WR, Kormos R, Griffith B. Cerebrovascular complications associated with the use of artificial circulatory support services. *Neurol Clin*, 11 (1993), 463–474.

63   Wagner WR, Johnson PC, Kormos RL, Griffith BP. Evaluation of bioprosthetic valve-associated thrombus in ventricular assist device patients. *Circulation*, 88 (1993), 2023–2029.

64   Icenogle TB, Smith RG, Cleavinger M, Vasu MA, Williams RJ, Sethi GK, Copeland JG. Thromboembolic complications of the Symbion assist device system. *Artif Organs*, 13 (1989), 532–538.

65   Clowes AW. Intimal hyperplasia and graft failure. *Cardiovasc Pathol*, 2 (1993), 179S–186S.

66   Clowes AW. Graft endothelialization: The role of angiogenic mechanisms. *J Vasc Surg*, 13 (1991), 734–737.

67   LoGerfo FW, Quist WC, Nowak MD, Crawshaw HM, Haudenschild CC. Downstream anastomotic hyperplasia. A mechanism of failure in Dacron® arterial grafts. *Ann Surg*, 197 (1983), 479–483.

68   Bush HL, Jakubowski JA, Hong SL, McCabe M, Deykin D, Nabseth DC. Luminal release of prostacyclin and thromboxane A_2 by arteries distal to small-caliber prosthetic grafts. *Circulation*, 70 (1984, Suppl. I), I-11–I-15.

69   Morgan AP, Dammin GJ, Lazarus JM. Failure modes in secondary vascular access for hemodialysis. *Amer Soc Artif Intern Organs*, 1 (1978), 44–52.

70   Burkel WE, Kahn RY. Biocompatibility of prosthetic grafts. In Stanley JC (Ed.), *Biologic and Synthetic Vascular Prostheses*. New York: Grune & Stratton, 1982, 221–247.

71   Dardik H, Baier RE, Meenaghan M, Natiella J, Weinberg S, Turner R, Sussman B, Kahn M, Ibrahim IM, Dardik II. Morphologic and biophysical assessment of long-term human umbilical cord vein implants used as vascular conduits. *Surgery*, 154 (1982), 17–26.

72   Canizales S, Charara J, Gill F, Guidoin R, Roy PE, Bonnaud P, Laroche G, Batt M, Roy P, Marois M, et al. Expanded polytetrafluoroethylene prostheses as secondary blood access sites for hemodialysis: Pathological findings in 29 excised grafts. *Can J Surg*, 32 (1989), 433–439.

73   Downs AR, Guzman R, Formichi M, Courbier R, Jausseran JM, Branchereau A, Juhan C, Chakfe N, King M, Guidoin R. Etiology of prosthetic anastomotic false aneurysms: Pathologic and structural evaluation in 26 cases. *Can J Surg*, 34 (1991), 53–58.

74   King MW, Zhang Z, Ukpabi P, Murphy D, Guidoin R. Quantitative analysis of the surface morphology and textile structure of the polyurethane Vascugraft arterial prosthesis using image and statistical analyses. *Biomaterials*, 15 (1994), 621–627.

75   Zhang Z, Guidoin R, King MW, How TV, Marois Y, Laroche G. Removing fresh tissue from explanted polyurethane prostheses: which approach facilitates physico-chemical analysis? *Biomaterials*, 16 (1995), 369–380.

76   Guidoin R, Chakfe N, Maurel S, How T, Batt M, Varois M, Gosselin C. Expanded polytetrafluoroethylene arterial prostheses in humans: Histopathological study of 298 surgically excised grafts. *Biomaterials*, 14 (1993), 678–693.

77   Topol EJ. Caveats about elective coronary stenting (Editorial). *N Engl J Med*, 331 (1994), 539–541.

78   Serruys PW, Strauss BH, Beatt KJ, Bertrand ME, Puel J, Rickards AF, Meier B, Goy JJ, Vogt P, Kappenberger L, Sigwart U. Angiographic follow-up after placement of a self-expanding coronary artery stent. *N Engl J Med*, 324 (1991), 13–17.

79   Anderson PG, Bajaj RK, Baxley WA, Roubin GS. Vascular pathology of balloon-expandable flexible coil stent in humans. *J Am Coll Cardiol*, 19 (1992), 372–381.

80   Anderson PG. Pathology of intravascular stents in man and experimental animals. In Waller BF (Ed.), *Coronary Artery Stenting*. Cambridge: Blackwell Scientific Publications, Inc., 1996.

81   van Beusekom HMM, van der Giessen WJ, van Suylen RJ, Bos E, Bosman FT, Serruys PW. Histology after stenting of human saphenous vein bypass grafts: Observations from surgically excised grafts 3 to 320 days after stent implantation. *J Am Coll Cardiol*, 21 (1993), 45–54.

82   Laborde C, Parodi JC, Clem MF, Tio FO, Barone HD, Rivera FJ, Encarnacion CE, Palmaz JC. Intraluminal bypass of abdominal aortic aneurysm: Feasibility study. *Radiology*, 184 (1992), 185–190.

83   Carter AJ, Laird JR, Farb A, Kufs W, Wortham DC, Virmani R. Morphologic characteristics of lesion formation and time course of smooth muscle cell proliferation in a porcine proliferative restenosis model. *J Am Coll Cardiol*, 24 (1994), 1398–1405.

84   Pantalos GM, Everett SD, Mohammad SF, Burns GL, Solen KA, Reynolds LO, Olsen DB. Quantification of perivalvular thrombus formation in blood pumps by polar coordinate mapping. *Artif Organs*, 14 (1990), 348–354.

85   Dewanjee MK, Solis E, Mackey ST, Lenker J, Edwards WD, Didisheim P, Chesebro JH, Zollman PE, Kaye MP. Quantification of regional platelet and calcium deposition on pericardial tissue valve prostheses in calves and effect of hydroxyethylene diphosphonate. *J Thorac Cardiovasc Surg*, 92 (1986), 337–348.

86   Parums DV, Cordell JL, Micklem K, Heryet AR, Gatter KC, Mason DY. JC70: A new monoclonal antibody that detects vascular endothelium associated antigen on routinely processed tissue sections. *J Clin Pathol*, 43 (1990), 752–757.

87   Albelda SM, Muller WA, Buck CA, Newman PJ. Molecular and cellular properties of PECAM-1 (endo-CAM/CD31): A novel vascular cell-cell adhesion molecule. *J Cell Biol*, 114 (1991), 1059–1068.

88   Miettinen M, Lindenmayer AE, Chaubal A. Endothelial cell markers CD31, CD34, and BNH9 antibody to H- and Y-antigens: Evaluation of their specificity and sensitivity in the diagnosis of vascular tumors and comparison with von Willebrand factor. *Mod Pathol*, 7 (1994), 82–90.

89   Pober JS, Cotran RS. Cytokines and endothelial cell biology. *Physiol Rev*, 70 (1990), 427–451.

90   Vane JR, Botting RM. Regulatory mechanisms of the vascular endothelium: An update. *Pol J Pharmacol*, 46 (1994), 499–521.

91   Cotran RS, Kumar V, Robbins SL. *Robbins Pathologic Basis of Disease*, 5th ed. Philadelphia, PA: W. B. Saunders, 1994, 75–80.

92   Junqueira LCU, Bignolas G, Brentani RR. Picrosirius staining plus polarization microscopy, a specific method for collagen detection in tissue sections. *Histochem J*, 11 (1979), 447–455.

93   Pickering JG, Boughner DR. Quantitative assessment of the age of fibrotic lesions using polarized light microscopy and digital image analysis. *Am J Pathol*, 138 (1991), 1225–1231.

94   Whittaker P, Kloner RA, Boughner DR, Pickering JG. Quantitative assessment of myocardial collagen with picrosirius red staining and circularly polarized light. *Basic Res Cardiol*, 89 (1994), 397–410.

95   Werkmeister JA, Peters DE, Ramshaw JA. Development of monoclonal antibodies to collagens for assessing host-implant interactions. *J Biomed Mater Res*, 23 (1989), 273–283.

96   Kodoba K, Schoen FJ, Jonas RA. Experimental comparison of albumin-sealed and gelatin-sealed knitted Dacron® conduits. *J Thorac Cardiovasc Surg*, 103 (1992), 1059–1067.

97   Cotran RS, Kumar V, Robbins SL. *Robbins Pathologic Basis of Disease*, 5th ed. Philadelphia, PA: W. B. Saunders, 1994, 30–31.

98   Schoen FJ, Levy RJ, Nelson AC, Bernhard WF, Nashef A, Hawley M. Onset and progression of experimental bioprosthetic heart valve calcification. *Lab Invest*, 52 (1985), 523–532.

99   Schoen FJ, Levy RJ, Hilbert SL, Bianco RW. Antimineralization treatments for bioprosthetic heart valves. *J Thorac Cardiovasc Surg*, 104 (1992), 1285–1288.

100 Webb CL, Schoen FJ, Flowers WE, Alfrey AC, Horton C, Levy RJ. Inhibition of mineralization of glutaraldehyde-pretreated bovine pericardium by $AlCl_3$. *Am J Pathol*, 138 (1991), 971–981.

101 Tomazic BB, Brown WE, Schoen FJ. Physicochemical properties of calcific deposits isolated from porcine bioprosthetic heart valves removed from patients following 2–13 years function. *J Biomed Mater Res*, 28 (1994), 35–47.

102 O'Brien K, Kuusisto J, Reichenbach DD, Ferguson M, Giachelli C, Alpers CE, Otto CM. Osteopontin is expressed in human aortic valvular lesions. *Circulation*, 92 (1995), 2163–2168.

103 Boström K, Watson KE, Horn S, Wortham C, Herman IM, Demer LL. Bone morphogenetic protein expression in human atherosclerotic lesions. *J Clin Invest*, 91 (1993), 1800–1809.

104 Demer LL. A skeleton in the atherosclerosis closet. *Circulation*, 92 (1995), 2029–2032.

105 DeLellis RA. In-situ hybridization techniques for the analysis of gene expression: Applications in tumor pathology. *Hum Pathol*, 25 (1994), 580–585.

106 Kraiss LW, Raines EW, Wilcox JN, Seifert RA, Barrett TB, Kirkman TR, Hart CE, Bowen-Pope DF, Ross R, Clowes AW. Regional expression of the platelet-derived growth factor and its receptors in a primate graft model of vessel wall assembly. *J Clin Invest*, 92 (1993), 338–348.

107 Peppas NA, Langer R. New challenges in biomaterials. *Science*, 263 (1994), 1715–1720.

108 Langer R, Vacanti JP. Tissue engineering. *Science*, 260 (1993), 920–926.

109 Epstein SE, Speir E, Unger EF, Guzman RJ, Finkel T. The basis of molecular strategies for treating coronary restenosis after angioplasty. *J Am Coll Cardiol*, 23 (1994), 1278–1288.

110 Riessen R, Isner JM. Prospects for site-specific delivery of pharmacologic and molecular therapies. *J Am Coll Cardiol*, 23 (1994), 1234–1244.

111 Nabel EG, Pompili VJ, Plautz GE, Nabel GJ. Gene transfer and vascular disease. *Cardiovasc Res*, 28 (1994), 445–455.

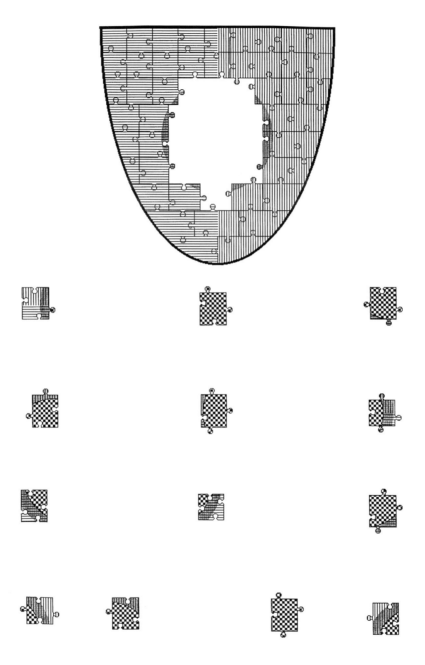

Section Eight

Hard Tissue Histology

Ulrich M. Gross

INTRODUCTION

In the past ten years, the field of biomaterials and implant-related histology has made great advances. This progress was made possible by the refinement of existing techniques and the development of new equipment and methods.

The types of techniques being used reveal trends in histological analysis. Therefore, the techniques used and the materials investigated in studies published in the *Journal of Biomedical Materials Research* during a three-year period have been compiled (see Table). It is interesting to note the considerable interest in in vivo studies, bone, and undecalcified tissue in PMMA blocks for light microscopical histology. It is also shown that the information which could be gained in the leading journal of biomaterials research does not contain sufficient information about the histological techniques used. This lack of information should be alleviated for the benefit of biomaterials research.

Chapter 44 discusses general aspects of hard tissue processing. General principles of implants containing bone dissection and documentation are outlined. Whereas the classical fixation, processing and staining methods held their position, the new immunohistochemical stains conquered ground and made possible the detection of specific macromolecules in various tissues of bone and organization tissue. The new technique of in situ hybridization has also become available for hard tissue analysis. It is anticipated that in situ PCR (polymerase-chain-reaction) will be available in the near future as well. There is progress in vital confocal microscopy and in scanning electron microscopy.

The special problems of permucosal loaded implants in an aggressive environment are covered in Chapter 45. Experimental models and histological evaluation are shown as a basis for clinical aspects; evaluation methods and future developments are also discussed.

Intra vitam staining techniques are widely used in experimental studies and to some minor extent in clinical practice. They are discussed in Chapter 46 along with radioactive tracers and polyphosphates.

Some special problems of quantitative morphology of the implant-bone interface are described and connected to the biomechanical function of experimentally and clinically applied implants in Chapter 47.

Microradiography and its practical implications for osteogramms are covered in Chapter 48.

The Usage of Histological Techniques as Published in the *Journal of Biomedical Research*, 1993–1995

JBMR	1993	1994	1995	sum
Volume	27	28	29	
Number of papers	30	23	22	75
In vitro studies	6	8	5	19
In vivo studies	25	16	19	60
Tissue				
Bone	21	15	21	57
Cartilage	2	4		6
Others	3	9	3	15
Fixation				
Formaldehyde	16	14	13	43
Glutaraldehyde	7	11	2	20
Ethanol	3	4	5	12
Decalcified	5	4	2	11
Undecalcified	7	3	16	26
Embedding				
PMMA	14	6	12	32
Polyester	4	10	5	19
Paraffin	2	4	1	7
Others		1		1
Sections				
Sawing microtome	9	10	7	26
Microtome	4	3	5	12
Grinding	2	1	6	9
LM	15	17	20	52
SEM	10	14	6	30
TEM	4	6	4	14
Materials				
Metal	9	6	11	26
HA	17	7	11	35
Glass	1	1	3	5
PGA/PLA	3	6	2	11
Others	3	3		6
X-rays	5	5	8	18

Chapter 44

Processing

Ulrich M. Gross

GROSS EXAMINATION

General Considerations

Experimental records of implant research should include: type of implant material, animal model, implantation site, surgical procedure, controls, evaluation methods, results, and all other pertinent information. Suggestions for documentation are given by the boards of various institutions (ISO/CEN [1], ASTM [2], BS [3], AFNOR, DIN). These suggested standards by panels in charge of assessment should provide an acceptable set of data.

Dissection Protocol (DP)

A detailed list of all procedures and observations for all specimens should be prepared in all cases. Some items that should be noted are: date and investigation title; name of the investigator; anatomical region; implantation period; pathological conditions (effusion, hematoma, induration, scar, color changes, etc.); specific tissues in which the specimens were located (e.g., compact bone, spongy bone, bone marrow, or soft tissues such as muscle, fat tissue, connective tissue, fasciae, tendons, synovia); relationship to joints, cartilage, and growth plates; and position of the implant in relation to special implant shape and design, as well as the relationship to vessels, nerves, gliding surfaces, and neosynovia. Information about biomechanical considerations (e.g., whether load was applied and transmitted to the implant) is invaluable. Some notion about the trimming of the specimen and a mark indicating the orientation (proximal, distal, medial, lateral, anterior or posterior) of the implant within the specimen or of the specimen within the tissue or organ is important for further preparation and for the eventual interpretation of the results.

In addition, a complete necropsy protocol should be prepared, and records of the retrieved tissue samples should include further fixation and histological evaluation. The basis for the techniques, documentation, reporting and retrieval should be the same as that of the necropsy of humans (4, 5). At the very least, specimens from the heart (left and right ventricles), both lungs, liver, spleen, kidneys, lymph nodes, and brain should be collected and stored in an appropriate fixative for further examination.

Macrophotography

Explants should be photographed immediately after removal from the recipients and prior to histological processing. This should be done at least with one explant out of a series of comparable specimens. Equipment for macrophotography is supplied by several reputable manufacturers. The skill of the photographer in arranging the best illumination is usually the most crucial point. Lenses used in macrophotography should be corrected for short focal distances so that the entire specimen is in focus and distortion is minimized. For macrophotography, translucent specimens, slides with cuts, diapositives, or X-ray films can be illuminated by positioning them on top of a transillumination chamber and subsequently photographed with a camera mounted on either a fixed tripod or a special stand. Macrophotography of whole bones, parts of the skeleton, or joints with synovia should be performed using two lamps for illumination, 500 watts each, positioned at a small angle to the surface of the specimen, to minimize spectral reflections. The background may be black or white or in color. Some equipment allows photography 1 : 1 by using a screw-on diopter lens or a macro lens. The diaphragm should be as small as possible to increase the depth of field. A metric scale and specimen identification number should be photographed with the specimen. In pictures for publication, the metric scale or the identification numbers may not be necessary.

The choice of film is wide for both black and white, and color. Films balanced for daylight will produce transparencies when using electronic flash. With tungsten lighting tungsten films can be used. Polaroid film is excellent when immediate prints are required; however, the image fades with longer storage.

Electronic recording of pictures on both macroscopical and microscopical levels is available. The storage of these documents on diskettes or other electronic measures has become quite common. In these pictures information can be directly inserted by a computer and the pictures evaluated from different aspects using morphometric programs [6].

Documentation

Documentation of all experimental studies should include at least the following items: the species, race, genetic conditions, sex, breeding conditions, housing, alimentation, age, the season, and body weight at the beginning and the end of the experiments. The clinical studies including surgical and autopsy specimens should be documented according to the suggestions given by ASTM [2] or ISO [1].

The implant materials should be clearly defined and described, including chemical composition, physical state, dimension, shape, surface structure (e.g., surface roughness), pores and the structure of pores (e.g., width, depth, and volume), preparation of the implant material, and mode of sterilization. This latter point should not be omitted since the procedures for sterilization are relevant to the destruction of biologically active molecules of bacteria, fungi, viruses or other organisms, implying that the surface properties of materials can be changed during this procedure (see Sections I and II and Chapters 18 and 33).

Operative procedures should be given in detail, including type of anesthesia, grade of sterility in performance of the operation, and experiment participants. The implantation procedure, the implantation site, special events during the operation (e.g., unusual bleeding or difficulty in accessing the implantation site), the method of hole preparation (with a burr drill or with a milling machine), cooling procedures (with saline or other solutions), the type of burr drills, the velocity (rpm) of burr drills, the means of inserting an implant, and other procedures should all be noted. The times of implantation, explanation, and processing of the specimen should be recorded. The clinical follow-up with X-rays and other methods should be documented. Section VI contains specific details about the operative procedures.

The choice of tissue fixation procedures requires documentation, such as immersion or perfusion fixation and the route of application. These procedures should be documented, including the diagrams, photographs, X-rays, fixative solution (pH, temperature and time), embedding, microtomy, and staining procedures.

The documentation could include the findings of light microscopy (LM), transmission electron microscopy (TEM), scanning electron microscopy (SEM), histochemistry, immunohistochemistry, in situ hybridization (ISH), energy-dispersive X-ray microanalysis (EDX), morphometry, and other analytic procedures. In each of these methods, the findings should be clearly described and separated from the interpretations and conclusions. Finally, a chapter should be prepared to summarize the experiment.

The time and work preparing documentation can be drastically reduced by using electronic data recording and processing. It has been shown that electronic data acquisition, administration, and evaluation is effective even in daily routine surgical pathology as well as in experimental pathology. Furthermore, the results of different experiments can be easily retrieved and then compared using well defined key words.

FIXATION

General Considerations

The choice of different fixatives depends on the purpose of the experiments and the intended methods for morphologic analysis, namely, light microscopy (LM). TEM, SEM, EDX, histochemical, immunohistochemical methods, intravital staining, microradiography, microangiography, autoradiography or in situ hybridization. There is a critical period after cessation of blood flow and prior to fixation of the cellular and extracellular components when cell and tissue death might occur. Such autolysis can be minimized by decreasing the reaction temperature in the tissue and by immediate fixation. The mode of reaction of a special fixative is determined by its chemical reactivity, concentration at the reaction site, temperature and the type of tissue fixed. General recommendations cannot be given for all fixatives, but only for special procedures dependent on the intended applications (LM, TEM, SEM). Fixation by perfusion rapidly distributes the fixative via the blood vessels, and so is superior to immersion fixation [7].

Dehydration of a specimen is another consideration in preparation for a microscopic study. If the specimen is to be embedded before sectioning, dehydration must be complete, especially for those media that are water-immiscible. Dehydration is usually accomplished by immersing in ethyl alcohol or acetone, with increasing concentrations up to absolute. Methanol has been used, but is not recommended for enzyme histochemistry [8]. Glycol methacrylate is water miscible, allowing specimen dehydration with 95% alcohol.

Fixation for Light Microscopy

Immersion and perfusion fixation can be carried out with formaldehyde solution (pH 7.2). The advantages are low costs and the possibility of keeping the specimens for weeks in the same solution. However, it must be remembered that during prolonged storage, decalcification can occur and disturb the structure and staining property of the decalcified tissues. Special techniques (e.g., tetracycline labeling) requires different fixation techniques [9]. Buffered formalin (or aqueous formaldehyde in methyl alcohol) is a common fixative used for light microscopy [10–14]. Gilbertson [14] found that use of formalin on mineralized samples lead to fracturing of the specimen: deep freezing was recommended. Other fixatives used are buffered glutaraldehyde [15], acetone for general microscopy and enzyme histochemistry [16, 17] and ethanol for tetracycline labeling [18, 19]. Ethanol and acetone are also used for dehydration. (Ethanol is sometimes used at 4°C for preservation of enzyme activity.) Acetone must be completely removed before embedding if methyl methacylate is used.

Fixation for Electron Microscopy

Perfusion fixation was found to be superior to immersion fixation. Perfusion is routinely done with a glutaraldehyde solution [3 percent (v/v)] in TES buffer solution (0.2 M, pH 7.35) [20] which was found to preserve cellular and extracellular structures better than formaldehyde solutions (pH 7.2).

Although use of osmium tetroxide is noted in literature as a second fixative [21], it was found that penetration was very slow, even for small specimens. Also, orientation of particles at the implant-tissue interface is difficult to discern due to the rather dark staining effect of osmium tetroxide.

Immersion fixation has been noted in literature, with 70–100 percent ethanol being the most common fixative [22-24]. Other immersion fixatives for EM preparation include buffered formaldehyde or Burkhardt's fixative [25], acetone and diethyl ether [26], and paraformaldehyde and glutaraldehyde [27].

Fixation of tissues and cell cultures for SEM can be done, for example, in the same manner as indicated for TEM with 3 percent glutaraldehyde in 0.02 M TES buffer, pH 7.35. Drying the cultured cells or tissues should be avoided, and the cultures should be rinsed with a buffer solution to avoid deposits on the cell surfaces prior to fixation.

Fixation for Histochemical Studies

Histochemical methods for demonstration of iron, periodic acid-Schiff (PAS)-positive material, or calcium using von Kossa's method can be applied when the material is fixed with formaldehyde or glutaraldehyde solutions. It is well known, however, that enzymatic activity is rapidly destroyed by such fixatives. Therefore, the specimens should be rapidly frozen in liquid nitrogen, then transferred to a cooled chamber for freeze drying in an appropriate apparatus. The enzymatic activity is well preserved with this method. Subsequently, the dried specimens, which should be as small as possible, are soaked in glycol methacrylate monomer at approximately 4°C. When the tissue is completely infiltrated with the monomer, polymerization is achieved at room temperature. The blocks with the undecalcified bone containing the implant can be sectioned with a sawing microtome.

The slides are immersed in the reaction solutions for demonstration of enzymatic activity which is not destroyed by the dehydration during freeze drying or polymerization of the glycol methacrylate monomer. A number of histochemical reactions can be performed, and excellent acid phosphatase activities can be shown. Immunohistochemical methods also seem to be relevant on slides prepared with this method, which is being further refined.

Other fixatives for histochemical studies include acetone and glutaraldehyde with paraformaldehyde [16, 17].

Perfusion Fixation

Perfusion fixation is a procedure in which the fixative is injected directly into the heart, aorta, or arteries. Veins can also be used; however, their valves inhibit the flow of the solution to the periphery. The critical stage of perfusion fixation is between cessation of blood flow and dispersion of the injected fixative solution. Perfusion of the fixative can be carried out immediately after perfusion with a balanced buffer or a saline solution. The use of a clearing buffer solution has been recommended to prevent intravascular blood clotting. Such rinsing is not always recommended because of the effects of ischemia and hypoxia on the tissue, which cannot be avoided by the rinsing. The tissues are fixed by perfusing with either buffered formaldehyde solution (pH 7.2) or buffered glutaraldehyde solution [20]. It is preferable to use a cold (4°C) solution to decrease the reaction temperature of metabolic processes and autolysis. Pressure is controlled by suspending the solution container 100 cm above the level of the operated animal. A syringe can also be used for injection with mild pressure. The insertion of the needle should be done quickly after the preparation of the heart, aorta, or artery with minimum disturbance of the blood flow of the anesthetized animal. The volume of solution for perfusion fixation should be in the order of 75 ml per 100 gm body weight when injecting into the heart. However, it is reasonable to perfuse via the abdominal aorta if the implants to be studied are located in the lower limbs; the procedure requires less solution, takes less time, and causes minimum trauma to the animal. This procedure has been recommended for rats and other small experimental animals, but can be modified for larger animals, including dogs and goats.

Perfusion fixation, although the most rapid method of fixing the tissues, may not be appropriate if multiple techniques are to be used. For example, if some implants or sections are to be utilized for mechanical testing and some for LM, or if LM and histochemical methods are to be combined, other methods of fixation or no fixation may be necessary.

Storage of Fixed Specimens

Prolonged storage of specimens prior to histological analysis presents a general problem and should be avoided by proper planning. Water-soluble material can be extracted when aldehyde solutions or buffers are used, and lipids are extracted when alcohols are used during storage, thus creating artifacts. Under no circumstances should the specimens be stored in a freezer below 0°C because ice crystals will develop and destroy cellular and extracellular tissue components.

Storage of previously fixed, small specimens for TEM for a few days in buffer solution at 4°C can be tolerated, but it is preferable to proceed with the embedding of the material after the rinsing of the fixed specimens in the appropriate buffer solution to remove the remaining fixative from the tissue. Larger specimens (e.g., femora or parts of the skeleton) can be stored in solutions especially developed for display of specimens in museums.

DECALCIFICATION

General Considerations

Decalcification procedures are widely used in histological routine; however, decalcification alters the structural integrity of the bone considerably. With modern plastic embedding methods and newer methods for sectioning, it is preferable not to decalcify the specimens but to cut the implants in situ within the hard tissues and to preserve their interface with the implants for histological analysis.

When soft biomaterials, which can be cut with a conventional microtome, are studied, decalcification, or more precisely, demineralization of the specimens can be accomplished with a considerable variety of procedures. Hard biomaterials encased in a bony implantation bed should be embedded in an appropriate polymer resin and cut with a sawing microtome without prior demineralization of the specimen. Soft biomaterials within bone can also be processed in the same manner without prior demineralization.

In principle, there are two types of procedures for demineralization of bone specimens: the use of acids and of chelating agents. Acidic solutions tend to destroy cellular and extracellular tissue components, and with prolonged exposure in the acidic solution, to give poor staining results. Procedures with chelating agents produce specimens that can be stained with better results, but they are time-consuming.

Decalcification Procedures

Hard tissues require complete fixation prior to any decalcification or demineralization procedure. After fixation in formaldehyde or in Schaffer's solution, the specimens should be made as small as possible and placed in a container with sufficient decalcification solution, applying constant agitation with a magnetic stirrer, so that the decalcification proceeds as quickly and uniformly as possible. Exposure to the decalcifying solution should be as short as possible, and should be checked daily for specimen hardness.

Decalcifying solution can contain hydrochloric acid, glacial acetic acid, nitric acid, formic acid, or citric acid in an aqueous or alcoholic solution. Different formulations that can be found in manuals for tissue processing are in routine use with more or less satisfying results. The use of the chelating agent ethylenediaminetetraacetic acid (EDTA) gives better results (e.g., 5.5 weight-percent aqueous solution of EDTA in a phosphate buffer, pH 7.4).

Accurate detection of the endpoint of decalcification is important because the specimen must complete microtomy but tissue damage should be avoided. Bending, squeezing, or probing the specimen with a needle are general methods of endpoint determination to determine specimen hardness; however these mechanical methods produce artifacts in the tissue and are unreliable.

Chemical methods cause precipitation of calcium oxalate from the decalcification solution. Ammonium hydroxide and ammonium oxalate are added to the solution to react with any calcium that was removed from the specimen. The decalcification solution is then changed and the test is repeated. When no precipitate is formed, decalcification is considered complete. A disadvantage is that near the end of decalcification, the precipitate becomes difficult to detect, which limits the accuracy of the test. In addition, chemical tests cannot be used when mineral acids (hydrochloric, sulfuric, or nitric) are used in high concentrations for decalcification.

The radiographic method produces visual evidence of demineralization. The procedure must be standardized to produce accurate results. The size of the specimen and X-ray exposure, film and the development are all variables. Specimens that have been fixed in Zenker's, Helly's or Heidenhains-Susa's solution will contain mercuric chloride and will yield false positive results.

EMBEDDING

General Considerations

Embedding of hard and soft tissue specimens within a matrix of wax or polymerized resin allows sectioning with a microtome at room temperature. The aim of the embedding is to bring tissue components with different density and hardness characteristics to the same density and hardness without shrinkage and to preserve the integrity of structures during sectioning. Therefore, the choice of embedding procedure depends on the properties of the implant material and adjacent tissue and on the type of microtome used. Early microscopic studies often used unembedded specimens for sectioning, and usually involved a great deal of hand grinding [28]; however, this method may not adequately preserve cellular integrity or soft tissue structures. Unembedded specimens are often used for microradiographic and metallographic studies because cells and soft tissues are not evaluated [14].

Unembedded and unfixed specimens that are snap frozen to avoid ice crystal formation can be cut with a cryostat microtome usually at a temperature between -15 and $-30°C$. Mineralized bone from teeth, however, is too hard and brittle to be cut properly with this procedure.

Embedding of Decalcified (Demineralized) Specimens

Demineralized specimens are usually dehydrated stepwise with alcohols of increasing concentration, cleared in xylene, infiltrated with paraffin wax, and cooled as blocks for sectioning on a sliding or rotary microtome. There is no fundamental difference in the embedding of decalcified specimens and soft tissues. Since decalcified hard tissues are considerably more dense than soft tissue, the time intervals for dehydration and infiltration steps must be increased by at least a factor of two. Since various bone densities are different, proper completion of the dehydration and infiltration in different specimens is critical and there are no generally accepted rules. Critical analysis of the results must be used to make the necessary corrections. These considerations are also true for undecalcified specimens that are to be embedded in resins, making them harder than those in paraffin or paraffin wax.

Embedding for Light Microscopy

The most common embedding media for light microscopy are Spurr's resin [29] and methyl methacrylate. Other media include glycol methacrylate and Epon 812 (Table 44-1). The advantages of Spurr's resin are in its low viscosity, resin hardness suited to bone, less shrinkage than other media, decreased time for polymerization with heat, and greater ease in sectioning. Its disadvantage is its toxicity, which mandates that appropriate precautions be observed during its use. In some countries Spurr's resin has been removed from the market due to its toxicity.

Advantages of methyl methacrylate are its effective penetration into the tissue, its clarity, and polymerization at room temperature and pressure. The known disadvantages are: lengthy and tedious preparation procedure, high incidence of air bubbles and overflowing upon excessive application of heat, and toxic fumes produced during polymerization.

Preparation time of the monomer can be reduced by the following methods:

1   Altering catalysts (benzoyl peroxide is usually used) [8, 30]
2   Addition of poly-methyl-methacrylate (PMMA) beads to monomer [12, 18]
3   Addition of heat (limited due to bubble formation) [22, 25]
4   Use of not-inhibited methyl methacrylate (eliminates time-consuming step of removing the inhibitor, hydroquinone) [8, 12]

It is possible to obtain methyl methacrylate without an inhibitor (from Matheson, Coleman, and Bell), which also reduces preparation time [13]. One problem is the embedding of PMMA-containing implants in resin without dissolution of the bone cement. To overcome this problem the use of the resin RL white or epoxy resin has been suggested [32]. Embedding

Table 44-1 Embedding for Light Microscopy

Medium	References	Comments
Methyl methacrylate	62	Thionin staining of osteoblasts mineralizing fronts and cement lines
Polymaster 1209AC	47	Rating of cutting artifacts
Methyl methacrylate	63	Overnight vacuum to prevent bubbles
Methyl methacrylate	67	Removal of PMMA with methyl-cello-solve and modified pentachrom stain
Epofix resin	41	Sections thickness 80 μm, no grinding or polishing
Glycol methacrylate	43	Undecalcified bone, water-miscible plastic, immunofluorescent stain
Saccharose acacia-gum snap frozen	70	Cryostat sections, immunohisto-chemical staining, bone marrow
Methyl methacrylate	64	Sawed sections ground to thickness 40 μm, paragon stain, morphometry
Methyl methacrylate	33	Energy-dispersive X-ray analysis
Methyl methacrylate	46	Morphometry, osteogenin, bone morphogenetic protein, calvaria
Modified methyl–methacrylate	65	Goldner's Masson trichrome stain
Epofix: epoxy resin	38	Bone cement PMMA is not affected
Technovit 7200 VCL	54	Photopolymerization of the blocks
Methyl and butylmethacrylate	34	Low temperature $-20°$C embedding enzyme and immunostaining
Glycol methacrylate	35	Enzyme histochemistry
Methyl methacrylate	36	Low temperature $-20°$C embedding enzyme activities maintained

of sections from otherwise embedded tissues is possible. Other techniques of analysis (e.g., EDX) are possible even after resin embedding [33].

Cclloidin has been used as an embedding medium for specimens that cannot withstand heat. Its major disadvantages are its long curing time (up to 8 weeks) and its difficulty in preparation. It has been found to be sufficient for small trabecular bone specimens [31]. Embedding in low temperatures (up to $-20°$C) allows for enzyme and immunohistochemistry [34, 35, 36].

Embedding for Transmission Electron Microscopy

The most important step for this embedding procedure is the penetration or diffusion of the embedding medium into the tissues. Diffusion processes are more easily achieved in soft versus dense or calcified tissue. The viscosity of the embedding medium plays an important role, achieving best results with low viscosity and high penetration [37, 38]. With prolongation of the time for diffusion or penetration, it is possible in some cases to gain acceptable results. The specimens should be as small as possible to assure that the entire tissue block is soaked evenly in the medium, and that penetration of the core is accomplished quickly.

Another critical step is the polymerization of the monomer using small specimens. During polymerization, an exothermic process, the increase in temperature might destroy tissue and cellular components. Small specimen size should assure the heat transfer to the vessel wall and the surrounding medium, assuring a temperature that does not exceed 40°C.

Another problem occurring during polymerization is the shrinkage of the polymer with respect to the monomer [12, 39]. For example, methyl methacrylate will have shrinkage factor of up to 20 percent of the original monomer volume; Araldite (Emscope Laboratories, Ashford, UK) has shown shrinkage as little as 2 percent [24]. Shrinkage causes artifacts, such as warping, voids, and tissue separation. Effects can be minimized if the size of the specimens and the vessels containing the embedding medium are as small as possible.

An additional known artifact of polymerization is the production of gas bubbles, often caused by moisture trapped in the specimen (if hydrophobic embedding media are used), although it can also be caused by over-heating or too rapid polymerization. Complete dehydration of the specimen is imperative. Large, undecalcified specimens used for sectioning with a special microtome are commonly dehydrated with alcohols and embedded with acrylates (a mixture of methylacrylate and butylacrylate). Methyl methacrylate may be used with or without an inhibitor and added PMMA [8, 18].

Araldite, acrylates, and Vestopal are commonly used embedding media for TEM. The best medium for implants into bone is Spurr's resin [29, 31]. Advantages and disadvantages are listed in the previous section. The greatest disadvantage of Araldite resin appears to be its high viscosity. Progressive mixtures of Araldite with xylene or propylene oxide decrease the viscosity and allow better infiltration of the specimen [23, 24]. In contrast, the water-miscible resin monomer Nanoplast polymerizes, producing triazin in which the tissue is enclosed [39]. The specimens must be small or saturation from the soaking may not be assured. The preparation of ultrathin sections is difficult due to the easy fracturing tendency of the specimens along the cell membranes and subcellular membranes which maintain their fat-containing structure.

It is also possible to use unfixed snap-frozen specimens for ultrathin sectioning and staining these cuts with special immunohistochemical procedures, providing considerable information.

Trimming of Specimen Blocks

Prior to cutting ultrathin sections for TEM, the tissue block has to be reduced to a size containing only the relevant structures. Therefore, most investigators prepare semithin sections (approximately 0.5 μm thick), and depending on the structures revealed in these sections, designation of an area of interest can be maintained by trimming superfluous areas. The staining of semithin sections can be performed with several methods (e.g., toluidine blue or Richardson's stain) that do not require removal of the embedding medium. Trimming of the blocks can be done with special equipment. However, this can present problems when hard and brittle implant materials are encased in the blocks. In such cases, it may be necessary to use diamond-coated blades, saws, or grinding machines to reduce implant materials close to the area of diagnostic interest: i.e., the interface between the implant material and surrounding tissues, particularly bone. It can be difficult if not impossible to produce sections without major artifacts if the implant material is not trimmed correctly. Accurate trimming is, therefore, an important step in the whole procedure for TEM analysis.

SECTIONING

General Considerations

Means of processing or, more specifically, sectioning an implanted bone depends upon implant material (soft filamentous carbon or hard cobalt chromium alloy), the type of bone (cortical or cancellous), the embedding media (Table 44-1), and the evaluation techniques that are to be utilized (LM, TEM, histochemistry, microangiography, autoradiography, fluorescence microscopy, ISH). Microtome sectioning of decalcified specimens can be done using routine methods and common sliding or rotating microtomes provided that no hard implant materials are present and the block matrix displays a hardness equal or similar to the hardness of the implant material. These methods can be accomplished with equipment available in all histological laboratories and produce results that are basic to microscopic anatomy and pathology. These 5–10 μm sections can be stained with a variety of methods to provide the basis for a biocompatibility evaluation. Disadvantages are that most of the mineralization information is lost and that only very soft implants or tissues with removed implants can be sectioned. Sectioning artifacts often result when implants are retained in the specimen. Methods of removing implants include chemical (e.g., acetone to remove bone cement), electrochemical (to remove metals) [40], or manual displacement of the implant. One must consider whether the interfacial tissue is disrupted during the removal procedure. Microscopic details may be removed along with the implant; this, however, can be reduced by pre-embedding of the specimen.

Undecalcified specimens with implants embedded in a hard matrix cannot be cut with either common sliding or rotary microtomes without damage to the microtome knife. For this purpose, special microtomes and saws are used, either with a low- or high-speed rotating disk or with an inner hole of the rotating disk [13, 15]. The cutting edges of these disks are preferably diamond-coated; however, other types of disks of carborundum crystals in a more-or-less hard bonding to the matrix of the disk can also be used (Table 44-2).

Microtome Sectioning of Decalcified or Undecalcified Specimens for Light Microscopy and TEM

There is a variety of commercially available microtomes for sectioning of decalcified or undecalcified specimens for light microscopy or TEM (Table 44-2). The results seem to be dependent on the appropriate embedding and trimming of the specimens and not so much on the type of microtome itself. Routine sectioning for light microscopy should be performed with a heavy-duty microtome and specially-adapted knives. Sectioning for TEM is performed with standard ultramicrotomes [41, 42]. The skill of the operator plays a major role in collecting thin or ultrathin sections of good quality.

Microtome Sectioning of Undecalcified Specimens for Light Microscopy and TEM

Heavy microtomes equipped with a specially hardened knife edge are adequate for sectioning of resin-embedded tissue blocks containing biomaterials with medium hardness [16]. The blocks should not exceed a diameter of 20 mm for the cutting plane.

There is no difference between cutting semithin and ultrathin sections of undecalcified and decalcified specimens, provided that glass knives of the ultratome are replaced by diamond knives whenever possible.

Table 44-2 Microtomes, Saws, Milling Attachments

Microtome	References	Medium	Block size	Thickness μm	Microtome type
Heavy-duty microtome, e.g., Polycut	43, 44, 45, 46, 62	PMMA, paraffin	25 × 20 × 7 cm	1–5	Sliding, motordriven
Ultramilling attachment, e.g., Polycut	63	PMMA	11 × 8 × 1.5 cm		Diamonded rotating head
Cryostat, e.g., Frigocut Reichert-Jung	70	Frozen	2 × 2 × 0.5 cm	10	Rotary automated
Reichert-Jung model K	8, 16, 25, 47, 65	PMMA		5	
Sorval JB-4	17, 65	GMA, paraffin, Spurr	12 × 16 mm	1–10	Rotary
Porter Blum	21, 23, 44	Epoxy resins			
Buehler Isomet	13, 50, 64	PMMA	7 mm	40	Circular saw
Exact band saw	34, 38, 42, 54	Epoxy resin, PMMA	3 × 2 cm	300	Diamonded band
Exact oscillating saw		PMMA, resins	4 × 4 × 1.5 cm	20	Rotating diamonded disk
Leitz sawing microtome	30, 49	PMMA, resins		20	Diamonded annular disk
Diamonded wire saw		PMMA, resins	5 × 5 × 10 cm	50	
Gillings Bronwill	11, 12, 15, 18, 19, 48	PMMA			
Ultramicrotome, e.g., LKB		Triazin, Epon, Spurr	2 × 2 mm	40 nm–2 μm	
Exact grinding machine	42	Resins, metals			Rotating carborundum disk

Heavier horizontal or vertical sledge microtomes (Table 44-2) can cut plastic-embedded (GMA, PMMA, Spurr's) mineralized bone that is not too large or dense. These microtomes are often made for specific embedding media. The method produces thin sections (1–5 μm) that generally have fewer artifacts than paraffin sections. Automated microtomes provide a slower, more uniform cutting force than manual ones.

The remaining problems are that the embedding material must have the proper hardness, the blocks must be trimmed to the right size and area of interest, and the blocks should not contain implant material too hard or too brittle to be cut with the diamond knife. The cutting angle must be optimized and adapted to the individual block. This procedure is highly dependent on acquired skills. Sometimes it is only necessary to turn the block in such a direction that the bone (soft tissue, osteoid, or chondroid) is cut prior to the interface and the implant material. In some cases, it is recommended to cut in a parallel direction to the interface. Only in rare cases is it preferable to cut the implant material first, then the interface, and lastly the bone or other tissues; this procedure would minimize cutting artifacts which might cause misinterpretation [47].

To cut semithin (0.5 μm) or ultrathin (60–80 nm) sections for TEM, commercially available ultramicrotomes are used with diamond knives instead of glass knives. In some

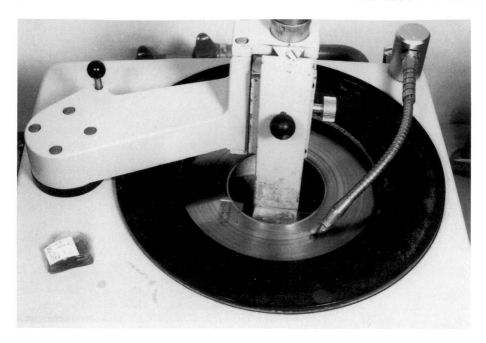

Figure 44-1 Sawing microtome. The diamonded edge of the rotating disk is pressed against a PMMA-block containing the specimen and mounted on the arm in the center of the hole. A glass or PMMA slide is glued on the block with cyanoacrylate instant bond to hold the section. Rinsing by tap water.

special cases, ion milling can be considered as a tool to reduce semithin sections to ultrathin sections suitable for TEM.

Machine Sectioning of Undecalcified Specimens

One method of obtaining relatively thin sections down to 20 μm from blocks with hard biomaterials in the specimen is to use a sawing microtome with an inner hole disk [30, 48]. This type of machine has a rotating cylinder on which a disk with an inner hole is mounted (Figure 44-1). The edge of the hole is coated with diamond powder in a supporting matrix. The block with the implant material surrounded by bone or other tissues is pressed by a supporting arm to the edge of the rotating disk and rinsed with cool tap water or saline solution. The thickness of the sections can be drastically decreased by mounting a coverslip glass or PMMA slide glued to the surface of the block with cyanoacrylate. With this procedure, the relatively thin section can be prevented from turning off the sectioning plane, and the thickness of the sections can be in the range of 20–50 μm. Additionally, the vertical movements and vibrations of the disk can be reduced by mild external pressure so that disruption of the block is prevented. The sections are then glued upside down, i.e., with the coverslip, onto regular glass or PMMA slides for further processing.

This type of sectioning can be accomplished with excellent results using relatively small specimens (diameter below 20 mm). Larger specimens are sectioned preferably with low or high speed saws (Table 44-2) that are equipped with a diamonded disk or band [42] providing thicker sections (thickness of 100–200 μm or even more) (Figures 44-2 and 44-3). The cutting edge can be lubricated with water [15], water and oil [22], kerosene, glycerol, or Buehler Isocut fluid [13]. These methods produce thick sections that can be

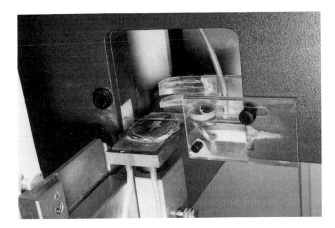

Figure 44-2 Diamonded band saw cutting through a PMMA-block containing a metal stem. The block is glued on the glass or plexiglass slide and this is held on a suction plate. Rinsing by cooling solution in the bottom of the tray.

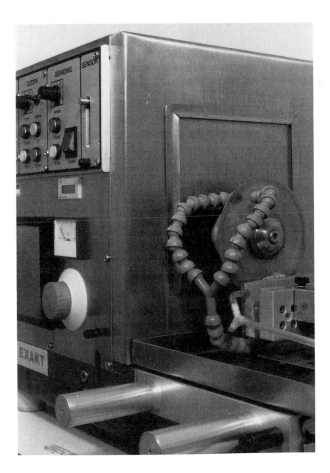

Figure 44-3 Oscillating saw. The diamonded rotating disk moves in the section plane and is rinsed by cooling solution in the tray. The PMMA-block with the specimen is glued on a plexiglass or glass slide and this is held by a suction plate.

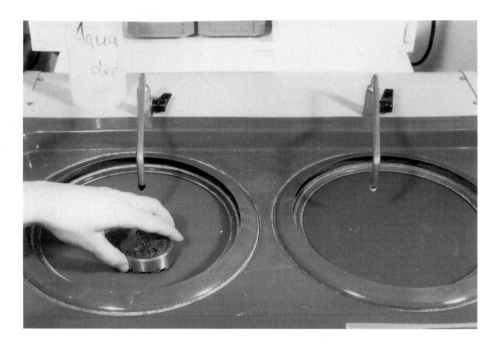

Figure 44-4   Simple grinding equipment. The section or block is mounted on a holder and moved by hand on top of a rotating disk with carborundum paper. Rinsing by tap water.

used for microradiography fluorescent microscopy or LM. A limited number of methods exist for surface staining these thick sections (Table 54-3). They allow direct visualization of the implant-mineralized tissue interface. However, the thickness of the plastic embedding media, implant, and tissue make critical evaluations at higher magnifications difficult. These sections have to be reduced in thickness by grinding.

Preparation of Ground Sections

Grinding and polishing (metallographic) methods (listed in Figure 44.4) are used to reduce the thickness of these sections and to remove sawing artifacts [47]. Various grits of silicone carbide paper, carborundum, or alumina, or glass roughened with these materials [31] are lubricated with oil [48], water [11, 18, 28, 55], alcohol [22], or liquid paraffin [24]. Such methods produce 30–50 μm sections that are more easily interpreted. This grinding can be done by hand, but it is time-consuming and needs skill for maintaining the integrity of the section [28].

The grinding can also be performed with a machine, usually with a rotating disk [14, 55] and with paste in which hard grains, e.g., silicone carbide, are the abrasive for the bone and the enclosed implant (Figure 44-5). Machine grinding can be done with multiple pastes of decreasing grain size, finally delivering a polished and rather flat surface of the section [18]. The section should be mounted on a support, e.g., a petrographic glass plate, with glue or tape, which can be removed by a solvent. The final product of this procedure can be a thin section appropriate for staining and light microscopic evaluation. The time necessary for this type of preparation is dependent on the equipment and also the skill of the individual. One possibility for reducing the preparation time is to use a

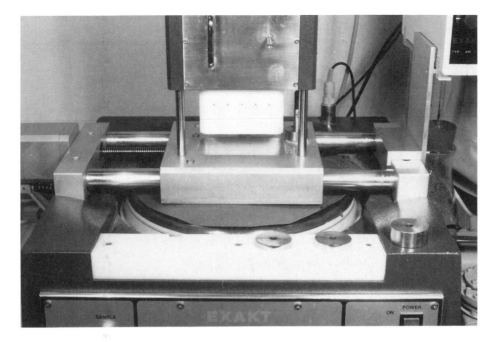

Figure 44-5 Automated grinding machine. The section is glued on a plexiglass or glass slide and mounted on a support which is moved against a rotating disk with carborundum paper on the bottom.

suction device to quickly mount the section on a porous metallic support or other types of slide holders. Smooth surfaces can also be prepared by milling machines which work with a rotating diamond instead of a knife in a heavy-duty microtome. There are usually advantages and disadvantages to each of these techniques. Often a combination of methods is needed to extract the most information about the histocompatibility of orthopedic implants.

STAINING

Staining Procedures for Light Microscopy

The most elegant modern technique uses unstained or fluorescent-dye-stained specimens in vital confocal microscopy [57, 58]. Block staining with basic fuchsin is easily performed by immersing the whole block of tissue including the implant into the dye solution prior to sectioning [59]. The disadvantage of this staining procedure is that a considerable time is required for diffusion of the dye into the tissues, and the result is only good if the sections are sufficiently thin. The histological evaluation can be difficult because the structures are not translucent enough and can be masked by dark red color in the case of fuchsin stain. Because of these disadvantages, block staining is not routinely used.

Methods of staining demineralized, paraffin-embedded bones for general morphology are similar to those described. These and other stains are utilized with plastic-embedded sections and provide information important for evaluating implants. Some staining methods and their results have been compiled in Table 44-3.

Table 44-3   Stains for Thick and Thin Sections, Surface Staining

Stain	References	Embedding media	Differentiates
Thick section			
Paragon	12, 13, 18, 21, 52	PMMA, Epon, Araldite	General morphology
Giemsa	30	PMMA, resins	General morphology
Alizarin red S-methylene blue	11	Spurr's	Calcium, Collagen
Acridine orange	51	Low melting point wax	Ribonucleic acid
Villanueva bone stain	56	Unembedded	Osteoid, bone
Thin section			
Hematoxylin and Eosin	8, 12, 25, 29, 43	Paraffin, Araldite, Spurr's	General morphology
Silver techniques	17, 43	PMMA, GMA	Collagen fibers, cartilage
Toluidine blue	25, 42	PMMA, GMA	Calcification front, osteoid, cement lines
Masson's trichrome	8, 31	PMMA, Spurr's	Collagen
Methylene blue	8, 17, 29, 60	GMA, Spurr's	General morphology, cartilage
Alcian blue	17, 67	GMA	Glycosaminoglycans
von Kossa	17, 31, 43, 61	PMMA, Spurr's	Mineral with calcium, bone, cartilage
Periodic acid Schiff	17, 43	PMMA, GMA	Glycogen, 1,2-glycols
Basic fuchsin	17, 61	PMMA, GMA, Spurr's	Soft tissue
Goldner	25, 65	PMMA	Collagen, muscle
Thionin	62	PMMA	Osteoblasts, cement lines

Undecalcified, thick sections can only be surface-stained, or more precisely expressed, stained in the surface layer without removal of the embedding medium [11, 30]. A prerequisite for this type of staining is that the embedding medium does not react with the dye. The Giemsa staining solution, which is available as a stock solution in every histological laboratory, is suitable for staining undecalcified sections embedded in methyl methacrylate (Figure 44-6B). The staining time is dependent on the concentration of the staining solution and can be chosen according to the result.

Surface staining can also be accomplished with other dyes or reactions [56, 59], e.g., periodic acid Schiff (PAS), toluidine blue, methenamine silver stain [66, 67], von Kossa stain [17, 61], Berlin blue or Perl's stain for iron, and a method for aluminum [68, 69].

Adequate surface staining results cannot be achieved with hematoxylin, hemalum, and other lacquer-forming dyes. In some cases, however, it has proved valuable to use acidic buffers for slight decalcification of the primarily undecalcified sections with remaining embedding medium prior to the staining of the slides with hemalum [43]. The result allows a rather clear demonstration of the cement lines of the osteons. Therefore, a whole range of staining effects can be achieved with comparatively simple and inexpensive procedures (Figure 44-6C and D). Unlike soft tissue staining methods that have long been developed and provide reproducible standardized results, hard tissue staining methods have only been developed recently and are rarely published in literature.

To enhance staining, deplasticized sections have been utilized. Spurr's sections have been deplasticized with sodium hydroxide in methanol or ethanol [31], bromide vapor and acetone, or sodium ethoxide [16]. Potassium hydroxide in ethyl alcohol has been used for an epoxy resin [44]. Methyl methacrylate has been removed with toluene [8], chloroform

[22], acetone [26], and cellosolve. Epon and Araldite sections have been deplasticized with potassium ethoxide; Araldite itself has been removed with bromide vapor (a dangerous procedure), then acetone. These methods are useful for thin sections (1–10 μm). There can be diffusion of the dye in the mounting medium holding the coverslip. Some mounting media are more compatible with a certain dye than others; the most stable combination must be determined experimentally. It may be necessary to use immersion oil to mount the coverslip and to remove it after microscopy. Difficulties may be encountered in applying some histological stains to glycol methacrylate sections. The polymer matrix can be stained by certain dyes, such as the azure II in Giemsa's method and the toluidine blue and others, thus obscuring details. Therefore, staining of nuclei is more accurately obtained by use of Gill's hematoxylin developed specifically for methacrylate sections.

Enzyme histochemical methods can be applied to frozen or freeze-dried and glycol methacrylate sections of bone and other tissues with implants [17, 70]. Sections of this type can be processed for enzyme activity, such as acid or alkaline phosphatase. The results are equivalent to those obtained with cryostat sections of soft tissues. In principle, it is expected that immunohistochemical procedures can also be applied to these sections. The antigenic sites are preserved after freeze drying, perfusion, and polymerization of the glycol methacrylate embedding medium. The antigenic sites can be set free by dissolving the embedding medium completely or partially with sodium methylate. Reactive sites are usually not completely destroyed by these procedures.

The *in situ* hybridization techniques for detection of transcripts, i.e., messenger ribonucleic acid (RNA), in cells are beginning to be elaborated and to provide new insight into the biochemical processes. Critical are proper fixation and inhibition of ribonucleases (RNAse), short decalcification to preserve the transcripts for reaction with the cDNA probes, and use of specially baked equipment to destroy RNAses [71–73]. An example for ISH is given in Figure 44-6A.

Staining Procedures for Electron Microscopy

Unstained, ultrathin sections can, in principle, be examined by TEM. The contrast of these sections, however, is low for cellular structures, whereas dense structures such as apatite crystals or collagen fibrils can be easily distinguished. The contrast of membranes, other cell constituents, and extracellular material can be augmented using osmium tetraoxide for fixation or by the use of uranyl acetate, lead citrate, or ruthenium red solutions for further contrast of ultrathin sections. Care must be taken to filter out precipitates in these solutions to minimize artifacts and other problems of TEM interpretation. An additional measure to avoid precipitation is to use only freshly prepared solutions. Generally, the staining procedures for TEM ultrathin sections of implant containing specimens do not differ from those used in every laboratory in which material is processed for TEM. The ultrastructural localization of intracellular antigens using protein-A gold-complex has been described [74]. This type of staining opens a wide field for the demonstration of various macromolecules in cells and in intercellular space by TEM.

SEM provides a powerful tool for the evaluation of implant-containing bone. The technical possibilities have been published recently [75]; therefore they are not repeated here. There are already quite a number of results with this technique [76]. The density of bone can be determined by backscattered mode in SEM, and the shape, orientation and size of mineral crystals by small-angle X-ray scattering (SAXS) [77].

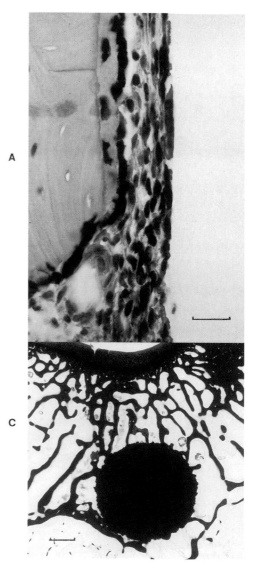

Figure 44-6 (A) *In situ* hybridization for procollagen a1(I) RNA 7 days after implantation of hydroxyapatite (HA) into the distal femur of female Chinchilla rabbits. HA was dissolved during EDTA decalcification. The red digoxygenin reaction product stains collagen-producing osteoblasts at the surface of inactive and negative bone, as well as fibroblasts up to the surface of HA. Counterstaining with Hemalaumn. Bar 37 μm. (B) Glass ionomer cement 4 years after insertion in the femur for fixation of an implant in a 85-year-old female patient and after recent fracture. Leached area of the glass ionomer cement (right), adjacent decalcified (osteoid) bone, and mineralized lamellar bone (left). On top inactive resorption zone in the bone and inflammatory reaction with macrophages (not in focus) containing abundant black particles supposedly derived from the metallic implant. Giemsa stain. Bar 100 μm.

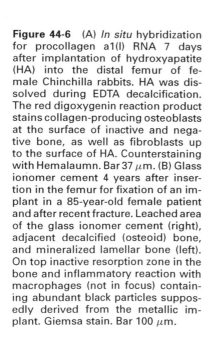

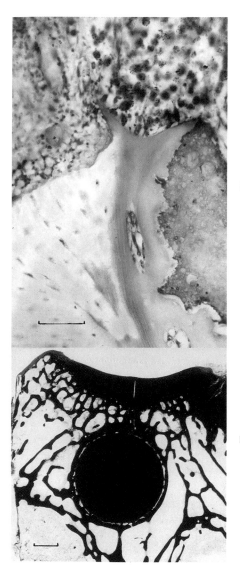

B

D

Figure 44-6 (*cont.*) (C) Commercial pure titanium cylinder 4 mm in diameter, surface roughness 100 μm by titanium plasma flame spray treatment, 168 days after implantation in the distal femur of a female Chinchilla rabbit. Insertion of bone trabeculae in the pores of the surface. Von Kossa and fuchsin staining. Small bubbles as artifacts. Bar 1mm. (D) Commercial pure titanium cylinder 4 mm in diameter, surface roughness 1 μm. 168 days after implantation in the distal femur of a female Chinchilla rabbit. Development of a bone ring fixed in the adjacent bone trabeculae on the external side and with small, footlike bone projections to the smooth, metallic implant surface. Von Kossa and fuchsin staining. Bar 1mm.

ACKNOWLEDGMENTS

The support of the biomaterials research group co-workers, P. D. Dr. C. Voigt, Dr. C. Müller-Mai, Th. Fritz, O. Majdani-Shabestari, M. Dilger-Rein, I. Borchert, and L. Jenkins, Clemson University, Clemson, SC, is acknowledged.

REFERENCES

1 ISO 10993-6. *Biological evaluation of medical devices—Part 6: Tests for local effects after implantation.* CH-1211. 1994, 1:11.
2 ASTM Designation F 561–587. Standard practice for analysis of retrieved metallic orthopaedic implants. In *Annual Book of ASTM Standards.* Philadelphia, PA: American Society for Testing and Materials, 1994, 115–118.
3 Recommendations for retrieval and examination of orthopaedic surgical implants and associated tissues. BS3531, Surgical implants–Part 22, 1988, 1–10.
4 Hutchins GM (Ed.). *Autopsy Performance and Reporting.* Northfield, IL: College of American Pathologists, 1990.
5 Coleman DL, King RN, Andrade JD. The foreign body reaction: An experimental protocol. *J Biomed Mater Res Symp,* 5 (1974), 65–76.
6 Sela J, Karasikov N, Amir D, Kedar Y, Schwartz Z. Ultrastructural computerized quantitative morphometry of extracellular organelles in calcifiying matrices. *J Comp Ass Micros,* 2 (1990), 203–210.
7 Rhinelander FW, Baragry RA. Microangiography in bone healing. *J Bone Joint Surg,* 44 (1962), 1273–1298.
8 Buijs R, Dogterom AA. An improved method for embedding hard tissue in PMMA. *Stain Tech,* 58 (1983), 135–141.
9 Frost HM. Tetracycline-based histological analysis of bone remodelling. *Calcif Tissue Res,* 3 (1969), 221–237.
10 Bergendahl G, Engfeldt B. Preparing material for microradiography. *Acta Pathol Microbiol Scand,* 49 (1960), 30–38.
11 Smith LG, Karaginanes MT. Histological preparation of bone to study ingrowth into implanted materials. *Calcified Tissue Res,* 14 (1974), 333–337.
12 Kenner GH, Henricks L, Gimenez G. Bone embedding technique with inhibited PMMA monomer. *Stain Technol,* 57 (1982), 121–126.
13 Steflik DE, McKinney RV, Mobley GL. Simultaneous histological preparation of bone, soft tissue and implanted biomaterials for light microscopic observations. *Stain Technol,* 57 (1982), 91–98.
14 Gilbertson EM. A method of preparation of undecalcified bone section. *Med Lab Sci,* 34 (1977), 89–91.
15 Seliger WG, Tietz WJ. The production of large epoxy embedded, 50 μm sections by precision sawing: A preliminary survey for ultrathin sectioning. *Stain Technol,* 49 (1968), 269–272.
16 Watts RH, Green D, Howells GR. Improvements in histological techniques for epoxy-resin embedded bone specimens. *Stain Technol,* 56 (1981), 155–161.
17 Horton WA, Dockery N, Sillence D, Rimoin DL. An embedding method for histochemical studies of undecalcified skeletal growth plate. *Stain Technol,* 55 (1980), 19–29.
18 Klawitter JJ, Hulbert SF. Application of porous ceramics for the attachment of load bearing internal orthopedic applications. *Biomed Mater Res Symp,* 2 (1971), 161–229.
19 Harris WH, Jackson RH, Jowsey J. The *in vivo* distribution of tetracycline in canine bone. *J Bone Joint Surg,* 44 (1962), 1308–1320.
20 Muhlrad A, Bab IA, Deutsch D, Sela J. Occurrence of actin-like protein in extracellular matrix vesicles. *Calcif Tissue Int,* 34 (1982), 376–381.
21 Spurlock BO, Skinner MS, Kattine AA. A simple rapid method for staining epoxy-embedded specimens for light microscopy with the polychromatic stain Paragon-1301. *Am J Clin Pathol,* 46 (1966), 252–258.
22 Jowsey J. The use of a milling machine for preparing bone sections for microradiography and microautoradiography. *J Sci Instr,* 32 (1955), 159–163.
23 Luft JH. Improvements in epoxy resin embedding methods. *J Biophys Biochem Cytol,* 9 (1961), 409–414.
24 McQueen CM, Monk IB, Horton PW, Smith DA. Preparation of undecalcified bone sections for auto- and microradiography. *Calcif Tissue Res,* 10 (1972), 23–30.
25 Savelkoul TJF, Viser WJ, Roelofs JMM. A rapid method for preparing undecalcified sections of bone for autoradiographic investigations with short-lived radionuclides. *Stain Technol,* 58 (1983), 1–5.
26 Woodruff LA, Norris WP. Sectioning of undecalcified bone. With special reference to radioautographic applications. *Stain Technol,* 30 (1955), 179–188.

27 Karnovski MJA. Formaldehyde-glutaraldehyde fixative of high osmolality for use in electron microscopy. *J Cell Biol*, 27 (1965), 137A–138A.

28 Frost HM. Preparation of thin undecalcified bone sections by rapid manual method. *Stain Technol*, 33 (1958), 273–277.

29 Spurr AR. A low-viscosity epoxy resin embedding medium for electron microscopy. *J Ultrastruct Res*, 26 (1969), 31–43.

30 Gross UM, Strunz V. Surface staining of sawed sections of undecalcified bone containing alloplastic implants. *Stain Technol*, 52 (1977), 217–219.

31 Johnstone JC, Tam CS. An improved histological method for undecalcified bone sections. *Med Lab Technol*, 30 (1973), 355–357.

32 Migheli-A, Attanasio A. Two methods for flat embedding sections in LR white cut from paraffin blocks. *Biotech Histochem*, 1 (1991), 89–92.

33 Åkesson K, Grynpas MD, Hancock RG, Odselius R, Obrant KJ. Energy-dispersive X-ray microanalysis of the bone mineral content in human trabecular bone: A comparison with ICPES and neutron activation analysis. *Calcif Tissue Int*, 55 (1994), 236–239.

34 Wolf E, Roser K, Hahn M, Welkerling H, Delling G. Enzyme and immunohistochemistry on undecalcified bone and bone marrow biopsies after embedding in plastic: A new embedding method for routine application. *Virchows Arch A Pathol Anat Histopathol*, 420 (1992), 17–24.

35 Islam A, Henderson ES. Glycol methacrylate embedding for light microscopy. I. Enzyme histochemistry on semithin sections of undecalcified marrow cores. *J Clin Pathol*, 40 (1987), 1194–1200.

36 Chappard D, Palle S, Alexandre C, Vico L, Riffat G. Bone embedding in pure methyl methacrylate at low temperature preserves enzyme activities. *Acta Histochem*, 81 (1987), 183–190.

37 Jowsey J, Kelly PJ, Riggs BL. Quantitative microradiographic studies of normal and osteoporotic bone. *J Bone Joint Surg*, 47 (1965), 785–806.

38 Jensen LN, Jensen JS, Gotfredsen K. A method for histological preparation of undecalcified bone sections containing acrylic bone cement. *Biotech Histochem*, 1 (1991), 82–86.

39 Bachhuber K, Frosch D. Melamine resins, a new class of water-soluble embedding media for electron microscopy. *J Microsc*, 1 (1983), 1–9.

40 Brown SA, Simpson J. Electrochemical dissolution of metallic implants prior to histologic sectioning. *J Biomed Mater Res*, 13 (1979), 337–338.

41 Wallin JA, Tkocz I, Levinsen J. A simplified procedure for preparation of undecalcified human bone sections. *Stain Technol*, 60 (1985), 331–336.

42 Donath K, Breuner G. A method for the study of undecalcified bones and teeth with attached soft tissues. The Säge-Schliff (sawing and grinding) technique. *J Oral Pathol*, 11 (1982), 318–326.

43 Franklin RM, Martin MT. Staining and histochemistry of undecalcified bone embedded in a water-miscible plastic. *Stain Technol*, 55 (1980), 313–321.

44 Imai Y, Sue A, Yamaguchi A. A removing method of the resin from epoxy-embedded sections for light microscopy. *J Electron Microsc*, 17 (1968), 84–85.

45 Harris WH, Travis DF, Frigerg V. The *in vivo* inhibition of bone formation by Alizarin Red S. *J Bone Joint Surg*, 46 (1964), 493–508.

46 Ripamonti U, Ma SS, Cunningham NS, Yeates L, Reddi AH. Reconstruction of the bone/bone marrow organ by osteogenin, a bone morphogenetic protein, and demineralized bone matrix in calvarial defects of adult primates. *Plast Reconstr Surg*, 91 (1993), 27–36.

47 Wood DJ, Mawhinney WH, Malcolm AJ, Stevens J. Technique for identifying cutting artefacts in sections of undecalcified bone biopsy specimens. *J Clin Pathol*, 43 (1990), 516–517.

48 Suzuki HK, Mathews A. Two-color fluorescent labeling of mineralizing tissues with tetracycline and 2,4-bis[N,N'-di-(carbomethyl)aminomethyl] fluorescein. *Stain Technol*, 41 (1966), 57–60.

49 Blencke BA. Erfahrungen mit dem Leitz-Sägemikrotom. *Leitz Mitt Wiss u Tech*, 6 (1975), 198–200.

50 Steflik DE, McKinney RV, Jr., Koth DL. Scanning electron microscopy of plasma-etched implant specimens. *Stain Technol*, 59 (1984), 71–77.

51 Bard DR, Dickens MJ, Edwards J, Smith AU. Studies on slices and isolated cells from fresh osteoarthritic human bone. *J Bone Joint Surg Br*, 56 (1974), 340–351.

52 Martin JH, Lynn JA, Nickey WM. A rapid polychrome stain for epoxy-embedded tissue. *Am J Clin Pathol*, 46 (1966), 250–251.

53 Roofe PG, Hoecker FE, Voorhees CD. A rapid bone sectioning technique. *Proc Soc Exp Biol Med*, 72 (1949), 619–622.

54 Rohrer MD, Schubert CC. The cutting-grinding technique for histologic preparation of undecalcified bone and bone-anchored implants. Improvements in instrumentation and procedures. *Oral Surg Oral Med Oral Pathol*, 74 (1992), 73–78.

55 Stürmer KM. Automatic grinding of undecalcified bone sections with exact adjustment of thickness. *Acta Anat Basel*, 103 (1979), 100–108.

56 Villanueva AR. A bone stain for osteoid seams in fresh, unembedded, mineralized bone. *Stain Technol*, 49 (1974), 1–8.

57 Boyde A, Wolfe LA, Maly M, Jones SJ. Vital confocal microscopy in bone. *Scanning*, 17 (1995), 72–85.

58 Greenberg G, Boyde A. Novel method for stereo imaging in light micrscopy at high magnifications. *Neuroimage*, 1 (1993), 121–128.

59 Frost HM. Staining of fresh undecalified thin bone sections. *Stain Technol*, 33 (1958), 135–146.

60 Bennett HS, Wyrick AD, Lee SW, McNeil JH. Science and art in preparing tissues embedded in plastic for light microscopy, with special reference to glycol methacrylate, glass knives and simple stains. *Stain Technol*, 51 (1976), 71–97.

61 Villanueva AR. Methods of preparing and interpreting mineralized sections of bone. *Proc 1st Workshop Bone Morphometry*, 1973; 341–357.

62 Derkx P, Birkenhager Frenkel DH. A thionin stain for visualizing bone cells, mineralizing fronts and cement lines in undecalcified bone sections. *Biotech Histochem*, 70 (1995), 70–74.

63 Sterchi DL, Eurell JA. A new method for preparation of undecalcified bone sections. *Stain Technol*, 64 (1989), 201–205.

64 Felsenfeld AJ, Harrelson JM, Gutman RA. A quantitative histomorphometric comparison of 40-micron-thick Paragon sections with 5-micron-thick Goldner sections in the study of undecalcified bone. *Calcif Tissue Int*, 34 (1982), 232–238.

65 Gruber HE. Adaptations of Goldner's Masson trichrome stain for the study of undecalcified plastic embedded bone. *Biotech Histochem*, 67 (1992), 30–34.

66 Movat HZ. Silver impregnation methods for electron microscopy. *Am J Clin Pathol*, 35 (1961), 528–537.

67 Olah AJ, Simon A, Gaudy M, Herrmann W, Schenk RK. Differential staining of calcified tissues in plastic embedded microtome sections by a modification of Movat's pentachrome stain. *Stain Technol*, 52 (1977), 331–337.

68 Maloney NA, Ott SM, Alfrey AC, Miller NL, Coburn JW, Sherrard DJ. Histological quantitation of aluminum in iliac bone from patients with renal failure. *J Lab Clin Med*, 99 (1982), 206–216.

69 Cole MB, Jr., Narine KR. Staining glycol methacrylate-embedded cartilage with triethyl-carbocyanin DBTC ("ethyl-stains all") with special reference to the interlacunar network. *Stain Technol*, 59 (1984), 323–333.

70 Falini B, Martelli MF, Tarallo F, Moir DJ, Cordell JL, Gatter KC, Loreti G, Stein H, Mason DY. Immunohistological analysis of human bone marrow trephine biopsies using monoclonal antibodies. *Br J Haematol*, 56 (1984), 365–386.

71 Voigt CF, Peljak P, Müller-Mai C, Herbst H, Gross UM. Topography of forming and resorbing cells on endosteal surfaces of the rabbit humerus by double-staining with *in situ* hybridization and tartrate-resistant acid phosphatase reaction: A new model to study the bone reaction to loading. *J Mater Sci: Mater Med*, 6 (1995), 279–283.

72 Wilcox JN. Fundamental principles of *in situ* hybridization. *J Histochem Cytochem*, 41 (1993), 1725–1733.

73 Neo M, Voigt DF, Herbst H, Gross UM. Analysis of osteoblast activity at biomaterial-bone interfaces by *in situ* hybridization. *J Biomed Mater Res*, 30 (1996), 485–492.

74 Roth J, Bendayan M, Orci L. Ultrastructural localization of intracellular antigens by the use of protein A-gold complex. *J Histochem Cytochem*, 26 (1978), 1074–1081.

75 Boyde A, Jones SJ. Scanning electron microscopy of bone: Instrument, specimen, and issues. *Microsc Res Techn*, 33 (1996), 92–120.

76 Orr RD, De Bruijn JD, Davies JE. Scanning electron microscopy of the bone interface with titanium, titanium alloy and hydroxyapatite. *Cells and Materials*, 3 (1992), 241–251.

77 Fratzl P, Groschner M, Vogl G, Plenk H, Jr., Eschberger J, Fratzl-Zelman N, Koller K, Klaushofer K. Mineral crystals in calcified tissues: A comparative study by SAXS. *J Bone Miner Res*, 7 (1992), 329–334.

78 Smith SC, Kunishima DH, Simon TM, Ohland KJ, Jackson DW, Aberman HM. A novel accelerated tissue processing technique for use with large specimens of bone containing biomaterials. *J Histopath*, submitted.

ADDITIONAL READING

1 Sheehan DC, Hrapechak BB. *Theory and Practice of Histotechnology*. St. Louis, MO: Mosby, 1980.

2 Luna LG. *Manual of Histologic Staining Methods of the Armed Forces Institute of Pathology*. New York: McGraw-Hill, 1968, 62–65.

3 Wilkinson DG. *In Situ Hybridization—A Practical Approach*. London: Oxford University Press, 1992.

4 Schenk R. Zur histologischen Verarbeitung von unentkalkten Knocken. *Acta anat*, 60 (1965), 3–19.

APPENDIX

Preparation of Calcified Bone for Light Microscopy

I   Fix in buffered formaldehyde according to Lillie, pH 7.2–7.4
  A. Composition:

1. Distilled water	900 ml
2. NaH_2PO_4	4 g
3. Na_2HPO_4	6, 5 g
4. 37 percent formaldehyde	100 ml
B. Immerse to fix femur of rabbits	7 days
femur of rats	3–4 days
	at 4°C

II   Rinse in tap water 12 hrs

III   Dehydrate with ethanol 70 percent, 80 percent, 90 percent, 96 percent and 2 × 100 percent, 3–7 days each step.
  Defat: Aether Chloroform 1 + 1
  Aether-Chloroform-Methylmethacrylate 3–7 days each

IV   Infiltrate at 4°C in methyl methacrylate
  Composition:
  1. Methyl methacrylate (Merck Co. No. 800 590) 1800 ml
  2. Dibutyl phthalate (Merck Co. No 800 919) 180 ml
  3. α, α-diazoisobutyronitrile (Fluka Nr. 11630), 2 × 3–7 days

V   Polymerize in glass tubes with methyl methacrylate at 40°C for 48 hrs

VI   Prepare sawed sections with the sawing microtome (Leitz 1600, Leitz, Wetzlar)
  A. Thickness of sawed sections 30–50 μm.
  B. Fix on coverslips with cyanoacrylate glue (Instantbond, M. Langnas, Berlin)

VII   Rinse with Sörensen phosphate buffer for 30 min, clean the surface with dry linen.
  A. Surface stain with Giemsa stain
  1. Composition
    a) 50 ml Giemsa solution (Merck Co., No. 9204)
    b) 50 ml Sörensen phosphate buffer, pH 7.4
  B. Composition for Sörensen buffer
  1. a) 97.150 g $Na_2HPO_4 \cdot 2H_2O$
    b) 16.525 g KH_2PO_4
  2. Adjust to pH 7.4. Solution in 5 liters of distilled water; prepare the solution by adding the second salt after the first salt is completely diluted. Otherwise crystalline material will be obtained.

VIII   Rinse the distilled water
  A. Dehydrate: with ethanol, xylene
  B. Embed: DePeX (Serva 18243)

Automated Tissue Embedding [78]

I   Tissue blocks are fixed, trimmed as small as possible, labelled, bagged and placed in a tissue processor (e.g., Shandon Hypercenter XP tissue processor).

A. 70% Reagent Alcohol (95% ethanol and 5% methanol)	4 hrs
B. 95% Reagent Alcohol	4 hrs
C. 95% Reagent Alcohol	6 hrs
D. 100% Reagent Alcohol	8 hrs
E. 100% Reagent Alcohol	6 hrs
F. 100% Reagent Alcohol	18 hrs
G. Xylene	6 hrs

H.	Xylene	8 hrs
I.	100% Reagent Alcohol	10 hrs
J.	100% Reagent Alcohol	24 hrs
K.	50% Alcohol, 50% Technovit 7200	24 hrs
L.	Technovit 7200	48 hrs
M.	Technovit 7200	48 hrs
N.	Technovit 7200 + 1%BPO	48 hrs

    1. Step 14 is performed in a vacuum dessicator at −900 mbar using Technovit 7200 with 1% benzoyl peroxide (BPO) added.

    2. Photo-polymerization by 2 hours yellow, 10 hours blue light in a Histolux (Exact Inc.) with the lid open. This is followed by:

O. 24 hours in an oven at 50°C to complete polymerization.

Preparation of Sections for Light Microscopy and Histochemistry

I Embedding in glycol methacrylate

  A. Perfuse and fix (30 min) in buffered formaldehyde according to Lillie

  B. Rinse in TES-buffer (Merck Co., No. T1375) for 24 hr (4°C)

  C. Gradual dehydration to 100 percent ethanol (each step 45 to 60 min)

  D. Composition of glycol methacrylate

    1. Uncatalyzed solution A

      a) Glycol methacrylate (Fluka Co. No. 641 70) 160 ml

      b) 2-Butoxyethanol (Fluka Co., No. 20400) 32 ml

      c) The mixture of both can be stored for sereral months at 4°C.

    2. Catalyzed solution A

      a) Uncatalyzed solution A 100 ml

      b) Benzoyl peroxide (Merck Co., No. 801 641) 0.9 ml

      c) The mixture can be stored for several weeks at 4°C (dark glass bottle)

    3. Solution B

      a) Polyethylene glycol 400 (Merck Co, No. 807 485)

      b) N-N-Dimethylaniline (Merck Co., No. 803 060) 1 ml

      c) The mixture can be stored at 4°C (dark jar).

    4. After dehydration, the bone material is stored for 3 days in catalyzed solution A at 4°C in the desiccator.

  E. Embed bone material in plastic jars with a mixture of

    1. 30 parts catalyzed solution A

    2. 1 part solution B.

    3. Polymerize for approximately 1 hr

    4. All solutions of the glycol methacrylate should be used at room temperature.

  F. Prepare sawed sections on a sawing microtome Leitz 1600 (Leitz, Wetzlar).

    1. Thickness of sections 30–50 μm.

    2. Fix sections on cover slips with cyanoacrylate Instantbond (M. Langnas, Berlin).

    3. Rinsing with Sörensen phosphate buffer for approximately 30 min.

  G. For phosphatase reaction see "Method for the Detection of Alkaline and Acid Phosphatase in Mineralized Bone Embedded in Glycol Methacrylate."

II Freeze-dried bone tissue

  A. Place unfixed bone fragments immediately in liquid nitrogen.

  B. Transfer to the freeze dryer, drying for approximately 1 week. Vacuum 0.6 atm at −4°C.

  C. Infiltration for 3 days and polymerization as described above (step II, D4). Dried specimens are to be transferred immediately into solution A.

Method for Detection of Alkaline and Acid Phosphatase in Mineralized Bone Embedded in Glycol Methacrylate

I   Alkaline phosphatase
  A. Incubation medium
   1. Naphtol-AS-BI-phosphate, (Sigma Co., No. 2250), 20 mg, dissolved in 0.5 ml dimethylformamide
   2. Tris-HCl buffer pH 8.9–9.4, 50 ml
   3. Fresh hexazotized Neufuchsin, (Merck Co., No. 4041), 0.5 ml
  B. Thoroughly mix all three components, filtrate, adjust to pH with 1 N or 0.1 N NaOH.
  C. Incubation time for 30–50 μm sections for 20–40 min.
  D. Rinse, embed with glycerin gelatin (Merck Co., No. 9242).
  E. Reaction product: red
  F. Nuclear staining with Gill's hematoxylin
  G. Hexazotized Neufuchsin
   1. 4 percent sodium nitrite, (Merck Co., No. 6549) 0.25 ml
   2. 4 percent Neufuchsin 0.25 ml
  H. Mix solution in separate vessels until yellow coloration appears.
   1. percent Neufuchsin: 4 g Neufuchsin in 100 ml 2 N HCl, store of the $NaNO_2$ at 4°C for a maximum of 1 week.

II Detection of Acid Phosphatase (Tartrate resistant) in Undecalcified Bone
  A. Fixation in formaldehyde according to Lillie pH 7.4, 15–30 min
  B. Rinse in acetate buffer pH 5
    Acetate buffer: 0.2 M Sodium.acetate
    Acetate buffer +0.2 M Acetic acid
  C. Incubation medium
   1. Acetate buffer pH 5,   50 ml
   2. Hexazotized para-rosaniline:
      4 % Sodium nitrite   2 ml
      4 % p-rosaniline freshly prepared   2 ml
   3. Naphtol-AS-BI-phosphate, 20 mg diluted in 0.5 ml dimethylformamide
   4. Stir the 3 components very well and filtrate
   5. Adjust to pH 5–5.5
   6. Add 0.28% tartrate
   7. Incubate for 1 hour
  D. Rinse in distilled water, two changes. Keep specimen in formaldehyde (Lillie) overnight.
  E. Rinse with water from the tap.
  F. Embed in glycerin gelatin.

Hematoxylin According to Gill

I	Distilled water	365 ml
II	Ethylene glycol	125 ml
III	Anhydrous powdered hematoxylin	2 g
IV	Sodium iodate ($NaJO_3$), weigh out accurately	0.2 g
V	$Al_2(SO_4)_3 \cdot 16H_2O$	40.25 g
VI	Citric acid	0.5 g
VII	Stain can be used after 1 hour of mixing.	

Scott's Tap Water Substitute

I   Distilled water   1 liter

II	Magnesium sulfate	10 mg
III	Sodium bicarbonate	2 mg

Staining Schedule for Gill's Hematoxylin

I   Place slides into hematoxylin for 10 min.
II Rinse in distilled water.
III Blue in Scitt's tap water substitute for 3 min.

Detailed Procedure for Preparation of TEM Sections from Bone or Cartilage

I   Removal of tissue
   A. Fixative: 4 percent glutaraldehyde (Sigma Co., No. G-5882) in 0.1 M cacodylate buffer, pH 7.2 30 min
   B. Preparation of bone, cutting 1 mm thick sections by low-speed diamond saw. Postfixation for at least 90 min, 30 min rinsing, store in cacodylate-buffer.

II Processing for electron microscopy (TEM)
   A. Rinse specimen with 0.1 M cacodylate-buffer, pH 7.2 three times, 10 min. each.
      1. 0.2 M stock cacodylate buffer:
         a) Sodium cacodylate   10.7 g
         b) H_2O 200 ml
      2. Adjust to pH 7.2 with 0.1 M HCl
      3. Fill up volume to 250 ml
      4. Dilute volume of stock solution with an equal volume of H_2O (1 parts distilled water, 1 part buffer).
   B. Postfixation with 1 percent OsO_4 in cacodylate buffer for 90 min at 4°C (3 volumes of working buffer solution with 1 volume of 4 percent OsO_4).
   C. Rinse specimen with 0.1 M cacodylate three times 10 min. each.
   D. Dehydration

1. 70 percent ethanol	20 min
2. 80 percent ethanol	20 min
3. 90 percent ethanol	20 min
4. 95 percent ethanol	20 min
5. 100 percent ethanol three times	20 min
6. Propylene oxide (PO) three times	15 min

   E. Infiltration in a mixture of Epon resin and PO: 3 parts PO + 1 part Epon 30 min.
                                                    1 part PO + 1 part Epon overnight
      1. Epon resin
         a) Stock solution I
            62 ml Epon (Serva, No. 21045) 100 ml
            DDSA (2 · Dodecenylsuccinic acid anhydride)
            b) Stock solution II 100 ml Epon 89 ml MNA (Methylnadic anhydride) (Serva, No. 29452)
      2. Stir in a beaker Sol. I and Sol. II at a 6 + 4
         volumetric ratio 2 min.
      3. Add: DMP-30 (Tris-dimethylaminomethylphenol) Serva Co., No. 36975 1.5 %
      4. Stir for 4 min.
      5. Excess resin can be stored at 4°C for a few days in a beaker sealed with Parafilm and hermetically wrapped in a nylon bag. For reuse leave package at room temperature for 30 min before unwrapping the nylon bag.
   F. Transfer to Epon for 1 hour, 2 times

    G. Embed in Epon resin in a flat capsule with the surface of the specimen facing downward at 65°C overnight in a vacuum embedding device.

III Sectioning

    A. Trim set block to the smallest possible size that contains the whole specimen.

    B. Prepare 1.0 μm thick sections and stain with methylene blue (Richardson stain).

    C. Choose desired area for TEM examination and trim block accordingly.

    D. Prepare ultrathin sections with a diamond knife. Float sections in water. Copper grids are preferable.

    E. Stain with uranyl acetate and lead citrate.

Richardson Staining for Semithin Sections

I Preparation of solution I and II

    A. 1 percent periodic acid (Merck Co., No. 524 in distilled water (1 g/100 ml)

    B. 1 percent azure II (Merck Co., No. 9211 in distilled water.

    C. 1 + 1 mixed = Mallory's azure II = solution I

    D. 1 percent methylene blue in 1 percent Borax = sodium borate, otherwise the staining is too pale).

    E. 1 g sodium tetraborate, (Merck Co., No 6308) dissolved in 100 ml distilled water, followed by addition of 1 g methylene blue (Merck Co., No. 1283) = solution II

II Mixture of equal volumes of solution I and II and addition of a "dash" of saccharose.

Preparation Technique of Tissue Cultures for Scanning Electron Microscopy

I Preparation of tissue cultures: Removal of medium from tissue culture. Rinse with TES buffer (twice, 4 min each). TES = (N-Tris [Hydroxymethyl] methyl-2-amino-ethane sulfonic-acid) Sigma No. T-1375

    A. Composition:

       1. 0.04 M TES buffer

       2. TES 27.5 g

       3. NaCl 47.0 g

       4. distilled water 2750 ml

       5. adjust to pH 7.35 and fill up to 3 l.

II Fixation with 3 percent glutaraldehyde in TES–buffer 15 min at 4°C. Rinse with buffer TES (three times, 10 min each at 4°C). Dehydrate with ethanol 30, 50, 70, 80, 90, and 100 percent, 5 min each time.

III Transfer into HMDS (Hexamethyldisilazane), Sigma Co., No. H–4875, 3 exchanges, 10 min each.

IV Air-dry overnight under fume hood.

V Store in a desiccator for at least 2 days. Sputtering: Mounting of specimens on a holder with silver print. After having reached the vacuum coating for 1–2 min (current 20–25 mA), coat thickness about 400 Å.

Preparation Technique of Bone for Scanning Electron Microscopy (SEM)

See also: Section TEM; Technique for SEM of Tissue Cultures

I Fix in 4 percent glutaraldehyde for 2–3 hours at 4°C.

II Rinse specimen with 0.1 M cacodylate buffer pH 7.2 three changes, 10 min each.

III Dehydrate in ethanol 30, 50, 70, 80, 90, 95, and 2 × 100 percent, 30 min each.

 IV Transfer into HMDS (hexamethyldisilazane) under fume hood 3 changes, 30 min each.
 V   Air-dry under fume hood overnight.
 VI Store in a desiccator for at least 2 days.
 VII Mount on to aluminum holders with silver print.
 VIII Sputtering.

Preparation of Calcified Bone and Bone Cement for Light Microscopy

 I   Fix in buffered formaldehyde according to Lillie, pH 7.4.
 II   Rinse in water from the tap for at least 4 hours.
 III Dehydrate with ethanol 70, 80, 90, 96, and 2 × 100 percent. 3–5 hrs. each
 IV   Infiltrate with L.R. White at room temperature 2–3 changes for 2–3 hours each or leave overnight.
 V   Polymerization: It is important to cool the molds in a bath of cold water to disperse the heat produced by the exothermic reaction. JB-4 type molds or glass containers can be used.
 a) Place the specimen into the mold.
 b) Prepare the embedding resin (one drop accelerator per 10 ml of resin, stir well). The specimens should be completely covered by the resin.
 c) Better results are obtained when oxygen is excluded by covering with polyethylene foil.
 d) Polymerization within 10–20 min.
 VI   L.R. White, hard grade, London Resin Company Ltd.

Staining Hard Materials for Light Microscopy

 I   Paragon method for thick sections
 A. Soak 6 min at 50°C in distilled water.
 B. Soak 3–10 min in Paragon at 50°C.
    Composition: 50 ml 30 percent ethanol,
    0.365 g toluidine blue O. 0.134 g basic fuchsin.
 C. Rinse 5 sec in distilled water at 22°C.
 D. Rinse 15 sec in 1 percent acetic acid ethanol at 22°C.
 E. Rinse 5 sec in 99 percent ethanol at 22°C.
 II   Modified Masson's Stain for Thick Sections
 A. Stock Solution A
    1. 1 g Ponceau de xylidine 1 g
    2. Distilled water 100 ml
 B. Stock Solution B
    1. Acid fuchsin 1 g
    2. Distilled water 100 ml
 C. Working Solution
    1. 9 ml solution A, 3 ml solution B, 120 ml, 0.2 percent acetic acid.
    2. Mix and filter before use.
 D. Aniline Blue Working Solution
    1. Dissolve 2.5 g aniline blue in 100 ml distilled water to which 2 ml glacial acetic acid has been added.
    2. This working solution may be reused many times if filtered before each use.
 III Von Kossa/Fuchsin staining
 A. Put sections in aqua dest, mop up.
 B. 5 percent silver nitrate solution 10–15 min

    1. Composition:
       a) silver nitrate (Merck Co., No. 1512) 5 g
       b) distilled water up to 100 ml
C. Rinse in distilled water three times for 5 min each.
D. Soda formol mixture 3–5 min
    1. Composition:
       a) 2.5 g Sodium carbonate (Merck Co., No 6392)
       b) 37.5 ml aqua dest
       c) 12.6 ml formaldehyde, 37 percent
E. Rinse in tap water, 10 min
F. sodium thiosulfate-pentahydrate, (Merck Co. No. 6516) 5 percent 5 min
G. Rinse in tap water. 10 min
H. Acid Fuchsin (Merck Co., No. 5231), 20–30 min
    1. Composition:
       a) 2 g acid Fuchsin
       b) 100 ml aqua dest
       c) 1 ml acetic acid
I. rinse in tap water
J. dehydrate in ethanol
K. xylene
L. mount in DePeX (Serva 18243)

Chapter 45

Special Aspects of the Permucosal Interface

John A. Jansen

THE SPECIAL CLINICAL CHALLENGE
OF THE INTEGUMENT-PENETRATING IMPLANT

A permucosal implant is defined as an object made of a synthetic material which is inserted into the alveolar bone and permanently penetrates the oral mucosa through a surgically created defect. A percutaneous implant is an object made of a synthetic material which generally is placed subcutaneously and permanently penetrates the skin. Only for certain applications, like the attachment of maxillofacial prostheses, are percutaneous implants fixed into skeletal bone.

Both permucosal and percutaneous implant systems are characterized by a permanent connection between the interior and exterior of the body. Via this connection, bacteria, debris, and antigenous material can penetrate into the tissues. Therefore, the formation and maintenance of an effective seal in the area where the implant penetrates the skin or mucosa is essential for the long-term success of such devices.

HISTOLOGICAL ANATOMY OF THE PERCUTANEOUS
AND PERMUCOSAL IMPLANT INTERFACE

A short review of the histological anatomy of natural percutaneous structures will provide a greater understanding of the tissue reaction around the integument-penetrating devices.

Teeth are the best-documented example of a naturally occurring, permanent, percutaneous passage [1]. Teeth perforate the gingiva which comprises that portion of the oral mucosa that covers the alveolar jaw bone and surrounds the neck of the teeth. It consists of connective tissue and stratified squamous epithelium. The connective tissue of the gingiva contains collagen fiber bundles, the so-called gingival fibers. These fibers perpendicularly attach to the tooth, thereby tightly fastening the gingiva to the tooth. In combination with the periodontal ligament, the connective tissue structure between the tooth root and alveolar jaw bone, they provide firmness and strength to the gingiva to withstand mechanical stresses. At the permucosal passage, the gingival epithelium invaginates for approximately 1 mm, forming the gingival sulcus. At the bottom of this sulcus, the epithelium is connected with the tooth by means of special cell structures called hemidesmosomes. In periodontal disease, the collagenous connective tissue fibers, periodontal ligament, and alveolar jaw bone are gradually broken down. This results in epithelial migration and mobility of the involved tooth, finally leading to tooth loss.

It is important to realize that percutaneous/permucosal implants, unlike natural percutaneous structures, are artificial devices. Therefore, some of the naturally occurring functional components are missing. Still, there is a similarity in soft tissue histology [2, 3, 4].

Light microscopic studies of the soft tissue surrounding successful implants show an apparently normal keratinized and non-keratinized oral sulcular and junctional epithelium against the implant post. The depth of the sulcus and the distance over which the junctional epithelium extends along the implant are the same as for natural teeth. The underlying connective tissues show a low-grade type of inflammation similar to inflammatory reactions seen in the gingival tissues around natural teeth. The very moderate character of this inflammatory reaction is supposed to limit the apical proliferation of the junctional epithelium.

Transmission electron microscopic studies reveal the existence of an epithelial attachment at the junctional epithelium-implant interface. The attachment is mediated by hemidesmosomes along the cell membrane facing the implant, and a lamina basalis, composed of a lamina lucida and a lamina densa, between the implant surface and the epithelial cell membrane. Underneath the epithelial junction, the collagen fibers in the connective tissue are predominantly oriented in a circular direction parallel to the implant surface. However, some studies showed that the surface topography of the implant can affect the orientation of the collagen fibers to a more or less perpendicular direction to the implant surface [5].

PATHOLOGICAL FINDINGS ASSOCIATED WITH PERCUTANEOUS/PERMUCOSAL IMPLANTS

Histological evaluation of the soft tissues surrounding failing skin/gingiva-penetrating implants demonstrates aspects quite different from those of successful implants. Histological examination reveals a persistent inflammation of the connective tissue, deep pockets, downward growth of epithelial cells, and no evidence of the development of an epithelial attachment to the percutaneous implant post [2, 3, 4].

Two major mechanisms, avulsion and infection, contribute to this pathological destruction of the permucosal-cutaneous seal [6]. In avulsion, mechanical stresses applied on the percutaneous device cause breakage of tissue bridges at the level of the epidermis and dermis. Depending on the severity of these stresses, this leads to the formation of microhematomata. These microhematomata induce focal inflammatory processes and consequently loss of connective tissue. Both the inflammatory response and the presence of blood around the device are a fertile soil for bacteria and can therefore lead to infection with subsequent failure of the percutaneous implant. The mechanical stresses can be divided in two groups, i.e., intrinsic and extrinsic stress factors. Retraction of the scar tissue surrounding the exit-site and surface migration of the epithelium are considered to be intrinsic stress factors. They are directly related to tissue growth and cell maturation. The extrinsic stresses acting on the percutaneous device are defined as those forces applied either to the skin or the implant by the external environment. They are directed either laterally, axially or torsionally.

In infection, the sinus tract development around the device often creates access for bacterial invasion into the cutaneous tissue. After insertion of the percutaneous device an initial superficial colonization around the exit-site occurs. Local conditions that allow bacterial invasion, such as trauma or pressure necrosis at the exit-site, can then result in infection. In addition, several other factors influence the occurrence of infection, e.g., the surgical approach used for the insertion of the percutaneous device, bacterial contamination during surgery, the state of the host defense mechanism, the quality of the postoperative care, and the personal hygiene of the recipient. The risk of infection is also influenced by the diameter of the implant at the exit-site, the duration of implantation and the presence of clotting around the implant site. When infection occurs, the subcutaneous tissue will form a thick capsule, infiltrated with inflammatory cells around the infected implant. Most of these inflammatory cells are polymorphonuclear leucocytes. The epidermal migration is inhibited and located adjacent to the tissue capsule. When infection cannot be controlled, loss of connective tissue surrounding the percutaneous implant will occur, eventually leading to extrusion of the device. Due to the decreased chances for infection, a direct bone-implant contact is considered to be the preferable situation for clinical success with permucosal implants [2, 3, 4]. However, even with proper bony fixations, such enossal implants will still fail if the gingiva-implant attachments are disturbed.

HISTO-TECHNOLOGICAL CHALLENGES OF THE PERCUTANEOUS/PERMUCOSAL EXIT SITE

Histological evaluation provides essential insights into the characteristics of implant materials which create an effective skin/gingiva seal. However, studies of the interface between skin/gingiva and actual implant are hampered by technical problems, because most percutaneous and permucosal implants are manufactured of hard solid metals and ceramics or soft polymers. The extreme difference in hardness between the implant material, the tissue, and the embedding material causes the bond between implant and tissue to be disrupted easily during the histological sectioning process, thus destroying very relevant information.

For the light microscopical sectioning of implant-containing specimens, this problem can be avoided by the use of special sectioning techniques: the "sawing-grinding" technique as developed by Donath [7], and the modified inner circular "sawing" technique as developed by van der Lubbe and Klein [8].

The equipment necessary for the sawing-grinding method (Exakt-cutting-grinding-system®, Exakt Apparatebau, Norderstedt, Germany) consists of a precision-guided, diamond-coated band saw and an automatic grinding machine. With the band saw, a first cut is made through the polymerized block. On the exposed tissue-implant surface, a microscope slide is glued. This slide is mounted again in the band saw using a vacuum slide holder. Subsequently, a planoparallel section is cut of a thickness between 50–200 μm. This section is thinned down to a thickness of 5 to 10 μm with the grinding machine. Finally, the section is stained. For the staining, the usually employed (although limited) staining procedures available for plastic embedded tissues can be used.

For the modified inner circular sawing technique, a horizontal innerlock saw microtome (Meprotech BV, Heerhugowaard, The Netherlands) is used which allows for some adjustments, i.e., freedom of movement of the saw blade, balanced rotation mechanism, and thickness of sectioning. To prepare sections, the polymerized tissue/implant block is fixed in the specimen holder and a first cut is made to expose the implant surface. After staining the exposed specimen surface with basic fuchsin, Giemsa or methylene blue, a glass coverslip is fixed on the sample surface with cyanoacrylate-based glue. After drying, the coverslip, with the attached tissue/implant, is sawed off the block using a 1:1(V/V) mixture of glycerine and water as cooling liquid and lubricant. The sections obtained have a consistent thickness between 5–10 μm. Finally, a glass slide is glued against the section.

Using these methods, it is possible to make thin sections of implant material and surrounding tissue without damaging the interface. Both methods have their merits. For example, the sawing-grinding technique results in sections of an occasionally very high quality. On the other hand, the sawing technique is less elaborate (no grinding or polishing) and allows the preparation of a series of sections from the same implant/tissue specimen. After the sectioning procedure, the obtained sections can be investigated by light microscopy.

For the preparation of transmission electron microscopical (TEM) sections, the earlier indicated sectioning difficulties can be solved by employing thin film coating techniques [9] or electrochemical dissolving methods [10]. Thin metal or ceramic films can be obtained on polymer implants by means of vacuum vapor or sputter deposition. Of such implants, ultra-thin TEM sections, containing the metal or ceramic interface with the periimplant tissues, can be prepared. Electrochemical dissolving methods are based on polymer paraffin embedding of tissue specimens, followed by removal of the metallic implant by electrochemical dissolution in low concentrations of perchloric acid (3–5%). After complete removal, the specimens are reembedded and ulrathin sections for TEM are prepared.

Apart from the electrochemical technique, calciumphosphate ceramic implants within polymer blocks can be removed by decalcification in 5% nitric acid.

Despite encouraging results with these methods, it has to be emphasized that TEM preparation and evaluation is very time-consuming and complicated, with frequently disappointing technical results.

CURRENT APPROACHES

Current developments are focussed on improving the tight seal between the skin/gingiva and implant, a prerequisite for the success of penetrating implants. Four factors are considered to be important:

1   Chemical and physical properties of the implant materials.
2   Surface geometrical properties of the implant materials.
3   Mechanical stresses, generated at the percutaneous implant-skin interface by the relative movement between implant and skin.
4   Surgical procedure.

Given the influence of the physico/chemical properties, it is generally accepted that the used material has to be biocompatible. Therefore, titanium and hydroxyapatite ceramic are the preferred materials for the manufacturing of the percutaneous implant part [11, 12].

Besides these bulk properties, the chemical surface composition is an important factor. Currently, for example, silver films are applied on percutaneous catheters because of their antimicrobial activity [13].

Furthermore, the surface geometrical properties of an implant can influence the final tissue reaction. Recent studies demonstrated that microtextured implant surfaces can reduce the inflammatory response and fibrous capsule formation at the implant-tissue interface [14].

Mechanical stresses are another cause for percutaneous implant failure. To reduce these interfacial stresses, many designs have been investigated, including micro- or macroporous cuffs or flanges to anchor the implant. The purpose of this porosity was to allow ingrowth of connective tissue, resulting in a strong mechanical link with the device. However, almost all designs eventually failed due to the inability to obtain well vascularized connective tissue inside the pores of the anchor. Instead, the pores were filled with inflammatory cells. Recently, two new concepts have been proposed which may solve this problem. First, Heimke [15] suggested the use of subcutaneous anchors with a gradient in elastic properties (flexible at the edges to stiff in the center). Jansen et al. [16] described the use of flexible titanium fiber mesh for the fabrication of the soft-tissue-anchored implant component. In addition, based on experience with oral implants, they introduced a two-stage surgical procedure. During the first surgical session, the subcutaneous implant part which is not exposed to loading conditions was inserted. After a healing period of 6 weeks to 3 months, the permanent skin penetration was created, allowing subsequent loading.

In contrast to percutaneous devices, it should be noted that the occurrence of gingival interface stresses is not such a problem for the bone-anchored permucosal implants if a proper bone response is obtained [2, 3, 4]. The importance of this implant-bone anchorage can be derived from the observed difference in survival rate between implants inserted into the maxilla and into the mandible (96.7% in the mandible and 70.6% in the maxilla). A limited bone-implant contact is held responsible for this difference. Therefore, most of the research in permucosal implants is focused on improvement of the bone-healing response, e.g., by using "bioactive" implant materials, biomechanically designed implant systems and surface treatment procedures.

REFERENCES

1   Schroeder HE. *Oral Structural Biology*. Stuttgart, Germany: Thieme Verlag, 1991.
2   Schroeder A, Sutter F, Buser D, Krekeler G. *Orale Implantologie*. Stuttgart, Germany: Thieme Verlag, 1994.
3   Mish CE (Ed.). *Contemporary Implant Dentistry*. St. Louis: Mosby, 1993.
4   Block MS, Kent JN (Eds.). *Endosseous Implants for Maxillofacial Reconstruction*. Philadelphia, PA: W. B. Saunders, 1995.
5   Campbell CE, von Recum AF. Microtopography and soft tissue response. *J Invest Surg*, 2 (1989), 51–74.
6   von Recum AF, Park JB. Permanent percutaneous devices. *CRC Crit Rev Bioeng*, 5 (1981), 37–77.
7   Donath K, Brenner G. A method for the study of undecalcified bones and teeth with attached soft tissues. *J Oral Pathology*, 11 (1982), 318–326.
8   van der Lubbe HBM, Klein CPAT, de Groot K. A simple method for preparing thin histological sections of undecalcified plastic embedded bone with implants. *Stain Technology*, 63 (1988), 171–177.
9   Jansen JA, de Wijn JR, Wolters-Lutgerhorst JML, van Mullem PJ. Ultrastructural study of epithelial cell attachment to implant materials *J Dent Res*, 64 (1985), 891–896.
10 Bjursten LM, Emanuelsson L, Ericson LE, Thomsen P, Lausmaa J, Mattson L, Rolander V, Kasemo B. Method for ultrastructural studies of the intact tissue-metal interface. *Biomaterials*, 11 (1990), 596–601.
11 Bardos DJ. Titanium and titanium alloys. In *Concise Encyclopedia Medical and Dental Materials*. Oxford: Pergamon Press, 1990, 360–365.
12 Aoki H, Akao M, Shin Y, Tsuzi T, Togawa T. Sintered hydroxyapatite for a percutaneous device and its clinical application. *Medical Progress through Technology*, 12 (1987), 213–220.
13 Sioshansi P. New processes for surface treatment of catheters. *Artif Organs*, 18 (1994), 266–271.
14 von Recum AF, van Kooten TG. The influence of micro-topography on cellular response and the implications for silicone implants. *J Biomat Science-Polymer Edition*, 7 (1995), 181–198.
15 Heimke G. Percutaneous implants. *Adv Mater*, 3 (1991), 108–110.
16 Jansen JA, van der Waerden JPCM, de Groot K. Development of a new percutaneous access device for implantation in soft tissues. *J Biomed Mater Res*, 25 (1991), 1535–1545.

Chapter 46

Intra Vitam
Staining Techniques

Berton A. Rahn

A histological section represents only one moment in the entire process of biological re-actions during the incorporation of a biomaterial into calcified tissues. In order to provide a complete image of a dynamic process, intra vitam staining techniques aim at providing information on the functional status of tissues and producing a record of the biological history of these tissues. This decreases the need to capture and analyze a larger series of consecutive single moments, and thus helps to reduce the number of experimental animals and the amount of work involved.

Site, amount, and the chronology of bone formation are important factors in under-standing implant incorporation in the skeletal system. A prerequisite for the involved bi-ological processes is a functioning circulation in the environment to a biomaterial. Both aspects, mineralization and circulation, can, to some extent, be addressed by intravital staining techniques.

VISUALIZATION OF HARD TISSUE CIRCULATION

The presence or absence of vessels near biomaterials may already provide clues about the acceptance of the material in a biological environment. Thus important information can be gained by their visualization. Filling vessels with microparticles like India ink [1, 2, 3], barium sulphate [4, 5, 6], Monastral Blue [7] or Berlin blue [3, 5], or using polymerizing substances [5, 8, 9, 10, 11, 12] demonstrates the accessibility of the filled circulatory area and provides preparations that help to understand the three-dimensional relationships of the vascular tree. The functional capacity of vessels filled by the particles, however, is not addressed by these techniques. A further limitation consists in the fact that not all vessels are completely filled; thus sections without the contrast medium may even be observed in a normally supplied area. While the presence of the filling material in a vessel proves an open circulatory pathway, its absence is not necessarily indicative of a deficient circulation in a specific vessel.

Microspheres [13, 14], visualized by autoradiography of attached isotopes or by a fluorescing component are transported by physiologic circulation. This method thus can be considered to be an intravital staining technique. Due to their size, the microspheres are trapped in capillaries, the vessels become blocked, and microcirculation will be altered, which is a limitation of the method.

Need and Relevance

The surgical access required for implantation always leads to a certain interference with circulation in the environment of an implant. All biological reactions occurring after implantation of a biomaterial are based on the access of nutrients, which in turn depends on an intact circulation. Information on the circulatory status of the peri-implant tissues, on the amount of interference with blood supply, and on the recovery of the damaged area could thus facilitate the interpretation of a histological observation. Techniques revealing the actual perfusion conditions are required. These techniques could become especially helpful in the case of compact bone, where complete functional re-attachment to the circulatory network may require up to several months, since new vessels only get access in connection with relatively slow intracortical remodelling processes.

Factors Affecting Test and Evaluation Methods

To provide information on the functional status of local circulation, the interference of the techniques with afferent or efferent circulatory pathways has to be minimized. This requirement is best met by the use of water-soluble, diffusible dyes, usually administered intravenously, which mix with the blood. They are distributed by the bloodstream to the sites of intact circulation. Such dyes may diffuse beyond the capillaries, thus not only indicating the functioning of the corresponding vessels, but also indicating the status of supply to the respective areas.

Tests and Evaluation Methodologies

In vivo staining of tissue perfusion using water-soluble dyes is of practical importance and has found clinical applications (Disulphine Blue, Fluorescein) in diagnosis and planning of surgical procedures. Procion Red, a substance restricted to animal experimentation, may serve similar purposes while offering certain technical advantages.

Disulphine Blue   Disulphine Blue is the monosodium salt of anhydro-4,4'-bis (diethylamino) triphenylmethanol 2″, 4″-disulfonic acid, available as a 6.2 percent sterile solution (ICI, Imperial Chemical Industries). It has been used clinically to assess the extent of burn injuries [15] or for demarcation of bone sequestra [16] at a dosage of 0.25 to 0.5 ml per kg of body weight. For animal experimentation [16, 17], the powder (Merck No. 121444) is dissolved in distilled water, and the pH is adjusted to 7.2–7.4 by adding NaOH. The intravenous administration of 2.5 ml/kg of a 6.2 percent solution is still tolerated well. For preterminal administration, the dosage may even be increased by using a fully saturated solution (approximately 12 percent). Perfused tissues stain in a deep blue, making the substance well suited for macroscopic observations. The staining remains visible for about a day, which in patients may be cosmetically disturbing. For observation and for photography in the light microscope, a diffuse illumination reduces the contrast of the surrounding tissues and allows for better visualization of the blue stain. On a microscopic level the resolution of Disulphine Blue stain routinely is limited to the size of Haversian canals. Under optimal conditions, the resolution may be extended to single osteocytes. Because the attachment of Disulphine Blue to tissues is not very stable, special processing techniques are required (see below).

Fluorescein   Fluorescein, synthesized in 1871, was administered to study eye fundus pathology in 1910 [18], disturbed circulation after frostbite injury was assessed by its intravenous injection [19], and the technique was extended to the microscopic level for bone specimens [20]. Its fluorescence is best excited with blue light. A typical filter set (Zeiss) for selective excitation includes an exciter filter BP 485, a beam splitter FT 510, and a barrier filter LP 520, eventually supplemented by an additional barrier filter KP 540.

The resolution easily reaches the level of osteocytes and their canaliculi (Fig VII / 3 / 2). Fluorescein has the advantage of being barely visible under normal light, which makes the dye suited for work in patients. It is clear that only preparations which conform to the corresponding regulations should be used. For animal work, the dye is prepared by dissolving 10 g of Fluorescein Sodium (Siegfried, Zofingen, Switzerland) in 100 ml of a phosphate buffer (30 ml of Na_2HPO_4 (11.876 g / 1000 ml) and 70 ml of KH_2PO_4 (9.078 g / 1000 ml)). Fluorescein is administered at a dosage of 100 mg / kg. Like Disulphine Blue, Fluorescein is not very stably attached to tissues; thus its proper visualization depends on similar special processing techniques.

Procion Red Procion dyes, originally developed for the staining of textiles, have widely been used to label bone apposition [21, 22, 23]. They are fixed to the nonmineral phase of the bone and remain at their site after decalcification. Procion Red (H-8BN, Zeneca Specialties, Manchester, Greta Britain) is dissolved in demineralized water (5 g / 100 ml) and administered intravenously at a dose of 100 mg / kg. The stain remains visible in living animals for several days. The attachment to tissues is stable. It resists various chemicals used during histological processing and does not leak out significantly in aqueous solutions. Since the stain only gives low contrast in white light, it requires fluorescence techniques for optimal results (Figure 46-1). Procion Red can be made visible by excitation over a relatively broad spectrum. A selective excitation is based on green light; a typical filter set

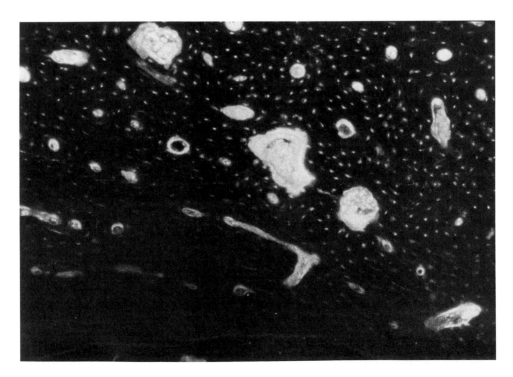

Figure 46-1 In vivo staining of bone perfusion. Haversian canals, resorption spaces, and osteocytes are stained in areas which are accessible to circulation and its related perivascular perfusion. Circulation of the inner portion of the cortex was interrupted during insertion of an intramedullary implant (bottom). In consequence the intravitally administered dye does not gain access to the tissues and cells in the zone of disturbed vascular supply. The fluorescence technique produces high contrast between stained structures and the dark background. (Intravital Procion Red staining, methacrylate embedding, 60 micrometer undecalcified saw cut, incident light fluorescence, green light excitation.)

(Zeiss, Oberkochen, Germany) includes an exciter filter BP 546, a beam splitter FT 580, and a barrier filter LP 590. Resolution spans from the macroscopic aspect to the osteocytes and their canaliculi, if adequate light microscopic fluorescence techniques and (for the highest resolution) confocal laser scanning microscopy are used.

The preparation of water-soluble dyes for injection is unproblematic. Undissolved particles are removed by filtration. In order to avoid any alterations to the dye, sterilization is performed by filtration. Injection or infusion is performed slowly, taking advantage of the dilution effect to minimize adverse reactions. After a circulation time of five minutes, the dye usually is distributed homogeneously enough in the tissues to permit a distinction between perfused and non-perfused regions. The time available for diffusion determines penetration depth into the areas deprived of functioning vessels. Diffusion starts at the beginning of the injection and continues after harvesting of the specimen. In order to reach comparable results, the duration of diffusion has to be kept reproducible. Freezing of the specimen reduces diffusion significantly, but a storage of more than a few days in a freezer gradually leads to drying artifacts which reduce the quality of the histological section.

The attachment to tissues for some of these water-soluble dyes (Disulphine Blue, Fluorescein) is not very strong, which results in significant dilution and loss of staining if processing is based on aqueous solutions. The dye can be preserved in situ by immediate freezing, and subsequent freeze-drying, of the specimen. While still under vacuum, the vessel containing the dried specimen is flooded with xylene. Xylene is replaced stepwise by methylmethacrylate or any other non-aqueous substance used for polymer embedding, using the substance-specific protocols. Saw cuts of 60 micrometers can be used for routine sectioning. Compact bone may as well be cut fresh, without any embedding, to a thickness of approximately 100 micrometers. The diamond charged saw blade is lubricated with cutting oil (VC-50 cutting oil, Leco Corporation, St. Joseph, MO). For immediate microscopy the sections are mounted in immersion oil. To obtain a more definitive mount, the sections may be soaked in cutting oil until the initially opaque sections become transparent. Then they are transferred to xylene to replace the cutting fluid, and final mounting may use any non-fluorescing routine mounting medium.

With all three dyes, gross specimens present clear differences between supplied and non-supplied bone; the border zones may show a gradual transition from stained to unstained. This represents the transport of the dye by diffusion into an area in which the vascular network is not functioning.

In white light, the contrast between the dye and its surroundings decreases the thinner the stained structure gets. Visualization by fluorescence techniques provides a better contrast, because the stained structure stands out, shining on a dark background. The intensity of fluorescence may reach such a high level in an opaque medium that fine structures become invisible. Reduction of the thickness of the section may improve the situation; optimal detail is obtained by confocal laser scanning microscopy with its narrow field of illumination. This technique permits a penetration in plastic-embedded bone to a depth of 70 micrometers and gives the possibility of three-dimensional reconstruction.

Evaluation is directed towards assessment of stained sites in relation to implants, to other tissue components, and to formative and resorptive activities in bone. Quantitative measurements of perfused and nonperfused areas may be performed, using either interactive methods or techniques based on videodigitizing and computerized image processing. Interpretation is based on observing whether or not the dye has found access to a specific tissue area. The quantification of gradual differences by densitometry is theoretically possible, but superimposure effects may be disturbing in 60-100-micrometer-thick sections.

Critical Problems and Directions for Future Evaluations / Research

Diffusion in bone follows the bone channels (Havers, Volkmann, and canaliculi). The molecular weight of the described water-soluble stains is several times higher than of, e.g., a glucose molecule. As a working hypothesis one could assume that nutrients may be able to reach a cell if the dye is reaching it. No proof for this hypothesis is available yet. Physico-chemical interactions of the dyes with tissues may additionally influence their distribution, and in vital tissues an active transport mechanism has to be postulated, since the dyes are found in osteocytes and canaliculi thirty seconds after intravenous injection, while diffusion in isolated bone specimens proceeds with a speed of a fraction of a millimeter in a few hours.

Recommendations and Conclusions

The perfect dye which fulfills all requirements is not available. A compromise has to be found, whereby the selection has to be based on the specific strengths and weaknesses of the corresponding substance.

Disulphine blue is specially suited for macroscopic investigations, less for high resolution. Fresh sections may undergo immediate photographic documentation, using normal lighting conditions. The dye is not firmly attached to tissues; therefore, special precautions have to be taken to preserve the stain during processing. Since its visualization is not based on fluorescence techniques, Disulphine Blue, in contrast to Fluorescein and Procion Red, is fully compatible with bone-labelling fluorochromes.

Fluorescein, like Disulphine Blue, is not strongly attached to the tissues; its preservation becomes difficult. The staining results in a high resolution, providing details of osteocytes and canaliculi with normal fluorescence techniques. The combination with bone fluorochromes excludes the use of Calcein and DCAF, which fluoresce in the same spectral range, so the substances would mutually camouflage each other. A nicely contrasting combination could be obtained by Xylenol Orange and Fluorescein, with the limitation, that Fluorescein requires special processing techniques.

Procion Red presents a stable attachment to tissues, thus permitting normal histological processing. In thick sections the overall intensity reaches such a high level that it overwhelms finer details. To obtain a high resolution, thin sections or the use of confocal laser scanning microscopy are required. In combining Procion Red with bone fluorochromes, the problem of mutual camouflaging arises with Alizarin and Xylenol Orange. A perfectly contrasting color combination is given by the green fluorescence of the bone-seeking fluorochrome Calcein and the diffusible dye Procion Red. A complete separation of the two colors can be obtained by using the selective filter combinations specific for each fluorochrome, and both fluorochromes can be shown together under broad band blue light excitation.

LABELLING OF HARD TISSUE FORMATION

Historically the first observations on intravital bone stainings were made at the end of the 16th century [24]; in the 18th century peroral staining by madder found experimental use [25, 26], and madder was later replaced by its main staining component, the industrially produced Alizarin red. Many of the basic investigations on bone formation and bone remodelling have been carried out by means of Alizarin vital staining [27, 28, 29]. Occasionally this substance is still used, especially since fluorescence techniques have led to a reduction of dose [30] and thus of toxicity. Porphyrins [31, 32, 33], substances fluorescing in the red to orange range, have served the same purpose, but toxic side effects have limited their wider use.

Need and Relevance

The formation of lamellar bone occurs with a speed of one to two micrometers per day; resorption takes place at a speed of approximately 60 micrometers per day. Modelling and remodeling is then a concerted action of both processes, formation and resorption. Microradiographs produced from undecalcified sections allow for a rough discrimination between old and new bone since the mineral content of newly formed bone is initially low. For the evaluation of implant materials, additional information on site, amount, chronology, speed, and direction of the mineralization process would be important for judging the success of the procedure. Dynamics of the mineralization process can be assessed by multiple labelling, whereby the accretion rate can be determined by measuring the amount of bone formed in the time interval between the multiple administrations of the dye. Preferably the labelling substance should be strongly attached to the matrix of the bone, thus guaranteeing a long-term presence in the mineralized structure. Two types of bone-labelling substances can be distinguished, those which are attached to the organic component and those linked to the mineral phase.

Factors Affecting Test and Evaluation Methods

Those intravital dyes which show an affinity to the mineral phase are substances which are able to form chelate complexes with apatite. After administration of these dyes they are distributed by circulation to every accessible site. It is possible that they temporarily influence the serum level of calcium. They are attached to available binding sites, while the non-bound excess is excreted. In calcifying tissues, accessible binding sites [34] are osteocyte lacunae, resorption sites, mineralizing sites (cartilage, bone formation, necrotic foci), and mechanically injured surfaces. Since accessible binding sites already exist at the time of administration of the dye, labelling occurs in a retrograde manner. A high concentration peak of the injected dye is maintained for several hours, resulting for practical applications in a minimal interval of approximately one day to permit discrimination between two labels in a bone which is formed at full accretion rate. Due to the affinity of these substances to bone during the mineralization process, however, it has been claimed that they themselves might influence osteogenesis and fracture healing [35, 36], but this side effect seems not to be linked to the chelating effect [37, 38, 39].

The other type of labelling substances, those which are linked to the organic component and which are characterized by their persistence after decalcification, have to be interpreted as passive indicators of the mineralization process since they seem to be walled in during osteogenesis.

Visualization of many of the dyes is based upon their fluorescence. On the dark background at a lower dose a better contrast can be obtained by this technique than in white light. For routine purposes, the incident light technique has demonstrated its superiority, mainly attributable to a higher intensity.

Tests and Evaluation Methodologies for Chelate-Forming Dyes

Alizarin Complexone Alizarin Complexone [40] (Fluka, Buchs, Switzerland, No. 05590) is based on Alizarin, with the addition of an iminodiacetic acid group. Its fluorescence appears in a deep red, although histological processing may alter it towards orange. The dose for parenteral administration is 30 mg / kg. For preparation, 3g are dissolved in 80 ml of demineralized water, NaOH is added to a pH of 7.2–7.4, and then water is added to 100 ml. The excitation maximum is found at 550 nm, the emission maximum at 640 nm. Green light excitation produces a maximum, but Alizarin Complexone can be excited over a broad spectral range.

Calcein Calcein (Fluka, Buchs, Switzerland, No. 21030) or, alternatively DCAF [41], are both derivatives of fluorescein, containing two iminodiacetic acid groups. Their intense fluorescence requires a low dose of 5mg / kg. A solution is prepared by dissolving 0.5g in 80ml of demineralized water, adjusting pH to 7.2–7.4 by addition of NaOH, and adding water to 100 ml. The emission maximum was observed at 530 nm, the excitation maximum at 495 nm. A typical filter set (Zeiss) includes an exciter filter BP 485, a beam splitter FT 510, and a barrier filter LP 520.

Calcein Blue Calcein Blue [42] (Fluka, Buchs, Switzerland, No. 21040) is a fluorochrome originally developed for the determination of calcium, strontium, and barium, containing an iminodiacetic acid group. Its emission maximum is at 445 nm, the excitation maximum at 375 nm. It requires ultraviolet excitation exclusively, a typical filter set (Zeiss) including an exciter filter BP 365, a beam splitter FT 390, and a barrier filter LP 390. Its blue fluorescence, not very strongly contrasting to the autofluorescence of bone, fades rapidly under excitation, making it a less desirable fluorochrome (Figure 46-2).

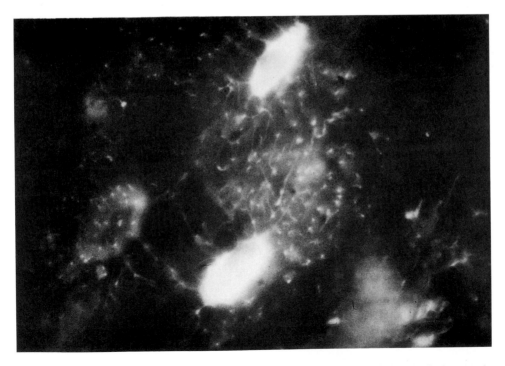

Figure 46-2 Intravital staining of osteocytes and their canaliculi. Intracortical perfusion can be traced into areas far beyond the perivascular spaces. On the dark background even the perfusion of osteocyte canaliculi, structures of one micrometer and less, can be visualized. (Intravital Fluorescein staining, methacrylate embedding of freeze-dried specimen, 60 micrometer undecalcified saw cut, incident light fluorescence, blue light excitation.)

Tetracyclines   Tetracyclines [43, 44, 45] are the only bone labels to be used legally in humans. As a dose for labelling, the highest permitted single or multiple doses, as indicated by the manufacturer for clinical purposes, will produce sufficient intensities in fluorescence (Figure 46-3). Depending on measurement conditions, an excitation maximum is found between 350 and 400 nm; the emission maximum is around 520 nm. Optimal filter sets cover a broad spectrum from ultraviolet to blue on the exciter side. Tetracyclines, because of their affinity to calcifying tissues, are used as a carrier for Technetium-99m and are used for autoradiography, for instance in the identification of necrotic cells [46].

Xylenol Orange   Xylenol Orange [47] (Fluka, Buchs, Switzerland, No. 95615) is another reactive dye containing two iminodiacetic acid groups responsible for the chelating properties. The dose for parenteral administration is 90 mg / kg, prepared by adding 9g of the substance to 80ml of demineralized water, adjusting the pH to 7.2–7.4 by adding HCl, and then adding water to 100 ml. The emission maximum is found at 610 nm and the exitation maximum at 580 nm, with a side maximum at 460 nm. Broad band blue excitation provides good results. Selective excitation is obtained by a filter set (Zeiss) including an exciter filter BP 546, a beam splitter FT 580, and a barrier filter LP 590.

Combinations   Multicolor combinations of fluorochromes [22, 34, 48, 49] facilitate the interpretation of subsequent labellings. Since an appropriate balance of intensities of the different fluorochromes is reached by adjusting the dose, the above doses could serve

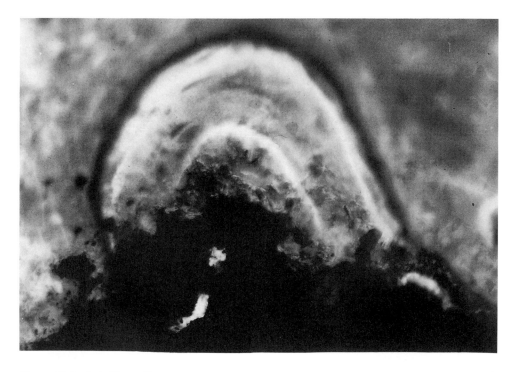

Figure 46-3   Labelling of bone deposition on a titanium surface. New bone deposition, as visualized by double tetracycline labelling, must have started directly on the surface of a titanium plasma-coated titanium surface, since the youngest structure, the dark-stained osteoid seam (Fuchsin) is found far from the implant surface. (Intravital tetracycline labelling, block staining of specimen with Basic Fuchsin, methacrylate embedding, 60 micrometer undecalcified saw cut, incident light fluorescence, blue light excitation.)

as starting points. Optimal filter sets include on the excitation side a broad range from ultraviolet to blue, and a barrier filter which transmits the entire visible spectrum. The type of filter set may have a significant influence on color balance as well. The evaluation includes qualitative as well as quantitative aspects. Distances between single labels or between labels and implants or other landmarks may be measured; areas can be determined or the sequence of different colors may indicate the direction of the mineralization process.

Tests and Evaluation Methodologies for Organic Matrix Markers

Procion dyes [21] have been used as markers in bone formation. Their binding is to the organic matrix of bone, not to the mineral phase, which makes these stains resistant to decalcification. Lead acetate is injected at a dose of 4 mg / kg, bound in mineralizing tissues, and identified after being transformed into the black lead sulfide [50]. The stain is resistant to various procedures in histological processing including decalcification and does not require facilities for undecalcified histology. Both labelling procedures seem to be based on a passive inclusion of the substance during the mineralization process.

Tests and Evaluation Methodologies for Radioactive Tracers

Radioactive tracers are not stains in the strict sense of the word, since they are not directly visible in histologic sections. They are visualized in their target structure by autoradiographic exposure of a contacting photographic emulsion. It would be beyond the scope of this chapter to deal with technical details, but since these techniques might supplement other in vivo procedures a few possibilities are mentioned.

Bisphosphonates   Polyphosphates show a high affinity to mineralizing tissues [51]. They are found in regions of intense bone turnover. Technetium-99m may be complexed to such compounds, resulting in autoradiographs of excellent resolution [52]. Their use has been described for the evaluation of ceramic implants in bone [53].

Labelled Bone Components   It seems logical to monitor the process of mineralization by tracing its main components. Calcium 45 [54] and other isotopes may be considered. The site of radioactive calcium deposition seems not to be absolutely identical with the site of simultaneously injected fluorochromes [55, 56].

Other Tracers   Strontium-85 shows a deposition behavior similar to that of calcium; Fluorine-18 [57] shows a skeletal affinity. Short-term uptake of isotopes used for bone scanning seems rather to be related to regional blood flow rather than to the rate of osteogenesis [57]. Labelled implant components may be of interest in tracing the path of degradation products of resorbable implants.

Critical Problems and Directions for Future Evaluations / Research

The influence on bone formation described for tetracyclines cannot be completely discounted. It seems, however, that it does not lead to a permanent damage, and the effect seems to be less pronounced for the other chelating agents.

Heating will destroy the labelling capacity of these substances. Sterilization therefore has to be performed exclusively by filtration. This process in addition retains eventual undissolved particles.

A fading of fluorescence under excitation can be observed, leading additionally to some color shifts. Except for Calcein Blue, fading is not a major problem, since sufficient time is provided for photomicrography and evaluation. It is advisable to take the photographs on a small magnification first to avoid burn-ins by the condensed illumination at higher magnifications.

RECOMMENDATIONS AND CONCLUSIONS

For routine applications, a tricolor labelling protocol using Calcein, Xylenol Orange, and a tetracycline is appropriate. General guidelines on when to administer the labelling substances cannot be given. The dates of labellings, labelling intervals, and eventual repetitions of the same fluorochromes have to be determined specifically with respect to the research question asked by the experimental design. Often an experienced researcher knows to expect the most prominent activities. The labelling protocol then has to address these critical times.

If labels have to be separated by selective excitation, then only the combination of the green fluorescence of Calcein with Xylenol Orange is adequate. Tetracyclines in their emission spectrum overlap strongly on both sides, green and orange, and thus cannot be completely separated from the other colors.

Continuous labelling over an extended period of time is best performed perorally, whereby the fluorochromes can be added to the drinking water. This technique is especially efficient if the total amount of mineralization has to be determined over a certain period of time. Calcein and Xylenol Orange have been tested for this purpose [58]. The combination of these two fluorochromes is especially suited for selected excitation, videodigitizing, and automated image analysis.

REFERENCES

1   Szabo K, Csanyi K. Eine modifizierte Tuscheinjektionsmethode zur Darstellung embryonaler Gefässe in der Ratte. *Mikroskopie*, 38 (1981), 319–324.
2   Mitchell J, Evans H. An Indian ink / gelatin perfusion technique for the demonstration of intracerebral blood capillaries by light and electron microscopy. *Med Lab Sci*, 35 (1978), 393–395.
3   Schöntag H, Schöttle H, Kruse HP, Langendorff H. Die Technik der Gefässdarstellung mit Gelatine unter besonderer Berücksichtigung intraossärer Arterien.*Unfallchir*, 5 (1979), 105–109.
4   Rhinelander FW, Baragry RA. Microangiography in bone healing. I. Undisplaced closed fractures. *J Bone Jt Surg*, 44A (1962), 1273–1298.
5   Crock HV. *The Blood Supply of the Lower Limb Bones in Man*. Edinburgh: Livingstone, 1967.
6   Van de Berg A, Dambe TL, Schweiberer L. Angiographische und mikroangiographische Technik an der Tibia des Hundes. *In Angiographie und ihre Fortschritte*. Stuttgart: Thieme, 1972.
7   Joris I, DeGirolami U, Wortham K, Majno G. Vascular labelling with Monastral blue B. *Stain Technol*, 57 (1982), 177–183.
8   Matsusaka T, Fujibayashi T. Ultrastructural specialization appearing on the plastic cast of ocular blood vessels. *J Clin Electron Microsc*, 7 (1974), 3–4.
9   Matsusaka T. Angioarchitecture of the choroid. *Japan J Ophthalmol*, 20 (1976), 330–346.
10 Schlüter O. Organinjektionen mit Acrylharz zur Korrosionspräparation. *Präparator*, 8 (1962), 83–90.
11 Schummer A. Ein neues Mittel (Plastoid) und Verfahren zur Herstellung korrosionsanatomische Präparate. *Anat Anz*, 81 (1935), 177–200.

12 Lenz P. Zur Technik der Gefässdarstellung im Kiefer-Gesichtsbereich mittels Plastoid. *Stoma*, 24 (1971), 210–218.

13 Tothill P. Bone blood flow measurements. *J Biomed Eng*, 6 (1984), 251–256.

14 Okubo M, Kinoshita T, Yukimura T, Abe Y, Shimazu A. Experimental study of measurement of regional blood flow in the adult mongrel dog using radioactive microspheres. *Clin Orthop*, 138 (1979), 263–270.

15 Tempest MN. A new technique in the clinical assessment of burns. *Trans Ass Industr Med Off*, 11 (1961), 22–26.

16 van Dooren J, Verdonk R, Uyttendaele D, de Groote W, Vercauteren M, Claessen, H. Disulphine blue as a diagnostic aid in the demarcation of bone sequestra. *Acta Orthop Belg*, 44 (1978), 797–808.

17 Gunst M, Suter C, Rahn B. Die Knochendurchblutung nach Plattenosteosynthese. Eine Untersuchung an der intakten Kaninchentibia mit Disulfinblau-Vitalfärbung. *Helv Chir Acta*, 46 (1979), 171–175.

18 Crismon J, Fuhrman F. Studies on gangrene following cold injury. V. The use of fluorescein as an indicator of local blood flow: Fluorescein tests in experimental frostbite. *J Clin Invest*, 26 (1947), 268–276.

19 Maumenee A. Fluorescein angiography in the diagnosis and treatment of lesions of the occular fundus. *Trans Ophthal Soc UK*, 88 (1968), 529–556.

20 Rahn B. *Die Fluorochromierung von Knochenanbau und-zirkulation*. Bern: Swiss Academy of Natural Sciences, 1984, 33–40.

21 Prescott GH, Mitchell DF, Fahmy H. Procion dyes as matrix markers in growing bone and teeth. *Am J Phys Anthrop*, 29 (1968), 219–224.

22 Solheim T. Pluricolor fluorescent labelling of mineralizing tissue. *Scand J Dent Res*, 82 (1974), 19–27.

23 Seiton E, Engel M. Reactive dyes as vital indicators of bone growth. *Am J Anat*, 123 (1969;1), 373–391.

24 Mizaldus A. Centuriae IX. Memorabilium. Frankofurti, 1599. Cited in Gottlieb, 1914 (see reference 27).

25 Belchier J. An account of the bones of animals being changed to a red color by aliment only. *Phil Trans*, 39 1(1736), 287–288. Reprinted in *Clin Orthop*, 40 (1965), 3.

26 Belchier J. A further account of the bones of animals being changed to a red color by aliment only. *Phil Trans*, 39 (1736), 299–300. Reprinted in *Clin Orthop*, 40 (1965), 4.

27 Gottlieb B. Die vitale Färbung der kalkhaltigen Gewebe. *Anat Anz*, 46 (1914), 179–194.

28 Hoyte D. Alizarin red in the study of the apposition and resorption of bone. *Am J Phys Anthropol*, 29 (1968), 157–178.

29 Baer M, Ackerman J. *A Longitudinal Vital Staining Method for the Study of Apposition in Bone*. New York: Springer, 1966, 81–92.

30 Adkins K. Alizarin red as an intravital fluorochrome in mineralizing tissues. *Stain Technol*, 40 (1965), 69–70.

31 Fikentscher R, Fink H, Emminger E. Untersuchungen an Knochen wachsender Säugetiere nach Injektion verschiedenartiger Porphyrine. *Virchows Archiv*, 287 (1933), 764–783.

32 Marique P. Aspects histologiques de la calcification dans le rachitisme experimental. Un nouveau détecteur du calcium: l'hématoporphyrine. *Rév Belg Path*, 30 (1964), 369–375.

33 Coutelier L, Dhem A, Vincent J. La microscopie de fluorescence dans l. Étude de l'ossification endochondrale. *Bull Acad Roy Med Belg*, 3 (1963), 675–689.

34 Olerud S, Lorenzi G. Triple fluorochrome labelling in bone formation and bone resorption. *J Bone Jt Surg*, 52A (1970), 274–278.

35 Gudmundson C. Oxytetracycline-induced fragility of growing bones. An experimental study in rats. *Clin Orthop*, 77 (1971), 284–289.

36 Gudmundson C. Oxytetracycline-induced disturbance of fracture healing. *J Trauma*, 11 (1971), 511–517.

37 Franklin T. The effect of chlortetracyline on the transfer of leucine and ribonucleic acid to rat-liver ribosomes in vitro. *Biochem J*, 90 (1964), 624–628.

38 Graf E, Benz G. Toxicity of streptomycin and terramycin, and influence on growth and developmental time of drosophila melanogaster. *Experientia*, 26 (1970), 1339–1341.

39 Holmes I, Wild D. The synthesis of ribonucleic acid during inhibition of escherichia coli by chlortetracycline. *Biochem J*, 97 (1965), 277–283.

40 Rahn B, Perren S. Alizarinkomplexon-Fluorochrom zur Markierung von Knochen-und Dentinanbau. *Experientia*, 28 (1972), 180.

41 Suzuki H, Mathews A. Two-color fluorescent labeling of mineralizing tissues with tetracycline and 2,4-BIS[N,N'-DI-(carbomethyl)aminomethyl] fluorescein. *Stain Technol*, 41 (1966), 57–60.

42 Rahn B, Perren S. Calcein blue as a fluorescent label in bone. *Experientia*, 26 (1970), 519.

43 Milch R, Rall D, Tobie J. Bone localization of the tetracyclines. *J Nat Cancer Inst*, 19 (1957), 87–91.

44 Frost H, Villanueva A, Roth H, Stanisavljevic S. Tetracycline bone labeling. *J New Drugs*, 1 (1961), 206–216.

45 Frost H, Villanueva A. Tetracycline staining of newly forming bone and mineralizing cartilage in vivo. *Stain Technol*, 35 (1959), 135–138.

46 Dewanjee MK. Autoradiography of live and dead mammalian cells with 99mTc-Tetracycline. *J Nucl Med*, 16 (1975), 315–317.

47 Rahn B, Perren S. Xylenol orange, a fluorochrome useful in polychrome sequential labelling of calcifying tissue. *Stain Technol*, 46 (1971), 125–129.

48 Rahn B. Polychrome fluorescence labeling of bone formation. Instrumental aspects and experimental use. *Zeiss Information*, 85 (1976), 36–39.

49 Rahn B, Perren S. Die mehrfarbige Fluoreszenzmarkierung des Knochenanbaus. *Chem Rundschau*, 25 (1975), 12–15.

50 Schneider B. Lead acetate as a vital marker for the analysis of bone growth. *Am J Phys Anthropol*, 29 (1968), 197–200.

51 Rohlin M, Hammarstroem L. Whole-body autoradiography of 99m Tc-labelled pyrophosphate and related compounds in young rats. *Acta Radiol*, 18 (1976), 319.

52 Tilden R, Jackson J, Enneking W, DeLand F, McVey J. 99mTc-polyphosphate: Histological localization in human femurs by autoradiography. *J Nucl Med*, 14 (1973), 576–578.

53 Patka P, den Hollander W, den Otter G, Heidendal G, de Groot K. Scintigraphic studies to evaluate stability of ceramics (hydroxyapatite) in bone replacement. *J Nucl Med*, 26 (1985), 263–271.

54 Lacroix P. Autoradiographies du tissu osseux spongieux. *Experientia*, 8 (1952), 426.

55 Dixon A, Hoyte D. A comparsion of autoradiographic and alizarin techniques in the study of bone growth. *Anat Rec*, 145 (1963), 101–113.

56 Hammarstroem L. Different localization of tetracycline and simultaneously injected radiocalcium in developing enamel. *Calcif Tiss Res*, 1 (1967), 229–242.

57 Genant HK, Bautovich GJ, Sing M. Bone-seeking radionuclides: An in vivo study of factors affecting skeletal uptake. *Radiology*, 113 (1974), 373–382.

58 Rahn BA, Bacellar FC, Trapp L, Perren SM. Methode zur Fluoreszenz-Morphometrie des Knochenanbaus. *Akt Traumatol*, 10 (1980), 109–115.

ADDITIONAL READING

1 Allen L, Kirkendall W, Snyder W, Frazier O. Instant positive photographs and stereograms of ocular fundus fluorescence. *Arch Ophthal*, 75 (1966), 192–198.

2 Armstrong W, Engstroem A, Paul K. Porphyrins and bone. *Scand J Clin Lab Invest*, 14 (Suppl., 1962), 7–11.

3 Brash J. Vital staining of bone with hydroxyanthraquinone derivatives. *J Anat*, 74 (1939), 141.

4 Guilbault G. *Practical Fluorescence. Theory, Methods, and Techniques*. New York: Marcel Dekker, 1973.

5 Haitinger M. *Fluorescenz-Mikroskopie. Ihre Anwendung in der Histologie Chemie*. Leipzig: Akademische Verlagsgesellschaft, 1938.

6 Hansen P. Spectral data of fluorescent tracers. *Acta Histochem*, 7 (Suppl., 1967), 167–180.

7 Lunde PK, Michelsen K. Determination of cortical blood flow in rabbit femur by radioactive microspheres. *Acta Physiol Scand*, 80 (1970), 39–44.

8 Mendes M, Pritzker K. Optimizing multiple fluorochrome bone histodynamic markers. *Bone*, 14 (1993), 537–543.

9 Modis L, Petko M, Foeldes I. Histochemical examination of supporting tissues by means of fluorescence. *Acta Morph Acad Sci Hung*, 172 (1969), 157–166.

10 Piattelli A, Trisi P, Passi P, Piattelli M, Cordioli G. Histochemical and confocal laser scanning microscopy study of the bone-titanium interface: An experimental study in rabbits. *Biomaterials*, 15:3 (1994), 194–200.

11 Silvermann DG, Myers B. *Surgical Uses of Fluorescein*. New York: Praeger Scientific, 1985.

12 Schoutens A, Bergmann P, Verhas M. Bone blood flow measured by 85Sr microspheres and bone seeker clearances in the rat. *Am J Physiol*, 236 (1979), H1–H6.

13 Smith J, Gass J, Justice J. Fluorescence fundus photography of angioid streaks. *Brit J Ophthal*, 48 (1964), 517–521.

14 Tothill P, MacPherson J. Limitations of radioactive microspheres as tracers for bone blood flow and extraction ratio studies. *Calcif Tiss Int*, 31 (1980), 261–265.

15 Trapp L. Ueber Lichtquellen und Filter für die Fluoreszenzmikroskopie und über die Auflichtfluoreszenzmethode bei Durchlichtpräparaten. *Acta Histochem*, 7 (Suppl., 1967), 328–338.

16 Udenfriend S. *Fluorescence Assay in Biology and Medicine*. New York: Academic Press, 1962.

Chapter 47

Quantitative Morphology of the Implant-Bone Interface

Ulrich M. Gross

OVERVIEW

The mathematical basis for bone sterology and morphometry was formulated in 1847 by the French geologist Delesse, who analyzed minerals. The Delesse principle [1] states that the volume fraction V_{Vi} of a component i in tissue can be estimated by measuring the area fraction A_{Ai} of a random section occupied by transsections of i:

$$V_{vi} = A_{Ai}$$

Given this fundamental relationship, the pioneers of bone morphometry elaborated on a considerable set of parameters to describe the structure of cortical and spongy bone. The derivation of the equations are given in a number of excellent overviews [1–6]. In clinical histopathology, the method of bone morphometry is widely used in the analysis of iliac crest biopsies, where the most important parameters describe bone structure, bone deposition, and bone resorption. The procedures are published extensively and are, therefore, not repeated here [7]. These methods can be applied to the quantitative evaluation of the implant-bone interface.

For an accurate assessment of an implant material inserted in bone, quantitative morphometry should be used to measure the different tissues at the interface [8]. In principle, bone, osteoid (unmineralized bone), chondroid (cartilage similar bone precursor), and soft tissue with or without bone marrow can be found at an implant interface. The quality of an implant material that is inserted in bone can be defined by its ability to bond or to contact with bone. Therefore, the percentage of bone at the interface characterizes the capacity of an implant material for bone bonding or contact, and provides the most important parameters. Since some materials can inhibit bone development or mineralization [9–11], not only bone but also other tissues are of interest. Their length or area at the interface should be recorded. The percentage of such tissue at the interface of a material in a bony implantation bed represents an additional and important parameter for the assessment of the material and its biological response.

Four valuable parameters of bone morphometry for the evaluation of bonding in the vicinity of implants in bone are:

1   Bone volume (V_V) occupied by mineralized bone as a fraction of the total unit volume;
2   Bone-specific surface (S_V) giving the area of the bone surface per unit volume of bone;
3   The ratio of the bone surface area to its volume;
4   The orientation of the bone trabeculae with respect to the implant.

The volume of bone adjacent to the implant ($V_V\%$), which reflects the biomechanical stability of this area, is a parameter that gives information on the dynamics of bone formation and can be measured in follow-up studies. The volume of newly deposited bone in an operative bone defect provides insight into the dynamics of bone repair. The particular volume of other tissues (osteoid, chondroid, soft tissue) in the original bone defect can supply additional information on the inhibiting or stimulating influence of the implant material, especially when surface-reactive or absorbable material is used. This consideration demonstrates, for example, the potential of surface reactive materials to deliver constituents that increase or inhibit bone differentiation and osteoid mineralization.

The volume of a given constituent (bone, osteoid, chondroid, soft tissue) can be described further by the surface density [$S_V(\text{mm}^2/\text{mm}^3)$]. Low values for this parameter signify rather dense component structures, whereas high values indicate a comparatively uneven and structured surface.

The volume for the specific surface which represents the density of the structural component can be calculated from the surface density and the respective volume, or S/V (mm^2/mm^3). This can also be calculated for the different tissue components mentioned above.

The orientation of the bone—especially of bone trabeculae—reflects the geometry of the surrounding bone and the biomechanical situation [12–16]. The orientation of bone trabeculae can be orthogonal, parallel or oblique to the implant surface, which helps interpret the principal stresses and other biomechanical values in the surroundings of an implant [17]. Bone geometry was successfully used in computer-assisted design (CAD) and in establishing finite element method (FEM) calculations for interpretation and prediction of biomechanical data [18, 19]. With the improvement of image resolution and precision in computer tomography (CT) and nuclear magnetic resonance (NMR) techniques, biomechanical predictive diagnostics for the quality of the implant bone interface will be possible [20, 21].

An implantation bed can be located in cortical bone, in trabecular bone, in the marrow cavity, or in operative defects for these three different structures. Morphometric evaluation should be separate for these different histological locations because the percentage of bone at the interface and the bone volume density, among other parameters, can provide very different results [8, 22–26].

Further subdivision of areas under morphometric investigation should be considered under special circumstances [27]. For example, in the case of a square-shaped implant in a cylindrical drill hole, geometrical incompatibility is obvious. The transverse sections through the implant and its vicinity demonstrate at least four segments in which the distance from the implant to the preexisting bone varies considerably. Since bone development starts normally at the edge of the preexisting bone, the filling of the operative defect with bone would be dissimilar to an implant shaped differently. Bone bonding begins at the implant corners and later at the center of the implant plane. Biomechanical influences are assumed to be operative in the development of bone bonding and so there can be stress concentration at the implant edges. Implant materials that inhibit or stimulate bone development can be better characterized by measuring the structures in a defined zone around the implant. In this way, more information can be collected on the physico-chemical properties of the implant material than by measuring the whole segment [11].

Methods and equipment for the morphometry of implants inserted into bone are identical with those used in ordinary bone morphometry, e.g., iliac crest biopsies. The equipment can be very simple, using point and linear intersection counting grids. However, this equipment requires a time-consuming procedure and is seldom used routinely. Semiautomatic counting with a computer is much easier and saves time as shown in a study where electron microscopic subcellular organelles in the bone-implant interface provided data on the host response [28].

Radiographs, autoradiographs, or stained sections of specimens which provide a picture can be scanned and digitalized, then highlighted for specific morphological features such as color or brightness, and calculated for the whole area or volume. In correcting the artifacts in a picture, it is important to have interaction with the researcher. An advantage is that the investigator must decide critically what type of structure should be measured.

The fully automatic counting sets are not recommended for morphometry of implants inserted into bone because they require very high uniformity of sectioning and staining, which is usually not achieved. Furthermore, the machine may automatically record mistakes or misinterpretations due to artifacts in the section.

Reference values of parameters for compact and trabecular bone are accessible in standard books of bone morphometry [1–6].

The interpretation of findings is difficult for experiments with implants of different chemical and structural features since there are no generally accepted normal or control values. Standards must be established through the analysis of species-, age-, and sex-related standard implants and implantation sites. The reliability of results can be defined with at least the mean values and the stand errors of the mean. Using these preliminary results, the number of experimental animals and slides to be analyzed may be determined in order to achieve reliable results. Application of more elaborate statistical methods provides an expanded basis for interpretation and improvement of future investigations. Results collected from different implant materials in similar implantation sites can be compared, and the advantages of a given implant material over another material can be assessed.

REFERENCES

1   Weibel ER, Elias H. *Quantitative Methods in Morphology*. New York: Springer-Verlag, 1967.
2   Anderson C. *Manual for the Examination of Bone*. Boca Raton, FL: CRC Press, 1982.
3   Recker RR. *Bone Histomorphometry: Techniques and Interpretation*. Boca Raton, FL: CRC Press, 1983.
4   Jowsey J. *The Bone Biopsy*. New York: Plenum Press, 1977.
5   Schenk R. Zur histologischen Verarbeitung von unentkalktem Knochen. *Acta Anat*, 60 (1975), 3–19.
6   Delling G. *Endokine Osteopathien*. Stuttgart, Germany: Fischer-Verlag, 1975.
7   Frost HM. Tetracycline-based histological analysis of bone remodeling. *Calc Tis Res*, 3 (1969), 211–237.
8   Gross U, Müller-Mai C, Fritz T, Voigt C, Knarse W, Schmitz HJ. Implant surface roughness and mode of load transmission influence periimplant bone structure. *Advances in Biomaterials*, 9 (1990), 303–308.
9   Gross UM, Strunz V. The anchoring of glass-ceramics of different solubility in the femur of the rat. *J Biomed Mater Res*, 14 (1980), 607–618.
10 Gross UM, Brandes J, Strunz V, Bab I, Sela J. The ultrastructure of the interface between a glass ceramic and bone. *J Biomed Mater Res*, 15 (1981), 291–305.
11 Gross UM. Biocompatibility, the interaction of biomaterials and host response. *J Dent Edu*, 52 (1988), 798–803.
12 Vander Sloten J, Van der Perre G. Trabecular structure compared to stress trajectories in the proximal femur and the calcaneus. *J Biomed Eng*, 11 (1989), 203–206.
13 Hert J. A new explanation of the cancellous bone architecture. *Funct Dev Morphol*, 2 (1992), 15–21.
14 Turner CH. On Wolff's law of trabecular architecture *J Biomech*, 25 (1992), 1–9.
15 Fiala P, Hert J. Principal types of functional architecture of cancellous bone in man. *Funct Dev Morphol*, 3 (1993), 91–99.
16 Goldstein SA, Goulet R, McCubbrey D. Measurement and significance of three-dimensional architecture to the mechanical integrity of trabecular bone. *Calcif-Tissue-Int*, 53 (1993; Suppl. 1), 127–133.
17 Van Rietbergen B, Huiskes R, Weinans H, Sumner DR, Turner TM, Galante-JO. ESB Research Award 1992. The mechanism of bone remodeling and resorption around press-fitted THA stems. *J Biomech*, 26 (1993), 369–382.

18   Huiskes R, Weinans H, Grootenboer HJ, Dalstra M, Fudala B, Sloof TJ. Adaptive bone-remodeling theory applied to prosthetic-design analysis. *J Biomechanics*, 20 (1987), 1135–1150.

19   Mattheck C. Engineering components grow like trees. *Mat wiss.Werkstofftech*, 21 (1990), 143–168.

20   Keaveny TM, Hayes WC. A 20-year perspective on the mechanical properties of trabecular bone. *J Biomech Eng*, 115 (1993), 534–542.

21   Gluer CC, Wu CY, Genant HK. Broadband ultrasound attenuation signals depend on trabecular orientation: an in vitro study. *Osteoporos Int*, 3 (1993), 185–191.

22   Cowin SC, Sadegh AM, Luo GM. An evolutionary Wolff's law for trabecular architecture. *J Biomech Eng*, 114 (1992), 129–136.

23   Hollister SJ, Kikuchi N, Goldstein SA. Do bone ingrowth processes produce a globally optimized structure? *J Biomech*, 26 (1993), 391–407.

24   Mihalko WM, May TC, Kay JF, Krause WR. Finite element analysis of interface geometry effects on the crestal bone surrounding a dental implant. *Implant-Dent*, 1 (1992), 212–217.

25   Hämmerle CHF, Olah AJ, Schmid J, Flückiger L, Gogolewski S, Winkler JR, Lang NP. The biological effect of natural bone mineral on bone neoformation on the rabbit skull. *Clin O Impl Res*, 1995.

26   Brunski J. The influence of force, motion, and related quantities on the response of bone implants. In Fitzgerald R, Jr. (Ed.), *Non-Cemented Total Hip Arthroplasty*. New York: Raven Press Ltd., 1988, 7–21.

27   McCabe JT, Bolender RP. Estimation of tissue mRNAs by in situ hybridization. *J Histochem Cytochem*. 41, 1777–1783

28   Sela J, Karasikov N, Amir D, Kedar Y, Schwartz Z. Ultrastructural computerized quantitative morphometry of extracellular organelles in calcifying matrices. *J Comp Ass Micros*, 2 (1990), 203–210.

ADDITIONAL READING

1   Baak JPA, Oort J. A *Manual of Morphometry in Diagnostic Pathology*. New York: Springer-Verlag, 1983.

2   Boyde A, Jones SJ, Aerssens J, Dequeker J. Mineral density quantitation of the human cortical iliac crest by backscattered electron image analysis: Variations with age, sex, and degree of osteoarthritis. *Bone*, 16 (1995), 619–627.

3   Cheung RCY, Gry C, Boyde A, Jones SJ. Effects of ethanol on bone cells in vitro resulting increased resorption. *Bone*, 16 (1995), 143–147.

Chapter 48

Microradiography

Dieter G. Eschberger
Josef Eschberger

Microradiography is a technology in which a specimen, e.g., a section of embedded material, is microscopically examined employing X-rays instead of visible light. Visualization and quantification of the radiation-produced images can be achieved by three methods: scintillation, fluorescence, and the blackening of photosensitive (silver) emulsions. Photographic reproduction is the simplest approach with a sufficient resolution and can be readily correlated with other histological data. This accounts for its preferred use in medical research. Scintillation and fluorescence are less suitable for quantification and will not further be discussed in this paper.

NEED AND RELEVANCE

Histology employing visible light microscopy broadly includes the study of cellular and tissue structure. Microradiography documents concentrations of known elements in tissue sections and can therefore be used to investigate mineral densities or visualize borders between different elements such as tissue/implant interfaces. The method can be combined with conventional histology to show mineral densities with respect to cellular bounds. For special tasks like locating a specific element [1], monochromatic X-rays can be applied. Microradiography is a good choice for the study of bone reactions to implant materials because bone proliferation adjacent to metal implant surfaces and the quality of newly formed bone can both be evaluated. Measurement of the size of the mineral-free area around foreign material provides an effective and reproducible means of quantifying tissue compatibility (Figure 48-1). If an implant (an auditory ossicle implant, for example), is designed to stimulate connective tissue formation only, then microradiography can be used to detect undesirable bone contacts.

FACTORS AFFECTING TESTS AND EVALUATION METHODS

X-Ray Generation

X-rays used in microradiography have a wavelength from 10 nm to 4 pm. They are generated in high vacuum when an electron beam hits a target, with the resulting electromagnetic waves radiating out of the vacuum tube through a window. The spectrum of the emitted rays is determined by the energy of the beam, the material of the target, and the permeability of the window. The shortest and most energetic wavelength depends on the applied accelerating voltage and is described by

$$\lambda_{\min} \text{ (nm)} \approx 1.2367/\text{kV [2]}.$$

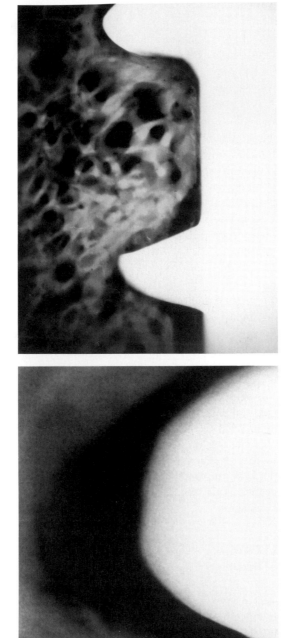

Figure 48-1 Bone-implant interfaces. In the left microradiograph (100X) a gap can be seen between the implant (light area) and the structured bone. In the right picture (10X) bone has reached the metallic surface of a screw after about six months after implantation. The newly formed bone is of high quality, suggesting good biocompatibility.

744

Beyond the continuous x-rays generated in form of "Bremsstrahlung" in the Coloumb field of the nuclei of the target, there are also characteristic x-rays emitted. These are produced by electrons scattered from their shell by the electron beam and replaced by energy-releasing electrons of a higher level. The energy difference between the orbits defines the radiation maximas that have consequently been named $K\alpha$, $K\beta$, $L\alpha$, and so forth.

The choice of the anode-material is very important for good results. A chromium anode is used for procedures requiring longer waves. A copper emits its x-rays in narrowly focused bundles of medium wavelengths and allows the emission of almost monochromatic x-rays, especially when additional metal foil-filters are introduced into the x-ray path. The tungsten anode works uniformly well over the entire wave spectrum.

The intensity of the x-ray emission can be modified by changing the current provided to the electron beam. Consequently the wavelength is adjusted with a voltage-regulator and the x-ray density with a current regulator. The product of current intensity and exposure time, expressed in milliampere-seconds (mAs), can be regulated by either component. This is important for microradiographic equipment that does not provide for regulation of the current intensity and only allows variation of the exposure time.

X-Ray Absorption

X-ray absorption depends on the spectrum and energy of the rays and the composition and thickness of the investigated object; it is generally nonlinear. Absorption using monochromatic x-rays relates to the exponential function of the negative product of specimen thickness and absorption coefficient. The latter is a function of the x-ray wavelength and the atomic number of the atoms of the specimen and is independent of their chemical bonds.

The influence of wavelength is not continuous because the absorption of very soft rays is almost exclusively produced by the photoelectric effect. Additionally, absorption maxima can be found when an x-ray quantum lifts an electron from its shell into the continuum. These atomic-number-dependent absorption (K, L, M . . .) edges are like fingerprints of the radiated elements and can be used to identify them. They can also lead to severe artifacts in quantitative microradiography.

X-Ray Equipment

Currently no optical lens systems are available for x-rays. Magnification is therefore more difficult than in conventional microscopy. Two solutions are practicable: magnification by projection and post-magnification of a photographic contact picture.

In projection microradiography, a bundle of x-rays coming from a point-sized source is passed through the specimen in a manner similar to that of a projection apparatus. The film, which is placed behind the specimen, shows an enlarged projected image. The advantage of this method is that a conventional film can be used because the subsequent magnification can be kept to a minimum. Major disadvantages are the lack of focus that increases with magnification, the very limited size of the specimen, and the long distance between x-ray source and film causing considerable absorption by air. Consequently, projection microradiography can only satisfy minimal resolution requirements and does not allow for quantitative analysis.

In contact microradiography, the specimen is close to the photosensitive film. Therefore the focal spot size has only a minimal effect on the focus of the picture. The only disadvantage is the need of very fine-grain emulsions, because of the subsequent microscopical magnification. Such emulsions have only poor sensitivity, requiring long exposure times of up to half an hour.

Any x-ray machine that allows voltage reductions down to at least 15 kV and has a sufficiently small focal spot can be used for microradiography. Specialized microradiographic equipment is also available. Currently three principal types exist.

In the first type, the specimen and the film are introduced into the x-ray tube and exposed under high vacuum. This equipment is only suitable for small specimens and operates at voltages of 3–6 kV. Its primary advantage is the ability to use very long waves because there is no air-dependent absorption. It is required for contrast documentation of elements with low atomic numbers (including sulphur), but it is not suitable for mounted bone/implant material specimens.

The second type (for example, Faxitron, Faxitron X-Ray Corporation, Buffalo Grove, IL) has voltage and current regulators and a non-changeable anode consisting of tungsten or copper. The focal distance can be varied within limits. This equipment is suitable for routine work, but it is usually too small for the investigation of larger specimens or whole implants.

Equipment of the third type is actually built for x-ray but can be easily adapted for microradiography. It has an exchangeable x-ray tube with variable anode materials and an optical bench with devices for film and specimen mounting. Its only disadvantage is the need of a darkroom, since it has no light protection device.

Adjustment of the X-Ray Equipment

The choice of the (main) x-ray wavelength is very important for good results. Due to higher absorption, pictures of better contrast are achieved by use of longer waves, but, as mentioned before, the absorption of a defined wave-length depends on the ordinal atomic number of the radiated element. To avoid problems with absorption by atmospheric air, especially when larger objects are examined requiring longer distances between the x-ray tube and the specimen, the voltage must be increased, or work must be conducted under vacuum.

In quantitative analysis, special care should be taken to avoid absorption edges. Because of the large magnifications involved, special attention must be given to focusing. The anode focal spot should be kept as small as possible; the specimen should be thin and placed close to the film. With increasing tube distance from the film, these factors have less effect and the picture generally grows sharper (Figure 48-2).

The focal spot size is predetermined by the available tube and cannot be varied, and the focus-film distance is predetermined by the size of the specimen. Consequently, the factors that can be optimized are the film-specimen, the specimen thickness, and the film emulsion thickness. We use a special device which presses a thin polyvinyl chloride film onto the specimen and underlying film by means of a vacuum, thus reducing the film-to-specimen distance to a minimum (Figure 48-2, left). Moving the vacuum plate in small circles blurs eventual density inconsistencies of the x-ray beam. Unfortunately a suitable commercial apparatus for this purpose is not available.

Choice of Film, Exposure and Development

The film material chosen for microradiography should give sufficient structural resolution to allow magnifications of at least up to 100 times. The film should be as thin as possible. We use high-resolution 1A Kodak (Eastman Kodak Company, Rochester, NY) film that meets

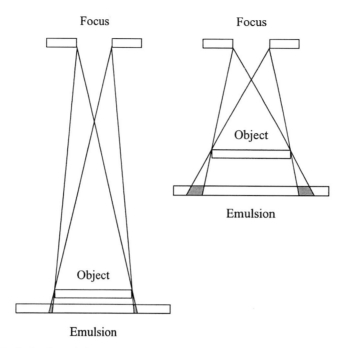

Figure 48-2 Optimization of the microradiographic unit. The hatched areas correspond to the geometric, unfocussed area. The left set-up has minimal distance between the specimen and the emulsion, and the picture is sharply defined. In the right drawing, the specimen (object) is placed some distance from the emulsion, thus producing a magnified but poorly defined picture. The smaller focal distance contributes considerably to the problem.

all of these requirements. Kodak spectroscopic plates can also be used, but in our experience they do not give the same high-quality results. Detailed information can be obtained from the manufacturer.

Exposure times must be determined empirically, since exposure meters are not available for microradiography. The radiation density of x-rays decreases with the square of the distance. Additionally, with low voltage, air absorption can become considerable, requiring the exposure time to be increased significantly. Because of the fine-grain nature of the light-sensitive emulsion which is required for the subsequent magnification, exposure times of up to half an hour are needed for microradiography with such emulsions.

The degree of film blackening during increasing exposure times follows an S-shaped curve (Figure 48-3). For quantitative analyses, the film exposure must be adjusted for utilization of the almost-linearly-ascending middle part of the curve (between A and B). Though the pictures obtained in the curved and flat parts of the function are not suitable for quantitation, they show beautiful contrasts and are therefore often used in publications (Figure 48-4).

The correct range of film blackening can be tested by irradiating an aluminium step-wedge with 10–15 steps using various wavelengths and exposure-times. The settings are correct if the aluminium equivalents of the specimen are in the middle range of the curve. The appropriate focal distance can be found by irradiating a fluorescent foil to show the diameter of the x-ray bundle. It should be large enough to avoid focusing problems.

The film developer's prescribed development times and the film manufacturer's suggested temperatures are suitable for almost all purposes. However, to achieve optimal results, an individual calibration of the whole film-process is necessary: To calibrate the process,

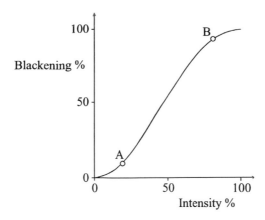

Figure 48-3 Blackening function (schematic). The blackening of an emulsion increases with intensity of radiation or duration of exposure. The correlationship is nearly linear only between the two points marked A and B. Left to A and right to B the curve has a form that leads to a "contrast distortion," causing unpredictable results in quantification. Longer wavelengths utilize a greater range on the curve, which of course is desirable, until either A or B or both are exceeded and the film is "overcharged."

unexposed film sections are developed in a series of increasing time periods. The optimal development time is the one just before the first grey haze can be detected. This process should be repeated with each new film material.

The developer is prepared on the day of use, and the film is developed under constant temperature. During manual development, the film should be agitated gently every 10–15 seconds. After a quick water rinse, the film is fixed and rinsed again. Automated developing equipment simplifies the process, but should also be calibrated as described above.

The dried films are mounted with a neutral mounting medium on glass slides with the emulsion side up toward the cover glass.

TEST AND EVALUATION METHODOLOGIES

Evaluation

A microradiograph is a planar representation of the mineral distribution in the specimen. Because hard tissue sectioning methodology at present does not readily allow serial sections, two-dimensional microradiographs must be used to determine all parameters, even three-dimensional ones, by two-dimensional stereology. They are evaluated in a similar manner to conventional x-rays of body regions: the lighter the area on the film, the greater the mineral content in the corresponding tissue section area.

A microradiograph of a bone of an adult person shows a characteristic distribution of grey values. The osteoid forms a fine, dark rim around a uniformly light area, which corresponds to the normally mineralized bone. Small, light zones of very high mineralized bone represent the oldest areas of the bone section, the intermediate lamellae. Low-mineralized zones of bone formation predominate in the young bone; in the older bone, the high-mineralized zones prevail. Disease or injury anywhere in the skeletal system leads to an alteration of the mineral distribution of the whole system, mostly in the medium mineralization ranges. After the healing of the insult an equilibrium is achieved, which normally differs a little from the primary mineral distribution. All changes of the mineral structure occur at the cost of the "normal" bone, which consequently decreases.

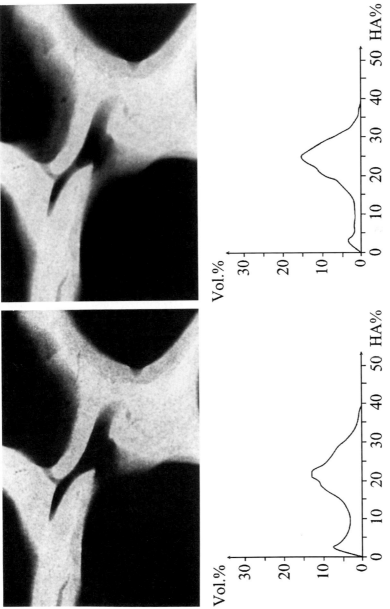

Figure 48-4 Microradiographs of spongy bone at various wavelengths. The left radiograph of a spongy bone sample using 7 kV and tungsten anode has greater contrasts, and the blackening is partly not in the linear section of the blackening function. The corresponding histogram (below) shows increased bone formation (between 0–8% HA) and bone-remodelling (10–24% HA) at the cost of normal-mineralized bone (26–32% HA). The right radiograph of the same area using 12kV has considerably less contrast. The film exposure has been adjusted to the middle part of the blackening curve. The histogram shows a quite normal mineral distribution with no signs of increased bone turnover.

Because microradiography shows only mineralized tissue, the borderline between un-mineralized osteoid and marrow is invisible, since it lies between two non-mineralized structures. This is especially important in the case of defective mineralization, in which the absorption of broad osteoid seams does not differ from the absorption of bone marrow.

Quantitative Methods

The x-ray absorption of an element at a defined wavelength is described by its absorption coefficient. The appropriate values can be found in the *International Tables for X-ray Crystallography* [3]. The absorption increases exponentially with the thickness of the element. Under identical conditions (voltage setting, anode material, exposure, focal distance), the absorption coefficients allow the comparison of different elements. That means that the concentration of a certain element can be evaluated by comparison of its x-ray absorption with that of another element with known concentration.

The element of interest in the bone is calcium; its ideal reference material is aluminum. The ratio of the absorption coefficients at a wavelength of 100 pm is 0.651; at 154 pm (copper $K\alpha$ radiation), 0.585 [3]. The calcium concentration at a certain location can be determined by measuring the absorption and comparing it with that of an aluminium step-wedge which is radiated together with the specimen. We use a three-step reference that allows sufficient interpolation. The step-wedge can be easily made of strips of aluminium foil of constant thickness. The thickness must be measured as accurately as possible since it has direct influence on the accuracy of the whole measurement. This can be achieved by using the specific weight. Some strips are cut and glued together with a low-viscosity adhesive with an offset of about 0.5 mm.

The step-wedge is positioned close to the specimen to minimize artifacts from inconsistent radiation densities and x-rayed on a high-resolution film. The exposure time must be carefully chosen to make best use of the linear part of the blackening curve. As mentioned before, a reference with 12–15 steps is needed for first tests until an appropriate setting is reached, after which three to five steps are sufficient.

The numerical equivalents of the grey values are determined with a photometer microscope. The mean value of each step of the reference represents the aluminum absorption at the known thickness of this step. The latter can be expressed as an absolute value or as volume percentage relative to a maximal thickness. By interpolation each grey value can be assigned to an aluminum concentration. The absolute amount of calcium at a certain location is calculated by multiplication with a correction factor that is defined by the ratio of the absorption quotients. The relative concentration in volume percent can be determined after measuring the thickness of the specimen at the same point with a micrometer.

Osteogramm

Based on the works of Ericsson [2] we developed a method in our laboratory that allows the quantitative analysis of the mineral distribution in a specimen in the form of an "osteogramm" [4].

First a 100-mm-thick ground section of a PMMA-embedded bone is x-rayed together with a three-step aluminum step-wedge at 12–30 kV on Kodak high-resolution SO-343 film. The distribution of grey levels is then measured using a photometer microscope (Leitz MPV2, Ernst Leitz, Wetzlar, Germany) with a computer-controlled scanning table. The mean values of the three steps and the background are used to define a third-degree function that describes the correlation between the grey-values and the mineral content. The point of highest mineral density in the bone section is searched and its hydroxyapatite content determined after measuring the thickness at that point in the original specimen with a micrometer. Then the specimen is ground to 20–30 μm to reduce the influence of three-dimensional structures, and a second microradiograph is made and scanned in the microscope. Bone marrow components are eliminated from analysis under videoscope control, leaving only the mineralized tissues. The points with the highest densities are considered to have the same maximum mineral density that has been determined in the first step. After subtraction of the background, each grey value can be correlated with a defined volume percentage of hydroxyapatite.

The mineral distribution of each point in the measured area is calculated and graphically and numerically represented as a histogram. Additional parameters including bone volume and surface are determined by two-dimensional stereometry. The final data presentation is called an "osteogramm" (Figure 48-5).

The diagram of mineral distribution in normal bone shows a typical division into five segments. The first segment correlates with bone formation, the second and third with remodelling, the fourth with normal mineralized bone, and the fifth with high-mineralized

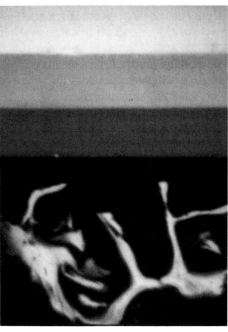

Maximum hydroxyapatite:	37.55	HA%
Average hydroxyapatite:	24.48	HA%
Bone volume:	23.80	Vol.%
Relative surfaces:	3.47	mm^2/mm^3
Specific surfaces:	15.46	mm^2/mm^3
Bone formation:	8.51	Vol.%
Bone remodelling:	33.15	Vol.%
Normal-mineralized bone:	47.40	Vol.%
High-mineralized bone:	10.94	Vol.%

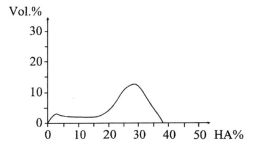

Figure 48-5   Microradiograph and osteogramm of a healthy iliac crest, condensed form. The microradiograph has been made at 12 kV and demonstrates the use of the aluminium step-wedge. The mean grey levels of the three steps are used to calculate the maximum absolute hydroxyapatite content of the densest (= brightest) area of a 100 μm bone ground section which has been placed close to the reference. This value is used for the calibration of a second microradiograph of the same specimen ground to 30 μm.
Additional structure parameters are calculated including average hydroxyapatite (average hydroxyapatite in the whole mineralized tissue), bone volume (ratio of mineralized part to total volume), relative surfaces (areas of bone/marrow interfaces relative to total volume) and specific surfaces (areas of bone/marrow interfaces relative to total mineralized volume).
Bone formation represents the amount of tissue which has a mineralization from >0–8% HA, bone remodelling >8–24% HA, normal-mineralized >24–32% HA, high-mineralized >32% HA. The values can be calculated using smaller histogram steps resulting in a curve like that shown below.

bone. Increased bone formation leads to a shift of the curve to the left with a higher first peak. Increased bone turnover can be diagnosed by an increased middle part at the cost of the normal and highly mineralized tissue. Osteoporosis shows almost no change in the curve (only in some cases a slight shift to the right) but it does show as a significant loss of bone.

CRITICAL PROBLEMS AND DIRECTIONS FOR FUTURE RESEARCH

Choice of the Specimen Thickness

The adequate preparation of the specimen in a suitable thickness is very important for reliable results. We use $100\,\mu$m ground sections for the determination of the absolute values because this reduces the influence of the thickness measurement. At this dimension an error of 1 μm is equivalent to 1% accuracy, which is acceptable; at 20 μm it would be five times as high. Increasing the thickness over the size of the bone trabecules leads also to erroneous results, so a thickness of 100 μm has proven to be a good compromise.

For stereology the thickness must be reduced as far as possible to reduce the influence of oblique surfaces that simulate areas of low mineral densities. Ideally it should be less than 10 μm which in fact is not realistic for ground sections, so a thickness of 20–30 μm is fairly suitable.

Future Improvement of the Equipment

The photometer used for measuring the grey values can of course be replaced by a video camera to speed up the scanning process. However, video cameras have a very limited grey resolution of normally only 256 steps, whereas the resolution of a photometer is nearly unlimited. Furthermore, the field illumination of a video camera is uneven, which requires the use of a correction matrix that needs adjustment for every change in light conditions. These problems do not arise with the use of a scanning microscope, because the microradiograph is moved in an exactly defined measuring system.

RECOMMENDATIONS AND CONCLUSIONS

Microradiography plays an important role in the evaluation of hard tissues. It can supply objective and quantitative data on bone mineralization, bone loss, and hydroxyapatite deposition. Information about effects at the bone/implant interface can be gained at the microscopic level. It should be preferred to methods like backscatter-imaging in SEM whenever effects beyond the surface of the specimen are of interest.

REFERENCES

1   Neumann K. Anwendung von Röntgenlicht für histochemische Untersuchungen. In Graumann W, Neumann K (Eds.), *Handbuch der Histochemie*, 1/1. Stuttgart, Germany: Gustav Fischer Verlag, 1958, 346.
2   Ericsson SC. Quantitative microradiography of cementum and abraded dentine. *Acta Radiol*, 246 (1965), 12–14.
3   Lonsdale K (Ed.). *International Tables for X-ray Crystallography*, Vol. III. Physical and Chemical Tables. Birmingham, UK: The Kynoch Press, 1962.
4   Eschberger J, Hartenstein H. Bestimmung der quantitativen Verteilung von Hydroxylapatit im Knochengewebe. *Mikroskopie*, 33 (1977), 2–10.

ADDITIONAL READING

1 Baud CA, Bang S. Microscopic and submicroscopic localisation of F in fluorotic bones. *IADR Abstracts*, 49 (1971), 72.
2 Baud CA, Lee HS. X-ray diffraction study of carbonat incorporation in vivo into bone mineral substance. *J Dent Res*, 49 (1970), 689.
3 Bergman G. Combined microradiographic and autoradiographic investigations on carious teeth. *J Dent Belge*, 50 (1959), 75–85.
4 Bergman G, Engfeldt B. Benvävnadens Biologi. Nordisk Klinisk. *Odontologi*, 1 (1960).
5 Bergman G, Lind PO. A quantitative microradiographic study of incipient enamel caries. *J Dent Res*, 45 (1966), 5.
6 Bloebaum RD, Lauritzen RS, Skedros JG, Smith EF, Thomas KA, Bennett JT, Hofmann AA. Roentgenographic procedure for selecting proximal femur allograft for use in revision. *Arthroplasty*, 8:4 (1993), 347–360.
7 Engström A. Microradiography. *Acta Radiol*, 31 (1949), 503–521.
8 Engström A. Use of soft x-rays in the essay of biological material. *Progr Biophys Chem*, 1 (1950), 164–196.
9 Engström A, Lindström B. The properties of fine grained photographic emulsions used for microradiography. *Acta Radiol*, 35 (1951), 33.
10 Engström A, Wegstedt L. Equipment for microradiography with soft roentgen rays. *Acta Radiol*, 35 (1951), 345.
11 Ericsson SC. Quantitative microradiography of cementum and abraded dentine. *Acta Radiol*, 246 (1965), 12–14.
12 Eriksen T, Koch R, Nautrup CP. Microradiography of the feline marginal periodontium with a microfocal high-resolution x-ray system. *Scand J Dent Res*, 102:5 (1994), 284–289.
13 Eschberger J. Das Osteogramm. *Acta Med Austr*, 32 (1984), 19.
14 Eschberger J, Eschberger D. Revitalisierung der Oberschenkelkopfnekrose. *Acta Med Austr*, 40 (1988), 22.
15 Eschberger J, Eschberger D: Veränderungen der Mineralverteilung im Beckenkamm menschlicher Patienten nach Knochenbrüchen. *Acta Med Austr*, 38 (1988), 24.
16 Eschberger J, Eschberger D, Haveletz H, Czitober K, Klaushofer K, Kovarik J, Plenk Jr. H, Willvonseder R. Mineraldichteverteilung im Knochengewebe bei Hyperparathyreoidismus. *Acta Med Aust*, 23 (1982), 6.
17 Eschberger J, Hartenstein H. Bestimmung der quantitativen Verteilung von Hydroxylapatit im Knochengewebe. *Mikroskopie*, 33 (1977), 2–10.
18 Fratzl P, Roschger P, Eschberger J, Abendroth B, Klaushofer K. Abnormal bone mineralization after fluoride treatment in osteoporosis: A small-angle x-ray scattering study. *J Bone Miner Res*, 9:10 (1994), 1541–1549.
19 Goby P. Micro-radiography. *Arch Roentg Rays*, 18 (1913), 247–250.
20 Grampp W, Hallen O. Microphotometry in x-ray contact microscopy. *Exper Cell Res*, 19 (1960), 83.
21 Henke BL, Lundberg B, Engström A. Conditions for optimum visual and photometric contrast in microradiograms. In Cosslett VE, Engström A, Pattee HH (Eds.), *X-ray Microscopy and Microradiography*. New York: Academic Press, Inc., 1957.
22 Jowsey J. The use of the milling machine for preparing bone sections for microradiography and microautography. *J Scient Instr*, 32 (1955), 159.
23 Jowsey J, Kelly PJ, Riggs BL, Bianco AJ, Scholz DA, Gershon-Cohen. Quantitative microradiographic studies of normal and osteoporotic bone. *J Bone and Joint Surg*, 47A (1965), 785.
24 Jönsson E. *Absorptionsmessungen im langwelligen Röntgengebiet und Gesetz der Absorption*. Dissertation, Uppsala, Sweden, 1928.
25 Lagerweij MD, de Josselin de Jong E, ten Cate JM. The video camera compared with the densitometer as a scanning device for microradiography. *Caries Res*, 28:5 (1994), 353–362.
26 Lippert K, Eschberger J, Eschberger D. Veränderungen des An- und Umbaues am gesamten Skelettsystem der Ratte nach Solitärfraktur. *Acta Med Austr*, 35 (1986), 4.
27 Neumann K. Anwendung von Röntgenlicht für histochemische Untersuchungen. In Graumann W, Neumann K (Eds.), *Handbuch der Histochemie*, 1/1. Stuttgart, Germany: Gustav Fischer Verlag, 1958, 346.
28 Newbrun E, Brudevold F, Mermagen H. A microroentgenographic investigation of demineralized enamel, comparing natural and artificial lesions. *Oral Surg*, 12 (1959), 576–584.
29 Rückert H. A quantitative x-ray microscopical study of calcium in the cementum of teeth. *Acta Odont Scand*, 25 (1958).
30 Rowland RE, Jowsey J, Marshall JH. Microscopic metabolism of calcium in bone. Microradiographic measurements of mineral density. *Radiol Res*, 10 (1959), 234.
31 Schwarz N, Schlag G, Thumher M, Eschberger J, Dinges HP, Redl H. Fresh autogeneic, frozen allogeneic, and decalcified allogeneic bone grafts in dogs. *J Bone Joint Surg* [Br], 73:5 (1991), 787–790.

32 Schwarz N, Schlag G, Thurnher M, Eschberger J, Zeng L. Decalcified and undecalcified cancellous bone block implants do not heal diaphyseal defects in dogs. *Arch Orthop Trauma Surg*, 111:1 (1991), 47–50.
33 Soni NN, Brudevold F. Microradiographic and polarized-light studies of initial carious lesions. *J Dent Res*, 38 (1959), 1187–1194.
34 van Strijp AJ, Buijs MJ, ten Cate JM. Contact microradiography of dentine under wet conditions to prevent lesion shrinkage. *J Caries Res*, 29:2 (1995), 107–110.
35 Victoreen JA. The calculation of x-ray mass absorption coefficients. *J Appl Physics*, 20 (1949), 1141.
36 Yoshino M, Imaizumi K, Miyasaka S, Seta S. Histological estimation of age at death using microradiographs of humeral compact bone. *Forensic Sci Int*, 64 (1994), 191–198.

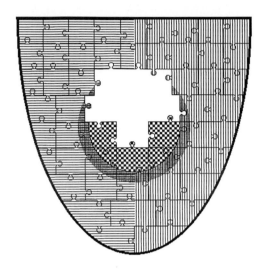

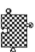

Section Nine

Regulations

William A. Morton

INTRODUCTION

The U. S. Food and Drug Administration (FDA) is the regulatory agency primarily responsible for the regulation of medical devices and the materials from which they are constructed. This regulatory authority was initially granted to the FDA under the 1976 amendments to the U. S. Food, Drug and Cosmetic Act. The medical device provisions of the Act were further modified in 1990 and 1992. Congress has periodically reviewed FDA implementation of the Act. Under the authority of the Act, the FDA has published an extensive series of regulations affecting the medical device industry from early feasibility preclinical and clinical studies to product manufacturing and marketing.

While the legislation and implementing regulations focus primarily on the finished medical devices, the research, evaluation, and manufacturing of biomaterials are regulated on the basis that such materials are components of medical devices. In recent years, FDA has issued a series of draft guidance documents related to the evaluation and testing of biomaterials. Some of these guidance documents relate to the general evaluation of materials, while others relate to specific devices. In addition, the FDA has extensive inspection and enforcement powers to assure compliance with the Medical Device Amendments. The FDA's actions can range from simply refusing to accept test data to criminal prosecution for noncompliance with regulatory requirements. Therefore, it is important that researchers have an understanding of the regulations and the importance of compliance with these regulations relating to their work.

Chapters 49–51 discuss these regulations and how they relate to the preclinical and clinical testing of biomaterials and devices as well as the manufacturing and marketing of finished devices. Chapter 52 discusses the need to protect the rights of human subjects involved in medical device research and testing and the regulatory requirements aimed at protecting those rights.

Chapter 49
Legal Aspects

Mark A. Heller
Louise N. Howe

INTRODUCTION

Under the Food, Drug, and Cosmetic Act (the Act) [1], the United States Food and Drug Administration (FDA) has authority to protect the public from unsafe or ineffective devices. That authority is comprehensive and covers devices before they reach the marketplace and thereafter. Materials in devices typically raise safety questions and may also raise device effectiveness questions. The Act, through its device investigation, classification and approval provisions, intends to provide a reasonable assurance of device safety and effectiveness for each product that is commercially distributed. Through its general controls, e.g., the Act's misbranding and adulteration provisions, device safety and effectiveness is monitored and ensured by extensive product experience reporting, facility inspections and numerous enforcement options for the FDA, ranging from criminal prosecution to product recall.

In this maze of comprehensive regulation, devices, including the materials used to make them, are subject to significant FDA oversight. The following describes the many authorities that may apply to materials that are a part of devices. Depending on the context, these authorities can apply to each person in the distribution chain of a device.

HISTORY OF FDA's AUTHORITY TO REGULATE MEDICAL DEVICES

The Federal Food, Drug, and Cosmetic Act of 1938 [2] provided the first authority to the FDA to regulate devices because of Congress' increasing concerns about fraudulent or quack devices. The statute did not provide for premarket clearance of medical devices, largely reflecting Congress' belief that such products played little role in health care. Instead, Congress prohibited shipment of adulterated or misbranded devices and authorized enforcement against such products to protect consumers primarily from economic injury. As device technology developed, and devices, e.g., heart valves, became more important to health care, the FDA realized that devices should be subject to more comprehensive regulation, including premarket review. In the 1960s, the FDA began to creatively apply its drug premarket review authority to devices, requiring drug premarket approval of products that appeared to be devices [3].

In the early 1970s, Dr. Theodore Cooper, then Undersecretary for Health of the Department of Health, Education, and Welfare, published the so-called "Cooper Report," which evaluated literature reports on devices and made recommendations of the type of legislation that was necessary to protect the public. Ultimately, Congress responded, and in 1976, the FDA received its first premarket review authority specific to devices. The Medical Device Amendments of 1976 (MDA) set forth a three-class device classification scheme, classifying devices by risk and by the controls that would be necessary to provide a reasonable assurance of safety and effectiveness. The riskiest devices were classified into class III and were intended to undergo product-by-product premarket approval before marketing. Devices for which performance standards could be established, which were too risky to be regulated under class I controls, were placed into class II. The least risky devices were placed into class I because premarket approval or complying with standards before marketing were unnecessary to assure product safety and effectiveness.

The MDA classified devices that were in commercial distribution prior to May 28, 1976, the enactment date of the amendments, through classification recommendations from expert advisory panels, and FDA notice and comment rulemaking. Devices first marketed after May 28, 1976, were classified by the FDA after receiving reports under section 510(k) of the Act at least 90 days prior to intended commercial distribution. If a device subject to such a report was "substantially equivalent" to a pre-amendment device (one in commercial distribution prior to May 28, 1976) then it would be classified and regulated the same as the "predicate" device. This meant that if a new device were substantially equivalent to a "predicate" device, it could be marketed immediately unless the predicate device were subject to a premarket approval requirement. However, if a new device were not equivalent to a predicate, it would automatically be placed in class III and would need FDA's approval before marketing.

The MDA also amended the definition of device and gave the FDA authority to promulgate regulations governing good manufacturing practices and adverse experience reporting. Although Congress' intent was to create substantial premarket entry hurdles to ensure device safety and effectiveness, in practice the FDA has reviewed the vast majority (about 98 percent) of devices through the more abbreviated 510(k) premarket notification process.

In 1990, Congress enacted the Safe Medical Devices Act (SMDA) [4], which codified the FDA's premarket review practices and added emphasis to the FDA's post-marketing regulation of medical devices. The SMDA also added documentation requirements to the 510(k) process (i.e., summaries of substantial equivalence for public disclosure or statements committing submitters to make 510(k) information available upon request), and mandated greatly increased device experience reporting to the agency. The law also required tracking and postmarket surveillance for certain types of devices; authorized the FDA to require reports of voluntary device removals and corrections after promulgating regulations; and provided the FDA with mandatory administrative recall, PMA suspension and civil penalty authority. The SMDA also added a new regulatory category, combination products, to cover products which fit under more than one of the Act's definitions of drug, device or biologic. Finally, the SMDA expanded the FDA's GMP authority to include pre-production design validation.

In 1992, Congress enacted the Medical Device Amendments which built on the SMDA and made a few refinements to that act.

OVERVIEW OF DEVICE REGULATION

The FDA's Device Jurisdiction

Definition of a Device   The Act's definition of "device" is the starting point for device regulation because it is the FDA's jurisdictional basis for regulating such products. The definition is contained in Section 201(h) of the Act, 21 USC 321(h), and states that a device is:

> an instrument, apparatus, implement, machine, contrivance, implant, in vitro reagent, or other similar or related article, including any component, part, or accessory, which is—
>
> **(1)**   recognized in the official National Formulary, or the United States Pharmacopoeia, or any supplement to them,

(2) intended for use in the diagnosis of disease or other conditions, or in the cure, mitigation, treatment, or prevention of disease, in man or other animals, or

(3) intended to affect the structure or any function of the body of man or other animals, and

which does not achieve it primary intended purposes through chemical action within or on the body of man or other animals and which is not dependent upon being metabolized for the achievement of its primary intended purposes.

The first part of the definition identifies devices as things, i.e., "instrument[s], apparatus[es]," and items that are integral to creating such things, i.e., "component[s], part[s] or accessor[ies]." The definition's first criterion, i.e., inclusion in standard compendia, has not been relied on by either the FDA or the courts as an exclusive basis for jurisdiction. The second criterion, which defines devices as things intended to diagnose diseases or conditions (such as pregnancy), or to cure, mitigate or treat diseases in man or other animals, is the most relied-upon basis to establish the FDA's device authority over a medical product. The third criterion defines devices as things intended to affect the structure or function of the body. It is difficult to imagine a product that affects a disease state or condition of the body and which achieves its primary purposes through physical action which would not act on a body structure or function. Interestingly, this criterion applies even when diseases or pathologies are not present. The last portion of the definition is intended to separate devices from drugs because their respective definitions are so similar [5]. Devices are those things that achieve their primary intended purpose through physical and not chemical and metabolic means, which are exclusive to drugs. However, a device that contains a drug will still be a device if the drug action is secondary to the device's primary physical action. Importantly, the intended use of a product is critical to determining if it is a device.

Combination Products   While the device definition was drafted to more clearly distinguish between devices and drugs, many products have components which span the device and drug definitions. For example, a dental barrier performs a device function, but when it is impregnated with an antibiotic, it performs both a device and drug function. These products are now regulated as combination products under Section 503(f) of the Act, 21 USC 353(f). Because the FDA was highly inefficient in regulating these products, often significantly delaying product jurisdiction decisions or requiring multiple reviews by different centers, Congress in the SMDA required the agency to designate a component of the FDA to take primary jurisdiction for regulation of a combination product. To ensure FDA action, the agency was required to issue regulations establishing the procedures for determining product review responsibility over a combination product within one year of the 1990 law's enactment. These regulations are contained in Part 3 of the Code of Federal Regulations [6]. The FDA also has developed intercenter agreements which reflect voluntary accommodations between the centers regarding regulation of combination products. When conflicts exist regarding product designations or the identification of the center with responsibility for a product's regulation, FDA regulations establish the agency's ombudsman as the arbiter between an applicant and the FDA.

Classification System   The classification system originally put in place by the 1976 amendments remains the principal way that the FDA determines the level of regulation for devices to ensure devices' safety and effectiveness. Devices are classified into one of three classes, I, II, or III, depending upon the degree of risk they are believed to present, and the level of regulation necessary to ensure safety and effectiveness. The three classes are subject to progressively more comprehensive requirements.

Class I contains the most innocuous devices such as tongue depressors and dental floss. These devices are subject to the "general controls" of the Act, i.e., the Act's misbranding and adulteration provisions, device registration and listing, banned device authority, consumer notification and recall, product reporting, and good manufacturing practices. Devices in all classes are subject to general controls. For class I devices, there is either enough information to conclude that the device's safety and effectiveness can be assured by general controls alone, or a device "is not purported or represented to be for a use in supporting or sustaining human life or for a use which is of substantial importance in preventing impairment of human health, and does not present a potential unreasonable risk of illness or injury" [7].

Class II devices are those which cannot be classified into class I because the general controls themselves are insufficient to provide reasonable assurance of the safety and effectiveness of the device and there is sufficient information to establish "special controls" to provide such assurance for these devices [8]. Class II devices present a broad range of risk, but enough is known about them that the general controls and "special controls," which can include performance standards (such as conformance of a biomaterial with an ASTM standard), are enough to reasonably assure safety and effectiveness. "Special controls," particularly guidelines, have no independent enforcement status under the Act. As a result, as a practical matter, general controls are also the primary means by which class II devices are regulated.

Class III devices (1) are those for which there is insufficient information to demonstrate that either the general controls or special controls will provide a reasonable assurance of safety and effectiveness and (2) are purported or represented to be for a use in supporting or sustaining human life or for a use that is of substantial importance in preventing impairment of human health or (3) present a potential unreasonable risk of illness or injury. Class III devices thus present the most risk and in addition to the general controls of the Act are subject to product-by-product premarket approval by the FDA before they can be marketed. Premarket approval is a process of rigorous scientific testing and regulatory review to reasonably assure the safety and effectiveness of a device. For class III devices subject to PMA approval requirements, a manufacturer must submit a premarket approval application to the FDA for approval before marketing. FDA regulations define the content of PMAs [9] and FDA authority to approve or deny such applications [10].

PREMARKET REGULATION

Investigation of Devices

The FDA provides an exemption from all device-related requirements of the Act in order to allow unapproved or uncleared devices to be distributed in interstate commerce so that their safety and effectiveness can be studied and ascertained [11]. The regulations governing these investigational device exemptions (IDEs) are contained in 21 C.F.R. Part 812. There are two main categories of device investigations, "significant risk" device investigations (SR) and "nonsignificant risk" device investigations (NSR). An example of a significant risk device investigation would be one involving a respiratory ventilator, whereas a nonsignificant risk device study would be one involving a denture repair kit. Significant risk device investigations are subject to a full-blown application and approval procedure through the FDA, whereas nonsignificant risk device investigations may be approved through an abbreviated clearance procedure by an institutional review board (IRB) without FDA involvement. FDA regulations only define "significant risk" devices [12]. Any investigation that is not a "significant risk" device investigation is a nonsignificant risk device investigation.

An SR investigation requires approval of an application submitted to the FDA. The application must contain a detailed investigational plan as well as manufacturing and quality control information and other detailed and general information [13]. An NSR investigation merely requires IRB approval of the study, after submission of an explanation why the device is not a significant risk device, and a commitment to compliance with labeling, reporting and other requirements [14]. Both types of investigations require various recordkeeping and reporting, as well as informed consent of subjects. Promotion and commercialization of investigational devices is prohibited [15].

An IDE would permit the shipment of an unapproved device containing a new material for clinical evaluation.

Premarket Approval

The MDA of 1976 established the FDA's premarket approval review process for all class III post-amendment and transitional medical devices (transitional devices are those which were regulated as drugs prior to the 1976 amendments) and certain class III pre-amendments devices. Any manufacturer of a class III device subject to a PMA regulation must submit a PMA and receive an approval order from the FDA for the device before marketing.

The FDA has specific and substantial content and format requirements for PMAs [16]. The PMA must contain, among other things, a description of the intended use of the device, clinical and non-clinical safety and effectiveness data and a detailed summary of the data contained in the PMA. The FDA usually requires at least one well-controlled clinical investigation to demonstrate a class III PMA device's safety and effectiveness. Once a PMA is submitted, the FDA files it for review if it meets the content requirements for PMAs. The PMA then progresses to a full substantive review. If the PMA is not filed, the applicant must submit the PMA anew, provide additional information, or challenge the FDA's decision. Once the PMA is filed, the FDA has 180 days to conduct the substantive review, but as a practical matter, this 180-day period is never met. The FDA must use expert panels to assist it in its substantive review of the PMA, unless the product review issues have already been addressed by the panel [17]. After panel review is complete, the FDA must approve or deny approval of the application. The FDA may impose conditions of approval that must be complied with after an approval. Review of FDA approvals and denials of approval of PMAs may be obtained by an applicant, although this has rarely been done [18].

Premarket Notification

Premarket notification was intended as a classification process for devices brought to market after the 1976 amendments. However, in practice it has become a product clearance process by which the FDA reviews safety and effectiveness of devices and clears them for marketing. Premarket notification, also known as "510(k)" because of the section of the Act requiring a notification before marketing, requires those who wish to market a device to notify the FDA of that intent at least 90 days prior to commercially distributing the device [19].

A principal part of the notification is a statement of what class the submitter believes is appropriate for the submitter's device and an argument that the device is "substantially equivalent" to a legally marketed device classified in the designated class (the "predicate" device). A newer device is substantially equivalent to a predicate device if it has the same intended use and technological characteristics as the predicate, or the same intended use and different technological characteristics from the predicate but information submitted in the 510(k) demonstrates that the device is as safe and effective as the predicate and does not raise different questions of safety and effectiveness than the predicate device does [20]. If technological characteristics differ because of differences in materials, the FDA will require data demonstrating the biocompatibility and effectiveness of the new device's material, unless the material is well characterized and understood and its biocompatibility is well known.

Premarket Notification (510(k)) and Premarket Approval–Materials Testing

Biomaterials issues are relevant in the context of 510(k)s and PMAs because the FDA will not clear or approve a medical device if any of its biomaterial components present unresolved safety issues. Biological evaluation is required "to determine the potential toxicity resulting from contact of the component materials of the device with the body [21].

For clearance or approval, biomaterials cannot directly, nor via their release: (1) produce adverse local or systemic effects; (2) be carcinogenic; or (3) produce adverse reproductive and developmental effects [22]. Manufacturers of products that contain materials that are not well characterized and understood must submit toxicology data (or reference such data in master files held by others, if appropriate) to the FDA showing that the benefits from the product exceed potential risks from the biomaterials' interactions with the body.

The safety of device biomaterials depends upon their chemical characteristics and the nature, degree, frequency, and duration of their exposure to the body. Because device characteristics and intended effects differ, the toxicity tests that the FDA requires vary depending upon the particular product. Therefore, the FDA suggests that manufacturers consult the agency's reviewing division for the appropriate tests and that, if necessary, reviewers consult Office of Device Evaluation toxicologists [23]. To date there are no device-specific toxicity test guidances. However, the FDA's biomaterials guidance document contains both an FDA-modified matrix that designates the type of testing needed for various categories of medical devices and a flow chart entitled "Biocompatibility Flow Chart for the Selection of Toxicity Tests for 510(k)s" (see Figure 49-1). According to the agency, this flow chart will be applicable to some, but not all, PMAs [24].

The toxicity testing that the FDA recommends is based upon standards from the ISO matrix for biological evaluation of medical devices, with some modifications. The matrix has two tables, one containing "Initial Evaluation Tests for Consideration" (see Table 50-1) and the other containing "Supplemental Evaluation Tests for Consideration" (see Table 49-1). The "Initial Evaluation Tests for Consideration" are cytotoxicity, sensitization, irritation or intracutaneous reactivity, systemic toxicity, sub-chronic toxicity, genotoxicity, implantation, and hemocompatibility. "Supplemental Tests for Consideration" include chronic toxicity, carcinogenicity, reproductive/developmental, and biodegradation.

The matrix categorizes devices based upon the biomaterials' types of body contact. The three categories are surface devices (skin, mucosal membrane, and breached or compromised surfaces), external communicating devices (blood path or indirect, tissue/bone/dentin communicating, and circulating blood), and implant devices (tissue/bone, and blood). Each category has three subcategories based on duration of body contact: limited (24 hours or less), prolonged (more than 24 hours up to 30 days) and permanent (greater than 30 days). For the other device categories, the FDA designates which tests are useful to determine toxicity. The FDA labels these tests as either "ISO Evaluation Tests for Consideration" or "Additional Tests Which May Be Applicable." For example, for surface devices affecting mucosal membranes permanently, the ISO suggests initial tests for cytotoxicity,

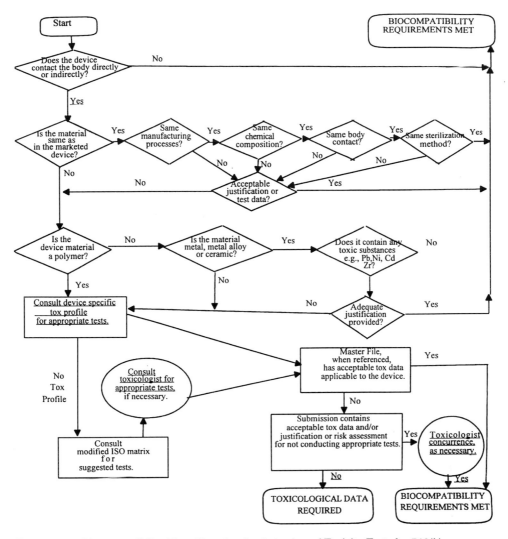

Figure 49-1 Biocompatibility Flow Chart for the Selection of Toxicity Tests for 510(k)s.

sensitization, irritation or intracutaneous reactivity, sub-chronic toxicity and genotoxicity. A supplementary test which may be applicable is chronic toxicity.

The guidance document is relevant to 510(k) clearance. Thus, if a manufacturer establishes that the biomaterial it is using is technologically the same as the predicate's, i.e., it has the same manufacturing process, chemical composition, body contact and sterilization method, it should not need to conduct toxicity tests [25]. The FDA will frequently accept certification of conformance to an ASTM or other voluntary standard as sufficient proof of the biomaterial's safety and effectiveness. If, on the other hand, the device contains a biomaterial that is either not well-characterized or not well-known and understood by the agency, the FDA will likely require toxicity tests in accordance with the guidance document's FDA-modified ISO matrix in order to establish device safety and effectiveness. FDA reviewers are advised to use their scientific judgment in requiring tests to demonstrate substantial equivalence for devices made of "materials that have been well characterized chemically and physically in the published literature and have a long history of safe use" [26].

Table 49-1   Suplementry Evaluation Tests for Consideration

Device categories		Contact duration A-Limited (= 24 h) B-prolonged (24 h to 30 days) C-permanent (>30 days)	Chronictoxicity	Carinogenicity	Reproductive/Developmental	Biodegradation
Surface devices	Skin	A				
		B				
		C				
	Mucosal Membrane	A				
		B				
		C	o			
	Breached or compromised surfaces	A				
		B				
		C	o			
External communicating devices	Blood path, indirect	A				
		B				
		C	x	x		
	Tissue/bone/dentin communicating	A				
		B				
		C	o	x		
	Circulating blood	A				
		B				
		C	x	x		
Implant Devices	Tissue/bone	A				
		B				
		C	x	x		
	Blood	A				
		B				
		C	x	x		

x = ISO Evaluation tests for consideration
0 = Additional Tests which may be applicable

Products that have 510(k) clearance may also require toxicity testing. A new 510(k) is required by the FDA if a manufacturer intends to make a major change in new intended use for a cleared product or wants to change the product in a manner that could significantly affect the device's safety and effectiveness [27]. Changes that could significantly affect a device's safety and effectiveness include a "significant change or modification in design, material, chemical composition, energy source, or manufacturing process" [28]. The FDA has circulated a draft guidance document setting forth analytical schemes to assist manufacturers in determining when such product or labeling changes require a new premarket notification [29]. Material changes are specifically addressed in the draft guidance document.

Changes in materials can trigger the requirement to file a new premarket notification. Additionally, changes in materials must be assessed to determine whether they also constitute other types of changes which may require new premarket notifications, such as major labeling or technology or performance specification changes. If a materials change also constitutes a change in performance specifications, the change must be analyzed under both the materials and performance specification logic schemes (see Figures 49-2 and 49-3). If a change in material type or formulation is made to an implant and the changed material is likely to contact body tissues and fluids, the FDA believes that a 510(k) is normally required because of the potential for new interactions of the device material on the body [30].

The interactions or effects of new materials can critically affect a device's safety or effectiveness. If, on the other hand, the material change was made to a component or part of the implant that is not likely to contact body tissues or fluids, e.g., changes in the interior material of an implantable electric stimulator, such as a single chamber cardiac pacemaker, a 510(k) is normally not required. In such a case, a new premarket notification would not be required because the new material would be sealed from ingress of body fluid or tissues. However, such a change might require a 510(k) for reasons other than the biocompatibility of the new material, such as new performance implications.

If the change in material is not to an implant but to a "limited exposure" or "prolonged exposure" device as described in ISO-10993, and the material of the affected part of the device is likely to contact body tissues or fluids, a 510(k) is usually required if the matrix states that additional testing is required. If such additional testing is not required, a 510(k) will likely not be required for this change.

If a manufacturer changes the vendor of a raw material from which the device is made, a 510(k) will not be required if the manufacturer purchases the material against a materials specification. Such a specification requires that the performance characteristics of the raw materials be related to the intended performance characteristics of the device. Ensuring conformance to such a specification may involve biomaterials testing of the new vendor's raw material. Importantly, this approach is limited to merely changing vendors but not materials.

POSTMARKET REGULATION

Misbranding and Adulteration

The Act's adulteration and misbranding provisions are general controls which provide the FDA's basis to enforce the law against substandard or potentially substandard devices. The FDA enforces these provisions to ensure safe and effective products by removing them from commercial availability either by seizing the product or enjoining its distribution.

The Act defines misbranded devices in numerous ways, including that their labeling is false or misleading in any particular [31], the labeling fails to contain adequate directions for use [32], a premarket notification requirement has not been met [33], or orders requiring reports, consumer notifications or recalls are not satisfied [34]. The Act also defines adulterated devices in various ways, including failures to have a required PMA [35], failures to manufacture devices in accordance with GMPs [36], or failures to comply with the requirements of an investigational device investigation [37].

Under Section 301 of the Act, misbranding and adulterating a device and receiving, delivering or introducing such a device into interstate commerce are prohibited acts. Section 301 is the basis for enjoining or criminally prosecuting law violators under the Act. Injunctions under Section 302 of the Act and misdemeanor and felony prosecutions under Section 303 of the Act specifically reference violations of Section 301. Product seizures under Section 304 depend upon findings that devices are misbranded or adulterated.

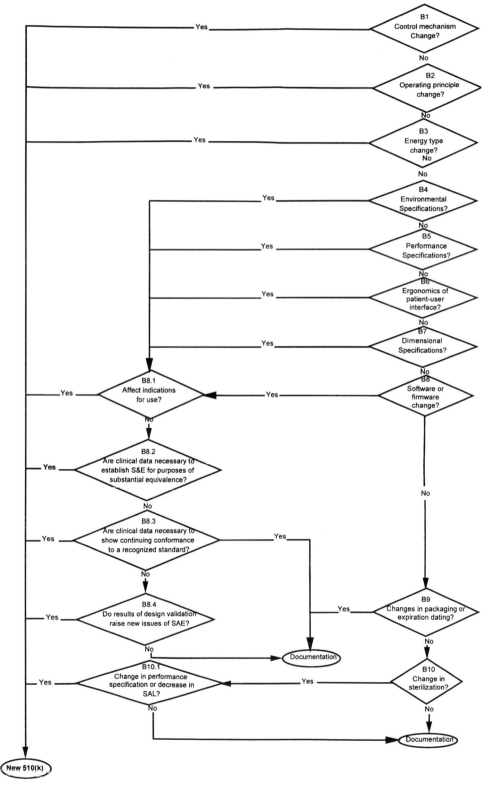

Figure 49-2 Scheme for analysis of technology or performance change.

768

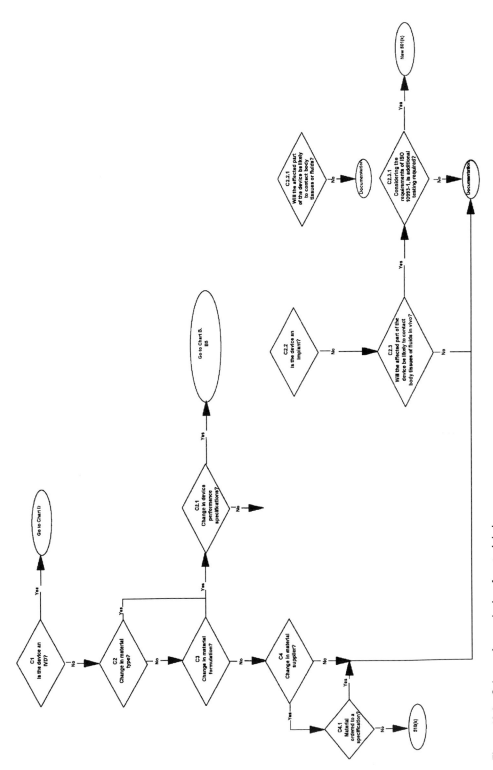

Figure 49-3 Scheme for analysis of material change.

Inspection and Enforcement Authorities

Under Section 704 of the Act, the FDA has comprehensive inspection authority. The agency may enter facilities where devices are "manufactured, processed, packed or held" [38]. FDA inspection of a facility with restricted devices may extend to "all things therein (including records, files, papers, processes, controls and facilities)" [39]. However, inspections of devices that are not restricted are narrower and the FDA is not authorized to have access to financial data, certain sales data, pricing data, and certain personnel data even if the device is restricted [40]. Although there are some limits to FDA access to records, access must be provided to all documents associated with IDEs and records required to be kept under Section 519, which includes medical device reports (MDRs).

The FDA has substantial enforcement authority over devices. The Act's enforcement provisions include both administrative and judicial remedies. The agency's enforcement remedies include administratively detaining devices [41], administrative mandatory recalls when a device would cause serious adverse health consequences or death [42], administrative mandatory notification of device users when a device presents an unreasonable risk of substantial harm to the public health [43], administrative civil penalties [44], judicial injunctions (which can shut down an entire business) [45], judicial device seizures [46], and criminal prosecutions, which can involve incarceration for individuals and substantial fines for companies and individuals [47].

In pursuing its remedies, the FDA is aided by the presumption of interstate commerce. Because interstate commerce is presumed, the FDA needs to show it when seeking an injunction, seizure or criminal prosecution involving a medical device. The presumption may be rebutted, but this is difficult because components, including materials, typically have interstate contact, which suffices for establishing interstate commerce.

PARTICULARLY IMPORTANT DEVICE COMPLIANCE REQUIREMENTS

Good Manufacturing Practices

The good manufacturing practice regulations outline for manufacturers' obligations which include manufacturing and related practices designed to ensure consistent product quality [48]. In other words, GMPs require procedures and practices that will permit manufacturers to translate a device design into a finished product in a highly predictable way. While GMPs are critical to a device PMA approval and, according to the FDA, must be in place before a device with a 510(k) may be marketed, GMP inspections mostly take place after the marketing of a product. Manufacturers of finished devices are subject to GMPs and are responsible for ensuring the appropriateness of any biomaterials that are incorporated into their devices.

If a device is otherwise safe and effective, compliance with GMPs will help ensure the device's performance by requiring that it be manufactured in a reproducible and consistent manner. However, the GMPs themselves will not make a device safe and effective. The current GMP regulation sets forth two levels of compliance—for critical and non-critical devices. The proposed GMP regulation may obviate this distinction [49]. The GMP regulation intends to create a closed loop or total systems approach. Every step in the manufacture of a device must be specified and controlled and provide feedback that is incorporated into the manufacturing process. The system extends from customer requirements to device development and production, customer use, feedback and corrective action.

A basic GMP requirement is that an organizational structure and sufficient qualified personnel exist to ensure GMP compliance, and that a quality assurance program is established [50]. The GMP regulation further contains requirements governing cleanliness and maintenance of buildings and equipment; environmental control of buildings; control of components, production and processes, including the writing, implementation and control of manufacturing specifications and processing procedures; control of packaging and labeling; control of holding, distribution and installation of devices; device evaluation; and recordkeeping, including device master records, history records and complaint files.

In 1990, the SMDA authorized the FDA to add "pre-production design validation (including a process to assess the performance of a device but not including an evaluation of the safety or effectiveness of a device)" to the GMP regulation [51]. This enabled the FDA to move one step back in the manufacturing process, to cover the original design process for devices. The requirements regarding pre-production design validation will require manufacturers to create a process to originate and evaluate a device's design by appropriate laboratory, bench and other testing to assure that the device's design is adequate for its intended use. Of course, this will include evaluation of the adequacy and appropriateness of the materials used in the device.

In March 1996, the FDA issued two guidance documents regarding design controls [52]. These are intended to be applicable to process and product development. The FDA explains that "[d]esign controls are a set of interrelated techniques and activities that apply to the design process to ensure that design process objectives are met" [53]. Design controls directly include consideration of materials to be used in a device.

Reporting

Medical device reporting is the FDA's eyes and ears in the marketplace. It is the FDA's primary means of determining the performance of marketed products. In 1990, the SMDA greatly expanded the scope of the Act's reporting authorities. The SMDA shifted the premarket approval emphasis of MDA by accepting the FDA's reliance on premarket notification reports for product clearance and by beefing up device experience reporting to the FDA to facilitate the removal of unsafe products from use.

The medical device reporting regulations require manufacturers to report to the FDA whenever they receive or otherwise become aware of information that reasonably suggests that one of their marketed devices may have caused or contributed to a death or serious injury, or has malfunctioned and the device or any other device marketed by the manufacturer would be likely to cause or contribute to a death or serious injury if the malfunction were to recur [54]. Thus, medical device reports provide FDA with a means of monitoring the performance of marketed devices.

Additionally, SMDA granted the FDA authority to require reports of adverse experiences from device user facilities, such as hospitals, nursing homes, and other health care facilities (but not doctors' offices) [55]. Congress believed user reporting was necessary because such facilities did not routinely report serious illnesses, serious injuries, or deaths to the FDA. The SMDA also requires distributors to file reports with manufacturers regarding adverse experiences [56]. Furthermore, the SMDA gave the FDA the authority to require manufacturers, importers and distributors to report health-related device corrections or removals from the market [57].

Finally, the SMDA required that manufacturers of permanent implants, life-sustaining or life-supporting devices, and other devices that potentially present a serious risk to human health to conduct mandatory postmarket surveillance and monitor the experience with such devices after distribution [58]. The FDA also has discretion to require postmarket surveillance if the agency feels it is necessary to protect the public health or provide safety or effectiveness data for the device [59].

The SMDA also provided the FDA with mandatory and discretionary tracking authority that requires device manufacturers to follow certain devices from their first distribution to the ultimate user [60].

REFERENCES

1 21 USC § 301 et seq.
2 Pub. L. No. 75-717, 52 Stat. 1040 (1938), as amended, 21 USC § 301 et seq.
3 See *United States v. An Article of Drug . . . Bacto-Unidisk*, 394 U.S. 784 (1969). In *Bacto-Unidisk*, the Supreme Court held that an antibiotic sensitivity disk used as a laboratory screening test to help determine the proper antibiotic drug to administer was a drug within the Act and thus subject to preclearance requirements, even though good arguments supported the product being classified as a device. The Court emphasized that the Act should be "given a liberal construction consistent with the Act's overriding purpose to protect the public health." 394 U.S. 784, 798.
4 Pub. L. No. 101-629, 104 Stat. 4519 (1990).
5 See § 201(g) of the Act, 21 USC § 321(g).
6 21 C.F.R. Part 3.
7 § 513(a)(1)(A)(ii) of the Act, 21 USC § 360c(a)(1)(A)(ii).
8 Originally, the safety and effectiveness of class II devices were to be assured by general controls and performance standards, but the FDA never promulgated a performance standard. As a result, Congress in 1990 replaced the performance standard concept with that of "special controls."
9 See 21 C.F.R. § 814.20.
10 See 21 C.F.R. § 814.45.
11 § 520(g) of the Act, 21 USC § 360j(g).
12 21 C.F.R. § 812.3(m).
13 See 21 C.F.R. § 812.20.
14 See 21 C.F.R. § 812.2(b).
15 See 21 C.F.R. § 812.7.
16 See 21 C.F.R. § 814.20.
17 See § 515(c)(2) of the Act, 21 U.S.C. § 360e(c)(2).
18 See § 515(d)(3) of the Act, 21 U.S.C. § 360e(d)(3).
19 § 510(k) of the Act, 21 USC § 360(k).
20 See § 513(i) of the Act, 21 U.S.C. § 360c(i).
21 FDA Bluebook Memorandum #G95, *Use of International Standard ISO-10993, Biological Evaluation of Medical Devices Part-1: Evaluation and Testing*. This FDA guidance document modifies *International Standard 10993, Biological Evaluation of Medical Devices Part 1: Evaluation and Testing*. The FDA states that it will use the ISO-10993 Standard Part 1 in lieu of the Tripartite Biocompatibility Guidance to harmonize biological response testing with the requirements of other countries. FDA Bluebook Memorandum, #G95-1, page 2.
22 *Id.* Part I of the ISO 10993 standard contains guidance for selecting which tests to use to evaluate biomaterial safety. Most of the other eleven parts of the ISO standard deal with methods to conduct the tests.
23 *Id.*
24 *Id.*
25 FDA Bluebook Memorandum, #G95-1.
26 *Id.*
27 21 C.F.R. § 807.81(a)(3).
28 21 C.F.R. § 807.81 (a)(3)(i).
29 Deciding When To Submit a 510(K) for a Change to an Existing Device, Draft #2, August 1, 1995.
30 Under GMPs, manufacturers are responsible for assessing the possibility that a change in material may affect the performance of a device.
31 § 502(a) of the Act, 21 USC § 352(a).
32 § 502(f)(1) of the Act, 21 USC § 352(f)(1).
33 § 502(o) of the Act, 21 USC § 352(o).
34 See§ 502(t), 21 U.S.C. § 352(t).
35 § 501(f)(1)(A) of the Act, 21 USC § 351(f)(1)(A) for preamendment devices after a call for PMAs,

or § 510(f)(1)(C), 21 USC § 351(f)(1)(C) for transitional devices, which were regulated as drugs prior to the Medical Device Amendments of 1976.

36 § 501(h) of the Act, 21 USC § 351(h).
37 See § 501(i), 21 U.S.C. § 351(i).
38 § 704(a) of the Act, 21 USC § 374(a).
39 § 704(a) of the Act, 21 USC § 374(a).
40 Most devices are not restricted. To date, only certain PMA devices are restricted. The FDA also contends that hearing aids (a class I device) are also restricted.
41 § 304(g) of the Act, 21 USC § 334(g).
42 § 518(e) of the Act, 21 USC § 360h(e).
43 § 518(a) of the Act, 21 USC § 360h(a).
44 § 303(g) of the Act, 21 USC § 333(g).
45 § 302 of the Act, 21 USC § 332.
46 § 304 of the Act, 21 USC § 334.
47 § 303(a) of the Act, 21 USC § 333(a).
48 See 21 C.F.R. Part 820.
49 See 58 Fed. Reg. 61952 (November 23, 1993).
50 21 CFR § 820.20 and § 820.25.
51 § 520(f)(1)(A) of the Act, 21 USC § 360j(f)(1)(A).
52 The guidance documents are: (1) *Do It By Design, An Introduction to Human Factors in Medical Devices*, U.S. Department of Health and Human Services, Public Health Service, Food and Drug Administration, Center for Devices and Radiological Health. Draft: March 1, 1996; and (2) *Design Control Guidance for Medical Device Manufacturers*, Draft: March 1, 1996.
53 *Do It By Design.*
54 § 519(a) of the Act, 21 USC § 360i(a).
55 § 519(b) of the Act, 21 USC § 360i(b).
56 § 519(a)(9) of the Act, 21 USC § 360i(b)(9).
57 § 519(f)(1) of the Act, 21 USC § 360i(f)(1).
58 See § 522(a) of the Act, 21 USC § 360l(a).
59 § 522(a) of the Act, 21 USC § 360l(a).
60 See § 519(e) of the Act, 21 USC § 360i(e).

Chapter 50

Preclinical Testing Guidelines

Arthur A. Ciarkowski
Edward Mueller

This chapter gives an overview of FDA's regulatory process for medical devices, explain the practical implications of the current regulatory system, and describe how the system specifically affects biomaterials used in the manufacture of medical devices. The regulation of biomaterials is an often confusing area for developers of new medical devices.

REGULATION OF MEDICAL DEVICES AND BIOMATERIALS

Medical Device Regulation Overview

The history of regulatory requirements in the last two centuries shows a great increase in both the numbers and the types of strictures. Table 50-1 plots a time line of important events in the regulation of medical devices.

While the Food and Drug Administration (FDA) was established in 1906, it was not until the Federal Food, Drug and Cosmetic Act (FD&C Act) of 1938 that the FDA obtained regulatory powers over medical devices. The law, however, was limited in its scope. The FDA could only take action against an individual or company if they marketed a dangerous device or made false claims. Under the expanded human drug authority conferred by the 1962 amendments to the FD&C Act, some devices were regulated as drugs.

With the continual advancement in medical technology came findings of patient injuries. These findings were published in the Cooper Report of 1970 [1] and became the basis of the Medical Devices Amendments of 1976 [2].

In the years since passage of the landmark law, Congress has twice modified the 1976 law. The most substantive action occurred in 1990 with Congressional approval of the Safe Medical Devices Act [3]. This amendment increased the requirements for FDA scrutiny of medical devices and broadened the FDA's enforcement powers including the use of civil penalties for violations of the FD&C act.

Statutes, Regulations, and Policies

Taken as a whole, current authorities afford the FDA with control over virtually all life phases of a medical device, from conception throughout its useful life. FDA device regulation, however, primarily focuses on the premarket testing, manufacture, and post-market experience of devices. In practical terms, this entails stratifying devices on the basis of risk and applying commensurate regulatory control, a process known as classification.

Based on the laws enacted by the United States Congress, the FDA has developed a device regulatory program that consists of manufacturer registration; product listing; premarket evaluation of newly emerging devices and oversight of clinical investigations that generate data necessary to support market applications; post-market requirements such

Table 50-1   Regulatory Events

Year	Regulatory event
1906	FDA Established
1938	Food, Drug & Cosmetic Act enacted into law
1966	Fair Packaging & Labeling Act
1970	Cooper Report (basis of medical device amendments)
1974	Bureau of Medical Devices & Diagnostics Product Group formed to regulate devices using drug provisions of the act
1976	**Medical Device Amendments**
1978	Good Manufacturing Practices Regulation Published
1980	Investigation Device Exemption Regulation Published
1982	Center for Devices and Radiological Health formed from the Bureau of Medical Devices and the Bureau of Radiological Health
1990	**Safe Medical Devices Act**
1992	Amendments to delay tracking requirements and to adjust reporting requirements

as product tracking and product performance studies; manufacturing controls, known as Good Manufacturing Practices (GMP) and site inspections by agency personnel to verify compliance with these requirements; and the reporting of adverse device-related incidents by manufacturers and users.

BIOMATERIAL POLICIES

Many believe that the FDA regulates all materials used in medical devices, in addition to regulating the device itself. Hence, the FDA is regularly asked, "How do I get my biomaterial approved by the FDA?" and "How do I get a list of the approved materials for use in medical devices?" The answers to these questions depend entirely on the intended application of the materials. The FDA regulates the end product (medical device), not the materials from which it is made. The FDA does not approve biomaterials. Therefore, the FDA does not maintain a list of approved biomaterials, nor does it provide guidance on how to get a biomaterial approved for general application. There are, however, cases in which a biomaterial is the end product, e.g., PMMA bone cement, block silicone, injectable collagen, etc. In these cases, the claims made for the material by the manufacturer are for specific applications and the manufacturer has provided adequate in vitro and in vivo testing to demonstrate the safety and efficacy for those applications.

The FDA does, however, provide premarket evaluation guidance for a wide variety of medical devices. While this guidance does, in some instances, address materials considerations, it is fundamentally directed at demonstrating safety and effectiveness of specific devices.

Since the FDA does not evaluate or approve device materials per se, but does approve devices in regard to their safety and effectiveness, a safe biological response to the material is obviously an important aspect of the review process.

Biocompatibility

Biocompatibility encompasses the elements of toxicology, surgical technique, implant design, motion, mechanics, porosity, surface properties, biorecognition, processing, handling, and storage conditions. The list of tests to evaluate biocompatibility is extensive and lengthy.

Table 50-2 Authorities Regulating Biomaterials

Statute	Purpose	Regulation	Applicable section
510	Good Laboratory Practices	21 CFR 58	All
510(k)	Premarket Notification	21 CFR 807	807.87(f),(g),(h)
514	Voluntary Standards	21 CFR 861	All
515	Premarket Approval	21 CFR 814	814.20
518	Recall	21 CFR 7	518(b) "state-of-the-art"
520(f)	Good Manufacturing Practices	21 CFR 820	All
520(g)	Investigational Device Exemption	21 CFR 812	812.27(a) and (b)(3)
		21 CFR 813	812.25 (d)
		21 CFR 50	
		21 CFR 56	
706	Color Additives	21 CFR 70	All
		21 CFR 71	
NEPA*	Environmental Impact	21 CFR 25	25.22(a)(18) and 25.31 Exclusions under 25.24(e)(4) or (5) and 25.23(c)

*National Environmental Policy Act of 1969 (NEPA)

The tests and procedures discussed in other chapters of this book are an excellent starting place in developing a testing plan. Some of the tests that exist are critical to evaluating the biocompatibility of a material in a particular application, while other tests yield no useful information. Therefore, it is necessary to understand the material selected and the circumstances of its use before doing an evaluation. The same material selected for different applications will require different testing plans. Fundamental principles of biological testing are provided in Table 50-3.

Biological Evaluation

Biological evaluation of medical devices is performed to determine the potential toxicity resulting from contact of the component materials of the device with the body. The device materials should not either directly or through the release of their material constituents (i) produce adverse local and systemic effects, (ii) be carcinogenic, or (iii) produce adverse reproductive and developmental effects. Therefore, evaluation of any new device intended for human use requires data from systematic testing to ensure that the benefits provided by the final product will exceed any potential risks produced by device materials.

When selecting the appropriate tests for biological evaluation of a medical device, one must consider the chemical characteristics of device materials, and the nature, degree, frequency and duration of its exposure to the body. Table 50-4 presents terminology for the duration of implant contact with tissues. In general, the tests include: acute, sub-chronic and chronic toxicity; irritation to skin, eyes and mucosal surfaces; sensitization; hemolysis; thrombogenicity; genotoxicity; carcinogenicity; and, effects on reproduction including developmental effects. However, depending on varying characteristics and intended uses of devices as well as the nature of contact, these general tests may not be sufficient to demonstrate the safety of some specialized devices. Additional tests for specific target organ toxicity, such as neurotoxicity and immunotoxicity, may be necessary for some devices. For example, a neurological device with direct contact with brain parenchyma and cerebrospinal fluid (CSF) may require an animal implant test to evaluate its effects on the brain

Table 50-3   Fundamental Principles of Biological Testing

No.	Fundamental principle	Elements
1	Selection of Device Material	Formulation, Additives, Contaminants, Impurities, and Physical, Chemical & Toxicological Properties
2	The Final Product	Materials of Manufacture, Additives, Process Contaminants, Degradation Products, Residual Chemicals, Leachable Chemicals, and Interactions
3	Selections of Tests Based on Materials and Tissue Contact	* Nature * Degree * Duration * Frequency
4	Tests must be conducted according to recognized GLPs and be evaluated by competent informed persons	
5	Data and findings should be presented in a manner that would allow independent conclusions	
6	Changes must be evaluated with respect to possible changes in toxicological effects and need for additional testing	Source, specification of materials, composition, manufacturing process, physical configuration, intended uses, and sterilization process
7	Other available information, clinical and non-clinical, should be considered for overall evaluation	

parenchyma, susceptibility to seizure, and effects on the functional mechanism of choroid plexus and arachnoid villi to secrete and absorb CSF. The specific clinical application of the new device determines which tests are more appropriate.

In 1986, the FDA, Health and Welfare Canada, and Health and Social Services UK issued the *Tripartite Biocompatibility Guidance for Medical Devices*. This Guidance has been used by FDA reviewers, as well as manufacturers of medical devices, in selecting appropriate tests to evaluate the adverse biological responses to medical devices. Since that time, the International Standards Organization (ISO), in an effort to harmonize biocompatibility testing, developed a standard for biological evaluation of medical devices (ISO 10993). The scope of this 12-part standard is to evaluate the effects of medical device materials on the body. The first part of this standard, *Biological Evaluation of Medical Devices: Part 1: Guidance on the Selection of Tests*, provides guidance for selecting the tests to evaluate the biological response to medical devices. Most of the other parts of the ISO Standard deal with appropriate methods to conduct the biological tests suggested in Part 1 of the standard.

ISO 10993, Part 1 and the FDA-Modified Matrix   The ISO Standard, Part 1 uses a guidance approach to test selection that is very similar to the currently-used Tripartite Guidance, including the same seven principles. It also uses a tabular format (matrix) for laying out the test requirements based on the various factors discussed above. To harmonize biological response testing with the requirements of other countries, the FDA will apply the ISO Standard, Part 1, in the review process in lieu of the Tripartite Biocompatibility Guidance.

Table 50-4   Duration of Contact

Duration of contact	Category
up to 24 hours	Limited Exposure
24 hours to 30 days	Prolonged
greater than 30 days	Permanent

The FDA reviewed the differences between the Tripartite Guidance and the ISO 10993-Part 1. Differences between the two documents on the definitions for duration of contact and other factors were minor and will have little impact on FDA requirements for most of the devices in the selection of tests. However, the FDA believes that the suggested tests in the matrix, based on the *type* of tissue contact, may not be adequate to evaluate certain device categories. For instance, for the category of "surface devices contacting mucosal membranes with permanent contact" (e.g., IUDs), the ISO Standard would not require acute and chronic systemic toxicity. The FDA notes that the ISO Standard acknowledges these kinds of discrepancies and states that additional tests not listed in the matrix of the standard may be required for certain categories of devices. In keeping with the inherent flexibility of the ISO Standard, the FDA modified the matrix to accommodate certain types of necessary testing.

The FDA expects that manufacturers will consider the additional tests for certain categories of devices suggested in the FDA-modified matrix. This does not mean that all the tests suggested in the modified matrix are essential and relevant for some devices. In addition, the device manufacturers are advised to consider tests to detect chemical components of device materials which may produce pyrogenic reaction. The FDA believes that if ISO 10993-1 is used by persons who are knowledgeable in its provisions and who consider additional tests suggested, it should generate adequate biological data to meet FDA requirements.

Characterization

Some devices are made of materials that are well characterized chemically and physically and have a long history of safe use. For the purposes of demonstrating the substantial equivalence of such devices, it may not be necessary to conduct all the tests suggested in the FDA guidance. FDA reviewers are advised to use their scientific judgment in determining which tests are required for the demonstration of substantial equivalence. In such situations, the manufacturer must document the use of a particular material in a legally marketed predicate device or a legally marketed device with comparable patient exposure.

Mechanical Evaluation

A mechanical failure of a device is usually serious. When the device is a life-supporting device, an evaluation of the mechanical properties of the material in its final design is critical (see Chapters 1–6). A review of some device failures underscores the need to evaluate the specific application, material selection, and device design and select appropriate tests to evaluate the safety of the material in its final configuration.

The fatigue of the strut on the Shiley 60° c/c and 70° c/c valves (Shiley, Inc., Irvine, CA) demonstrates the need to understand how the selection of a material impacts on its manufacturability. Haynes 25 was selected in these designs. While this material is excellent in some applications, the ability to weld and shape the material during manufacturing was not highly reproducible.

Some of the biological heart valves developed in the early 1970s used plastics for the stent of the valve. Some of these plastics were subject to plastic deformation. In their clinical application, the pulsatile forces acting on the stents over time deformed the stents until the heart valves became stenotic.

Microcatheters used for spinal anesthesia used radioopaque material that decreased the tensile strength of the plastic selected for the catheter. Under certain conditions, patient movement caused the disks of the spine to close on the catheter, and the catheter fractured upon extraction. The use of a radioopaque material was not warranted since the amount of material, the size of the catheter, and shielding of the bone made the x-ray visualization of the catheter impossible.

In the mid-1980s, the Duromedic heart valve (Baxter, Irvine, CA) was recalled by the manufacturer because of fractures in the pyrolytic carbon. During the examination of these failures, two lessons were learned. The first lesson was that classical fatigue testing did not apply to these glassy ceramics. To understand the reliability of these materials under the pulsatile pressures applied during clinical use, the field of fracture mechanics and testing to estimate the critical crack growth size of faults in the material were necessary. The second lesson was that the selection of grid size and boundary conditions for finite element testing is important in understanding the stress distribution. In the original analysis, the grid size was large and localized stress points were missed.

In the 1990s, the Telectronic's J-lead (Telectronics Pacing Systems, Englewood, CO) was recalled because a stiffening wire fractured and then migrated out of the sheath of the lead wire. In the original testing, the duration of the cyclical testing selected for the test was inadequate to evaluate the durability of the device under long-term use.

Sterilization, Packaging and Shelf Life

The sterilization (see Chapter 15), type of packaging, and the duration of time and environment during shipping and storage can affect the biomaterial properties. For example, polypropylene hollow fibers that are gamma sterilized quickly degrade over time. While tests of plasma flux through the fibers before and after sterilization showed no change, the fibers themselves degrade as they sit on the shelf waiting to be used.

When selecting a material for a device, information about how it will be sterilized, how it will be packaged, and how long it will remain on the shelf before use are important considerations. Once this information is ascertained, appropriate tests can be done to evaluate the performance of the device and to properly label the device for the user.

Color Additives

Devices that contain color additives may be affected by additional regulations. Section 21 CFR 70 requires a petition for listing and certification of color additives, and 21 CFR 73 lists those color additives exempt from certification. If the biomaterial contains a color additive, the FDA can be contacted regarding the requirements for listing and certification of the color additive.

Most polymers contain additives, such as mold release agents, plasticizers, and other agents, used in the usual manufacturing of devices. It is presumed that the preclinical testing of biomaterials is done with the biomaterial as it is used in the device. When additives change the characteristic of the biocompatibility of the plastic or leach into the body, additional tests may be needed to demonstrate the safety of the device. The tests must measure the maximum concentration of the additive that the device presents to the patient, determine the concentration of the additive that causes some biological effect, and show that the maximum exposure to the patient is less than the "no effect" level.

Environmental Impact

As part of the National Environmental Policy Act of 1969, the FDA must consider the environmental impact of a new device on the environment. The environmental impact assessment is listed in 21 CFR 25. This provision applies primarily to new products reviewed under the PMA provision and not to products that are determined to be substantially equivalent under Section 510(k).

Exclusions to the environmental impact are listed under Section 25.23(c) and Sections 25.24(e)(4) and (5). The exclusions apply to almost all new medical devices, but the exclusions are not automatic. Manufacturers should review these exclusions in the light of the materials and chemical byproducts in the manufacture of the device. Based on this review, the appropriate exclusion and supporting information can be submitted in a PMA application to satisfy these requirements.

Good Laboratory Practice Requirements

The Good Laboratory Practice (GLP) regulations (21 CFR 58) prescribe practices for conducting "nonclinical laboratory studies" designed to support applications for research or market permits for a number of FDA-regulated products, including medical devices for human use. Non-clinical laboratory studies include any in vitro and in vivo experiments or tests in which a test article is studied in a test system, including animals under laboratory conditions to determine the safety of the device [4, 5].

The GLP regulations apply only to a segment of preclinical studies, depending on the purpose of the study. If the development of a device could be categorized (such as basic and exploratory research, evaluation of concept, studies of safety for human use, clinical trials, process validation studies, and quality control studies), GLP regulations would only apply to the studies that have the purpose of studying safety for human use. All of the biological and mechanical evaluation testing discussed in this chapter fall into the safety category and must comply with the GLP regulations.

Tests that must comply with GLP regulations must adhere to the provisions for organization and personnel, facilities, equipment, testing facilities operation, test and control articles, protocols for and conduct of a nonclinical laboratory study, records and reports, and disqualification of testing facilities. If these test data are submitted to the FDA and do not conform to the GLP regulations, the FDA may not accept the data as valid.

Other Regulations Concerning the Use of Animals

If preclinical studies use animals, the research facility conducting the animal studies may be subject to the Animal Welfare Act and the Health Research Extension Act of 1985 in addition to the GLP requirements (see Chapter 29). Generally, those facilities that conduct animal research under a federal contract or grant must comply with the Animal Welfare Act and the Health Research Extension Act if an NIH award is received for the research. If either act applies, the research facility must identify each animal it handles and keep records on the origin and disposition of each animal. It must also follow federal standards for humane care and treatment of animals. These include housing, handling, feeding, watering, sanitation, ventilation, transportation, and protection against extremes of heat, cold, and weather. Animals must also receive proper veterinary care, and incompatible animals must be separated from each other. Some of these concerns are addressed in the guideline for the human use of animals in research prepared by the National Institutes of Health [6].

Enforcement of the Animal Welfare Act is carried out by the United States Department of Agriculture (USDA), principally through its Animal and Plant Health Inspection Service. The inspection authorities for the Animal Welfare Act and the GLP regulation are complementary. The USDA inspection is directed toward ensuring the *humane care* of animals used in research, whereas the FDA inspection is directed toward ensuring the *quality of data* obtained from safety experiments that involve animals.

PRACTICAL CONSIDERATIONS

When to Submit a New Application

At the time that this chapter is being written, there is little concrete guidance on when to submit a new application. General guidance for each type of application is discussed below, but these criteria will certainly be revised in the near future. The FDA is currently working with the Health Industry Manufacturers Association (HIMA) to establish when a 510(k) application is required when a change is made to the device. Congress is also considering changes to the medical device amendments, and the language of proposed legislation may impact the deadline by which a revised device must receive premarket evaluation by the FDA. The best advice is to contact the agency when device changes are being considered.

Premarket Notification (510(k))   When a change is made to an existing device, which requires a 510(k) application for market clearance, the criteria for when to submit a new 510(k) are stated in the 510(k) regulation in 21 CFR 807.81(a)(3). A premarket notification must be submitted when:

> The device . . . is about to be significantly changed or modified in design, components, methods of manufacture, or intended use. The following constitute significant changes or modifications that require a premarket notification:
>
> **(i)**   A change or modification in the device that could significantly affect the safety or effectiveness of the device, e.g., a significant change or modification in design, material, chemical composition, energy source, or manufacturing process.
> **(ii)**   A major change or modification in the intended use of the device.

The key phrase here is "could significantly affect the safety or effectiveness of the device." In this regard, judgment must be applied on a case-by-case basis to evaluate the circumstances of use, the intended use, and the magnitude of change made to the device. Reaching a decision is a process, not a simple "yes" or "no" decision. Even when the agency releases guidance on this matter, the guidance will only provide landmarks to make the decision process by manufacturers and by the FDA more consistent. In all cases, this process should be followed, and the facts of the case and the decision reached documented.

Premarket Application (PMA)   For devices approved through the PMA application process, the requirements for submitting a PMA supplement are contained in 21 CFR 814.

The Office of Device Evaluation has a policy guide (Blue Book Memoranda) stating that a PMA supplement must be submitted when a change to the device is being made and testing (bench, animal, or human) must be completed to assure that the device performs according to specifications. For most implanted devices a new PMA supplement must be submitted when a change or modification in the material of a device is made. For example, PMA supplements have been evaluated for an alternate material in a pacemaker, changes in the material used in a heart valve sewing ring, changes in supplier of material for a heart valve, using a different bonding material in a coronary catheter, and changes in the thickness and tensile strength of coronary catheters.

Submitting Information

Once characterization, biological, mechanical, and environmental tests are conducted, the amount of information collected can be overwhelming. The information can be equally overwhelming to the FDA staff who are assigned to review the application. How the information is organized, displayed, and interpreted affect the speed of the review process.

The Health Industry Manufacturers Association (HIMA) did a case study of information submitted for 510(k) review (the Model 510(k) Project). Those applications that featured a well-structured format, an index pointing to critical information in the application, and data clearly displayed in tables and charts were completed in less time than other applications of comparable complexity.

Organization is key to any application especially when the application is lengthy and/or complex. It is not uncommon that a page of critical data or information is overlooked in an application that is volumes thick when the organization of the application is poor or when it lacks a table of contents or index. Manufacturers can save time spent in answering requests for additional information by taking time to organize the application.

When FDA review staff are reviewing an application, they are usually more interested in viewing, examining, and analyzing the data and information in the application and reaching their own conclusions. Lengthy texts with little data to support the claims of the document are difficult to review and often raise questions. Whenever possible, the data should be displayed in tables or charts for easy visualization. Sometimes it is even advisable to submit spreadsheets on a computer disk when the tables are large. It is usually beneficial to contact the review group and discuss the optimal means of presenting complex and lengthy data.

Standards, Performance Standards and Special Controls

From a regulatory point of view, there is a distinction among the terms standard, performance standard, and special control. The agency does not issue standards, but does depend on standards developed by professional organizations to evaluate the safety and effectiveness of a device.

The agency can issue performance standards, but no performance standards have been promulgated by the agency to date for medical devices. Under the original medical device amendments, a device could be classified into class II if a performance standard could be developed. The Safe Medical Devices Act of 1990 revised the definition of a class II device by allowing the classification of a device into class II if a special control can be developed.

Special controls are those controls, such as performance standards postmarket surveillance, patient registries, guidelines, recommendations, data, device labeling, and others, that provide reasonable assurance of device safety and effectiveness that cannot be provided by general controls, yet are sufficient to obviate the need for submission of a PMA application. When a device was classified, the risks associated with each device was itemized.

Testing for New versus Existing Materials

For existing materials, the entire battery of characterization, mechanical, and physical testing does not always need repeating. Test data from a materials supplier can be used in an application. If a supplier has submitted test data in a master file, then this information can be referenced in the device application. In all cases, however, the test data need to apply to the intended use of the device. In one instance, a manufacturer referenced a master file for material characterization and biological test data for an implanted device. When the master file was reviewed by FDA staff, the master file contained test data on contact of the material with milk. There were no test data to show that the material was biocompatible with tissue or blood.

CRITICAL ISSUES FOR FUTURE EVALUATION AND RESEARCH

One of the problems with the current state of knowledge about biomaterials and of the regulatory structure is that it is difficult to define when enough testing and data are enough. The biocompatibility and performance testing requirements often address potential rather than real problems. This posture evolves from a lack of specific feedback on the performance of materials when used in various applications. When a problem with a device is identified, there is often insufficient data to specify whether the manufacturing process, the method of use, the condition of the patient, or the biomaterial contributed to the failure of the device.

An important focus of the FDA's future activities in medical devices is risk assessment. There is a great need in the device area to weigh a product's risks against its benefits. In some cases the calculation is reasonably straightforward, e.g., comparing the morbidity and mortality of a damaged heart valve with the use of a prosthetic valve. For many other devices, the relationship is more convoluted. How does one measure the benefits of a breast implant? How does one measure the risks of a material like silicone gel or oil, when its basic toxicology and pharmacokinetics is still uncertain? Straightforward or convoluted, the process is difficult.

To confound the issue, societal messages associated with risk assessment are mixed and inconsistent. Many people have been led to believe that no amount of risk from a medical product is acceptable, and that the government's role is to guarantee that the products it regulates are risk-free. That view is quite unrealistic, and greatly hampers the ability to communicate effectively about risk/benefit issues.

With regards to biomaterials and risk/benefit decision-making, the FDA needs a systematic means for evaluating/comparing clinical performance against in vitro assessments of material and device characteristics and properties. As in medicine, biomaterials biocompatibility assessments are not absolute measurements but are very much comparative evaluations. Imperative in such an approach is the use of consistent (standardized) methods of evaluation and a common knowledge base.

A direction the FDA is currently exploring involves development of a compendium of knowledge about the performance and potential risks of specific biomaterials in specific environments. Such a compendium could be a resource for both manufacturers and

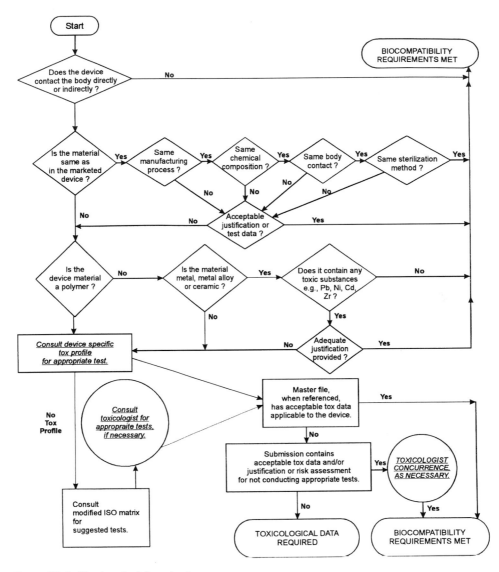

Figure 50-1 Testing decision chart.

government, particularly to streamline and improve the quality and consistency of the product approval process. The compendium is envisioned to be a network of existing databases which would relate device applications of biomaterials to clinical performance, materials properties and testing methods and standards. Initially, the FDA is trying to construct a series of tables and a controlled vocabulary to identify in a consistent manner the materials used in the many implantable devices. This would form the basis for a device/biomaterial dictionary which could provide links to library, industrial and other databases (Figure 50-1).

A second project proposed by the FDA involves the development of standard reference biomaterials with the National Institute of Standards and Technology (NIST). Initially, the FDA is developing with NIST a family of calcium phosphate materials which are loosely referred to as hydroxyapatite.

Table 50-5   List of Standards/Specifications

ASTM Standard	ISO Standard	Title
F138, F139	ISO 5832-1	Metallic materials Part 1: Wrought stainless steel
F67	ISO 5832-2	Metallic materials Part 2: Unalloyed titanium
F136	ISO 5832-3	Metallic materials Part 3: Wrought titanium 6-aluminum
F136	DIS 5832-3	Metallic materials Part 3: Wrought titanium 6-aluminum
F75	ISO 5832-4	Metallic materials Part 4: Cobalt-molybdenum casting alloy
F90	ISO 5832-5	Metallic materials Part 5: Wrought cobalt-chromium tungsten-nickel alloy
F562	ISO 5832-6	Metallic materials Part 6: Wrought cobalt-nickel-chromium molybdenum alloy
F799, F961	ISO 5832-7	Metallic materials Part 7: Forged and cold-forged cobalt-chromium-nickel-molybdenum alloy
F563	ISO 5832-8	Metallic materials Part 8: Wrought cobalt-nickel-chromium-molybdenum tungsten-iron alloy
F1314	DIS 5832-9	Metallic materials Part 9: Wrought high nitrogen stainless
F451	ISO 5833-1	Acrylic resin cements Part 1: Orthopedic applications
F451	DIS 5833-1	Acrylic resin cements Part 1: Orthopedic applications
F648	ISO 5834-2	Ultra-high molecular weight polyethylene Part 1: Powder form
	ISO 5834-1	Ultra-high molecular weight polyethylene Part 2: Molded forms
F543	DIS 5835	Metal bone screws with hexagonal drive connection, spherical undersurface of head, asymmetrical thread—Dimensions
F543	ISO 5836-1	Metal bone screws—Dimensions Part 1: Screws with asymmetrical thread, spherical under-surfaces
F786	ISO 5836-4	Metal bone plates Part 4: Holes and slots corresponding to screws with symmetrical thread and conical under-surfaces
F339	ISO 5837-1	Intramodullary nailing systems Part 1: Intramodullary nails with cloverleaf or V-shaped cross-section
F366, F453, F454	ISO 5837-2	Intramodullary nailing systems Part 2: Modullary pins
F366	ISO 5838-1	Skeletal pins and wires Part 1: Material and mechanical requirements
F366	DIS 5838-2	Skeletal pins and wires Part 2: Steineann skeletal pins—Dimensions

Table 50-5 (*Continued*)

ASTM Standard	ISO Standard	Title
F366	DP 5838-3	Skeletal pins and wires—Dimensions
		Part 4: Kirschner skeletal pins—Dimensions
	ISO 5839	Orthopaedic joint protheses—Basic requirements
	ISO 5840	Cardiovascular implants—Cardiac valve prostheses
	DIS 5840	Cardiovascular implants—Cardiac valve prostheses
	ISO 5841-1	Cardiac pacemakers
		Part 1: Implantable ventricular pacemakers
	DIS 5841-1	Cardiac pacemakers
		Part 1: Implantable pacemakers
	ISO 5841-2	Cardiac pacemakers
		Part 2: Reporting of the clinical performance of populations of pulse generators
F898	DIS 5841-3	Cardiac pacemakers
		Part 3: Low profile connectors for implantable pacemakers
F603	ISO 6018:1987	Orthopaedic implants—General requirements for marking, packaging and labelling
F603	ISO 6474:1981	Ceramic materials based on alumina
	DP 6474	Ceramic materials based on high purity alumina
F382	DIS 6475	Metal bone screws with asymmetrical thread and spherical under-surface—Mechanical requirements and test methods
	ISO 6475-1	Metal bone screws—Mechanical requirements and methods of test
		Part 1: Screws with asymmetrical thread, variable fitting (spherical), stainless steel
	ISO 6475-2	Metal bone screws—Mechanical requirements and methods of test
		Part 2: Screws with asymmetrical thread, constant fitting (spherical), stainless steel
	ISO 7197	Neurosurgical implants—Sterile, single-use hydrocephalous shunts and components
	DP 7198-1	Cardiovascular implants—Tubular vascular prostheses
		Part 1: Synthetic vascular prostheses
	DP 7199	Cardiovascular implants and artificial organs—Extracorporeal gas/blood exchangers
	ISO 7206-1	Partial and total hip joint prostheses
		Part 1: Classification, assignation of dimensions and requirements
	ISO 7206-2	Partial and total hip joint prostheses
		Part 2: Bearing surfaces made of metallic plastics materials
	ISO 7206-3	Partial and total hip joint prostheses
		Part 3: Determination of endurance properties of stemmed femoral components without application of torsion
	ISO 7206-4	Partial and total hip joint prostheses
		Part 4: Determination of endurance properties of stemmed tonsorial components with application of torsion
	DP 7206-5	Partial and total hip joint prostheses
		Part 5: Determination of resistance to static load of the head and neck of stemmed femoral components

(Continued)

Table 50-5 (*Continued*)

ASTM Standard	ISO Standard	Title
	DP 7206-6	Partial and total hip joint prostheses Part 6: Determination of endurance properties of the head and neck of stemmed femoral components
	DP 7206-7	Partial and total hip joint prostheses Part 7: Endurance performance of stemmed femoral components
	ISO7207-1:1985	Partial and total knee joint prostheses Part 1: Classification definitions and designation of dimensions
F116	ISO 8319-1	Orthopaedic instruments—Drive connections Part 1: Keys for use with screws with hexagon socket heads
F116	ISO 8319-2	Orthopaedic instruments—Drive connections Part 2: Screwdrivers for single slot head screws, screws with cruciate slot and cross-recessed head screws
F787	DIS 8615	Fixation devices for use in the ends of the femur in adults
	ISO 8637	Hemodialysers, hemofilters and hemoconcentrators
	DIS 8638	Extracorporeal blood circuit for hemodialysers, hemofilters and hemoconcentrators
F564	ISO 8827	Staples with parallel legs for orthopedic use—General requirements
F565	ISO 8828	Guidance on care and handling of orthopedic implants
F543	ISO 9268	Metal bone screws with conical under-surface of head—Dimensions
F367	ISO 9269	Metal bone plates—Holes and slots corresponding to screws with conical under-surface
	ISO/TR 9325	Partial and total hip joint prostheses— Recommendations for simulators for evaluation of hip joint prostheses
	ISO/TR 9356	Partial and total hip joint prostheses—Guidance for laboratory evaluation of change of form of bearing surfaces
F601	DP 9683	Fluorescent penetrant inspection of metallic implants
F629	DP 9684	Radiographic testing of cast metallic implants
F382	DIS 9686	Method for testing bending strength and stiffness of bone plates
	ISO/TR 9686	Usage of terms "valgus" and "varus" in orthopedic surgery
	DIS 9713	Neurosurgical implants—Self-closing intracranial aneurysm clips
F340	DIS 9714-1	Orthopedic drilling instruments Part 1: Drill bits, taps and countersink cutters
F748	DIR 9966	Biocompatibility - Selection of biological test methods for materials and devices
	DP 10310	Neurosurgical implants—Marking and packaging of implantable neural stimulators
F643, F644	DP 10334	Malleable wires for use as sutures or for other applications
	ISO 8548-1:1989	Prosthetics and orthotics—Limb deficiencies Part 1: Method of describing limb deficiencies present at birth

Table 50-5 (*Continued*)

ASTM Standard	ISO Standard	Title
	DP 8548-2	Prosthetics and orthotics—Limb deficiencies
		Part 2 Method of describing lower limb amputation stumps
	DP 8548-3	Prosthetics and orthotics—Limb deficiencies
		Part 3: Method of describing upper limb amputation stumps
	ISO 8549-1:1989	Prosthetics and orthotics—Vocabulary
		Part 1: General terms for external limb prostheses and external orthoses. Bilingual Edition
	ISO 8549-2:1989	Prosthetics and orthotics—Vocabulary
		Part 2: Terms relating to external limb prostheses and wearers of these prostheses. Bilingual Edition
	ISO 8549-2:1989	Prosthetics and orthotics—Vocabulary
		Part 3: Terms relating to external orthoses. Bilingual Edition
	DP 10328-1	Prosthetics—Structural testing of lower limb prostheses
		Part 1: Test configuration for single point loading
	DP 10328-2	Prosthetics—Structural testing of lower limb prostheses
		Part 2: Test samples for single point loading
	DP 10328-3	Prosthetics—Structural testing of lower limb prostheses
		Part 3: Test methods for single point loading

RECOMMENDATIONS AND CONCLUSIONS

The characterization, biological testing, and performance data on materials is an important part of an application for premarket evaluation by the FDA. In planning tests to evaluate the biocompatibility of a material, the intended use of the device will determine the level of testing and data needed to support the safety and effectiveness of the device. When there are questions regarding the types of testing or test methods, voluntary standards and guidance materials—including the information in this book—are a good starting point (see Table 50-5). When further assistance is needed, appropriate individuals in the FDA can be contacted for additional information and guidance.

REFERENCES

1 U. S. House of Representatives. Conference Report 94-853, 1976, 10–12.
2 Medical Device Amendments of 1976, Federal Food, Drug and Cosmetic Act as Amended and Related Laws. O-248-576QL3, 1990.
3 The Medical Device Amendments of 1976, as Further Amended by the Safe Medical Devices Act of 1990.
4 Good Laboratory Practice Regulations Management Briefing: Post Conference Report. Rockville, MD: Federal Drug Administration, August, 1979.
5 *Implementation of Good Laboratory Practices*. Washington, DC: American Chemical Society, 1994.
6 *Public Health Service Policy on Humane Care of Laboratory Animals*. Washington, DC: U.S. Department of Health and Human Services, 1992, 325–945.

ADDITIONAL READING

1   Basile EM. In Estrin NF (Ed.), *Overview of Current FDA Requirements for Medical Devices*. New York: Marcel Dekker, 1990.

2   Basile EM, Prease AJ. Compiling a successful PMA application. In Estrin NF (Ed.), *The Medical Device Industry*. New York: Marcel Dekker, 1990, 245–264.

3   Canty EL. Complying with the IDE regulation. In Estrin NF (Ed.), *The Medical Device Industry*. New York: Marcel Dekker, 1990, 273–282.

4   *Premarket Approval Manual*. FDA 87-4214, 1986.

5   *Investigational Device Exemptions—Regulatory Requirements for Medical Devices*. FDA 89-4159, 1989.

6   *Premarket Notification: 510(k)—Regulatory Requirements for Medical Devices*. FDA 90-4158, 1990.

7   *Highlights of the Safe Medical Devices Act of 1990*. FDA , 1991.

8   Preamendments Class III Devices; Strategy Document; Availability. *Federal Register*, Vol. 59, No. 87, May 6, 1994, 23731–23732.

9   The Gray Sheet: Proposed Calls for PMAs on Seven Devices Planned by FDA in 1994. May 9, 1994, 14–17.

10 Holstein HM. How to submit a successful 510(k). In Estrin ND (Ed.), *The Medical Device Industry*. New York: Marcel Dekker, 1990, 227–244.

11 Munsey RR, Holstein HM. FDA/GMP/MDR inspections: Obligations and rights. In Estrin ND (Ed.), *The Medical Device Industry*. New York: Marcel Dekker, 1990, 367–386.

12 O'Reilly JT. *Food and Drug Administration*. New York: McGraw-Hill Book Company, 1979.

13 Stigi JF, Kohler KC. U.S. and foreign requirements: A legal overview. In Estrin ND (Ed.), *The Medical Device Industry*. New York: Marcel Dekker, 1990, 855–888.

14 Yahiro MA. The Food and Drug Administration's MEDWatch program: Adverse events for orthopedic devices in 1993. 1994.

Chapter 51
Clinical Trials of Medical Devices

Diane E. Minear

OVERVIEW

The Federal Food, Drug, and Cosmetic Act, as amended (the Act), identifies the requirements, prohibited acts, and penalties associated with the introduction of medical devices into interstate commerce. The provisions of the Act are enforced by the U. S. Food and Drug Administration (FDA; see Chapter 50). Although the controls implemented by the Act are extensive, as discussed in Chapter 50, this chapter will review those portions of the statute and the regulations which are relevant to clinical trials of medical devices. Regulations implementing the Act have been promulgated by FDA and are found in Title 21 of the Code of Federal Regulations (21 CFR).

Those regulations having the greatest impact on the conduct of clinical trials for medical devices are Part 50 which discusses the protection of human subjects in clinical investigations, Part 56 which describes the functions and operations of an institutional review board (IRB), and Part 812 which describes the requirements and responsibilities associated with an Investigational Device Exemption (IDE). The protection of human subjects and IRB functions are discussed in Chapter 52. This chapter will focus on the regulatory issues associated with an IDE. Most medical devices must be either cleared or approved by FDA prior to commercial distribution in the United States, through either the premarket notification (510(k)) or premarket approval (PMA) process. The determination of the type of marketing application to be submitted and the possibility of required clinical data is based primarily on the classification of the device.

DEVICE CLASSIFICATIONS

All medical devices may be classified into one of three classification categories according to the relative degree of control that is considered necessary in order to provide reasonable assurance of the safety and effectiveness of the device.

Class I

"General Controls" are considered adequate to provide reasonable assurance of the safety and effectiveness of these devices. Examples of such general controls are found in the provisions of the Act, and include registration and listing requirements, premarket notification [510(k)] requirements, prohibitions against banned devices, notification requirements regarding repair, replacement, or refund for a commercially distributed device which presents an unreasonable risk of substantial harm to the public health, record keeping and reporting requirements, good manufacturing practices, and prohibitions against adulteration and/or misbranding. Many class I devices now have been exempted from the 510(k) premarket notification requirement.

Class II

In addition to the general controls described above, "Special Controls" are required to provide the necessary assurance of the safety and effectiveness of these devices. Examples of such special controls include, but are not limited to, performance standards, postmarket surveillance, patient registries, and guidelines developed and disseminated by FDA (including guidelines for the submission of clinical data in premarket notification submissions.) Expanded indications for use and increased sophistication of many class II devices have led to increased requirements for clinical trial data in 510(k) submissions.

Class III

General Controls and Special Controls are not considered adequate to assure the safety and effectiveness of these devices. Therefore, valid scientific evidence supporting the safety and effectiveness of the device must be submitted in a premarket approval application (PMA). This evidence must include adequate and well-controlled clinical studies of the device. If the device is completely new and unique in design, function, or intended use, the PMA must be approved by FDA prior to commercial distribution of the device.

FDA has not yet called for the PMAs for some of the class III devices which were marketed prior to the enactment of the Medical Device Amendments of 1976. Nevertheless, these devices will ultimately either be reclassified or require PMA approval to continue in commercial distribution.

INVESTIGATIONAL DEVICE EXEMPTIONS

Recognizing that clinical data would be required for some new devices prior to their commercial distribution, Congress included provisions in the Act for exemptions from certain of the Act's requirements, in order to allow for clinical investigations of either new devices or new intended uses of devices. Section 520(g) of the Act therefore provides exemptions for devices for investigational use. These exemptions are commonly referred to as the Investigational Device Exemptions (IDE)s. The stated purpose of this portion of the Act is "to encourage, to the extent consistent with the protection of the public health and safety and with ethical standards, the discovery and development of useful devices intended for human use and to that end to maintain optimum freedom for scientific investigators in their pursuit of that purpose."

The remainder of this chapter discusses the requirements for clinical trials of devices as detailed in the IDE regulation (21 CFR 812) and the PMA regulation (21 CFR 814). Regulations regarding institutional review boards (IRBs), protection of human subjects, and informed consent are discussed in Chapter 52.

IDE REGULATION—GENERAL PROVISIONS

The regulation regarding the shipment of medical devices for investigational purposes, i.e., in order to confirm the safety and effectiveness of a device for its intended use in a human (clinical) trial, is found in 21 CFR, Part 812, and is referred to as the IDE (Investigational Device Exemption) regulation. This regulation applies to the clinical trials of investigational devices, regardless of the classification of the device. Nevertheless, some investigations are exempt from the IDE requirements.

Scope

The IDE regulations define the required procedures for the conduct of clinical trials which are investigating the safety and effectiveness of devices. An approved IDE allows a sponsor to ship an investigational device to a clinical investigator in order to obtain clinical safety and effectiveness data, and exempts the sponsor from complying with most sections of the Act that apply to commercially distributed devices.

The IDE regulations do not apply to bench (performance) testing or preclinical (animal) testing. Regulations affecting preclinical testing, such as the Good Laboratory Practices (GLP) regulations, were discussed in Chapter 50.

Applicability

The IDE regulations apply to all clinical investigations of devices, although some investigations are exempted from the regulations and some (non-significant risk studies) are subject only to abbreviated requirements. The regulations apply to studies conducted by a single investigator who may sponsor his or her own study, as well as to studies conducted at multiple investigational sites that may be sponsored by a manufacturer or others.

Exempted Investigations

The IDE Regulations do not apply to investigations of the following categorics of devices: (1) Devices (other than transitional devices) which were in commercial distribution prior to May 28, 1976, or which have been determined to be substantially equivalent to such devices, when used or investigated in accordance with the indications in labeling accepted by FDA for the particular device. (Transitional devices are those which were regulated as drugs prior to May 28, 1976. Although these devices were declared by the act to be class III, some of these devices have since been reclassified to class II.) (2) Diagnostic devices, if the testing is noninvasive, does not require an invasive sampling procedure that presents significant risk, does not by design or intention introduce energy into a subject, and is not used as a diagnostic procedure without confirmation of the diagnosis by another, medically established diagnostic product or procedure. (3) Devices undergoing consumer preference testing, testing of a modification, or testing of a combination of two or more devices in commercial distribution, as long as the testing is not for the purpose of determining safety or effectiveness and does not put subjects at risk. (4) Devices intended solely for veterinary use. (5) Devices shipped solely for research on laboratory animals and which are so labeled. (6) Custom devices, unless the device testing is being used to determine either safety or effectiveness for commercial distribution of the device.

There are limits set on certain exemptions; in the case of a class II or class III device which is either a preamendment device (i.e., was in commercial distribution prior to May 28, 1976), or has been found to be substantially equivalent to a preamendment device, the device must have an approved IDE beginning on the date stipulated by an FDA regulation or order that calls for the submission of premarket approval applications for an unapproved class III device, or establishes a performance standard for a class II device. Such devices remain investigational and subject to the IDE regulations unless and until they either receive PMA approval, or conform to the required performance standard, whichever applies. (To date, no performance standards have been adopted by FDA and it appears unlikely that class II devices will be subjected to this requirement.)

Significant/Nonsignificant Risk Devices

The degree of risk associated with a device determines the degree of regulatory requirements imposed under the IDE regulations. A "significant risk device" is any device which when used in the course of a clinical investigation, presents a potential for serious risk to the health, safety, or welfare of a subject. Examples of such devices specifically mentioned in the IDE regulation include implants, life supporting/sustaining devices, and devices "of substantial importance in diagnosing, curing, mitigating, or treating disease, or otherwise preventing impairment of human health" [21 CFR 812.3(m)].

The determination of whether or not a device being used in a clinical study is "significant risk" or "nonsignificant risk" is usually made by the IRB reviewing the study. If multiple investigational sites are involved, all IRBs must be in agreement that the study is non-significant risk. When an IRB determines that a device is a significant risk device, and the sponsor had proposed that the IRB consider the device to be non-significant risk, the sponsor must notify FDA of the IRB's determination within 5 working days after first learning of the IRB's determination. In these cases, FDA will normally provide guidance or render an opinion with respect to the significant risk vs. non-significant risk of the device. Although FDA normally relies upon the IRB to make the significant risk/non-significant risk determination, the Agency may use its regulatory discretion to overrule IRB decisions.

Non-significant risk device studies do not require submission of a formal IDE application to FDA. The IDE is considered to be approved if the sponsor has obtained IRB approval (from all participating sites) which concurs with the non-significant risk determination. Nevertheless, such studies are required to comply with labeling, informed consent, monitoring, reporting, and record-keeping requirements of the IDE regulation. Furthermore, even if a formal IDE is not required by FDA, it is usually advantageous for the sponsor to contact the appropriate reviewing group at FDA to confirm the type and amount of clinical data that may be required in the marketing application for a particular device.

Labeling

Investigational devices (or their immediate package) must be labeled with the following statement: "CAUTION—Investigational device. Limited by Federal (or United States) law to investigational use." The label must also comply with the requirements of the labeling regulation (21 CFR 801), in identifying the contents, quantity of contents, name and address of the manufacturer, and all relevant contraindications, hazards, adverse effects, interfering substances or devices, warnings, and precautions. The labeling may not include any false or misleading statement and may not suggest that the device is safe or effective for the purposes for which it is being investigated.

Prohibition of Promotion and Commercialization of the Device

Sponsors, investigators, and/or their representatives may not promote or test market an investigational device until after FDA has approved the device for commercial distribution. Furthermore, sponsors, investigators, and representatives of the device may not represent the investigational device as being either safe or effective for the purposes for which it is being investigated. FDA does not prevent investigators from publishing or presenting study results in scientific journals or at scientific meetings; however, such presentations should be made with the above concerns in mind.

The investigational device may not be commercialized by either: (1) charging a price for the device which exceeds the costs of manufacturing, researching, developing, and handling the device, or (2) unduly prolonging the investigation (especially after learning that the study data demonstrate that the device is not safe and effective for the intended use for which it is being studied.) It is unusual for FDA to question the charges for investigational devices since the costs of research and development of the device generally far exceed the price which will be charged for the device. Consideration of reimbursement issues frequently influences sponsor decisions in this area. The Health Care Financing Administration (HCFA) and FDA have mutually established reimbursement codes for investigational devices with two basic categories of investigational devices being defined. *Category A: Experimental/Investigational Devices* includes those class III investigational devices which have never been cleared for marketing and for which no PMA for any indication for use has ever been approved, as well as class III devices which have undergone significant modification for a new indication for use. These devices are not eligible for medicare reimbursement. *Category B: Non-experimental/Investigational Devices* are all devices being investigated to support a determination of substantial equivalence to a legally marketed device, nonsignificant risk device investigations, and the majority of class III device investigations [1].

Import and Export Issues

Foreign manufacturers cannot directly export investigational devices from a foreign country to the United States; they must have a U. S. agent who will act as the sponsor of the U. S. clinical investigation of the device.

The Act requires a person exporting an investigational device from the United States to a foreign country to have FDA approval to do so, and to comply with the other statutory requirements for export. However, FDA's current policy is that if the device is the subject of an approved IDE (or exempt from such requirements), and will be marketed or used in clinical trials in the foreign country for the same intended use as that in the approved IDE, no prior approval is necessary, if the exporter complies with the remaining statutory requirements for export. These include that the device: (1) accords to the specifications of the foreign purchaser, (2) is not in conflict with the laws of the country to which it is intended for export, (3) is labeled on the outside of the shipping package that it is intended for export, and (4) is not sold or offered for sale in domestic commerce. Since the right to export an IDE-approved device without prior FDA approval is a matter of policy rather than regulation, manufacturers should confirm that the policy is still current prior to exporting investigational devices. If FDA withdraws approval of the IDE or the sponsor terminates any or all parts of the investigation because unanticipated adverse device effects present an unreasonable risk to subjects, exportation of the investigational device may continue only with FDA approval [2].

Export restrictions have been further eased by the FDA Export Reform and Enhancement Act, which became law on April 26, 1996. This new law allows for a device not approved in the U.S. to be exported to any country in the world if the product complies with the laws of the country to which it is exported and if it has valid marketing authorization in any one of certain developed countries, as follows: Australia, Canada, Israel, Japan, New Zealand, Switzerland, South Africa, and any country in the European Union or the European Economic Area.

IDE APPLICATIONS

A sponsor of a significant risk device investigation must submit three copies of an IDE application to the FDA and receive approval before beginning the investigation. IRB review and approval need not be obtained prior to submitting the IDE to the FDA. Many sponsors choose to get the FDA approval first, since any changes to the investigational plan, as recommended or required by FDA, will routinely need to be approved by the IRB as well. The application is submitted to: Center for Devices and Radiological Health, IDE Document Mail Center (HFZ-401), Food and Drug Administration, 9200 Corporate Boulevard, Rockville, MD 20850. This address may change over time and should be confirmed prior to mailing/shipping the document.

Contents of the Application

There is no standardized form available from the FDA for submitting the IDE. The document must be prepared by the sponsor according to the requirements found in 21 CFR, Part 812, and must be submitted in the following order:

   (1)   The name and address of the sponsor.
   (2)   A complete report of prior investigations of the device.
This report must include all prior clinical, animal, and laboratory testing of the device. (The information provided must be comprehensive and adequate to justify the proposed investigation.) With regard to any nonclinical laboratory studies, the sponsor must identify if all such studies have been conducted in compliance with applicable requirements in the good laboratory practice (GLP) regulations [3], and if not, a stated reason for the noncompliance. The report must also include a bibliography of *all* publications (whether adverse or supportive), that are relevant to an evaluation of the safety or effectiveness of the device, with copies of all published and unpublished adverse information. The sponsor must summarize any other unpublished information that is known or reasonably obtainable regarding the device that is relevant to an evaluation of the safety or effectiveness of the device.
   (3)   The investigational plan. Although the regulation allows for submission of a "summary" of the investigational plan if the IDE has been reviewed by an IRB, there is also a caveat which allows the Agency to request a complete investigational plan. The complete investigational plan is invariably required, and should be submitted in the initial application to avoid delay of the approval process for the IDE. The investigational plan must include the following information in order:
   (a)   *Purpose.* The name and intended use of the device and the objectives and intended duration of the investigation.
   (b)   *Protocol.* A written protocol describing the methodology to be used and an analysis of the protocol demonstrating that the investigation is scientifically sound. The protocol

should be carefully and thoroughly designed to include appropriate regulatory endpoints for assessing the safety and effectiveness of the device for its intended use. Whenever possible, the study design should incorporate an appropriate control group(s) and blinding of investigators or evaluators. A complete summary of the statistical methodology that will be used to analyze the data also should be included. Without these elements, the FDA is unlikely to sanction the scientific soundness of the study.

(c) *Risk Analysis.* A description and analysis of all increased risks to which subjects will be exposed by the investigation; the manner in which these risks will be minimized; a justification for the investigation; and a description of the patient population, including the number, age, sex, and condition. (Statistical support for the selected sample size should be included.)

(d) *Device Description.* A description of each important component, ingredient, property, and principle of operation of the device and of each anticipated change in the device during the course of the investigation.

(e) *Monitoring Procedures.* The sponsor's written procedures for monitoring the investigation and the name and address of the study monitor.

(f) *Device Labeling.* Copies of all labeling for the device must be included. This includes package labels, printed information which will be on the actual device, and Directions for Use. As previously discussed, the precaution statement identifying that the device is investigational must be included.

(g) *Consent Materials.* Copies of all forms and informational materials to be provided to subjects to obtain informed consent. The informed consent form must include all of the required elements and any additional applicable elements of 21 CFR, Part 50 [4].

(h) *IRB Information.* A list of the names, locations, and chairpersons of all IRBs that have been or will be asked to review the investigation, and a certification of any action taken by any of those IRBs with respect to the investigation. If the investigational sites have not been selected at the time of the submission of the IDE, this should be stated, in which case, the IRB information need not be provided.

(i) *Other Institutions.* The name and address of any/each institution at which a part of the investigation may be conducted that has not been identified in paragraph (h) above.

(j) *Additional Records and Reports.* A description of records and reports that will be maintained on the investigation in addition to those prescribed in the IDE regulation. It is advisable to include copies of the standardized data collection forms that will be used to document the study, even in draft form, if they are available. The forms add a level of credibility to the study, and FDA reviewers who are experienced with a particular type of study may be able to provide valuable input respecting the design of the data collection forms.

(4) Manufacturing information.
A description of the methods, facilities, and controls used for the manufacture, processing, packing, storage, and, where appropriate, installation of the device, in sufficient detail so that a person generally familiar with good manufacturing practices (GMPs) can make a knowledgeable judgment about the quality control used in the manufacture of the device.

(5) Investigator information.
An example of the agreement(s) to be entered into by all investigators to comply with investigator obligations of the IDE regulations, and a list of the names and addresses of all investigators who have signed the agreement. The sponsor must certify that all investigators who will participate in the investigation have signed the agreement, that the list of investigators includes all the investigators participating in the investigation, and that no investigators will be added to the investigation until they have signed the agreement. If all of the investigators have not been selected, the list should include those who have been selected (if any), and the certification should state that all investigators who will participate in the investigation *will* have signed the agreement and that no investigators will be added to the investigation until they have signed the agreement.

(6) Sales information.

If the device is to be sold, the amount to be charged for the device, and an explanation of why sale does not constitute commercialization. If the device is not to be sold, this should be stated.

(7) Environmental impact assessment.

An environmental impact assessment describing the potential environmental impact of manufacturing and investigating the device must be included or a claim for categorical exclusion from this requirement, which states that: "Devices shipped under this Investigational Device Exemption are intended to be used for clinical studies in which waste will be controlled or the amount of waste expected to enter the environment may reasonably be expected to be nontoxic" [5].

(8) Other information.

This includes any other relevant information that FDA requests for review of the application. Guidance documents are available from FDA for some types of studies and may identify specific additional information that the Agency wants to review. Also, contacting the appropriate review staff in advance of submitting the IDE application can frequently be helpful in determining additional information that may be required for a specific device.

FDA Action on Applications

Upon receipt of an original IDE application, FDA provides a written acknowledgment of receipt of the document and provides the sponsor with the date of receipt of the document and the assigned document number for the application. Since there is a brief thirty-day review period for IDE applications, for all subsequent amendments and supplements to the IDE, FDA notifies the sponsor in writing of the date the application was received when it sends the letter of response. The IDE application is assigned a unique document number which begins with the letter "G" followed by a six-digit identifier; the first two numbers reflect the year in which the IDE application was submitted, while the last four numbers reflect the chronological order in which the application was received by the FDA during that year. For example, G960152 would be the document number assigned to the 152nd original IDE application received by FDA in 1996. Thirty days after the date of receipt FDA will notify the sponsor of its decision regarding the application. Legally, the sponsor may begin the investigation thirty days after the application has been received, if FDA has not responded. However, sponsors should contact the reviewing branch prior to proceeding with an investigation, particularly if there has been no communication with FDA during the review period and no approval letter has been received, since the response may be delayed in the mail and may not be an approval.

FDA has three choices for responding to the IDE application. First, FDA may approve the investigation as proposed by the sponsor. Second, FDA may approve the investigation with modifications; this is known as conditional approval since the Agency places certain "conditions" on the sponsor for proceeding with the study. If the sponsor does not agree to the conditions, then the study is automatically disapproved and may not proceed. Lastly, FDA may disapprove the study.

FDA may disapprove (or subsequently withdraw approval of) an IDE application if it finds that: (1) There has been a failure to comply with any requirement of the IDE regulation or the act, any other applicable regulation or statute, or any condition of approval imposed by an IRB or FDA; (2) the application or a report contains an untrue statement of a material fact, or omits material information required by the IDE regulation; (3) the sponsor fails to respond to a request for additional information within the time prescribed by FDA;

(4) there is reason to believe that the risks to the subjects are not outweighed by the anticipated benefits to the subjects and the importance of the knowledge to be gained, or informed consent is inadequate, or the investigation is scientifically unsound, or there is reason to believe that the device as used is ineffective; (5) It is otherwise unreasonable to begin or to continue the investigation owing to the way in which the device is used or the inadequacy of: (a) the report of prior investigations, (b) the manufacturing process of the device in some particular, or (c) the monitoring and review of the investigation.

If FDA disapproves an IDE application, or proposes to withdraw approval of an application, FDA will notify the sponsor in writing. The disapproval order (or notice of a proposed withdrawal of approval) will contain a complete statement of the reasons for this action and a statement that the sponsor has an opportunity to request a hearing regarding this matter. In the case of a study already in progress, the opportunity for a hearing will be provided before actual withdrawal of approval unless FDA has determined that continuing the investigation represents an unreasonable risk to the public health.

Addendums to the IDE

Additional submissions that describe revisions or changes made in the investigation *prior* to approval of the IDE are referred to as *amendments* to the IDE. FDA often has taken a very broad interpretation of its authority to disapprove an IDE. This has resulted in the submission of multiple amendments to some IDE applications prior to their being approved. Each amendment to the IDE triggers another 30-day review cycle and another official response from the Agency. Some of these delays can be eliminated by providing complete and adequate information in the initial application. Other delays, however, may be due to philosophical differences regarding the investigational plan and may be less easily resolved. This underscores the importance of communicating with the appropriate FDA review staff prior to submitting the IDE in order to determine any areas of concern for the Agency staff and how best to respond to those concerns.

Additional submissions regarding the investigation made to FDA *following* approval of the IDE application are referred to as IDE *supplements*. All correspondence, reports, and revisions or changes to the investigation are recorded as individual supplements to the IDE. If a sponsor or investigator proposes a change to the investigational plan that may affect the scientific soundness of the study, or the rights, safety, or welfare of subjects, the sponsor must first submit a supplement to the FDA and obtain FDA approval (as well as IRB approval for changes affecting the rights, safety, or welfare of a subject) prior to implementing that change in the study. In the case of a deviation from the investigational plan that is made in order to protect the life or physical well-being of a subject in an emergency, the sponsor must notify FDA of the deviation within five working days after learning of the incident.

Confidentiality of Data and Information

Generally, FDA will not disclose the existence of an IDE (unless its existence has previously been publicly disclosed or acknowledged by the sponsor) until FDA approves or clears the product for marketing. If the existence of an IDE file has not been publicly disclosed or acknowledged, no data or information in the file are available for public disclosure, with two exceptions. First, FDA will make publicly available (upon request) a detailed summary of information that was the basis for an order approving, disapproving, or withdrawing approval for an IDE for a banned device. Such a summary would include information on any adverse effect on health caused by the device. (Currently, the only device to be banned by FDA is "prosthetic hair fibers.") Second, upon request or on its own initiative, FDA may disclose to an individual on whom an investigational device has been used, a copy of a report of adverse device effects relating to that use. Safety and effectiveness information in the IDE file, including test protocols, adverse reaction reports, consumer complaints, etc., can be made publicly available after the device is cleared or approved for marketing. In this case all trade secret or confidential commercial or financial information will not be disclosed, including manufacturing information, production, sales, distribution information, quantitative or semiquantitative formulas.

RESPONSIBILITIES OF SPONSORS

Sponsors are responsible for selecting qualified investigators and providing them with the information they need in order to conduct the investigation properly, including copies of the investigational plan and the report of prior investigations of the device. They must also ensure that there is proper monitoring of the study by qualified persons, that IRB approval is obtained and appropriately maintained at each investigational site, and that the IRB(s) and FDA are promptly informed of significant new information about the investigation. They must control the shipment of investigational devices to the participating investigators and ensure that all investigators are complying with the investigator agreement, investigational plan, and all applicable regulations. They must maintain all appropriate records of the study and submit any required reports to investigators, IRBs, and FDA.

Unanticipated Adverse Device Effects

The sponsor must immediately conduct an evaluation of any unanticipated adverse device effects. If the sponsor determines that an unanticipated adverse device effect presents an unreasonable risk to subjects, the sponsor must terminate all investigations or parts of investigations presenting that risk within 5 days of making the determination and within 15 days of being notified of the unanticipated device effect. A study, or part of a study, which has been terminated requires IRB approval in order to be resumed (and FDA approval if it is a significant risk device study).

RESPONSIBILITIES OF INVESTIGATORS

Investigators must ensure that the investigation is conducted according to the signed agreement, the investigational plan, any conditions imposed by the IRB and/or FDA, and applicable FDA regulations for protecting the rights, safety, and welfare of the study subjects, as well as for the control of the devices under investigation. They must also ensure that informed consent (21 CFR, Part 50) is obtained from all subjects, that required study records are appropriately completed and maintained, and that required reports are submitted to the sponsor, IRB, and FDA.

Investigators may determine whether or not potential subjects would be interested in participating in an investigation, but may not obtain informed consent or allow any subject to participate before obtaining IRB approval (and FDA approval for a significant risk device study). For an approved study, the investigator must supervise the use of the investigational device and ensure that it is only used by authorized personnel for appropriate purposes of the study. The investigational device may only be used on subjects under the investigator's supervision. Upon completion/termination of the investigator's participation in the study, the investigator must return to the sponsor any remaining supply of the device or must otherwise dispose of the device as the sponsor directs.

RECORDS AND REPORTS

For clinical investigations of both significant risk devices (requiring formal FDA approval) and non-significant risk devices (requiring IRB approval), the investigator(s) and sponsor must maintain accurate, complete, and current records relating to the study, and must submit complete, accurate, and timely reports. There are multiple types of records and reports required of both the sponsor and investigator; these record-keeping and reporting requirements are monitored and enforced by the sponsor, the IRB, and FDA. In addition to the records and reports specified below, sponsors and investigators must maintain and/or submit any additional records and reports stipulated by either a reviewing IRB or FDA regarding any aspect of their particular investigation.

Investigator Records and Reports

Correspondence Records   Investigators must maintain records of all correspondence relating to the study. This correspondence may be with another participating investigator, an IRB, the sponsor, a monitor, or FDA.

Device Records   Records of receipt, use, or disposition of a device must be kept that identify: a) the type and quantity of the device, the dates of its receipt, and the batch number (or device code number), b) the names of all persons who received, used, or disposed of each device, c) the number of and reason for devices being returned to the sponsor, or repaired, or otherwise disposed of.

Patient Records   Case histories of subjects exposed to the device must be accurately and completely recorded. The case history records must include documentation of informed consent (or documentation justifying failure to obtain informed consent), all relevant observations made during the study (including previous medical history, results of diagnostic tests, adverse device effects, and the condition of the subjects at follow-up), and a record of the exposure of each subject to the investigational device, including the date and time of each use, and any other (related) therapy.

Protocol Records   The protocol must be kept on record with documents showing the dates of and reasons for each deviation from the protocol.

Unanticipated Device Effects Report   A report of any unanticipated device effect must be submitted to the sponsor and the reviewing IRB as soon as possible and at least within 10 working days of the date the investigator first learns of the effect.

Withdrawal of IRB Approval Report   An investigator must report to the sponsor within 5 working days, if the reviewing IRB withdraws approval for his/her part of the investigation.

Progress Reports   The investigator must submit progress reports on the investigation to the sponsor, monitor, and IRB at least yearly.

Report of Deviations from the Investigational Plan or Failure to Obtain Informed Consent   If an investigator must deviate from the investigational plan to protect the life or physical well-being of a subject in an emergency and/or if an investigational device is used without obtaining informed consent, the investigator must report such deviation and/or use of the device to the sponsor and the IRB within 5 working days of the event.

Final Report   Investigators must submit a final report of the investigation or their part of the investigation to the IRB and the sponsor within 3 months of the termination or completion of their part of an investigation.

Sponsor Records and Reports

Correspondence Records   Sponsors must maintain records of all correspondence relating to the study; such correspondence may be with another sponsor, a monitor, an investigator, an IRB, or FDA.

Device Records   Such records will include documentation of both shipment (including type and quantity of devices shipped, name and address of consignee, date of shipment, and batch or code number) and disposition (including batch or code number of any devices returned to the sponsor for repair or disposal, or separately disposed of by the investigator or someone else, and the reasons for and method of disposal).

Investigator Agreement Records   Copies of all signed investigator agreements must be kept on file by the sponsor.

Nonsignificant Risk Device Study Records.   The sponsor must maintain in one consolidated file available for FDA inspection the following records: the name and intended use of the device, the objectives of the investigation, justification for why the device is not a significant risk device, the name and address of each investigator and his/her reviewing IRB, a description of the applicability of GMPs to the manufacture of the device, all adverse device effects and complaints, and any other information specified by FDA.

Adverse Device Effects Records   These records document all adverse device effects (whether anticipated or not) as well as all complaints.

Unanticipated Adverse Device Effects Report   The results of any evaluation of an unanticipated adverse device effect must be reported to FDA and to all participating investigators and their IRBs within 10 working days of the sponsor first being notified of the effect. Additional reporting on a given incident may be required at FDA's discretion.

Withdrawal of IRB or FDA Approval Report   If either an IRB or FDA withdraws approval of an investigation or part of an investigation, the sponsor must notify all participating investigators and their IRBs and/or FDA as appropriate. Such reports must be made within 5 working days of the sponsor being notified of any such withdrawal of approval.

Current Investigator List Report   A sponsor of an approved significant risk device IDE must submit to FDA, at 6-month intervals, and beginning 6 months after FDA approval, a current list of the names and addresses of all investigators participating in the investigation.

Progress Reports   At least yearly, the sponsor must prepare and submit a progress report on the conduct of the study to all IRBs reviewing the study, as well as to FDA (if it is a significant risk device).

Recall and Device Disposition Reports   Within 30 days of a request, sponsors must notify FDA and any reviewing IRB of any request (including the reason for the request) for an investigator to return, repair, or otherwise dispose of any units of a device.

Informed Consent   When a sponsor receives any report from an investigator regarding use of the device without prior informed consent, a copy must be submitted to FDA within 5 working days of receiving such a report.

Final Report   For a significant risk device study, the sponsor must notify FDA within 30 working days of the completion or termination of an investigation, and must submit a final report to FDA and all participating investigators and their IRBs within 6 months of study completion or termination. For a non-significant risk device study, the final report must be submitted to the reviewing IRBs within 6 months of completion or termination of the study.

Records Custody and Retention

Investigators and sponsors must maintain the required records of an investigation during the entire investigation and for a period of two years after either the date of termination or completion of the study, or the date that the records are not longer required for purposes of supporting a marketing application for a class III device, whichever is later. Investigators or sponsors may withdraw from the responsibility to maintain records for the required period of time if they transfer custody of the records to another person who accepts responsibility for the records in conformance with the entire IDE regulation, including making the records available for inspection by FDA.

INSPECTIONS AND BIORESEARCH MONITORING

A sponsor or an investigator (who has authority to grant access) must permit authorized FDA employees to enter and inspect any establishment where investigational devices are held (including any facility where devices are manufactured, processed, packed, installed, used, or implanted or where records of results from use of devices are kept). A sponsor, IRB, investigator, or anyone acting on behalf of such persons must permit authorized FDA employees to inspect and copy all records relating to an investigation. If FDA has reason to suspect that adequate informed consent was not obtained, or that records required to be submitted by the investigator to the sponsor or IRB have not been submitted or are incomplete, inaccurate, false, or misleading, the investigator must permit authorized FDA employees to inspect and copy records that identify subjects. All such inspections should be conducted at a reasonable time and in a reasonable manner by the FDA.

The Division of Bioresearch Monitoring in FDA's Center for Devices has grown significantly in recent years and IDE investigational sites are now routinely inspected prior to approval of a PMA. Use of this enforcement tool has resulted in numerous warning letters issued to investigators, IRBs, and sponsors, as well as recommendations for disapproval of marketing applications.

PROPOSED RULES

Proposals for revisions to the current IDE regulation have been published in the Federal Register and are pending final rule. Nevertheless, FDA has implemented by policy certain requirements of these new rules.

Disqualification of Clinical Investigators

The FDA has proposed to revise its IDE regulation to include provisions for disqualification of clinical investigators. Such provisions are intended to support consistent bioresearch monitoring regulations for all products regulated by FDA and to improve the remedies available to deal with clinical investigator misconduct. The proposed rule (21 CFR 812.119) identifies the purposes of disqualification of an investigator who has violated the regulations, which are to: (1) preclude the investigator from conducting clinical investigations subject to requirements under the act unless and until it becomes likely that said investigator will abide by the regulations or that such violations will not recur; and (2) exclude the consideration of any clinical investigations which have been conducted in whole or in part by the investigator, in support of applications for IDE or PMA approval from FDA, until such time as it becomes likely that the investigator will abide by the regulations. The proposed regulation is consistent with similar regulations imposed for drug and biologic clinical investigations and details the administrative procedures associated with this process, such as the opportunity for a hearing, consent agreements, and requirements for reinstatement of a disqualified investigator [6].

Financial Disclosure by Clinical Investigators

FDA has proposed to implement 21 CFR 54 and 21 CFR 812.110(e) to address the issue of Financial Disclosure by Clinical Investigators. This requirement will apply to most clinical studies involving human subjects. The agency is proposing to require that sponsors either certify to the absence of certain financial interests of clinical investigators or disclose those financial interests when clinical studies are submitted to FDA in support of a marketing application. Failure to provide either a certification or disclosure statement in appropriate documents could result in the agency refusing to file the application. This new requirement is based on recognition that certain financial arrangements between clinical investigators and product sponsors, or the personal financial interests of clinical investigators, can potentially bias the outcome of clinical trials [7].

CGMP Requirement

Although devices being evaluated under an IDE were previously exempt from conformance with current good manufacturing practices (CGMP) requirements, manufacturers conducting IDE studies were required to manufacture the devices used in the studies under a state of control. The new section 820.30 of the final CGMP would require manufacturers to implement design controls for all class II and class III devices, as well as some class I devices. FDA believes that it is reasonable to expect manufacturers who design medical devices to develop the designs complying with design control requirements and that imposing such requirements is necessary to adequately protect the public from potentially dangerous devices. Therefore, IDE devices are not exempt from 21 CFR 820.30, "Design Controls" in the Quality System regulation [8].

Humanitarian Device Exemption

The Safe Medical Devices Act (SMDA) of 1990 amended the Federal Food, Drug, and Cosmetic Act and included a provision for exempting humanitarian devices from the effectiveness requirements of sections 514 (special controls) and 515 (premarket approval) of the Act if the agency finds that: (1) the device is designed to treat or diagnose a disease or condition that affects fewer than 4,000 individuals in the U.S.; (2) the device is not available otherwise and there is no comparable device available to treat or diagnose the disease or condition; and (3) the device will not expose patients to unreasonable or significant risk, and the benefits to health from the use outweigh the risks. The purpose of this provision was to encourage the discovery and use of devices that would benefit fewer than 4,000 individual in the United States. Devices granted an exemption may only be used at facilities that have an established IRB which approves the use of the device. An exemption may be granted only for an initial period of 18 months but may be subsequently extended. However, the initial exemption may only be granted in the 5-year period beginning on the date that an implementing regulation for this part of the act takes effect. FDA has not yet published a humanitarian device exemption regulation.

IDE POLICIES AND GUIDELINES

Multiple guidance documents are available from FDA to assist manufacturers in the interpretation of various requirements of the IDE regulation. Examples of these include the Guideline for Monitoring Clinical Studies (a copy of this guidance is included in the approval letter for each original IDE application), Guidance on Significant Risk and Nonsignificant Risk Device Studies, Suggested Format for IDE Progress Reports, Guidance on the Emergency Use of Unapproved Medical Devices, Guidance on Notices of Availability of Investigational Devices, Guidance on the Applicability of the GMP Regulation to IDEs, and Guidance on Feasibility Studies. All of these guidance documents are available from FDA and all are incorporated into FDA's Investigational Device Exemptions Manual. This manual can be obtained by contacting FDA's Division of Small Manufacturers' Assistance (DSMA) at 1-800-638-2041, or by writing: Superintendent of Documents, U.S. Government Printing Office, Washington, D.C. 20402, and requesting Document Number: GPO 017-012-00337-1. The following text and Tables 1–4 summarize this information.

Feasibility Studies

FDA recognizes the importance of providing flexibility in the review of IDE applications for feasibility studies, as long as the subjects' safety and welfare are assured. These studies are useful when a device involves a new device design or technology and the sponsor wishes to conduct an initial limited clinical study to confirm the design and operating specifications, or to test the study protocol or evaluation tools prior to beginning an extensive (or pivotal) clinical trial. Since the results of feasibility studies may lead to the determination that the device is unsuitable for further development or must be redesigned for further development, review of some parts of the application, e.g., prior investigations, investigational plan, and

Table 51-1   Investigator and Sponsor Responsibilities for Maintaining Records

	Records	Maintained by Investigator	Maintained by Sponsor
Significant Risk Device	• All Correspondence Pertaining to the Investigation	√	√
	• Shipment, Receipt, Disposition	√	√
	• Device Administration and Use	√	–
	• Subject Case Histories	√	–
	• Informed Consent	√	–
	• Protocols and Reason for Deviations from Protocol	√	–
	• Adverse Device Effects and Complaints	√	√
	• Signed Investigator Agreements	–	√
	• Membership/Employment/Conflicts of Interest	–	–
	• Minutes of Meetings	–	–
Non-significant Risk Device	• Name and Intended Use of Device	–	√
	• Brief Explanation of Why Device Does Not Involve Significant Risk	–	√
	• Name and Addresses of Investigator(s) and IRBs	–	√
	• Degree GMPs Followed	–	√
	• Informed Consent	√	–
	• Adverse Device Effects and Complaints	–	√

Source: Investigational Device Exemptions: Regulatory Requirements of Medical Devices, Food and Drug Administration (1989).

manufacturing information, may be less stringent than for a pivotal trial. Generally, the focus of the review for feasibility studies is on the device's potential risk to subjects. Early interaction with FDA can help to establish rapport with the review group and identify the degree of information that may be required for such an application.

Refusal to Accept Policy

As a means to more effectively utilize review resources and to improve the timeliness of the device evaluation process, FDA has established a Refuse to Accept Policy for IDEs. Immediately following receipt of a new IDE application, a threshold determination regarding the quality of the submission is made in order to determine whether or not the application merits substantive evaluation by FDA scientists. An IDE Checklist is used by reviewing divisions to provide uniformity in determining the acceptability of IDE submissions and is included below.

Expedited Review

FDA believes it is in the interest of the public health to review marketing applications (PMAs and 510(k)s) for certain devices in an expedited manner. Expedited review will

Table 51-2   Responsibilities for Preparing and Submitting Reports for Non-Significant Risk Devices

Type of report	Report prepared by	
	Investigators for	Sponsors for
Unanticipated Adverse Effect Evaluation	Sponsors and IRBs	FDA, Investigators and IRBs
Withdrawal of IRB Approval	Sponsors and IRBs	FDA, Investigators and IRBs
Progress Report	N/A	IRBs
Final Report	N/A	IRBs
Inability to Obtain Informed Consent	Sponsors and IRBs	FDA
Withdrawal of FDA Approval	N/A	IRBs and Investigators
Recall and Device Disposition	N/A	FDA and IRBs
Significant Risk Determinations	N/A	FDA

Source: Investigational Device Exemptions: Regulatory Requirements of Medical Devices, Food and Drug Administration (1989).

generally be considered when an application offers evidence of a potential for clinically meaningful increased benefit compared to the existing alternatives, or when the new medical device promises to provide a revolutionary advance (not incremental advance) over currently available modalities. Granting of expedited review means that the marketing application receives priority review before other pending PMAs and 510(k)s. Each reviewing division at FDA will identify those applications which merit expedited review, either during the IDE stage, through pre-submission meetings with the applicant, or through a preliminary evaluation of the submitted application [9].

CLINICAL DATA IN PREMARKET APPROVAL APPLICATIONS

Because a clinical trial of an investigational device is intended to evaluate the safety and effectiveness of the device, the clinical data most often is incorporated into a premarket approval application (PMA). 21 CFR, Part 814 is the implementing regulation stipulating the requirements for a PMA. With respect to the requirements for clinical data, the regulation states that the application must include a summary of the clinical investigations submitted in the application, including a discussion of subject selection and exclusion criteria, study population, study period, safety and effectiveness data, adverse reactions and complications, patient discontinuation, patient complaints, device failures and replacements, results of statistical analyses of the clinical investigations, contraindications and precautions for use of the device, and other information from the clinical investigations as appropriate. A discussion demonstrating that the data and information in the application constitute valid scientific evidence and provide reasonable assurance that the device is safe and effective for its intended use must also be included, as well as a discussion of the risk and benefit considerations related to the device (including any adverse effects of the device on health). Valid scientific evidence is defined by FDA as "evidence from well-controlled investigations, partially controlled studies, studies and objective trials without matched controls, well-documented case histories conducted by qualified experts, and reports of significant human experience with a marketed device, from which it can fairly and responsibly be concluded by qualified experts that there is reasonable assurance of the safety and effectiveness of a device under its conditions of use."

Table 51-3   Responsibilities for Preparing and Submitting Reports for Significant Risk Devices

Type of report	Report prepared by	
	Investigators for	Sponsors for
Unanticipated Adverse Effect Evaluation	Sponsors and IRBs	FDA, Investigators and IRBs
Withdrawal of IRB Approval	Sponsors	FDA, Investigators and IRBs
Progress Report	Sponsors, Monitors and IRBs	FDA and IRBs
Final Report	Sponsors and IRBs	FDA, Investigators and IRBs
Emergencies (Protocol Deviations)	Sponsors and IRBs	FDA
Inability to Obtain Informed Consent	Sponsors and IRBs	FDA
Withdrawal of FDA Approval	N/A	IRBs and Investigators
Current Investigator List	N/A	FDA
Recall and Device Disposition	N/A	FDA and IRBs
Records Maintenance Transfer	FDA	FDA
Significant Risk Determinations	N/A	FDA

Source: Investigational Device Exemptions: Regulatory Requirements of Medical Devices, Food and Drug Administration (1989).

There is reasonable assurance that a device is safe when it can be determined, based upon valid scientific evidence, that the probable benefits to health from use of the device for its intended uses and conditions of use, when accompanied by adequate directions and warnings against unsafe use, outweigh any probable risks. The evidence must adequately demonstrate the absence of unreasonable risk of illness or injury associated with the use of the device for its intended uses and conditions of use.

There is reasonable assurance that a device is effective when it can be determined, based upon valid scientific evidence, "that in a significant portion of the target population, the use of the device for its intended uses and conditions of use, when accompanied by adequate directions for use and warnings against unsafe use, will provide clinically significant results."

The plan or protocol for a study and the report of the results of a well-controlled investigation must include: (1) a clear statement of the objectives of the study; (2) a method of subject selection that provides adequate assurance that the subjects are suitable for the purposes of the study, provides diagnostic criteria for the condition to be treated or diagnosed, provides confirmatory laboratory tests where appropriate and, in the case of a device to prevent a disease or condition, provides evidence of susceptibility and exposure to the condition against which prophylaxis is desired; (3) a method of assigning the subjects to test groups, if used, in such a way as to minimize any possible bias; (4) a method of selecting subjects that assures comparability between test groups and any control groups of pertinent variables such as sex, severity or duration of the disease, and use of therapy other than the test device; and (5) an explanation of the methods of observation and recording of results utilized, including the variables measured, quantitation, assessment of any subject's response, and steps taken to minimize any possible bias of subjects and observers. A comparison of the results of treatment or diagnosis with a control must be provided in such a fashion as to permit quantitative evaluation. The precise nature of the control must be specified and an explanation provided of the methods employed to minimize any possible bias of the observers and

Table 51-4   Original IDE Checklist for Administrative Review

Filing review elements	Yes (Present omission justified)	No (Inadequate omitted)
I. Screening Information:		
A. Is the investigation within the categories of investigations that are not exempt from the IDE regulation under 812.2(c)?		
B. Is this a significant risk device investigation? (21 CFR 812.3(m) and 812.20(a)(1))		
C. If there has been an Integrity Investigation, has the ODE integrity officer given permission to proceed with review? (If no integrity investigation, check yes)		
D. U.S. sponsor, address, telephone number and contact person identified? (Note: IDE application will not be approved without a U.S. sponsor.) (21 CFR 812.18(a))		
II. Format for submission:		
A. Table of contents (21 CFR 812.20(b))		
B. Submission clearly paginated		
C. 3 copies included (21 CFR 812.20(a)(3))		
III. Required elements for application		
A. Report of prior investigations (Are the following items present in the application?) (21 CFR 812.27)		
1. Report of clinical, animal and laboratory testing		
2. Bibliography of all relevant publications		
3. Copies of published and unpublished adverse information		
4. Summary of all other unpublished information		
5. Statement whether nonclinical tests comply with GLP regulation or justification for noncompliance		
B. Investigational Plan (21 CFR 812.25)		
1. Purpose: Are the following items clearly defined?		
a. Name and intended use of the device		
b. Objectives of the investigation		
c. Duration of the investigation (Example: specify months and years)		
2. Protocol: Are the following items present?		
a. Written protocol describing methodology including:		
i. objectives, hypothesis to be tested, or question to be answered		
ii. description of the type of trial (i.e., controlled/open, double-blind/single-blind, etc.)		
iii. detailed description of the conduct of the trial		
iv. description of statistical methods		
v. case report forms		

(Continued)

Table 51-4   (*Continued*)

Filing review elements	Yes (Present omission justified)	No (Inadequate omitted)

3. Risk Analysis: Are the following items present in the application?
  a. Description and analysis of all risks to subjects
  b. Justification for the investigation		

4. Description of the Device: Are the following items present?
  a. Description of each important component, ingredient and property
  b. Principle of Operation
  c. Copies of all labeling for the device		

5. Monitoring Procedures: Are the following items present?
  a. Written procedures for monitoring
  b. Name and address of the individual(s) who will monitor the study		

C. Manufacturing Information (21 CFR 812.20(b)(3)) Does the application contain a description of methods, facilities and controls used for:
  1. Manufacturing
  2. Processing
  3. Packing
  4. Storage
  5. Installation		

D. Investigator Information (21 CFR 812.20(b)(4): Are the following items included?
  1. Example of investigator agreement in accordance with 21 CFR 812.43(c)
  2. Certification that all participating investigators will or have signed the agreement and that no investigator will be added until the agreement is signed (21 CFR 812.20(b)(5))		

E. Sales Information (21 CFR 812.7(b)): Is the following information provided?
  1. Is the device to be sold?
  2. Explanation of why sale does not constitute commercialization		

F. Labeling (21 CFR 812.5) Is a sample of the proposed labeling complete and included in the submission?		
G. Informed Consent Materials (21 CFR 50.20 and 812.25(g)) Are *all* forms and informational materials to be presented to the subjects submitted?		

H. Environmental Impact Assessment (21 CFR 25.31 and 812.20(b)(9)): Has the sponsor provided:
  1. An environmental impact assessment describing the potential environmental impact of manufacturing and investigating a device
  2. A claim for categorical exclusion from the requirement		

Table 51-4 (*Continued*)

Filing review elements	Yes (Present omission justified)	No (Inadequate omitted)
RECOMMENDATION		
Do in-depth review_____ Prepare incomplete letter		
REVIEWED BY:		
(Reviewer's Signature)		
BRANCH: _____ DIVISION:		
DATE:		
CONCURRENCES BY:		
(Supervisor's Signature)		
DATE:		

analysts of the data. Level and methods of "blinding," if appropriate and used, are to be documented. Generally, four types of comparisons are recognized: (1) no treatments, (2) placebo control, (3) active treatment, and (4) historical controls [10]. Of these four types of controls, FDA seems to be least comfortable with the use of historical controls, particularly since historical control group patients rarely can be matched to treatment group patients.

The clinical section of the PMA must include detailed descriptions of the entire study and the study results. The sponsor must assure that all clinical studies submitted in the PMA application were conducted in conformance with the IRB and informed consent regulations, as well as with the IDE regulation, or if not, a stated reason for the noncompliance.

In recent years, FDA has required this level of clinical data in PMA submissions in order to provide reasonable assurance of the safety and effectiveness of a new class III medical device. Preliminary meetings and discussions with the FDA review staff and use of device-specific guidance documents can be critical to the success of the overall process. It is therefore clear that the conduct of a clinical trial under an IDE must be thoughtfully planned and carefully designed in order to assure that the results of the investigation will support a PMA application, and underscores the importance of the concept that before designing the clinical trial for the IDE, the requirements for the PMA must first be clearly defined.

REFERENCES

1 Federal Register. Vol. 60, No. 181 (September 19, 1995), 48417–48425.
2 Lucas JE, Cardamone TE. *Export of Medical Devices, A Workshop Manual*. FDA 95-4227, CDRH (HFZ-265).
3 21 CFR, Part 58—Good Laboratory Practice for Nonclinical Laboratory Studies.
4 21 CFR, Part 50—Protection of Human Subjects.
5 21 CFR 25.24(e)(7).
6 Federal Register. Vol. 58, No. 192 (October 6, 1993), 52144.
7 Federal Register. Vol. 59, No. 183 (September 22, 1994), 48708.
8 Federal Register. Vol. 60, No. 141 (July 24, 1995), 37856–37858.
9 Expedited Review Guidance, ODE Blue Book Memorandum, #G89-2, October 25, 1989.
10 21 CFR 860.7(f)(1).

ADDITIONAL READING

1   Heller MA. *Guide to Medical Device Regulation*. Washington, DC: Thompson Publishing Group, Inc., 1995.
2   Mohan K, Sargent HE. Clinical trials, an introduction. *Medical Device & Diagnostic Industry*, 18:1 (1996), 114–119.
3   Hurley FL, West DL. The logistics of conducting clinical studies. *Medical Device & Diagnostic Industry*, 18:5 (1996), 112–120.

Chapter 52

Protection of Human Subjects

Marien E. Evans

INTRODUCTION

For nearly fifty years, since the end of World War II, the ethics of the use of humans as the subjects of biomedical research have been the topic of discussion, argument, guidelines, pronouncements and, finally, laws and regulations. This chapter addresses, briefly, the history of human experimentation; some of the abuses, reports of which gave impetus to a congruence of the competing interests of ethicists and scientists; evolution of governmental awareness of the need to protect human subjects while encouraging needed research; and current federal regulations which reflect that awareness.

EVOLUTION OF GOVERNMENTAL AWARENESS

Biomedical experimentation using humans as subjects is not a twentieth-century phenomenon. Throughout history, man has been aware of the need for innovation in medical treatment. Egyptians were recorded as having experimented with vivisection on condemned prisoners in the first century [1]. Other notable examples of human experimentation include the eighteenth-century smallpox study conducted by Zabdiel Boylston involving the inoculation of individuals with unattenuated small pox virus. Of the 247 persons inoculated, 6 died [2]. Also in the eighteenth century, an English surgeon was found liable for damages to his patient after subjecting the patient to an experimental procedure. The surgeon was found to have deliberately re-broken his patient's leg in order to assess the efficacy of a device intended to provide for a better healing process [3]. In the early 1900s, Walter Reed's infection of volunteers with malaria received mostly positive public responses [4].

Until the present century and the development of statistical tools, however, deliberate therapeutic manipulation, or the controlled study, was relatively rare [5]. With statistical tools came abuses which led, ultimately, to governmental intervention to protect the subjects of human experimentation.

In 1945, the world was shocked to learn of the experiments on persons in concentration camps which were revealed during the prosecution of Karl Brandt and others by the Nuremberg Military Tribunal [6]. During the 1960s and 1970s other reported abuses further demonstrated the need for control of human experimentation. In the mid-1960s, it was reported that human cancer cells had been injected into the bodies of twenty-two patients of the Jewish Chronic Disease Hospital (JCDH) in Brooklyn, New York. The investigators had not obtained consent from the elderly patients because they feared an emotional response on the part of the patients as well as their refusal to participate in the study. Despite the existence of a human research committee at JCDH, investigators did not submit the protocol to the committee for approval. Further, the investigators did not seek or obtain the approval of several attending physicians prior to injecting the cancer cells [7]. In the Willowbrook studies, investigators deliberately infected institutionalized, mentally retarded children with viral hepatitis in order to study the course of the disease in institutionalized persons [8].

In the early 1970s, the Tuskegee study came to public attention. The study, which was initiated in the 1930s by the United States Public Health Service, was a long-term study of untreated syphilis. Two groups of African American males were involved in the study. One group consisted of men diagnosed with syphilis. The other group was deemed to be syphilis-free. No treatment for syphilis was provided to members of either group, even after penicillin therapy became available in the 1950s, although the disease course was monitored frequently [9].

In 1972, newspapers reported that scientists supported with National Institutes of Health funds were perfusing decapitated fetal heads to study ketone metabolism. The existence of this project contributed to a moratorium on all fetal research [10].

These studies are but a few of the more widely discussed abuses of subjects of human experimentation and demonstrate the need for protection of human subjects of biomedical investigations.

Early efforts to control experimentation on humans included peer pressure and litigation. These efforts were largely unsuccessful. For instance, Zabdiel Boylston's plan to inject individuals with live smallpox virus was condemned by the medical establishment. Despite the reaction of his peers, Boylston went forward with the experiment. Perhaps the support of Cotton Mather, the well known churchman, had a greater influence on Boylston than the opinion of his medical colleagues [11]. Similarly, legal actions for negligence instituted after the failure of unorthodox or experimental procedures seemed to have scant preventative effect [12].

The abuses in human experimentation described above occurred after the development of the Nuremberg Code, the first of more than thirty-three sets of guidelines and codes of ethics directed towards the protection of human subjects of biomedical research [13]. The Nuremberg Code, which emerged from the Allied War Council trials, consisted of ten points, the most important of which may be summarized as requiring: voluntary participation by a subject who is fully informed of the details of the study, including but not limited to the risks involved; provision for the subject's withdrawal from the study at any time with impunity; the elimination of all unnecessary risks in the design of the research, by prior animal studies if appropriate; research benefits, to either the subject or to society at large, outweighing the risks to the subject; research conducted by a competent researcher [14].

In 1962, fifteen years after the development of the Nuremberg Code and in response to the thalidomide tragedy, Congress enacted amendments to the Food Drug and Cosmetic Act [15]. The amendments, as well as the regulations promulgated in 1963 by the Food and Drug Administration (FDA), mandated that consent be obtained from human beings engaged in Investigational New Drug (IND) research. Those regulations were amended in 1966 to include the Nuremberg and Helsinki requirements for obtaining *fully informed consent* [16]. Later, the FDA required approval by Institutional Review Committees [17].

In 1964, the World Medical Association issued the Helsinki Declaration relative to the rights of subjects of human experimentation [18]. The American Medical Association and the United States Public Health Service (USPHS) in 1966 [19], as well as the FDA regulations of 1963, all adopted requirements which substantially reflected the Nuremberg principles.

The 1966 USPHS requirements regulated the use of human subjects in so called extramural research, i.e., research funded through contracts, grants and awards from the USPHS. The requirements were developed because of the lack of uniformity and control of human experimentation and such cases as the JCDH matter described above [20]. The USPHS required an assurance of prior review of research proposals by an institutional committee to assure an independent determination of: (1) the adequacy of protection of the rights and welfare of the individuals involved as subjects; (2) the appropriateness of the method of obtaining informed consent; and (3) the risks and potential medical benefit of the investigation [21]. Subsequently, USPHS published *The Institutional Guide to DHEW Policy On The Protection Of Human Subjects* in l974 [22].

During the next several years, DHEW and its successor agency, the Department of Health and Human Services (DHHS), promulgated extensive regulations relative to human subjects of biomedical research [23]. Additionally, Congressional enactment of the National Research Act of 1974 [24] and the Medical Device Amendments of 1976 [25] provided additional impetus to the development of a framework within which ethical experimentation with human subjects could be conducted. The National Research Act established the National Commission for the Protection of Human Subjects of Biomedical and Behavioral Research (National Commission) with direction to develop guidelines for the ethical conduct of human research. The National Commission identified a set of principles which were published in the Belmont Report. Those principles may be generally categorized as respect for persons, beneficence, and justice. The concept of respect involves two principles of ethical behavior. First, competent persons must be permitted the opportunity to provide prior, uncoerced, informed consent before becoming research subjects. Second, persons whose competence is diminished may participate in research only if additional protections are provided for them.

The principle of beneficence mandates that the risks of a research project be reasonable in light of the expected benefits, and that the possibility of risk be minimized and the possibility of benefit be maximized to the extent possible, consistent with good research design. The principle of justice demands that the benefits and risks of research be distributed equitably among the community in which the research is conducted [26]. In addition, the National Commission developed recommendations relative to the conduct of research with children (l972), prisoners (1977), psychosurgery (1977), institutionalized mentally infirm (1978), the establishment of Institutional Review Boards (IRBs) (1978), and research involving fetuses, pregnant women and in vitro fertilization (1978). The recommendations relative to IRBs, fetuses, pregnant women and in vitro fertilization have been incorporated into DHHS regulations at 45 CFR part 46, and FDA regulations at 21 CFR part 50. Additionally, the FDA has promulgated basic IRB and informed consent regulations similar to those promulgated by DHHS. FDA regulations apply only to research conducted with investigational new drugs, devices, and biological and radiological products [27]. DHHS regulations apply, with certain exceptions, to "all research involving human subjects conducted, supported or otherwise subject to regulation by any federal department or agency which takes administrative action to make the policy applicable to such research... except that each department or agency may adopt such procedural modifications that may be appropriate from an administrative standpoint" [28].

In 1978, Congress enacted Public Law 95-622 which established another commission to provide advice concerning the conduct of human research [29]. This commission, the President's Commission for the Study of Ethical Problems in Medicine and Biomedical and Behavioral Research, was directed to further study the ethical principles of biomedical research, the implementation of federal regulations, and the delivery of health care within the United States [30]. The President's Commission produced several reports and published *The Official IRB Guidebook* [31]. As had previous commissions and task forces, the President's Commission strongly recommended that the various federal agencies develop a uniform set of regulations governing the conduct of human research [32]. To the extent practicable, as demonstrated by the DHHS and FDA regulations referred to above, federal agencies have responded to such recommendations.

CURRENT REGULATORY FRAMEWORK

Responsibility for protecting human subjects of biomedical and behavioral research has, for the most part, been placed in the hands of the institutions at which the research is to be conducted. This responsibility has been placed in the hands of the IRB with general monitoring by the appropriate federal agency. Any research (defined as a systematic investigation designed to lead to generalizable knowledge) involving humans as subjects must be submitted to an IRB for approval prior to the initiation of the research [33]. In certain cases, IRBs which are not affiliated with institutions (free-standing IRBs) have been approved to review and approve research [34].

This discussion will focus on DHHS regulations, assuming that federal regulations regarding the protection of human subjects have been reconciled. Differences in the regulations will be described where appropriate.

Assurances

Institutions which support the conduct of human research covered by DHHS regulations or financed or conducted by a federal agency must file with the department or agency head an assurance that it will comply with the DHHS policy in the conduct of the particular research. In the alternative, an institution may submit to and obtain approval of a "general assurance" from the Office for Protection from Research Risks (OPRR), the agency within DHHS which is responsible for monitoring research projects and for providing technical assistance to IRBs. The assurance must contain, minimally: (1) a description of the institutional principals which govern the protection of the rights and welfare of human subjects who participate in any and all research conducted or supported by the institution; (2) the fact that one or more IRBs have been established in accordance with DHHS policy with adequate meeting space and support; (3) a list of the IRB membership, together with the members' qualifications and relationships to the institution and the other IRB members; (4) written procedures for the IRB's conduct of initial and continuing review of research and for reporting the IRB findings and actions to the investigator and the institution; (5) written procedures for reporting to the IRB, the institution, and the agency head any risks to the subjects or to others which had not been anticipated and any instances of serious non-compliance with DHHS policy or IRB requirements, or of termination of the project.

The assurance is evaluated by OPRR (or department head if appropriate) in accordance with specific criteria to determine whether the institution will adequately protect the rights and welfare of research subjects. After approval of the assurance, the institution is required to certify that each individual research study, not otherwise exempt, has been reviewed and approved by the IRB. Federal agencies may not support research projects unless the institution certifies that the studies have been reviewed and approved by the IRB [35]. Since the FDA does not support research, it does not require the submission of assurances *per se*. However, the FDA will not accept data supporting an IND or an IDE unless the clinical investigations have been reviewed and approved by an IRB [36].

IRB Membership

The regulations require that the IRB's membership consist of no fewer than five members whose backgrounds and qualifications are sufficiently diverse to permit thorough review of the research generally conducted at the institution. The experience and expertise of the members must be such that they are sensitive to gender issues, community attitudes, institutional commitment, applicable regulations and law and standards of professional conduct. If an IRB regularly reviews projects involving special populations, it may involve one or more persons who are experienced in working with that population, e.g., pediatricians, if children are frequent subjects. Selection of the members may not be gender-biased; that is, the membership should not consist of a single sex, and the board must include at least one member who is not otherwise affiliated with the institution and who is not related to any other member. Such members are often referred to as "public members." At least one IRB member must be a scientist and the primary concern of at least one member must be in a non-scientific area. Any member who has a conflicting interest in a protocol being reviewed by the IRB must not participate in consideration of the proposal, although she or he may provide information requested by the IRB. Of course, IRBs may invite individuals with expertise in special areas to assist in evaluating projects, but those individuals may not vote with the IRB [37].

General Requirements for IRB Review

In performing their duties, IRBs are required to follow the policies set forth in their approved assurances. Except in the case of "expedited review," the IRB must review the research proposal at a regularly convened meeting of at least a majority of the members. Approval of a majority of the members present is required.

No prescription exists for the frequency of meetings, although the requirement of at least annual continuing review of projects would mandate at least annual meetings [38]. An IRB may approve, disapprove or require modifications of proposed projects. An IRB's disapproval of a project is final; although institutional officials may further review the project, they may not validly approve a project which the IRB has disapproved. They may, however, disapprove a project which the Board has approved [39].

An IRB must require that the information provided to subjects as part of the informed consent process complies with regulation 45 CFR, s 46.116, discussed below. The IRB may require the provision of additional information to the subject if the members determine that such information would enhance the protection of the subject's rights and welfare. Documentation of informed consent shall be required unless the IRB waives the requirement in accordance with the conditions set forth in s. 46117 (c) of the regulations. Those conditions include a finding that either (1) the consent form would be the only record linking the subject to the research and that the primary risk of the research would be a breach of confidentiality; or that (2) the research presents no more than minimal risk of harm to the subject and involves no procedure for which written consent would not otherwise be obtained. Minimal risk is defined as meaning that the probability and magnitude of harm or discomfort anticipated in the research are no greater in and of themselves than those ordinarily encountered in daily life or during the performance of routine physical or psychological examinations or tests [40]. The FDA regulations permit the waiver of documentation of informed consent only if the research involves minimal risk to the subject and involves no procedures for which written consent would otherwise be obtained [41]. As discussed below, FDA regulations also provide for the conduct of clinical investigations in the absence of informed consent in certain situations [42]. Both DHHS and FDA regulations permit the IRB to require investigators to provide subjects with a written statement regarding the investigation in the event of a waiver [43].

Expedited Review

The Secretary of DHHS and the FDA have published in the Federal Register lists of categories of research which may be approved by an IRB by an expedited procedure. These lists are updated periodically in the Federal Register. The IRB may use expedited procedures to review the research which appears on the list and are found by the reviewers to involve no more than minimal risk to the subject. Minor changes in previously approved research may also be approved as the result of an expedited review. The expedited review may be performed by one or more experienced IRB members designated by the chairperson, or by the chairperson him/herself. In any event, the reviewer may not disapprove the research. Only the full Board is authorized to disapprove the research after a complete review [44]. IRB procedures should provide for referral to the full Board of protocols about which the reviewers have concerns over approving through the expedited process.

Criteria for IRB Approval

In order to approve a research proposal, an IRB must make seven specific findings relative to the proposal [45]. Those findings are: (1) that risks to subjects are minimized by the use of procedures consistent with sound research design and which do not unnecessarily expose the subject to risk, and where possible, by using procedures already being performed on the subjects; (2) that risks to subjects are reasonable in relation to anticipated benefits, if any, and the importance of the knowledge to be gained (only the risks of the research are to be considered, not risks and benefits of therapies the subject would otherwise receive); (3) that the subjects are selected equitably, taking into account the purpose of the investigation, the setting in which it will take place and the vulnerability of any of the subjects involved; (4) that informed consent will be sought from prospective subjects or their legally authorized representatives, which is a court or other body or individual authorized by applicable law to consent to the subject's participation in the study [46]; (5) that informed consent will be documented in accordance with regulations; (6) that where appropriate, adequate provisions are made in the protocol for monitoring data collection; (7) that adequate provisions are made to protect the subject's privacy and the data's confidentiality, and if vulnerable populations are involved, that additional protections are provided.

IRBs, or their institutions, are required to maintain records of IRB activities, including copies of proposals, consent documents, progress reports, and minutes of IRB meetings together with the votes taken as well as discussions held. The records must also contain a list of the IRB membership and procedures, documentation of continuing review, and correspondence relative to the projects, as well as statements of any new findings provided to subjects. These records must be available to inspection by federal officials. If an institution fails to maintain such records or refuses to permit inspection, DHHS may withdraw support of the project or deny support for future projects [47]. Also, the FDA may refuse to accept data collected in support of test articles and it may disqualify the IRB [48].

Informed Consent

As discussed earlier in this chapter, the doctrine of informed consent in the research setting evolved, in great part, because of the reported abuses of patients' rights, and is directed towards the voluntary and informed decision of individuals to participate in the research process. The doctrine has been refined and codified in federal regulations [49]. Except under circumstances described later in this chapter, no individual may be involved in research covered by federal regulations unless the investigator has obtained legally effective informed consent from the prospective subject or a representative. The information must be provided under circumstances such that the prospective subject or representative has adequate time to come to a reasoned decision about participating. The information must be presented in language comprehensible to the prospective subject or representative—in the native language if appropriate. The IRB should be aware of any communication problems which might be anticipated. The information may not contain any language which may result in, or appear to result in, the subject's waiving any legal rights or releasing the investigator, the institution or its agents from liability for negligence.

The basic elements of informed consent may be summarized as follows: (1) a description of the study, including the fact that it is research, the scientific principles involved, and the duration of the subject's participation; (2) a description of any reasonably foreseeable risks or discomforts involved; (3) a description of any expected benefits; (4) information about any advantageous alternative treatment which might be available; (5) a statement concerning the confidentiality of information; (6) a statement relative to compensation or medical treatment available if greater than minimal risk is involved; (7) the names of persons to contact about the subject's rights and research-related injury; and (8) a statement that participation is voluntary and that refusal to participate or withdrawal from the study will not jeopardize any rights or benefits to which the subject is entitled [50].

Where appropriate, the IRB may require that additional information is provided to the prospective subject or representative. That information may include: (1) a statement that the procedure may involve risks which are currently unforeseeable; (2) a description of the circumstances under which the subject's participation may be terminated unilaterally by the investigator; (3) any additional costs to the subject because of the experimental aspects of the study; (4) the consequences of the subject's decision to withdraw from the study and the procedure for terminating participation; (5) a statement that any significant findings that might impact on the subject's desire to continue participation in the study will be provided; and (6) the approximate number of subjects to be involved in the study [51]. The additional requirements for vulnerable populations will be discussed below.

Exceptions to the Requirement for Informed Consent

Both FDA and DHHS regulations allow for exceptions to the requirement of obtaining informed consent from prospective subjects under very specific conditions. As of this writing, FDA regulations permit the use of test articles and devices in clinical investigations without prior consent under circumstances where obtaining such consent is deemed not to be feasible by both the investigator and a physician who is not otherwise associated with the investigation. Both individuals must certify that: (1) the human subject is in a life-threatening situation necessitating use of the test article; (2) informed consent can not be obtained because of the inability to communicate with or to obtain legally effective consent from the subject; (3) insufficient time is available to obtain consent from the subject's representative; and (4) no approved or generally recognized alternative therapy which would offer the same or a greater likelihood of saving the subject's life is available [52].

If time does not permit contacting an independent physician because of the emergent nature of the subject's condition, the test article may be used without such consent. However, within 5 working days of the use of the article, a written review and evaluation must be conducted by an independent physician. Documentation of the need and review must be submitted to the IRB within 5 days of use of the article [53].

The DHHS does not make similar provisions in its regulations for research which does not fall under the authority of the FDA. As previously discussed, DHHS regulations permit waiver of informed consent only where minimal risk is involved. For several years, IRBs utilized a "deferred consent" procedure in circumstances in which the FDA regulations did not apply, but informed consent could not be obtained from subjects or their representatives. This deferred consent process, which has not been sanctioned by either the FDA or OPRR, relied upon obtaining consent from the subject or representative after the treatment. The subject or representative was asked to ratify use of the treatment after the fact and to agree to continuation of the therapy [54].

In response to concerns articulated by numerous organizations, individuals and IRBs over the constraints against evaluating current medical practices relative to, for example, emergency treatment of head injuries, the FDA in September 1995 proposed new rules which when finalized will amend 21 CFR, s 50.24 and 21 CFR parts 312 and 812 to permit the conduct of clinical investigations when obtaining informed consent is not feasible. The amendments would allow for such investigations if the IRB, with a licensed physician concurring, finds that the human subjects are in life-threatening situations, available treatments are unproven or unsatisfactory, and the collection of valid scientific information is most beneficial. Obtaining consent may not be feasible because the medical condition prevents the subject from giving consent, time does not permit obtaining consent from a representative and the emergence of the condition could not have been predicted so that consent could have been obtained in advance. Additionally, the IRB must find that the research is in the best interest of the subject, the risks are reasonable, and the research could not, practically, be conducted in absence of the waiver.

Additional protections of the rights and welfare of the subject must be monitored. For example, an IRB will be expected to consult with representatives of the communities from which subjects will be selected. Before beginning the study, the investigator or the sponsor will be required to publicly disclose information sufficient to describe the study, its risks and benefits. Upon completion of the study, the results must be publicly disclosed. An independent board will be established to monitor subject safety and data collected. The IRB must also review and approve a consent document to be used where feasible. As soon as possible, the subject, the representative or family member will be informed of the nature of the study and of the right to terminate participation in the study.

Protocols involving the proposed exceptions must be performed under separate INDs or IDEs, even if they would be covered under existing INDs or IDEs. It must be clearly noted in the IND or IDE that subjects who would not be able to provide consent will participate in the project [55].

Documentation of Informed Consent

Federal regulations require that investigators document that informed consent has been obtained. Such documentation may be accomplished by providing the subject or representative with a document ("consent form") which fully encompasses the elements of informed consent. The document may be read to the subject or representative; however, ample opportunity must be provided for the subject or representative to read the document before signing it. The IRB may also approve the use of a "short form" which states that the elements of informed consent have been presented orally. A witness must observe this presentation and the IRB must approve a written summary of the information to be presented to the subject or representative. The subject or representative need only sign the short form, but the witness must sign both the short form and the summary. Copies of both the short form and the summary are to be provided to the subject or representative [56]. As noted previously, DHHS regulations currently permit the IRB to waive the documentation requirement when the only link between the subject and the research is the consent document, the principle risk is a breach of confidentiality, only minimum risk is involved and the subject agrees to the waiver [57].

Special Populations

Certain individuals who may become the subjects of biomedical investigations, by virtue of their ages, mental capabilities or life situations, are exquisitely susceptible to exploitation. In recognition of this vulnerability, federal agencies have promulgated additional requirements designed to further protect the rights and welfare of children [58], and prisoners [59] and to assure the ethical conduct of research involving fetuses, pregnant women and human in vitro fertilization [60].

Additional Protections Relative to Fetuses

In 1975, HEW promulgated its initial regulations governing research with fetuses [61]. Those regulations have been amended as recently as 1994 [62], and impose conditions in addition to those discussed above. The FDA has no final regulations analogous to the DHHS regulations.

DHHS itself has assumed a greater degree of responsibility relative to research involving fetuses, pregnant women and in vitro fertilization by the establishment of "Ethical Advisory Boards." Such boards are established by the Secretary with a membership competent to address medical, legal, societal, ethical and related issues. The Ethical Advisory Board renders advice as to the ethical issues raised by experimentation proposed to be conducted under these regulations. The board may establish categories of research which need not be submitted for its review as well as categories which, absent review and approval from the board, may not be funded by DHHS [63].

Additionally, IRBs which review such research have the added responsibility of determining that sufficient consideration has been given to the methods of selecting prospective subjects so that the onus does not fall on a single population. Also, IRBs must evaluate the procedures for monitoring the consent process and, where appropriate, that monitoring may be performed by the IRB itself or by subject advocates observing the consent process. Another additional responsibility is that of monitoring the progress of the research activity to determine whether any risks have surfaced. IRBs may also be assigned additional tasks by the Secretary [64].

General Requirements

Investigators who intend to conduct research involving fetuses, pregnant women, or *in vitro* fertilization are obligated to ascertain that appropriate animal studies or studies involving non-pregnant women have been completed. Unless the purpose of the study is to address the mother's medical needs or those of the particular fetus, the risk to the fetus may not be greater than minimal and the risk is the least possible for achieving the purposes of the study. Investigators are not permitted to participate in any decisions regarding: the timing of termination of the pregnancy; the method of termination of the pregnancy; or the determination of the viability of the fetus. Great care must be taken to insure that no change in the abortion procedure which would involve more than minimal risk to the mother or to the fetus may be introduced for the purposes of the study. Finally, no compensation or other inducements may be offered to a woman to induce her to terminate her pregnancy for research purposes [65].

Pregnant Women as Research Subjects

Unless the research is directed towards the woman's medical needs and the risk to the fetus will not exceed that necessary to address those needs or risk to the fetus is minimal, pregnant women may not be involved in research. Both parents must be legally competent to give informed consent and the information provided must include any potential harm to the fetus. Consent from the father need not be obtained if the research is intended to benefit the mother, if the father is unavailable, if his identity or whereabouts is unknown or if the pregnancy was the result of rape [66].

Fetuses Ex Utero

Unless the purpose of the research is to enhance the potential for survival of the fetus, or the research will not risk the viability of the fetus, and the purpose of the study is to obtain vital medical information which can not otherwise be obtained, ex utero non-viable fetuses may not be the subject of research [67]. If the fetus is viable, it is an infant and any research is governed by regulations pertinent to children [68]. Research involving non-living fetus or fetal tissue is governed by applicable State and local law [69].

Research Involving Prisoners

Because of the potential for abusing the rights of incarcerated individuals, special additional requirements have been adopted by both DHHS and FDA relative to research involving that population. Because of the special circumstances, a different definition of minimal risk is applied. Minimal risk, for the purpose of these regulations, is "the probability and magnitude of physical or psychological harm that is normally encountered in the daily lives or in the routine medical, dental or psychological evaluations of healthy persons" [70].

A majority of the members of IRBs which review research projects that contemplate enrolling prisoners as subjects may not have an affiliation with the prisons involved, and at least one member of the Board must be a prisoner or a prisoner representative. The IRBs have the additional responsibilities of insuring that the research involves the study of the causes, effects and processes of incarceration, or of prisons as institutional structures, or of prisoners as incarcerated persons. No more than minimal risk may be involved and no more than minimal inconvenience may be caused to the subjects. IRBs must also determine that possible advantages to the subjects are not so great that they impair the prisoner's ability to weigh the risks against those advantages. The risks involved must be commensurate with the risks that would be acceptable to non-prisoner volunteers. Selection of the subjects must be fair and without intervention from prison authorities. Parole boards may not take into account the fact that a prisoner has participated in research in deciding whether to grant parole. IRBs must insure that participants are informed of any need for care following conclusion of the study [71].

In addition to studies of the sociological aspects of prisons, prisoners may be involved in studies which have a reasonable probability of improving the health and well-being of the prison population. In such cases, the Secretary consults with appropriate experts before deciding whether the studies may take place [72].

Special Protections for Children

Children are particularly vulnerable as research subjects because their ages, emotional and intellectual capacities, and educational levels constrain their abilities to comprehend the effect of research. In addition, they are not legally competent to provide consent to participation in research studies. Therefore, pursuant to DHHS regulations, IRBs are required to insure that the special protections are in place before approving studies involving children. The protections include obtaining the assent (not merely lack of objection) of the child, if the IRB deems the child capable of assenting to participate, as well as the permission of one or both parents or a guardian [73]. Children may participate in research involving more than minimal risk only if the risk is justified by the expected benefit to the child, the risk/benefit ratio is at least equal to that of alternative therapies, and assent and permission are obtained [74]. Minimal risk for children is that inherent in actual or expected medical, dental, psychological, social or educational situations [75]. A study which would expose children to a minor increase over minimal risk may be approved only if the study would provide generalizable knowledge about the child's own condition and is vitally important to understanding that condition [76]. Under certain circumstances, with the approval of the Secretary, studies offering no potential benefit to the participating children may be conducted if the study has a reasonable potential for providing an understanding of or treatment for children's illnesses [77].

Wards of the state or other agency may not participate in research which is not of direct benefit to them, unless, in addition to other requirements, the study is related to their status as wards, the majority of the children involved are not wards, and an advocate is appointed to act on behalf of the children [78].

SUMMARY

This chapter deals with the need for protection of the rights and welfare of human subjects of biomedical research, and the development by the federal government of procedures and regulations to insure those protections. The cogent regulations are summarized and discrepancies between FDA and DHHS regulations are noted. This chapter does not discuss state and local requirements which, if more restrictive than the analogous federal requirements, must be followed.

REFERENCES

1 Brady J, Johnson A. The evolution of regulatory influences on research with human subjects. In *Human Subject Research*. New York: Plenum Press, 1982, 3.
2 Moore D. Therapeutic innovations: Ethical boundaries in the initial clinical trials of new drugs and surgical procedures. *Daedulus*, 98 (1969), 502.
3 *Slater v Baker and Stapleton*, 2 Wilson K.B. 339, 95 Eng. Rep. 860 (1767).
4 Brady J, Johnson A. The evolution of regulatory influences on research with human subjects. In *Human Subject Research*. New York: Plenum Press, 1982, 3.
5 Brady J, Johnson A. The evolution of regulatory influences on research with human subjects. In *Human Subject Research*. New York: Plenum Press, 1982, 4.
6 *U.S. v Karl Brandt, et al.* Trials of War Criminals Before Nuremberg Military Tribunals Under Control Council Law, No. 10. The Medical Case, Vol. 2 (1947).
7 Hyman v. *Jewish Chronic Disease Hospital*, 206 NE 2d 338 (1965).
8 Hersey N, Johnson R. *Human Experimentation and the Law*. Baltimore, Maryland: Aspen Systems, 1976, 8–9.
9 Hersey N, Johnson R. *Human Experimentation and the Law*. Baltimore, Maryland: Aspen Systems, 1976, 9.

10 Brady J, Johnson A. The evolution of regulatory influences on research with human subjects. In *Human Subject Research*. New York: Plenum Press, 1982, 6.

11 Brady J, Johnson A. The evolution of regulatory influences on research with human subjects. In *Human Subject Research*. New York: Plenum Press, 1982, 3.

12 *Carpenter v Baker*, 60 Barb 481 (NY 1871).

13 *U.S. v Karl Brandt, et al.* Trials of War Criminals Before Nuremberg Military Tribunals Under Control Council Law, No. 10. The Medical Case, Vol. 2 (1947).

14 *U.S. v Karl Brandt, et al.* Trials of War Criminals Before Nuremberg Military Tribunals Under Control Council Law, No. 10. The Medical Case, Vol. 2 (1947).

15 P.L. 87-781, 21 USC 355, *et seq.*

16 Curran, WJ. Governmental regulation of the use of human subjects in medical research: The approach of two federal agencies. *Daedulus*, 98 (1969), 542–594.

17 Curran, WJ. Governmental regulation of the use of human subjects in medical research: The approach of two federal agencies. *Daedulus*, 98 (1969), 542–594.

18 World Medical Association. Recommendations guiding doctors in clinic research. *British Medical Journal*, 196:2.

19 Curran, WJ. Governmental regulation of the use of human subjects in medical research: The approach of two federal agencies. *Daedulus*, 98 (1969), 542–594.

20 Brady J, Johnson A. The evolution of regulatory influences on research with human subjects. In *Human Subject Research*. New York: Plenum Press, 1982, 3.

21 Hersey N, Johnson R. *Human Experimentation and the Law*. Rockville, MD: Aspen Systems, 1976, 8–9.

22 *The Institutional Guide to DHEW Policy on Protection of Human Subjects*. Washington, DC: Department of Health Education and Welfare, 1971.

23 39 FR 30618, August 25, 1974.

24 Pub. Law 93-348.

25 Pub. Law 92-295.

26 44 FR 23193, April 18, 1979.

27 60 FR 49088, September 21, 9295.

28 45 CFR s. 46.101.

29 Pub. Law 95-622.

30 Pub. Law 95-622.

31 The Official IRB Guide Book. Washington, DC: Office for Protection from Research Risk, 1982.

32 60 FR 49086, September 21, 1995.

33 45 CFR s. 46.101; 21 CFR s.50.1.

34 45 CFR s. 46.103.

35 45 CFR s. 46.103.

36 21 CFR s. 56.103.

37 45 CFR s. 46.107; 21 CFR s. 56.107.

38 45 CFR s. 46.109; 21 CFR s. 56.109.

39 45 CFR s. 46.112; 21 CFR s. 56.112.

40 45 CFR s. 46.102 (i).

41 21 CFR s. 56.109 (c).

42 21 CFR s. 50.23 (a), (b).

43 45 CFR s. 46.117 (c) (2); 21 CFR s.56.109 (3).

44 45 CFR s. 46.110; 21 CFR s. 56.110.

45 45 CFR s. 36.116; 21 CFR 50.24

46 45 CFR s. 46.102 (c); 21 CFR s. 50.3 (m).

47 45 CFR s. 46.123.

48 21 CFR s. 56.120, *et. seq.*

49 45 CFR s. 46.117; 21 CFR s. 50.20.

50 45 CFR s. 46.116; 21CFR s.50.25.

51 45 CFR s. 46.116 (b); 21CFR s. 50.25 (b).

52 21 CFR s. 50.23

53 21 CFR s. 50.23 (c).

54 60 FR 49088, September 21, 1995.

55 60 FR 49094, 49095, September 21, 1995.

56 45 CFR s. 46.117; 21 CFR s.50.27.

57 45 CFR s. 46.117 (c).

58   45 CFR s. 46.401, *et. seq.*
59   45 CFR s. 46.301, *et. seq.*; 21 CFR s.50.40, *et. seq.*
60   45 CFR s. 46.201, *et. seq.*
61   40 FR 33528, August 8, 1975.
62   59 FR 28276, June 1, 1995.
63   45 CFR s. 46.204.
64   45 CFR s. 46.205.
65   45 CFR s. 46.206.
66   45 CFR s. 46.208.
67   45 CFR s. 46.208.
68   45 CFR s. 46.209.
69   45 CFR s. 46.210.
70   45 CFR s. 46.303 (d); 21 CFR s. 50.44.
71   45 CFR s. 46.305; 21CFR s. 50.48.
72   45 CFR s. 46.306.
73   45 CFR s. 46.408.
74   45 CFR s. 46.405.
75   45 CFR s. 46.406 (b).
76   45 CFR s. 46.406.
77   45 CFR s. 46.407.
78   45 CFR s. 46.409.

ADDITIONAL READING

1   Fost N, Robertson JA. Deferring consent with incompetent patients in an intensive care unit. *IRB Review of Human Subject Research.* 2 (1980), 5–6.
2   Levine R. Commentary: Deferred consent. *Controlled Clinical Trials*, 12 (1991), 546–550.
3   Olson CM. The letter or spirit; consent for research in CPR. *JAMA*, 271 (1994), 1445–1447.
4   Informed consent– Legally effective and prospectively obtained. *OPRR Reports–Human Subject Protections.* 93:3 (1993).
5   Levine R. Research in emergency situations; the role of deferred consent. *JAMA*, 273 (1995), 1300–1302.
6   Sprung C, Winnick B. Informed consent in theory and practice: Legal and medical perspectives on the informed consent doctrine and a reconceptualization. *Critical Care Medicine*, 17 (1989), 1346–1354.
7   Rosoff A. *Informed Consent*. Rockville, MD: Aspen Publishing, 1981.

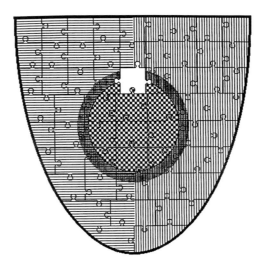

Section Ten

Clinical Trials

Stephen R. Ash

INTRODUCTION

The development of new biomaterials and new devices is requiring more resources, more time, and more patience than ever. It was once sufficient to develop a new material, substitute it for a similar component in a medical device, perform some in vitro tests, test the new device in a short, nonrandomized clinical trial to prove safety (often under IRB approval), and submit a 510(k) application to the FDA with sufficient justification for safety of the new material. A similar "friendly IRB" pathway was possible for most new devices. Only those materials and devices which were implanted long-term and were life-supporting (Class III devices, by FDA definition) required clinical trials proving efficacy as well as safety. The 510(k) route to achieve approval to market a device "substantially similar" to a prior device was considerably simpler than the Pre-Market Approval (PMA) route to market a truly new device.

With the Medical Device Act of 1990, the requirement for clinical trials for all 510(k) devices was expanded, and the nature of these clinical trials was defined. All 510(k) applications for Class II and Class III devices now require clinical trials to justify that *safety* and *efficacy* of the device is similar to previously marketed devices. Further, these clinical trials must be performed in a *randomized, prospectively-controlled* manner, meaning that some patients receive treatment by prior devices, and other patients receive treatment with the new device. The mathematical analysis needed to assure that treated and control patient groups are similar is not defined, but need for this analysis is implied. Finally, the classification of a device depends not upon its own intrinsic risk, but upon the risk of priorly marketed devices. A device will be considered Class II if the indication for use is the same as a prior Class II device, and Class III if the indication is the same as a prior Class III device. In essence, the FDA has made the 510(k) and PMA routes to market devices similar, has made randomized, prospectively controlled studies the only allowed structure, and blunted the difference between Class II and Class III devices.

Since adequate clinical trials are now more narrowly defined and more frequently required, their design is more important than ever. The chapters in this section address the following critical issues: Chapter 53, the logical approach to patient selection, including means to assure similar features in treated and control groups; Chapter 54, the different phases of device testing as defined by the FDA, and methods to adjust the protocol to be appropriate with each phase of the testing; Chapter 55, the general considerations and limitations of clinical testing; Chapter 56, the malpractice risk in clinical trials and how to minimize this risk; and Chapter 57, the control of release of information to the public during a clinical trial.

Chapters 54, 55, and 57 are reprinted with only minor adjustments by the editor. These chapters reflect enduring, patient-related issues in clinical device testing that should be the concern not only of the investigative clinician but also of the implant design team.

Chapter 53

Patient Selection

Ronald L. Wathen

Chapters 55 and 56 represent a new thrust into education of the biomedical professional involved in materials or device development for human use. Background or support literature therefore is scant, there being only one prior publication identified which deals with the problem of patient selection for clinical trials similar to the purpose and manner described here. Since the scope of this prior publication involved only artificial kidney (dialyzer) testing [1], it was of limited help in preparing this new approach. There is one journal [2] available which deals with clinical trials. However, this journal is mainly concerned with the testing of drugs, the theory and practice of which are not necessarily germane to materials or device testing.

Thus, the development of a logical approach to patient selection and utilization in device testing meets almost a singular need. The approach must include an orderly examination of general concerns (e.g., age, gender, race, cultural background), as well as severity of illness, degree of help conferred by a given device, medical perspective on devices, criteria for patient selection, and the practical aspects of informed consent. Some of these issues are so straightforward that they require little comment, while others, perhaps not so obvious to the nonphysician biomedical professional, require extensive treatment. Because of my background in the theory and application of hemodialysis therapy, the I have drawn heavily on personal experiences in device development as they relate to treatment of kidney failure.

Finally, clinical trials of materials or devices, more often than not, require a team effort, minimally including both engineer and physician. The team may additionally consist of allied health professionals, such as a skilled nurse, social worker, and dietitian.

DEMOGRAPHIC FACTORS

As a single factor concerning entry of a patient into a clinical trial, age is important because of legal aspects attributable to being a minor. Parent(s) or guardian(s) may speak for a minor, in which case the age factor largely becomes a medical rather than a legal issue. The investigator, whenever possible, should obtain written consent from both parents (living together or not, biological or not) or guardian(s) (there may be more than one) before entry of a minor into a trial. The intent of informed consent is to inform all, including the minor patient. Inclusion of the minor in a trial may not be desirable, if the patient is so young as to lack adequate cognitive (comprehension) or language (expression) skills.

There are less obvious constraints imposed by age of the recipient of a material or device. The investigator, for example, may not feel comfortable working with patients who are too young to be able to understand what is happening. Conversely, if the patient is elderly, the investigator might question the correctness of applying an unproved device to such a patient for fear of foreshortening any useful time left to the patient. One must weigh both purpose and expectation for a device when considering age as a factor. Implicit in age, also, is whether or not the patient is capable of self-care. This ability may be the crucial factor to achieving a favorable outcome in clinical trials.

More often than not, age to adulthood correlates with the size of the patient. Therefore, if the device to be tested is physically large and cumbersome and requires implantation, then a child is far less likely to be a reasonable subject that an adolescent or adult. There are situations, however, where device testing in the very young, based on the intent of the device, is highly desirable. An example might be the testing of the artificial "ear"; several types and models are currently available or under trial. The desirability of testing artificial ears in the very young emanates here from the fact that, if successful, the patient will be far more likely to develop language skills, the very lack of which was indicated above as a subtle, but not absolute, contraindication for device testing.

Gender may require little attention when considering device testing; e.g., if a hearing deficit can be attenuated or corrected with application of an artificial "ear," then both sexes would benefit equally. Financial productivity, because of the expense incurred by utilization of the device, was a major consideration in the early (pre-Medicare) days of artificial kidney therapy, a time when this treatment could still be considered to be in its clinical trial stage. Thus, historically, the middle-aged housewife with no dependent children (and, similarly but irrespective of gender, the very young and the very old) was far less likely to be considered for dialysis therapy than was the young adult, fiscally productive male with a family to support. With well over 100,000 male and female patients maintained by dialysis in the United States today, one can safely assume that such therapy is beyond both the clinical trial and the discriminatory stage. Fortunately, patient selection today for clinical trials must be passed upon by the local Institutional Review Board, not by a "life or death" committee.

There are body habitus considerations regarding the sex of the individual. For instance, if a device is to be implanted in the arm or connected to blood vessels or placed inside the chest or burrowed into the skull or gums of the patient, then, generally speaking, in the initial throes of a study, the larger adolescent or adult male will prove an easier (and safer) recipient for device implantation and manipulation. A device typically undergoes size reduction as it goes through development so that, ultimately, gender diminishes in importance in the patient selection process.

There are otherwise few gender-dependent physiological or anatomical constraints in device testing other than where the device is considered gender-specific (e.g., male penile or female breast prostheses). Experience with breast prostheses also underscores the seriousness, sometimes disastrous outcome, of materials and device use. The major manufacturer of silicone prosthetic devices (Cordis-Dow) was forced into bankruptcy in 1995 due to lawsuits emanating from the (still presumed) immunologic complications which have ostensibly occurred in thousands of prothesis recipients after years of prolific use of the silicone material. Interestingly, male silicone penile prostheses have not been similarly associated with immunologic disorders.

There are presently no apparent major considerations of race relevant to device or materials testing. Of course, one could conjecture development of an intra- or extra-corporeal device used to treat a hemoglobin disorder such as sickle cell anemia, a disease found predominantly in the Black race. Clearly, to test such a device, one would have to seek out patients of the appropriate race. Similarly, though not a racial consideration, to develop a device for treatment of Tay-Sachs disease, a lipid storage abnormality of metabolism, patients of Jewish or eastern European ancestry would be needed for testing. These examples are of additional importance because they again emphasize age considerations; because of their severity, living patients with these diseases are likely to be minors, not adults.

An intra- or extra-corporeal device used in the treatment of disease is generally divorced from racial considerations. Illustrating this would be a device that could be used in the treatment of anyone of a number of leukemias, these being blood dyscrasias which are generally without racial predilection. However, age, again, becomes a major consideration, since leukemias are broadly divided into childhood and adult forms which, moreover, may require totally different therapeutic strategies. Ideally, blood dyscrasias, congenital metabolic disorders and many other illnesses will someday become amenable to gene manipulative therapy, once transcription of the human genome is complete and we learn how to use the information. Such therapy may still require intra- or extra-corporeal materials and device considerations.

Cultural heritage and religious preference are frequently fused in social definition, more because of the impact of religion than heritage. Examine the cultural differences between a highly educated, urban bank president and a little-educated backwoods laborer. Both may be Fundamentalists/Pentecostalists of the Christian faith. Both, for example, may be Jehovah's Witnesses. Because of the differences in educational backgrounds, each can be anticipated to rationalize religious viewpoints differently. But in this instance, because of secular inflexibility, each can also be expected to rebuke blood or blood-product transfusions and, often, cadaveric organ transplantation. It would be uncommon, however, for one of the Jehovah's Witness faith, particularly the more urban individual, to renounce application of an artificial life-sustaining device, since it is not comprised of blood products.

Social or educational deprivation, not religious preference, are often major considerations in device testing; i.e., ignorance can breed skepticism and fear, if not paranoia. The investigator must never appear condescending; the appropriate choice of words is of utmost importance in written and verbal communication in order to elicit trust. Ideally, the clinical trials investigator and team should have access to patients crossing all educational and social strata to fully evaluate a given material or device.

SEVERITY OF PATIENT DISEASE

There are numerous classifications regarding the type and severity of illness. Every subspecialty in medicine has its favorite method of classification (e.g., the American Heart Association classification for the cardiac patient, the Arthritis Foundation for the arthritic patient, or the American Diabetes Association for the diabetic patient). For device testing, it is recommended that the rather simple classification of terminally ill, seriously ill, and functionally impaired be adopted, the latter being intended also to identify patients for specific male and female prosthetic devices such as penile and breast implants where psychological impairment is sometimes the apparent predominating disorder. Such a generic approach provides the philosophical underpinning for device testing, irrespective of the type of illness or organ system involved. Thus, the terminally ill patient is awaiting death, the severely ill may be very limited and suffer repetitive hospitalizations but death can be forestalled, and the functionally impaired may exist without significant medical intervention. In the order given, examples might include the inoperable lung cancer patient, the chronic renal failure patient, and the deaf/blind patient.

Many people are born with congenital illnesses, presenting as either inherited metabolic disorders or structural deformities, including absence of certain nervous system functions, such as vision, hearing, or motor coordination. People so burdened often work hard to minimize their deficiency to the point that, frequently, the handicap, even if severe, may be largely ignored or, perhaps, even suppressed in the patient's mind. To illustrate this, a 29-year-old white male, with muscular torso and arms but wheelchair-bound since birth because of spina bifida (a disorder of the spinal cord), related that he had recently placed third among wheelchair contestants in a 13-mile mini-marathon, in fact, nearly tying the winning (normal) runner! This feat is additionally spectacular because the patient also had been surviving for more than 5 years on hemodialysis with all of its attendant inadequacies. Spina bifida frequently results in end-stage renal disease due to neurogenic bladder complications.

It is necessary that the subject view a defect as a disability in order to be receptive to device trials that might reduce the disability. Obviously, a totally blind or deaf individual, whether or not congenital, is likely to be receptive to being a test subject to restore either of these crucial senses, even if only partially. It can be speculated, however, that there are few people with a withered arm or leg who would endure amputation of the afflicted extremity, no matter how contorted or functionally ineffective, to submit to a trial with a new life-like, even highly functional prosthesis.

The patient with an acquired infirmity or illness (e.g., traumatic amputation of a limb, traumatic blindness or deafness, life-threatening cancer or leukemia, or end-stage heart, kidney or liver disease) is likely to view such defects differently from the patient with a congenital defect because the former will have a reference point, i.e., the prior state of normalcy. Even while maintaining an apparently bright psychological outlook, however, such patients may voice futility over efforts to compensate their infirmities by artificial means. Passive-dependent attitudes of patients with acquired chronic illnesses or afflictions are well recognized within the medical community.

For severe, particularly acquired, disorders where death is imminent, the patient's outlook may also be pervaded by a "What have I got to lose?" attitude. It is all too easy for a clinical trials team to take advantage of such patients. Complete, almost bone-jarring, honesty must be maintained regarding the possible outcome(s) regarding the nature of the illness; the patient must be fully informed concerning the potential of severe injury, even death, in relation to the material or device being tested. Submission to a clinical trial may also prove to be a subtle, passive suicide attempt on the part of the severely afflicted, terminally ill patient. It is not for the team to pass moral judgments on such situations but to recognize that they exist. Whenever possible, the legal next-of-kin or representative should be present during any major discussions with the seriously or terminally ill prospective test subject. This will minimize the risk for later confusion within the patient's family, if not malpractice complaints.

DEGREE OF HELP CONFERRED BY DEVICE

When considering the degree of help conferred by a device, one often must reckon first with the imminence of death. Imagine, for example, the patient with end-stage heart disease who is hospital-bound and completely bedridden, being maintained with intravenous drugs and nutrients and perhaps a ventilating machine. The patient's physician(s) might conclude that life cannot be maintained without these assists and that in spite of them, multi-organ failure is developing secondary to underperfusion with blood. The decision may then be made to implant an essential (life-giving) device, an artificial heart, with the intent in mind possibly of maintaining the recipient until an appropriate cadaveric donor heart becomes available for transplantation. This scenario is becoming increasingly common today.

The above discussion immediately brings to mind Barney Clark, the recipient of one of the most dramatic materials and device tests in the history of medicine (i.e., the first human recipient of an artificial heart). Fiscal and other issues surrounding the Barney Clark episode are published elswhere [3, 4]. The outcome for Barney Clark illustrates the irreversibility a test can impose. Once the recipient's heart was surgically removed to make room for insertion of the artificial heart, there remained no other immediate life-giving alternative for the patient. Furthermore, because the artificial heart evoked severe systemic disease (multiple thrombo-emboli or blood clots), the patient's remaining potential alternative of cadaveric heart transplantation rapidly dissipated. After 112 medically tempestuous days, Barney Clark was declared dead.

In using the first artificial heart test as an example, it must rightfully be added that, with concurrence of the FDA and all involved, the investigator purposefully chose this patient because he was considered too old and medically unsuited for cadaveric heart transplantation. Nevertheless, the illustrative aspects of the example remain valid.

There are many examples of quasi-essential (life-sustaining) artificial support systems or devices used in modern medicine. Chief among them remains the artificial kidney. Annually, large numbers of patients are treated with either hemodialysis or peritoneal dialysis for acute, reversible kidney failure. While peritoneal dialysis does not necessarily require a machine in its application, it does require synthetic materials and manufactured solutions. The prefix "quasi" indicates that if other but timely measures are taken by the physician, dialysis can often be avoided. However, dialysis or artificial kidney therapy for acute or transient kidney failure, even when not absolutely required to avoid death from uremia, is frequently called upon today because it may increase the chances of survival. At a minimum, dialysis permits greater latitude in patient management (e.g., fluids, nutrients, and medications can be administered more easily and safely). The causes of acute reversible kidney failure are nearly legion, but success in treating this problem with return of patients to a normal existence grows yearly. Dialysis is now such an expected and common therapy that obtaining the routine hospital informed consent is occasionally overlooked before its application. Similarly, use of respiratory or ventilatory assist devices has achieved equal stature in the treatment of acute respiratory failure.

Another even more successful example but of an intra-corporeal system being employed with growing frequency in the treatment of specific (electrical) malfunctions of the heart is the cardiac pacemaker. Such devices are now often geared to biventricular pacing of the heart and, being programmable, can respond by increasing heart rate automatically to meet exercise needs. It is estimated that about one million Americans currently have permanent pacemakers and that over 400 new patients per million members of the population received pacemakers in 1993 [5]. Such devices have become so sophisticated that cardiologists must now receive special training in their application.

The above systems are obviously comprised of materials and devices and may be used on a chronic life-giving basis for irreversible organ failure or disease. Of these examples, again, one of the still most commonly employed extra-corporeal system is the artificial kidney. However, this therapy, in spite of nearly 30 years of large-scale clinical application, still has many inadequacies associated with it when used on a chronic basis [6]. The reasons are not always apparent, but a symposium on hypersensitivity reactions during hemodialysis clearly indicates that materials-related problems contribute to some of the inadequacies of this therapy [7]. The artificial kidney also demonstrates that a long time frame of months to years may be required before toxicity of a material or device becomes manifest. Such observations may be missed entirely in acute, short-term applications where the patients may be severely ill with many obscuring problems.

There are numerous examples of nonessential (life-independent) materials or devices. These run the gamut from teeth and hip prostheses to breast and penile implants, to the artificial ear, to attempts at constructing an electronic eye, and, more recently, to attempts at replacing spinal cord and peripheral nerve functions with computerized electronic devices in paralyzed patients. Although more comfortable and meaningful living may be ascribed to use of many devices, none in this category is essential to life. It is, therefore, implicit in the testing or utilization of such devices that they do no additional harm to the patient or test subject. However, this is not always the case. For example, consider the hip prosthesis. Even after years of trials and now general use in the surgical community, hip prosthetic materials, though much improved today, continue to be a long-term problem because of stress or corrosive deterioration. Moreover, on insertion of the hip prosthesis, a relentless vigil must be kept until wound healing is complete in order to avoid disastrous infections. Infectious complications may leave the patient much worse off, even dead.

DEVICE-RELATED PERSPECTIVE
(POTENTIAL VERSUS REAL ASSISTANCE)

Whether physician or engineer, the investigator should always be on guard against his or her personal bias. Every effort should be extended to avoid overselling a device when discussing it with a trial subject or, for that matter, anyone else. If months or even years have been expended in developing a device, particularly if by the investigator, bias may be inescapable. The investigator will likely be perceiving mostly the *potential* for the material or device.

A useful technique for combating bias, though not perfect because of team loyalty, is to have the skilled nurse introduce the device concept to the patient first and, then, following an appropriate time interval, for the investigator to make his own presentation to the patient. This has an additional advantage in that the time lapse gives the patient or responsible family member or representative more opportunity to digest the information. Better questions can be anticipated regarding the device, concerning its advantages and disadvantages. Unfortunately, there is as yet no perfect method for explaining to patients the risks and hazards of a new material or device to be tested. A "Catch 22" can also prevail. If there is no historical information of any consequence upon which to base a discussion, then one must experiment to assess the qualities of the device. As tests occur and as success, guarded as it may be, becomes apparent, the presentation will become more patent, if not encompassing.

Paradoxically, the patient may be the least reliable of all in assessing the quality of life bestowed by a new device; the patient's emotional response may be unwarranted when results are viewed objectively by the investigator and the team. There is a placebo effect even in device testing. Information may even be suppressed that is critical to survival not only of the device but of the patient, as well. Such suppression may also occur unwittingly because the subject may not know or recognize critical problems. This underscores the need for an ongoing, iterative patient educational process during clinical trials. It is necessary to see the patient often for examination of the device and the patient, including periodic assessment of device function, if feasible. The patient's desire for success may exceed the investigator's; *real* perspective may escape both for a period of time.

On the whole, the peer community generally comprises the most critical group. This may be true for a variety of reasons, but hinges heavily on the purpose and construction of materials or device and the method of introduction. If the purpose or construction are outlandish enough to gain only derogatory comments or if the introduction is made with fanfare but shows little scientific awareness, then the investigator can expect lack of enthusiasm or acceptance by his or her peers (see Chapter 59). Such approaches create an uphill struggle and, frequently, also resentment amongst individual members of the investigator's own clinical trials team.

It behooves the clinical trials investigator to guide the team in quiet work until valid data can be organized and appropriately presented for scrutiny by the peer community. The best method of establishing a balanced scientific perspective is publication of results in peer-reviewed scientific journals before formal introduction to the public at large. This has the distinct advantage of letting the peer community know that the investigator and clinical trials team have critically analyzed their own data and presented conclusions in an unbiased a manner as possible. One should avoid, at all costs, compromise of personal integrity and the appearance of fanaticism regarding the device being tested.

The lay community is a combination of the least, and yet often the most, severely critical of devices used in medicine. It is usually the final judge regarding benefit to patients. This may be because the lay community is related to or becomes the patient pool from which test subjects eventually arise. Media handling of device information is presented elsewhere in the text (see Chapter 59). However, in attempts at establishing meaningful rapport between the investigator or clinical trials team and the lay community and to avoid the risk of overstating the issue, one must minimize the use of any misinterpretable or misrepresentative statements or claims.

FUNCTIONAL INTENT OF DEVICE

Building on the foregoing discussion, it is now apparent that devices for patients can be assigned to the broad categories of (a) substitutes for failed bodily functions or (b) vehicles for treatment of underlying disease. Though potential for confusion exists, distinguishing between these two major categories is helpful in formulation of device ideas relative to the selection of patients. Distinguishing between categories is not meant to define necessity for maintenance of life of a given patient but achievement, realized or not, in completeness of concepts.

Substitutes for failed bodily functions are reasonably obvious and include the artificial heart, blood, kidney, ear, eye, hip, leg, arm, etc. The essentialness of these examples underscores whether or not toxicity and durability of materials are major considerations. Examples of vehicles for therapy might include a wearable, programmable insulin pump for subcutaneous insulin administration in the diabetic patient, implantable insulin or heparin delivery systems used in diabetic and hypercoaguable patients, and wearable or implantable devices for administration of intravenous nutrients in patients with absent small intestines or for administration of chemotherapeutic agents to cancer and leukemic patients.

The potential for progression from therapeutic vehicle to functional substitute becomes apparent when considering, for example, an insulin pump, an otherwise open-loop device unresponsive to direct changes in blood glucose. Such devices only approximate an artificial pancreas, albeit in only one of this gland's many functions. Suppose, however, the pump could be tied to a glucose sensor (see Chapter 29) and the combination positioned so as to infuse insulin into the portal vein. Suddenly, the now complex device takes on the aspects of being a "truer" artificial pancreas, i.e., a *functional* substitute.

INCAPACITATION DUE TO DISEASE

Many diseases can be manifest in global or wide-spread systemic illness or remain limited to single-organ dysfunction. Prime examples of the latter would be disease limited to the eye or ear. Less obvious, on the other hand, is the fact that disease involving the kidneys, for example, may only involve the kidneys and no other organs directly or the kidney disease may be the result of and complicated by systemic illness, as well. Patients with disease restricted to the kidney may develop total kidney failure in a silent, almost imperceptible manner.

Far too commonly, kidney disease may be catastrophic in its presentation with associated systemic effects; the patient may have been obviously ill for some time and finally presents in a uremic state. Prime examples of such patients are those who suffer from autoimmune, immune, and toxic diseases (e.g., systemic lupus erythematosis, poststreptococcal glomerulonephritis, acute tubular necrosis, respectively). It may be difficult to imagine that patients with end-stage liver or heart disease can present similarly, but they do. Therefore, it is important for the investigator to recognize that just replacing the failed organ's function may or may not tend to all problems incumbent to failure of the organ, *per se*.

COGNITIVE STATUS OF PATIENT

The extent of the patient's illness may determine his/her cognitive status. Delirious, even combative, behavior is commonly associated with active thrombotic thrombocytopenia purpura. Equally common is that improvement of brain function may be the first sign of successful therapy in such patients. Because plasmapheresis (membrane filtration of whole plasma with concomitant replacement with fresh plasma proteins) is frequently utilized for the treatment of this illness in its acute stages, one may be faced with the dilemma of obtaining informed consent in circumstances where the patient may be totally incoherent but where the incoherence may remit with as little as one therapeutic session.

The responsible family member(s) or representative(s) must be contacted for informed consent, if at all possible. If attempts at contact of responsible individuals are unsuccessful and therapy with a device is known to have a high probability of success, then therapy may be commenced on an emergency basis without informed consent. It is necessary to emphasize, here, that success must have some assuredness before commencing therapy without informed consent. Application of a device in such situations assumes prior knowledge and should never be attempted in treatment of a disease where there is no historical information and where outcome is not known to be favorably influenced with reasonable predictability. Such decisions weigh heavily on the investigator.

In either of the above circumstances, it is a good practice after the patient has regained composure to have the patient also sign the informed consent, even though *post facto*. The patient may have a recurring problem and it is sometimes necessary to obtain a "standing" informed consent. One must anticipate relapses and future treatments for many diseases.

A patient's mental status with either acute or chronic illness may vacillate between extremes of depression and euphoria. Such statements are qualifiers; if severe enough, as in a state of delirium, they may be associated with legally definable mental incompetence. In the throes of catastrophic illness, it is frequently impossible to ascertain whether or not the mental state of the patient is acute or chronic, baseline or altered. Family members or representatives can be helpful, if they have current knowledge of the patient. Depending on the purpose and objective of device testing, one may or may not wish to be involved with either the acutely or chronically mentally incompetent patient.

Regardless of the device application, there are other factors that may specifically affect cognitive status. These may be summarized as language barriers. Such barriers may be due to age (either the very young or the very old patient), to nationality (the investigator and the patient may not speak the same language), or to congenital (cerebral palsy) or acquired (stroke victim) central nervous system deficits. Considerable time and patience may be necessary to gain some comprehension. Family members or long-term acquaintances as well as interpreters may have to be relied upon to appreciate the subject's idiosyncrasies in comprehension.

ORGAN SYSTEM INVOLVEMENT

Depending upon the vocation or psychological makeup of a patient, the absence of a single digit might assume proportions of extreme importance in one individual (a pianist), much as would complete debilitation from a severe neuromuscular disorder in another (anyone). Disregarding vocational and psychological considerations, the involved organ system frequently predetermines the risks and hazards to the patient in device testing. Thus, it is almost inconceivable that an artificial heart would not pose greater risks and hazards to the patient in device testing than would an "artificial ear." This issue must be borne in mind from the commencement of device development through completion of clinical trials. This is undoubtedly one reason why today small, implantable, electrically driven ventricular assist devices are gaining a foot-hold as opposed to the more global concept of an artificial heart. Such devices are typically implanted in the aorta to assist cardiac output and are used to carry the patient through to cadaveric heart transplantation.

In considering those bodily functions that might ultimately be amenable to partial or total replacement, one can conceptualize a hierarchy of risks and hazards based on the need for invasiveness, types of materials required, and structure of the device, all coupled with the biochemical or physiological function of the organ system to be substituted. In an elementary fashion, the rank order of (decreasing) difficulty in construction and risks and hazards for functional substitutes of organ systems might be as follows: cardiac, hepatic, pulmonary, renal, neuromuscular, pancreatic, skeletal, visual, and auditory. This hierarchy may be modified, disputed or altered for individual perceptions. A final determinant may also be whether or not functional demand is continuous or intermittent.

INFORMED CONSENT AND ITS
PRACTICAL ASPECTS

The concept of informed consent is treated more extensively elsewhere in this text (Chapters 51, 53, 54, and 58). The task at hand is defining construction, application, and disposition. It is necessary that informed consent follows the format required by FDA regulations. Inherent in construction of informed consent is attention to (a) word choice (simple, understandable words without jargon or double meaning), (b) brevity (without compromise of completeness), (c) honesty (statements on cosmetic attributes of device and complications, including possible death, must be made), (d) alternatives (frequently these exist in the form of other already approved and marketed devices), and (e) immutability (as a legal instrument, the informed consent must be considered unchangeable, without agreement to change by local or FDA Institutional Review Boards).

Generally, reading of the informed consent to, or with, the patient should be a physician-investigator responsibility, if for no other reason than the legal aspects of performing clinical trials. Adequate time must be devoted to the reading. It is good practice to have the nurse first spend time with the potential subject and go over the document. The informed consent should be left with the potential test subject or responsible individual and time should elapse before the physician-investigator approaches the subject (or representative) for rereading the document. It is also good practice to encourage double signing of the informed consent, this being by the prospective test subject and spouse or next-of-kin. Additional time should elapse, if feasible, and the document again read and signed by the same persons. It is necessary always to have a witness present, whether family member, allied health professional unrelated to the clinical trials team, or a close friend of the patient.

After reading of the informed consent and with all necessary signatures affixed, the informed consent must be filed in multiple locations. These minimally include with the patient, in the patient's chart, and in the investigator's FDA or project file, and with a sponsor if different from the investigator. Such completeness in filing of the informed consent is necessary also to accommodate an FDA audit.

REFERENCES

1 *Evaluation of Hemodialyzers and Dialysis Membranes*. DHEW Publication No. (NIH) 77-1294. Washington, DC: U. S. Department of Health, Education and Welfare, 1977.
2 *Controlled Clinical Trials*. Baltimore, MD: Elsevier Science, 1984.
3 Devries WC, Anderson JL, Joyce LD, et al. Clinical use of the total artificial heart. *N Engl J Med*, 310:5 (1984), 273–278.
4 Galletti PM. Replacement of the heart with a mechanical device. *N Engl J Med*, 310:5 (1984), 312–314.
5 Kusumoto FM, Goldschlager N. Medical progress: Cardiac pacing. *N Engl J Med*, 334:2 (1996), 89–98.
6 Gotch FA, Krueger KK (Eds.). Proceedings of a conference on adequacy of dialysis. *Kidney Internatl*, 7 (1975, Suppl. 2), S1–S269.
7 Wathen R L, Klein E. Symposium on Hypersensitivity in Hemodialysis. *Artif Organs*, 8:3 (1984), 270–272.

Chapter 54

Multiphasic Device Testing

Ronald L. Wathen

WHY CLINICAL TRAILS?

Regulatory controls concerning device development are discussed in depth elsewhere in this text (see Section IX). In brief, the Federal Drug Administration (FDA) recognizes three classes of devices based upon perceived increasing risks and hazards for the patient: Classes I, II, and III (see Chapter 53). Many Class II and most Class III medical devices need clinical trials either to demonstrate substantial equivalency to a preamendment device, including safety and effectiveness [510(k) requirements] or to support a premarket approval application (PMA) following exercise of an investigational device exemption (IDE). Excellent graphic presentations for device pathways to market have been published by Morton [1] and the FDA [2]. To conduct an investigation of a significant risk device under an IDE, the sponsor (manufacturer or investigator) must obtain both FDA and local institutional review board (IRB) approval. In the case of a PMA, the FDA usually requires the manufacturer to conduct a postmarket surveillance study after initiating marketing. This type of study is oriented toward ensuring the safety of the device when used in large scale. Once devices, irrespective of class, have been authorized for marketing, the manufacturers must continue mandatory device reporting (MDR) of complications as long as the device is marketed. Implicit in the MDR regulation is that distribution of a device may be stopped if the safety or effectiveness comes into serious doubt.

In none of the device legislation or regulations, although clinical trials may be required, is it stated how a device should be tested, what form the tests should take, how many devices should be tested, what patient considerations should be entertained, etc. Why, then, should effort be made to describe a three-phase scheme for clinical trials testing of a device when no regulations exist that make this a requirement? The answer is simple. There are many complications that can result from device use, some obvious and others extremely esoteric or obscure. Only clinical trials provide a proper vehicle for determining the safety and effectiveness associated with clinical application of the device before large-scale use. However, most people involved in device development, investigators and manufacturers alike, adhere to the clinical trials format that follows, albeit to varying degrees. Appreciation of both scientific methodology and empathy are deeply imbedded in our medico-industrial community. After discussing general considerations pertinent to devices and animal trials, this chapter establishes a logical clinical trials sequence for device testing that could be applied to most devices.

GENERAL CONSIDERATIONS

Purpose, Implantation Surgery, Biocompatibility, and Self-Care Capability

Researchers considering clinical trials need to be able to articulate the purpose of the materials or device in terms of medical need. In addition to defining this attribute of a device, the purpose will also largely dictate the site implanation, extent of surgery required for implanation, ability to repair the device in situ, and difficulty in removal should failure occur.

One cannot overemphasize the importance of choosing the appropriate site for implantation of a device. Flexibility in choice of site may falsely appear to exist. An example might be an implantable percutaneous device attachable to an artery and a vein, permitting blood access for hemodialysis, intravenous feeding, or chemotherapy without necessity of painful venipuncture. Size of the device might be such that it could be implanted either in the lower or upper arm. However, an additional and simple consideration may restrict the implanation site to the upper arm. The lower arm undergoes frequent and extensive pronation and supination, setting up shear forces that might forecast failure due either to exit site erosion or clotting because of torsion or irritation of the attached blood vessels. The medial aspect of the patient's thigh might prove a better site for such implantation; however, in this location, there is potential for infection around the device by rectal and genital soiling of the perineum. Thigh implantation of such a device might also impose cosmetic and coital constraints, particularly in the female.

More often that not, the purpose of the device will nearly mandate the site of implantation. For instance, the anatomy of the chest and great vessels is such that an artifical heart would require a sternal approach and placement in the mediastinum. Similarly, a joint prosthesis obviously has to supplant the diseased joint. Exteriorized components of the artificial ear, on the other hand, could be implanted in the neck or even beneath the clavical with electrodes running subcutaneously to the point of penetration into the cochlea. However, the correct location was established behind and in close proximity to the real ear. This position allows for immobilization of the device by imbedding in the mastoid bone and allows the shortest possible electrode path.

One of the difficulties in device development and testing is to appreciate the fact that failure can, and will, occur. Failure may be partial or complete. If partial, it is necessary to have adequate perspective in developing a device to anticipate the need for repair in situ, if this is at all possible. Thus, the example of a blood access might include a self-sealing plastic septum that is penetrated each time access to the bloodstream is warranted. The septum might develop a leak from laceration or scouring with a needle adapter used for penetration. Should this occur, the septum should be replaceable without need of surgery or harmful effects to the patient.

The first human implantation of an artificial heart demonstrated that even something as complex as the artificial heart could be repaired while in the patient. Early in the patient's course, a materials failure occurred in a part of the device. Because such a possibility was anticipated in design, the failed portion of the device was replaceable in situ. However, unlike the simpler example given above of the blood access device, the patient was returned to the operating room for repeat sternotomy under general anesthesia, causing far greater discomfort and risk for the patient. In parallel to the blood access and artificial heart, comparable increasing levels of patient discomfort and risk are apparent for repair of an artificial ear and hip, respectively.

The need to remove a failed device may provoke fear and apprehension in the patient. This is particularly true if major surgery and/or anesthesia is required for removal. There are several factors to consider when need for removal presents: first, patient apprehension; second, the device, if implanted in (or surrounded by) soft tissue, may become badly encased in scar tissue, making removal actually more difficult than insertion; and, third, the degree of complications (e.g., infection) may be such that a second device cannot be substituted in the same implant site as used for the first, at least for some time, regardless of the patient's desire. Need for removal is perhaps not such a critical issue for a blood access device where alternative sites can usually be established. However, imagine the consternation provoked by bacterial infection of the mediastinum for the artificial heart or in the juxtaposed pelvic bone or joint space of the artificial hip recipient. The former literally may have no recourse. while the latter, as indicated previously, may suffer serious consequences from a wound infection.

One of the axioms of materials and device testing is that infection may not clear, even with the most advanced antibiotic therapy available, as long as prosthetic materials are retained in the patient. Testament to this axiom is repeated daily in the practice of nephrology, wherein a device as simple as the plastic catheter for peritoneal dialysis may have to be removed to achieve control of otherwise intractable bacterial peritonitis.

Studies aimed at establishing biocompatibility of materials and device must precede human implantation of a device and show no evidence of overt materials toxicity (see Section III). Such evaluation is not mandatory before animal trials. However, should animal trial success with a device be poor, one would have difficulty in determining whether failure was due to device design, test design, direct toxicity of materials, or animal-species-related incompatibility (see Chapter 31).

The induction of hypersensitivity reactions by materials are dealt with elsewhere in this text (see Chapter 18). The local allergic reaction to materials in the in vivo setting is particularly bothersome with percutaneous devices. This may appear as a sterile inflammatory reaction at the exit site that may abate with time. Eosinophil and giant cell infiltration will occur around a device if the materials, additives, or bonding agents are allergenic. Currently, such a tendency apparently does not totally preclude human use of some materials; however, it is my opinion that any material chosen should not provoke a sterile inflammatory reaction at the implantation site. At a minimum, such a reaction prejudices the long-term qualitative nature of the scarring process. A more reasonable goal for any device, percutaneous or not, would be the allowance of normal tissue ingrowth in the area surrounding the device. Tissue ingrowth with minimum scar formation will provide a better antibacterial interface.

It is appropriate also to evaluate the adequacy of the human test subject in self-care. Failure of the subject in proper self-care may be critical to the outcome of device testing. This is particularly true where the device makes contact with or traverses the body surface. All humans do not bathe daily, or adequately when they do bathe; all do not brush their teeth routinely or adequately; all do not clean body orifices routinely or adequately; in short, some people are totally unkempt, and this increases the skin and orifice bacterial burdens, sometimes with alarming species of bacteria. Patients may have other undesirable habits, such as alcohol, tobacco and/or illicit drug consumption. The net result of poor hygiene and bad habits, particularly when combined, is usually infectious complications during device testing. The underlying disease that is being treated or palliated with a device may already be the cause for a compromised immune system. While patients with poor self-care or who have chemical addiction(s) may make poor test subjects. They do provide the acid test regarding quality of the device tested. The investigator should assess the importance of this aspect of device testing to the device in question.

Acute and Chronic Animal Studies

Purpose In terms of a completed but not fully developed device, the overall purpose of animal trials, whether acute or chronic, is to approximate the human circumstance (see Section VI). Acute trials are more oriented toward determination of unsuspected toxicity, while simultaneously affording in vivo observation for need of design change. Chronic trials, on the other hand, are generally oriented toward assessment of materials intregrity. One must remember the necessity for (a) selection of an appropriate test animal (size relative to device is a major determinant); (b) sterile, aseptic conditions for surgical implantation; (c) maximum cleanliness in the animal housing area; (d) ability to monitor device function in the animal; and (e) weight and/or growth (general health status) of the test animals. If the device exits through the skin, then the exit site must be monitored frequently for evidence of infection, i.e., purulent drainage and/or wound dehiscence.

Need for Reentry into Animal Trials   Reentry into animal trials may become necessary at any point in any phase of human trials. Reasons include appearance of unsuspected toxicity of the materials or device or recognition of need for major changes in design or materials. Untoward toxicity or need for design or materials changes do not necessarily stop human testing, as the problems may only be suspected and not well defined. Animal trials may be reentered and run in parallel to continuing human trials.

Comparableness of Animal and Human Trials   Animal trials usually do not adequately mimic or parallel human experience with a device. However, this should in no way suggest that animal trials are not warranted; they are always required with new materials or devices before human trials. This failure to parallel human experience has many probable causes. Depending upon whether the device is in contact with circulating blood, a hollow cavity, bone, skin, or the external surface of the animal, species differences in the makeup of blood and body constituents and the ability to combat infection count heavily in failure of animal and human trials to be comparable.

Simpler aspects of animal trials accounting for this lack of comparableness are frequently overlooked in the zealous approach to device testing. First, the test animal is almost invariably healthy or should be; certainly, the test animal is unlikely to manifest the disease process being treated with the device in the human subject. The interpretation of results of device testing must incorporate these critical differences between human and animal trials. Second, the laboratory animal does not have the capability of self-care in personal hygiene. While of less critical importance for testing of internalized devices, any device in contact directly or indirectly with the exterior of the animal may be preordained to failure due to either self-mutilation or infectious complications at the site. Only imperfect ways of dealing with these problems are available. Frequently, devices that fare poorly in animal trials, particularly if due to infectious complications, may do superbly in human studies if the test subjects exhibit adequate self-care practices.

PHASE I CLINICAL TRIALS

Type of Patient Selected

Degree of Patient Incapacitation   In addition to trial design, the investigator, as well as the sponsor and manufacturer, should devote considerable attention to patient selection. There are few events more disheartening in the commencement of a clinical trial than to discover that the patients of proper qualification thought to be available are not. Months before the anticipated commencement of testing, patient availability should be determined. The selection process hinges, first, on the type of illness to be treated and, second, on the degree of incapacitation to be attacked with the device.

Reliability and Accessibility of Selected Patients   After determining the availability of patients with the type and degree of illness sought, the investigator should establish reliability and accessibility of the patients. Reliability evaluation may require comment from other team members, particularly nurses and social workers, to assess patient compliance and the ability to self-care. Furthermore, in evaluation of a Class III device that has life-and-death implications in terms of malfunction, patient accessibility is paramount in the selection process. A patient who lives several hundred miles away and cannot obtain appropriate emergency help, should need arise, should not be selected for trial of an artificial organ high in the hierarchy. The terminally or seriously ill patient may wish to relocate clinical trials, whereas it is less likely that the functionally impaired would agree to do so. However, the need for relocation to allow close follow-up may be for only a short time, of several days or weeks, in which case many patients may agree to this inconvenience, irrespective of the nature of the affliction.

Close Cooperation with Institutional Review Board (IRB) and Sponsor and Manufacturer   The commencement of patient selection activities assumes that a study protocol, inclusive of proper documentation regarding the materials or device and informed consent, has been developed and submitted to the IRB. Such a document is inherently an aggregate result of efforts by the investigator, the sponsor, and the manufacturer. If the process of clinical trials is sufficiently entrained, the opportunity now presents for informal discussions with potential test subjects to ensure further that an adequate patient population exists. It is appropriate at this time for the sponsor and manufacturer, if different from the investigator, to be present at the initial device implantations, and frequently through all implantations in Phase I if the device is sufficiently complex. Once the protocol and informed consent have been accepted by the local IRB, and the FDA if it is a significant risk device, patients should be approached with the informed consent. Once signed, Phase I trials can begin.

Coordination of Investigator and Sponsor and Manufacturer Efforts

Documentation   The assembling of research data (documentation of events), is probably the most laborious, yet most important, aspect of performing a clinical trial. It is necessary early on for the investigator and sponsor and manufacturer to agree on the type and extent of data to be obtained. One usually overestimates capabilities and underestimates ultimate need in this regard, but it is important to have available proper data storage forms or flowsheets. These must be continually updated during the course of study. In addition, one should have a computer available with software to permit ease of storage and rapid retrieval of data. Data are obtained first in hard copy for permanent storage, entered into computer storage, and then, with the proper format, printed periodically during the study for discussion by the investigator, the team, and the sponsor and manufacturer.

Communication   The proper storage of data and continued, frequent surveillance of test subjects promotes calm communication with the sponsor and manufacturer of a device (i.e., surprises, otherwise buried in the hard copy data flies that only surface with periodic, in-depth study of accumulated data, can be avoided). This minimizes emergency (and harried) communication with the sponsor and manufacturer over a problem just discovered but which may have been there all along. Also, frequent planned meetings with the sponsor and manufacturer to assess data in a leisurely fashion and view representative test subjects help to minimize surprises and misinformation.

Avoidance of Frustration   Many clinical trials start off with the best of intentions only to dwindle to total unproductivity because of loss of faith and frustration among the investigator and the sponsor and manufacturer. The uninitiated clinical trials investigator must also become aware of one, seemingly unavoidable, frustration: the investigator's company contact or research liaison may change with some frequency. This occurs because the person assigned to the task may relocate within or without the manufacturer's organization. A rapid change in company personnel may signal that the manufacturer's interest in the project has subsided or that emphasis has shifted to other products or investigators. Most often, this is not the case because the capital investment in a given project is likely to be substantial. The industrial work force simply tends to change more rapidly than does that of the medical community. One way to combat this problem is to insist on assignment of more than one liaison person to the clinical trials program. When manufacturing personnel assigned to a project do change, it is absolutely necessary that the investigator do his or her share in quickly educating and updating the new representative.

Conclusion of Phase I

Patient Number and Specified Stop Date   Implicit in Phase I device testing is the use of small numbers of patients, perhaps only 10 or 12. This is because Phase I is a time for intense observation of the patients for signs and symptoms of occult toxicity of materials and of the device for functional integrity. To maintain an orderly approach in device testing, it is necessary to agree on a maximum number of test subjects that can be followed appropriately by the investigator. Since the numbers of patients will be small, it is desirable to anticipate a stop date, after which no further Phase I trials will be performed.

On termination of Phase I trials, some time should be allowed to elapse before considering commencement of Phase II trials. This permits determination of any additional untoward side effects, disruption of wound healing, confidence in functional integrity of a device, etc. During this time lapse, continued close follow-up of patients should occur.

PHASE II CLINICAL TRIALS

Validity of Original Informed Consent

The results of Phase I trials must be viewed carefully to ascertain whether or not alteration of the original informed consent is advisable. It may have been determined in Phase I experience that the informed consent was not practical or easily understood. The experience may suggest to the investigator that additional complications have to be listed or that functional limitations, heretofore unsuspected, became apparent and have to be noted. Completion of Phase I trials is an ideal time for adjustment in protocol, if warranted, and any such change must also be noted in the informed consent.

In any event, if the informed consent is altered by the investigator, the revised informed consent must be presented to the IRB, and, if it is a significant risk device, to the FDA, for formal acceptance. When the amended informed consent is accepted, copies should be forwarded to the sponsor and manufacturer, if different from the investigator. An amended informed consent should be denoted by inscribing the revision number and the date of the latest revision on all pages.

Increase in Patient Numbers and Relaxation of Entry Criteria

Use of Less Severely Ill Patients   Frequently terminal or seriously ill patients are the first entered into a protocol. This is because (1) maximum benefit to patients is desired secondary to device assist; (2) the risks and hazards of the device are such that use of only severely ill patients can be justified; or (3) the degree of improvement to be expected is unknown and, therefore, the device might be unwarranted in less-affected patients. These three considerations may simultaneously occupy the minds of the investigator and sponsor and manufacturer. Once the true benefit to be derived from a device and the risks and hazards are identified, it is logical to increase the numbers of test patients while simultaneously relaxing entry criteria. This assumes the device in question has proper merit. This is the appropriate time to prepare for an enlargement of experience beyond just the primary investigator's environment.

Preparation for an Enlarged Experience   Critical alterations in protocols and reporting forms must be made so that they are usable by multiple groups. Crude user's manuals or guides should be generated to assist the added trials centers. The format for data recording and reporting must be rationalized and be made constant from group to group in preparation for greater patient numbers.

The ultimate number of patients required for a Phase II study is highly variable, being largely device-dependent. Using the artificial ear as an example, an aggregate of six centers, each contributing five patients to attain a total of 30 patients under study, might be reasonable. Assuming no comparable device already exists and is marketed, the artificial ear is a Class III device. Moreover, it has electrical requirements with electrodes penetrating areas close to brain substance, and the percutaneous portion of the device increases the chance of osteomyelitis; all are features potentially of substantial risks and hazards for the user and require standards of performance.

Addition of Trial Centers and Coordination of Multiple Investigators   Both the original Phase I investigator and the sponsor and manufacturer will probably know of potential additional investigators. The primary investigator, if the Phase I investigator, is likely to be thinking of who is the best scientifically, and, while this feeling may be shared, thoughts will now be arising within the sponsor and manufacturer's organization concerning marketing strategies. Therefore, the manufacturer may be searching for potential, not necessarily scientifically based, device users to provide enlargement of the clinical trials. A compromise will be reached as to who the additional investigators will be. A mixture of scientifically based and general medical users will result as both the primary investigator and the manufacturer select additional investigators.

Enlargement to the Phase II level must anticipate greater difficulty in obtaining creditable data regarding performance and complications. Therefore, it is necessary to establish a broadened study group with a strong infrastructure. It is reasonable for the primary investigator to have considerable authority regarding patient selection or rejection and, if the need arises, to reject a secondary investigator if performance is not adequate. The primary investigator must negotiate this authority early in the interaction with the sponsor and manufacturer. If such precautions are not taken, then the ability to generate scientifically sound data is compromised and the goal of being able to withstand peer scrutiny may be compromised. Acceptance by the peer community is very important.

The Phase II primary investigator should anticipate need for travel to the centers involved, certainly in the beginning stages of Phase II trials. Furthermore, the investigator must anticipate, if not require, frequent telephone conferencing with the multiple secondary investigators. Updated data forms and flowsheets should be mailed on a monthly basis to the primary investigator. This investigator, in turn, should transmit cumulative data for all test centers to each participating investigator. Finally, the Phase II investigators should plan to meet in a central location, perhaps twice yearly depending on the length of the study, to discuss results. The sponsor and manufacturer must be prepared to underwrite costs necessary to establish this structure. The assigned company personnel must also visit the secondary investigators as often as is necessary or feasible and participate in the combined meetings for discussion of results.

Conclusion of Phase II, Continued Patient Observation   Like Phase I trials, Phase II trials should end as near as possible to a predetermined time and with a predetermined numer of patients. Again, there should be a waiting period before progression to the next trial phase. During this time interval, intense surveillance of all patients should be continued, including those carried forward from Phase I as well as those added in Phase II trials.

The device under study should now be approaching, or have achieved, a marketable state. There may well be future generations of the device, but the device, as it stands, should be close to release for general use. The data acquired should support the contention that the device performs as specified and is safe within the limits outlined. If the consensus is that plans to market the device are justified, then the sponsor and manufacturer should have utilized observations in Phase II for developing comprehensive instruction manuals for implantation and use of the device.

Adequacy of Informed Consent   Additional considerations of the informed consent now become important, if continued (Phase III) trials are indicated or desired. It is probable that the informed consent will now be generally satisfactory and few, if any, changes will have to be made.

PHASE III CLINICAL TRIALS

Submission to FDA with or without Phase III Clinical Trials

It is probably reasonable to state that either a PMA or 510(k) could be achieved for almost any device by completing either Phase I or Phase II Clinical trials, depending on the nature of the device. Logic mitigates for inclusion of Phase III trials for most Class III and many Class II devices. No matter how simple their function, devices may provoke obscure, difficult-to-identify systemic effects in the user. In addition, deterioration of materials may take a surprisingly long period to become identifiable. This is compounded by the fact that some manufacturers begin in-depth device testing without conviction of need. As soon as the device in question appears acceptable and marketable, the manufacturer may, correctly or not, begin to develop plans for recovery of investment and, ultimately, the development of profit, while simultaneously dismantling the (expensive) clinical trials organization.

It requires the collective wisdom of many highly dedicated people, i.e., investigators, allied health professionals, patients, and manufacturers, alike, to determine if esoteric, undesirable problems exist. Then, for most devices, can the determination be considered infallible? The millions of dollars spent annually in malpractice claims, recalls, and loss of business because of perceived inferior practices, all factors subtracting from the profit line, suggest that the best investment a manufacturer can make regarding a marketable (or marketed) device is in Phase III clinical trials. The foregoing discussion is not meant to imply that a device cannot, or should not, under any circumstances be marketed simultaneously during Phase III clinical trials if FDA authorization for marketing has been obtained. If this were the case, the expense of development would be staggering, and, importantly, many patients would be deprived unnecessarily of the utilization of a device critical to their functioning, if not their survival.

Continuance into Phase III Clinical Trials

Adjustments in Protocol and Informed Consent   Because of the anticipated larger numbers of patients and investigational centers, final efforts should be expended in making sure the protocol can be adhered to properly by the necessarily less-scientific community to be involved. Similarly, all instructional materials should be made as succinct and readable as possible. Any minor changes in informed consent should also be reckoned with before commencing Phase III trials. All FDA regulations should be adhered to, and all investigational files should be kept at a level amenable to FDA audit.

Estimates of Necessary Patient Numbers   Because of the carry-forward of patients remaining from Phase I and Phase II trials, it is difficult to estimate the numbers of patients required. For the Class II device, it would be reasonable to double the number of patients under study. For Class I devices, assuming trials are even entered into, the number could be much larger. For certain Class III devices, and particularly when one considers the severity of diseases these devices may be used to treat, a far smaller number of patients would satisfy both Phase II and III testing.

The Infrastructure of the Phase III Clinical Trials   Infrastructure of the Phase III clinical trials should be largely as defined for Phase II trials. At Phase III, however, it may be reasonable to consider a three-tiered system; thus, based on the pyramidal growth in investigators, there should be the primary, the secondary, and now the tertiary levels of investigators. A similar monitoring system for collection of data should be in place. However, because of the numbers of professionals now involved, some alteration in group meetings and interaction with the sponsor and manufacturer should be anticipated. Certainly, fewer meetings among all involved would be reasonable, and the attention paid by the sponsor and manufacturer to the tertiary level centers could be considerably less than the attention given to those involved in Phase II trials. The entire system should be more reliant on collection and processing of data forms developed for this purpose, with the primary investigator and/or the sponsor and manufacturer being the repository for data and data processing.

Phase III Trial Period   The length of time needed for Phase III trials is obviously device-dependent and not easily estimated. Where in the hierarchy of organ dysfunction the device enters and whether or not its use is constant or intermittent are factors of considerable importance. The requirements for the majority of devices would be satisfied by less than a year of observation, while others might require two to three years, and still others, an indeterminant period of time. In developing a Phase III clinical trial program for a given device, again, a large measure of common sense must be utilized by all involved to arrive at a reasonable time frame. Intense surveillance of residual patients from Phases I and II should end with the termination of Phase III clinical trials.

THE PERPETUAL CLINICAL TRIAL

The Manufacturer's Responsibility

Continued In-house Data Collection and Adherence to FDA Manufacturing Regulations   Manufacturers are required by federal regulation (the GMPs) to maintain an in-house system for data collection regarding user complaints and complications. The physician or allied health professional generally acts as the user intermediary in reporting, and the reliability is probably highly variable. Many manufacturers maintain a hot line or toll-free telephone number for this purpose. Significant value can be placed on such a system because it provides the manufacturer with indirect measures of quality control and insight for continued improvements in device design and production. Such a system also allows the manufacturer to hear a complaint before the FDA is informed. Thus, the manufacturer can act in good faith by reacting in-house to a complaint, as well as reporting a device failure or problem to the FDA if required under the MDR regulations.

Such a system, in conjunction with a less formal and less expensive observation of residual patients from Phase III trials for an indeterminant time, provides an effective means of device monitoring.

The Successful Device Is the Ultimate Goal of the Manufacturer

The perspectives of the investigator, the patient, the scientific (peer) community, and the lay community have been examined in this chapter. To this list must be added the manufacturer's perspective.

The fundamental assumptions should be made that manufacturers are honest, forthright, and not involved in deceptive practices. It is clear that the manufacturer is as interested as anyone in development of a highly functional, safe device. Achieving this, along the methods developed in this chapter, will allow satisfaction of the manufacturer's profit motive, with the further assumption that there is public demand for the device and that the device is amenable to economical production. All involved in the sequence of events to this point must realize that the making of profit is truly the final (bottom line) statement. Frequently, the academic professional seems disturbed by the profit motive concept. However, until such time that profit ceases to be a driving force in the marketplace, future device development will depend on it.

REFERENCES

1   Morton WA. Regulatory Pathways to the Market: An Overview. *Int Soc Artif Organs*, 6:4 (1982), 463–470.
2   Regulatory Requirements for Medical Devices. A Workshop Manual. Publ. No. FDA83-4165. Washington, DC: U. S. Department of Health and Human Services-FDA, 1983.

Chapter 55

Design of Clinical Trials

Richard A. Ward
Thomas A. O'Connor
Pippa M. Simpson

GENERAL ASPECTS OF CLINICAL TRIAL DESIGN

Clinical trials are the principal means of evaluating new therapeutic interventions. Although the design and execution of these trials are based mainly on common sense and an understanding of clinical medicine, the recent proliferation of articles on statistical techniques in medical journals indicates that statistical considerations are also important. To that end, a clinical investigator should seek a biostatistician's help early in the planning of any trial. However, before seeking such a collaboration, the investigator needs to know how statistics, properly applied, can help a correct conclusion be reached in a clinical trial. This chapter aims to provide this understanding. For more specific information, the reader is referred to books by Pocock [1] and Friedman et al. [2] and to a growing group of journals in biostatistics and clinical trials. These include *Biometrics*, *Controlled Clinical Trials*, and *Statistics in Medicine*. In addition, some clinical journals, such as *The New England Journal of Medicine*, now carry regular articles on clinical trial methodology.

In designing a clinical trial, an investigator must focus on two important criteria. First, the trial must address a clinically significant question. Most clinical trials are costly in terms of both money and resources, and the decision to conduct a clinical trial should be made only after careful consideration of whether or not an answer to the question(s) posed merits the effort required to obtain the answer. Second, the trial must be designed in such a way that the chances of reaching the correct conclusion are optimized. This will involve selecting an appropriate sample size, choosing a design that will not allow the results to become confused or confounded by factors other than those of primary interest, collecting the data efficiently and accurately, and analyzing the data using appropriate statistical and clinical approaches. All of these aspects are covered in some detail in this chapter. From the discussion, it will be seen that all these processes are interwoven. Such interrelationships should be understood before commencing a trial or, especially, when changes are contemplated in the planned design while the trial is in progress.

In considering the design of clinical trials for biomaterials, it is important to recognize the role of three factors in shaping the form of such trials. First, it must be recognized that clinical trials of biomaterials, per se, are essentially never performed. Rather, a medical device, which may contain one or more biomaterials, is the subject of the clinical trial. Consequently, the examination of a given biomaterial in a clinical trial will depend on the nature of the device in which it is utilized. For example, stainless steel may be used in devices intended for permanent implantation (e.g., a hip prosthesis), long-term, but not permanent, application (e.g., a fracture fixation plate and screws), or transient use (e.g., needles for venipuncture). Although the material is the same in each case, the design of the clinical trials will vary because of the different life expectancy and function of the device being evaluated.

The second factor that will influence the design of a clinical trial is its purpose. A clinical trial may be performed to answer one of two types of questions, those pertaining to basic information on how a device functions under idealized conditions and those relating to a decision on the effectiveness of a device under routine clinical conditions. Schwartz and Lellouch [3] have described these categories of questions as the "explanatory" and "pragmatic" approaches, respectively. The final trial design will reflect which of these general questions the investigator wishes to ask. Trials asking both types of question may be necessary in the evolution of a device.

Finally, the clinical trial of a medical device may also be governed by the regulatory requirements of the Food and Drug Administration (FDA). Many clinical trials involve new or modified devices and are performed with a view to obtaining data required to gain approval from the FDA for marketing of the device. The Medical Device Amendments of 1976 charge the FDA with determining the safety and efficacy of medical devices. These regulations require that valid scientific evidence be produced to allow a determination of whether or not there is reasonable assurance that a medical device is safe and effective. Valid scientific evidence is defined to consist principally of well-controlled investigations. In addition, the device regulations divide devices into three different categories on the basis of their perceived potential risk, and the degree of testing required for the devices in the three categories differs substantially. To a large extent, FDA regulations require that the applicability of a given biomaterial in a particular circumstance be clearly established in the preclinical stage of testing; however, final confirmation of safety and efficacy must be established in clinical trials.

Consideration of the objectives of a clinical trial from the biomaterial point of view must be predicated on these three factors: the nature of the device, the overall purpose of the study, and any relevant regulatory requirements. It is with this background that the design of clinical trials is considered in the following sections of this chapter.

FORMULATING THE QUESTION

Establishment of Objectives

Sackett and Gent [4] have suggested that many of the disagreements that occur over the interpretation of results from a clinical trial arise from ambiguities in the questions posed in formulating the trial. Thus, the first important step in designing a clinical trial is to enunciate clearly the objective(s) of the trial. In doing so, the investigator must be certain there is reasonable expectation that the objective(s) can be met, that the objective is appropriate, and that the objective is unambiguous. In most cases, there will be more than one objective. For example, the clinical trial of a new membrane blood oxygenator may be needed in order to obtain the data required for premarket approval by the FDA. What is the objective of such a trial? Put simply, this is an example of a "pragmatic" trial used to demonstrate the safety and efficacy of the oxygenator under routine conditions of use. However, in terms of designing a trial, this is clearly too vague an objective. A little thought reveals that this broad, single objective can be resolved into multiple objectives, including (a) is gas transfer adequate to maintain blood oxygenation and acid-base status in the normal range under the projected conditions of use; (b) is there trauma to the cellular elements of blood; and (c) does the device elicit any immunological or hematological response? From this list, one must choose what are considered to be the most important questions; these become the primary objectives of the trial. Using this example, one might choose the demonstration of adequate gas transfer to be the primary objective. The trial will then be designed to meet this objective. Secondary objectives may be addressed, but the design may not guarantee that they will be satisfactorily answered.

Selection of Outcome Variables

Once the objectives of a clinical trial have been determined, the outcome variables can be selected. It should be possible to measure the chosen variables accurately, and they should afford the investigator the maximum ability to discriminate (i.e., the change in a variable as a result of the experimental treatment should be large compared with the errors inherent in measuring the variable). If qualitative determinants, such as rating scales, must be used, there must be prior assurance that they will provide consistent data for the length of the trial. For example, if a questionnaire is to be completed periodically by a patient to assess changes in mobility after implantation of an artificial joint, the investigator must assure that the patient's response to the questionnaire is predominantly a function of changes in mobility, not of changes in the patient's general feeling of well-being or of the investigator's influence, and that repeated completion of the questionnaire does not condition the patient's response.

In selecting variables, it is important to ensure that those selected provide both necessary and sufficient data to answer the question(s) posed by the investigator. In practice, even if a preliminary study is conducted, it is difficult to determine the correct amount of data to collect. Obviously, insufficient data collection will result in a failure to meet the objectives of the trial, while excessive data collection will waste resources without adding to the conclusions reached. In reaching a decision, two issues always arise. First, is the accuracy and precision with which a variable can be measured sufficient to answer the question posed? Second, is acquisition of the data logistically feasible? If the answer to either of these questions is negative, the objectives of the trial may need to be revised.

Selection of outcome variables is inexorably linked to a consideration of the length of the trial and the frequency with which the variables are to be sampled. For given outcome variables, the frequency of observation and the length of the trial must be sufficient to provide a reasonable expectation that the objective(s) of the trial can be met. In designing a clinical trial, the investigator does not have the benefit of hindsight in selecting outcome variables and determining the frequency of sampling or the length of the trial. However, the success of the trial will depend, in large part, on correct decisions being made in advance; therefore, an investigator must maximize his chances of success by utilizing all available information, such as prior in vitro or animal studies and clinical experience, in making these decisions. In some cases, pilot studies may be required to finalize the trial design.

SELECTING A SAMPLE TO ANSWER THE QUESTION

Determination of Sample Size

In any clinical trial, the investigator must be reasonably assured that the number of patients likely to complete the trial is sufficient to allow the primary objectives of the trial to be correctly met. A prospective estimation of the number of patients required for a given trial should, therefore, be an integral part of the process of trial design. Inclusion of too few patients in the trial can result in a failure to demonstrate significant differences where they exist [5], whereas inclusion of too many patients is clearly wasteful of time and resources and may result in a trial that cannot be completed in a reasonable time.

In determining the optimal sample size for a comparative study, the investigator must consider several factors. First, he/she must decide what difference in the value of the outcome variable(s) must be detected in order to claim therapeutic benefit; i.e., what change would be clinically significant? This decision must be based, in part, on knowing the variation associated with measurement of the outcome variable. Second, the investigator must decide with what confidence he/she wishes to exclude the possibility that a difference in treatments is due to chance or that a negative result is real and not due to chance.

The traditional approach to determination of sample size is based on these considerations, and details of the methods used can be found in standard statistical texts [6, 7]. Fleiss [7] also included tables, and Clark and Downie [8] have developed graphs that can be used to find the required sample size. Calculations of sample size quickly demonstrate that large sample sizes are required to detect small changes between treatments. As a consequence, prospective performance of such calculations can prevent the investigator from embarking on a study for which he/she does not have the time, money, or patient base to complete successfully.

These methods are generally satisfactory for short-term studies of two treatments with limited outcome variables. However, they may be inadequate for long-term studies, for trials with several treatments, or when multiple outcome variables are to be considered. An approach has been developed [9] that accounts for dropouts, a frequent problem in long-term trials, and recently methods were reviewed [10] that address other problems associated with long-term clinical trials. Methods for estimating sample size when more than two treatments are to be compared or when multiple outcome variables are to be used have also been suggested [11].

Elimination of Bias

The goal of any clinical trial is to produce a finding that can be transferred to the appropriate population of patients at large. In order to extend results from a small study group to a larger patient population, the investigator must take steps to avoid bias in the study. Different techniques may be used to avoid bias, depending on its source. Randomization is generally used to avoid bias in the sampling process. A control group, equivalent in all aspects to the study group, may be used to avoid bias arising from extraneous effects on the variables of interest. Finally, to avoid bias in the measurement of variables due to the patient's or the investigator's preconceptions, blinding is used to conceal the nature of the treatment from the patient and/or the investigator. These techniques—randomization, controls, and blinding—are discussed in the following sections.

Randomization   Patients, who meet the entry requirements for the trial, should be randomly allocated into groups using, for example, tables of random numbers [12]. Usually, randomization of a patient to a particular group does not occur until after the patient has consented to participate in the trial. The concept of randomization can raise difficulties for some investigators in that a physician may feel that he or she needs to be in control of the treatment [13, 14]. Randomization is especially difficult in situations where death may be the result of not choosing the best treatment.

In sampling to create one or more groups, it may be necessary that patients in all groups possess certain attributes. In this circumstance, the groups should be randomly selected from a larger group first selected to possess these attributes. This is known as prestratification. Prestratification can also be combined with blocking; that is, from each group, a subgroup can be selected to receive a treatment with the other members of the group serving as controls.

Controls Controls can take several forms: another treatment in the same patient, another treatment in another group of patients treated concurrently, baseline observations made in the same patient before and/or after treatment, or historical baseline data in another group of patients. The choice of a trial design usually determines the type of controls to be used. However, it has been suggested [15, 17] that use of historical or other external controls may predispose to false-positive results, and their use should be approached with caution. Having made this decision, the next important step is to ensure that differences between the control and treatment groups are reduced to a minimum. At first sight, this would appear a trivial problem where the patients serve as their own controls. However, an effect carried over from a previous treatment can give rise to differences between the control and treatment groups, and these must be considered in the statistical analysis of the trial.

Blinding Blinding the patient, the investigators, and the treatment staff, collectively or individually, to which treatment the patient is receiving can help minimize the effect of preconceptions. Blinding of the investigator to which treatment the patient will receive eliminates the possibility that such knowledge will influence whether or not the investigator approaches a patient or that the investigator's attitudes will inadvertently influence whether or not the patient will consent to participate in the study. However, blinding requires that the investigator obtain consent without being able to tell the patients which treatment they will receive, and some feel that this limits the number of patients available for a study both because the investigator is uncomfortable with the randomization process and because patients are uncomfortable with the uncertainty over which treatment they will receive. To mitigate this problem, Zelen [18] has formulated the "double-consent randomized design" or pre-randomization approach to clinical trials. This technique performs randomization before obtaining consent, thus allowing the investigator to tell patients which treatment they would receive if they consent to participate in the trial. However, because the assumptions behind pre-randomization are questionable, use of the technique should be considered only if conventional randomization fails to yield sufficient patients for the trial [13].

Although blinding is possible with some types of devices [19], total, or even partial, blinding is often impossible, and the investigator must rely predominantly on selection of proper controls and randomization.

Choice of a Study Design

There are many possible designs for clinical studies [20]. However, for controlled clinical studies, designs are based on the concepts of randomization and controls. For studies over time, the roles of cross-over and parallel designs have been reviewed recently [21–23], and these are discussed below. Ensuing sections in this chapter discuss possible modifications to cross-over and parallel designs to deal with some problems associated with them.

Cross-Over Designs In cross-over designs, each patient receives two or more treatments in sequence, and outcomes in the same patient are contrasted. By this means, the effect of patient characteristics can be eliminated from the comparison. This can be important when interpatient variation is large relative to intertreatment differences. In such situations, a cross-over design, based on a smaller sample, will give the same statistical information as most other designs based on a larger sample that do not compare a patient's results under one treatment against the same patient's results under another.

In designing a cross-over trial, the investigator must consider the method of treatment assignment, order effects, and the definition of cross-over point. Care must be exercised in assigning the order of treatments. To minimize the placebo effect often observed by starting a treatment of any kind, equal numbers of patients must begin the trial with each of the treatment options under study, and the order of treatments should be randomized thereafter. This maneuver also offers some protection against one type of order effect, temporal changes unrelated to the trial, due to spontaneous waxing and waning of the disease state.

For a comparison between two treatments, patients should meet the same predetermined criteria as they enter each treatment. Failure to meet this requirement may be the result of a second type of order effect, carry-over from one treatment to the next. Random sequencing of treatments offers some protection from this source of error, and there are some modified cross-over designs that allow for a few types of carry-over effect [24]. However, in general, it is better to insert a period of nontreatment between each treatment period.

The cross-over point in a cross-over trial should be predetermined and based on time of treatment; other determinants are usually scientifically less defensible. If possible, neither the observer nor the patient should know when the point of cross-over occurs; that is, they should be blinded.

A major problem with cross-over designs arises if any sample points are lost due to dropout or implausible measurements. In such cases, analysis becomes much more difficult. Moreover, a cross-over design may simply not be feasible. For example, in a trial of a hip prosthesis or a heart valve, a crossover design cannot be implemented.

Self-Controlled Designs   Designs in which a single treatment is compared with control data in the same patient (self-controlled designs) have many similarities to cross-over studies but have some additional limitations associated with them [21]. In some circumstances, the nature of the device being tested may force the investigator to adopt a self-controlled trial design. This is particularly true early in the evolution of a device where alternative treatments may not exist. Examples include the first hip prostheses, artificial limbs, and intraocular lenses. Another circumstance is when the device is intended for use in a situation where failure to use the device would result in certain death. For example, the first hemodialyzers developed for the treatment of end-stage renal failure would have fallen into this category. In these circumstances, a control group in the usual sense is clearly ethically unacceptable.

In addition to all of the considerations discussed above for cross-over trials, there are further limitations associated with self-controlled trials. These arise, in the main, from the reduced control the investigator has over the design of the trial. First, the types of observation made during the control period and the treatment period may differ considerably, and, second, the patients studied in the trial may come from a restricted population. Self-controlled designs are frequently used for the initial trials of new devices. Such trials often involve patients who have proved refractory to conventional therapies and/or who may have far-advanced disease. In such circumstances, one may question whether or not the trial provides a fair test of the new device. This was clearly of concern in interpreting the results of the first implant of a total artificial heart [25] and has been raised in the discussion of extracorporeal immunoadsorption therapies for the treatment of patients with malignancies [26]. In contrast to comparative trials of mature devices in which a limited number of clinical outcome variables may be monitored, multiple parameters may be measured to assess device function in the early stages of device development. This requires use of more complex multivariate statistical methods in analyzing the data from the study.

Parallel Designs In parallel designs, patients are assigned to one of two or more groups. The groups are then treated concurrently, with each group receiving a different treatment. Parallel study designs are often more suited to clinical trials of medical devices than are cross-over designs. However, the fact that treatments are now being compared between two or more groups of different patients requires consideration of factors, other than the specific treatment, that may influence the outcome of the trial. For example, the success of an artificial ear may depend on whether or not the recipient has been totally deaf since birth or has become deaf after developing speech recognition. If one group in a trial of two artificial ears contains a disproportionate number of subjects totally deaf since birth (this can occur even with random assignment), the results obtained in that group may be inferior to those obtained in the other group because of this imbalance and not because of any inherent inferiority of the device. Such confounding factors are known as "covariates" or "prognostic factors." In addition to randomization between groups, prestratification may be necessary to deal with the problem of imbalance in covariates. Some adjustment may also be possible during analysis of the data, but it is preferable to adopt a method of allocating patients to the trial groups that minimizes any imbalance in the covariates.

Sequential Designs In some circumstances, not all patients required for a trial will be available for entry at the initiation of the trial; patients will continue to be added to the study population as suitable candidates become available. This presents a special dilemma. As the investigator assesses the trial results with time, he/she may find that a statistically significant result has been obtained before the scheduled termination of the trial. This poses two problems. The first is the ethical question of whether or not patients should continue to be treated by an inferior therapy once a superior one has been identified, and the second is whether or not resources should continue to be expended on a trial for which a result is considered known. This dilemma has led to the development of the sequential trial design [27].

In essence, sequential trials are not based on a predetermined sample size; rather, the final sample size depends on the outcome of individual patients. As results accumulate, they are periodically analyzed and, depending on the outcome of the analysis, the trial continues, with more data collection, or it is terminated with the primary objectives answered. In addition to addressing the ethical dilemma described above, sequential designs can reduce the total number of patients required for a trial. However, sequential designs are a relatively recent development, and some technical issues relating to decisions on termination and when testing should be done remain to be fully elucidated. Many variations lie between sequential trials, with no fixed sample size, and the ordinary situation of a predetermined sample size. A recent review [24] discusses developments in this area.

COLLECTING THE DATA

Patient Inclusion-Exclusion Criteria

Once a study design has been selected, the investigator must establish criteria by which potential subjects for the trial will be identified. The first step in this process is to carefully define the medical criteria that identify the patient as a candidate for the treatment to be studied. For any device, these criteria may differ depending on whether the trial is following the "explanatory" or the "pragmatic" approach. The use of idealized conditions in the former may lead to more stringent criteria being established than in the latter, where more routine clinical conditions obtain. The criteria selected may also reflect the stage of evolution of the device, with more restrictive criteria being set in the early stages of development, particularly with high-risk devices. On occasion, the final criteria may reflect ethical, as well as clinical, considerations. Whatever criteria are selected, they should include a requirement that the presence of the disease state to be treated has been unequivocally established in the patient. Having determined that the patient meets the medical criteria, the next criterion is that the patient will consent to participate in the trial after being fully informed of its nature. The concepts and regulations governing informed consent are described elsewhere in this handbook and will not be discussed further in this chapter.

In recruiting patients for a trial, the investigator must endeavor to screen out subjects who, for a variety of reasons, are unlikely to complete the trial or be compliant with the protocol. A clear understanding of the responsibilities of patient and investigator must be reached, usually during the process of obtaining informed consent. Elimination of poorly compliant patients may help to reduce experimental error and increase the discriminatory power of the trial. However, in establishing criteria for exclusion in a trial, the investigator must consider whether the results obtained on a select group of subjects will be applicable to the wider patient population who must ultimately be treated by the device. Furthermore, the exclusion criteria must not be so restrictive that they preclude being able to recruit sufficient subjects for the trial. An analytical approach to patient exclusion criteria has been proposed [28]. For more details on patient selection, see Chapter 53.

The Clinical Monitor

Even the most carefully designed clinical trial may be designed to fail if the execution of the trial is not carefully managed. Central to a well-managed trial is a clear definition of the responsibilities of each member of the investigational team and designation of a clinical monitor whose task is to oversee the trial, ensuring that protocols are followed and that all data are accurately recorded [29]. The importance attached to clinical monitors is indicated by their mandatory requirement in device trials conducted under the FDA's investigational device exemption regulations. In clinical trials of medical devices conducted under these regulations, clinical monitors have several well-defined functions. These include ensuring that the investigators follow the trial protocol according to signed investigator agreements, evaluating any adverse effects that may be encountered and reporting their results to the FDA, controlling the distribution of devices to the trial centers, and ensuring that unused devices are disposed of properly upon completion of the trial. The choice of a clinical monitor may be one of the most critical decisions in assuring the successful outcome of a well-designed trial.

Multicenter Trials

All the problems associated with conducting a clinical trial of a medical device are magnified severalfold if the trial involves more than one trial center. Multicenter trials require the establishment of a management team, usually under the aegis of the trial sponsor, whose task is to oversee the conduct of the trial. This team, which includes the principal investigator and trial monitor, must assure that all centers follow the trial protocol, collate data, and generally maintain communication between the various trial centers. In addition to these logistical concerns, other problems can arise in multicenter trials, including variation in laboratory tests and differences in clinical assessment from one physician to another. Furthermore, multicenter trials can involve a considerable increase in expense over a trial conducted at a single trial center. However, in spite of their inherent problems, multicenter trials often represent the only practical approach for evaluating devices intended for relatively few patients. Some appreciation of the complexities of a large multicenter study involving medical devices can be obtained from the reports of the National Cooperative Dialysis Study sponsored by the Artificial Kidney-Chronic Uremia Program of the National Institutes of Health in the late 1970s [30].

Data Collection

Well-planned mechanisms for data collection are necessarily an integral part of any clinical trial [29]; the larger and more complex the trial, the more important these methods of data collection become. Data collection usually occurs on two levels, recording of discrete data items on individual patients and consolidation of these individual data records into an overall data base for the trial.

A form should be carefully designed to record the discrete data items [31]. Individual data should be recorded by hand on the forms, although data may also be recorded in clinical or research laboratory notebooks. The form should be easy to fill out and encourage legibility and accuracy. In designing the form, questions should be formulated so that only a fixed number of alternative answers are possible. This avoids the subjective element in interpreting data. However, in practice, inclusion of some open-ended questions may be necessary. After the data on these forms has been transferred to the trial's central data base, they should be filed to allow for subsequent rechecking of data and/or audit by regulatory agencies. This is mandatory if the trial of a device is conducted under FDA regulations, such as an investigational device exemption. Increasingly, central trial data bases are being computerized. This can facilitate data collection from the various sites of a multicenter trial through remote computer terminals as well as expediting ongoing data analysis. In any event, the central data base should be designed to allow the investigator to assess easily the status of the trial at any time.

Continued assessment of the trial data provides a means of quality control for the trial and brings to the investigator's attention unanticipated findings, which may influence the conduct of the trial. The extent and complexity of the quality control mechanisms will be predicated on the size and length of the trial. In long-term or multicenter trials, quality control of the data base and of data collection procedures is of the utmost importance, and appropriate mechanisms should be included in the scheme of trial management. Such procedures should include review of selected individual data forms, comparison of computer records with the original data forms or laboratory notebooks, isolation and investigation of outlying values, and checks on data transfer to the central data base for failure to enter or double entry. Some of these checks must be performed manually, while others can be incorporated into the computer's database management program; some can be a routine part of the handling of each data item, while others must be part of periodic audits. In spite of all precautions, some data will be found to be missing or inaccurate, and procedures to deal with this must be incorporated into the trial management plan.

Analysis of the Data

The motivation of a clinical trial is to demonstrate the validity of a conjecture of the investigator, for example, that one device is superior to another, or that intervention with a device causes a change in some parameter. This conjecture is termed the alternative hypothesis. Complementing the alternative hypothesis is the null hypothesis that covers the possibility of no difference or no change. In the statistical theory of hypothesis testing, it is necessary to argue by contradiction. Thus, the null hypothesis is assumed to be true. A test is then made to see whether or not the data support rejection of the null hypothesis. The type of test chosen will depend on the type of data collected and the assumptions that can be made about the data. Depending on which test is selected, a value can be calculated which, in turn, leads to a P value. The P value is the probability of the observed result occurring if the null hypothesis were true. Hence, if this probability is low (for example, $P < 0.05$ or a 5% chance) the investigator will usually decide to reject the null hypothesis because, otherwise, a very unlikely event has occurred. Before making a test, it may be decided that if the P value is smaller than some value, α, then the null hypothesis will be rejected. This value, α, is called the significance level. If the null hypothesis is rejected, then the alternative hypothesis is implicitly accepted. In addition to the P value, which is the probability of erroneously rejecting the null hypothesis, the power of a test can be calculated. The power of a test relates to the probability of erroneously accepting the null hypothesis. Clearly, if a test results in acceptance of the null hypothesis, then the power of the test should be examined.

The assumptions about the variables will range from simple to complex and will lead to different statistical tests. For example, when testing only one variable that measures the difference between two devices, a nonparametric sign test is appropriate if only minimal criteria are met, whereas the more well-known Student's t test can be used where classic statistical theory applies. A discussion of statistical tests and their relationship to assumptions is beyond the scope of this chapter and will really need an expert biostatistician's aid. Nevertheless, the background to the choice of an appropriate test has been reviewed [32] and details on the use of the various tests can be found in standard statistical texts [6, 7, 12].

In interpreting the statistical analysis of results from a clinical trial, it is important to differentiate between statistical significance and clinical significance. Statistically significant results are not always clinically significant; a small difference in an outcome variable can be statistically significant, particularly if the number of observations is large, but may be of no clinical importance. The converse is also true; if the sample size is very small, the results may be clinically significant even though statistical significance cannot be demonstrated. The investigator must never lose sight of the real purpose of many clinical trials, that is, to demonstrate that one treatment affords the patient a clinically superior outcome to another.

Selection of tests should occur before the data are collected. For example, to calculate the required sample size, the tests, the required significance level, and the acceptable power must be chosen in advance. In a clinical situation, a trade-off can be made between the sample size, the test, the significance level, the power, and the magnitude of the detectable difference. Ideally, the methods of statistical inference and the design for a clinical trial can be predetermined. In practice, there is often an iterative process involved in which, as the data are collected, they are examined and used as a basis for modification of previous decisions. For example, as estimates of the variability of the data improve, a more precise calculation of the necessary sample size is possible. Alternatively, it may be found, in looking at the data, that very different tests are needed than those originally selected. For example, an unexpected confounding factor may need to be allowed for by a covariate analysis, or a much more attractive event might occur where the results are so clear that no statistical test is needed. Thus, exploring the data at all stages of a trial is an integral part of the clinical trial.

PRESENTATION OF RESULTS

Essentially, the final stage in a clinical trial is publication of the results, whether this be in a peer-reviewed journal, a submission to the FDA, or some other forum. In preparing data for publication, the investigator must strive to present a convincing argument to the wider clinical and scientific community. Many investigators sell their trials short by failure to adhere to proper reporting standards in presenting their data, and this situation may be exacerbated by journal editors in their attempts to shorten manuscripts [33, 34]. Two recent publications [33, 35] have provided guidelines for the presentation of clinical data, including minimum requirements, and these are recommended to the investigator planning a clinical trial. Because it is frequently not possible to obtain required data retrospectively, it should be evident that consideration of data presentation should occur during the planning of a trial, before any data are collected.

REFERENCES

1   Pocock SJ. *Clinical Trials: A Practical Approach*. New York: Wiley Medical, 1983.
2   Friedman LM, Furberg CD, DeMets DL. *Fundamentals of Clinical Trials*. Boston: John Wright, 1981.
3   Schwartz D, Lellouch J. Explanatory and pragmatic attitudes in therapeutic trials. *J Chronic Dis*, 20 (1967), 637–648.
4   Sackett DL, Gent M. Controversy in counting and attributing events in clinical trials. *N Engl J Med*, 301 (1979), 1410–1412.
5   Freiman JA, Chalmers TC, Smith H, et al. The importance of beta, the Type II error and sample size in the design and interpretation of the randomized control trial. *N Engl J Med*, 299 (1978), 690–694.
6   Snedecor GW, Cochran WG. *Statistical Methods*. Ames, IA: Iowa State University Press, 1967.
7   Fleiss JL. *Statistical Methods for Rates and Proportions*. New York: Wiley, 1981.
8   Clark CJ, Downie CC. A method for the rapid determination of the number of patients to include in a controlled clinical trial. *Lancelot*, 2 (1966), 1357–1358.
9   Schork MA, Remington RD. The determination of sample size in treatment-control comparisons for chronic disease studies in which drop-out or non-adherence is a problem. *J Chronic Dis*, 20 (1967), 233–239.
10 Donner A. Approaches to sample size estimation in the design of clinical trials — A review. *Stat Med*, 3 (1984), 199–214.
11 Lachin JM. Sample size determinations for $r \times c$ comparative trials. *Biometrics*, 33 (1977), 315–324.
12 Armitage P. *Statistical Methods in Medical Research*. Oxford, UK: Blackwell Scientific, 1971.
13 Ellenberg SS. Randomized designs in comparative clinical trials. *N Engl J Med*, 310 (1984), 1404–1408.
14 Taylor KM, Margolese RG, Soskolne CL. Physicians' reasons for not entering eligible patients in a randomized clinical trial of surgery for breast cancer. *N Engl J Med*, 310 (1984), 1363–1367.
15 Sacks H, Chalmers TC, Smith H. Randomized versus historical controls for clinical trials. *Amer J Med*, 72 (1982), 233–240.
16 Sacks HS, Chalmers TC, Smith H. Sensitivity and specificity of clinical trials. Randomized versus historical controls. *Arch Intern Med*, 143 (1983), 753–755.
17 Bailar JC, Louis TA, Lavori PW, et al. Studies without internal controls. *N Engl J Med*, 311 (1984), 156–162.
18 Zelen M. A new design for randomized clinical trials. *N Engl J Med*, 300 (1979), 1242–1245.
19 Dwosh IL, Giles AR, Ford PM, et al. Plasmapheresis therapy in rheumatoid arthritis: A controlled, double-blind, crossover trial. *N Engl J Med*, 308 (1983), 1124–1129.
20 Bailar JC, Louis TA, Lavori PW, et al. A classification for biomedical research reports. *N Engl J Med*, 311 (1984), 1482–1487.
21 Louis TA, Lavori PW, Bailar J, et al. Crossover and self-controlled designs in clinical research. *N Engl J Med*, 310 (1984), 24–31.
22 Brown BW. The crossover experiment for clinical trials. *Biometrics*, 36 (1980), 69–79.
23 Lavori PW, Louis TA, Bailar JC, et al. Designs for experiments — Parallel comparisons of treatment. *N Engl J Med*, 309 (1983), 1291–1299.
24 Louis TA, Mosteller F. Timely topics in statistical methods for clinical trials. *Ann Rev Biophys Bioeng*, 11 (1982), 81–104.
25 DeVries WC, Anderson JL, Joyce LD, et al. Clinical use of the total artificial heart. *N Engl J Med*, 310 (1984), 273–278.

26 Bensinger WI, Buckner CD, Clift RA, et al. Clinical trials with staphylococcal protein A. *J Biol Resp Modif*, 3 (1984), 347–351.

27 Armitage P. *Sequential Medical Trials*. New York: Wiley, 1975.

28 Donner A. The exclusion of patients from a clinical trial. *Stat Med*, 1 (1982), 261–265.

29 Marinez YN, McMahan CA, Barnwell GM, et al. Ensuring data quality in medical research through an integrated data management system. *Stat Med*, 3 (1984), 101–111.

30 Lowrie EG, Laird NM (Eds.). Co-operative dialysis study. *Kidney Int*, 23 (1983, Suppl. 13).

31 Wright P, Haybittle J. Design of forms for clinical trials. *Brit Med J*, 2 (1979), 529–530, 590–592, 650–651.

32 Ambler S. Statistical analysis of clinical trial data. In Johnson FN, Johnson S (Eds.), *Clinical Trials*. Oxford, UK: Blackwell Scientific, 1977.

33 DerSimonian R, Charette LJ, McPeek B, et al. Reporting on methods in clinical trials. *N Engl J Med*, 306 (1982), 1332–1337.

34 O'Fallon JR, Dubey SD, Salsburg DS, et al. Should there be statistical guidelines for medical research papers? *Biometrics*, 34 (1978), 687–695.

35 Altman DG, Gore SM, Gardner MJ, et al. Statistical guidelines for contributors to medical journals. *Brit Mcd J*, 286 (1983), 1489–1493.

Chapter 56

Malpractice Risk
in Clinical Trials

Robert J. Pristave
Scott Becker
Scott P. Downing

INTRODUCTION

The purpose of this chapter is to provide the investigator with guidelines for minimizing malpractice risks with human subjects. First, we focus on the general approach investigators should take in conducting investigations with human subjects. Some practical considerations are provided for minimizing malpractice risk from the investigator's point of view, highlighting the importance of documenting research strategy and the organization and conduct of clinical trials.

This chapter also provides an outline of the legal obligations imposed upon the investigator by law and reviews the investigator's duty to observe proper procedures and standards of practice in order to avoid malpractice liability. An overview of the law of strict liability is given, and strategies are outlined for the investigator to take in order to limit his liability in light of the application of principles of strict liability to the manufacturer of the biomaterial or device.

GENERAL APPROACH
TO CONDUCTING INVESTIGATIONS

Documentation of Research Strategy

In the contemporary environment for medical research, the impatient investigator may look upon the complex array of requirements to be met in order to gain approval for human experimentation as arbitrary barriers to his or her progress. The prudent investigator, in contrast, will recognize the requirements imposed by law and ethical principles as helpful guidelines for his or her protection as well as for the protection of the human subject's interests.

An investigator who wishes to minimize malpractice risk will recognize that the documentation or "record" relevant to a clinical trial has many components and extends back in time to early planning and research results. Elements of documentation may include research applications, records reviewing group actions, research notebooks, progress reports, publications, applications to institutional approval for human experimentation and applications for Food and Drug Administration (FDA) Investigational Device Exemption (IDE). Throughout the phases of an investigation, the availability of clear and complete documentation will prove to be a valuable resource in subsequent steps. For example, the background, research plan, and prior research results summarized in a grant application will also be useful for preparation of applications for approval by the institutional human research committee or the FDA. When an investigator prepares documentation for an additional step, he or she should also address any criticisms or shortcomings noted in the previous record. For instance, if the record of review raises certain questions or points of doubt, especially about human applications, these issues should be directly addressed.

At the outset of development of a new biomaterial or device, the investigator should plan to document his or her research and development strategy in a logical and stepwise fashion with respect to the ultimate application in humans. The necessity to document thoroughly and clearly the strategy at each step is essential. An important factor to document is how the new material or device differs from the current accepted practice regarding a biomaterial or device. The record should demonstrate the logic of selection of certain bench tests to validate elements of the new and different behavior or properties of the new biomaterial or device. Consequently, it would be advantageous to show comparative tests with accepted materials or devices (i.e., a positive control). Similarly, the documentation of the specific animal trials undertaken should demonstrate the new biomaterial's or device's overall performance as well as compare its behavior and properties with those of existing biomaterials or devices. Hopefully, both bench and animal tests will show equivalent or superior performance of the new material or device in terms of both selected properties and/or overall performance.

Prior to undertaking a clinical trial, the investigator should be able to demonstrate by his or her record of prior results that the biomaterial or device will (a) perform the proposed function, (b) operate at a reliability level suitable for human application, and (c) have a low probability of harm to a research subject, based on all existing information. The last two points are a matter of judgment; hence, the investigator's case will be strengthened by objective opinions made by other "experts."

An investigator will benefit from periodic consultation with his colleagues and other persons who are experts in the field. Such consultation is likely to improve the quality of science, sharpen the experimental approach, and lead to the development of other data useful for evaluating the appropriateness of human experimentation. Generally, some expert review of a project intending to use human subjects will occur upon submission of applications for funding to various granting agencies. The investigator will also seek the advice of others prior to critical reviews in order to increase the objectivity of his/her presentations and documentation. Similarly, because expertise of review groups may be limited, an investigator may wish to consult others, especially with respect to matters of judgment such as the appropriate time (in the development of the overall data base) to initiate clinical trials. In summary, additional consultations with appropriate experts in the field can broaden peer acceptance of the proposed clinical trial and strengthen the investigator's record.

Thus, the development of good documentation dealing with the research strategy, the scientific issues to be tested, and the logic of the research sequence will serve as factors to reduce the risk of malpractice in a clinical trial of a new biomaterial or device. This goal may be achieved in two ways. First, the conscious process of developing the careful record will tend to lessen the probability of overlooking a critical factor. Second, the availability of a carefully gathered, logical account of the investigation will provide an excellent factual base for defense against potential malpractice actions.

ORGANIZATION AND CONDUCT OF A CLINICAL TRIAL

While many aspects of the conduct of a clinical trial may have some bearing on malpractice risk, two factors seem of importance. The first relates to the clear definition of the scientific issues that are the subject of the trial and the boundaries of "new" practice, as compared to conventional practice. Medical care for a patient participating in a clinical trial may consist of a number of components, only one of which is experimental. Therefore, written descriptions of the trial, patient consent forms, etc., should make clear the bounds of the trial. Similarly, clear descriptions of the particular scientific issues being studied are of importance. Such descriptions will lessen the possibility of third persons broadening the area of experimentation in the mind of a subject or other party. A further reason for defining limits to the scientific questions under study is that the background data gathered in bench and animal trials will have relevance only to limited questions. The logical justification of the clinical trial will be confined to the designated selected areas. Such descriptions will again lessen the probability of a third person viewing the trial much more broadly or loosely.

The investigator interested in minimizing malpractice risk should take particular care in defining and operating a system for monitoring patient safety. In large-scale trials, guidelines of the National Institutes of Health require that an independent patient safety committee be appointed for monitoring patient safety. In small-scale studies, the institutional review board (IRB) often assumes a continuing role in monitoring patient safety. Monitoring of longer-term trends in an individual patient or experimental group of patients can be effectively accomplished with an alert expert or an outside group or committee. If the scale of the trial does not permit use of such a group, the investigator may wish to provide such a function in some other manner. Monitoring longer-term patient safety with expert, unbiased observers helps minimize malpractice risk.

Monitoring short-term or acute individual patient safety is a different matter. The patient's own physician is the responsible person. If a physician is also the principal investigator of a clinical trial, he or she may be considered to have a biased point of view. Therefore, an investigator planning a clinical study may design the protocol so that he or she will not assume direct responsibility for any individual patients in the study. Patient monitoring and short-term safety would be arranged through a colleague, who would have only patient responsibility and not be directly concerned with the conduct of the trial. Such a procedure eliminates the factor of potential bias on the part of the investigator. Thus, provision for short-term patient care or monitoring by an unbiased physician is another means of minimizing malpractice risk [1].

LEGAL RESPONSIBILITIES OF INVESTIGATORS

Overview of Procedural Guidelines

Institutions and individual investigators conducting research and experimentation have a duty to oversee research performed on human subjects. Review by an IRB and/or the Food and Drug Administration (FDA) should be seriously considered. Generally, researchers have the option to obtain either IRB review and approval (for non-significant risk devices) or FDA review and approval (for significant risk devices). It should be noted, however, that the FDA will require IRB approval prior to giving its approval. With respect to the composition of the IRB membership, at least some members of the IRB should be experienced in the general area of research and the specific topic under investigation. Nevertheless, it is virtually impossible for all of the IRB members to be experienced in a medical topic because the committee should generally contain community members who are not physicians.

The IRB should press for details about the need for research on human subjects; proof that answers are not already available; the exact procedure to be used; anticipated hazards and risks; the procedure for selecting subjects; potential for therapeutic benefit versus mere research value; emergency precautions that will be available; experimental facilities;

the procedure for obtaining proper consents; record-keeping; definition of terms such as "terminal"; elimination of any aspects of consent; proof that potential benefits outweigh the risks; assurance of impartiality of the investigator; proper follow-up means for the IRB; and availability of treatment for complications.

The investigator should adopt procedures for review of work in progress to ensure that safety standards and procedures are followed throughout experimentation. This requires constant monitoring of the subject(s) under experimentation and the investigators.

The investigator must maintain comprehensive records. Under some grants, open records may have to be available for inspection. Finally, if the investigation is subject to federal or state regulation, the investigation must adopt a system whereby regulatory bodies or grant agencies are assured of compliance with applicable rules.

Finally, the most crucial feature of institutional and investigatory supervision is ensuring that informed consent is obtained from the human subject.

Procedures for Obtaining Consent from Human Subjects

Independent and institutional investigators should adopt procedures to ensure consent of subjects in writing. Three elements must be present for a valid informed consent, whether given by the subject or his authorized representative. They include (a) the communication of sufficient information to enable the making of an intelligent decision regarding the course of care; (b) a determination by the investigator and witness that the subject or subject's authorized representative has capacity to understand the information and to decide freely to participate in the experiment; and (c) the expression of consent or the refusal to consent to the proposed investigation.

Informed Consent   The first element requires communicating to the subject sufficient information to reach an intelligent decision regarding participation in the study. There appear to be differences between informed consent for medical or surgical treatment, informed consent for clinical research primarily for treatment, and informed consent for clinical research primarily for the advancement of scientific knowledge. The investigator should obtain the fullest informed consent from subjects for whom no benefit from the research is expected [2]. The courts have not fully addressed the extent to which a subject should be informed of procedures and risks where the research is primarily for the advancement of scientific knowledge [3]. However there appears to be a duty to provide a full description of procedures and risks involved.

In *Halushka v. University of Saskatchewan* [4], a 21-year-old student agreed to participate in a medical research project that involved a comparative study of anesthetics. As a consequence of his participation, he suffered a cardiac arrest. Although consent to treatment had been obtained, the investigator described the nature of the procedure and the risks in general (not specific) terms. The court noted that in research situations, as compared to therapeutic medical ones, investigators have as great a duty, if not a greater one, to give fair and reasonable explanations of proposed treatments and their risks. In addition, the court stressed that in research there can be no exceptions to the disclosure requirements.

Furthermore, at least one court has determined that physicians must disclose to their subjects pecuniary gain that may result from their scientific research. In *Moore vs. Regents of the University of California* [5], physicians treating a patient suffering from hairy-cell leukemia used the patient's cells obtained from his removed spleen, blood, and bone marrow for research to devise a cell line to treat various forms of leukemia. The physicians failed to inform the patient that they intended to perform research with his removed cells, and neglected to inform the patient of the patent which they subsequently obtained on the new cell line. The court found that the physicians violated the patient's legally protected interest in being fully informed prior to medical procedures when the physicians failed to disclose their economic interest in the patient's cells. The court held that a physician must disclose personal interest unrelated to the patient's health, whether research or economic, that may affect the physician's professional judgment; the failure to do so would give rise to a cause of action for performing medical procedures without informed consent [5].

Generally, a physician using experimental or innovative medical procedures is obligated to make a reasonable disclosure of hazards involved in medical treatment [6]. This disclosure requires a fair explanation of procedure risks and benefits. In *Nathanson v. Klein*, although a patient's consent to treatment had been obtained, the consent was considered invalid because the patient was not informed of the risks of the probable consequences of radiation therapy [6].

However, what constitutes reasonable disclosure is a complex issue. In *Canterbury v. Spence* [7], a 19-year-old male who ultimately suffered paralysis of the intestines from a laminectomy was not told by his neurosurgeon of this uncommon, but possible, complication of the operation. The court overruled the traditional majority rule of disclosure based upon customary standards of disclosure in a physician's community. Instead, the court stated:

> The patient's right of self-decision shapes the boundaries of the duty to reveal. That right can be effectively exercised only if the patient possesses enough information to enable an intelligent choice. The scope of the physician's communications to the patient, then, must be measured by the patient's need, and that need is the information material to the decision [7].

The court recognized, however, that the physician has no obligation to communicate dangers that are commonly known or already known by the patient or have no bearing on the patient's decision to accept or reject treatment. In addition, the court noted two exceptions from the rule of disclosure: (a) when in an emergency situation the patient's decision cannot be obtained and harm from failure to treat is greater than threat from the proposed procedures, and (b) when the disclosure of risks upsets the patient so seriously that the treatment or patient is harmed [8]. It is less likely, however, that therapeutic privilege will be used as a viable defense in the future because the American Medical Association's (AMA) current ethical code emphasizes honesty with patients, a departure from the old code that said a physician could withhold information from patients if it was in their interests [9]. In addition, the therapeutic defense is less likely to be available when the use of experimental or investigational procedures are involved.

Grants administered by the federal government under the auspices of the Department of Health and Human Services require that investigators follow a specified procedure in obtaining consent from human subjects [10]. Informed consent must contain the following components (see also Chapter 51):

1 A statement that the study involves research, an explanation of the purposes of the research and the expected duration of the subject's participation, a description of the procedures to be followed, and identification of any procedures that are experimental.

2 A description of any reasonably foreseeable risks or discomforts to the subject.

3 A description of any benefits to the subject or to others that may reasonably be expected from the research.

4 A disclosure of appropriate alternative procedures or courses of treatment, if any, that might be advantageous to the subject.

5 A statement describing the extent, if any, to which confidentiality of records identifying the subject will be maintained.

6   For research involving more than minimal risk, an explanation as to whether any compensation and an explanation as to whether any medical treatments are available if injury occurs and, if so, what they consist of, or where further information may be obtained.

7   An explanation of whom to contact for answers to pertinent questions about the research and research subjects' rights and whom to contact in the event of a research-related injury to the subject.

8   A statement that participation is voluntary, that refusal to participate will involve no penalty or loss of benefits to which the subject is otherwise entitled and that the subject may discontinue participation at any time without penalty or loss of benefits to which the subject is otherwise entitled.

When appropriate, one or more of the following additional elements of information shall also be provided to each subject:

9   A statement that the particular treatment or procedure may involve risks to the subject (or to the embryo or fetus, if the subject is or may become pregnant) that are currently unforeseeable.

10   Anticipated circumstances under which the subject's participation may be terminated by the investigator without regard to the subject's consent .

11   Any additional costs to the subject that may result from participation in the research .

12   The consequences of a subject's decision to withdraw from the research and procedures for orderly termination of participation by the subject .

13   A statement that significant new findings developed during the course of the research that may relate to the subject's willingness to continue participation will be provided to the subject .

14   The approximate number of subjects involved in the study [10].

Capacity to Consent   The second element of consent concerns capacity to consent to or refuse treatment. An individual participating in research must have the legal capacity to give consent. The individual must be capable of fully exercising his or her ability to make choices and understanding information. First, this includes being legally capable of understanding the information communicated (the investigator-subject conference), and, second, reaching an intelligent decision regarding participation in the experimental procedure. Generally, legal incompetency results from the subject's legal status as opposed to whether or not the person actually can make an intelligent decision to participate in the research. Legal incompetence typically includes the following: minors, the unconscious, the institutionalized mentally retarded, as well as those adjudicated insane or incompetent [10]. To the extent that an individual is incapable of giving consent because of medically or legally declared incompetence, state law governs the extent of authority of a legal representative or guardian to consent for incompetent individuals. The use of a witness is very important in this context because the witness' signature affirms the patient's lack of capacity to provide his/her own consent.

Voluntary Consent   The third element of consent concerns the expression of consent. To be effective, consent must be given without coercion or deceit. If the subject is coerced to give consent to a procedure and the investigator's coercive techniques are responsible for the subject's consent, then the investigator has obtained an involuntary and invalid consent.

Voluntary consent means individuals have a right to give consent knowingly and freely to be research subjects. It also means that these individuals have the right to refuse participation or to withdraw from the study at any time without recriminations [2]. In addition, rewards should not be so great that they constitute undue influence. The rewards should not be so large that they diminish the subject's ability to appraise risks accurately and, consequently, diminish his or her will for self-preservation [2, 11].

Documentation of Consent   Another important part of the informed consent process is documentation in the medical record and investigator's records in order to provide a lasting record of the subject's or authorized representative's consent or refusal to consent. The investigator should clearly document the general circumstances of the informed consent conference in the subject's medical record. Any signed consent form should be included in the medical record. Although the extent of the documentation obviously depends upon the complexity of the procedure and the degree of risk involved, sound and reasonable documentation should include:

1   A statement that an informed consent conference was conducted by the physician with the patient or his/her authorized representative
2   The name(s) and identity of the person(s) involved in the conference, including witnesses.
3   An indication of the extent of the competency of the patient and the reasons for discussing the proposed procedure with or obtaining consent from someone other than the patient.
4   A general and brief summary of the information conveyed and discussed.
5   The reasons for making limited disclosures to the patient or his/her authorized representative.
6   Unusual observations or circumstances necessitating certain actions on the part of the physician.
7   Such other information as may be useful in the future.
8   A record of any consultations obtained regarding the patient's condition and competency [12].

In clinical investigation primarily for scientific knowledge, the AMA's *Ethical Guidelines for Clinical Investigation* require without exception that consent be in writing, either from the subject or a legally authorized representative [13].

At the federal level, regulations regarding documentation of informed consent for research have been carefully spelled out [10].

Other variations on the documentation of informed consent include the following:

1   A statement on the consent form, beneath that of the subject, which investigators sign ensuring that they have explained the study to the subject.
2   An attempt to assess the subject's understanding by asking him/her to restate the informed consent information in his/her own words.
3   An attempt to assess the subject's understanding by adding a questionnaire to the consent form to assess his/her understanding of informed consent (known as a two-part consent form) [14].

Another variation in constructing a consent form is the three-part form that includes a complete description of the study, space for subjects to describe the study in their own words, and several objective questions about important parts of the study.

Legal consent can be given without signing a consent form. However, a written document does ensure a permanent record of what was agreed to and will minimize malpractice risk should the issue arise.

Subjects may, however, change their minds and verbally rescind a written consent at any time. Any procedure done on subjects in which there is inadequate consent or in which subjects withdraw their consent has been considered by the courts to be a battery or negligence [2].

Generally, it is improper to limit liability by obtaining a waiver from the subject on either a consent form or separate document. For the most part, courts will find such waivers invalid. In the *Halushka* case [4], the subject was asked to sign an informed consent statement that released the chief investigators and their associates, as well as technicians, the hospital board, and the University of Saskatchewan, from all responsibility and claims related to the procedures. The Court held that the waiver was legally unenforceable.

Strict Liability and the Investigation Utilizing Medical and Experimental Equipment or Biomaterials

General Theories of Strict Liability versus Negligence   The majority of decisions dealing with medical device products liability have been based on the negligence theory of recovery. This is the breach of a duty to exercise reasonable care. However, courts have been willing to apply strict liability to manufacturers. The opposite is true when the doctrine is urged against doctors and hospitals. Strict liability is based upon the unreasonable danger of a defective product to the user.

Negligence is the traditional method of recovery in tort. However, it is often difficult to prove in medical device situations against doctors and hospitals because of the difficulty faced in accurately testing the equipment. Negligence claims have been successful, however, against the manufacturer based on design, assembly, testing, advertising, education, and use [15]. Although recovery under negligence theories have not always been successful in medical device cases, such theories have been used in the majority of litigation.

When an injured patient seeks recovery under either a warranty or tort theory, the first question asked is whether privity of contract is required. This question is especially important in medical device actions because usually more than two parties are involved. A normal transaction usually involves the sale of the product from the manufacturer to either a doctor, an investigator, or hospital. The device is in turn used by the ultimate consumer, a patient or human subject. Normally, the patient will have no direct dealing with the manufacturer or the distributor and thus, will not have privity of contract [16]. Privity of contract is a doctrine which, when applied, generally requires that in order for a party to hold another party liable for injuries that the first party sustains from a product, the two parties in question must have entered into a contract regarding that product (e.g., for the sale and purchase of the product). Lack of privity may result in an injured patient or human subject being unable to sue a manufacturer or distributor of a device which injures such patient or subject.

The law has evolved in both the tort and warranty areas so that now recovery may be obtained without privity in most situations [15]. The fact that privity is usually not required should be a point of particular interest to doctors afraid of being drawn into products liability actions.

Investigators may be able to avoid being unnecessarily drawn into litigation if it is fairly clear that the injury occurred from a defect in the product rather than from malpractice. If privity of contract were still applicable, the subject would be forced to sue the investigator first, and the investigator would in turn have to sue the manufacturer. Major decisions seem to indicate that the doctrine of strict liability will be restrained to the manufacturer in most situations and that a showing of negligence is required against the doctor and hospital, in order to include them in the action [16]. Once again, the investigator or owner of the medical instrument is often joined as a defendant in malpractice actions for failure to inspect for defects. The institutional investigator, because it is a permanent owner of the device and has continuous control over it, is held to a somewhat higher inspection standard than physicians. Hospitals and institutional investigators have been liable for failure to discover patent defects, such as frayed electrical wiring, and they are required to make periodic examinations and tests for latent defects. If such defects are reasonably discoverable, they will be held liable [16]. The institutional investigator may also be held per se liable for negligently supplying defective equipment and the reasonably foreseeable dangers resulting from defects.

Minimizing Malpractice Risks in the Use of Medical Devices in Light of Law of Strict Liability   If, in experimentation, the clinician can prove that his procedures and methodology were not the cause of the subject's injury, the investigator may be able to prove that all injury was due from a defect in the medical device proposed for use by the manufacturer.

From a practical point of view, both the individual and institutional investigator are both responsible for training the assisting personnel in the proper use of such equipment. The manufacturer in almost all instances will supply a manual that describes how to assemble and use its product. The manufacturer's representatives will also visit the hospital and conduct training exercises for the investigator to educate him in the correct use of their products. Certainly all personnel who will be involved with the equipment should attend these sessions. It is also recommended that diagrams supplied by the manufacturer for setting up and operating the equipment be followed precisely. The investigator and the institutional investigator's representatives should be present for all testing. Whenever equipment is suspected of being defective, the device and its ancillary components should be isolated from properly functioning equipment, packed, and stored in a clean secure area. All documents associated with the device, including shipping vouchers should be reviewed. The manufacturer should also be asked to provide its own documentation for a particular device based on the lot number (if applicable), including quality assurance, quality control, and other in-house testing documents [17].

Practically all reputable manufacturers of biomedical equipment have developed well conceived protocols for isolating and identifying potential problems with their equipment. Accordingly, they have built specialized circuitry to accomplish this task. An outside consultant called to assist an institutional investigator case by case most probably will not have the same resources at his disposal as does the equipment manufacturer. Thus, if the manufacturer agreed to permit outside representatives of the investigators and the institutions to view their testing, it would seem that testing by the manufacturer under appropriate observation offers the best opportunity for determining conclusively the source of the defect.

An aggressive strategy regarding biomedical equipment problems must be followed. Simply returning suspect equipment unaccompanied to the manufacturer for testing is not sufficient to protect the interest of the hospital and physicians. Human subjects who are injured by equipment failure often survive, but are unable to function in any substantial way, and seven-figure settlements or court judgments are frequent. Thus, taking the steps necessary to maximize the likelihood that the injury will be attributed to the responsible party is essential [17].

REFERENCES

1   Goldsmith LS, Rheingold PD. Experimentation. In Goldsmith LS (Ed.), *Liability of Hospitals and Health Care Facilities*, Vol. 67. New York: Practicing Law Institute, 1983.

2   Silva MC. Informed consent in human experimentation. *Trial. Association of Trial Lawyers of America*, 1980, 38–39.

3   Wecht CH. *Medical Ethics and Legal Liability*. New York: Practicing Law Institute, 1976, 72.

4   *Halushka v. University of Saskatchewan*, 52 W.W.R. 608 (Sask. 1965).

5   *Moore vs. Regents of the University of California*, 793 P.2d 479 (Cal. 1990).

6   *Nathanson v. Klein*, 186 Kan. 393, 350 P.2d 1093 (1960), *aff'd on rehearing*, 187 Kan. 186,354 P.2d 670 (1960).

7   *Canterbury v. Spence*, 464 F.2d 772,786 (D.C. Cir. 1972).

8   Knapp TA, Huff RL. Emerging trends in the physician's duty to disclose: An update of *Canterbury v. Spence*. *J Legal Med*, 3 (1975), 41–45.

9   American Medical Association, *Code of Medical Ethics*, 1994. § 8.08.

10 Basic HHS Policy for Protection of Human Research Subjects, 45 CFR § 46.116 (1983); 45 C.F.R. § 46.117 (1981).

11 Annas GJ, Glantz LH, Katz BF. *Informed Consent to Human Experimentation: The Subject's Dilemma*. Cambridge, MA: Ballinger, 1977, 112.

12 Roberts BK, Simon JL. Informed consent. In *Representing Health Care Institutions and Professionals*, Vol. 2. Chicago: Illinois Institute for Continuing Legal Education, 1980, 14–24.

13 American Medical Association, *Code of Medical Ethics*, § 2.07.

14 Downs FS, Fleming JW. *Issues in Nursing Research*. New York: Appleton-Century-Crofts, 1979, 122–124.

15 Prosser WL, Keaton WP. The Law of Torts, 5th ed. West, 1984, § 98.

16 Noblett P. An overview of litigation concerning products liability and medical devices. *Amer J Trial Advocacy*, 5 (1981), 309–317.

17 Borovetz H. Biomedical equipment problem: Strategy for the hospital and physician. *Hospital Newsletter*, 1:11 (1984), 1.

Chapter 57
Information for the Public

Stephen R. Ash

FACTORS INFLUENCING EVALUATION
OF A MEDICAL DEVICE

An unsettling fact of clinical research is that it remains, after all planning and efforts, essentially research. The effectiveness of a device can never be fully known until it has been tested in clinical trials. Even if the device is remarkably effective and safe in tests on normal or diseased animals, it is not certain that it will function in patients with clinical diseases for long periods of time. Even in clinical studies, side effects and complications of devices may be difficult to separate from catastrophic effects of diseases themselves. Clinical tests of biomaterials are especially difficult, because the success of the materials may depend upon the device in which they are used.

Disease considerations aside, the appraisal of risk versus benefit of medical devices is a complex task, creating difficulty in achieving a meaningful clinical trial protocol. The issues and risks and hazards of a device are difficult to convey, as well, even to a patient familiar with his disease and its outcome. Moreover, the meaning of "statistical significance" is difficult to convey to all concerned (i.e., researchers, physicians, and patients alike). After either a good or bad result with a device, "personal experience" tends to overshadow statistical analysis of a large group of patients, and maintaining objectivity is exceedingly difficult for both the individual patient and the physician. The importance of a clinical trial, the risks, and the value of conclusions are even more difficult to convey accurately to the public at large than to physicians and patients. The first success or failure of a device is usually considered newsworthy, while the findings of long-term, multiple-center, randomized clinical trials seem to cause much less excitement. Isolated occurrences and experiences always make better "copy" than tables and graphs.

In the medical community, the first report of efficacy or safety of a device is usually viewed with skepticism. The proper "position" of a medical device, its utility, and risk and hazards are eventually determined through the published opinion of a variety of specialists. This decision process takes several years, and, even in the medical community, there are certain oscillations in opinion concerning new medical devices and drugs. Public response to a new device or drug typically goes through four phases. After an initial phase of skepticism, there is a "honeymoon" phase in which the device is overutilized. There is then a period of dissatisfaction or disappointment, as experience spreads concerning the device and as complications occur. Finally, the device is used in a manner appropriate to its effectiveness and safety. The proper indications are defined, and more appropriate patient selection occurs. These phases could also describe the responses of a single patient, after implantation and utilization of a new device. In early phases of use, even highly educated physicians have varying opinions concerning the usefulness of a new device. It can hardly be expected, therefore, that the press and public will have a more accurate opinion.

PREVENTING RELEASE OF INFORMATION

Public awareness of a device may occur at any of the phases of the research and development. Most new medical devices and biomaterials begin in a rather quiet way. A scientist perceives a problem in the present status of such materials or devices. The scientist then decides whether there are resources to solve or study the problem. A biomaterials scientist may be reviewing medical devices, looking for applications of a particular material or new research technique. If a possible advantage or difference of a material is perceived, the scientist then proceeds to produce and test the material. Often an NIH grant may be prepared next or a corporate sponsor may be approached for research support. In addition to funding research, technical assistance may be offered by a corporate sponsor.

Companies are particularly secretive about their supported research and collaborations. Proposal reviews by NIH are conducted in confidence. Certain portions of a grant request may specifically be labeled confidential. However, reviewers do not sign strict nondisclosure agreements, and new information may be conveyed to scientific colleagues in grant review panels. The press is usually, and fortunately, unaware of this early stage of research.

After initial tests of materials biocompatibility, the researcher proceeds to animal tests. In vitro or in vivo results may be published at this time. First journal publications are generally not considered "newsworthy" by the press, if they involve animals. The researcher or a physician may then plan a clinical trial of this new device, submitting to review by an institutional review board (IRB) and, if necessary, the Food and Drug Administration (FDA).

Requests for permission for human clinical trials rarely receive notice by the press. Notable exceptions have included the artificial "heart" implantation in Utah, in which the hospital IRB delayed the first implantation. Affirmative action by an IRB usually receives less notice than a denial. Institutional review board review is an unfortunate time for a decision to become "politicized." Press notice and public awareness is essentially equivalent to political pressure of one sort or another. During IRB assessment of a study request, every effort should be made to avoid publicity of either a positive or negative decision.

RELEASE OF INFORMATION

Even after the first clinical trial of a device is performed, it is still desirable to avoid publicity. The trial results of the first device test, either positive or negative, are essentially meaningless from a scientific standpoint. As clinical trials expand, multiple centers may become involved, and the trial period becomes longer. The risk of public exposure becomes greater. Nonetheless, to maintain scientific credibility, it is important to avoid widespread publicity. Publicity at this point, quite surprisingly, may be to the detriment of supporting companies. In 1974, Reemtsma and Maloney published a satirical paper in the New England Journal of Medicine. In this paper, they pointed out that the press usually overrates the initial success and potential benefit of any new drug or medical device [1]. Inside information within a company (often incomplete) has usually caused the company's stock value to increase before the clinical trials of a device even start. At the time of the clinical trial or introduction of a device, the press detects news of the device. The public then becomes aware of the device at about the same point the medical community learns of its limitations. For investors interested in medical companies, Reemtsma and Maloney suggest that they "sell short" a company's stock whenever news of a new product of that company reaches the market. Within a few months, any problems of the device become apparent, and the company stock value will almost surely begin to fall. Several new product introductions justified the conclusions of the authors [1]. Recent examples of new products whose stock effect would fit the Reemtsma-Maloney law include: Oraflex, Zomax, the laserscope, ventricular assist devices, insulin infusion pumps, interferon, and erythropeoitin.

Choice of Public Medium

It would seem, in general, that release of information to the media is contrary to the directions of good science. What, then, is the best approach to supplying the necessary knowledge of devices to the public? It is preferable that the inventors of devices remain totally silent until the clinical trial and product introduction phases are completed. Especially with investor capital and entrepreneurial backing, it is best to avoid or minimize press coverage until the device is widely accepted and tested. To do otherwise can actually be detrimental to the company, although a potential benefit to the short-term investor. Interviews by electronic media generally are more risky and less thorough than those of newspapers and weekly magazines. The amount of text in television interviews is rarely more than 200 or 300 words. The visual images used convey more information than the background statements. The choice of images by the station editor may slant the interview to be either entirely positive or entirely negative. The scientist or clinical investigator must always ask himself/herself the question, "What is the *need* of the public to know about this device?" When that need appears to be great, the interviewing source should be carefully screened. It is best for the interviewee to request the right to review an article or preview a video before it is published. Of the thousands of news reporters in the United States, only about 100 are fulltime science writers [2]. Providing written material to the reporter is essential in order to avoid technical inaccuracies. One might present a typed, short description of the nature of the research project, including demographic details concerning the research team (names of co-workers and their institutions). At the time of the interview, one should hand the reporter the summary and indicate what material is essential for inclusion in the article. It is sometimes necessary to *insist* that the article include the names of co-workers. The enjoyable and short book by Gastel gives other hints for a successful interview and methods for assisting the seriously interested reporter [2].

CORRECTING MISINFORMATION

Occasionally, the level of misinformation concerning the value of a device may become intolerable. At this point, the investigator recognizes that the misinformation of the public and physician could lead to real harm to patients. It may even prove advisable to help correct misinformation by contacting someone from a public medium different from the original medium. Thus, if a television interview gives an overly negative or positive opinion, this may be partially corrected by an interview with a newspaper. There is a pride in journalism, akin to the pride in the medical profession. It is unlikely that one television station will criticize another or one newspaper criticize another. Reporters and editors are much more sensitive to impressions created by their media than are scientists or physicians. In general, the press of free countries has an honest, altruistic motivation. Reputable reporters desire to correct any misrepresentation at the earliest possible moment.

DEVICE JUSTIFICATION

The final importance of a medical device is established by the benefit derived by the general population of patients. Premature press announcements sacrifice potential good for a large number of patients by contributing to excessively high and overuse of devices. The highest compliment to the scientist or physician, and the greatest justification of a device, comes from the general use of a device by colleagues in their patients, not from press releases.

If a device truly provides patient benefits, then proper release of information to the media regarding a device may have resultant advantages for the investigator. Such advantages may assist in gaining further monetary support for continued device development through industrial/federal funding or through donations. Future patients will, thereby, share in this advantage.

REFERENCES

1   Reemtsma K, Maloney JV, Jr. The economics of instant medical news. *N Engl J Med*, 290 (1974), 429–442.
2   Gastel B. *Presenting Science to the Public*. Philadelphia, PA: ISI Press, 1983.

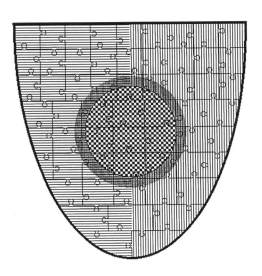

Index

(t, table; f, figure)

strain energy in, 542
surface area in, 543
ultimate compressive or tensile stress in, 540
volume ratio in, 543
yield compressive or tensile strength in, 540–541
Osteocompatibility, implantation sites in
advantages and disadvantages of, 549t
cranium, 551
intramedullary, 550–551
intramuscular and subcutaneous, 551
mandible, 551
subchondral, 551
transcortical, 547–550
Osteocompatibility, testing in
functional properties in, 552–553
nonfunctional properties in, 539–551
Osteocyte, intravital staining of, 733f
Osteogramm, 750–752
Osteolysis, from particulate material, 241, 247
Otology, animal model for, 477
Outcome variable selection, 851
Out-of-plane properties
of laminates, 53–54
in shear tests, 55–56
Oxidative degradation, of UHMWPE, 246
Ozone, for sterilization, 259

P
P value, 858
Pacemaker, cardiac, 833
Packaging, preclinical testing of, 780
Paraffin
processing and embedding with, 588–590
sectioning of, 592–593
staining of, 594
Parallel design, 855
Particulate material, 241–250
articulating surface conformity differences on, 246
biocompatibility issues of, 247
effects of, 241–244
energy dispersive X-ray microanalysis (EDX) for, 248
metal wear particles in, 246–247
particle isolation methods for, 249
particle morphology and response to, 244–247
particle quantity-based response to, 246
particle size-based response to, 245–246
in surface topography, 229
testing methods for, 247–250
ultrastructural examination for, 248–249
in vivo examination of, 249–250
Particulate-leaching, in tissue engineering, 390

Patch method, repeated, 280–281
Pathogen, transport of, 499
Patient
attitude of, 832
cognitive status of, 836
informed consent of (*see* Informed consent)
Patient selection
for clinical trials (*see* Clinical trials, patient selection for)
incapacitation degree on, 842
IRB in, 843
reliability and accessibility in, 842–843
Patterned substrates, in biomimetic materials, 216
PC. *see* Phosphatidylcholine
PDS, 100t
Peer community, in clinical trials, 834–835
PEG (polyethylene glycol)-monomethacrylates, graft co-polymerization of, 210–211
Penicillin, 328
Pentobarbital, in general anesthesia, 484
for euthanasia, 512
PEO. *see* Polyethylene oxide (PEO)
Peptide coupling, PEO as spacer arms in, 215
Peptides, cell adhesion, 213
Peracetic acid, 259
Percutaneous access, for biosensors, 455
Perfusion fixation, 693–695
Peri-implant zone, 571
clinical assessment of, 575–576
Perimucosal tissue, 571
Peritoneum, implant studies in, 496
Permeability
in drug-plastic interactions, 269
hydraulic, 413–414
Permeation, in drug-plastic interactions, 269
Permucosal interface, 721–725
avulsion in, 722
current approaches in, 724–725
exit site challenges in, 723–724
histological anatomy of, 721–722
infection in, 722–723
maxilla *vs.* mandible implants in, 725
mechanical stresses in, 724
pathological findings in, 722–723
procollagen in situ hybridization in, 708f, 709f
special challenges of, 721
success factors in, 723
Peroxidase-antiperoxidase method, 651
Perturbation, in biosensors, 439
PET (polyethylene terephthalate). *see* Polyethylene terephthalate (PET)
PGE2. *see* Prostaglandin E2 (PGE2)
pH, of culture mediums, 327
Phagocytosis, 601–602
aminopeptidase in, 633